Encyclopedia of Intensive Care Medicine

Jean-Louis Vincent and Jesse B. Hall (Eds)

Encyclopedia of Intensive Care Medicine

Volume 1

A–C

With 716 Figures and 450 Tables

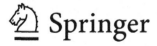 Springer

Editors
Jean-Louis Vincent
Head Dept of Intensive Care
Erasme Hospital (Free University of Brussels)
Route de Lennik 808
1070 Brussels
Belgium

Jesse B. Hall
University of Chicago Medical Center
5841 S. Maryland Ave.
MC 6076
Chicago, IL 60637
USA

ISBN 978-3-642-00417-9   e-ISBN 978-3-642-00418-6
Print and electronic bundle under ISBN 978-3-642-00419-3
DOI 10.1007/978-3-642-00418-6
Springer Heidelberg Dordrecht London New York

Library of Congress Control Number: 2012931922

Printed on acid-free paper

Springer is part of Springer Science+Business Media (www.springer.com)

List of Contributors

N. I. ABATE
Internal Medicine – Endocrinology
University of Texas Medical Branch
Galveston, TX
USA

ADEEL ABBASI
Emergency Medicine
Hospital of the University of Pennsylvania
Philadelphia, PA
USA

KAREEM R. ABDELFATTAH
Division of Burns, Trauma, and Critical Care
Department of Surgery
UT-Southwestern Medical Center
Dallas, TX
USA

BENJAMIN S. ABELLA
Department of Emergency Medicine and Department of
Medicine, Pulmonary, Allergy, and Critical Care Division
Hospital of the University of Pennsylvania
Philadelphia, PA
USA

EDWARD ABRAHAM
Department of Medicine
University of Alabama
Birmingham, AL
USA

GIHAN ABUELLA
Department of General Intensive Care
St. George's Hospital
London
UK

CHARLES A. ADAMS JR.
Department of Surgery
Rhode Island Hospital
Providence, RI
USA

RAEANNA C. ADAMS
Department of Surgery
Vanderbilt University Medical Center
Nashville, TN
USA

BASHEAL M. AGRAWAL
Department of Neurological Surgery
University of Wisconsin
Madison, WI
USA

OMAR AHMAD
Department of Emergency Medicine
University of British Columbia Critical Care, Emergency
and Trauma Medicine, Royal Columbian Hospital
New Westminster, BC
Canada

HESHAM M. AHMED
Division of Acute Care Surgery
UMDNJ-RWJMS, Robert Wood Johnson University
Hospital
New Brunswick, NJ
USA

KEVIN S. AKERS
Department of Medicine
Brooke Army Medical Center
Fort Sam Houston, TX
USA

JAMEEL ALI
Division of General Surgery
St. Michael's Hospital University of Toronto
Toronto, ON
Canada

AHMED M. AL-MOUSAWI
Department of Surgery
University of Texas Medical Branch and Shriners
Hospital for Children
Galveston, TX
USA

N. Al-Subaie
Department of Intensive Care
St. George's Hospital
London
UK

Jaffar A. Al-Tawfiq
Speciality Internal Medicine
Saudi Aramco Medical Services Organization
Kingdom of Saudi Arabia

Nagesh S. Anavekar
Department of Cardiology
The Northern Hospital
Melbourne
Australia

Caesar A. Anderson
University of Pennsylvania, Hyperbaric Medicine
San Diego, CA
USA

Kenton L. Anderson
Emergency Medicine
Duke University Medical Center
Durham, NC
USA

Ronald Anderson
MRC Unit for Inflammation and Immunity, Department
of Immunology, Faculty of Health Sciences
University of Pretoria, and Tshwane Academic Division
of the National Health Laboratory Service
Pretoria
South Africa

Martin K. Angele
Department of Surgery
Klinikum Grosshadern
Munich
Germany

Devashish J. Anjaria
Department of Surgery
UMDNJ-New Jersey Medical School
Newark, NJ
USA

Djillali Annane
General ICU
Raymond Poincaré Hospital (APHP)
University of Versailles SQY
Garches
France

David R. Anthony
Emergency Medicine Residency
New York-Presbyterian Hospital
New York, NY
USA

Massimo Antonelli
Istituto di Anestesiologia e Rianimazione, Policlinico
Universitario A. Gemelli
Università Cattolica del Sacro Cuore
Rome
Italy

Anastasia Antoniadou
Fourth Department of Internal Medicine
University General Hospital ATTIKON
Athens
Greece

Christopher T. Aquina
Division of Acute Care Surgery
UMDNJ-RWJMS, Robert Wood Johnson University
Hospital
New Brunswick, NJ
USA

Yaseen M. Arabi
Intensive Care Department
King Saud Bin Abdulaziz University for Health Sciences
King Abdulaziz Medical City
Riyadh
Kingdom of Saudi Arabia

Y. Asencio
Department of Anesthesia and Intensive Care Unit
La Timone Hospital
Marseille
France

JUAN A. ASENSIO
Department of Surgery
University of Miami Miller School of Medicine
Ryder Trauma Center
Miami, FL
USA

RÜDIGER AUTSCHBACH
Clinic for THG Surgery
University of Aachen
Aachen
Germany

MICHELLE BAACK
Department of Pediatrics
University of Iowa Children's Hospital
Carver College of Medicine
Iowa City, IA
USA

HILARY M. BABCOCK
Department of Internal Medicine
Washington University, School of Medicine
St. Louis, MO
USA

JAY P. BABICH
Division of Gastroenterology, Hepatology, and Nutrition
Winthrop University Hospital
Mineola, NY
USA
and
School of Medicine
State University of New York
Stony Brook, NY
USA

DANIEL DE BACKER
Department of Intensive Care
Erasme University Hospital
Free University of Brussels
Brussels
Belgium

DAVID BACON
General Intensive Care Unit
St. George's NHS Trust
London
UK

JOAN R. BADIA
Unitat de Vigilancia Intensiva Respiratòria
Servei de Pneumologia, Institut Clínic del Tórax
IDIBAPS and CIBER de enfermedades respiratorias
Hospital Clínic de Barcelona
Barcelona
Spain

SEAN M. BAGSHAW
Division of Critical Care Medicine
University of Alberta
Edmonton, AB
Canada

CHRISTOPHER C. BAKER
The Isidore Cohn
LSU Health Sciences Center – LSUHSC
New Orleans, LA
USA

JONATHAN BALL
General Intensive Care Unit
St. George's Hospital & Medical School
University of London
London
UK

MANSOOR N. BANGASH
Barts and the London School of Medicine and Dentistry
Intensive Care Unit Royal London Hospital
London
UK

LUIGI BARBERIS
Dipartimento di Anestesiologia e Rianimazione
Università di Torino
Turin
Italy

ADRIAN BARBUL
Department of Surgery
Sinai Hospital of Baltimore and the Johns Hopkins
Medical Institutions
Baltimore, MD
USA
and
Department of Surgery
Hackensack University Medical Center
Hackensack, NJ
USA

CARLTON C. BARNETT JR.
Rocky Mountain Regional Trauma Center
Denver Health Medical Center
Denver, CO
USA

JOSEPH B. BARNEY
Division of Pulmonary, Allergy and Critical Care
University of Alabama at Birmingham
Birmingham, AL
USA

TYLER W. BARRETT
Department of Emergency Medicine
Vanderbilt University
Oxford House
Nashville, TN
USA

JOEL M. BARTFIELD
Department of Emergency Medicine
Albany Medical College
Albany, NY
USA

GIANLUIGI LI BASSI
Department of Pulmonary and Critical Care Medicine
Hospital Clinic
Barcelona
Spain

JANE BATT
Division of Respirology, Department of Medicine
Keenan Research Centre of the Li Ka Shing Knowledge
Institute, St. Michael's Hospital
University of Toronto
Toronto, ON
Canada

ANDREW M. BAUER
Department of Neurological Surgery
University of Wisconsin
Madison, WI
USA

WERNER BAULIG
Institute of Anesthesiology
University Hospital Zurich
Zurich
Switzerland

BRIGITTE M. BAUMANN
Department of Emergency Medicine
Cooper University Hospital
Camden, NJ
USA

DANIEL G. BAUSCH
Department of Adult Infectious Diseases
Tulane University Health Sciences Center
New Orleans, LA
USA

KATHRYN M. BEAUCHAMP
Department of Neurosurgery
Denver Health Medical Center
University of Colorado School of Medicine
Denver, CO
USA

BRETT F. BECHTEL
Department of Emergency Medicine
Vanderbilt University
Oxford House
Nashville, TN
USA

JENNIFER BECK
St. Michael's Hospital
Toronto
Canada

RICHARD H. BEIGI
Department of Obstetrics, Gynecology and
Reproductive Sciences
Magee-Womens Hospital of the University of Pittsburgh
Medical Center
Pittsburgh, PA
USA

THOMAS BEIN
Leiter Operative Intensivstation
Universitätsklinikum Regensburg
Regensburg
Germany

MARIA L. BELALCAZAR
Department of Internal Medicine
The University of Texas Medical Branch
Galveston, TX
USA

VENKATESH BELLAMKONDA-ATHMARAM
Department of Emergency Medicine
The George Washington University Medical Center
Washington, DC
USA

GIACOMO BELLANI
Department of Perioperative Medicine and Intensive
Care A.O. Ospedale S. Gerardo
University of Milan-Bicocca
Monza
Italy

SCOTT E. BELL
Department of Neurosurgery
School of Medicine
University of Colorado Health Sciences Center
Denver, CO
USA

GIUSEPPE BELLO
Istituto di Anestesiologia e Rianimazione
Policlinico Universitario A. Gemelli
Università Cattolica del Sacro Cuore
Rome
Italy

RINALDO BELLOMO
Department of Intensive Care
Austin Hospital
Heidelberg, Melbourne, VIC
Australia

DENIS D. BENSARD
Department of Acute Care Surgery Denver Health
Medical Center
University of Colorado School of Medicine
Denver, CO
USA

METTE M. BERGER
Adult Intensive Care Medicine Service and Burn Center
CHUV (University Hospital)
Lausanne
Switzerland

FRANCESCA BERNABÈ
Department of Perioperative Medicine, Intensive Care
and Emergency
Cattinara Hospital, Trieste.
University School of Medicine
Trieste
Italy

KRISHNENDU BHADRA
Division of Pulmonary Disease and Critical Care
Medicine
University of Vermont College of Medicine
Burlington, VT
USA

PARITA BHUVA
Division of Neurocritical Care
Departments of neurology
University of Virginia
Charlottesville, VA
USA

B. J. BIEMOND
Academisch Medisch Centrum
Universiteit van Amsterdam
Amsterdam
The Netherlands

B. KIRKE BIENEMAN
Department of Radiology
Saint Louis University School of Medicine
St. Louis, MO
USA

WALTER L. BIFFL
Department of Surgery
Denver Health Medical Center
Denver, CO
USA

LLUIS BLANCH
CIBER Enfermedades Respiratorias, ISCiii, Spain and
Critical Care Center
Hospital de Sabadell
Corporacio Parc Tauli, Sabadell
Spain

FRANK BLOOS
Department of Anesthesiology and Intensive Care
Medicine
Jena University Hospital
Jena
Germany

STIJN BLOT
Department of General Internal Medicine & Infectious
Diseases
Ghent University Hospital
Ghent
Belgium

KEITH BONIFACE
Department of Emergency Medicine
The George Washington University Medical Center
Washington, DC
USA

JORDAN BONOMO
Departments of Emergency Medicine and Neurosurgery
University of Cincinnati
Cincinnati, OH
USA

DANIEL G. BOUTSIKARIS
Intensive Care Unit
University of Maryland
Mount Airy, MD
USA
and
Combined Emergency Medicine/Internal
Medicine/Critical Care Program
Baltimore, MD
USA

ARIANNE BOYLAN
Department of Neurosurgery
University of Colorado Denver
School of Medicine
Denver, CO
USA

DEES P. M. BRANDJES
Department of Internal Medicine
Slotervaart Hospital
Amsterdam
The Netherlands

RICHARD D. BRANSON
Division of Trauma and Critical Care
University of Cincinnati
Cincinnati, OH
USA

PETER G. BRINDLEY
Division of Critical Care Medicine
University of Alberta Hospitals
Edmonton, AB
Canada

L. D. BRITT
Department of Surgery
Eastern Virginia Medical School
Norfolk, VA
USA

ANUPAMA G. BRIXEY
Division of Pulmonary/Critical Care Medicine
Vanderbilt University Medical Center
Nashville, TN
USA

ITZHAK BROOK
Departments of Pediatrics and Medicine
Georgetown University School of Medicine
Washington, DC
USA

PATRICK D. BROPHY
Department of Pediatrics
University of Iowa Children's Hospital
Carver College of Medicine
Iowa City, IA
USA

CALVIN A. BROWN III
Department of Emergency Medicine
Brigham and Women's Hospital
Boston, MA
USA

PATRICIA D. BROWN
Department of Medicine
Wayne State University
Detroit, MI
USA

CHARLES S. BRUDNEY
Department of Anesthesiology
Duke University Medical Center
Durham, NC
USA

AMY E. BRYANT
Infectious Diseases Section
Veterans Affairs Medical Center, Boise, ID
University of Washington School of Medicine
Seattle, WA
USA

DANIEL BURKHOFF
Department of Medicine
Columbia University
New York, NY
USA

CLAY COTHREN BURLEW
Department of Surgery
Denver Health Medical Center
University of Colorado Denver
Denver, CO
USA

JONATHAN L. BURSTEIN
Emergency Medicine
Harvard University
Boston, MA
USA

JOHN H. BURTON
Department of Emergency Medicine
Carilion Clinic Virginia Tech Carilion School of Medicine
Roanoke, VA
USA

CHRISTIAN BYHAHN
Department of Anesthesiology, Intensive Care
Medicine, and Pain Management
J.W. Goethe-University Hospital Center
Frankfurt
Germany

PIETRO CAIRONI
Dipartimento di Anestesiologia
Terapia Intensiva e Scienze Dermatologiche
Università degli Studi
Milan
Italy

DIANE P. CALELLO
Department of Emergency Medicine
Morristown Memorial Hospital
Morristown, NJ
USA

JAUME CANET
Department of Anaesthesiology and Postoperative
Care Unit
Hospital Universitari Germans Trias i Pujol
Badalona, Barcelona
Spain

MAXIME CANNESSON
Department of Anesthesiology & Perioperative Care
School of Medicine
University of California
Irvine, CA
USA

ABELARDO CAPDEVILA
French Authority For Health
Haute Autorité de santé
Saint-Denis, La Plaine Cedex
France

E. CARLESSO
Dipartimento di Anestesiologia
Terapia Intensiva e Scienze Dermatologiche;
Università degli Studi
Milan
Italy

JEAN CARLET
French Authority For Health
Haute Autorité de santé
Saint-Denis, La Plaine Cedex
France

JORDI CARRATALÀ
Infectious Disease Department
Hospital Universitari de Bellvitge, Institut
d'Investigacions Biomèdiques de Bellvitge (IDIBELL)
L'Hospitalet de Llobregat
Barcelona
Spain
and
Department of Clinical Sciences
University of Barcelona
Barcelona
Spain

STEVEN E. CARSONS
Division of Rheumatology, Allergy and Immunology
Winthrop–University Hospital
Mineola, NY
USA
and
Stony Brook University School of Medicine
Stony Brook, NY
USA

DIEGO CASTANARES-ZAPATERO
Department of Critical Care Medicine
Saint-Luc University Hospital-Louvain Medical School
Brussels
Belgium

MAURIZIO CECCONI
Department of Intensive Care
St. George's Hospital
London
UK

JORGE CERDÁ
Division of Nephrology
Albany Medical College
Albany, NY
USA

JAMES D. CHALMERS
Centre for Inflammation Research
Queens Medical Research Centre
Edinburgh, Scotland
UK

HOWARD R. CHAMPION
Uniformed Services University of the Health Sciences
Bethesda, MD
USA

JEFFREY CHAN
Cardiology
VA San Diego Healthcare System
San Diego, CA
USA

M. CHANDALIA
Internal Medicine – Endocrinology
University of Texas Medical Branch
Galveston, TX
USA

VIKAS P. CHAUBEY
Department of Critical Care Medicine
University of Calgary and Calgary Health Region
Calgary, AB
Canada

IRSHAD H. CHAUDRY
Center for Surgical Research and Department of Surgery
University of Alabama at Birmingham
Birmingham, AL
USA

ESTHER H. CHEN
Department of Emergency Medicine
San Francisco General Hospital
San Francisco, CA
USA

ALFRED B. CHENG
Department of Emergency Medicine
Hospital of the University of Pennsylvania
Philadelphia, PA
USA

DAVIDE CHIUMELLO
U.O. Anestesia e Rianimazione
Dipartimento di Anestesia, Rianimazione (Intensiva e
Subintensiva) e Terapia del Dolore
Fondazione IRCCS Ca' Granda - Ospedale Maggiore
Policlinic
Milan
Italy

JULIE P. CHOU
Department of Internal Medicine
University of Calgary
Calgary, AB
Canada

ANAN CHUASUWAN
Department of Critical Care Medicine
University of Pittsburgh School of Medicine
Scaife Hall
Pittsburgh, PA
USA

WILLIAM G. CIOFFI
Department of Surgery
Rhode Island Hospital
Providence, RI
USA

G. Citerio
Neuroanesthesia and Neurointensive Care Unit
Department of Perioperative Medicine and
Intensive Care
San Gerardo Hospital
Monza
Milan
Italy

William R. Clark
Gambro Renal Products
Lakewood, CO
USA
and
Nephrology Division
Indiana University School of Medicine
Indianapolis, IN
USA

C. Coccia
Department of Critical Care Medicine
National Institute for Cancer "Regina Elena"
Rome
Italy

Thomas H. Cogbill
Department of Surgery
Gundersen Lutheran Medical Center
La Crosse, WI
USA

Edmond Cohen
Anesthesiology and Cardiothoracic Surgery
Mount Sinai Medical Center
New York, NY
USA

J. Cohen
Royal Brisbane Hospital
Brisbane, QLD
Australia

Mitch Cohen
Department of Surgery
University of California
San Francisco, CA
USA

Keri A. Cohn
Divisions of Emergency Medicine and Infectious
Diseases
Children's Hospital Boston
Harvard Medical School
Boston, MA
USA

Raul Coimbra
Division of Trauma, Surgical Critical Care, and Burns
Department of Surgery
University of California
San Diego School of Medicine
San Diego, CA
USA

David W. Collins
The Prince of Wales Hospital
Randwick, NSW
Australia

Alexander L. Colonna
Wake Forest University Baptist, Medical Center
Medical Center Boulevarde
Winston-Salem, NC
USA

Christopher B. Colwell
Department of Emergency Medicine
Denver Health Medical Center
Denver, CO
USA

Alain Combes
Service de Réanimation Médicale
Institut de Cardiologie, Groupe Hospitalier
Pitié–Salpêtrière
Paris Cedex
France
and
Université Pierre et Marie Curie, Paris Universitas
Paris
France

David C. Cone
Department of Emergency Medicine
Yale University
New Haven, CT
USA

JOHN B. CONNEELY
Department of Surgery
National University of Ireland
Dublin 2
Ireland

ANDREW K. P. CONNER
Indiana University School of Medicine
Indianapolis, IN
USA

MICHAEL D. CONNOLLY
Department of Surgery
Rhode Island Hospital
Providence, RI
USA

MIHAI A. CONSTANTINESCU
Department of Plastic and Hand Surgery
University Hospital Bern and University of Bern
Bern
Switzerland

LAURA A. COOLEY
Department of Adult Infectious Diseases
Tulane University Health Sciences Center
New Orleans, LA
USA

CRAIG M. COOPERSMITH
Department of Surgery
Emory University School of Medicine
Atlanta, GA
USA

JEREMY CORDINGLEY
Adult Intensive Care Unit
Royal Brompton Hospital
London
UK

HOWARD L. CORWIN
Departments of Medicine and Anesthesiology
Dartmouth–Hitchcock Medical Center
Lebanon, NH
USA

MARIA GABRIELLA COSTA
Department of Anesthesia and Intensive Care Medicine
Medical School of the University of Udine
University of Udine
Udine
Italy

TODD W. COSTANTINI
Division of Trauma, Surgical Critical Care, and Burns
Department of Surgery
University of California
San Diego School of Medicine
San Diego, CA
USA

CLAY C. COTHREN
The Department of Surgery
Denver Health Medical Center
University of Colorado School of Medicine
Denver, CO
USA

DOUGLAS B. COURSIN
Departments of Anesthesiology and Medicine
University of Wisconsin School of Medicine and
Public Health
Madison, WI
USA

DANIEL B. CRAIG
Denver, CO
USA

MECHEM C. CRAWFORD
Philadelphia Fire Department
University of Pennsylvania
Philadelphia, PA
USA

JACQUES CRETEUR
Department of Intensive Care
Erasme University Hospital
Université Libre de Bruxelles
Brussels
Belgium

ROSELLE CROMBIE
Department of Surgery
Yale University School of Medicine
New Haven, CT
USA

Jovany Cruz
Department of Neurosurgery
Baylor College of Medicene
Houston, TX
USA

Caitlin Curtis
Clinical Science Center University of Wisconsin
Hospital and Clinics
Madison, WI
USA

Ramsey J. Daher
Division of Nephrology and the Center for Immunity
Inflammation and Regenerative Medicine
University of Virginia Health System
Charlottesville, VA
USA

Martin Damm
Department of Anesthesiology and Intensive
Care Medicine
University Hospital Carl Gustav Carus, University of
Technology of Dresden
Dresden
Germany

Andrew Davenport
Department of Nephrology & Transplantation
Royal Free Hospital
London
UK

James W. Davis
Department of Surgery
Community Regional Medical Center
University of California – UCSF
Fresno, CA
USA

Stefan De Hert
Department of Anesthesiology
Academic Medical Centre
University of Amsterdam
Amsterdam
The Netherlands

Inneke E. De laet
Department of Internal medicine
Ghent University Hospital
Ghent
Belgium

Barbara De Meuter
Medical Director Cardiac ITU
Hartcentrum Hasselt
Hasselt
Belgium

Bart De Moor
Department of Nephrology
Jessa ziekenhuis
Hasselt
Belgium

Jan J. De Waele
Department of Critical Care Medicine
Ghent University Hospital
Ghent
Belgium

Charles D. Deakin
Department of Anaesthetics
Southampton University Hospital NHS Trust
Southampton
UK

Anthony J. Dean
Division of Emergency Ultrasonography
Department of Emergency Medicine
Hospital of the University of Pennsylvania
Philadelphia, PA
USA

Edwin A. Deitch
Department of Surgery
UMDNJ-New Jersey Medical School
Newark, NJ
USA

Giorgio Della Rocca
Department of Anesthesia and Intensive Care Medicine
Medical School of the University of Udine
University of Udine
Udine
Italy

ROLF DEMBINSKI
Klinik für Operative Intensivmedizin
Universitätsklinikum Aachen
Aachen
Germany

DEMETRIOS DEMETRIADES
University of Southern California
Los Angeles, CA
USA

ANEET DEO
Division of Nephrology
Tufts Medical Center
Boston, MA
USA

FRANCIS DEROOS
Emergency Medicine
Hospital of the University of Pennsylvania
Philadelphia, PA
USA

CLIFFORD S. DEUTSCHMAN
Department of Anesthesiology and Critical Care
(AJR, CSD)
University of Pennsylvania School of Medicine
Philadelphia, PA
USA

PRASAD DEVARAJAN
Department of Nephrology and Hypertension
Cincinnati Children's Hospital Medical Center
University of Cincinnati
Cincinnati, OH
USA

ABHAY DHAND
Division of Infectious Diseases
Department of Medicine
New York Medical College
Valhalla, NY
USA

MANUEL DIBILDOX
Department of Surgery
University of Texas Medical Branch and Shriners
Hospital for Children
Galveston, TX
USA

ROCHELLE DICKER
University of California
San Francisco, CA
USA

EDWARD T. DICKINSON
Department of Emergency Medicine
Hospital of the University of Pennsylvania Ground
Ravdin
Philadelphia, PA
USA

JENNIFER M. DICOCCO
General Surgery Resident
University of Tennessee Health Science Center
Memphis, TN
USA

DEBORAH B. DIERCKS
Department of Emergency Medicine
University of California Davis Medical Center
Sacramento, CA
USA

ANA CRISTINA DIOGO
Intensive Care Unit
Hospital dos Capuchos, CHL-ZC, E.P.E
Lisbon
Portugal

BRADLEY P. DIXON
Division of Nephrology and Hypertension
Cincinnati Children's Hospital Medical Center
Cincinnati, OH
USA

REBECCA M. DODSON
Department of Surgery
Sinai Hospital of Baltimore and the Johns Hopkins
Medical Institutions
Baltimore, MD
USA

GORDON S. DOIG
Northern Clinical School
University of Sydney
Sydney
Australia

JESSICA A. DOMINGUEZ
Department of Anesthesiology
University of Colorado Denver School of Medicine
Aurora, CO
USA

STÉPHANE Y. DONATI
Service de Réanimation Polyvalente
Hôpital Font-Pré
Toulon
France

CHARLES G. DURBIN JR.
Anesthesiology and Surgery
University of Virginia
Charlottesville, VA
USA

A. BRENT EASTMAN
Scripps
San Diego, CA
USA

RAUL EASTON-CARR
Department of Emergency Medicine
Olive View-UCLA Medical Center
Sylmar, CA
USA

JONATHAN R. EGAN
The Children's Hospital at Westmead
Westmead
Australia

PETER Q. EICHACKER
Critical Care Medicine Department
Clinical Center
National Institutes of Health
Bethesda, MD
USA

TAREK EID
Oregon Health and Sciences University
Portland, OR
USA

ITORO ELIJAH
Department of Surgery, Medical Branch
University of Texas
Galveston, TX
USA

ALI EL-SOLH
Medical Research
VA Western New York Healthcare System
Buffalo, NY
USA

E. WESLEY ELY
Division of Pulmonary and Critical Care Medicine
Center for Health Services Research
Vanderbilt University Medical Center
Nashville, TN
USA
and
Veteran's Affairs Geriatric Research Education Clinical
Center (GRECC) of the VA Tennessee Valley Healthcare
System
Nashville, TN
USA

TOBY M. ENNISS
Wake Forest University Baptist Medical Center
Medical Center Boulevarde
Winston-Salem, NC
USA

DANIEL W. ENTRIKIN
Department of Radiology and Internal Medicine
Section on Cardiology
Wake Forest University School of Medicine
Winston-Salem, NC
USA

SCOTT K. EPSTEIN
Tufts University School of Medicine
Pulmonary Critical Care and Sleep Medicine
Tufts Medical Center
Boston, MA
USA

SILVANO ESPSOSITO
Dipartimento di Malattie Infettive
Seconda Università degli Studi di Napoli
Naples
Italy

ANTHONY L. ESTRERA
Department of Cardiothoracic and Vascular Surgery
The University of Texas Medical School at Houston
Houston, TX
USA

TIMOTHY C. FABIAN
Surgery – General
University of Tennessee Health Science Center
Memphis, TN
USA

MATTHEW E. FALAGAS
Alfa Institute of Biomedical Sciences (AIBS)
Marousi, Athens
Greece
and
Department of Medicine
Henry Dunant Hospital
Athens
Greece
and
Department of Medicine
Tufts University School of Medicine
Boston, MA
USA

VITO FANELLI
Dipartimento di Anestesiologia e Rianimazione
Università di Torino
Turin
Italy

BRENNA M. FARMER
Division of Emergency Medicine
Weill Cornell Medical Center
New York, NY
USA

CHRISTOPHER FEE
Department of Emergency Medicine
University of California
San Francisco, CA
USA

CHARLES FELDMAN
Division of Pulmonology, Department of Internal
Medicine, Charlotte Maxeke Johannesburg Academic
Hospital, and School of Clinical Medicine
University of the Witwatersrand
Parktown, Johannesburg
South Africa

DAVID V. FELICIANO
Department of Surgery
Emory University School of Medicine
Grady Memorial Hospital
Atlanta, GA
USA

NIALL D. FERGUSON
Interdepartmental Division of Critical Care Medicine
Department of Medicine
Division of Respirology
University Health Network and Mount Sinai Hospital
University of Toronto
Toronto, ON
Canada

MASSIMO FERLUGA
Department of Perioperative Medicine, Intensive Care
and Emergency
Cattinara Hospital, Trieste.
University School of Medicine
Trieste
Italy

ARNY A. FERRANDO
Center for Translational Research in Aging and
Longevity
DWR Institute on Aging
Little Rock, AR
USA

JASON FERRIES
Division of Pulmonary and Critical Care Medicine
University of California, Davis School of Medicine
Sacramento, CA
USA

MARINO S. FESTA
The Children's Hospital at Westmead
Westmead
Australia

J. MATTHEW FIELDS
Department of Emergency Medicine
Thomas Jefferson University
Philadelphia, PA
USA

FREDERICK FIESSELER
Department of Emergency Medicine
Morristown Memorial Hospital
Morristown, NJ
USA

JOHN FILDES
Department of Surgery
University of Nevada School of Medicine
Las Vegas, NV
USA

KEVIN W. FINKEL
The Division of Renal Diseases and Hypertension
The University of Texas Medical School
Houston, TX
USA

GREGORY W. FISCHER
Adult Cardiac Anesthesia, Anesthesiology and
Cardiothoracic Surgery
Mount Sinai Medical Center
New York, NY
USA

JONATHAN I. FISCHER
Division of Emergency Ultrasonography
Department of Emergency Medicine
Hospital of the University of Pennsylvania
Philadelphia, PA
USA

MICHELLE A. FISCHER
Penn State Hershey
Hershey Medical Center Emergency Medicine
Hershey, PA
USA

STUART M. FLECHNER
Glickman Urological and Kidney Institute
Cleveland Clinic Lerner College of Medicine
Cleveland, OH
USA

NICK FLETCHER
Department of Anaesthesia and Intensive Care
St. George's Hospital
London
UK

MICHAEL A. FLIERL
Department of Orthopaedic Surgery
Denver Health Medical Center
University of Colorado School of Medicine
Denver, CO
USA

DANA FORMAN
Department of Surgery
Community Regional Medical Center
University of California – UCSF
Fresno, CA
USA

MARIE FRÖBERG
Department of Anesthesia & Intensive Care Medicine
Karolinska University Hospital Huddinge
Stockholm
Sweden

JACOB FREEMAN
Department of Neurosurgery
University of Colorado
Denver, CO
USA

ERIC R. FRYKBERG
Department of Surgery
University of Florida Health Science Center
Jacksonville, FL
USA

DAVID F. GAIESKI
Department of Emergency Medicine
Hospital of the University of Pennsylvania
Philadelphia, PA
USA

OGNJEN GAJIC
Department of Intensive Care Medicine
Mayo Epidemiology and Translational Research in
Intensive Care (METRIC)
Mayo Clinics
Rochester, MN
USA

MARCELO GAMA DE ABREU
Department of Anesthesiology and Intensive Care
Medicine
University Hospital Carl Gustav Carus
University of Technology of Dresden
Dresden
Germany

RICHARD L. GAMELLI
Stritch School of Medicine
Loyola University Medical Center
Maywood, IL
USA

MICHAEL T. GANTER
Institute of Anesthesiology
University Hospital Zurich
Zurich
Switzerland

JAVIER GARAU
Department of Medicine
Hospital Mutua de Terrassa
Terrassa, Barcelona
Spain

CAROLINA GARCIA-VIDAL
Infectious Disease Department
Hospital Universitari de Bellvitge, Institut
d'Investigacions Biomèdiques de Bellvitge (IDIBELL)
L'Hospitalet de Llobregat
Barcelona
Spain

JOSÉ GARNACHO-MONTERO
Intensive Care Unit
Hospital Universitario Virgen del Rocío
Sevilla
Spain

SUSAN GARWOOD
Department of Anesthesiology
Yale University School of Medicine
New Haven, CT
USA

LUCIANO GATTINONI
Dipartimento di Anestesia, Rianimazione e Scienze
Dermatologiche. Fondazione IRCCS Cà Granda -
Ospedale Maggiore Policlinico
Università degli Studi di Milano
Milan
Italy

GERD G. GAUGLITZ
Department of Dermatology and Allergology
Ludwig-Maximilian-University
Munich
Germany

DIMITRIOS GEORGOPOULOS
Department of Intensive Care Medicine
University Hospital of Heraklion
University of Crete
Heraklion
Crete
Greece

VICTOR E. A. GERDES
Department of Internal Medicine
Slotervaart Hospital
Amsterdam
The Netherlands

R. T. NOEL GIBNEY
Division of Critical Care Medicine
University of Alberta Hospital
Edmonton, AB
Canada

C. GIUSSANI
Neurosurgery
San Gerardo Hospital
Monza
Milan
Italy

JESSIE S. GLASSER
Department of Medicine
Brooke Army Medical Center
Fort Sam Houston, TX
USA

STUART L. GOLDSTEIN
Department of Pediatrics
Baylor College of Medicine Texas Childrens Hospital
Houston, TX
USA

EDUARDO GONZALEZ
Denver Health
Denver, CO
USA

BRENT P. GOODMAN
Mayo Clinic College of Medicine
Mayo Clinic Arizona
Scottsdale, AZ
USA

ANTHONY GORDON
Imperial College London
Critical Care Unit, Charing Cross Hospital
London
UK

MUNISH GOYAL
Department of Emergency Medicine
Washington Hospital Center
Washington, DC
USA

VICENTE H. GRACIAS
Division of Acute Care Surgery
UMDNJ-RWJMS, Robert Wood Johnson University
Hospital
New Brunswick, NJ
USA

M. SEAN GRADY
Department of Neurosurgery
Hospital of the University of Pennsylvania
Philadelphia, PA
Philadelphia

ROBERT S. GREEN
Department of Anesthesia, Division Critical Care Med.
and Department of Emergency Medicine, QEII Health
Sciences Centre, VG Site
Capital Health and Dalhousie University
Halifax, NS
Canada

CESARE GREGORETTI
Intensive Care Unit, Dipartimento di emergenza e
accettazione
Azienda Ospedaliera CTO-CRF-ICORMA
Turin
Italy

HOWARD A. GRELLER
North Shore University Hospital
Manhasset, NY
USA

JAMES H. GRENDELL
Division of Gastroenterology, Hepatology, and Nutrition
Winthrop University Hospital
Mineola, NY
USA
and
School of Medicine
State University of New York
Stony Brook, NY
USA

DONALD GRIESDALE
Department of Anesthesia & Program of Critical
Care Medicine
Vancouver General Hospital and the University
of British Columbia
Vancouver, BC
Canada

LIVIU-ADELIN GULDFRED
Department of Otolaryngology and Head
and Neck Surgery
Rigshospitalet
Copenhagen
Denmark

OLIVER L. GUNTER
Department of Surgery
Vanderbilt University Medical Center
Nashville, TN
USA

KALPALATHA K. GUNTUPALLI
Baylor College of Medicine
Ben Taub General Hospital
Houston, TX
USA

MIKKO HAAPIO
Division of Nephrology
HUCH Meilahti Hospital
Helsinki
Finland

SAMIR H. HADDAD
Intensive Care Department
King Abdulaziz Medical City
Riyadh
Kingdom of Saudi Arabia

DAVID J. HAK
Denver Health
Denver, CO
USA

MARK HAMILTON
Department of Intensive Care
St. George's Hospital
London
UK

CHRISTIAN A. HAMLAT
Department of Surgery
Harborview Medical Center
Seattle, WA
USA

PETER M. HAMMER
Department of Surgery
University of Pennsylvania School of Medicine
Philadelphia, PA
USA

E. MARK HAMMERBERG
Department of Orthopaedic Surgery, Denver Health
Medical Center
University of Colorado School of Medicine
Denver, CO
USA

SONJA HANSEN
Charité Campus Benjamin Franklin
Institute of Hygiene and Environmental Medicine
Charité – University Medicine
Berlin
Germany

STEPHAN JÜRGEN HARBARTH
Charité Campus Benjamin Franklin Infection Control
Program, Division of Infectious Diseases
Geneva University Hospitals and Medical School
Geneva
Switzerland

BRIAN G. HARBRECHT
Department of Surgery
University of Louisville
Louisville, KY
USA

JEFFREY N. HARR
Department of Surgery
Denver Health Medical Center
University of Colorado School of Medicine
Denver, CO
USA

CHARLES E. HARTFORD
Department of Surgery, Division of Pediatric Surgery
(The Children's Hospital)
University of Colorado at Denver and Health Sciences
Center
Aurora, CO
USA

CHRISTIANE S. HARTOG
Department of Anesthesiology and Intensive Care
Medicine
Jena University Hospital
Jena
Germany

PER-OLOF J. HASSELGREN
Department of Surgery
Beth Israel Deaconess Medical Center, Harvard Medical
School
Boston, MA
USA

JOHN E. HEFFNER
Department of Medicine
Providence Portland Medical Center
Oregon Health and Science University
Portland, OR
USA

J. Claude Hemphill III
Department of Neurology
San Francisco General Hospital University of California
San Francisco, CA
USA

Ulf Hemprich
Department of Anesthesiology
University of Rochester School of Medicine and
Dentistry
Rochester, NY
USA

Dietrich Henzler
Division of Critical Care
Dalhousie University and QEII Health Sciences Center
Halifax, NS
Canada

Stefan Herget-Rosenthal
Department of Nephrology
University of Duisburg-Essen
Duisburg
Germany

David N. Herndon
Department of Surgery
University of Texas Medical Branch and Shriners
Hospital for Children
Galveston, TX
USA

Margaret S. Herridge
Toronto General Hospital
University Health Network
Toronto, ON
Canada

Dean Hess
Respiratory Care
Massachusetts General Hospital
Boston, MA
USA

Russ Hewson
Barts and The London NHS Trust
Intensive Care Unit Royal London Hospital
London
UK

Christoph E. Heyde
Department of Orthopaedic Surgery
University of Leipzig
Leipzig
Germany

Caitlin W. Hicks
Cleveland Clinic Lerner College of Medicine
Cleveland, OH
USA
and
Howard Hughes Medical Institute–National Institutes
of Health Research Scholar
National Institutes of Health
Bethesda, MD
USA

Adam T. Hill
Department of Respiratory Medicine
Royal Infirmary and University of Edinburgh
Edinburgh, Scotland
UK

Nicholas S. Hill
Department of Pulmonary, Critical Care and Sleep
Medicine
Tufts-New England Medical Center
Boston, MA
USA

A. L. Hoefnagel
Department of Anesthesiology
University of Rochester School of Medicine and
Dentistry
Rochester, NY
USA

Christoph K. Hofer
Institute of Anaesthesiology and Intensive Care
Medicine
Triemli City Hospital Zurich
Zurich
Switzerland

Brian K. Hogan
Department of Medicine
San Antonio Military Medical Center
Fort Sam Houston, TX
USA

JUDD E. HOLLANDER
Department of Emergency Medicine
University of Pennsylvania
Philadelphia, PA
USA

HITOSHI HONDA
Department of General Internal Medicine and Infectious
Diseases
Teine Keijinkai Medical Center
Teine, Sapporo
Japan

WALDEMAR HOSCH
Department of Radiology
Heidelberg University Hospital
Heidelberg
Germany

ERIC A. J. HOSTE
Department of Internal Medicine
Ghent University Hospital
Ghent
Belgium

ANDREW A. HOUSE
Division of Nephrology
London Health Sciences Centre
London
Canada

TJASA HRANJEC
Department of Surgery
University of Virginia Health System
Charlottesville, VA
USA

LAURENCE HUANG
Division of Pulmonary and Critical Care Medicine and
HIV/AIDS Division
University of California
San Francisco School of Medicine
San Francisco General Hospital
San Francisco, CA
USA

ZHONGPING HUANG
Department of Mechanical Engineering
Widener University
Chester, PA
USA

W. GREGORY HUNDLEY
Department of Internal Medicine, Section on Cardiology
and Department of Radiology
Wake Forest University School of Medicine
Winston-Salem, NC
USA

OLIVER L. HUNG
Department of Emergency Medicine
Morristown Memorial Hospital
Morristown, NJ
USA

RYAN T. HURT
Division of General Internal Medicine
Mayo Clinic
Rochester, MN
USA
and
Departments of Medicine, Physiology & Biophysics
University of Louisville School of Medicine
Louisville, KY
USA

MUSTAFA HUSSAIN
Department of Surgery
NYU Langone Medical Center
New York, NY
USA

MUHAMMAD N. IQBAL
Cardiology
VA San Diego Healthcare System
San Diego, CA
USA

ROBERT A. IZENBERG
San Francisco General Hospital and Trauma Center
Department of Surgery
University of California
San Francisco, CA
USA

LA SCIENYA M. JACKSON
Department of Surgery
UCSF/Fresno University of California
San Francisco/Fresno, Community Regional Medical
Center
Fresno, CA
USA

NATTAPONG JAIMCHARIYATAM
Division of Pulmonary and Critical Care Medicine
Department of Medicine
Chulalongkorn University
Bangkok
Thailand

DAVID H. JANG
Department of Emergency Medicine
New York University
New York, NY
USA

MARC G. JESCHKE
Department of Surgery
Division of Plastic Surgery University of Toronto
Sunnybrook Research Institute
Toronto, ON
Canada

ARUN JEYABALAN
Department of Obstetrics, Gynecology, and
Reproductive Sciences
University of Pittsburgh School of Medicine
Pittsburgh, PA
USA

AARON M. JOFFE
Department of Anesthesiology and Pain Medicine
University of Washington
Harborview Medical Center
Seattle, WA
USA

JEFFREY JOHNSON
Denver Health Medical Center
University of Colorado Denver
Denver, CO
USA

DARYL JONES
Department of Intensive Care
Austin Hospital
Heidelberg, Melbourne, VIC
Australia

JANEEN R. JORDAN
University of Colorado
Denver, CO
USA

SARAH E. JUDKINS
Rocky Mountain Regional Trauma Center
Denver Health Medical Center
Denver, CO
USA

THOMAS JUNGHANSS
Section Clinical Tropical Medicine
Department of Infectious Diseases
Heidelberg University Hospital
Heidelberg
Germany

GREGORY J. JURKOVICH
Department of Surgery
Harborview Medical Center
Seattle, WA
USA

ANDERS KALLNER
Department of Clinical Chemistry
Karolinska University hospital
Stockholm
Sweden

TSUYOSHI KANEKO
Department of Cardiothoracic and Vascular Surgery
The University of Texas Medical School at Houston
Houston, TX
USA

NEETA KANNAN
Department of Critical Care Medicine
University of Pittsburgh School of Medicine
Pittsburgh, PA
USA

LEWIS J. KAPLAN
Department of Surgery
Yale University School of Medicine
New Haven, CT
USA

CONSTANTINE KARVELLAS
Divisions of Gastroenterology and Critical Care
Medicine
University of Alberta
Edmonton, AB
Canada

JOHN KASHANI
Department of Emergency Medicine
Morristown Memorial Hospital
Morristown, NJ
USA

JEFFRY L. KASHUK
Division of Trauma, Acute Care and Critical Care Surgery
and Section of Acute Care Surgery
Penn State Hershey Medical Center
Hershey, PA
USA

SANDRA L. KAVALUKAS
Department of Surgery
Sinai Hospital of Baltimore and the Johns Hopkins
Medical Institutions
Baltimore, MD
USA

CHRISTIAAN KEIJZER
Department of Anesthesiology
Academic Medical Centre
University of Amsterdam
Amsterdam
The Netherlands

JOHN A. KELLUM
Department of Critical Care Medicine
University of Pittsburgh School of Medicine
Pittsburgh, PA
USA

GILI KENET
Thrombosis Unit
The Israel National Hemophilia Center
Tel-Hashomer
Israel

F. KERBAUL
Department of Anesthesia and Intensive Care Unit
La Timone Hospital
Marseille
France

JEREMY KILBURN
Department of Medicine
Washington University School of Medicine
St. Louis, MO
USA

FERNANDO J. KIM
Denver Health Medical Center
Department of Surgery (Urology)
Denver, CO
USA

JOCELYN T. KIM
David Geffen School of Medicine
University of California
Los Angeles, CA
USA

WILLIAM A. KNIGHT
Emergency Medicine
University of Cincinnati
Cincinnati, OH
USA

M. MARGARET KNUDSON
Department of Surgery
University of California
San Francisco, CA
USA

MARIN H. KOLLEF
Department of Medicine
Washington University School of Medicine
St. Louis, MO
USA

JAY L. KOYNER
School of Medicine and Medical Science
University College Dublin
Dublin
Ireland

ROSEMARY A. KOZAR
University of Texas Health Science Center
Houston, TX
USA

ROBERT KRAFT
Department of Surgery
Medical Branch University of Texas
Galveston, TX
USA

JOHN P. KRESS
Department of Medicine, Section of Pulmonary and
Critical Care
University of Chicago
Chicago, IL
USA

KENNETH A. KUDSK
Division of General Surgery
Clinical Science Center University of Wisconsin
Madison, WI
USA

HRISHIKESH S. KULKARNI
Baylor College of Medicine
Ben Taub General Hospital
Houston, TX
USA

MATTHEW KUTCHER
Department of Surgery
University of California
San Francisco, CA
USA

SONIA LABEAU
Faculty of Medicine and Health Sciences
Ghent University
Ghent
Belgium

DAVID LAMBERT
Department of Emergency Medicine (KMW) and
Environmental Medicine (DL)
University of Pennsylvania
Philadelphia, PA
USA

THOMAS LANGER
Dipartimento di Anestesiologia, Terapia Intensiva
e Scienze Dermatologiche
Università degli Studi di Milano, Fondazione IRCCS
Ospedale Policlinico, Mangiagalli e Regina Elena
Milan
Italy

STEPHEN E. LAPINSKY
Interdepartmental Division of Critical Care
Department of Medicine
Mount Sinai Hospital
University of Toronto
Toronto, ON
Canada

SUSAN M. LAREAU
Department of Obstetrics, Gynecology and
Reproductive Sciences
Magee-Womens Hospital of the University of Pittsburgh
Medical Center
Pittsburgh, PA
USA

JULIUS LARIOZA
Division of Infectious Diseases
Baystate Medical Center
Springfield, MA
USA

PIERRE-FRANÇOIS LATERRE
Department of Critical Care Medicine
Saint-Luc University Hospital-Louvain Medical School
Brussels
Belgium

KEVIN B. LAUPLAND
Department of Critical Care Medicine
University of Calgary and Calgary Health Region
Calgary, AB
Canada

MARTINE LEBLANC
Service de néphrologie
Hôpital Maisonneuve-Rosemont Centre hospitalier
affilié à l'Univ. de Montréal
Montréal, QC
Canada

ANNA M. LEDGERWOOD
Department of Surgery
Wayne State University
Detroit, MI
USA

ANDIE S. LEE
Department of Infectious Diseases and Microbiology
Division of Medicine
Royal Prince Alfred Hospital and University of Sydney
Sydney
Australia
and
Charité Campus Benjamin Franklin Infection Control
Program, Division of Infectious Diseases
Geneva University Hospitals and Medical School
Geneva
Switzerland

ANDREW G. LEE
Department of Radiology
University of Calgary
Calgary, AB
Canada

JONG O. LEE
Department of Surgery
Medical Branch University of Texas
Galveston, TX
USA

CEDRIC W. LEFEBVRE
Emergency Medicine
Wake Forest University School of Medicine
Winston Salem, NC
USA

SEBASTIANO LEONE
U.S.C. Malattie Infettive
Ospedali Riuniti
Bergamo
Italy

ANDREW S. LEVEY
Division of Nephrology
Tufts Medical Center
Boston, MA
USA

MARCEL M. LEVI
Department of Medicine
Academic Medical Center
University of Amsterdam
Amsterdam
The Netherlands

DONALD P. LEVINE
Department of Medicine
Wayne State University
Detroit, MI
USA

MITCHELL M. LEVY
Brown University School of Medicine
Rhode Island Hospital
Providence, RI
USA

PHILLIP D. LEVY
Department of Emergency Medicine
Wayne State University
Detroit, MI
USA

RICHARD J. LEVY
Division of Anesthesiology and Pain Medicine (RJL)
Children's National Medical Center
Washington, DC
USA
and
Stavropoulos Sepsis Research Program (AJR, RJL, CSD)
University of Pennsylvania School of Medicine
Philadelphia, PA
USA

DAVID LEWINSOHN
Portland VA Medical Center
Portland, OR
USA

LUCAS LIAUDET
Adult Intensive Care Medicine Service and Burn Center
CHUV (University Hospital)
Lausanne
Switzerland

ELAINE CHIEW-LIN LIEW
Department of Anesthesiology
Keck School of Medicine of the University of Southern
California
Los Angeles, CA
USA

RICHARD W. LIGHT
Division of Pulmonary/Critical Care Medicine
Vanderbilt University Medical Center
Nashville, TN
USA

TOM LIM
Department of Internal Medicine
University of Calgary
Calgary, AB
Canada

CATHARINA F. M. LINSSEN
Department of Medical Microbiology
University Hospital Maastricht
Maastricht, AZ
The Netherlands

HAROLD LITT
Department of Radiology
University of Pennsylvania
Philadelphia, PA
USA

OLLE LJUNGQVIST
Department of Surgery
Örebro University Hospital
Örebro
Sweden

CLARA LLUBIÀ
Department of Anaesthesiology and Postoperative
Care Unit
Hospital Universitari Germans Trias i Pujol
Badalona, Barcelona
Spain

DILEEP N. LOBO
Division of Gastrointestinal Surgery
Nottingham Digestive Diseases Centre NIHR Biomedical
Research Unit, Nottingham University Hospitals
Queen's Medical Centre
Nottingham
UK

PHILIP LoBUE
Division of Tuberculosis Elimination
Centers for Disease Control and Prevention
Atlanta, GA
USA

IAN LOFTUS
St. George's Healthcare NHS Trust
London
UK

JOSÉ A. LORENTE
CIBER de Enfermedades Respiratorias
Hospital Universitario de Getafe
Universidad Europea de Madrid
Madrid
Spain

UMBERTO LUCANGELO
Department of Perioperative Medicine, Intensive Care
and Emergency
Cattinara Hospital, Trieste.
University School of Medicine
Trieste
Italy

CHARLES E. LUCAS
Department of Surgery
Wayne State University
Detroit, MI
USA

GINA LUCKIANOW
Department of Surgery
Yale University School of Medicine
New Haven, CT
USA

THOMAS LUECKE
Department of Anesthesiology and Critical Care
Medicine
University Hospital Mannheim
Mannheim
Germany

CARLOS M. LUNA
Department of Internal Medicine
Hospital de Clinicas
Universidad de Buenos Aires
Banfield, Buenos Aires
Argentina

CHARLES-EDOUARD LUYT
Service de Réanimation Médicale
Institut de Cardiologie Groupe Hospitalier
Pitié-Salpêtrière
Paris
France

JOSEPH P. LYNCH III
Division of Pulmonary, Critical Care Medicine, Allergy,
and Clinical Immunology
The David Geffen School of Medicine at UCLA
Los Angeles, CA
USA

LUKE MACYSZYN
Department of Neurosurgery
Hospital of the University of Pennsylvania
Philadelphia, PA
Philadelphia

SHELDEN MAGDER
Critical Care Division
McGill University Health Centre
Royal Victoria Hospital
Montreal, QC
Canada

DUSHYANT MAHARAJ
Department of Obstetrics & Gynaecology
University of Otago
Wellington South
New Zealand

RONALD V. MAIER
Department of Surgery
Harborview Medical Center
Seattle, WA
USA

ALAN S. MAISEL
VA San Diego Healthcare System
University of California Cardiology Section
San Diego, CA
USA

NIMA MAJLESI
Department of Emergency Medicine
Morristown Memorial Hospital
Morristown, NJ
USA

MARK A. MALANGONI
Department of Surgery
MetroHealth Medical Center
Cleveland, OH
USA

MANU L. N. G. MALBRAIN
Intensive Care Unit
Ziekenhuis Netwerk Antwerpen Hospital Campus
Stuivenberg
Antwerp
Belgium

KATHERINE MANDELL
Department of Surgery
Harborview Medical Center
Seattle, WA
USA

LIONEL A. MANDELL
McMaster University Hamilton Health Sciences
Henderson
Hamilton, ON
Canada

PAUL E. MARIK
Pulmonary and Critical Care Medicine
Thomas Jefferson University
Philadelphia, PA
USA

ANTONELLA MARINO
U.O. Anestesia e Rianimazione, Dipartimento di
Anestesia, Rianimazione (Intensiva e Subintensiva) e
Terapia del Dolore
Fondazione IRCCS Ca' Granda - Ospedale Maggiore
Policlinic
Milan
Italy

THOMAS J. MARRIE
Department of Medicine
University of Alberta
Edmonton, AB
Canada

Eric M. Massicotte
Division of Neurosurgery
University of Toronto
University Health Network Toronto Western Hospital
Toronto, ON
Canada

Brittany Matava
Department of Orthopaedic Surgery
Denver Health Medical Center
University of Colorado School of Medicine
Denver, CO
USA

Ricardo Matos
Unidade de Cuidados Intensivos Polivalente (UCIP)
Hospital de St. António dos Capuchos - Centro
Hospitalar de Lisboa Central, E.P.E.
Lisbon
Portugal

Kenneth L. Mattox
Department of Surgery
Baylor College of Medicine
Ben Taub General Hospital
Houston, TX
USA

Clive May
Howard Florey Institute
University of Melbourne
Parkville
Victoria
Australia

John C. Mayberry
Trauma/Critical Care
Oregon Health & Science University
Portland, OR
USA

Konstantin Mayer
Department of Internal Medicine II
University of Giessen Lung Center
Giessen
Germany

Stephen A. McClave
Division of Gastroenterology, Hepatology and Nutrition
University of Louisville School of Medicine
Louisville, KY
USA

James McCord
Henry Ford Hospital Center
Detroit, MI
USA

Erin McDonough Grise
Emergency Medicine
University of Cincinnati UC Health Emergency Medicine
Cincinnati, OH
USA

Michelle K. McNutt
University of Texas Health Science Center
Houston, TX
USA

Norman E. McSwain Jr.
Department of Surgery
Tulane University School of Medicine
New Orleans, LA
USA

C. Crawford Mechem
Department of Emergency Medicine
Hospital of the University of Pennsylvania
Philadelphia, PA
USA
and
Philadelphia Fire Department
Philadelphia, PA
USA

Gabriel A. Mecott
Division of Plastic Surgery
Universidad Autonoma de Nuevo Leon
Monterrey, NL
Mexico

Wouter Meersseman
Department of General Internal Medicine
University Hospital
Leuven
Belgium

ZIAD A. MEMISH
Ministry of Health
Riyadh
Kingdom of Saudi Arabia

NATALIA MENDOZA
Center for Clinical Studies
Houston, TX
USA
and
El Bosque University
Bogota, Colombia
Canada

DAVID K. MENON
Department of Anaesthesiology
University of Cambridge & Addenbrooke's Hospital
Cambridge
UK

ARES KRISHNA MENON
Klinik f. Thorax-, Herz-, Gefäßchirurgie
Klinikum der RWTH
Aachen
Germany

J. WAYNE MEREDITH
Wake Forest University Baptist, Medical Center
Medical Center Boulevarde
Winston-Salem, NC
USA

ELISABETH MEYER
Charité Campus Benjamin Franklin
Institute of Hygiene and Environmental Medicine
Charité – University Medicine
Berlin
Germany

MINI MICHAEL
Department of Pediatrics, Renal Section
Baylor College of Medicine
Texas Children's Hospital
Houston, TX
USA

ARGYRIS MICHALOPOULOS
Department of Critical Care Medicine
Henry Dunant Hospital
Athens
Greece
and
Alfa Institute of Biomedical Sciences (AIBS)
Marousi, Athens
Greece

FREDERIC MICHARD
Director, Medical Strategy
Edwards Lifesciences
Nyon
Switzerland

CHADWICK D. MILLER
Department of Emergency Medicine
Wake Forest University Baptist Medical Center School
of Medicine
Winston-Salem, NC
USA

MELISSA A. MILLER
Pulmonary and Critical Care Medicine
Medical Center Drive
Taubman Center
Ann Arbor, MI
USA

ANGELA M. MILLS
Department of Emergency Medicine
University of Pennsylvania
Philadelphia, PA
USA

JOSEPH P. MINEI
Division of Burns, Trauma, and Critical Care
Department of Surgery
UT-Southwestern Medical Center
Dallas, TX
USA

MARY K. MIRANOWSKI
Nestlé Health Care Nutrition

CHRISTOPHER H. MODY
Departments of Internal Medicine and Microbiology
Immunology and Infectious Disease
University of Calgary
Calgary, AB
Canada

BERTON R. MOED
Department of Orthopaedic Surgery
Saint Louis University School of Medicine
St. Louis, MO
USA

WILSON MOLINA
Denver Health Medical Center
Department of Surgery (Urology)
Denver, CO
USA

BRUCE A. MOLITORIS
Division of Nephrology, Department of Medicine
Indiana University School of Medicine
Indianapolis, IN
USA

XAVIER MONNET
Medical Intensive Care Unit, Bicêtre Hospital
Assistance Publique – Hôpitaux de Paris and Paris-Sud
University
Le Kremlin-Bicêtre
France

A. MONTCRIOL
Department of Anesthesia and Intensive Care Unit
La Timone Hospital
Marseille
France

ERNEST E. MOORE
Department of Surgery
Denver Health Medical Center
University of Colorado Denver
Denver, CO
USA

FREDERICK A. MOORE
Department of Surgery
The Methodist Hospital
Houston, TX
USA

HUNTER B. MOORE
University of Vermont College of Medicine
Burlington, VT
USA

LAURA J. MOORE
Department of Surgery
The Methodist Hospital Research Institute
Houston, TX
USA

GREGORY J. MORAN
Department of Emergency Medicine
Olive View-UCLA Medical Center
Sylmar, CA
USA

RUI P. MORENO
Unidade de Cuidados Intensivos Polivalente, Hospital
de Santo António dos Capuchos
Centro Hospitalar de Lisboa Central, E.P.E
Lisbon
Portugal

MARINA S. MORGAN
Department of Medical Microbiology
Royal Devon & Exeter Foundation NHS Trust
Exeter, Devon
UK

ALISON MORRIS
Division of Pulmonary, Allergy, and Critical Care
Medicine
University of Pittsburgh School of Medicine
Pittsburgh, PA
USA

ANDREW M. MORRIS
Mount Sinai Hospital and University Health Network,
University of Toronto
Toronto, ON
Canada

JOHN A. MORRIS JR.
Department of Surgery
Vanderbilt University Medical Center
Nashville, TN
USA

KATIE MORRISON
Center for Clinical Studies
Houston, TX
USA

RYAN P. MORRISSEY
Central Texas Poison Center
Scott & White Memorial Hospital
Temple, TX
USA
and
New York City Poison Control Center
New York University Medical Center and Bellevue
Hospital Center
New York, NY
USA

PETER F. MOUNT
Austin Research Institute
Austin Hospital
Heidelberg, VIC
Australia

NATHAN T. MOWERY
Wake Forest University Baptist, Medical Center
Medical Center Boulevarde
Winston-Salem, NC
USA

J. PAUL MUIZELAAR
Department of Neurological Surgery
University of California
Davis, CA
USA

ASHLEY MULL
Department of Emergency Medicine
Denver Health Medical Center
Denver, CO
USA

RICHARD J. MULLINS
Department of Surgery
Oregon Health & Sciences University
Portland, OR
USA

BRYN E. MUMMA
Department of Emergency Medicine
University of California Davis Medical Center
Sacramento, CA
USA

CLINTON K. MURRAY
Department of Medicine
San Antonio Military Medical Center
Fort Sam Houston, TX
USA

PATRICK T. MURRAY
School of Medicine and Medical Science
University College Dublin
Dublin
Ireland

RAGHAVAN MURUGAN
Department of Critical Care Medicine, The CRISMA
(Clinical Research, Investigation, and Systems Modeling
of Acute Illness) Center
University of Pittsburgh School of Medicine
Pittsburgh, PA
USA

JOHN G. MUSCEDERE
Department of Medicine
Kingston General Hospital
Kingston, ON
Canada

KURT G. NABER
Technical University
Straubing, Munich
Germany

JOHN TOBIAS NAGURNEY
Department of Emergency Medicine
Massachussets General Hospital
Harvard Medical School
Boston, MA
USA

PAYAM NAHID
University of California, San Francisco
San Francisco, CA
USA

LENA M. NAPOLITANO
Department of Surgery
University of Michigan, 1C340A-UH, University Hospital
Ann Arbor, MI
USA

BARNETT R. NATHAN
Division of Neurocritical Care
Departments of Neurology
University of Virginia
Charlottesville, VA
USA

LEWIS S. NELSON
New York City Poison Control Center
New York University Medical Center and Bellevue
Hospital Center
New York, NY
USA

CARLA NESTER
Department of Pediatrics
Division of Pediatric Nephrology, Dialysis &
Transplantation
University of Iowa Children's Hospital
Carver College of Medicine
Iowa City, IA
USA

LINDSAY E. NICOLLE
Department of Internal Medicine/Medical Microbiology
University of Manitoba/Health Sciences Centre Section
of Infectious Diseases
Winnipeg, MB
Canada

LISE E. NIGROVIC
Division of Emergency Medicine
Children's Hospital Boston
Harvard Medical School
Boston, MA
USA

NICOLÁS NIN
CIBER de Enfermedades Respiratorias
Hospital Universitario de Getafe
Universidad Europea de Madrid
Madrid
Spain

LORETTA NORTON
Graduate Program in Neuroscience
University of Western Ontario
London, ON
Canada

MELISSA NYENDAK
Oregon Health and Sciences University
Portland, OR
USA

BLANCA OCHOA
Baylor College of Medicine
Houston, TX
USA

JUAN B. OCHOA
Trauma and Surgical Critical Care
University of Pittsburgh Medical Center
Pittsburgh, PA
USA

GAGE M. OCHSNER
Savannah, GA
USA

DAVID N. O'DWYER
Department of Respiratory Medicine
St. Vincent's University Hospital
Dublin
Ireland

MARK D. OKUSA
Division of Nephrology and the Center for Immunity,
Inflammation and Regenerative Medicine
University of Virginia Health System
Charlottesville, VA
USA

DEAN OLSEN
Medical Toxicology and Emergency Medicine
New York City Poison Control Center
Manhattan, NY
USA

JAMES C. O'NEILL
Department of Emergency Medicine
Wake Forest University Baptist Medical Center
Winston-Salem, NC
USA

EDMUND ONG
Department of Infection and Tropical Medicine
Royal Victoria Infirmary
Newcastle upon Tyne
UK

OSITA I. ONUGHA
Department of Surgery
Stanford University
Stanford, CA
USA

DAVID OSMAN
Service de Réanimation Médicale
CHU Bicêtre, AP-HP
Université Paris-Sud
Le Kremlin-Bicêtre
France

GEORGES OUELLET
Service de néphrologie
Hôpital Maisonneuve-Rosemont Centre hospitalier
affilié à l'Univ. de Montréal
Montréal, QC
Canada

KAGAN OZER
Denver Health Medical Center
University of Colorado Denver, School of Medicine
Denver, CO
USA

H. LEON PACHTER
Department of Surgery
NYU Langone Medical Center
New York, NY
USA

JOSÉ ARTUR PAIVA
UAG da Urgência e Cuidados Intensivos
Hospital Sao Joao and Medical School
University of Porto
Porto
Portugal

PAUL M. PALEVSKY
Renal Section
VA Pittsburgh Healthcare System
Pittsburgh, PA
USA
and

Renal–Electrolyte Division
Department of Medicine
University of Pittsburgh School of Medicine
Pittsburgh, PA
USA

NOVA L. PANEBIANCO
Department of Emergency Medicine
University of Pennsylvania
Philadelphia, PA
USA

NEESH PANNU
Division of Nephrology
Department of Medicine University of Alberta
Edmonton, AB
Canada

PETER J. PAPADAKOS
Department of Anesthesiology
University of Rochester School of Medicine and
Dentistry
Rochester, NY
USA

LAURENT PAPAZIAN
Service de Réanimation médicale, Assistance Publique
Hôpitaux de Marseille, URMITE CNRS-UMR 6236
Université de la Méditerranée Aix-Marseille II
Marseille
France

GIDEON PARET
Safra Children's hospital, Sheba Medical Center
Tel Hashomer
Israel

TANYALAK PARIMON
Pulmonary and Critical Care Division
Department of Medicine
Veterans Affairs Medical Center, Boise, ID
University of Washington School of Medicine
Seattle, WA
USA

MARGARET M. PARKER
Department of Pediatrics
Stony Brook University Medical Center
Stony Brook, NY
USA

AMBICA PARMAR
Division of Critical Care Medicine
University of Alberta
Edmonton, AB
Canada

MATTEO PAROTTO
Istituto di Anestesia e Rianimazione
Dipartimento di Farmacologia e Anestesia
Università degli Studi di Padova
Padova
Italy

DAVID A. PARTRICK
Division of Pediatric Surgery
The Children's Hospital
University of Colorado School of Medicine
Denver, CO
USA

JOSE L. PASCUAL
Division of Traumatology, Surgical Critical Care and
Emergency Surgery
University of Pennsylvania Health System
Philadelphia, PA
USA

MEHUL PATEL
Division of Infectious Diseases, Department of Medicine
University of Toronto and University Health Network
Toronto, ON
Canada

W. FRANK PEACOCK
Department of Emergency Medicine
The Cleveland Clinic Cleveland Clinic Foundation
Cleveland, OH
USA

RUPERT M. PEARSE
Barts and The London School of Medicine and Dentistry
Intensive Care Unit Royal London Hospital
London
UK

MARCUS PECK
Department of Intensive Care
St. George's Hospital
London
UK

ANDREW B. PEITZMAN
Department of Surgery
University of Pittsburgh School of Medicine
Pittsburgh, PA
USA

PAOLO PELOSI
Department of Ambient, Health and Safety
Università degli Studi dell'Insubria
Varese
Italy

MARIANO ALBERTO PENNISI
Istituto di Anestesiologia e Rianimazione
Policlinico Universitario A. Gemelli
Università Cattolica del Sacro Cuore
Rome
Italy

J. M. PEREIRA
UAG da Urgência e Cuidados Intensivos
Hospital Sao Joao and Medical School
University of Porto
Porto
Portugal

RUI PEREIRA
Unidade de Cuidados Intensivos Polivalente (UCIP)
Hospital de St. António dos Capuchos - Centro
Hospitalar de Lisboa Central, E.P.E.
Lisbon
Portugal

AZRIEL PEREL
Department of Anesthesiology and Intensive Care
Sheba Medical Center
Tel Aviv University
Tel Aviv
Israel

JEANMARIE PERRONE
Department of Emergency Medicine
Hospital of the University of Pennsylvania
Philadelphia, PA
USA

ANTONIO PESENTI
Department of Perioperative Medicine and Intensive
Care A.O. Ospedale S. Gerardo
University of Milan-Bicocca
Monza
Italy

ALOIS PHILIPP
Leiter Kardiotechnik
Universitätsklinikum Regensburg
Regensburg
Germany

BARBARA J. PHILIPS
St. George's University of London
London
UK

JASON M. PHILLIPS
Denver Health Medical Center
Department of Surgery (Urology)
Denver, CO
USA

CLAUDE PICHARD
Unité de Nutrition
Hôpitaux Universitaires de Genève
Geneva
Switzerland

FREDRIC M. PIERACCI
Trauma and Acute Care Surgery
Department of Surgery
Denver Health Medical Center
University of Colorado Health Sciences Center
Denver, CO
USA

JESSE M. PINES
Center for Health Care Quality
Departments of Emergency Medicine and Health Policy
George Washington University
Washington, DC
USA

SARAH E. PINSKI
Department of Orthopaedic Surgery
Denver, CO
USA

DIDIER PITTET
Infection Control Programme
University of Geneva Hospitals
Geneva
Switzerland

LUCIDO L. PONCE
Department of Neurosurgery
Baylor College of Medicine
Houston, TX
USA

ANNE-CORNÉLIE J. M. DE PONT
Academisch Medisch Centrum
Academisch Ziekenhuis bij de Universiteit van
Amsterdam
Amsterdam
The Netherlands

LAURA J. PORRO
Department of Surgery
University of Texas Medical Branch and Shriners
Hospital for Children
Galveston, TX
USA

JOSEPH A. POSLUSZNY JR.
Department of Surgery
Loyola University Medical Center
Maywood, IL
USA

NIKHIL PREMCHAND
Department of Infection and Tropical Medicine
Royal Victoria Infirmary
Newcastle upon Tyne
UK

SUSANNA PRICE
Department of Intensive Care
Royal Brompton Hospital
London
UK

SEAN PRIMLEY
Denver Health Medical Center
Department of Surgery (Urology)
Denver, CO
USA

JANE M. PROSSER
Department of Emergency Medicine
Weill Cornell Medical Center
New York, NY
USA

J. JAVIER PROVENCIO
Cerebrovascular Center and Neuroinflammatory
Research Center
Cleveland Clinic/NC30
Cleveland, OH
USA

JOHN R. PROWLE
Department of Intensive Care
Austin Hospital
Melbourne
Australia

SRINI PYATI
Division of Veterans Affairs
Duke University Medical Center
Durham, NC
USA

PRASANNA SIMHA MOHAN RAO
Cardiothoracic and Vascular Surgery
Sri Jayadeva Institute of Cardiovascular Sciences and
Research
Malleswaram, Bangalore
India

RON H. RAWLINGS
Department of Anesthesiology
Duke University Medical Center
Durham, NC
USA

SUNIL S. RAYAN
Scripps
La jolla, CA
USA

KONRAD REINHART
Department of Anesthesiology and Intensive Care
Medicine
Jena University Hospital
Jena
Germany

DANIEL K. RESNICK
Department of Neurological Surgery
University of Wisconsin
Madison, WI
USA

STEVEN REYNOLDS
UBC Department of Medicine
Royal Columbian Hospital
New Westminster, BC
Canada

STUART F. REYNOLDS
Division of Critical Care Medicine
University of Alberta Hospitals
Edmonton, AB
Canada

ANDREW RHODES
Department of Intensive Care
St. George's Hospital
London
UK

ZACCARIA RICCI
Department of Pediatric Cardiac Surgery
Bambino Gesù Children's Hospital
Rome
Italy

AARON RICHMAN
Institute of Terrorism Research and Response
Philadelphia, PA
USA

JAMES RIDDELL IV
Department of Internal Medicine
Division of Infectious Diseases
University of Michigan Health System
Ann Arbor, MI
USA

JOHN T. RIEHL
Geisinger Medical Center Orthopaedics
Danville, PA
USA

CLAUDIA S. ROBERTSON
Department of Neurosurgery
Baylor College of Medicine
Houston, TX
USA

BRYCE R. H. ROBINSON
Division of Trauma and Critical Care
University of Cincinnati
Cincinnati, OH
USA

JOSÉ RODOLFO ROCCO
Clementino Fraga Filho University Hospital
Federal University of Rio de Janeiro
Rio de Janeiro
Brazil

ADAM ROMANOVSKY
Division of Critical Care Medicine
University of Alberta
Edmonton, AB
Canada

CLAUDIO RONCO
Department of Nephrology
St. Bortolo Hospital
Vicenza
Italy

ANDREA O. ROSSETTI
Service de Neurologie
Centre Hospitalier Universitaire Vaudois (CHUV-BH07)
Lausanne
Switzerland

COLEMAN ROTSTEIN
Division of Infectious Diseases
Department of Medicine
University of Toronto and University Health Network
Toronto, ON
Canada

BRIAN H. ROWE
Department of Emergency Medicine
University of Alberta
Edmonton, AB
Canada

ANDREW K. ROY
School of Medicine and Medical Science
University College Dublin
Dublin
Ireland

GRACE S. ROZYCKI
Emory University School of Medicine
Chief of Trauma/Surgical Critical Care/Emergency
General Surgery Department of Surgery
Atlanta, GA
USA

ALBERT J. RUGGIERI
Department of Anesthesiology and Critical
Care (AJR, CSD)
University of Pennsylvania School of Medicine
Philadelphia, PA
USA

SAMIR G. SAKKA
Department of Anesthesiology and Intensive Care
Medicine, Medical Center Cologne-Merheim
University Witten/Herdecke
Cologne
Germany

EDGARDO S. SALCEDO
Division of Traumatology, Surgical Critical Care and
Emergency Surgery
University of Pennsylvania Health System
Philadelphia, PA
USA

CHRISTIAN SANDROCK
Division of Pulmonary and Critical Care Medicine
University of California, Davis School of Medicine
Sacramento, CA
USA

ARTHUR SANFORD
Stritch School of Medicine
Loyola University Medical Center
Maywood, IL
USA

BABAK SARANI
Departments of Surgery
University of Pennsylvania The Trauma Center at Penn
Philadelphia, PA
USA

TODD SARGE
Beth Israel Deaconess Medical Center/Harvard Medical
School
Boston, MA
USA

ANGELA SAUAIA
Colorado School of Public Health
University of Colorado Denver
Aurora, CO
USA

LINA MARIA SAUCEDO
Department of Pulmonary and Critical Care Medicine
Hospital Clinic
Barcelona
Spain

JUDY SAVIGE
Department of Medicine
University of Melbourne Northern Hospital
Melbourne, VIC
Australia

ROBERT G. SAWYER
Department of Surgery
University of Virginia Health System
Charlottesville, VA
USA

HUGO SAX
Infection Control Programme
University of Geneva Hospitals
Geneva
Switzerland

THOMAS M. SCALEA
Shock Trauma Center
University of Maryland School of Medicine
Baltimore, MD
USA

DANIEL SCHEURICH
Department of Internal Medicine
Washington University, School of Medicine
St. Louis, MO
USA

MARCUS J. SCHULTZ
Laboratory of Experimental Intensive Care and
Anesthesiology (L·E·I·C·A)
Academic Medical Center, University of Amsterdam
Amsterdam
The Netherlands

C. WILLIAM SCHWAB
Department of Surgery
University of Pennsylvania School of Medicine
Philadelphia, PA
USA

SABINO SCOLLETTA
Department of Surgery and Bioengineering
Cardiothoracic Anaesthesia and Intensive care,
University Hospital Le Scotte
Siena
Italy

MARC M. SEDWITZ
Scripps
Chief of Staff, Scripps Memorial Hospital, La Jolla.
Attending General and Vascular Surgeon, Scripps
La Jolla, CA
USA

RAGHU R. SEETHALA
Department of Anesthesiology, Perioperative and Pain
Medicine
Brigham and Women's Hospital
Boston, MA
USA

WAHIDA SEKANDAR
Cardiology
University of California
San Diego, CA
USA

PARHAM SENDI
University Clinic for Infectious Diseases
University Hospital Bern and University of Bern
Bern
Switzerland

P. W. Serruys
Director of the Department of Interventional Cardiology
Thoraxcenter
Erasmus Medical Centre
GD, Rotterdam
The Netherlands

Jos J. Settels
BMEYE BV
Amsterdam, BE
The Netherlands

Kiarash Shahlaie
Department of Neurological Surgery
San Francisco Veterans Affairs Medical Center
University of California
San Francisco, CA
USA

Sajid Shahul
Anesthesia and Critical Care
Beth Israel Deaconess Medical Center
Harvard Medical School
Boston, MA
USA

Haim Shapiro
Critical Care Medicine and Institute for Nutrition
Research
Rabin Medical Center Beilinson Hospital
Petah Tikva
Israel

Asif Sharfuddin
Division of Nephrology
Department of Medicine
Indiana University School of Medicine
Indianapolis, IN
USA

Tarek Sharshar
General Intensive Care Unit
Raymond Poincaré Teaching Hospital (AP-HP)
University of Versailles Saint-Quentin en Yvelines
Garches
France

Andrew Shaw
Department of Anesthesiology
Duke University Medical Center
Durham, NC
USA

Yahya Shehabi
Clinical School, University New South Wales
The Prince of Wales Hospital
Randwick, NSW
Australia

Suzanne M. Shepherd
Department of Emergency Medicine
Hospital of the University of Pennsylvania
Philadelphia, PA
USA

Richard D. Shih
Department of Emergency Medicine
Morristown Memorial Hospital
Morristown, NJ
USA

Catherine T. Shoff
Pulmonary/Critical Care/Sleep Medicine
Uniformed Services University of Health Sciences
Lackland AFB, TX
USA

William H. Shoff
Department of Emergency Medicine
Hospital of the University of Pennsylvania
Philadelphia, PA
USA

Andrew F. Shorr
Division of Pulmonary and Critical Care Medicine,
Georgetown University School of Medicine
Washington Hospital Center
Washington, DC
USA

Chuin Siau
Division of Respiratory Medicine
Department of Medicine Changi General Hospital
Singapore
Singapore

MICHAEL E. SILVERMAN
Department of Emergency Medicine
Morristown Memorial Hospital
Morristown, NJ
USA

FIONA SIMPSON
Clinical Senior Lecturer in Intensive Care
Northern Clinical School
University of Sydney
Sydney
Australia
and
Department of Intensive Care
Royal North Shore Hospital
St. Leonards, NSW
Australia

CARRIE A. SIMS
The Trauma Center at Penn
Philadelphia, PA
USA

CHRISTER A. SINDERBY
St. Michael's Hospital
Toronto
Canada

KAI SINGBARTL
Department of Critical Care Medicine
University of Pittsburgh
Pittsburgh, PA
USA

BEN SINGER
Department of Intensive Care
St. George's Hospital
London
UK

PIERRE SINGER
Critical Care Medicine and Institute for Nutrition
Research
Rabin Medical Center Beilinson Hospital
Petah Tikva
Israel

DANIEL J. SKIEST
Division of Infectious Diseases
Baystate Medical Center
Springfield, MA
USA

HEATHER E. SKILLMAN
Pediatric Critical Care Dietitian
The Children's Hospital
Aurora, CO
USA

ANNIE L. SLAUGHTER
University of Colorado School of Medicine
Denver, CO
USA

LEO SLAVIN
Cardiology
University of California
San Diego, CA
USA

WADE R. SMITH
Geisinger Medical Center Orthopaedics
Danville, PA
USA

MARCEL SOESAN
Department of Internal Medicine
Slotervaart Hospital
Amsterdam
The Netherlands

MITCHELL C. SOKOLOSKY
Emergency Medicine Medical Center Boulevard
Wake Forest University Baptist Medical Center
Winston-Salem, NC
USA

OTHMAN SOLAIMAN
Interdepartmental Division of Critical Care Medicine
Department of Medicine
Division of Respirology
University Health Network and Mount Sinai Hospital
University of Toronto
Toronto, ON
Canada

R. Sonneville
General Intensive Care Unit
Raymond Poincaré Teaching Hospital (AP-HP)
University of Versailles Saint-Quentin en Yvelines
Garches
France

Lorenzo Del Sorbo
Dipartimento di Anestesiologia e Rianimazione
Università di Torino
Turin
Italy

Olan A. Soremekun
Emergency Medicine
University of Pennsylvania Health System
Philadelphia, PA
USA

Gina Soriya
Department of Emergency Medicine
Denver Health Medical Center
Denver, CO
USA

Karina M. Soto-Ruiz
Dorrington Medical Associates
Houston, TX
USA
and
School of Medicine
Universidad Autonoma de Baja California
Tijuana
Mexico

C. de Sousa
Cardiology Department
Hospital Pulido Valente
Lisbon
Portugal

Donat R. Spahn
Institute of Anesthesiology
University Hospital Zurich
Zurich
Switzerland

David A. Spain
Chief of Acute Care Surgery
Department of Surgery
Stanford University
Stanford, CA
USA

Dominic W. K. Spray
Anaesthetics and Intensive Care
St. George's Hospital
London
UK

Pierre Squara
CERIC – ICU
Clinique Ambroise Paré
Neuilly-sur-Seine
France

Nattachai Srisawat
Department of Critical Care Medicine
University of Pittsburgh School of Medicine
Pittsburgh, PA
USA

Philip F. Stahel
Department of Orthopaedic Surgery and
Department of Neurosurgery,
Denver Health Medical Center
University of Colorado School of Medicine
Denver, CO
USA

Renee D. Stapleton
Division of Pulmonary Disease and Critical Care
Medicine
University of Vermont College of Medicine
Burlington, VT
USA

Andrew Stephen
Department of Surgery
Rhode Island Hospital
Providence, RI
USA

DENNIS L. STEVENS
Infectious Diseases Section
Veterans Affairs Medical Center, Boise, ID
University of Washington School of Medicine
Seattle, WA
USA

ROBERT D. STEVENS
Departments of Anesthesiology Critical Care Medicine,
Neurology, Neurosurgery, and Radiology
Johns Hopkins University School of Medicine
Baltimore, MD
USA

MARIJA STOJKOVIC
Section Clinical Tropical Medicine
Department of Infectious Diseases
Heidelberg University Hospital
Heidelberg
Germany

MICHAEL SUGRUE
Department of Surgery
Letterkenny General Hospital
Letterkenny, Co Donegal
Ireland

DERRICK SUN
Department of Neurosurgery
Denver Health Medical Center
University of Colorado School of Medicine
Denver, CO
USA

BENJAMIN SUN
Emergency Department
University of California, Los Angeles/West Los Angeles
Veterans Affairs Medical Center
Los Angeles, CA
USA

DANIEL TALMOR
Department of Anesthesia and Critical Care Medicine
Beth Israel Deaconess Medical Center Harvard Medical
School
Boston, MA
USA

ADDY TAN
Department of Anaesthesia
National University Hospital
Singapore
Singapore

CHARLES TATOR
Krembil Neuroscience Centre
Toronto Western Hospital
Toronto, ON
Canada

JEAN-LOUIS TEBOUL
Service de Réanimation Médicale
CHU Bicêtre, AP–HP
Université Paris–Sud
Le Kremlin–Bicêtre
France

TIFFANY TELLO
Urology
Denver Health Medical Center/UCHSC
Denver, CO
USA

RICHARD E. TEMES
Rush University Medical Center
Illinois
USA

ERWIN R. THAL
Department of Surgery
UT Southwestern Medical Center
Dallas, TX
USA

RONAN THIBAULT
Service d'Hépato–gastro–entérologie et Assistance
Nutritionnelle
UMR 1280 Physiologie des Adaptations Nutritionnelles,
CHU Nantes, CRNH Nantes, IMAD Université de Nantes
Nantes
France
and
Unité de Nutrition
Hôpitaux Universitaires de Genève
Genève
Switzerland

GRIET VAN THIELEN
Department of Intensive Care
Royal Brompton Hospital
London
UK

ASHITA J. TOLWANI
Department of Medicine
University of Alabama at Birmingham
Birmingham, AL
USA

MARCIE TOMBLYN
H. Lee Moffitt Cancer Center & Research Institute,
Department of Blood and Marrow Transplantation
Associate Professor of Oncologic Sciences, USF
Tampa, FL
USA

ANTONI TORRES
Department of Pulmonary and Critical Care Medicine
Hospital Clinic
Barcelona
Spain

NICOLE T. TOWNSEND
University of Colorado Health Sciences Center
Denver, CO
USA

DONALD D. TRUNKEY
Department of Surgery
Oregon Health & Science University
Portland, OR
USA

PETER I. TSAI
Department of Surgery
Baylor College of Medicine
Houston, TX
USA

STEPHEN K. TYRING
Departments of Dermatology
University of Texas and Center for Clinical Studies
Houston, TX
USA

S. UDDIN
Department of Intensive Care
King's College Hospital
London
UK

AYTEKIN UNLU
Division of Trauma Surgery and Surgical Critical Care
DeWitt Daughtry Family Department of Surgery
Medical Director for Education and Training
International Medical Institute
University of Miami Miller School of Medicine
Ryder Trauma Center
Miami, FL
USA

ADITYA UPPALAPATI
Department of Critical Care Medicine
University of Pittsburgh School of Medicine
Pittsburgh, PA
USA

DANIEL Z. USLAN
David Geffen School of Medicine
University of California
Los Angeles, CA
USA

FRANCO VALENZA
Dipartimento di Anestesiologia, Terapia Intensiva e
Scienze Dermatologiche
Università degli Studi di Milano, Fondazione IRCCS
Ospedale Policlinico, Mangiagalli e Regina Elena
Milan
Italy

MARCO VALGIMIGLI
Director of the Cath. Laboratory
University of Ferrara, Cardiovascular Institute
Arcispedale S. Anna Hospital
Ferrara
Italy

ERIC C. M. VAN GORP
Department of Internal Medicine
Slotervaart Hospital
Amsterdam
The Netherlands

MATTHIJS VAN WISSEN
Department of Internal Medicine
Slotervaart Hospital
Amsterdam
The Netherlands

TODD F. VANDERHEIDEN
Department of Orthopaedic Surgery
Center for Complex Fractures and Limb Restoration
Denver Health Medical Center
University of Colorado School of Medicine
Denver, CO
USA

DOMINIQUE VANDIJCK
Faculty of Medicine and Health Sciences
Ghent University
Ghent
Belgium

KRISHNA K. VARADHAN
Division of Gastrointestinal Surgery
Nottingham Digestive Diseases Centre NIHR Biomedical
Research Unit, Nottingham University Hospitals,
Queen's Medical Centre
Nottingham
UK

JOSEPH VARON
Dorrington Medical Associates
Houston, TX
USA
and
The University of Texas Health Science Center at
Houston, and The University of Texas Medical Branch at
Galveston. Memorial Hermann Hospital
Texas Medical Center
Houston, TX
USA

ELISA VEDES
Department of General Intensive Care
St. George's Hospital
London
UK

ANA VELEZ
Division of Infectious Diseases and International
Medicine
Department of Medicine
Tampa, FL
USA

GEORGE C. VELMAHOS
Division of Trauma, Emergency Surgery, and Surgical
Critical Care
Massachusetts General Hospital
Harvard Medical School
Boston, MA
USA

BALA VENKATESH
Department of Critical Care, Endocrinology and
Metabolism Research Unit
University of Queensland, and Princess Alexandra and
Wesley Hospitals
Brisbane, QLD
Australia

JUAN M. VERDE
Division of Trauma Surgery and Surgical Critical Care
DeWitt Daughtry Family Department of Surgery
Medical Director for Education and Training
International Medical Institute
University of Miami Miller School of Medicine
Ryder Trauma Center
Miami, FL
USA

ANTOINE VIEILLARD-BARON
Intensive Care Unit
University Hospital Ambroise Paré
Boulogne
France
and
Faculté de Médecine Paris Ile de France Ouest
Université de Versailles Saint Quentin en Yvelines
France

CHRISTOPHE VINSONNEAU
Mixt ICU
Marc Jacquet Hospital
Melun
France

GORAZD VOGA
Medical ICU
General Hospital Celje
Celje
Slovenia

KATHLEEN M. VOLLMAN
Advancing Nursing
Northville, MI
USA

ELENA VOLPI
Department of Internal Medicine and Sealy Center on
Aging
The University of Texas Medical Branch
Galveston, TX
USA

PASCAL VRANCKX
Medical Director Cardiac ITU
Hartcentrum Hasselt
Hasselt
Belgium

FLORIAN M.E. WAGENLEHNER
Clinic for Urology, Pediatric Urology and Andrology
Justus-Liebig-University
Giessen
Germany

MATTHEW J. WALL JR.
Department of Surgery
Baylor College of Medicine
Houston, TX
USA

SAMUEL WALLER
Department of Neurological Surgery
University of Colorado School of Medicine
Denver, CO
USA

KRISTY M. WALSH
Department of Emergency Medicine (KMW) and
Environmental Medicine (DL)
Hospital of the University of Pennsylvania
Philadelphia, PA
USA

LI WAN
Department of Intensive Care and Medicine
Austin Hospital
Melbourne
Australia

DAVID K. WARREN
Division of Infectious Diseases
Department of Medicine
Washington University School of Medicine
Saint Louis, MO
USA

CHRISTOPHER M. WATSON
Division of Trauma and Acute Care Surgery
Palmetto Health
Columbia, SC
USA

LINDSAY-RAE B. WEITZEL
Department of Anesthesiology, Critical Care
University of Colorado Denver, Translational
PharmacoNutrition Laboratory (TPN Lab) Anschutz
Medical Campus
Aurora, CO
USA

XIAOYAN WEN
Department of Critical Care Medicine
University of Pittsburgh School of Medicine
Pittsburgh, PA
USA

JULIA A. WENDON
Liver Intensive Therapy Unit
Institute of Liver Studies
Kings College Hospital
London
UK

JAN WERNERMAN
Department of Anesthesia & Intensive Care Medicine
Karolinska University Hospital Huddinge
Stockholm
Sweden

J. P. J. Wester
Department of Intensive Care Medicine
Onze Lieve Vrouwe Gasthuis
HM
Amsterdam
The Netherlands

Derek S. Wheeler
Division of Critical Care Medicine
Cincinnati Children's Hospital Medical Center
Cincinnati, OH
USA
and
The Kindervelt Laboratory for Critical Care Medicine
Research
Cincinnati Children's Research Foundation
Cincinnati, OH
USA

Lars Widdel
Department of Neurosurgery
University of Colorado Denve Health Medical Center
Denver, CO
USA

Lara Wijayasiri
Department of Anaesthesia
St. George's Hospital
London
UK

Eelco F. M. Wijdicks
Department of Neurology
Mayo Clinic
Rochester, MN
USA

Anna Wilkes
Department of Surgery
Hunter New England Area Health Network
Newcastle, NSW
Australia

Brian H. Williams
Division of Burns, Trauma, and Critical Care,
Department of Surgery
UT Southwestern Medical Center
Dallas, TX
USA

Beau Willison
Center for Clinical Studies
Houston, TX
USA

Sarah L. Wingerter
Division of Emergency Medicine
Children's Hospital Boston, Harvard Medical School
Boston, MA
USA

Ken R. Winston
Department of Neurosurgery
University of Colorado
Denver, CO
USA

Michael E. Winters
Intensive Care Unit
University of Maryland
Mount Airy, MD
USA
and
Combined Emergency Medicine/Internal Medicine/
Critical Care Program
University of Maryland School of Medicine
Baltimore, MD
USA

Kevin Winthrop
Oregon Health and Sciences University
Portland, OR
USA

Paul P. E. Wischmeyer
University of Colorado at Denver School of Medicine
Aurora, CO
USA

David H. Wisner
Department of Surgery
University of California
Sacramento, CA
USA

Jens-Peter Witt
Neuro Spine Program, Department of Neurosurgery
University of Colorado Hospital
Colorado, CO
USA

Max V. Wohlauer
Department of Surgery, Denver Health Medical Center
University of Colorado School of Medicine
Denver, CO
USA

Robert R. Wolfe
Center for Translational Research in Aging and
Longevity
DWR Institute on Aging
Little Rock, AR
USA

Hector R. Wong
Division of Critical Care Medicine
Cincinnati Children's Hospital Medical Center
Cincinnati, OH
USA
and
The Kindervelt Laboratory for Critical Care Medicine
Research
Cincinnati Children's Research Foundation
Cincinnati, OH
USA

Gary P. Wormser
Division of Infectious Diseases
Department of Medicine
New York Medical College
Valhalla, NY
USA

Christopher R. Wyatt
Emergency Medicine
Case Western Reserve University Metro Health Medical
Center
Cleveland, OH
USA

Wei Xiong
Departments of Anesthesiology Critical Care Medicine
and Neurology
Johns Hopkins University School of Medicine
Baltimore, MD
USA

Nektaria Xirouchaki
Department of Intensive Care Medicine
University Hospital of Heraklion
University of Crete
Heraklion, Crete
Greece

Yang Xue
Cardiology
VA San Diego Healthcare System
San Diego, CA
USA

D. Dante Yeh
Department of Surgery
University of California
San Francisco, CA
USA

Andrew D. Yeoman
Liver Intensive Therapy Unit
Institute of Liver Studies
Kings College Hospital
London
UK

G. Bryan Young
Department of Clinical Neurological Sciences
University of Western Ontario
London, ON
Canada

Lester Young
Clinical Fellow in Hand Surgery
Denver Health Medical Center
University of Colorado Denver, School of Medicine
Denver, CO
USA

Behrouz Zand
Baylor College of Medicine
Ben Taub General Hospital
Houston, TX
USA

ALEXANDER ZARBOCK
Department of Anesthesiology and Surgical Critical
Care Medicine
University of Münster
Münster
Germany

SACHA ZEERLEDER
Department of Immunopathology
Sanquin Research at CLB and Landsteiner Laboratory
of the AMC
Amsterdam
The Netherlands
and
Department of Hematology
Academic Medical Center
University of Amsterdam
Amsterdam
The Netherlands

MARYA D. ZILBERBERG
School of Public Health and Health Sciences
University of Massachusetts
Amherst, MA
USA
and
EviMed Research Group, LLC
Goshen, MA
USA

ANDREAS ZOLLINGER
Institute of Anaesthesiology and Intensive Care
Medicine
Triemli City Hospital Zurich
Zurich
Switzerland

A

A1M

▶ Serum and Urinary Low Molecular Weight Proteins

AAA

▶ Abdominal Aortic Aneurysm: Diagnosis and Management

AAST Spleen Injury Scale

The American Association for the Surgery of Trauma sponsored an expert panel that described five categorizes of progressively more severe spleen injury which correspond to prognosis, and have been used to guide decisions regarding nonoperative management.

Abbreviated Injury Scale

Howard R. Champion
Uniformed Services University of the Health Sciences, Bethesda, MD, USA

Synonyms
The Abbreviated Injury Scale has no synonyms. It is commonly known by its acronym (AIS), however, with versions noted by year, for example, AIS 2005

Definition

Injury Severity Scoring
▶ Injury severity scoring systems are used to measure the impact of injury both in terms of physical damage and of response of the body to that damage. Anatomic scores describe the force applied to the body and indicate site of injury and extent of damage. Physiologic scores (discussed elsewhere) attempt to summarize the body's response to injury (e.g., changes in blood pressure, respiratory rate, and responsiveness).

Injury severity scores are used to characterize injury severity and predict patient outcome; to aid health-care personnel in making triage and patient management decisions; in objective assessment of prehospital, trauma center, and trauma system care; and in clinical research, quality assurance/improvement, and resource allocation. Anatomic scores are used to compare injuries for the purposes of quantifying outcomes for quality assurance and epidemiologic studies. The AIS is one of the most commonly used anatomic scoring systems.

Abbreviated Injury Scale (AIS)
The AIS is a method of ranking anatomic injury in nine body regions along a six-point scale of severity. Promulgated in 1971 by the Association for the Advancement of Automotive Medicine (AAAM) in response to the growing number of worldwide vehicular injuries and deaths, it provided for the first time a simple, standardized vocabulary for describing injuries and a numerical method for ranking and comparing injuries by severity [1]. At present, the AIS is still used as a primary measure of injury severity in clinical research, trauma registries, government, academia, and industry [2].

AIS severity	
1	Minor
2	Moderate
3	Serious
4	Severe
5	Critical
6	Maximal (currently untreatable)

AIS Components
AIS 2005, Update 2008, the most recent version, comprises six values, a dot, a one-digit severity code, and eight optional values (see Table 1). The injury descriptor

Jean-Louis Vincent & Jesse B. Hall (eds.), *Encyclopedia of Intensive Care Medicine*, DOI 10.1007/978-3-642-00418-6,
© Springer-Verlag Berlin Heidelberg 2012

comprises the six digits to the left of the dot; this pre-dot code contains values indicating AIS body region injured, type of structure injured, specific anatomic structure injured, and level of injury. The post-dot code contains the severity score, and may also contain optional descriptors indicating location of injury, whether it was intentional or unintentional, cause of injury, etc. Example injuries coded in AIS 2005 Update 2008 (using all but the optional components) are parsed out in Table 2.

Abbreviated Injury Scale. Table 1 AIS components

Code	Description
Pre-dot code	
1	AIS body region/chapter: (1) head, (2) face, (3) neck, (4) thorax, (5) abdomen/ pelvis, (6) spine, (7) upper extremities, (8) lower extremities, (9) external/burns, (0) other trauma
2	Structure type: (1) whole area, (2) vessels, (3) nerves, (4) internal organs, (5) skeleton, (6) skin
3, 4	Specific anatomic structure: (00–99), for example, 30 = femur
5, 6	Level of injury: (00–99), e.g., 01 = proximal portion of bone
Post-dot code	
7	Injury severity: (1) minor, (2) moderate, (3) serious, (4) severe, (5) critical, (6) maximal (currently untreatable), (9) unknown
Optional post-dot codes	
8, 9	Injury location: Side and aspect of injury location (01–99)
10, 11	Injury location: Used with 8, 9 for more specific location information (00–99)
12	Volition: 0 = non-intentional, 1 = intentional (0–1)
13, 14	Cause of injury (01–99)
15	0 or specific situations (e.g., infant seat) (0–?)

Of the components of the AIS, the severity score (first post-dot code) is the most widely used and reflects injury severity by body region along a six-point ordinal scale ranging from minor to untreatable. Severity scores are determined via expert consensus using the criteria of threat to life, permanent impairment, treatment period, and energy dissipation [2]. The severity score component is the feature for which the AIS is most well known and was the starting point for the expanded versions that followed as the AIS evolved.

Evolution of the AIS: 1971–Present

The initial iteration of the AIS contained five body region classifications (head/neck, chest, abdomen, pelvis/extremities, and general) and a dictionary of 73 blunt injuries, with each assigned a severity score ranging from 1 (minor) to 6 (maximal, untreatable). The scores were determined by a group of experts who ranked each injury based on threat to life, permanent impairment, treatment period, and energy dissipation. Since its introduction, the AIS has been revised and updated several times (Table 3). The dictionary listing grew from its original 73 descriptions of primarily blunt injury to approximately 500 by the time the 1976 version was published to more than 2,000 descriptors by AIS 2005 Update 2008.

AIS 1985 marked an important shift in the AIS progression. Not only were penetrating injury descriptions included, but numeric codes designating specific injuries were added (the pre-dot code) and initial attempts to indicate injury location were made [3]. In AIS 1990, more than 100 injury descriptors (particularly head injuries) were added, the pre-dot code was expanded from five to six digits, and computerized injury location analysis by body chapter was made available.

Use of AIS in Risk Analysis

The AIS has been shown to be a good predictor of mortality. An analysis of National Trauma Data Base

Abbreviated Injury Scale. Table 2 Explanations of AIS 2005 codes for sample injuries

Pre-dot code							Post-dot code
AIS 751251.2: Simple humerus shaft fracture							
7	5	1	2	5	1	•	2
Upper extremity	Skeletal injury	Humerus		Fracture type (simple, oblique, or transverse)			Moderate severity
AIS 140692.5: Penetrating injury to cerebrum > 2 cm deep							
1	4	0	6	9	2	•	5
Head	Organ	Cerebrum		Penetrating injury (depth of penetration)			Critical injury

Abbreviated Injury Scale. Table 3 Evolution of the AIS (Adapted from [4])

Revision year	Description
1971	• Original AIS • Standardized system for classifying type and severity of vehicle crash injuries • 73 injuries classified
1975–1976	• First injury coding dictionary (~500 injuries and severity levels 1–6) published • AIS adopted as standard for US crash investigation teams
1980	• Injury dictionary tripled in scope • Injury descriptions improved • Brain injury section updated
1985	• Nonimpact injury descriptions included • Increased specificity of injury descriptions, especially thoracic and abdominal • Unique code assigned to each injury for computerization • Descriptors for coding penetrating injuries added
1990	• Expanded descriptions • Coding guidelines developed for standardization • Descriptors useful for nonfatal outcome determinations added • Further expansion of penetrating injury descriptors • Inclusion of pediatric injuries • Numerical identifier system improved
1998	• Clarification of 1990 version • Linked with the Organ Injury Scale (OIS)
2005	• Dictionary expanded to ~2,000 injury descriptors • Enables precise location of injury using numerical identifier system • Addresses injury bilaterality • Includes blast and other nonmechanical injuries • Linked with the Orthopedic Trauma Association Fracture Classification System (FCS) • Maps to AIS-98 • Includes optional injury locators (e.g., aspect, side)
2005-Military	• Enables coding of external injuries from multiple fragment wounds • Includes codes for soft-tissue fragment wounds • Includes descriptors for blast overpressure lung injury • Includes descriptors for injuries due to explosions
2005 update 2008	• Includes additional codes (multiple fractures of orbit, palate, appendix) • Includes clarifications for certain codes

(NTDB, which contains data on patients presenting to US trauma centers) data from 181,707 patients with single injuries revealed mortality risk ratios that clearly increased with AIS severity (Fig. 1) [4].

The AIS is an ordinal scale with values assigned in rank order of increasing severity. Therefore, the mortality risks at each severity level are not consistent, i.e., mortality risk is not evenly distributed across each severity level. For example, the increase in mortality between AIS 4 and 5 (23.5%) is much greater than the increase between AIS 1 and 2 (0%) [5]. This reveals that lower AIS scores are influenced by factors other than mortality [4]. Further, the same score may represent a different mortality risk depending on body region. For example, an AIS 3 injury to the head/neck has a different risk of mortality than an AIS 3 injury to the extremities. These limitations, which are echoed in morbidity risk assessment as well, make the AIS insufficiently sensitive to discern changes at the same severity level within and among body regions, particularly when evaluating effects of interventions. Because a myriad of anatomic scoring systems (a prime example being the Injury Severity Score [ISS]) are based on the AIS, its limitations are magnified when these derivative scores are calculated.

AIS-Based Scoring Systems

As discussed above, the AIS is best suited for characterizing single injuries but does not reliably characterize

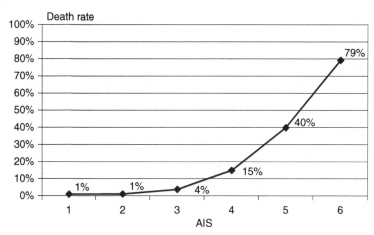

Abbreviated Injury Scale. Figure 1 Correlation between AIS 1990 severity and mortality (NTDB data) [4]

multiple injuries by summarizing severity (e.g., AIS 3 + AIS 4 = 7, with 24% mortality, but AIS 5 + AIS 2 = 7, with 54% mortality). The ISS was introduced in 1974 as a summary measure of injury severity that would take into account the contribution to mortality of second and subsequent injuries. Perhaps the most ubiquitous ► injury severity score, the ISS (see separate entry) has been described as the "gold standard" of severity scoring. The ISS uses six rather than the nine AIS body regions and is calculated by (1) squaring the three highest AIS scores in three different body regions (which do not exactly correspond to AIS body regions), and (2) adding the three values to obtain a total that falls along an ascending scale of severity from 1 (minor) to 75 (maximally injured). The simplicity of the ISS is one of its best features, enabling quick calculation of injury severity from a simple list of patient injuries. A variation called the New Injury Severity Score (NISS) was developed to improve the ability of the ISS to predict mortality by considering the three highest AIS values regardless of body region. Other AIS-based systems include the Anatomic Profile (AP, an equation containing summary scores of all severe injuries) and the Modified Anatomic Profile, which consists of components of the AP combined with ► maximum AIS (MAIS) scores across all body regions.

AIS Variations

- Maximum AIS (MAIS)

  The MAIS is the highest AIS severity score when multiple injuries are present. It has been used for many years as an effective abbreviated method for assessing overall injury severity and probability of survival. The MAIS is a simple, reliable indicator of outcome that is used extensively in vehicle crash, general morbidity/mortality, and combat injury classification

Abbreviated Injury Scale. Table 4 Characteristics of the AIS [4]

Simple	Straightforward method of ranking injuries by severity
Standardized	Injury descriptions use standardized terminology
Versatile	Usable for many causes of injury
Flexible	Suitable for small and large data-collection efforts
Anatomic	Injury descriptions organized anatomically, not physiologically
Unique	Each score reflects one injury
Independent	Each score is a single time-independent value
Current	Each score represents current injury, not its sequelae
Expanded	Each score reflects morbidity as well as mortality
Singular	Each score reflects injury severity in an adult with no co-morbidities
Relative	Injury severity relative to importance to whole body

and analysis. Although a myriad of scoring systems have been developed to estimate injury probability, the more basic questions of survivability and general injury severity following vehicle crashes are answered using the MAIS. The MAIS is used throughout the world and is the primary indicator of injury severity in vehicle crash injury research. It is frequently used as a measure of injury severity in cases of multiple injuries and is used in US Department of Transportation (DOT) databases and analyses.

- AIS 2005-Military
  Since the addition of descriptors for coding penetrating injuries with the AIS 1985 edition, researchers have had a tool for evaluating both blunt and penetrating injuries. These codes, however, did not adequately describe commonly seen penetrating combat injuries such as soft-tissue fragment wounds, high-velocity penetration, and/or bilateral and multiple injuries resulting from improvised explosive devices (IEDs). To address these issues, ▶ AIS 2005-Military was developed to code combat injuries, especially explosion-related injuries. AIS 2005-Military codes were derived by identifying each combat injury that is more severe than the corresponding civilian injury, and increasing the AIS code by one or two increments of severity.

Characteristics

The AIS is characterized as "…*an anatomically based, consensus derived, global severity scoring system that classifies each injury in every body region according to its relative importance on a 6 point ordinal scale*" [4]. Its distinguishing features are listed in Table 4.

References

1. Committee on Medical Aspects of Automotive Safety (1971) Rating the severity of tissue damage. JAMA 215:277–286
2. Expert Group on Injury Severity Measurement. Discussion document on injury severity measurement in administrative datasets. May 5, 2005. http://www.cdc.gov/nchs/data/injury/DicussionDocu.pdf. Accessed 17 Mar 2010
3. Gennarelli TA, Baker SP, Bryant TW et al (1985) Abbreviated Injury Scale 1985 Revision. American Association for Automotive Medicine, Arlington Heights
4. Gennarelli TA, Wodzin E (2006) AIS 2005: A contemporary injury scale. Injury 37:1083–1091
5. Copes WS, Champion HR, Sacco WJ et al (1988) The injury severity score revisited. J Trauma 28:69–77

Abbreviated Laparotomy

▶ Abdominal Trauma, Damage Control
▶ Damage Control Surgery
▶ Open Abdomen

ABCDEs

▶ Initial Trauma Management, ABCs

Abdominal Aortic Aneurysm

▶ Vascular, True Aneurysms

Abdominal Aortic Aneurysm: Diagnosis and Management

Nova L. Panebianco
Department of Emergency Medicine, University of Pennsylvania, Philadelphia, PA, USA

Synonyms

AAA; Triple-A

Definition

As we age, the walls of the abdominal aorta weaken and become prone to dilatation. While there is no strict definition, it is widely accepted that the abdominal aorta is considered aneurismal once the maximal diameter reaches 3 cm or greater, or, when there is an infrarenal to suprarenal diameter ratio greater than 1.2–1.5 [1]. Abdominal aortic aneurysms (AAAs) are most commonly located in the distal aorta, inferior to the renal arteries. A true AAA involves all layers of the tunica, otherwise it is a pseudoaneurysm. Most commonly, AAAs are fusiform in morphology involving the vessel as a whole. However, less commonly, a saccular aneurysm including only part of the aortic circumference is formed. Most AAAs are asymptomatic until their moment of rupture.

Epidemiology

Abdominal Aortic Aneurysms are the tenth most common cause of death in men over 55 and the incidence of disease is increasing in Western Countries. A ruptured AAA is often a catastrophic event with a mortality rate as high as 85% and an estimated 9,000–15,000 deaths in the USA per year. Even for those who present urgently without evidence of shock have a mortality rate approaching 50%. The elective operative 30-day mortality rate is much less dismal with endovascular repair mortality rates as low as 1.4% and open repair rates as low as 4.7% [1].

Evaluation/Assessment

Signs and Symptoms

Without screening, the majority of patients with AAA do not know they have the condition. Sir William Osler wrote, "Aneurysm of the abdominal aorta is very often diagnosed when not present, and when present the symptoms may be so obscure that the nature of the trouble is overlooked." The clinical triad of hypotension, abdominal or back pain, and a pulsatile abdominal mass seen in acute rupture is unreliable and occurs in only 25–50% of patients. Patients can present with vague abdominal pain, back pain, syncope, limb ischemia, and flank pain among other symptoms that carry a broad differential diagnosis. The signs and symptoms of a ruptured AAA may depend on the location of rupture. Eighty percent of infrarenal AAA rupture posteriorly into the retroperitoneal cavity, manifesting typically with back pain and hypotension. In some patients, the limited space of the retroperitoneum allows for tamponade of the bleeding, providing time for surgical repair. Anterior wall rupture typically results in intraperitoneal bleeding. This type of tear often causes severe abdominal pain and rapid cardiovascular collapse from hypovolemic shock. Approximately 4% of AAAs leak slowly into the retroperitoneum, with no signs of hemodynamic instability, and thus do not raise the red flags of a catastrophic leak. These patients are particularly at risk for misdiagnosis of renal colic, musculoskeletal back pain, or nonspecific abdominal pain.

Imaging: Ultrasound Versus Computer Tomography (CT)

In a meta-analysis of AAA surveillance it was found that abdominal ultrasound can reliably visualize the abdominal aorta in 99% of people (Figs. 1–3) [1]. Abdominal ultrasound is relatively inexpensive, noninvasive, and does not expose the patient to ionizing radiation, making it an excellent surveillance tool for the presence of AAA. Its drawbacks include that imaging is operator dependent, and while ultrasound is excellent for the detection of AAA, it cannot reliably be used to determine the presence or abscess of retroperitoneal rupture. However, in the scenario of acute rupture, an unstable patient and an ultrasound positive for the presence of AAA is enough to activate the operating room.

CT of the abdomen is very sensitive for AAA. In addition, it provides information regarding the extent of the lesion, which may aid the operative strategy

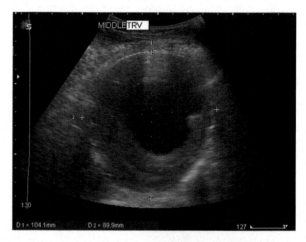

Abdominal Aortic Aneurysm: Diagnosis and Management.
Figure 2 Ultrasound of a AAA in transverse plane with anterior-posterior and horizontal calipers

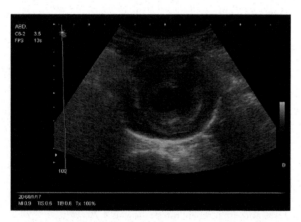

Abdominal Aortic Aneurysm: Diagnosis and Management.
Figure 1 Ultrasound of a AAA in transverse plane. Notice that the vessel lumen is relatively small secondary to surrounding plaque and thrombus. Measurements should be made from outer-wall to outer-wall to avoid underestimation of the size of the aorta

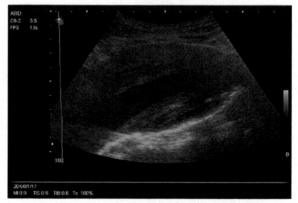

Abdominal Aortic Aneurysm: Diagnosis and Management.
Figure 3 Ultrasound of a AAA in longitudinal plane. Caliper measurements should not be made in this plane as a tangential measurement will underestimate the vessel size

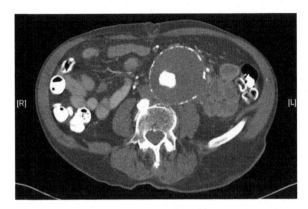

Abdominal Aortic Aneurysm: Diagnosis and Management.
Figure 4 CT of the abdomen reveals a AAA with calcifications in the vessel wall, intravascular thrombus, and small internal lumen diameter

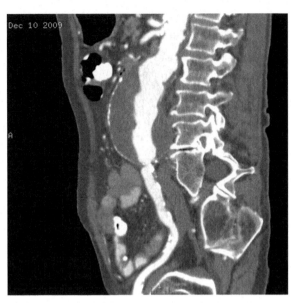

Abdominal Aortic Aneurysm: Diagnosis and Management.
Figure 6 CT of an AAA in coronal plane

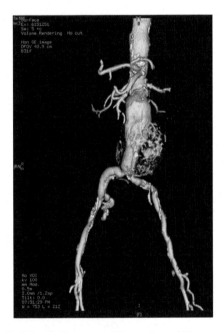

Abdominal Aortic Aneurysm: Diagnosis and Management.
Figure 5 CT angiogram of an AAA

(Figs. 4–6). Additionally, if AAA is not detected on CT scan it often provides the clinician with an alternative diagnosis. Its drawbacks include cost, the need for contrast, taking a potentially unstable patient out of the department, and exposure to ionizing radiation. In the stable patient, CT is warranted but one must remember that a leaking AAA can rupture at any moment.

Effectiveness/Tolerance/Pharecoeconomics

Screening

There is debate as to who should have screening for this condition, and once pathology is detected, what the appropriate surveillance intervals are. A screening exam for a given condition should have a high sensitivity, target the population most at risk for the condition, be cost-effective, and be well tolerated by the subject of the exam. Age 65 has been proposed as an ideal age to begin screening for AAA because 95% of patients dying of AAA rupture are older than 65 years, and future death from AAA is rare after a negative ultrasound result at this age [1]. In a Cochrane review "Screening for Abdominal Aortic Aneurysm" the authors determine that men aged 65–79 years who undergo ultrasound screening for AAA have a significant reduction in mortality. However, there was insufficient evidence to demonstrate benefit in women. The Multicenter Aneurysm Screening Study (MASS) in the Cochrane review describes a study of 67,800 men aged 65–74 years; half of the participants were invited to have ultrasound screening for AAA and the other half (the control group) were simply followed. They found that the risk of dying from an AAA over 4.1 years is reduced from 3.3/1,000 to 1.9/1,000 among those invited for screening. In other words, 710 men would need to be screened to prevent one death in this time frame.

The Emergency Department (ED) is a portal of care for the underprivileged and vulnerable populations.

It is conceivable that patients who use the ED for their primary care have less access to preventative services, and thus a higher rate of undetected AAA. Because of the high mortality rate of ruptured AAA and the curable nature of the disease when detected early, there is a clear public health incentive to capture these at-risk patients for screening. Ultrasound screening in the emergency department of asymptomatic high risk patients is a fast and accurate method for identifying patients with AAA who may benefit from follow-up or intervention. Screening for a disease can burden a population with the cost of the test and provoke anxiety in those being tested. Patients who received an ED ultrasound screening for AAA tolerated the study well, felt that it improved the quality of their care, and improved patient satisfaction. However, ED clinician sonographers reported that the ED was not an appropriate setting for AAA screening and would not recommend that other EDs adopt a routine AAA screening program because it reduced the operational efficiency of the ED [2].

Surveillance

The natural history of an AAA is typically slow steady growth followed by an acceleration in expansion. Small AAAs typically enlarge by 0.2–0.3 cm in diameter/year and rarely rupture before a diameter of 6.0 cm. Because of the increased risk of rupture, elective surgical repair is recommended for aneurysms greater than 5.5 cm. A statement from the Joint Council of the American Association for Vascular Surgery and Society for Vascular Surgery estimated the annual rupture risk according to AAA diameter [3]:

- Zero percent in aneurysms less than 4.0 cm in diameter
- 0.5–5% for those 4.0–4.9 cm
- 3–15% for those 5.0–5.9 cm
- 10–20% for those 6–6.9
- 20–40% for those 7.0–7.9
- 30–50% for those $\geq$8 cm in diameter

Maximum aortic diameter is the best determinant of the risk of rupture. In a study by Ernst, he found that during the 5 years following diagnosis, aneurysm rupture occurred in about 2% of aneurysms less than 4 cm and in 25% of aneurysms larger than 5 cm [1]. The rate of expansion tends to accelerate as the maximum diameter increases. In a review by Brady et al. [4] the rates of expansion from the UK Small Aneurysm trial are noted below:

- 0.19 cm per year for aneurysms 2.8–3.9 cm in baseline diameter

- 0.27 cm per year for those 4.0–4.5 cm in baseline diameter
- 0.35 cm per year for those 4.6–8.5 cm in baseline diameter

The average rate of expansion across all patients with a known AAA was 2.6 mm/year, however, there was a wide range of variability (95% reference range: 1.0–6.1 mm/year). Individuals that were self-reported smokers had 15–20% faster AAA expansion (by approximately 0.4 mm/year) than those who did not report active tobacco use. They offer a scientific basis for screening intervals in surveillance programs based on the criteria that less than 1% of patients would have an aneurysm that exceeded the 5.5 cm threshold at the subsequent visit. Using this criterion, the authors found that patients with AAA less than 4 cm could have rescreening at 24 months. Patients with AAA 4.1–5.0 cm could be safely returned for surveillance at 12-month intervals. Patients with AAA greater than 5.0 cm should be evaluated at 3-month intervals.

Risk Factors

Non-modifiable risk factors include age, male gender, and Northern European dissent. A history of smoking (current or historic) is the greatest risk factor for the presence of AAA, and active smokers are at increased risk for AAA expansion, rupture, and have a worse clinical prognosis. In fact, smoking was found to be the only modifiable factor associated with AAA expansion. Other variables significantly related to AAA include a history of angina, myocardial infarction, lower ankle-arm blood pressure ratio, higher maximum carotid artery stenosis, greater intima-media thickness of the internal carotid artery, higher creatinine, lower HDL levels, and higher LDL levels. There is a strong association of cardiovascular risk factors, measures of clinical and subclinical atherosclerosis, and the prevalence of aneurysms [5]. This may be secondary to shared common risk factors such as tobacco, sedentary life style, and hypertension. Individuals with AAA are more likely to have cardiac disease and are more likely to experience a cardiac event putting them at risk for sudden death unrelated to their AAA.

While women are less likely to have AAA than men, they have rupture at smaller diameters. For example, women rupture at a rate four times greater than men for aneurysms 4.0–5.5 cm in diameter [4]. This may be because women have smaller vessel diameters than men, and thus a diameter of 6.0 cm represents a greater degree of dilatation in women than it does in men. Women account for one-third the number of AAA ruptures and almost as many deaths as men. Given that women have a longer life expectancy than men, and they are at equal risk of death from rupture, developing screening recommendations for women may be of value.

Treatment and After-care

Medical Therapy

Patients that are hemodynamically stable with AAA less than 5.5 cm, or who are not surgical candidates, may be medically managed. As stated above, smoking is the most important modifiable risk factor to prevent rupture. Smoking also puts one at risk for significant comorbidities including hypertension, ischemic heart disease, lung cancer, and stroke. Any patient actively smoking should be aggressively counseled as to the benefits of cessation.

It is common to treat individuals with AAA similarly to the way one would treat an individual with other cardiovascular risk factors including hypertension and dyslipidemia. In a small study of individuals with AAA, the portion of patients that were treated with a beta blocker had significantly lower expansion rates than those who did not receive a beta blocker (0.36 cm versus 0.68 cm per year). However, in the Cochrane review the authors discuss a subgroup report of people with aneurysms between 3.0 and 4.9 cm who participated in a double blind trial of the impact of propranolol versus placebo on the expansion rate of small AAAs. The trial was stopped after 2 years because the propranolol group had significantly higher rates due to difficulty breathing, decreased pulmonary function, and death [1]. In the paper by Gollegde et al. they report that patients with high cardiac risk on beta-blockers have a tenfold improved perioperative morbidity and mortality than those not on beta-blockers. Additionally, they report that the use of statins in perioperative patients improved the risk of stroke with 30 days of surgery from 11% to 3.7% [5]. Statin drug therapy has been shown to improve survival after AAA repair with a threefold reduction in risk of cardiovascular death [5].

Surgery

AAAs less than 5.5 cm in men have a low rate of rupture, less than 1% per annum, and elective surgery for aneurysms less than this size has not shown improved survival. Patients, however, who are symptomatic from their AAA should undergo repair, regardless of aneurysm diameter, as long as there are no major contraindications to surgery. While it is generally recommended that asymptomatic individuals do not consider elective surgery until after an AAA diameter of 5.5 cm, it may be beneficial in those patients whose aneurysm increases more than 0.5 cm diameter in 6 months [3]. The risk of mortality from elective surgery, however, is not insignificant at 1–5% and thus must be balanced with the risk of acute rupture. Most operative mortality and morbidity are secondary to cardiac events. The benefit of coronary artery revascularization before surgery remains unclear and there is no consensus on the optimum strategy for preoperative cardiac management in patients undergoing elective AAA repair.

Open surgical AAA repair requires general anesthesia, a large midline incision, and often an extended intensive care unit and hospital stay. The 30-day mortality rate of elective open repair is roughly 3–5%. The mortality rate is highest when surgery is performed by general surgeons (5.5%) and lowest when performed by vascular surgeons (2.2%). Additionally, the in-hospital mortality is related to the volume of procedures performed at the hospital. Not surprisingly, the more often the procedure is performed at the institution, the better the outcomes. Additional considerations should be given to the specific morbidities from surgery, which include left colon ischemia, renal failure (secondary to thromboembolic events) and, infrequently, paraplegia. Patients with significant comorbidities may not be ideal candidates for open AAA repair.

Endovascular repair uses the deployment of stent grafts typically via iliofemoral cannulation and has become a widely practiced alternative to open repair. The advantages are that the procedure is less invasive, has a more rapid recovery time, and has a lower perioperative mortality rate. Roughly 40–80% of AAAs are amenable to endovascular grafting based on the aneurysm anatomy. At this time, the long-term advantages of endovascular repair are unknown. A portion of the endovascular grafts fail, either by rupture or required conversion to open repair. In a study where over 1,000 patients were either randomized to open or endovascular repair (EVAR), there is no advantage to endovascular repair with respect to all cause mortality and quality of life compared to open repair. Within 4 years of randomization 41% of patients in the EVAR group had a postoperative complication versus 9% in the open repair group (hazard ratio 4.9, 95% CI 3.5 – 6.8, $P =$ 0.0001). There were no significant differences in health-related quality of life between the two groups after 12 months. Additionally, hospital costs were higher in the EVAR group out to 4 years [6]. The decision to have open repair versus EVAR ought to be considered on a case-by-case basis.

Prognosis

A ruptured AAA is a catastrophic event with 80–90% mortality. With early detection, AAA is a treatable disease with a relatively low mortality rate. Screening for AAA with abdominal ultrasound is a well tolerated, high yield, cost-effective way of preventing mortality from this condition. Addressing modifiable risk factors particularly smoking and cardiovascular disease, one can potentially improve outcomes. If surgery is required, the advantages and disadvantages to open or endovascular surgery should be determined on a case-by-case basis.

References

1. Cosford PA, Leng GC, Thomas J (2010) Screening for Abdominal Aortic Aneurysm (Review) Issue 7. The Cochrane Collaboration. Wiley
2. Hoffmann B, Um P, Bessman ES, Ding R, Kelen GD, McCarthey ML (2009) Routine screening of asymptomatic abdominal aortic aneurysm in high-risk patients is not recommended in emergency departments that are frequently crowded. Acad Emerg Med 16(11): 1242–1250
3. Brewster DC, Cronenwett JL, Hallett JW Jr et al (2003) Guidelines for the treatment of abdominal aortic aneurysms. report of a subcommittee of the joint council of the american association for vascular surgery and society for vascular surgery. J Vasc Surg 37:1106
4. Brady AR, Thompson SG, Fowkes GR, Greenhalgh RM, Powell JT (2004) Abdominal aortic aneurysm expansion: risk factors and time intervals for surveillance. Circulation 110:16–21
5. Golledge J, Powell JT (2007) Medical management of abdominal aortic aneurysm. Eur J Vasc Endovasc Surg 34:267–273
6. (September 2005) Endovascular aneurysm repair versus open repair in patients with abdominal aortic aneurysm (EVAR trial 1): randomized controlled trial. J Vasc Surg 42(3):592

Abdominal Cavity Infections

Jan J. De Waele
Department of Critical Care Medicine, Ghent University Hospital, Ghent, Belgium

Synonyms

Complicated intra-abdominal infections; Intra-abdominal infections; Peritonitis

Definition

"Abdominal cavity infection" or "intra-abdominal infection" usually refers to infections that spread to the peritoneum, the virtual space between the visceral and parietal peritoneum, and that usually originate from the gastrointestinal tract. They should be discerned from intra-abdominal solid organ infections, although these also may lead to peritonitis.

Peritonitis can be classified based on the origin (primary, secondary, and tertiary peritonitis) as well as on the extent of the process (localized or diffuse peritonitis).

In primary peritonitis, no evident source can be identified, and no anatomical disruption of the gastrointestinal tract is present; this includes spontaneous bacterial peritonitis (which is a typical complication in patients with liver cirrhosis and is considered to be the consequence of bacterial translocation through the bowel wall) continuous ambulatory peritoneal dialysis related peritonitis (which occurs in chronic renal failure patients with an indwelling intraperitoneal catheter) and rare conditions such as streptococcal peritonitis that occurs in young female patients. Secondary peritonitis is much more common and is the consequence of a local infectious process within the abdominal cavity, with or without a hollow viscous perforation, and can lead to localized or diffuse peritonitis. Tertiary peritonitis is increasingly observed in critically ill patients who survive an episode of secondary peritonitis; it is generally referred to as a persistent or recurrent peritonitis after initial adequate treatment for secondary peritonitis.

When the infection is contained within one of the abdominal quadrants, localized peritonitis is present; this may develop in diffuse peritonitis when it spreads to the rest of the abdominal cavity. When the process can be controlled by the inflammatory reaction of the peritoneum and omentum, an abscess may form.

The term "complicated" intra-abdominal infection often causes confusion and should be avoided in critically ill patients, as most (if not all) of these patients who require critical care have complicated abdominal infections with established MODS. In "uncomplicated" intra-abdominal infection, the infectious process is contained within a single organ, e.g., gastroenteritis or simple appendicitis and cholecystitis, and no anatomical disruption is present. In "complicated" intra-abdominal infection, the infectious process extends beyond the primary focus of the infection and enters the peritoneal space. Although patients with uncomplicated disease may present with (severe) sepsis symptoms, full-blown MODS rarely develops without the extension of the disease in the peritoneum.

The most common causes of cIAI are perforation (due to breakdown of a surgical anastomosis, a peptic ulcer, or after trauma), intestinal ischemia, cholecystitis, and postoperative abscesses. Special attention should be paid to patients with recent GI anastomoses, who develop organ dysfunction or require vasoactive drugs as the probability of leakage is higher in these patients.

Evaluation/Assessment

The care for the intensive care patient with cIAI has changed significantly in recent years. Due to improvements in critical care and surgical strategies, patients are more likely to survive the initial phase of critical illness, and are often left with complex residual abdominal situations including short bowel syndrome, enteric and pancreatic fistulas, and open abdomens. These patients are posing unique challenges for surgeons involved in the definitive repair of the injuries, but also make diagnosis and management of new abdominal complications difficult. Not only the patient, but also the infecting organisms are changing. Multidrug-resistant (MDR) organisms are posing important problems in most intensive care units, and as patients with cIAI have multiple risk factors for colonization and infection with MDR bacteria, antibiotic treatment has also evolved. The same is true for invasive candidiasis, but for these infections, new antifungal drugs have become available. Also, the increase in patient requiring bariatric surgery is expanding the spectrum of patients and complications in the ICU.

Clinical Signs and Symptoms

The diagnosis of abdominal cavity infections in the critically ill patient is often challenging. Medical history can often offer a clue and should always be checked, e.g., in patients with documented liver cirrhosis, and the diagnosis of primary peritonitis should be actively sought after when sepsis is present; similarly, in a patient with previous abdominal or gastrointestinal surgery, a local complication such as perforation or postoperative abscess should be excluded. Surgical history and especially information on previous abdominal surgery should be obtained, as well as exposure to antibiotics in previous months to identify patients at risk of infection with antibiotic resistant organisms.

Clinical signs and symptoms are the key to the diagnosis in most patients and usually consist of abdominal pain and a systemic inflammatory response, including fever, tachycardia, and tachypnea. On clinical examination, there may be localized or diffuse tenderness on palpation or even signs of peritoneal irritation such as rebound tenderness. Clinical examination of the abdomen can often help to locate the source of the infection and direct imaging studies to confirm the diagnosis. Sedation and analgesia may minimize or completely suppress local symptoms in the ICU patient.

The course of hospital-acquired intra-abdominal infections is often atypical, and may lead to considerable delay in recognition of the problem, especially in sedated patients. Also, concomitant infections may blur the clinical picture. When intra-abdominal infections affect hospitalized patients, it often involves a complication of a preexisting disease or a surgical intervention. The most common problem is anastomic leakage of enteric anastomoses. A low index of suspicion for anastomic leakage in patients after abdominal surgery who are treated for severe sepsis or septic shock is appropriate. Also in other patient categories, the possibility of complicated intra-abdominal infection should be considered when (severe) sepsis develops.

In patients after previous abdominal surgery, careful examination of the surgical wound and abdominal drains if present is mandatory. If obvious signs of gastrointestinal perforation such as gas, or intestinal content are present, re-exploration is necessary in case of recent surgery. If this occurs in the late postoperative course, the presence of ongoing contamination of the peritoneal cavity should be excluded, and management should be adapted accordingly.

Diffuse abdominal pain and generalized (rebound) tenderness often are signs of complicated peritonitis, and appropriate action should be undertaken. Additional imaging techniques are not always indicated in these patients as this may delay the definitive management, and these patients should be considered candidates for immediate surgery.

Imaging

The role of imaging techniques to guide the management of patients with (suspected) cIAI in the ICU is very important. It will not only help to confirm the diagnosis but also will guide surgical therapy.

Ultrasound can be a very useful tool to detect intra-abdominal fluid collections and may help to determine a safe location of diagnostic fine needle aspiration. The absence of fluid or other abnormalities on ultrasound does not exclude a cIAI at all.

Contrast-enhanced (orally, rectally, and, if necessary, intravenously) CT scan will detect most if not all abdominal mishaps. Signs may be subtle though, especially in the early stages of cIAI. The need for intravenous contrast is decided on after an unenhanced examination. As there may be overt signs of ongoing contamination dictating a surgical intervention on nonenhanced CT (see Fig. 1), and as the risk for contrast nephropathy is often significant, we do not advise to routinely give IV contrast at this stage. When the nonenhanced CT scan is equivocal or non-diagnostic, IV contrast should be administered. When suspected, immediate percutaneous drainage of abdominal collections should be available.

Diagnostic Strategy

Figure 2 summarizes our current diagnostic strategy in patients with suspected cIAI in the ICU. Ultrasound is

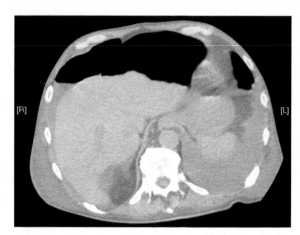

Abdominal Cavity Infections. Figure 1 Non-enhanced abdominal CT scan demonstrating free intraperitoneal air; explorative laparotomy confirmed intestinal perforation

used as an early screening technique and abdominal CT scan is performed when US or FNA is negative.

Treatment

In the context of intra-abdominal infections, adequate treatment is more than choosing the right antimicrobial. The choice of the procedure that controls the source of infection with minimal damage to the patient's physiology is important, and appropriate supportive treatment should be provided.

General Approach

Timely hemodynamic resuscitation and support of vital functions is important in the treatment of all types of infections. Patients with cIAI may be more prone to hypovolemiea due to the fluid loss in the GI system and reduced intake in previous days. Early administration of antibiotics also is an important element and should not be delayed if simultaneous source control cannot be obtained. However, as outcome will mainly be determined by the of source control of the infection, the focus should be on rapid diagnosis and above all definitive control of the source of the infection.

Antibiotics

The main objectives of antimicrobial therapy in the treatment of intra-abdominal infections are to prevent local and hematogenous spread, and to reduce late complications. Antibiotics should be administered upon the diagnosis, and intraoperative confirmation should not be awaited. Oral administration is to be avoided as absorption will usually be unreliable, and the effect may be

delayed. Patients with severe sepsis and septic shock may have altered physiology that requires higher doses of antibiotics; for some antibiotics, such as penicillins and carbapenems, extended or continuous infusion may be preferable.

In critically ill patients, the threshold for starting antibiotics may be lower as the delayed treatment of infections is associated with considerable morbidity and mortality. Still the decision to start antibiotic therapy should not be taken too lightly, and the duration of antimicrobial therapy should ideally be defined from the start of the treatment. Although only limited data are available, it appears that the overuse of antibiotics in this setting is considerable, resulting in unnecessary costs and, more importantly, increased resistance. The start of antibiotics should, on the other hand, not give the treating physicians a sense of security. If an intra-abdominal infection is present, source control is more important, and antibiotics alone will not be able to cure the patient in most cases.

Not all patients undergoing surgery for intra-abdominal infection need antimicrobial therapy, and this decision should be made intraoperatively by the surgeon. These patients will be treated following local guidelines to prevent wound infections. A number of diagnoses were identified that do not preclude the need for antibiotic treatment (Table 1).

Several schemes for antibiotic therapy have been proposed for the treatment of complicated intra-abdominal infections, and none these has proven to be superior (Table 2). These infections always require coverage for both gram-positive and gram-negative bacteria, as well as a drug active against anaerobe bacteria. In case of prior antibiotic exposure, a drug of the same antibiotic class should be avoided. Most importantly, the choice of empiric antibiotic treatment should be guided by the local resistance patterns that is expected and may include resistant gram-positive coverage; local guidelines should be developed and used accordingly.

Although there is no relation between the severity of an infection and the degree of antimicrobial resistance and the presence of nosocomial organisms in patients with cIAI, it may be prudent to initiate a broad spectrum antibiotic that also covers more resistant organisms such as Pseudomonas (see Table 2). Procurement of intraoperative samples is imperative in order to deescalate antibiotic treatment at a later stage.

Duration of Antibiotic Treatment

In case of intra-abdominal infections with prompt surgical intervention and adequate source control, antimicrobial therapy is generally recommended to continue

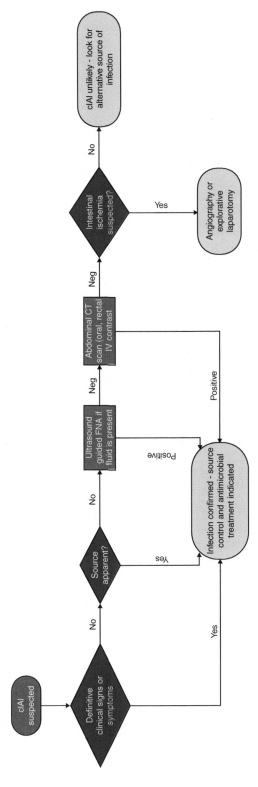

Abdominal Cavity Infections. Figure 2 Diagnostic approach in suspected cIAI

Abdominal Cavity Infections. Table 1 Conditions for which therapeutics antibiotics (>24 h) are generally not recommended

• Traumatic and iatrogenic small and large bowel enteric perforations operated on within 24 h (including intraoperative contamination)
• Gastroduodenal perforations operated on within 24 h
• Acute or and gangrenous appendicitis without perforation
• Acute and/or gangrenous cholecystitis without perforation
• Transmural bowel ischemia and necrosis from embolic, thrombotic, or obstructive vascular obstructive vascular occlusion without perforation or established peritonitis or abscess

Abdominal Cavity Infections. Table 2 Antibiotic treatment of cIAI

• **Recommended regimens: single agents**
• β Lactam/β lactamase inhibitor combinations: ampicillin/sulbactam[a], amoxycillin/clavulanic acid[a], ticarcillin/clavulanic acid[a], piperacillin/tazobactam
• Carbapenems: doripenem, ertapenem[a], imipenem, meropenem
• Quinolones: moxifloxacin[a]
• Tigecycline[a]
• **Recommended regimens: combination regimens**
• Cephalosporin based: cefazoline or cefuroxime + metronidazole[a], CF3 or CF4 + metronidazole
• Quinolone based: FQ + metronidazole
• Others: aztreonam + metronidazole

[a]Pseudomonas spp. not covered, not recommended for empiric treatment in nosocomial infections

for 5–7 days, and even shorter courses have been proposed. As a guideline for clinical practice, antimicrobial therapy for established infections can safely be stopped after resolution of clinical signs of infection. Once symptoms such as fever and leucocytosis disappear, and the patient tolerates enteral feeding, recurrent infection is not likely to occur. It should be added that in critically ill patients, the use of these clinical parameters is often not useful. In some cases, an abdominal CT scan is the only means to demonstrate resolution of the infection. Positive cultures from abdominal drains or open wounds should not solely be used to prolong treatment; colonization, often with organisms like coagulasenegative staphylococci,

fungi, and nosocomial gram-negative organisms, is common and can usually not be eradicated with antibiotic treatment.

In patients with persistent sepsis after initiation of antimicrobial therapy, antibiotic therapy should not merely be continued as this frequently points to failed source control or another focus of hospital-acquired infection. Repeat contrast examination and an active search for a persistent focus of infection should not be delayed.

In selected patients, prolonged antimicrobial therapy up to several weeks may be necessary, especially when source control is impossible or too risky to obtain; infected pancreatic necrosis is a typical example.

Source Control

The focus of the treatment of infections, including cIAI, currently is mostly on the management of organ dysfunction and antibiotic treatment. Let there be no misunderstanding, although these aspects are important, outcome is mainly determined by appropriate control of infection. Source control consists of all physical measures intended to eliminate a source of infection, to control ongoing contamination, and to restore premorbid anatomy and function. When applied to critically ill patients, the elimination of the source and the control over ongoing contamination are most important and determine early and long-term success of the treatment. Restoration of anatomy and complete function can be performed at a later stage when prolonging the surgical intervention is often harmful to the patient at the first operation.

Source control is based on three principles: drainage, debridement, and restoration of anatomy and function. All three principles are important as such, but in the individual patient, they can be applied independently and at different moments.

Drainage is defined as the evacuation the contents of an abscess. The efficiency of the drain is determined by its size and should allow complete evacuation of the abscess. If the abscess cannot be drained completely, source control will be unsuccessful. The use of additional drains can be considered in these patients, but some abscesses or infections cannot be drained adequately, with diffuse peritonitis as an example. In these patients, proper debridement of necrotic tissues or removal of gastrointestinal contents may be necessary.

Drainage of an abscess can be performed surgically or percutaneously, using ultrasound or CT scan. In critically patients, especially after previous abdominal surgery, percutaneous drainage (PCD) has become very popular. It can be successful provided that adequate drainage is possible, and no debridement or repair of anatomical structures is necessary. When percutaneous drainage fails or cannot be performed, for example, when multiple abscesses are present, surgical drainage is indicated.

Debridement or removing dead tissue and foreign material from the abdominal cavity is often necessary in case of cIAI. This can only be accomplished surgically, and the extent to which this should be done remains a controversial topic. Some surgeons favor a minimalistic approach, which consists of removing dead tissue and use gauze to remove any pus present, whereas others promote an aggressive approach of high volume peritoneal lavage and meticulously removing all fibrin adherents to the intestines or abdominal wall.

Restoration of anatomy and function is the final step in the management of intra-abdominal infections, and as such, often the goal of the surgical intervention. In most patients, it can be established at the first operation, but in some patients, it needs to be delayed until the condition of the patient allows a sometimes lengthy procedure and until tissue healing is adequate. In some patients, this delay of a definitive procedure can take months, and the patient may even be discharged home before reconstruction is finalized.

The application of source control in critically ill patients is often delayed. This is most often due to failure to recognize the disease and reluctance to intervene until diagnosis is confirmed. Sometimes patients are considered too sick to undergo surgery, and stabilization is desired first; in patients with diffuse peritonitis, these attempts will most likely be futile, and surgery should not be delayed. Resuscitation should be continued intraoperatively.

When choosing the means to obtain source control, benefits and risks for the patients at that particular moment should be carefully considered. The method that causes the least collateral damage to reach the goal at that moment should be preferred. Any intervention may cause bleeding and additional organ damage; impaired coagulation or previous abdominal procedures may be indications to prefer percutaneous over surgical abscess drainage. PCD can also be used as a temporizing strategy; definitive management is delayed until appropriate treatment is better tolerated by the patient. The role of the intensivist is essential to determine the optimal method to obtain source control in the critically ill patient – close interaction with the surgeon is mandatory.

There is an ongoing debate whether on-demand relaparotomy is better than planned relapatomy. A recent RCT could not show a mortality difference, but an on-demand approach was associated with decreased length of stay in the ICU and in the hospital. The number of laparotomies was significantly reduced, with percutaneous drainage procedures were more frequent in the on-demand group. Except for patients with suspected ongoing ischemia, an on-demand approach is to be preferred.

Fungal Infections

Candida species are often involved at some stage in ICU patients with cIAI, and mortality rates of 50–75% have been reported. Often it is difficult to distinguish infection from colonization. Predictive factors of Candida isolation are female gender, hemodynamic compromise, ongoing antimicrobial treatment, and upper GI-tract perforation. The high risk for candidiasis in these patients has led to an increased use of antifungal prophylaxis. Often, multiple risk factors for invasive candidiasis are present in patients with cIAI. Also, in a placebo-controlled trial, it was demonstrated that prophylaxis with fluconazole reduces the rate of intra-abdominal candidiasis in patients with gastrointestinal perforations and anastomotic leakage. Based on these considerations, prophylaxis in these high-risk patients is justified. Routine treatment of Candida isolated following surgery for cIAI, on the other hand, cannot be recommended in otherwise healthy patients.

Intra-abdominal Hypertension (IAH)

IAH has recently been identified as an important source of morbidity in the ICU. Due to fluid accumulation, ileus and bowel wall edema, critically patients with cIAI seem to be particularly at risk for IAH and abdominal compartment syndrome (ACS). Intra-abdominal pressure (IAP) measurement is imperative and can reliably be done in the ICU using the bladder as a route. Several techniques for IAP measurement have been described and are commercially available. Also intraoperatively, the possibility of subsequent ACS should be considered and open abdomen treatment used when necessary. When IAH develops, medical treatment options, including percutaneous drainage of fluid collections, nasogastric suctioning, or neuromuscular blockers, should be considered before surgical decompression is performed. If open abdomen treatment is necessary, all attempts should be aimed at early closure of the abdomen; prolonged open abdomen treatment is associated with increased complications and often requires planned hernia repair later.

Fistula Care

The presence of fistulas is often a challenging issue in patient with cIAI after previous gastrointestinal surgery. Fluid losses can be considerable, and in some patients, the use of antisecretory drugs may be indicated. The presence of fistula often prohibits enteral nutrition; however, the possibility of enteral nutrition should carefully be explored, and when necessary, nasogastric or biliary aspirate can be reinfused with the nutrition in the small bowel. Fistulas in patients with an open abdomen pose a particular challenge in this setting.

Effectiveness

Evaluation of Source Control Adequacy

As source control is the most important determinant of outcome, failure of source control should be detected as early as possible. Diagnosis however is more difficult than treatment in critically ill patients with again clinical examination being useless in most occasions. The clinical setting is most often typical with patients suffering from persistent organ dysfunction with elevated inflammatory markers. Pre- and postoperative factors such as the extent of peritonitis, the focus and etiology of the infection, and the type of contamination were found not to be associated with failed source control when postoperative variables associated with organ failure were entered in the model. Therefore, clinical signs and symptoms should be considered most important when failure of the source control procedure is suspected. Procalcitonin may also prove valuable in the early recognition of source control failure; persistently elevated PCT values have been associated with inadequate source control.

Tertiary Peritonitis

Tertiary peritonitis is peritonitis that persists or recurs at least 48 h after apparently adequate management of peritonitis after Often, it is the long-term consequence of failed or impossible source control. One of the particularities of tertiary peritonitis is the unsatisfying response to antimicrobial treatment, and the typical microbiology of nosocomial organisms. In this setting, colonization and infection are difficult to discriminate, and surgical treatment is often unsuccessful.

Prognosis

The prognosis of cIAI in the critically ill patients is mainly determined by underlying conditions and comorbities, severity of organ dysfunction at admission, and the adequacy of source control. In some conditions, it can be difficult if not impossible to obtain proper source control, and infected pancreatic necrosis or peritonitis due to duodenal perforation are typical examples; all too often, patients enter a vicious cycle of antibiotic resistance, inappropriate antibiotic treatment, and ongoing contamination of the peritoneum, and finally die.

References

1. Blot SI, Vandewoude KH, De Waele JJ (2007) Candida peritonitis. Curr Opin Crit Care 13(2):195–199
2. Dellinger RP, Levy MM, Carlet JM et al (2008) Surviving sepsis campaign: international guidelines for management of severe sepsis and septic shock: 2008. Intensive Care Med 34(1):17–60
3. Marshall JC (2004) Intra-abdominal infections. Microbes Infect 6(11):1015–1025
4. Schein M, Marshall J (2004) Source control for surgical infections. World J Surg 28(7):638–645
5. Solomkin JS, Mazuski JE, Baron EJ et al (2003) Guidelines for the selection of anti-infective agents for complicated intra-abdominal infections. Clin Infect Dis 37(8):997–1005

Abdominal Compartment Syndrome

Lewis J. Kaplan[1], Manu L. N. G. Malbrain[2]
[1]Department of Surgery, Yale University School of Medicine, New Haven, CT, USA
[2]Intensive Care Unit, Ziekenhuis Netwerk Antwerpen Hospital Campus Stuivenberg, Antwerp, Belgium

Synonyms

While there are no accurate synonyms, the term intra-abdominal hypertension (IAH) is often used to describe one of the two required key elements for the syndrome to occur – Intra-Abdominal Hypertension (IAH). IAH is defined as an intra-abdominal pressure (IAP) that persistently equals or exceeds 12 mmHg (see Intra-Abdominal Pressure Monitoring) [1]

Definition

The World Society of Abdominal Compartment Syndrome (www.WSACS.org) has derived a consensus statement with definitions of IAH and ACS [1]. The ACS is defined as an intra-abdominal pressure that exceeds 20 mmHg and is accompanied by an attributable organ failure. This definition acknowledges that the syndrome may occur with or without an abdominal perfusion pressure (APP) <60 mmHg. The APP can be calculated by subtracting the IAP from the mean arterial pressure (MAP), APP = MAP − IAP. The formula for APP is similar to the one used to assess intracranial pressure (ICP) and cerebral perfusion pressure (CPP = MAP − ICP) and also provides a therapeutic target for maintaining visceral perfusion when IAP is greater than 12 mmHg but less than 20 mmHg.

ACS may occur with primary or secondary IAH. Primary IAH is generally related to injury within the abdomino-pelvic region and mostly reflects blood or clot as the primary etiologic agents for increased IAP [1]. Secondary IAH on the other hand generally relates to extra-abdominal disease with capillary leak and the formation of large volume ascites that raises the IAP [2]. A common example is secondary IAH after Early Goal Directed Therapy driven plasma volume expansion for pneumonia complicated by septic shock. However, secondary IAH may also be related to intra-abdominal disease processes, usually infectious or ischemic in nature that result in visceral edema before or after surgical therapy and are also accompanied by ascites formation. Common surgical processes at-risk for secondary IAH include perforated diverticulitis, mesenteric ischemia, and necrotizing pancreatitis.

Treatment

Treatment of the ACS when it is diagnosed is dictated by the patient's physiologic status as well as the underlying cause of the syndrome. For instance, a trauma patient who has undergone a damage-control laparotomy for hepatic injury and who develops ACS 4 h postoperatively should be reexplored, have bleeding controlled, and a temporary abdominal wall closure reapplied (Fig. 1). Figure 1 represents a schematic of a method of achieving temporary abdominal wall closure. In contrast, the medical patient with pneumonia and ascites as the proximate cause of their ACS should be considered for percutaneous catheter

drainage of the ascites. In *both* circumstances, the therapeutic goal is to relieve IAH and restore venous return and cardiac performance to support end-organ oxygen delivery and utilization.

However, not all patients present for therapy with an established ACS. Many present with IAH that is progressive, and if left untreated, will result in the ACS. The management of patients with IAH is based on the following four principles: (1) specific procedures to reduce IAP and the consequences of ACS, (2) general support and medical management of the critically ill patients, (3) surgical decompression, and (4) optimization after surgical decompression. The WSACS has created an algorithmic approach to the medical management of such patients that may be practically utilized at the bedside (Fig. 2) [1]. This approach is based on five principles: (1) improvement of abdominal wall compliance, (2) evacuation of intraluminal contents, (3) evacuation of abdominal fluid collections, (4) correction of capillary leak and positive fluid balance, and (5) specific treatment to support end-organ function. Thus this approach recognizes the contributions of: (1) excessive fluid (especially crystalloid) administration on visceral edema and ascites formation, (2) inadequate sedation and analgesia of abdominal and thoracic wall muscular tone, (3) space occupying lesions in the abdominal cavity (including the enterally nourished intestine and gas filled colon), and (4) the role of

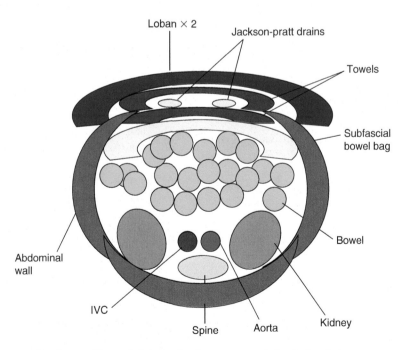

Abdominal Compartment Syndrome. Figure 1 Schematic of a temporary abdominal wall closure

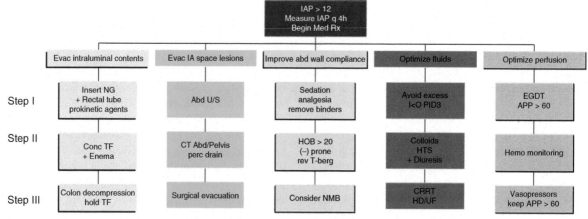

Abdominal Compartment Syndrome. Figure 2 Stepwise management of intra-abdominal hypertension

myocardial contractility and its assessment by flow-based volumetric monitoring in the genesis and management of IAH and the evolution of the ACS in at-risk patients (see ▶ Intra-Abdominal Pressure Monitoring).

Below are some recommendations that direct end-organ support in patients with IAH as well as those who have required therapy for the ACS:

Neurologic Function
- Because of the interactions between IAP, ITP, and ICP, accurate monitoring of IAP in head trauma victims with associated abdominal lesions is worthwhile.
- The presence of increased IAP can be an additional "extracranial" cause of intracranial hypertension in patients with abdominal trauma without overt cranio-cerebral lesions.
- Laparoscopy in the acute post-traumatic phase is more foe than friend and recent head injury should be considered a contraindication for laparoscopic procedures.
- The same principles are responsible for the development of idiopathic intracranial hypertension (pseudotumor cerebri) in morbidly obese patients.
- Weight loss by bariatric surgery is associated with improvements in ICP and CNS symptoms (although this is not an acute management strategy).

Respiratory Function
- IAH decreases total respiratory system compliance by a decrease in chest wall compliance, while pulmonary parenchymal compliance remains unchanged.

- Best PEEP should be set to counteract IAP while in the same time avoiding over-inflation of already well-aerated lung regions. In some circumstances, Best PEEP = IAP, but IAP is not the sole determinant of Best PEEP and flow-based monitoring should be considered to optimize PEEP titration.
- The ARDS consensus definitions should take into account PEEP and IAP values (as well as other relevant factors such as gas flow rate, ventilator mode, waveform, and inspiratory time).
- During lung protective ventilation, *in the setting of IAH*, consideration should be made to increasing the limits for the *transmural* plateau pressures below 35 cm H_2O. In order to use this formula, one must convert the mmHg of IAP to cm H_2O pressure using the conversion factor of 1.36.
  - Pplat™ = Pplat – IAP/2
- The PaOP criterion in ARDS consensus definitions is often not useful in patients with IAH and should be revised as most patients with IAH and secondary ALI/ARDS will have a PAOP above 18 mmHg.
- IAH increases extravascular lung water and thereby renders monitoring of extravascular lung water index (EVLWI) a potentially useful parameter in guiding fluid balance
- Body position affects IAP
  - Placing an obese patient in the upright position can cause ACS.
  - The abdomen should optimally hang freely during prone positioning instead of resting directly against a mattress, regardless of the pressure relief characteristics of the surface.

- Reverse Trendelenburg positioning may improve respiratory mechanics, but may decrease splanchnic perfusion, create subclinical tissue ischemia, and engender an ischemia-reperfusion injury with positional change that augments visceral edema and capillary leak.
- Consideration of neuromuscular blockade should balance the potentially beneficial effects on abdominal muscle tone resulting in decreased IAP and improved APP against the potentially detrimental effect on lung mechanics, peripheral neuromuscular function, pressure ulceration, and deconditioning that culminate in atelectasis, hypoxic pulmonary vasoconstriction, right ventricular ejection fraction decrease, and ultimately pulmonary superinfection in unventilated areas with nosocomial pathogens.
- The presence of IAH will lead to pulmonary hypertension via increased ITP with direct compression on lung parenchyma and vessels and via the diminished left and right ventricular compliance.
- The effect of IAP on parenchymal compression is exacerbated in cases of hypovolemia regardless of cause.

Cardiac Function

- Cardiovascular dysfunction and failure (low cardiac output) are commonly observed in patients with IAH or ACS.
- Accurate assessment and optimization of preload, contractility, and afterload is essential to restore end-organ perfusion and function.
- Our understanding of traditional hemodynamic monitoring techniques and parameters, however, must be reevaluated in IAH/ACS since pressure-based estimates of intravascular volume as pulmonary artery occlusion pressure (PaOP) and central venous pressure (CVP) are readily misinterpreted. Instead, strong consideration should be made to utilize flow-based monitoring techniques instead of relying on pressure-based modalities.
  - The clinician must be aware of the interactions between ITP, IAP, PEEP, and cardiac chamber filling pressures.
  - Misinterpretation of the patient's minute-to-minute cardiac status may result in the institution of inappropriate and potentially detrimental therapy, generally additional volume expansion.
  - Transmural™ filling pressures, calculated as the end-expiration value (ee) minus the ITP better reflect preload but require monitoring with an esophageal balloon device:

- CVP™ = CVPee – ITP
- PAOP™ = PAOPee – ITP
- A quick estimate of transmural filling pressures can also be obtained by subtracting half of the IAP from the end-expiratory filling pressure since abdomino-thoracic pressure transmission has been estimated to be around 50%.
  - CVP™ = CVPee – IAP/2
  - PAOP™ = PAOPee – IAP/2
- The surviving sepsis campaign guidelines targeting initial and ongoing resuscitation toward a CVP of 8–12 mmHg and other studies targeting a MAP of 65 mmHg should be interpreted with caution in case of IAH/ACS to avoid unnecessary over- and under resuscitation. These recommendations may be inappropriate in the case of patients who sustain injury but do not have sepsis as their diagnosis.
- Volumetric estimates of preload status such as right ventricular end diastolic volume index (RVEDVI) or global end diastolic volume index (GEDVI) may be especially useful because of the changing ventricular compliance and elevated ITP.
- Functional hemodynamic parameters such as stroke volume (SVV) or pulse pressure variation (PPV) may be useful in determining the need for plasma volume expansion to support volume responsive cardiac performance or the initiation of pressure agent administration; systolic pressure variation (SPV) may not hold similar clinical utility as it may be relatively insensitive to changes in stressed volume.
- The cardiovascular effects of IAH are aggravated by hypovolemia and the application of PEEP, whereas hypervolemia has a temporary protective effect in a similar fashion to plasma volume expansion in patients with evolving cardiac tamponade.
- Analogous to the widely accepted and clinically utilized concept of cerebral perfusion pressure, calculated as mean arterial pressure (MAP) minus intracranial pressure (ICP), abdominal perfusion pressure (APP), calculated as MAP minus IAP, has been proposed as a more accurate predictor of visceral perfusion and a potential end point for resuscitation.
  - APP = MAP – IAP
  - APP, by considering both arterial inflow (MAP) and restrictions to venous outflow (IAP), has been demonstrated to be statistically superior to either parameter alone in predicting patient survival from IAH and ACS.
  - A target APP of at least 60 mmHg has been demonstrated to correlate with improved survival from IAH and ACS.

Renal Function

– Decreased renal perfusion pressure (RPP) and renal filtration gradient (FG) have been proposed as key factors in the development of IAP-induced renal failure.
  - RPP = MAP – IAP
  - FG = GFP – PTP = (MAP – IAP) – IAP = MAP – 2*IAP
    - GFP = Glomerular Filtration Pressure
    - PTP = Proximal Tubular Pressure

Thus, changes in IAP have a greater impact upon renal function and urine production than will changes in MAP. It should not be surprising, therefore, that decreased renal function, as evidenced by development of oliguria, is one of the initial signs of IAH. Conversely, therefore, it behooves us as clinicians to be cognizant that elevated IAP and its effect on renal function is often the first sign of *impending ACS*. Other key points to remember are as follows:

– The prerenal azotemia seen in IAH is unresponsive to plasma volume expansion to a normal or supra-normal CO, or loop diuretics.
– Renal function may be improved by paracentesis of ascitic fluid and reduction in the IAP in patients with secondary ACS.
– Prompt reduction of IAP has dramatic beneficial effect on urine output in patients with primary and secondary ACS after trauma provided that the genesis of the oliguria is IAH associated decreased cardiac performance and decreased stroke volume and renal perfusion. In patients with ATN, decreases in IAP are not likely to augment urine flow.
– Within the capsule of the kidney, hematoma formation after injury may have an adverse affect on tissue perfusion causing a local renal compartment syndrome.

Hepatic Function

– Close monitoring and early recognition of IAH, followed by aggressive treatment may confer an outcome benefit in patients with liver disease.
– In this unique patient population, it may be useful to measure the plasma disappearance rate (PDR) for indocyanine green (ICG) as this correlates not only with liver function and perfusion but also with IAP. The authors recognize that the ability to do so is not universally available.
– Since cytochrome P_{450} function may be altered (diminished) in case of IAH/ACS, medication doses should be adapted accordingly.

– Within the capsule of the liver, hematoma formation following injury may have an adverse affect on tissue perfusion causing a local hepatic compartment syndrome.
– With increasing IAP there is decreased hepatic arterial flow, decreased portal venous flow, and increased portacollateral circulation. In turn, physiological effects include
  - Decreased lactate clearance
  - Altered glucose metabolism
  - Altered mitochondrial function

A common theme with all of the end-organ support measures is management of microcirculatory delivery and utilization of oxygen. Further data are needed to enable the clinician to better support end-organ function and avoid the downstream sequelae of IAH and the ACS. At present, when the ACS is recognized, management strategies become streamlined.

While abdominal decompression via a decompressive laparotomy is the gold-standard against which all other therapeutic undertakings for the management of established ACS are measured, many other methods of management have been proposed. The most effective of these alternative methods is percutaneous decompression when ascites is large in volume and may be the major etiology of the IAH and ACS. Other investigators have noted that a central feature of decompressive laparotomy is to enlarge the peritoneal cavity. Therefore, some have proposed a laparoscopic approach to increase the size of the peritoneal envelope by performing a component separation of parts expansion of the anterior abdominal wall. While technically possible, this is not a standard approach and requires a hemodynamically appropriate patient and a unique surgical skill set [3].

In a related circumstance, since IAH and the ACS may recur even in a patient with a temporary abdominal wall closure from progressive visceral edema and ascites, some have proposed routine application of a negative pressure device to create a fluid sump effect. The goal is to reduce visceral edema and evacuate ascites to reduce the likelihood of IAH. While some authors have identified success with this approach, it is unclear whether the utility of this approach stemmed from negative pressure or concomitant plasma volume reduction with diuretics or renal replacement techniques [3]. Nonetheless, as a means of managing the usually large volume of ascites, either a "home-made VAC" as in Fig. 1 or utilizing the KCI Corporation's proprietary VAC system provides effective transudate control. Furthermore, application of negative pressure across an open wound has been associated with a greater likelihood of primary fascial closure after injury or critical illness when a patient required an open abdomen management approach [4]; although this technique has also been related to a higher incidence of fistulae if applied improperly.

The reader should note that negative pressure management is ineffective for hemorrhage related IAH; hemorrhage should prompt reexploration that may be complemented by intra- or post-operative angiography and embolization. This technique is particularly effective for solid organ injury recurrent hemorrhage management. While most patients are reexplored in the OR, decompression may also be effectively and safely performed at the bedside in the ICU. At one of the author's (LJK) institutions, bedside reexploration is more the rule rather than the exception, as these patients are often unstable and on advanced ventilation rendering transport to the OR frankly dangerous. This trend follows the increased utilization of the ICU for a host of procedures including open as opposed to percutaneous tracheostomy, fasciotomy, or endoscopic gastrostomy placement, as well as planned abdominal or thoracic reexploration. Furthermore, these procedures may be safely performed without support staff from the OR in environments supplemented by nonphysician providers, residents, or fellows in addition to the Attending physician especially if the Attending is also a surgeon (e.g., in the USA, generally a trauma, general, and critical care surgeon).

Evaluation/Assessment

Effectiveness

The combination of intra-vesical pressure (IVP) monitoring and a high index of suspicion in an appropriate patient set for the development of IAH is highly effective and accurate (see ▶ Intra-Abdominal Pressure Monitoring). Combining IVP with organ failure evaluation is highly

effective as a means of determining the presence of the ACS. In fact, at present, there is no other reliable means of establishing that the syndrome is present and the cause of the patient's abnormal physiologic profile. Physical examination has been documented to be notoriously unreliable as a guide to IAP assessment [3].

The efficacy of decompressive laparotomy at relieving the ACS is 100%. However, one must remain vigilant for recurrence due to recurrent hemorrhage, visceral edema, gaseous hollow viscus distension, or ascites formation. The frequency of this diagnosis is directly related to the frequency of monitoring for IAH. A recent review noted that most ICUs do not have an established protocol for monitoring for IAH and the ACS. A sample protocol is attached (Fig. 3). Moreover, regardless of the efficacy of decompression at relieving the syndrome, organ failure may not readily improve, as an attributable organ failure is part of the definition of the syndrome. Additionally, the at-risk patient population is the identical group of patients in whom organ failure is likely to occur due to the underlying disease process that established hypoperfusion in the first place. Thus, acute lung injury, acute kidney injury, and the like are common prior to the syndrome occurring. The reader should recall that mortality directly correlates with an increasing number of organ failures. Importantly, an organ failure that is not incorporated into the Sequential Organ Failure Assessment score (SOFA) but is a direct reflection of IAH is GI failure [5]. GI failure may be readily recognized by the bedside provider as intolerance of enteral feedings whether they be elemental or non-elemental.

Tolerance

There is no tolerance of the ACS by the patient, and as such, the ACS should be regarded as a surgical emergency by the physician. Thus, emergent relief of the increased IAP is appropriate and required for management. Tolerance of the *aftermath* of decompressive laparotomy

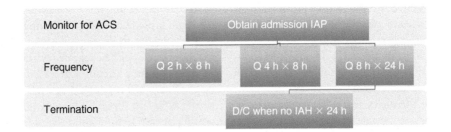

Notify MD for all IAP > 12

Abdominal Compartment Syndrome. Figure 3 Bladder pressure monitoring scheme

depends on whether or not the patient's abdominal wall may be primarily closed or not. This topic will be further explored in Aftercare but suffice it to note that the incidence of complications is vastly different between those able to undergo primary closure and those who require delayed reconstruction.

Pharmacoeconomics

The pharmacoeconomic impact of the ACS is currently unclear, but is generally believed to increase total healthcare costs as a result of intensive medical and surgical care. Nonetheless, certain observations are germaine to this topic. *First*, if left untreated, the ACS will result in death, the rapidity of which is related to the rate of progression of IAH. Of course, rapid death results in a lesser total economic expenditure for the healthcare system. *Second*, with increased awareness of the ACS, more patients (trauma, general surgery, vascular surgery, obstetrics, gynecologic oncology, and medical patients) are undergoing decompressive procedures. As a result, these patients remain alive to require care for their organ failure(s), as well as their acutely open abdomen. *Third*, these patients generally require intensive care management as well as relatively long general ward stays followed by rehabilitation facility inpatient care. Readmissions for complication management as well as reconstructive procedures further increase the healthcare system burden. *Fourth*, it is unclear how many of these patients return to gainful employment at present. There are no appropriately powered longitudinal studies to conclusively answer this financially relevant question. *Fifth* and finally, the system and physician reimbursement of these procedures and management is often regional and patient population specific depending on the local penetrance of appropriately insured, underinsured, and uninsured patients. As the US Centers for Medicare and Medicaid Services (CMS) threatens to not pay for the management of "complications," the reimbursement for providing the complex and intense care required by this critically ill patient population may garner a zero reimbursement, rendering this care increasingly difficult to support at all but large and financially successful institutions. If so, increased regionalization of specialty care may readily follow in the wake of the proposed CMS action, even if the CMS defined "complications" are not the direct result of inappropriate or ineffective physician or system care, but are instead commensals of the underlying disease process. At present, the US system is ill-prepared to handle the relocation of all such patients to regional resource centers due to lack of space, nursing staff, as well as appropriately trained surgeons.

The American Association for The Surgery of Trauma in conjunction with the American College of Surgeons Committee on Trauma has proposed a new designation and training program for surgeons who will provide trauma, general surgery, and critical care. This surgeon will be termed an Acute Care Surgeon. As current interest in trauma surgery and critical care is relatively low, the deliberate inclusion of emergency general surgery into the surgeon's purview may increase the appeal, stabilize the specialties' workload, and provide a cadre of appropriately trained surgeons to care for patients with progressive IAH and the ACS. While there are many hurdles to overcome to implement such a paradigm, training programs are being approved and the first trainees will soon graduate. The effectiveness and economic impact of these programs appear excellent at centers that have adopted such a model, but they have all been tertiary or quaternary referral academic training centers to date. Its impact in the community remains to be determined.

In Europe the socioeconomic burden of IAH and ACS patients is even more diverse. In some countries like the UK and The Netherlands, so-called abdominal rehabilitation or acute intestinal failure units have been formed under the auspices of the National Health Insurance (NHI) so that only doctors treating patients in those centers will be reimbursed, while in other countries no reimbursement or liberal reimbursement policies inconsistently apply.

After-care

Aftercare is identical to that of other critically ill patients with a few notable exceptions. Generally, patients with a temporary abdominal wall closure undergo abdominal cavity lavage every day or every other day during the early portion of their care as needed to evaluate injury, evacuate clot, or reduce bacterial burden to obtain adequate source control. The goal is to control the underlying disease process, while maintaining the fascial margins as close together as possible without allowing underlying adhesions or fistulas to develop and limit medial motion of the abdominal wall. The repeated washouts aid in limiting adhesions to the posterior aspect of the anterior abdominal wall and are augmented by placing a non-adherent barrier as far laterally under the anterior abdominal wall as possible at each reexploration (Fig. 1). A host of management methods to preserve fascial approximation exist and include the vacuum methods mentioned above, the application of a Wittman patch (two-layer hook and loop device) sewn to the fascia to progressively pull the fascia closer together, or other similar home-made device such as a piece of polypropylene mesh inside a bowel bag sewn to the fascia that is progressively tightened. Other methods such as a Bogota bag may provide temporary abdominal wall closure, but do not routinely provide for progressive fascial tightening (Fig. 4).

The rest of the aftercare will depend on whether or not the abdominal wall may undergo primary fascial closure or not. This key feature divides patients into two rather distinct groups based on length of stay, resource utilization, complications, and mortality. Patients who are able to undergo primary fascial closure generally do so within two weeks of having their abdomen opened or reopened. Increasingly, the primary fascial closure is buttressed with an underlay with a regenerative tissue matrix or a prosthetic mesh placed using nonabsorbable sutures creating a layered approach to closure (skin, subcutaneous tissue, fascia, mesh, and then abdominal contents). This technique has arisen from the observation that some of the patients who undergo primary closure present later with a ventral hernia, as well as the universal observation that all of these patients have some degree of protein-calorie malnutrition. Recall that the protein losses via the open abdomen are not measured, may be prodigious, and are not accounted for in the nutritional prescription. Thus, a buttress may help avoid wound failure; long-term data regarding outcome is currently being acquired. An alternative technique for those with closely opposed fascial margins that are unable to meet without tension is a variety of component release techniques, the review of which is beyond the scope of this chapter. These releases also utilize an underlay buttress closure technique in general, but some authors have successfully applied an overlay patch technique instead. These patients have similar courses to other ICU patients with respect to complications as adjusted for ICU length of stay.

Should the abdomen not be able to be primarily closed, delayed reconstructive techniques are required. Generally, but not universally, abdominal contents are constrained by applying an absorbable mesh constructed from polyglycolic acid (PGA) and sewn to either the fascia or skin using polyglycolic acid suture (Fig. 5). Quite commonly, the PGA mesh is then covered with a layer of Vaseline impregnated gauze to help prevent desiccation. This layer is then covered with a vacuum closure device, such as the KCI VAC to help draw the subcutaneous space together (Fig. 6). After granulation tissue begins to form, a split thickness skin graft (STSG) may be applied and then held in place with a VAC for 3 days prior to inspection. Alternatively, for heavily contaminated peritoneal spaces, no PGA mesh is applied and the STSG is directly

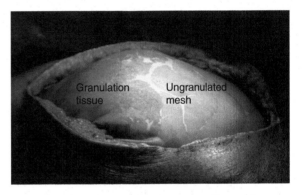

Abdominal Compartment Syndrome. Figure 5 PGA mesh temporary closure

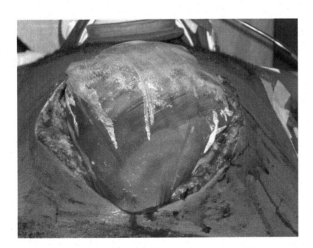

Abdominal Compartment Syndrome. Figure 4 Bowel bag and mesh temporary closure

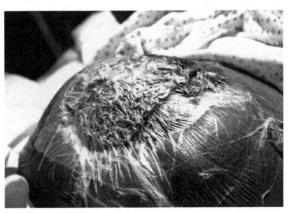

Abdominal Compartment Syndrome. Figure 6 KCI VAC temporary abdominal wall closure

applied to granulating bowel, omentum, or both and similarly held in place with a VAC.

Patients in this group generally have a longer ICU and total hospital length of stay than other patients with similar injuries or surgical diagnoses. This group is at increased risk for nosocomial infection, prolonged ventilator length of stay, tracheostomy, organ failure, and in particular enteroatmospheric fistula (EAF) and the occurrence of tertiary IAH as well as the "frozen abdomen." In particular, EAF is related to anastomoses that are not covered by vascularized tissue, multiple manipulations of friable tissue, and severe protein-calorie malnutrition as well as access sites for enteral feeding catheters. Therefore, long-term open abdomen patients may benefit from enteral access using nasojejunal tubes rather than catheters than cross the abdominal wall, especially since such catheters cross the rectus abdominous muscle rendering component separation difficult during later reconstruction. Mortality rates are increased with increased numbers of complications and organ failures in this group as well. A recent review of patients managed with an open abdomen at a high volume trauma center noted that readmission for infection and management of enteroatmospheric fistula was common, but manageable allowing excellent outcomes to be enjoyed. However, intense resource utilization was the rule for those who could not undergo primary fascial closure.

The maxim that "the longer one may wait prior to STSG removal and abdominal wall reconstruction the better" reflects the intense inflammatory response that underlies the reason that a patient has been managed with an open abdomen. Usually 9–12 months is a standard waiting period prior to undertaking the final reconstruction; generally patients have developed a giant ventral hernia by that time (Fig. 7). Such reconstructive procedures usually involved removing the STSG, employing a component separation of parts, abdominal wall release, and an underlay buttress reconstruction. Many of these patients also require restoration of GI continuity at the same operative sitting, thus making the use of prosthetic material for reconstruction more problematic than regenerative tissue matrixes with regard to infection. Involvement of a plastic surgeon with a focus on soft tissue reconstruction is often invaluable in this challenging patient population.

Prognosis

Since the mortality from unrelieved ACS approaches 100%, prognosis for survival is vastly improved with emergent relief. However, as noted above, the prognosis

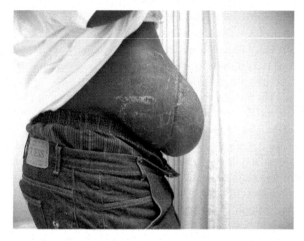

Abdominal Compartment Syndrome. Figure 7 Typical anterior abdominal wall giant ventral hernia

is often more related to concomitant organ failure, and less to the open abdomen itself. A recent review showed on average a mortality of 50% in these patients [6]. Instead, ACS is a marker for the severity of the primary disease process and its interplay with host defense and host inflammation. We are unfortunately in our infancy with regard to understanding the inflammatory response, let alone possessing a therapeutic tool with which to manipulate its complex interacting pathways. Nonetheless, since we are currently identifying the ACS as a combination of an increased IAP coupled with an attributable organ failure, we may be identifying it too late to abrogate other organ failures or progression of the attributable one. Ongoing investigation into renal biomarkers (like NGAL, cystatin C, and others) associated with AKI, or alveolar or plasma markers of pulmonary, gastrointestinal (citrulin), or other organ injuries may allow earlier identification of incipient organ failure, affording the clinician with an early warning signal that could trigger earlier decompression. Thus, much like the initial diagnosis of the syndrome, a firm grasp of the prognosis from ACS remains in flux.

Cross-References

▶ Burn Injury, Compartment Syndromes

References

1. Malbrain ML, Cheatham ML, Kirkpatrick A et al (2006) Results from the international conference of experts on intra-abdominal hypertension and abdominal compartment syndrome I. Definitions. Inten Care Med 32(11):1722–1732

2. Maxwell RA, Fabian TC, Croce MA, Davis KA (1999) Secondary abdominal compartment syndrome: an unappreciated manifestation of severe hemorrhagic shock. J Trauma 47(6):995–999

3. Betro G, Kaplan LJ (2009) Abdominal compartment syndrome. In: Ronco C, Bellomo R, Kellum JA (eds) Critical care nephrology, 2nd edn. WB Saunders, Philadelphia

4. Lui F, Sangosanya A, Kaplan LJ (2007) Abdominal compartment syndrome: clinical aspects and monitoring. Crit Care Clin 23:415–335

5. Malbrain ML, De Laet I (2008) AIDS is coming to your ICU: be prepared for acute bowel injury and acute intestinal distress syndrome. Inten Care Med 34(9):1565–1569

6. De Waele JJ, Hoste EA, Malbrain ML (2006) Decompressive laparotomy for abdominal compartment syndrome–a critical analysis. Crit Care 10(2):R51

Abdominal Pain

▶ Acute Abdominal Pain: General Approach
▶ Imaging for Acute Abdominal Pain

Abdominal Pressure

▶ Intraabdominal Pressure Monitoring

Abdominal Sepsis

▶ Peritonitis: Definitions of Primary, Secondary, and Tertiary

Abdominal Trauma

ANNIE L. SLAUGHTER[1], WALTER L. BIFFL[2]
[1]University of Colorado School of Medicine, Denver, CO, USA
[2]Department of Surgery, Denver Health Medical Center, Denver, CO, USA

Synonyms
Blunt abdominal trauma; Injury; Penetrating abdominal trauma; Torso trauma

Definition

Anatomy
Abdominal trauma is any injury to the abdominal wall or organs within the *abdominal cavity*. External landmarks for the abdomen are the transnipple line superiorly, the anterior axillary lines laterally, and the inguinal ligaments and pubic symphysis inferiorly. Between the anterior and posterior axillary lines, from the sixth intercostal space to the iliac crest, is the flank. The back is the region posterior to the posterior axillary lines, from the inferior tip of the scapulae to the iliac crests [1]. These landmarks are relevant primarily in terms of diagnostic evaluation for penetrating abdominal trauma.

The abdominal cavity contains three components – the *peritoneal cavity*, the *retroperitoneum*, and the *pelvic cavity* – and includes everything between the diaphragm superiorly, and the *pelvic floor* inferiorly. The upper peritoneal cavity is partially within the lower thoracic cage and is commonly referred to as the *thoracoabdominal region* [1]. It is covered by the lower portion of the bony thorax and contains the diaphragm, liver, spleen, stomach, and transverse colon. The lower peritoneal cavity contains the small bowel, portions of the ascending and descending colons, and the sigmoid colon. The retroperitoneal space is the region posterior to the peritoneal lining of the abdomen. It completely contains the abdominal aorta, inferior vena cava, iliac vessels, adrenal glands, kidneys, ureters, and bladder. In addition, the retroperitoneum contains part of the lower esophagus, the posterior aspects of the ascending and descending colon, as well as most of the pancreas, duodenum, and rectum. Many of the retroperitoneal and peritoneal organs are also found within the pelvic cavity, which also includes the female reproductive organs. The pelvic cavity is surrounded by the pelvic bones and rests on the pelvic floor.

Injury Mechanism
Blunt abdominal trauma refers to a direct blow or crushing mechanism that can injure organs or lacerate blood vessels in spite of an intact abdominal wall. Typically, blunt trauma results in multiple, widely spread injuries to organs less capable of an elastic deformation that might sustain impact [2]. Therefore, the most common organs injured in blunt trauma are the spleen (40–55%), liver (35–45%), and small bowel (5–10%) [1]. When surveying for blunt trauma, specific trauma mechanisms can suggest particular constellations of injuries. For example, frontal trauma often results in multisystem injury whereas collisions with side impact can fracture the pelvic ring and

rupture the diaphragm, but solid organ injury is typically limited to liver or spleen [2]. Keeping specific mechanisms in mind, presentation of certain injuries can suggest evaluation for other injuries that typically accompany them. *Shearing injury* is a form of blunt trauma that occurs when a shearing force is applied to a body part (e.g., following improper use of restraint devices), typically resulting in displacement or deformity. *Deceleration injury* is often the result of a collision with a stationary object or the ground (e.g., falls). In addition to injury to the body part directly colliding with the object, this mechanism may result in lacerations at the junction of fixed and mobile portions of organs. Lacerations of the liver and spleen at the site of their supporting ligaments are common sites for deceleration injuries.

Penetrating abdominal trauma refers to a mechanism by which an object (e.g., knife, bullet) penetrates the abdominal wall, often causing laceration of organs. Penetrating wounds are classified by weapon, or agent, and gunshot wounds are then further divided into low versus high velocity. Classification is important in determining the likelihood of involvement of structures lateral to the missile path. Additional injuries resulting from ricochet, fragmentation, and the transfer of kinetic energy are possible and should be considered whenever high-velocity gunshot wounds are encountered. It is also important to keep in mind that torso wounds below the nipple line and fractured ribs can likewise result in penetrating injury to abdominal structures, particularly the diaphragm, liver, and spleen. In general, penetrating trauma most commonly injures those organs with largest surface area when viewed from the front [2]. For stab wounds, the most likely organs involved are the liver (40%), small bowel (30%), diaphragm (20%), and colon (15%); while gunshot wounds injure the small bowel (50%), colon (40%), liver (30%), and major abdominal blood vessels (25%) [1].

Treatment

For adult patients with abdominal trauma, widely accepted indications for exploratory laparotomy include: hemodynamic instability with clinical evidence of intraperitoneal bleed (e.g., positive *focused abdominal sonography for trauma* (FAST), or *diagnostic peritoneal lavage* (DPL)), regardless of mechanism; gunshot wounds penetrating the peritoneal cavity; and stab wounds with evisceration or peritonitis [1, 3]. For hemodynamically stable patients without evidence of peritonitis, injuries to solid organs are managed nonoperatively in the majority of cases, while hollow viscera generally require operative repair. Although penetrating trauma is more often managed surgically, isolated solid organ injuries

following gunshot wounds are increasingly being managed nonoperatively.

Evaluation/Assessment

In the initial evaluation, the most important early decision to be made is whether exploratory laparotomy is emergently indicated [2, 3]. This may be determined on the basis of peritonitis on physical exam, or shock in the presence of penetrating abdominal trauma or blunt abdominal trauma with hemoperitoneum (see Diagnostic Evaluation, below). If the patient does not have immediate indications for laparotomy, further diagnostic evaluation is warranted. The physical exam is unreliable as altered mental status due to intoxication, central nervous systeminjury, severe associated injuries, or shock is common. Furthermore, the patient may lose a significant amount of blood into the abdominal cavity without shock or any signs of peritoneal irritation. As a result, overlooked and unrecognized abdominal injury continues to result in poorer outcomes and preventable death following trauma [1, 2].

Diagnostic Evaluation

There are a number of adjuncts to the physical exam that are useful to the clinician. These include devices, laboratory tests, endoscopy, and imaging studies.

Devices. Gastric tubes can be diagnostic as well as therapeutic. Decompression of the stomach can help avoid aspiration. In addition, the detection of blood in the gastric aspirate is a sign of esophageal or gastric injury and must be investigated. Urinary drainage catheters are important in the monitoring of organ perfusion and the response to resuscitation. In addition, the presence of hematuria is a sign of injury to the genitourinary system.

Laboratory tests. Serial monitoring of the blood hemoglobin concentration is important to detect occult bleeding before the patient develops shock. The *white blood cell count* is nonspecific in the first 24 h, but a progressively rising count $>20 \times 10^3/\text{mm}^3$ may be associated with hollow viscus injury. Another nonspecific test is the serum *amylase* level, which may be elevated in the setting of occult pancreatic injury [4]. *Urinalysis* may reveal microscopic hematuria, and aid in the diagnosis of genitourinary injury. *Arterial blood gas* provides a great deal of information. Metabolic acidosis may be a harbinger of ongoing shock, hemorrhage, or hollow viscus injury. A *diagnostic peritoneal lavage* is helpful to clarify an equivocal ultrasonographic exam or suspected hollow viscus injury (see below).

Endoscopy. Endoscopy may be employed to diagnose hollow viscus injuries to the esophagus, stomach, or duodenum in the presence of bloody gastric aspirate. Similarly, it is used to evaluate the integrity of rectosigmoid in the setting of severe pelvic fracture or penetrating pelvic trauma.

Imaging studies. During the primary survey, the *Focused Abdominal Sonographic examination for Trauma (FAST)* is performed; the identification of hemoperitoneum mandates laparotomy in the presence of shock, and should be further evaluated with computed tomographic (CT) scanning in a stable patient (see below). *Chest and pelvis radiographs* are an important component of the initial evaluation. Although not particularly sensitive or specific for significant abdominal injuries, these x-rays and can identify pneumoperitoneum, diaphragmatic rupture, or pelvic fractures. With advancing imaging technology and whole-body techniques, *CT scanning* is being used more and more broadly in trauma, supplanting plain radiography and arteriography for many applications. CT scanning is reserved for the stable patient without indication for immediate surgical intervention. It provides information about injuries to specific organs, allowing selection of patients for safe nonoperative management.

After-care

Following operative management ongoing resuscitation is critical to reverse shock. Patients who are being managed nonoperatively must be monitored for hemorrhage or missed hollow viscus injury. Recuperation from laparotomy takes a couple of weeks. Solid organ injuries that are managed nonoperatively have a low bleeding incidence over the first 2 weeks, with the spleen being the most likely to bleed after the first 2–3 days. The tensile strength of solid organs is returned to premorbid levels by 2–3 months, allowing safe return to vigorous activities.

Prognosis

There is little permanent morbidity following abdominal trauma. Most injuries can be repaired, with complete recovery. There are special circumstances, such as immune compromise in a splenectomized patient, or short bowel syndrome following extensive small bowel resection. Overall, however, the patient who avoids exsanguination, sepsis, or multiple organ failure is likely to recover fully.

References

1. American College of Surgeons Committee on Trauma (2008) Advanced trauma life support for doctors, 8th edn. American College of Surgeons, Chicago
2. Cothren CC, Biffl WL, Moore EE et al (2010) Trauma. In: Schwartz's principles of surgery, 9th edn. McGraw-Hill, New York
3. Biffl WL, Kaups KL, Cothren CC et al (2009) Management of patients with anterior abdominal stab wounds: a western trauma association multicenter trial. J Trauma 66:1294–1301
4. Biffl WL (2010) Trauma to the pancreas and duodenum. In: Mattox KL, Moore EE, Feliciano DV (eds) Trauma, 7th edn. McGraw-Hill, New York

Abdominal Trauma, Damage Control

CLAY COTHREN BURLEW, ERNEST E. MOORE
Department of Surgery, Denver Health Medical Center, University of Colorado Denver, Denver, CO, USA

Synonyms

Abbreviated laparotomy

Definition

The term "damage control" was coined by the US Navy during World War II, and was defined as those procedures and skills employed to maintain or restore the watertight integrity, stability, or offensive power in a warship. This military term is used today to describe the management of the surgical equivalent of a sinking ship. The concept was introduced by Stone et al. in 1983 [1] and promulgated by the Ben Taub General group [2]. The fundamentals of damage control surgery (DCS) are to limit the operation to essential interventions, namely, controlling hemorrhage, shunting major vascular injuries, and limiting enteric contamination, in patients who are dying due to the bloody viscous cycle (the lethal triad of hypothermia, coagulopathy, and acidosis) (Fig. 1) [3]. Aborting the operation enables one to return the patient to the surgical intensive care unit (SICU) for resuscitation and correction of the coagulopathy. Once physiologic restoration is complete, the patient is returned to the operating room for definitive repair of injuries.

Indications

A progressive and recalcitrant coagulopathy is the most common and compelling reason for an abbreviated laparotomy. Indications to limit the initial operation and institute damage control surgery techniques is a clinical decision, typically considering the objective signs of persistent temperature $<35°C$, arterial pH < 7.2, base deficit > 15 mmol/L, and INR or PTT $> 50\%$ of normal. The decision to abbreviate a trauma laparotomy is made intraoperatively as the patient's clinical course becomes

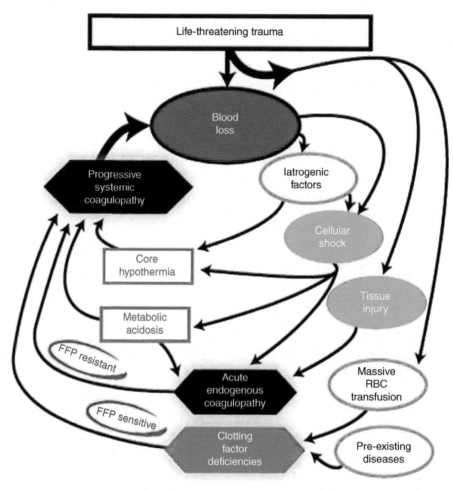

Abdominal Trauma, Damage Control. Figure 1 The bloody vicious cycle

defined. Laboratory results for the standard measurements of coagulation capability (i.e., INR, PTT, and platelet count) require approximately 30 min, so the decision to abort the full operative plan usually needs to occur before confirmatory evidence of the patient's physiologic derangements. The recent introduction of rapid thromboelastography may provide earlier objective measures to warrant damage control.

Application

The goal of damage control surgery is to control surgical bleeding, revascularize with shunts, and limit gastrointestinal spillage. The operative techniques employed are temporary measures, with definitive repair of injuries delayed until the patient is physiologically replete [2–5]. Controlling surgical bleeding while preventing ischemia is of utmost importance during DCS. Aortic injuries must be repaired using an interposition PTFE graft. Although celiac artery injuries may be ligated, the superior

mesenteric artery must maintain flow and the insertion of an intravascular shunt is advocated. Similarly, perfusion of the iliac system and infrainguinal vessels can be restored with a vascular shunt, delaying interposition graft placement until hours later. Venous injuries are preferentially treated with ligation in damage control situations, except for the suprarenal IVC. For significant injuries to the spleen, excision is indicated rather than attempting repair such as splenorrhaphy. Renal hematomas should not be explored unless actively expanding. For hepatic injuries, packing of the liver will usually tamponade bleeding. Translobar gunshot wounds of the liver are best controlled with balloon catheter tamponade, while deep lacerations can be controlled with Foley catheter inflation deep within the tract. Selective operative ligation of hepatic arteries and preperitoneal pelvic packing for recalcitrant bleeding should not be forgotten in this era of reliance on Interventional Radiology and angioembolization.

For thoracic injuries requiring DCS several options exist. For bleeding peripheral pulmonary injuries, wedge resection using a GIA stapler is performed. In penetrating injuries, pulmonary tractotomy is used to divide the parenchyma; individual vessels and bronchi are then ligated using a 3-0 PDS suture, and the tract is left open. Patients that sustain more proximal injuries may require pulmonary lobectomy or pneumonectomy to control bleeding. Cardiac injuries may be temporarily controlled using a running 3-0 prolene suture or skin staples. If this technique does not definitely control hemorrhage, pledgeted repair of the injury should be performed.

The second key component of DCS is limiting enteric content spillage. Small gastrointestinal injuries (stomach, duodenum, small intestine, and colon) may be controlled with a rapid whipstitch of 2-0 prolene. Complete transection of the bowel or segmental damage is controlled using a GIA stapler, often with resection of the injured segment. Alternatively, open ends of the bowel may be ligated using umbilical tapes to limit spillage. Pancreatic injuries, regardless of location, are packed and the evaluation of ductal integrity is postponed.

Although moving the patient from the operating room to the SICU for resuscitation is the goal, leaving the operating room too early is also problematic. One should ensure that the lack of hemostasis is due to coagulopathy rather than ongoing mechanical bleeding. Mechanical bleeding must be controlled before proceeding to the SICU, or the vicious cycle will only continue. One option is temporary closure of the abdomen with a towel clip (if bowel egress allows you to do so) for 30 min while allowing anesthesia and the blood bank to maximally correct the acidosis and coagulopathy (Fig. 2). The abdomen is then reopened and evaluated for control of mechanical bleeding, whether or not packs are actually needed, and a repeat look for any missed gastrointestinal injuries that need to be controlled.

Before transport to the SICU, the abdomen must be temporarily closed. Currently, ioban closure of the abdomen is performed for temporary closure (Fig. 3). In this technique, the bowel is covered with a fenestrated subfascial 1010 steri-drape (3M Health Care, St. Paul, MN) and two Jackson-Pratt drains are placed along the fascial edges; this is then covered using an ioban, allowing closed suction to control reperfusion-related ascitic fluid egress while providing adequate space for bowel expansion to prevent the abdominal compartment syndrome. Following normalization of physiologic parameters, typically after 12–24 h in the SICU, the patient is returned to the operating room for pack removal and definitive repair of injuries. Occasionally, ongoing bleeding will necessitate repeating the earlier steps of this algorithm and angiography should be considered in recalcitrant cases. Although patients ideally remain in the ICU for approximately

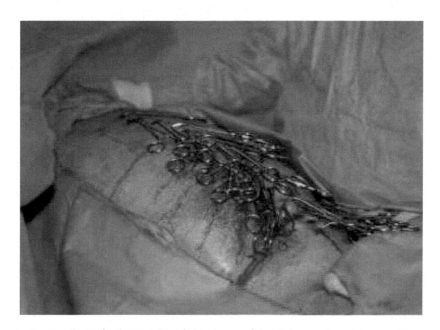

Abdominal Trauma, Damage Control. Figure 2 Towel clip closure of the abdomen allows intraoperative resuscitation of the patient

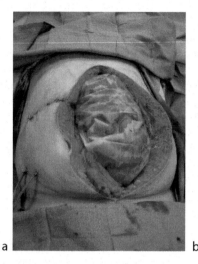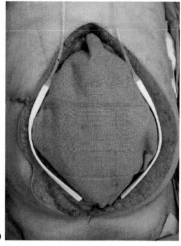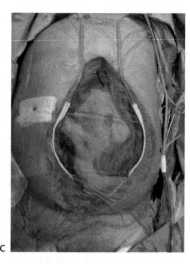

a   b   c

Abdominal Trauma, Damage Control. Figure 3 Temporary closure of the abdomen entails covering the bowel with a fenestrated 1010 drape (**a**), placement of JP drains and a blue towel (**b**), followed by ioban occlusion (**c**)

24 h during resuscitation and stabilization, early return to the operating room should be considered in patients with ongoing transfusion requirements despite correction of temperature and coagulation abnormalities.

References

1. Stone HH, Strom PR, Mullins RJ (1983) Management of the major coagulopathy with onset during laparotomy. Ann Surg 197:532–535
2. Burch JM, Ortiz VB, Richardson RJ et al (1992) Abbreviated laparotomy and planned reoperation for critically injured patients. Ann Surg 215:476
3. Moore EE (1996) Staged laparotomy for the hypothermia, acidosis, and coagulopathy syndrome. Am J Surg 172:405
4. Wyrzykowski A, Feliciano DV (2008) Trauma damage control. In: Feliciano DV, Mattox KL, Moore EE (eds) Trauma, 6th edn. McGraw-Hill, New York
5. Vargo DJ, Battistella FD (2001) Abbreviated thoracotomy and temporary chest closure: an application of damage control after thoracic trauma. Arch Surg 136(1):21–24

ABG

▶ Arterial Blood Gases Interpretation

Abscess

▶ Anaerobic Infections

Abscess, Epidural

PARITA BHUVA, BARNETT R. NATHAN
Division of Neurocritical Care, Departments of neurology, University of Virginia, Charlottesville, VA, USA

Synonyms

Intracranial epidural abscess; Spinal epidural abscess

Definition

Spinal epidural abscess (SEA) is a suppurative collection in the space surrounding the spinal cord located between the dura mater and the vertebral periosteum.

Spinal epidural infections are rare with an incidence of 0.2–2 cases per 10,000 hospital admissions. Most cases of SEA occur in patients aged 30–60 years. The most common risk factors for SEA are diabetes mellitus, followed by trauma, intravenous drug abuse, and alcoholism.

Treatment

Spinal epidural abscess is a neurosurgical emergency due to the potential for rapid deterioration to severe spinal cord dysfunction. The goal of surgery is immediate decompression and drainage. Posterior epidural abscesses are usually treated with decompressive laminectomy followed by irrigation through extradural drains for several days. In cases of anterior SEAs, anterior decompression is usually performed along with a partial or complete anterior or anterolateral corpectomy, because the infection usually extends to the vertebral column [1].

Antibiotic therapy should be based on the organisms most likely to be involved. An acceptable empiric regimen includes a third-generation cephalosporin along with an antistaphylococcal agent. If an organism or organisms are identified from culture, antibiotic therapy should be tailored based on susceptibility patterns. The adequate duration of antibiotic therapy for SEA has not been determined with certainty; however, a minimum of 6–8 weeks of treatment is the accepted standard of care, especially in cases managed medically. This recommendation is largely based on expert opinion and on the frequency of concomitant vertebral osteomyelitis seen in patients with SEA.

Evaluation/Assessment

The presenting signs and symptoms of a spinal epidural abscess can vary significantly. Back pain is the most common initial complaint. Other findings may include fever/chills, paresthesias, weakness, and difficulty ambulating. An established staging system outlines the progression of symptoms and physical findings:

Stage 1, back pain at the level of the affected spine
Stage 2, nerve-root pain radiating from the involved spinal area
Stage 3, motor weakness, sensory deficit, and bladder and bowel dysfunction and
Stage 4, paralysis [2]

Serologic tests are useful in the diagnosis and management of spinal epidural abscess. Essentially, all patients have an elevated erythrocyte sedimentation rate (ESR) on admission. An increased peripheral white blood cell count with a left shift is common.

Lumbar puncture is relatively contraindicated if spinal epidural abscess is suspected due to the risk of introducing purulent material into the subarachnoid space.

The diagnostic imaging of choice is a contrast-enhanced MRI. This imaging modality is highly sensitive, highly specific, and can accurately delineate the extent and location of the abscess. On T2-weighted image (T2WI)s, the hyperintense signal of the epidural mass can be differentiated from the non-enhancing thecal sac and neural elements. On CT, epidural abscess typically appears as a low attenuation extra-axial mass. On MRI, epidural abscesses have iso-signal on T1-weighted image and high signal on T2WI, with enhancement of the thickened dural surface.

Because most predisposing conditions allow for invasion by skin flora, *Staphylococcus aureus* causes about two thirds of cases. Less common causative pathogens include coagulase-negative staphylococci, such as *S. epidermidis* and gram-negative bacteria, particularly *Escherichia coli* and *Pseudomonas aeruginosa* [3].

After-care

Rehabilitation for any residual neurologic deficit may be necessary. This would include restrengthening programs and ambulation retraining. The many complications of spinal cord injury include bladder dysfunction, decubiti, supine hypertension, recurrent sepsis, and other problems.

Prognosis

The outcome of spinal epidural abscess is directly related to timely diagnosis. Patients diagnosed before the development of significant neurologic deficits fare better than those with weakness or paralysis for greater than 36–48 h at the time of diagnosis [4]. Other factors such as older age, septicemia, and greater degree of thecal sac compression are also associated with a worse outcome.

References

1. Kastenbauer S, Pfister HW, Scheld WM (1997) Epidural abscess. In: Scheld WM, Durack DT, Whitley RJ (eds) Infections of the central nervous system, 3rd edn. Raven Press, New York, pp 523–533
2. Darouiche RO (2006) Spinal epidural abscess. N Engl J Med 355 (19):2012–2020
3. Sendi P, Bregenzer T, Zimmerli W (2008) Spinal epidural abscess in clinical practice. QJM 101(1):1–12
4. Reihsaus E, Waldbaur H, Seeling W (2000) Spinal epidural abscess: a meta-analysis of 915 patients. Neurosurg Rev 23:175–205

Accelerated Recovery

► Enhanced Recovery After Surgery Intervention

Accessory Splenic Tissue

Naturally occurring heterotopic splenic tissue in the peritoneal cavity.

Acetaminophen Overdose

MICHAEL E. SILVERMAN, RICHARD D. SHIH
Department of Emergency Medicine, Morristown
Memorial Hospital, Morristown, NJ, USA

Synonyms

APAP; Tylenol

Definition

Acetaminophen overdose is the ingestion of supratherapeutic doses; this can be done as a one-time ingestion defined as acute overdose, or this can occur over extended periods of time, which is defined as chronic overdose.

Acute acetaminophen overdose causing toxicity is unlikely to occur in an acute ingestion in which less than 7.5 g is ingested in an adult or 140 mg/kg in a child [1].

Chronic acetaminophen overdose is the use of supratheraputic doses over an extended period of time. Nearly all reported cases of chronic acetaminophen toxicity involve patients who ingested supratheraputic doses and had factors that potentially predisposed them to acetaminophen-induced hepatic injury [1]. There is no clearly defined amount of acetaminophen ingested or duration of ingestion to define a chronic overdose.

There are multiple factors that likely increase your risk for toxicity to acetaminophen; they include chronic alcoholism, inducers of the enzyme P450 metabolic pathway, and malnutrition [1].

Treatment

N-acetylcysteine (NAC) in either intravenous or oral formulation is the treatment of choice for acetaminophen toxicity. Activated charcoal may be efficacious in the acute setting, it is most effective if given within 1–2 h after drug ingestion but may still have some efficacy if given in the first 4 h.

The Rumack–Matthew nomogram is utilized to assess patients for potential acetaminophen toxicity after a single ingestion. This nomogram utilizes a serum level of acetaminophen and the patient's time of ingestion [2]. If the patient's risk of acetaminophen toxicity is found to be either in the *possible* or *probable* risk, the antidote, n-acetylcysteine (NAC) is recommended for administration. N-acetylcysteine is most efficacious if used early after the acetaminophen ingestion and ideally within 8–10 h [2]. However, if the patient's time of ingestion is later than this time frame, NAC usage continues to have efficacy, albeit, not as great.

There are a number of presently utilized different NAC treatment protocols. The 20-h intravenous one appears to be most commonly utilized for uncomplicated cases of potential toxicity. This protocol involves the administration of an initial dose of 150 mg/kg over 15 min, followed by 50 mg/kg of NAC infused over the next 4 h. Over the remaining 16 h, an additional 100 mg/kg are administered as a constant infusion [1]. For patients with continued signs of toxicity after the 20 h period, some advocate continued NAC therapy. Other published protocols involve oral routes of NAC administration and longer durations of therapy. Controversy remains regarding the preferred route of NAC administration, duration of therapy, and when to discontinue therapy in complicated cases. The traditional 72-h oral NAC protocol is generally not completed for the entire duration in uncomplicated cases with negative follow-up acetaminophen levels and no liver function abnormalities.

In complicated cases of acetaminophen toxicity with ongoing hepatic toxicity, NAC therapy is continued beyond any predetermined time period. This is generally continued until the prothrombin time is near normal (PT < 1.5) [3]. For patients who do not develop liver failure but with elevated AST concentration, NAC may be continued until significant improvement, liver transplantation, or death [1]. However, these criteria for NAC discontinuation remain under debate.

Antiemetics may be necessary, especially when treating with the oral formulation of NAC, due to the nausea and vomiting associated with acetaminophen toxicity.

The decision whether to use oral or intravenous routes of administration rests with the clinician. Head-to-head comparisons have not been performed. However, observational studies involving both routes of administration suggest that either route is equally efficacious. Theoretical advantage for the oral route includes the decreased cost of the medication and potentially higher hepatic levels of NAC due to first-pass metabolism. In critically ill patients, the few studies available involve the use of intravenously administered NAC. Additionally, with possible decreased GI absorption in critically ill patients, the intravenous route would be preferred [4].

Few side effects are associated with the use of NAC. The most commonly reported adverse effects of intravenous acetylcysteine are anaphylactoid reactions, including rash, pruritus, angioedema, bronchospasm, tachycardia, and hypotension [4].

Evaluation/Assessment

A thorough history from patient, family, or other care providers can be helpful in determining events of ingestion, including amounts, timing and potential co-ingestions. Physical findings should be noted, although a complete physical examination is important in any potential overdose patient; in the setting of an acute acetaminophen overdose, there may be little if any abnormal initial physical examination findings. Right upper quadrant abdominal pain and tenderness may be present as acetaminophen-induced hepatotoxicity ensues.

Laboratory testing should include an acetaminophen level. Levels taken between 1–4 h can be difficult to interpret; however, an unmeasurable level at this time excludes a significant acute overdose. In an acute overdose patient, a measurable level drawn before 4 h mandates a repeat level at 4 h and needs to be assessed on the Rumack–Matthew nomogram. The nomogram can be used for levels up to 24 h post-ingestion [5].

In patients where it is unknown when the time of ingestion has occurred, liver transaminases should be measured. If there is an elevation of these tests, NAC should be administered regardless of what the measured acetaminophen level is. If the transaminases are negative with a negative acetaminophen level, toxicity is excluded.

In patients that demonstrate hepatoxicity, additional laboratory tests that are useful for assessing the degree of toxicity and prognosis include liver transaminases, prothrombin time, bilirubin level, serum glucose, serum blood urea nitrogen, serum lactate, serum creatinine, arterial pH, and individual clotting factor activity. Severe toxicity and increased mortality is seen in patients with metabolic acidosis, hepatic encephalopathy, elevated prothrombin times, and poor clotting factor activity [6].

Patients receiving intravenous acetylcysteine for severe hepatotoxicity need aggressive monitoring and supportive care provided in a critical care setting. Determining the length of NAC treatment in patients with severe hepatotoxicity can be difficult and is controversial. Most experts feel that NAC should be continued intravenously until encephalopathy resolves, there is no acidosis, the transaminases are improving, and the prothrombin time is improving.

One additional treatment modality available to severely poisoned patients is hepatic transplantation. A number of such patients have been successfully treated with this intervention. In one database, 40% of patients of liver transplants for drug-induced acute liver failure were due to acetaminophen [7]. An important factor involved in caring for severely acetaminophen-toxic patients is the rapidity that patients evolve from ingestion to hepatic toxicity to hepatic failure and death, if it occurs. One study revealed that acetaminophen-toxic patients that met criteria for liver transplantation developed surgical contraindications 30% of the time prior to transplant [8]. Given this, it is important to identify patients that are severely toxic and rapidly deteriorating for early referral for transplantation assessment.

Epidemiology

The incidence of acetaminophen toxicity continues to be one of the most common pharmaceutical ingestions as well as the most common cause of medication exposure toxicity. The 2008 Annual Report of the American Association of Poison Control Centers' National Poison Data System (NPDS): 26th Annual Report noted that the most common exposure-related fatalities by type was analgesics with acetaminophen being the most common as a single agent alone, followed by in combination [9].

After-care

Patients showing evidence of severe of significant liver toxicity or encephalopathy, and those at risk for hepatic failure may require ICU care. Consultation with a regional poison center, gastroenterologist (or hepatologist) consultant, and liver transplant center may be important to help plan treatment. As NAC is a very effective antidote, the vast majority of patients recover from their toxic ingestion. Once the medical issues have been resolved, if is important to assess any psychiatric issues that are present.

Prognosis

The prognosis of patients with acetaminophen overdose is based on their degree of liver dysfunction, as well as, the presence of additional comorbidities. Patients that do not develop significant liver toxicity have excellent prognoses. Patients who develop fulminant hepatic failure have significant morbidity and mortality. N-acetylcysteine therapy and liver transplantation may significantly reduce this mortality.

References

1. Rowden AK, Norvell J, Eldridge DL, Kirk MA (2006) Acetaminophen poisoning. Clin Lab Med 26:49–65
2. Wolf SJ, Heard K, Sloan EP, Jagoda AS (2007) Clinical policy: critical issues in the management of patients presenting to the emergency department with acetaminophen overdose. Ann Emerg Med 50:292–313
3. Fontana RJ (2008) Acute liver failure including acetaminophen overdose. Med Clin North Am 92(4):761–794
4. Heard K (2008) Acetylcysteine for acetaminophen poisoning. N Engl J Med 359:285–292

5. Rumack BH (2002) Acetaminophen hepatotoxicity: the first 35 years. J Toxicol Clin Toxicol 40:3–20
6. O'Grady JG, Alexander GJ, Hayllar KM, Williams R (1989) Early indicators of prognosis in fulminant hepatic failure. Gastroenterology 97:439–445
7. Mindikoglu AL, Magder LS (2009) RegevA Outcome of Liver Transplantation for Drug- Induced Acute Liver Failure in the United States:Analysis of the United Network for Organ Sharing Database. Liver Transpl 15:719–729
8. Bernal W, Wendon J, Rela M, Heaton N, Williams R (1998) Use and outcome of liver transplantation in acetaminophen-induced acute liver failure. Hepatology 27:1050–1055
9. Bronstein AC, Spyker DA, Cantilena LR, Green JL, Rumack BH, Giffin SL (2009) 2008 Annual Report of the American Association of Poison Control Centers' National Poison Data System (NPDS): 26th Annual Report. Clin Toxicol 47:911–1084

Acetylsalicylic Acid Overdose

▶ Salicylate Overdose

Ache

▶ Chest Pain: Differential Diagnosis

Acid Fast Bacilli (AFB)

Mycobacteria are aerobic bacteria with a specially adapted cell wall containing characteristic pepitdoglycolipids that render the bacteria somewhat resistant to gram staining. The term "acid fast bacteria (AFB)" refers to special procedures that allow for arylmethane dye uptake and retention, despite exposure to acid. Bacteria appear in a red–pink color by light microscopy.

Acid–Base

▶ Urine Electrolytes and Acid Base

Acid–Base Assessment

▶ Acid–Base Evaluation

Acid–Base Evaluation

Luciano Gattinoni[1], E. Carlesso[2], Pietro Caironi[2]
[1]Dipartimento di Anestesia, Rianimazione e Scienze, Dermatologiche. Fondazione IRCCS Cà Granda - Ospedale Maggiore Policlinico Università degli Studi di Milano, Milan, Italy
[2]Dipartimento di Anestesiologia, Terapia Intensiva e Scienze Dermatologiche; Università degli Studi, Milan, Italy

Synonyms
Acid–base assessment; Blood gas analysis

Definition
During the past years, different definitions of *acid* and *base* have been developed as shown in the following table [1]:

		Acid	Base
1887	Arrhenius	Hydrogen ion donor (aqueous medium)	Hydroxyl ion donor (aqueous medium)
1921	Van Slyke	Anion (apart from OH^-)	Cation (apart from H^+)
1923	Bronsted-Lowry	Hydrogen ion donor	Hydroxyl ion donor
1938	Lewis	Electron acceptor	Electron donor
1939	Usanovich	Cation donor, anion or electron acceptor	Anion donor, cation acceptor

The definition proposed by Arrhenius considers acid as a substance capable of dissociating in water that gives up hydrogen ions (H^+), while base as a substance that gives up hydroxide ions (OH^-). This definition, however, limits acids and bases to substances that can dissolve in water. The definition of Bronsted and Lowry includes even substances that are insoluble in water. The most general definition was introduced by Lewis, which defines an acid as an *electron-pair acceptor* and a base as an *electron-pair donor*. According to this definition, acids are also substances that do not contain any hydrogen atoms. Usanovich developed an even more general approach to acid–base theory that consolidated all the different approaches.

We may wonder, however, how these definitions are important in biology and medicine. For example, carbon dioxide, a compound of paramount importance in human physiology and acid–base equilibrium, per se, is not an acid; in contrast, when hydrated it behaves as such as it is transformed into carbonic acid. In general, we believe that the acid operational definition as proposed by Stewart in 1981 covers, in practice, all acid–base physiology and pathophysiology as encountered in biology and medicine. In fact, Stewart defined acid as any substance that added to a solution brings about an increase in hydrogen ion concentration of that solution, all the other independent variables remaining constant [2].

It must be pointed out that in solution the protons (H^+) are associated and react with the surrounding water molecules. This reaction is often represented by the hydronium ion (H_3O^+), while even this 1:1 relationship is not accurate. Moreover, the real behavior of solutions deviates from the ideal one because of the interactions between molecules. The ionic strength is a parameter that allows quantifying the effect of interionic interactions (molecular attraction and repelling). Ionic strength is computed as:

$$I = \sum_{i=1}^{n} [i] \times z_i^2 \tag{1}$$

where n denotes the number of ions in the solution, i denotes each specific ion in the solution, and z denotes the charge. Accordingly, greater is the ion concentration in solution and the ion charge, greater are the forces of attraction and repulsion, which are present in the solution. The relationship between concentration and activity is expressed as:

$$Activity = f \times concentration \tag{2}$$

where f denotes the activity coefficient. This indicates that activity and concentration are the same only in the case of extremely diluted solutions, where $f = 1$. Although the plasma ionic strength is not irrelevant (around 0.145 mmol/L) and the ion activity remarkably differs from their concentration (<0.76), in biology and medicine the activity is usually ignored as whatever change induced in physiological fluids by therapeutic interventions, such as hydratation or dehydratation or by the disease itself (if in limits compatible with life) do not modify remarkably the ionic strength. It is important to note, however, that pH, which is a key measurement for defining acidosis/alkalosis, measures the protons *activity* instead of their concentration. In fact, only the "active ions" may cross the glass electrode initiating the process finally leading to the pH measurement. In summary, although the pH measures the protons activity, all the derived computations involving

ions and pH refer to the concentration of the former instead of their activity.

Pre-existing Condition

Acid–Base Strength

Several substances acting as acids or bases are normally present in human plasma. As defined operationally above, an acid is a substance, which increases proton concentration in a solution. The strength of an acid (or a base) is the measurement of the tendency to release (dissociate) protons in solution, and is expressed as K_A. In fact:

$$K_A = \frac{[H^+] \times [A^-]}{[AH]} \tag{3}$$

The above equation set also the relationship between pH and pK. In fact:

$$\frac{K_A}{[H^+]} = \frac{[H^+]}{[AH]} \tag{4}$$

and in logarithmic form:

$$\log_{10} K_A - \log_{10}[H^+] = \log_{10}\frac{[A^-]}{[AH]} \tag{5}$$

as

$$-\log_{10}[H^+] = pH \tag{6}$$

and

$$-\log_{10} K_A = pK_A \tag{7}$$

it follows that:

$$pH = pK_A + \log_{10}\frac{[A^-]}{[AH]} \tag{8}$$

Indeed, greater is the K_A, lower is the pK_A and greater is the acid strength. In chemical textbooks an acid is usually defined as "strong" when its $pK_A << -2$. Therefore, strictly speaking, only few "strong acids" are actually present in the plasma, as hydrochloric acid ($pK_A = -9.3$) and sulfuric acid ($pK_A = -3$). Some other acids of biological importance, however, do have a pK_A between 2 and 4, which is greatly higher than the pK_A threshold for strong acid, as previously defined. For example, lactic acid has a pK_A equal to 3.8. At plasmatic pH, however, lactic acid is almost completely dissociated as the ratio $[A^-]:[AH]$ is 3981:1. Therefore, in medicine the concept of "strong acid," i.e., fully dissociated, must be considered relatively to the pH of the biological fluid. In contrast, weak acids are usually defined in medicine as those for which pK_A is between 6 and 7. In human plasma these are the carbonic acid ($pK \approx 6.1$), the phosphoric acid ($pK \approx 6.8$), and the imidazole groups of histidine residues of albumin (pK $\approx$ 6.8). These weak acids, in the traditional terminology, are named as *buffers*, as they may be present at plasmatic pH in their dissociated or undissociated forms, being their dissociated/undissociated ratio ranging between 4 and 20.

Determinants of Plasma pH

To understand the pH determinants it may be useful to reconstruct, step by step, the human plasma, which may be modeled as a water solution in equilibrium with the alveolar gases, in which acids and bases of different strength are mixed throughout. Let us assume that we want to prepare 1 L of solution resembling human plasma artificially. For the sake of simplicity we will consider only the compounds that are more relevant for the acid–base equilibrium.

Adding Strong Acids and Bases: Generation of Strong Ion Difference

The first step is to add 145 mmol of NaOH and 5 mmol of KOH to water. These two strong bases fully dissociate in water, and in the solution will be present 150 mmol of positive "strong ions" (145 mmol of Na^+ and 5 mmol K^+) as well as 150 mmol of OH^-. As the ionic product for water, i.e., $K'w = [H^+] \times [OH^-]$ may be considered constant (at 37°C, 2.39×10^{-14}), the pH may be easily computed. In fact $[H^+] = K'w/150 = 1.59 \times 10^{-13}$ mol/L, and pH $= 12.798$. Of note, the strong bases generated positive strong ions. Let us now add 110 mmol of HCl, a strong acid. In the new solution will be present 150 mmol of positive strong ions, 110 mmol Cl^- (strong negative ion), and 40 mmol OH^- (as 150 mmol OH^- + 110 mmol H^+ will produce 110 mmol H_2O and 40 mmol of OH^-). The difference between the positive strong ions and the negative strong ions is called, by Stewart, strong ion difference (SID) [2]. In this new solution the $[H^+] =$ $K'w/40 = 5.98 \times 10^{-13}$ mol/L and pH $= 12.224$. It must be stressed that SID may only be changed by removing strong ions, primarily through the kidney, or adding strong ions (metabolism and food). Note that SID may also be seen as the difference between strong bases and strong acids.

Adding Fixed Weak Acids (Buffers or A_{TOT})

Now let us add to the solution weak acids whose functional pK_A is between 6 and 7. According to Stewart's terminology, weak acids are named as A_{TOT} [2], while according to the traditional terminology, they are named as buffers. The most important weak acids in plasma are phosphoric acid and albumin (both at $pK_A \approx 6.8$). The albumin molecule includes amino acid residues, which

behave as strong acid or base, and other residues which behave as a weak acid. In particular, at plasmatic pH, arginine and lysine ($pK_A \approx 10$–12) always behave as strong bases, so that the $-NH_2$ residues are present only as $-NH_3^+$. On the contrary, the $-COOH$ residues of aspartatic and glutamic acid ($pK_A \approx 4.4$) are always present in their dissociated form $-COO^-$. The net charge due to the difference of strong acids and bases present in albumin molecule is -21 Eq/mol, independent on the pH value. From this point of view, albumin may be considered a strong acid. On the other hand, the molecule of albumin presents also 16 imidazole groups in the histidine residues ($pK_A \approx 6.8$), which are in the range of weak acids, thereby acting as buffers. Now we will add to our solution, characterized by SID 40 mEq/L and $[OH^-]$ 40 mEq/L, further 40 g albumin and 2 mEq of phosphate. These are equivalent to ≈ 17.8 mmol of A_{TOT}. The small part of A_{TOT}, which is undissociated at pH of 12.224 will react with part of the 40 mmol of OH^- according to the following reaction:

$$[AH] + [OH^-] = [A^-] + [H_2O] \qquad (9)$$

As a result, the pH will slightly decrease down to 11.967, while the $[OH^-]$ will drop from 40 to 22.16 mEq/L.

Adding a Volatile Weak Acid

Let us now equilibrate the solution with alveolar gases, in which PCO_2 is equal to 40 mmHg. Gaseous CO_2 in part dissolves in water solution where it stays unmodified (CO_2 dissolved), while, in part, will react with water forming carbonic acid (H_2CO_3, pK ≈ 6.1). This well-known reaction, extremely accelerated by the carbonic anydrhase is summarized as follows:

$$CO_2 + H_2O \Leftrightarrow H_2CO_3 \Leftrightarrow HCO_3^- + H^+ \qquad (10)$$

Most of the protons produced will react (buffering action) with the dissociated form of A_{TOT}, accordingly to the following reaction:

$$[HCO_3^-] + [H^+] + [A^-] = [AH] + [HCO_3^-] \qquad (11)$$

The above equations explain why the buffer base, which (see below) is the sum of $[A^-] + [HCO_3^-]$, is independent of the CO_2 variation. In fact, if 1 mmol of protons is generated by the hydration of 1 mmol of CO_2, 1 mmol of bicarbonate is produced, while 1 mmol of A^- is consumed. However, the sum of $[A^-]$ and $[HCO_3^-]$ remains constant. Therefore, when CO_2 changes only the composition of buffer base changes, while its total value remains constant. The addition of CO_2 at 40 mmHg to our solution will result in a solution with SID 40 mEq/L, $[A^-] =$ 14.6 mEq/L, [AH] $= 3.95$ mmol/L, and pH $= 7.413$.

The Physicochemical (Stewart's) Approach [2]

Stewart's Independent Variables: SID

Step 1 – We may note that in the "preparation" of human plasma explained above, we have observed a change of pH at each step of the preparation. In the first step the pH was determined by the positive difference between the strong bases and strong acids, which generated an amount of OH^- equal to the observed difference. This strong ion difference (SID), therefore, is an independent variable that determines the pH (dependent variable).

Stewart's Independent Variables: ATOT

Step 2 – In the second step, we added a physiological amount of weak acids. The dissociation of part of these substances led to a decrease of $[OH^-]$, with an increase of protons and a further decrease of pH. The total amount of weak acids, indeed, is the second independent variable, which may affect the pH (whatever is the value of SID).

Stewart's Independent Variables: PCO₂/CO₂ Content

Step 3 – In the third step, we added another weak acid, the carbonic acid, which derived from CO_2 hydration. Adding this acid led, as a final result, to a further decrease of pH. Therefore, the PCO_2 or, more properly, the total CO_2 content is the third independent variable, which may affect the pH. What we have described so far is nothing else than what has been called the Stewart's approach or physicochemical approach to the acid–base equilibrium.

The Traditional Approach

Henderson–Hasselbach Equation

The traditional approach is based on CO_2 equilibrium, and relies on Henderson–Hasselbach equation [3] and the Van–Slyke equation [4]. The former tells us that pH is a function of the ratio between bicarbonate and PCO_2:

$$pH = pK + \log_{10} \frac{[HCO_3^-]}{\alpha \times PCO_2} \qquad (12)$$

where α denotes the solubility coefficient for CO_2. It is worth noting that the term $\alpha \times PCO_2$ is used as substitute for carbonic acid. As shown, the Henderson–Hasselbach equation is the specific application to the carbonic buffer pairs (HCO_3^-/H_2CO_3) of the general equation of acid dissociation (Eq. (8)). The problem of this equation is that it includes both PCO_2 (a marker of respiratory problems) and HCO_3^-, which depends either on PCO_2 (i.e., ventilation), or on metabolic alkalosis/acidosis, as we will see below.

Buffer Base and Base Excess

As the Henderson–Hasselbach equation is inadequate to assess metabolic acidosis/alkalosis, Singer and Hastings introduced the concept of *buffer base* [5] to rid off the problem of "respiratory" CO_2. Buffer base, in fact, is defined as the sum of the dissociated forms of fixed and volatile weak acids ($A^- + HCO_3^-$). As whatever change of PCO_2 changes the concentration of HCO_3^- stoichiometrically with the concentration of A^-, with the opposite sign (i.e., $\Delta[HCO_3^-] = -\Delta[A^-]$), their sum, the buffer base, remains constant and independent of CO_2 changes (see Eqs. (10 and 11)). Buffer base value may only change when strong acids or bases are added/removed, consuming/increasing both $[A^-]$ and $[HCO_3^-]$. To assess the metabolic acidosis/alkalosis Siggaard–Andersen introduced the concept of *base excess* [1] as the difference between actual and normal buffer base values. Therefore, to compute the base excess, we have to know which are the normal values (the reference) and to compute the actual buffer base. The normal values refer to an ideal situation in which, at 37°C, the PCO_2 = 40 mmHg, pH= 7.4 and plasma proteins (ATOT) = 70 g/L. In these conditions, the bicarbonate portion of the buffer base equals 24.8 mmol/L, as computed by Henderson–Hasselbach equation, while the $[A^-]$ portion of the buffer base = 17.2 mmol/L, resulting in a normal buffer base of $\approx$42 mmol/L. To compute the base excess the formula recommended by Clinical and Laboratory Standards Institute, conceptually similar to the Van Slyke equation, is as follows:

$$BE = \Delta[HCO_3^-] + \beta \times \Delta pH \qquad (13)$$

where β is the buffer power of non-carbonic buffers. To estimate β in vivo we have to consider subjects in which the base excess is normal (i.e., equal to 0). It follows that:

$$\beta = \Delta[HCO_3^-]/\Delta pH \qquad (14)$$

Changing the HCO_3^- by changing the PCO_2 through variation of ventilation it is possible to determine β according to Eq. (14). The β value has been determined by Siggaard–Andersen in 11 normal subjects and was found equal to 16.7 mmol/L [1]. This represents the change of A^- for a unitary change of pH. Now it should be easy to understand Eq. (13). The first part:

$$\Delta[HCO_3^-] = [HCO_3^-]_{actual} - 24.8 \qquad (15)$$

tells us how much of the buffer base variation is due to the bicarbonate changes.

The second part of the equation:

$$\Delta[A^-] = \beta \times (pH_{actual} - 7.4) \qquad (16)$$

tells us how much of the buffer base variation is due to the change of A^-. Indeed the formula:

$$BE = ([HCO_3^-] - 24.8) + \beta \times (pH - 7.4) \quad (17)$$

estimates the buffer base variations compared to normal in its two determinants, i.e., $[HCO_3^-]$ and $[A^-]$. It is worth noting that the value of β, which is properly defined as the buffer power of non-carbonic acids, relates to normal subjects. In intensive care, the concentration of A_{TOT}, primarily in its albumin content, is usually lower than normal and this should be associated with a decrease of β. In clinical practice, however, all these subtle differences are not taken into account.

Similarities and Differences Between Stewart's and Traditional Approach

After a brief exposition of the two main approaches to the evaluation of acid–base equilibrium, it is worth noting that the Stewart's approach and the traditional approach are, in a sense, similar. In fact, the independent variables regulating pH according to the Stewart's approach are all present in the traditional approach. Namely:

1. The SID is equal to the buffer base, which may be easily estimated from the actual base excess. In fact

$$BE = Buffer\ base_{actual} - Buffer\ base_{ideal}$$
$$= SID_{actual} - SID_{ideal} \quad (18)$$

2. The PCO_2 is equally considered an independent variable in the two approaches.
3. The A_{TOT} value is substituted, in the traditional approach, by the non-carbonic buffer power β. This is the only real difference between the two approaches: the Stewart's approach requires the understanding and the measure of A_{TOT}, while the traditional approach considers it (measured by β) constant (70 g/dL).

A schematic representation of the two approaches is presented in Fig. 1.

Application

Sources of Error in the Preanalytical Blood Gas Analysis

Blood gas analysis is the most widely applied methodology to assess the acid–base status of critically ill patients, for the diagnosis, the clinical treatment, and during the subsequent clinical follow-up. The absolute values of the measured parameters are crucial to perform a correct diagnosis and during the follow-up, especially in life-threatening conditions. The preanalytical phase plays

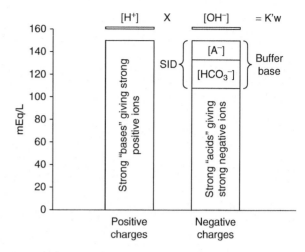

Acid–Base Evaluation. Figure 1 The figure shows an exemplificative gamblegram. SID denotes strong ion difference, $[A^-]$ the dissociated part of non-carbonic buffer concentration, $[HCO_3^-]$ the bicarbonate concentration, $[H^+]$ the proton concentration, $[OH^-]$ the hydroxyl ion concentration, and K'w indicates the ionic product of water. PCO_2 increase causes $[HCO_3^-]$ to increase, $[A^-]$ and $[OH^-]$ to decrease, while buffer base remains constant. As $[OH^-]$ decreases, $[H^+]$ increases to maintain K'w constant. This leads to a decrease of pH. Therefore, the final result increased PCO_2, decreased pH, unchanged buffer base (and base excess). This is called respiratory acidosis. On the other hand, if SID decreases, as an example increasing the negative strong ion column, this will cause a decrease of $[HCO_3^-]$, $[A^-]$ (buffer base), and $[OH^-]$. The $[OH^-]$ decrease is associated with $[H^+]$ concentration increase and pH decrease. This is typical of metabolic acidosis

a major role in the source of error in blood gas analysis. A typical preanalytical error is the presence of air bubbles in the blood sample. An air bubble of 0.5–1% left into the syringe for some minutes may seriously affect the pO_2 value measured. For what the storage is concerned, the collecting device, storage conditions, and time from the sample withdrawn to the analysis can cause significantly different measurements. When blood samples are collected in plastic syringes, they must be kept at room temperature and immediately analyzed. If the analysis is going to be delayed the sample should be stored in glass syringes and cooled with ice. The glass syringe is better than the plastic one for preserving arterial blood gas, especially for oxygen partial pressure determination. This phenomenon may be explained by the nanomaterial composition of the syringe itself. An excessive use of heparin solution as anticoagulant may cause dilution of the sample; therefore, it would be better to minimize the anticoagulant to sample volume ratio. The sample volume too can be a source of error if it is too small. This may affect the value of measured pO_2, BE of the total blood, and hemoglobin-related parameters, due to the analyzer used and to the fact that the plunger of the syringe is very close to the needle of the analyzer. Finally, the performance of precision of the analyzer has to be considered as it varies through the range of concentrations and values measured.

Directly Measured Variables

Hydrogen Ion Concentration: pH
As previously described, the pH, usually measured by glass electrode, expresses the activity of protons free in the plasma. A pH value of 7.4 corresponds to $[H^+]$ of $39.8{}^*10^{-9}$ mol/L, i.e., 39.8 *nanomoles per liter*. It is worth noting that this order of magnitude is one-million-time lower than the CO_2 or electolytes concentration, which are in the order of *millimoles per liter*. Normal values for arterial pH range from 7.35 to 7.45; pH values lower than 7.35 indicate acidemia and suggest a process called acidosis, while values greater than 7.45 indicate alkalemia and suggest a process called alkalosis.

Carbon Dioxide Tension (Arterial Carbon Dioxide Partial Pressure)
The partial pressure of CO_2 (PCO_2) measures the activity of CO_2 molecules dissolved into the plasma. PCO_2 is measured by the Stow–Severinghaus' electrode. Normal values of $PaCO_2$ range from 35 to 45 mmHg. The solubility coefficient is 0.0306 mmol/mmHg/L. Indeed, at 40 mmHg $PaCO_2$, CO_2 molecules dissolved as such into the plasma will amount to 1.224 mmol/L. As 1 mmol of gas occupies 22.414 mL, the normal amount of dissolved CO_2 corresponds to 27.4 mLCO2/L or to 2.74 mL. Of note 22.414 L is the volume of 1 mol of CO_2 in standard pressure/temperature condition, i.e., 760 mmHg and 0°C. The actual volume occupied by 1 mol of CO_2 at the body temperature of 37°C will be 25.455 L, according to the general equation of gases $PV = nRT$, in which $R = 0.08207$ L*atm/mol/K. A PCO_2 greater than 45 mmHg indicates hypercapnia and suggests a process called respiratory acidosis, while a PCO_2 lower than 35 indicates hypocapnia and suggest a process called respiratory alkalosis.

Electrolytes
The most important electrolytes, which participate in the formation of strong ion difference (SID) are sodium, potassium, and chlorine, which should be always assessed for a full understanding of acid–base equilibrium. In addition, lactate measurement is also indicated as it frequently causes a decrease of SID in critically ill patients. An exact computation of SID would require the analysis of all the strong ions present in the plasma. In practice, this is impossible and the electrolytes quoted above are sufficient for an "apparent" SID estimation in most clinical circumstances occurring in critically ill patients.

Weak Acids (A_{TOT}) and Buffers
The most important "weak acid," which contributes to buffer base in its dissociated form is albumin [2]. As discussed above the net charge of albumin at pH 7.4 is negative. Hypoalbuminemia is therefore associated, per se, with alkalosis. Although albumin concentration is usually expressed in terms of g/L or g/dL (normal values 40–50 g/L or 4–5 g/dL) in the acid–base context it must be considered in term of mmol/L (1 g/L = 0.38 mmol/L, normal values 15.2–19 mmol/L). Moreover, since what accounts for the buffer base is the dissociated form of albumin, it can be computed (in mEq/L) rearranging Eq. (8) and the conservation mass equation:

$$[A_{TOTAlb}] = [AH_{Alb}] + [A^-{}_{Alb}] \qquad (19)$$

as follows:

$$pH = pK_{Alb} + \log_{10} \frac{[A^-{}_{Alb}]}{[A_{TOTAlb}] - [A^-{}_{Alb}]} \qquad (20)$$

where $pK_{Alb} \approx 6.8$ and the footnote "Alb" denotes albumin.

The second weak acid, which contributes to the buffer base is the phosphate. Phosphate charge have two components: a fixed charge that functions as a strong ion (due to $PO_4{}^{3-}$ components) and a variable charge, which is responsible for the non-carbonic buffer behavior ($HPO_4{}^{2-}/H_2PO_4{}^-$ pair). Normal values of inorganic phosphorus are 0.81–1.4 mmol/L or 2.5–4.3 mg/dL, and its pK value is ≈ 6.8. The third weak acid, which contributes to the buffer base formation is the dissociated form of carbonic acid, i.e., bicarbonate, which will be discussed below.

The Computed Variables

Carbon Dioxide Content
The total CO_2 content (tCO_2) in plasma includes various species in which the CO_2 is present [1]:

$$\begin{aligned}[tCO_2] = &[dCO_2] + [HCO_3{}^-] + [CO_3{}^{2-}] \\ &+ [PrNHCOO^-] + [NaCO_3{}^-]\end{aligned} \qquad (21)$$

in which tCO_2 denotes the total CO_2, dCO_2 the dissolved form of CO_2, HCO_3^- bicarbonate, CO_3^{2-} the carbonate, $PrNHCOO^-$ the carbamino compound, and $NaCO_3^-$ denotes the sodium carbonate.

The three last species are usually ignored in human plasma and the $[tCO_2]$ provided by the blood gas machine is the sum of the $[dCO_2]$ and $[HCO_3^-]$. This amount, in normal plasma at pH 7.40, equals $1.224 + 24.8 = 26.02$ mmol/L, which is equivalent to 58.28 $mLCO_2$/dL. It is worth reminding that the total CO_2 content given by the blood gas machine refers to the CO_2 content of plasma and not of the whole blood. In fact, for the same PCO_2, the content of CO_2 into the red cells is lower than in plasma as the red cell pH is lower. The order of magnitude of the total CO_2 difference at similar PCO_2 between 1 L of plasma and 1 L of blood with a normal hematocrit is of 5–10 mmol/L, depending on PCO_2 and pH.

The primary variable derived from PCO_2 and pH measurement is the bicarbonate concentration. Rearranging the Henderson–Hasselbach equation:

$$[HCO_3^-] = 10^{pH-pK} * 0.0306 * PCO_2 \qquad (22)$$

The problem is the pK value. In some blood gas machine the algorithm for HCO_3^- computation includes the pK variations with pH. Some others use slightly different pK values. It is out of the purposes of this chapter to discuss the biochemistry of the carbon dioxide hydratation (see Siggaard–Andersen [1]). It is therefore sufficient to say that different blood gases machines, measuring exactly the same pH and PCO_2, may provide different values of HCO_3^- due to the differences of the implemented algorithms. The differences are minimal around the physiological pH and PCO_2 but may be as high as 2 mmol/L in case of severe alkalosis or acidosis. As in intensive care unit what is important is the trend of variables over time, if only one blood gas machine is employed this problem is irrelevant. It may become important if two blood gas machines with different implemented algorithms are used to follow the clinical course of a given patient.

Base Excess

The base excess (BE) is a parameter aimed to quantify the presence of strong acid (metabolic acidosis) or strong basis (metabolic alkalosis) either in the whole blood (in this case it is named as BE blood (BE(B)) or actual BE (ABE)) or in the extracellular fluid (named as extracellular BE (BEecf) or standard BE (SBE)). The difference is due to the presence of hemoglobin in the whole blood (a component of total weak acids [A_{TOT}] concentration). The BB of the whole blood, indeed, is higher than the BB of the

extracellular fluid, in which, by convention, hemoglobin contribution to the BB is assumed to be equal to 6 g/dL.

BE (positive and negative) is a measure of how much, *compared to the normal*, the BB is increased (alkalosis) or decreased (acidosis). Indeed the concept of BE implies the knowledge of a "normal reference state," i.e., what is the value of BB in standard condition. The reference state is the BB when $PaCO_2$ is 40 mmHg, the pH is 7.4 and the temperature is 37°C and the values of A_{TOT} (i.e., protein) is normal (70 gr/dL).

Normal BE is equal to 0 in arterial blood. It is important to note that the normal BE in the venous blood is ≈ 1.5 mmol/L greater than arterial one. This difference is not due to the "production" of positive bases in the venous side, but simply to an "artifact" related to the reference value. To exactly compute the venous BE the reference normal values should be the ones of the venous and not of the arterial blood, i.e., pH ≈ 7.38 instead of 7.4, and $[HCO_3^-] \approx 25.7$, instead of 24.8 mmol/L. These new reference values should be used in formula (17) to compute the exact base excess in the venous blood. Doing so, the BE will be the same both in arterial and venous side as it should be.

Strong Ion Difference

As discussed above, the apparent strong ion difference (SID) may be used in clinical practice, due to the impossibility of measuring all the ions present within the plasma. It must also be remembered that strong ion difference, buffer base, and BE are all related. In fact:

$$SID_{actual} \approx BE + 42mEq/L \approx [A^-] + [HCO_3^-] \qquad (23)$$

This is the reason why we believe that the Stewart's approach helps in understanding the acid–base equilibrium. In fact, if one of the above identities is not verified suggesting that unmeasured substances (either positive or negative ions) or even abnormal proteins are present within the plasma, the problem deserves attention and investigation. Normal SID should be around 42 mEq/L; its decrease indicates metabolic acidosis, while its increase indicates metabolic alkalosis.

Anion Gap

Anion gap is computed as the sum of the most representative positive strong ions ($[Na^+]+[K^+]$) minus the most representative negative strong ions ($[Cl^-]$) and bicarbonate. It is therefore a mixture between SID and carbonic buffer. In an ideal situation in which pH equals 7.4, PCO_2 40 mmHg and SID 42 mEq/L, the anion gap will be equal to 17 mEq/L, which is the amount of $[A^-]$ (albumin + phosphate). As each of the above normal values has its own standard deviation it follows that the "normal" anion gap ranges between 10 and 20 mEq/L when including potassium and 8–16 mEq/L when potassium is excluded. Since anion gap includes the bicarbonate, it depends in part on respiratory status, although an increase in bicarbonate due to CO_2 retention is usually associated, after few days, to a chloride decrease. As shown, also the anion gap is easily understandable mixing the traditional and the Stewart's approaches. The following relationships, in fact, hold true:

$$\text{Anion gap} \approx SID_{actual} - [HCO_3{}^-]$$
$$\approx BE + 42 - [HCO_3{}^-] \approx [A^-] \quad (24)$$

As anion gap is $\approx[A^-]$, it is easy to understand how the albumin, the primary component of A_{TOT}, may affect the anion gap. Normal anion gap with acidemia usually indicates that bicarbonate loss has been replaced by chlorine, while high anion gap with academia indicates that an "unknown negative ion" has "consumed" the bicarbonate, while the chlorine stays normal or even decreases.

References

1. Siggaard-Andersen O (1974) The acid-base status of the blood. Munksgaard, Copenhagen
2. Stewart PA (2009) Lulu.com, Amsterdam
3. Henderson LJ (1908) The theory of neutrality regulation in the animal organism. Am J Physiol 21:427–448
4. Siggaard-Andersen O (1977) The van Slyke equation. Scand J Clin Lab Invest Suppl 37:15–20
5. Singer RB, Hastings AB (1948) An improved clinical method for the estimation of disturbances of the acid-base balance of human blood. Medicine 27:223–242

Acinetobacter Bacteremia

▶ Acinetobacter Infections

Acinetobacter Central Venous Catheter Infection

▶ Acinetobacter Infections

Acinetobacter Cholangitis

▶ Acinetobacter Infections

Acinetobacter ICU-Acquired Infection

▶ Acinetobacter Infections

Acinetobacter Infections

ARGYRIS MICHALOPOULOS[1,2], MATTHEW E. FALAGAS[2,3,4]
[1]Department of Critical Care Medicine, Henry Dunant Hospital, Athens, Greece
[2]Alfa Institute of Biomedical Sciences (AIBS), Marousi, Athens, Greece
[3]Department of Medicine, Henry Dunant Hospital, Athens, Greece
[4]Department of Medicine, Tufts University School of Medicine, Boston, MA, USA

Synonyms

Acinetobacter ICU-acquired infection; Acinetobacter bacteremia; Acinetobacter ventilator-associated pneumonia; Acinetobacter urosepsis; Acinetobacter urine tract infection; Acinetobacter wound infection; Acinetobacter central venous catheter infection; Acinetobacter meningitis; Acinetobacter cholangitis; Acinetobacter peritonitis; Acinetobacter skin infection

Definition

Any nosocomial infectious disease owed to this specific Gram-negative pathogen is defined *Acinetobacter baumannii* infection. It is usually a hospital-acquired infection. It affects primarily critically ill patients of intensive care units, mainly in tropical climates.

Identity of Pathogen

The genus *Acinetobacter* consists of pleomorphic Gram-negative coccobacilli that are strictly aerobic, nonmotile, catalase positive, oxidase negative, nitrate negative, non-fermentative, sometimes difficult to decolorize, and frequently arranged in pairs. The word *Acinetobacter* originates from the Greek adjective "Akinetos" which means unable to move and the Greek noun "bacterion" which means rod. So, *Acinetobacter* means a nonmotile rod.

The genus *Acinetobacter* comprises 33 different types (species), of which 17 have been assigned valid. The term "*A. calcoaceticus – A. baumannii*" complex is often used to group the most clinically relevant species.

Acinetobacter spp. have been widely found in nature, mostly in water and soil. *A. baumannii* preferentially colonizes aquatic environments such as intravenous solutions. *A. baumannii* is most often associated with hospital-acquired infections and does not typically colonize healthy people. The main characteristic of *A. baumannii* is the capability to survive for weeks in the environment.

A. baumannii is commonly isolated from the hospital environment and hospitalized patients. *A. baumannii* isolates have been detected on hospital bed rails until 9 days after the discharge of an infected patient, suggesting that hospital equipments could serve as a secondary reservoir for the transmission of infection.

Sensitivity of Pathogen

A. baumannii is usually a multidrug-resistant (MDR) Gram-negative pathogen which has always been inherently resistant to multiple classes of antibiotics. Multidrug-resistant *Acinetobacter* is not a new or emerging pathogen. To date, some strains of *A. baumannii* have become resistant to almost all antimicrobial agents that are currently available.

Mechanisms of Resistance

Acinetobacter has a tendency to develop resistance to antimicrobials rapidly. Resistance mechanisms that are expressed frequently in strains of *A. baumannii* involve antimicrobial-degrading enzymes (β-lactamases including serine and metallo-β-lactamases, which confer resistance to carbapenems), efflux pumps and target modification, and cell-wall channels (porins). The acquisition of a MDR phenotype can be caused by mobile genetic elements such as plasmids, transposons, and integrons. Classes I and II integrons have been closely associated with MDR *A. baumannii* [1]. They are mostly acquired by contact with other bacteria, such as *Pseudomonas aeruginosa*. One example of integron transfer between *Pseudomonas* spp. and *A. baumannii* is the acquisition of the class I integron carrying the VEB-1 extended-spectrum ß-lactamase. *A. baumannii* can become resistant to quinolones through mutations in the genes *gyrA* and *parC* and can become resistant to aminoglycosides by expressing aminoglycoside-modifying enzymes. A recent report described a "resistance island" containing 45 resistance genes within the *Acinetobacter* genome. Resistance islands comprise one or more virulence genes located in a mosaic distribution within a large genomic region.

Pathogenicity and Virulence of *Acinetobacter*

Acinetobacter has emerged during the past 3 decades from an organism of questionable pathogenicity to an important pathogen for patients in hospitals worldwide. The factors influencing the pathogenicity of *Acinetobacter* were identified as the susceptibility of the host and the virulence potential of the organism, along with other factors, such as antimicrobial resistance and desiccation tolerance. Host factors include the immune status, particularly of patients in intensive care units, and the presence of foreign materials, such as central intravenous catheters. Many patients have lowered "colonization resistance" mainly owing to prolonged administration of multiple antibiotics. The recent availability of the full genome sequence of *A. baumannii* represents a huge opportunity to identify more specific virulence factors and establish their role in disease.

Virulence factors in *A. baumannii* include adhesions necessary for the formation of biofilm, the production of lipases which damage tissue lipids, and the elaboration of siderophores to scavenge iron and promote survival. In addition, the outer membrane of *A. baumannii* contains lipopolysaccharide (particularly S-form) which is a major stimulator of the immune response. This also confers resistance to the natural bactericidal action of human serum, thus promoting the survival of *A. baumannii* in the human bloodstream. Most strains of *A. baumannii* appear to produce a polysaccharide capsule that renders the cell surface more hydrophilic and enhances virulence.

Acinetobacter Colonization

Acinetobacter commonly colonizes patients in the intensive care unit (ICU) setting especially those who are hospitalized for prolonged period, who are intubated for prolonged period, and those who have central venous catheters, intravenous monitoring devices, surgical drains, or indwelling urinary catheters. In the ICU setting, digestive tract colonization is common, with rates as high as 40%. Wounds can be contaminated with dirt and debris containing *Acinetobacter* at the time of injury.

Acinetobacter Infection

Acinetobacter infections have been documented worldwide. They are more common in patients in tropical or subtropical climates. *Acinetobacter* infections occur almost exclusively in hospitalized patients. High-risk patients for development of an *Acinetobacter* infection are usually critically ill hospitalized for prolonged period in intensive care units. Numerous studies have supported that *A. baumannii* is the main genomic species associated with outbreaks of ICU-acquired infections in many settings.

The term "multidrug-resistant" (MDR) *A. baumannii* although does not have a standard definition universally acceptable is generally defined in the presence of carbapenem resistance or resistance to at least three classes of antimicrobials that would otherwise serve as treatment for *Acinetobacter* infections (e.g., cephalosporins, quinolones, aminoglycosides, and carbapenems). The term "pan-drug resistant, PDR" *Acinetobacter* has been used to describe strains of pathogen that are resistant to all standard antimicrobial agents (including polymyxins).

Multidrug-resistant (MDR) *A. baumannii* is a rapidly emerging pathogen in healthcare settings, where it causes infections that include bacteremia, pneumonia, meningitis, and urinary tract as well as wound infections mainly in tropical countries and during wars and natural disasters. Susceptibility of *A. baumannii* varies between countries, with some regions having an increased prevalence of MDR *A. baumannii*.

The most frequent infections due to *A. baumannii* are ventilator-associated pneumonia (VAP), central venous catheter–related infection, and bloodstream infection (bacteremia). VAP due to *Acinetobacter* occurs predominantly in critically ill ICU patients with history of diabetes mellitus, who require mechanical ventilation for prolonged period. VAP is often characterized by a late onset.

Acinetobacter Infections. Table 1

Main types of *Acinetobacter* infections
Ventilator-associated pneumonia (VAP)
Pneumonia/tracheobronchitis
Central venous catheter-related infection
Bloodstream infection (bacteremia)
Urinary tract infection
Wound infection
Meningitis
Ventriculitis
Cellulitis
Ocular infection
Native and prosthetic valve endocarditis
Osteomyelitis
Septic arthritis
Pancreatic abscess
Liver abscess

Type of Infections

Acinetobacter is associated with a broad spectrum of nosocomial infections, including VAP/pneumonia/tracheobronchitis, urinary tract infections that are urine catheter–associated, bloodstream infections, central venous catheter–related infections, wound infections, and meningitis that mainly occurs in colonized neurosurgical patients with external ventricular drainage tubes. Rarely, *Acinetobacter* causes other infections including cellulitis, ocular infections, native and prosthetic valve endocarditis, osteomyelitis, septic arthritis, and pancreatic and liver abscesses (Table 1).

The respiratory system is the most common site for *A. baumannii* infection. Hospital-acquired *Acinetobacter* pneumonia or VAP are frequently multi-lobar and complicated. Secondary bacteremia and septic shock are usually associated with a poor prognosis.

Risk Factors

Risk factors for hospital-acquired *Acinetobacter* infection include length of stay in the ward and in the ICU, previous mechanical ventilation for many days, previous infection necessitating treatment with broad-spectrum antibiotics, previous surgery, wounds, previous colonization with *Acinetobacter*, parenteral nutrition (TPN), and presence of intravascular devices. In a systemic review published in 2006, 55 studies were identified referring to *A. baumannii* (28 with case-control methodology and 27 outbreak investigations without case-control methodology). It was concluded that acquisition and spread of *A. baumannii* appear to be related to a large number of variables. Among the most important were deficiencies in the implementation of infection control guidelines and the prolonged use of multiple antimicrobials, especially broad-spectrum antibiotics, such as third-generation cephalosporins, quinolones, and carbapenems, in critically ill ICU patients who remain ventilated for many days [2].

Incidence of Nosocomial Infections

Over the past 2 decades, *Acinetobacter* infections have become an increasingly common nosocomial problem, especially in temperate climates. Over the past decade, the proportion of nosocomial infections caused by *Acinetobacter* spp. has increased worldwide. In the National Nosocomial Infections Surveillance System (NNISS) among Gram-negative bacilli isolated in ICU patients with pneumonia/VAP, *Acinetobacter* spp. ranked fourth (6.9%) during the period of 1986–2003, and it was the only Gram-negative organism with a significant increase in prevalence during the same period. *A. baumannii* is a common cause of late-onset VAP. The Surveillance and Control of Pathogens of Epidemic Importance (SCOPE) prospective surveillance study of nosocomial bloodstream infections (BSIs) classified *A. baumannii* as the tenth leading cause of bacteremia in the USA. In addition, there are also several reports from many countries worldwide suggesting that there is a substantial increase during the last decade in the incidence of nosocomial infections, predominantly due to Gram-negative isolates, mainly *A. baumannii*, *Klebsiella pneumoniae*, and *Escherichia coli*. Increased resistance in many classes of broad-spectrum antibiotics was also noted in *A. baumannii* hospital-acquired infections.

Treatment

Acinetobacter spp. is intrinsically MDR pathogen presenting with resistance to multiple antimicrobial agents. For this reason, the treatment should be carefully considered.

Medications to which *Acinetobacter* is usually sensitive include the following: polymyxins B and E (colistin), carbapenems, sulbactam, aminoglycosides, and tigecycline (Table 2). In general, first-, second-, and third-generation cephalosporins, macrolides, and most penicillins have little or no anti-*Acinetobacter* activity, and their use may predispose to *Acinetobacter* colonization.

Carbapenems still represent the treatment of choice, even if increasing carbapenem-resistant *Acinetobacter* isolates are reported worldwide. Doripenem, imipenem, and meropenem are equally active against carbapenemase-negative *A. baumannii* isolates. Although there are no randomized controlled studies on the treatment of *Acinetobacter* spp. infections, carbapenems have been considered the antimicrobial class of choice for the treatment of patients with severe nosocomial infections due to *A. baumannii*. Although they are considered to be the most effective antibiotics against *Acinetobacter* spp., an increasing number of carbapenem-resistant *Acinetobacter* isolates has been reported worldwide, thus reducing the existing therapeutic options. Carbapenems are inactive against *A. baumannii* isolates expressing plasmid-mediated carbapenemases [3].

Acinetobacter Infections. Table 2

Currently available antimicrobial classes/agents potentially effective against *Acinetobacter baumannii*
1. Sulbactam
2. Anti-pseudomonal penicillins
3. Anti-pseudomonal cephalosporins
4. Anti-pseudomonal carbapenems
5. Monobactams
6. Aminoglycosides
7. Fluoroquinolones
8. Tetracyclines
9. Glycylcyclines
10. Polymyxins

Recently, intravenous colistin which is polymyxin E has been administered in many ICUs worldwide for the treatment of hospital-acquired infections due to MDR *A. baumannii*. The increasing incidence of MDR *A. baumannii*, in addition to a lack of new antimicrobial agents, has revived interest in the utilization of colistin due to its good activity against this pathogen. Colistin is a potent antimicrobial polypeptide with specific activity against many Gram-negative bacilli. This agent was originally used in various parts of the world during the 1960s and 1970s, but it was not prescribed frequently during the 1980s and 1990s because of concerns about nephrotoxicity and neurotoxicity. However, given its potent activity against many Gram-negative bacilli, the role of colistin in serious nosocomial Gram-negative infections has been reappraised. Recently, colistin and polymyxin B have been used in various countries for the treatment of nosocomial infections due to *A. baumannii*. This is largely because many nosocomial isolates of *A. baumannii* are MDR and sometimes susceptible only to polymyxins. Most clinical studies investigating the use of polymyxins for the treatment of infections due to MDR Gram-negative bacilli refer to colistin (colistimethate sodium, colistin sulfomethate) rather than polymyxin B. Daily colistin dosing ranges from six to nine million international units in patients with normal renal function (usually divided in three doses). Especially for the management of VAP due to MDR *A. baumannii*, there are few reports indicating that aerosolized colistin may be a beneficial and safe additional therapeutic intervention.

Sulbactam is a ß-lactamase inhibitor which has specific intrinsic bactericidal in vitro activity against many MDR *Acinetobacter* strains, which is related to its affinity for penicillin-binding proteins. Sulbactam has been demonstrated to be effective against infections caused by moderately imipenem-resistant *Acinetobacter* isolates. The presence of a ß-lactam agent does not increase activity of sulbactam. In many countries, sulbactam is commercially available only in combination with ampicillin. It is given in a fixed 2:1 ratio of ampicillin/sulbactam every 6 h in patients with normal renal function. Earlier studies showed high in vitro susceptibility rates of *A. baumannii* isolates, including multidrug-resistant ones, to sulbactam or ampicillin/sulbactam combination. However, in recent studies, the antimicrobial activity of sulbactam against *A. baumannii* isolates has declined substantially. Still, sulbactam has been found active against a rather small proportion of carbapenem-resistant *A. baumannii* isolates.

Tigecycline, a glycylcycline with a theoretical broad spectrum of activity against susceptible and MDR

Gram-positive and Gram-negative pathogens, has been administered for the management of MDR *A. baumannii* infections. However, tigecycline has FDA approval only for complicated intra-abdominal, skin, and skin-structure infections. Large surveillance trials have shown high rates of susceptibility of *A. baumannii* to tigecycline. Tigecycline has been found to be active against minocycline-resistant, MDR, and imipenem-resistant isolates. However, there are recently a substantial number of reports indicating that tigecycline may not be consistently active against the imipenem-resistant isolates. The development of resistance in *A. baumannii* strains in tigecycline suggest that it should be always used in combination with other antimicrobial agents active against *Acinetobacter* spp. In addition, there are some recent clinical studies indicating poor clinical or microbiological outcomes with tigecycline therapy. Data from more studies are needed before tigecycline can be recommended for the treatment of MDR *Acinetobacter* infections.

Although mild to moderate infections may respond to monotherapy, serious *A. baumannii* infections should be treated with combination therapy. Bactericidal synergy occurs when several antimicrobials (e.g., carbapenem, sulbactam, tigecycline) are combined with an aminoglycoside, colistin, or rifampin. These therapeutic agents demonstrated in vitro synergism against *A. baumannii* infections. The presence of a ß-lactam agent in combination did not appear to contribute to the synergy.

Rifampin administered in combination with other antimicrobial agents, such as colistin, has been shown to be synergistic or additive against MDR isolates of *A. baumannii*. Rifampin may be a good alternative for the treatment of MDR *A. baumannii* infections, provided that the adequate dose is defined. However, the frequent development of high-level rifampin-resistant *A. baumannii* and the consequent risk of therapeutic failure suggest limitations of this regimen in clinical practice. By now, the best combination of rifampin in order to increase effectiveness and to avoid development of rifampin-resistant strains is not known.

The assessment of in vitro synergy of the combination of imipenem with a polymyxin against carbapenem-resistant *A. baumannii* strains has provided controversial findings. The combination of imipenem with rifampin, although synergistic in vitro, was not associated with clinical benefits in a small study. The combination of imipenem and tigecycline has not been shown to be synergistic. Regarding polymyxin-based combination regimens, the best studied one involves rifampin, which has shown synergistic in vitro activity against

multidrug-resistant *A. baumannii* strains in most studies, although not consistently.

VAP

Acinetobacter spp., a common pathogen in patients with VAP in some ICUs is becoming more resistant to first-line agents such as carbapenems. Sulbactam has good in vitro activity against *A. baumannii*; thus, the combination of ampicillin with sulbactam may be a good treatment alternative. In a retrospective study comparing the efficacy of imipenem/cilastatin and ampicillin/sulbactam in critically ill trauma patients with VAP due to *A. baumannii*, treatment efficacy was found to be similar in both groups. No statistically significant differences were found between the groups with regard to mortality, duration of mechanical ventilation, or length of ICU or hospital stay. In another randomized trial, critically ill patients with MDR *A. baumannii* VAP were randomly assigned to receive either 18/9 g or 24/12 g daily dose of ampicillin–sulbactam. There was no difference in clinical improvement between groups (66.7% and 64.3%, respectively). Bacteriological success was achieved in 77.8% of the study population, while the 14-day mortality rate was 25.9% and all-cause 30-day mortality rate was 48.1%.

A prospective study compared the effectiveness of colistin versus imipenem/cilastatin for the treatment of VAP due to MDR *A. baumannii*. VAP was considered clinically cured in 57% of cases in both groups. The VAP-related mortality rate was 38% in the colistin group versus 35.7% of imipenem group, while the in-hospital mortality rate was high in both groups (61.9% vs. 64.2%, respectively). There were no differences in clinical cure, in-hospital mortality rates, or toxicity. In another matched case-control study examining the safety and effectiveness of colistin compared with imipenem in the treatment of VAP caused by MDR *A. baumannii* or *P. aeruginosa*, a favorable clinical response occurred equally in both groups (75% in the colistin group compared with 71.7% in the imipenem group). During the antibiotic course, none of the patients in either group developed renal failure.

Bacteremia

In a retrospective cohort study of hospitalized (mainly critically ill) patients (*n*=39) with *A. baumannii* bacteremia, 64% of patients had bacteremia due to colistin-only-susceptible *A. baumannii* and 36% had bacteremia due to both colistin- and carbapenem-susceptible *A. baumannii* strains. All-cause mortality rate was 56% and 35.7%, respectively (*p*=0.22). The multivariate analysis showed that only exposure to fluoroquinolones was associated with development of a colistin susceptible-strain *A. baumannii* bacteremia.

In patients suffering from MDR *A. baumannii* bacteremia, the combination of a carbapenem and ampicillin–sulbactam was associated with a better clinical outcome than the combination of a carbapenem and amikacin or a carbapenem alone. The overall 30-day mortality rate was high (49%). In another study, the 30-day mortality rate of patients with imipenem-resistant *A. bacteremia* was higher compared with the control group (matched subjects with imipenem-susceptible *A. bacteremia*) (57.5% vs. 27.5%; $p = 0.007$). The rate of discordant antimicrobial therapy was higher in the imipenem-resistant group ($p < 0.001$). Some authors have found higher all-cause 30-day mortality associated with nosocomial bacteremia due to *A. baumannii* compared with bacteremia due to *K. pneumoniae*.

Central Nervous System Infections: Meningitis/Ventriculitis

A systematic review of the literature showed that 64 episodes of Gram-negative meningitis in both children and adults were treated with polymyxins administered intravenously and/or via the intraventricular or intrathecal route. Cure was achieved in 10 of 11 episodes of CNS infections (91%) due to *Acinetobacter* spp. The most common complication when a polymyxin was administered via the intraventricular or intrathecal route was the meningeal irritation. Regarding hospital-acquired meningitis caused by MDR or carbapenem-resistant *A. baumannii*, the available clinical experience with the use of ampicillin/sulbactam or other antibiotics is limited and rather nonconclusive. Treatment options against multidrug-resistant *A. baumannii* CNS infections seem to be limited.

Evaluation/Assessment

The main differential diagnostic problem presented by *Acinetobacter* is to differentiate colonization from infection. The pathological changes associated with *A. baumannii* infection are normally not distinguishable from those caused by other aerobic Gram-negative bacilli.

Effectiveness

A. baumannii has become a serious nosocomial pathogen due to its persistence in the hospital environment and its broad antimicrobial resistance patterns. Carbapenems, aminoglycosides, sulbactam, polymyxins (colistin and polymyxin B), tetracyclines, and tigecycline are often active against *A. baumannii* clinical isolates. However, carbapenem resistance or multiple-drug resistance in *Acinetobacter* spp. is at present an emerging problem worldwide. It should be noted that there are no randomized controlled trials on the treatment of patients with *Acinetobacter* spp. infections. In addition, it is not clear whether combination therapy is more effective than monotherapy against such infections. The optimal treatment for serious MDR *A. baumannii* infections and the role of combination therapy should be urgently addressed in randomized clinical trials.

Acinetobacter infections have become more difficult to treat owing to the emergence of MDR isolates which are resistant to many of the commonly prescribed antimicrobial agents. In addition, one more concern has been the acquisition of carbapenem resistance, mainly by means of class B and D carbapenemases. During the last years, *A. baumannii* present resistance to multiple antimicrobial agents, occasionally including polymyxins (colistin) and tigecycline [4].

In 2000, few *A. baumannii* isolates were resistant to carbapenems, with little impact in the hospital setting. By 2006, two carbapenemase-producing clones (SE and OXA-23 clone 1) spread in many hospitals. Of these, the OXA-23 clone 1 is only susceptible to polymyxins and tigecycline in vitro. Recently, a large number of class D OXA-type enzymes with activity against carbapenems were characterized in Europe, Japan, China, and Brazil. Some *Acinetobacter* isolates express class B metallo-ß-lactamases, such as VIM and IMP, which hydrolyze a broad array of antimicrobial agents, including carbapenems.

Although the controversy remains, ICU-acquired infections due to *A. baumannii* are associated with considerable attributable mortality. However, inappropriate antibiotic treatment is associated, among other factors, with mortality. Several studies evaluated the usefulness of diverse antimicrobial agents in cases of carbapenem-resistant *A. baumannii*. Some agents, such as sulbactam and colistin, have shown similar efficacy to imipenem, in the treatment of severe infections such as bacteremia, VAP, or meningitis. However, a significant proportion of patients die from nosocomial infections caused by *A. baumannii*. It should therefore be considered that, at present we do not have optimal treatment for *A. baumannii* nosocomial infections.

Well-designed clinical studies are necessary to answer questions relative to the effectiveness of combination therapy associated with fewer complications and lower rates of development of MDR or PDR *A. baumannii* strains.

Tolerance

The major adverse events of colistin are nephrotoxicity, neurotoxicity, and neuromuscular blockade leading to respiratory failure. However, several recent clinical studies found much less colistin-associated nephrotoxicity and neurotoxicity than originally reported. To avoid the adverse events, physicians should hydrate well their patients while maintaining a consistently satisfactory central venous pressure (CVP). In addition, if it is possible physicians should consider using alternative routes for colistin administration, including the inhaled and intraventricular routes. Colistimethate sodium (colistin) has been used via the respiratory tract or via the intraventricular route for the treatment of VAP or ventriculitis, respectively, due to MDR carbapenem-resistant *A. baumannii* with satisfactory results.

The most common adverse events associated with tigecycline are nausea (30%), diarrhea (16%), and vomiting (16%), which are usually mild or moderate in severity.

Pharmacoeconomics

Economic analyses performed in eight studies dealing with infections caused by extended-spectrum beta-lactamase-producing Enterobacteriaceae, MDR *P. aeruginosa*, and *Acinetobacter* spp. indicated that these resistant Gram-negative infections are associated with increased patient charges or hospital care costs. However, associations sometimes disappear in multivariate analyses after adjusting for significant variables in univariate analyses.

After-care

Persistent colonization of the respiratory tract with *A. baumannii* after improvement of patients with pneumonia may occur and lead to recurrence of the infection.

Prognosis

Mortality and morbidity rates remain high especially in critically ill patients with multiple organ failure treated in the ICU. Deaths due to *Acinetobacter* infections had risen from the 1990s onward. Collective findings from 21 relevant original studies and a meta-analysis, suggest that Gram-negative bacterial resistance increases the burden in the ICU as measured by mortality, length of stay, and charges [5]. Recently, severe ICU-acquired infections such as bacteremia or meningitis are associated with a mortality rate approximately 40%. However, mortality is increased mainly because of inappropriate therapy.

Nevertheless, because of limitations in the relative studies (e.g., small sample sizes, retrospective studies, failure to control for severity of illness before infection and exclusion of patients who are colonized but not infected with *Acinetobacter*, and inappropriate treatment), the exact attributable mortality of *Acinetobacter* infections and the burden of MDR or PDR *Acinetobacter* pathogens on patient outcomes still remain controversial. However, it should be emphasized that there are no randomized controlled trials comparing various antimicrobial treatment regimens of patients with pneumonia or VAP caused by *Acinetobacter* spp. Instead, only prospective or retrospective observational studies have been published. The discovery of new therapeutic agents coupled with randomized controlled clinical trials testing new agents or combinations of antibiotics targeting *Acinetobacter* spp. are urgently needed. Alternative treatment approaches, such as the antibiotic lock therapy and continuous intravenous antibiotic administration should be also carefully examined. In addition, greater emphasis should be given on the prevention of healthcare-associated transmission of MDR *Acinetobacter* infection. Well-designed research is also needed to determine the cost-effectiveness of appropriate empiric therapy with broad-spectrum agents active against resistant Gram-negative bacteria followed by de-escalation.

References

1. Munoz-Price LS, Weinstein RA (2008) *Acinetobacter* infection. N Engl J Med 358(12):1271–1281
2. Falagas ME, Kopterides P (2006) Risk factors for the isolation of multi-drug-resistant *Acinetobacter baumannii* and *Pseudomonas aeruginosa*: a systematic review of the literature. J Hosp Infect 64 (1):7–15
3. Pournaras S, Iosifidis E, Roilides E (2009) Advances in antibacterial therapy against emerging bacterial pathogens. Semin Hematol 46 (3):198–211
4. Matthaiou DK, Michalopoulos A, Rafailidis PI, Karageorgopoulos DE, Papaioannou V, Ntani G, Samonis G, Falagas ME (2008) Risk factors associated with the isolation of colistin-resistant gram-negative bacteria: a matched case-control study. Crit Care Med 36 (3):807–811
5. Shorr AF (2009) Review of studies of the impact on gram-negative bacterial resistance on outcomes in the intensive care unit. Crit Care Med 37(4):1463–1469

Acinetobacter Meningitis

▶ Acinetobacter Infections

Acinetobacter Peritonitis

▶ Acinetobacter Infections

Acinetobacter Skin Infection

▶ Acinetobacter Infections

Acinetobacter Urine Tract Infection

▶ Acinetobacter Infections

Acinetobacter Urosepsis

▶ Acinetobacter Infections

Acinetobacter Ventilator-Associated Pneumonia

▶ Acinetobacter Infections

Acinetobacter Wound Infection

▶ Acinetobacter Infections

Acquired Aneurysm

▶ Vascular, True Aneurysms

Acquired Immunodeficiency Syndrome

▶ HIV Infections
▶ HIV, Pneumonic Complications

ACT Analyzer

ACT analyzer provides the time in seconds from the activation of the sample until the beginning of a fibrin formation, named activated clotting time (ACT).

Active Surveillance Cultures

Universal or targeted microbiological screening cultures of patients on admission for the purposes of detecting asymptomatic MRSA colonization. Samples are usually collected from the anterior nares and other sites, including the perineum and wounds. In addition to specimens collected on admission, periodic specimens may be collected during hospital stay in high-risk patients who are not yet known to be colonized, to detect MRSA carriers who may have acquired the organism during their hospital stay.

Acute Abdomen

▶ Acute Abdominal Pain: General Approach

Acute Abdominal Pain: General Approach

ANGELA M. MILLS[1], ANTHONY J. DEAN[2]
[1]Department of Emergency Medicine, University of Pennsylvania, Philadelphia, PA, USA
[2]Division of Emergency Ultrasonography, Department of Emergency Medicine, Hospital of the University of Pennsylvania, Philadelphia, PA, USA

Synonyms
Abdominal pain; Acute abdomen; Peritonitis

Definition
In the United States, more patients seek emergency care annually for abdominal pain than for any other chief complaint. Abdominal pain accounted for eight million (7%) of the 119 million Emergency Department (ED) visits in 2006 [1]. The differential diagnosis is wide

and ranges from benign, self-limited diseases to life-threatening conditions requiring urgent intervention. A patient's demographic characteristics (e.g., age, sex, race/ethnicity, family history) may influence the incidence and clinical presentation of abdominal disease. Diagnosis may be difficult as various factors may obscure the clinical scenario and lead to a delay in diagnosis or a misdiagnosis. While the cause of abdominal pain may not always be identified, the clinician's role is to identify life-threatening causes and to narrow the differential diagnosis for further evaluation. Up to 40% of patients may be discharged with a diagnosis of nonspecific abdominal pain. This chapter will summarize general information and the approach regarding acute nontraumatic abdominal pain in adults with a focus on the history and physical examination. Imaging modalities utilized in the diagnosis of abdominal pain will be discussed in a separate chapter.

Differential Diagnosis

The initial evaluation of the patient with undifferentiated acute abdominal pain includes an assessment of the severity of illness, as patients with life-threatening disease may require resuscitation concomitant with their evaluation and workup. In some patients, the constellation of symptoms may point to a specific diagnosis. If they do not, the history and physical examination should be used to generate a focused and targeted workup, since indiscriminate testing has been shown to be of little utility to either rule in or exclude disease in patients with abdominal pain.

History

A thorough yet focused history is often the foundation of an accurate diagnosis. This includes a detailed understanding of the nature and course of the patient's symptoms combined with the past medical, surgical, and social history. Pain assessment should include onset, prior episodes, provocative, palliative and positional features, the quality of the pain, its region and patterns or radiation and referral, its severity, and temporal features such as whether it is intermittent or continuous, progressive, or waxing and waning. It may be helpful to remember these historical features (as listed) using the mnemonic "OPQRST."

Noxious stimuli from organs arising from the embryological gut are mediated by visceral fibers. Pain is usually perceived as dull, poorly localized, and in the midline. Foregut structures (lower esophagus, stomach, pancreas, liver, biliary system, proximal duodenum) produce pain in the epigastric region. For this reason, gallbladder inflammation, until it extends to the somatic fibers of the parietal peritoneum, is perceived in the epigastrium or lower chest and rarely in the right upper quadrant [2]. Midgut organs (remaining small bowel, proximal third of colon) generate pain perceived in the periumbilical area. This is the basis for the typical history of appendicitis with onset of pain in the periumbilical region, only localizing to the right lower quadrant when inflammation has extended to somatic nerve fibers of the parietal peritoneum. The hindgut structures (bladder, distal two-thirds of colon, intraperitoneal genitourinary organs) cause pain in the suprapubic area. Visceral pain fibers are triggered by distension, stretch, vigorous contraction, or ischemia. The retroperitoneal organs (aorta, kidneys) often cause back pain. Table 1 provides a differential diagnosis of major causes of abdominal pain by pain location.

Acute onset of severe pain should alert the clinician to an intra-abdominal catastrophe such as a vascular emergency (e.g., ruptured abdominal aortic aneurysm [AAA], aortic dissection). Occasionally perforated viscus, volvulus, mesenteric ischemia, and torsion may also cause pain of sudden onset, but more commonly symptoms develop

Acute Abdominal Pain: General Approach. Table 1 Differential diagnosis by location of acute abdominal pain

Diffuse pain	Abdominal aortic aneurysm, aortic dissection, appendicitis (early), bowel obstruction, gastroenteritis, ileus, mesenteric ischemia, metabolic acidosis, peritonitis, sickle cell crisis
Epigastric pain	Biliary colic, cholecystitis, gastritis, myocardial ischemia, pancreatitis, peptic ulcer disease
Right upper quadrant pain	Biliary colic, cholecystitis, hepatitis, hepatic abscess, hepatic congestion, herpes zoster, myocardial ischemia, right lower lobe pneumonia
Left upper quadrant pain	Gastritis, herpes zoster, left lower lobe pneumonia, myocardial ischemia, pancreatitis, peptic ulcer disease, splenic infarction, splenic distention or rupture
Right lower quadrant pain	Appendicitis, cystitis, diverticulitis, ectopic pregnancy, endometriosis, inflammatory bowel disease (ileitis), inguinal hernia, ovarian torsion, pelvic inflammatory disease, ruptured ovarian cyst, testicular torsion, ureteral calculi
Left lower quadrant pain	Cystitis, diverticulitis, ectopic pregnancy, endometriosis, inguinal hernia, ovarian torsion, pelvic inflammatory disease, ruptured ovarian cyst, testicular torsion, ureteral calculi

gradually. Thus, while severity of the patient's pain and underlying condition are often correlated, milder symptoms are never grounds for complacency since they do not exclude serious disease, especially in older patients.

Obtaining a history of radiation patterns and referral of pain may also be helpful. Diaphragmatic irritation, often from free intraperitoneal blood or a contiguous inflamed organ, may cause shoulder pain and is referred to as Kehr's sign. Biliary disease may lead to ipsilateral scapular pain, and acute ureteral obstruction may be associated with ipsilateral testicular pain. Pain radiation may also be a sign of disease progression such as with active aortic dissection or the passing of a ureteral stone.

The course of the patient's symptoms may also be helpful. Persistent worsening pain is concerning while pain which is resolving is often reassuring. While initially presenting as intermittent colicky pain, untreated small bowel obstruction causes increasingly severe constant pain as it progresses through the stages of distension, ischemia, inflammation, bacterial translocation, and necrosis. While symptomatic gallstones have traditionally been said to cause "colicky" pain, the symptoms actually described by patients with this condition, while episodic, usually last 5–16 h in a constant crescendo-decrescendo pattern.

Pain which is exacerbated with jarring movements such as walking or coughing suggests peritonitis. Biliary colic may be induced by eating. Upper abdominal pain worsened with eating may also suggest a gastric peptic ulcer while that relieved with eating may suggest a duodenal ulcer.

Abdominal diseases cause a variety of associated symptoms within and outside the abdomen. Unfortunately, the common associated symptoms of anorexia, nausea, vomiting, and diarrhea are neither sensitive nor specific in the diagnosis of abdominal pain. Anorexia is only reported in 68% of patients with appendicitis, with even lower rates among the elderly [3]. Vomiting may be present in almost any abdominal disease. In surgical conditions, pain often precedes vomiting. When vomiting precedes pain some degree of reassurance is warranted, since this is more often seen with self-limiting conditions such as gastroenteritis. In small bowel obstruction, the length of time prior to the onset of emesis may suggest the degree as well as the level of obstruction. Large bowel obstruction usually presents very indolently with vomiting occurring late in the course, or not at all. Important constitutional symptoms include fever and cardiopulmonary symptoms, and those relating to dehydration. Syncope may be caused by an etiology stemming from the chest (e.g., pulmonary embolism, aortic dissection) or the abdomen (e.g., ectopic pregnancy, abdominal aortic aneurysm).

Genitourinary tract diseases, especially pelvic inflammatory disease, endometriosis, and ovarian pathology in women, cause lower abdominal pain. Testicular torsion frequently presents with poorly localized abdominal pain, nausea, and vomiting, especially among children. Chronic prostatitis may also be poorly localized causing nonspecific back pain, malaise, and fever. In pregnant women the enlarging uterus may itself lead to pain and also interfere with the recognition of diseases in other abdominal organs due to their dislocation. For these reasons, and due to the high prevalence of genitourinary diseases, a careful menstrual, sexual, and genitourinary history is essential in the evaluation of abdominal pain.

Past Medical History

Prior surgical exploration of the abdomen is perhaps the most important part of the medical history since it reveals diseases that may be recurrent as well as being the commonest cause of bowel obstruction. Many chronic medical conditions (diabetes, cancer) and medications (steroid and nonsteroidal anti-inflammatory drugs, antineoplastic agents) impair the immune response leading to both increased susceptibility to intra-abdominal infections and impaired ability to detect them. A social history might prompt investigation of any of the many possible gastrointestinal (GI) complications of alcohol abuse.

Physical Examination

In the physical examination well-appearing patients, particularly older ones, may have serious abdominal pathology causing their pain. Thus, while fever suggests an infectious etiology, acute appendicitis presents without an elevated temperature in approximately one third of cases and in the majority of patients with acute cholecystitis [3]. Conversely, while tachypnea and tachycardia are frequently present in any painful condition, they may be essential clues to suggest metabolic acidosis due to ischemic bowel, diabetic ketoacidosis, or a pulmonary process contiguous with the diaphragm.

The abdominal examination, while often guiding the seasoned clinician in the workup and sometimes providing clues to the diagnosis, has many limitations. Inter-rater agreement regarding findings in ED patients with acute abdominal pain is only moderate in most of the exam components. Even in patients subsequently determined to have surgical abdominal conditions, inter-rater agreement is only fair [4].

Abdominal wall and flank inspection includes evaluation for surgical scars, masses, and a skin examination for rash (e.g., herpes zoster), signs of liver disease (e.g., caput medusa), and hemorrhage (e.g., Grey Turner's sign of flank ecchymoses indicating retroperitoneal bleeding, Cullen's sign of umbilical discoloration with intraperitoneal hemorrhage). Percussion of the distended abdomen may distinguish between bowel distension (tympany) and ascites (shifting dullness). Auscultation is often of limited diagnostic utility in the emergency evaluation of abdominal pain.

Palpation of the abdomen is primarily used to localize abdominal tenderness, detect abdominal guarding, and identify peritonitis. As such, palpation should consist of light and sensitive palpation to identify regions of maximal tenderness. Patients with voluntary guarding, or abdominal wall muscular contraction in anticipation or in response to palpation, may be asked to flex their knees and hips to decrease this contraction. Initial palpation of non-painful areas with progression to areas of pain may also aid in the examination. In contrast, deep palpation, traditionally required to physically palpate intra-abdominal organs and detect abnormal masses, is an anachronism in the age when these conditions can be much more accurately identified by widely available diagnostic imaging modalities. As such, deep palpation causes severe discomfort without any justifying diagnostic utility and has no place in a modern clinician's physical examination.

Peritonitis is suggested by rigidity, or involuntary guarding or reflex spasm, of the abdominal wall. However, the detection of peritoneal irritation, while of primary importance, is also subject to the inherent limitations of the physical examination of the abdomen. In older adults, abdominal wall muscular laxity may undermine this finding. Rebound tenderness is elicited by gentle abdominal pressure for approximately 20 seconds with sudden release. Rebound tenderness is present if greater pain is perceived on release than with direct pressure. Some authors condemn this test as unnecessarily painful while others have found it to be highly reliable. The positive likelihood ratio in patients with rebound tenderness varies greatly in appendicitis and is completely nondiscriminatory in the diagnosis of acute cholecystitis [2, 3].

Hernias should be sought in both men and women. Examination in a standing position may reveal a hernia not observed in the supine position. AAA is suggested by a mass that is both pulsatile and expansile (the latter finding lessens the likelihood of misidentification of a mass overlying the aorta), while the femoral pulses may be unequal with aortic dissection. While the rectal examination has been demonstrated to be of limited value in the assessment of abdominal pain, there may be utility in the evaluation of intestinal ischemia, gastrointestinal hemorrhage, and colon cancer. A pelvic examination in women and genitourinary examination in men may add relevant information to the clinical picture.

Analgesia and the Abdominal Examination
Historically, the early use of analgesia in patients with acute abdominal pain was thought to mask signs of peritonitis and potentially delay diagnosis and operative intervention. Multiple well-designed randomized controlled trials have conclusively demonstrated that the use of analgesia in acute abdominal pain does not lead to adverse outcomes [5]. Thus, the timely and judicious use of analgesia in abdominal pain patients who have been assessed and request symptom control should be a standard of care.

Cross-Reference to Disease
Critically ill patients with abdominal pain need immediate attention, stabilization, and resuscitation prior to diagnosis. Critical illness may be heralded by abnormal vital signs, sudden severe onset, or evidence of systemic involvement, with the elderly, immunocompromised, and those with comorbidities being the most susceptible. The usual management of critically ill patients prioritized by the "ABC's" should be applied. The clinician should be particularly vigilant in caring for patients with impaired ability to communicate whether due to cognitive impairment, intoxication, dementia, psychiatric illness, or language barriers. Hypotension due to vomiting, diarrhea, or hemorrhage is often evident from the history, but may also be due to third spacing of fluids from an intra-abdominal inflammatory process.

While diagnostic imaging is discussed elsewhere, the salient features of ultrasonography and computed tomography (CT) should be mentioned briefly in this overview. Bedside ultrasonography has many uses in the early management of critically ill patients with abdominal pain. Intravascular volume status can be rapidly assessed by evaluation of the inferior vena cava and cardiac function, and aortic aneurysms can be identified, as well as ascites and massive intraintestinal fluid collections associated with complete bowel obstruction or ileus. In unstable female patients of childbearing age, ruptured ectopic pregnancy or hemorrhagic ovarian cyst can be identified.

Abdominal CT has radically altered the proportion of patients with abdominal pain who can receive rapid, accurate, and timely diagnosis of abdominal pain within the course of a single ED encounter. There are CT findings that are moderately to highly accurate in identifying the majority of common abdominal conditions. However, CT has important drawbacks including preparation time, expense, contrast and radiation exposure, financial and manpower burdens, removal of the patient from the resuscitation area, and the need for 24-h availability of imaging specialists for interpretation.

Regardless of the imaging technology, clinicians should bear in mind that despite their extraordinary diagnostic power, none is much more than 90% accurate in diagnosing most abdominal conditions, so that with a high pretest clinical suspicion, patients with negative exams should be kept for a period of watchful waiting similar to that much more widely utilized in the "Pre-CT" era.

Laboratory Testing

While laboratory tests are often utilized in the assessment of acute abdominal pain, all diagnostic tests have significant false negative and false positive rates. Abnormal tests (e.g., temperature, lactate, white blood cell [WBC] count) are increasingly likely to be truly positive the further they deviate from the norm. Conversely, as noted above, an unremarkable value does not rule out disease. In particular, the WBC count has been shown to have limited utility in the evaluation of the three commonest causes of abdominal pain: appendicitis, biliary tract disease, and nonspecific abdominal pain. No laboratory finding accurately rules in or rules out the diagnosis of acute cholecystitis [2].

A urinalysis may assess for urinary tract infection and hematuria. Serum lipase has been shown to be more helpful in confirming or excluding the diagnosis of pancreatitis than serum amylase. In patients with liver disease, a prothrombin time may help determine severity of disease. In women of reproductive age, a urine pregnancy test should be obtained to determine whether ectopic pregnancy or non-pregnancy causes are the focus of gynecological concern. If there is a suspicion for pelvic infection, cervical cultures for chlamydia and gonorrhea should be obtained.

Consultation and Disposition

Emergency department or intensive care unit care encompasses early resuscitation, timely diagnosis, and prompt consultation when indicated. Surgical, gynecologic, or gastroenterological consultations may be necessary for further management of a patient's condition. High-risk patients with acute abdominal pain may warrant special consideration. In patients where the diagnosis remains in question, a period of continued observation may be necessary to assess disease progression or resolution. Patients who are not ill and have no clear etiology of their abdominal pain may be discharged from the ED with 24-h follow-up with their primary care provider. Discharge instructions should be clear and provide defined indications for return to the emergency department as well as a clear follow-up plan.

Conclusion

Abdominal pain is a common reason for patients seeking emergency care and a frequent cause of hospitalization. Prompt recognition of critically ill patients is necessary for simultaneous resuscitation and diagnostic evaluation. While laboratory testing is often not helpful when routine, it may be useful when guided by the history and physical examination. Clinicians should be mindful of certain patient populations where critical illness may not be immediately recognized including older adults, patients with altered immunologic response, and patients with altered cognitive function.

References

1. Pitts SR, Niska RW, Xu J et al (2008) National Hospital Ambulatory Medical Care Survey: 2006 emergency department summary. Natl Health Stat Report Aug 6(7):1–38
2. Trowbridge RL, Ruttconski NK, Shojania KG (2003) Does this patient have acute cholecystitis? JAMA 289:80–86
3. Wagner JM, McKinney WP, Carpenter JL (1996) Does this patient have appendicitis? JAMA 2786:1589–1594
4. Pines J, Uscher Pines L, Hall A et al (2005) The interrater variation of ED abdominal examination findings in patients with acute abdominal pain. AJEM 23:483–487
5. Manterola C, Astudillo P, Losada H et al (2007) Analgesia in patients with acute abdominal pain. Cochrane Database Syst Rev (3):CD005660

Acute Acalculous Cholecystitis

▶ Cholecystitis

Acute Asthma

CHRISTOPHER R. WYATT
Emergency Medicine, Case Western Reserve University
Metro Health Medical Center, Cleveland, OH, USA

Synonyms

Acute severe asthma; Asthma attack; Asthma exacerbation; Status asthmaticus

Definition

Asthma is a chronic inflammatory disorder of the airways in which many cells and cellular elements play a role in the inflammatory response. In particular, mast cells, eosinophils, T lymphocytes, macrophages, neutrophils, and epithelial cells are all involved. Neutrophils are especially prominent in sudden onset, fatal exacerbations, and in occupational asthma and in patients who smoke. In susceptible individuals, this inflammation causes recurrent episodes of coughing (particularly at night or early in the morning), wheezing, breathlessness, and chest tightness. These episodes are usually associated with widespread but variable airflow obstruction that is often reversible either spontaneously or with appropriate treatment [1].

The pathophysiologic hallmark of asthma is a reduction in airway diameter caused by smooth muscle contraction (bronchoconstriction), vascular congestion, bronchial wall edema, and increased mucous production with impaired mucociliary clearance precipitated by various inflammatory cascades. This reduction in airway diameter results in increased airway resistance and decreased airflow. Bronchoconstriction occurs due to allergic or non-allergic stimuli. Common stimuli include viral respiratory infections, exercise, environmental conditions, indoor antigens, occupational exposure, pharmaceutical agents, endocrine factors, and emotional stress.

Asthma exacerbations are acute or subacute episodes of progressively worsening shortness of breath, cough, wheezing, and chest tightness or some combination of these symptoms. Exacerbations are characterized by decreases in expiratory airflow that can be documented and quantified by simple measure of lung function such as spirometry or peak expiratory flow rates (PEFR).

Treatment

The best strategy for management of asthma is early treatment of asthma exacerbations. Clinicians and patients must recognize early signs of worsening asthma and take prompt and appropriate actions. Early indicators of an asthma exacerbation include changes in symptom control and severity demonstrated by increase use or decrease responsiveness to rescue short-acting beta-agonists (SABA) and worsening objective PEFR measurements. The goal of treatment is to rapidly reverse airflow obstruction, ensure adequate oxygenation, and relieve inflammation. Signs of worsening asthma should prompt intensification of therapy, often including a short course of systemic steroids, removal or withdrawal from allergens and precipitating irritants, and communication between patient and clinician about any serious deterioration in symptoms. Failure of these early measures should elicit an urgent or emergent care evaluation.

Pre-hospital management – including outpatient clinic evaluation and emergency transport – should include administration of oxygen to relieve hypoxemia in moderate or severe exacerbations, and should encourage standing orders for albuterol administration. Prolonged pre-hospital transport should consider protocols to include ipratropium bromide and systemic corticosteroids.

The acute management of asthma exacerbations in the emergency setting has the same goals. The clinician should assess the severity of the exacerbation with lung-function measures compared to patient's best or clinical predictors (if possible), relieve hypoxia, reverse airflow obstruction, and decrease inflammation. The response to therapy should be monitored. Adjunctive therapies should merit consideration in severe exacerbations unresponsive to initial treatment, and may decrease the likelihood for intubation.

The categories of medications used in the treatment of acute asthma include beta-adrenergic agonists, anticholinergics, and glucocorticoids. Adjuncts include magnesium sulfate, and heliox.

Selective $beta_2$-receptor agonists are the preferred initial rescue medication for acute bronchospasm. In about 60–70% of patients, response to three administered doses in the emergency department will be sufficient for patient discharge, and most patients will have a significant response after the first dose. Beta-agonists act on $beta_2$-receptors to stimulate the enzyme adenylate cyclase. This enzyme converts intracellular adenosine triphosphate (ATP) into cyclic adenosine monophosphate (cAMP), increasing its level and activity. Through complex protein-related interactions this results in bronchial smooth muscle relaxation, as well as inhibits mediator (inflammatory) release and promotes mucociliary clearance. Inhaled short-acting beta-agonists include albuterol and levalbuterol (the R-enantiomer of albuterol). Systemic beta-agonists include epinephrine and terbutaline. There has been no proven benefit to parenteral beta-agonists over inhaled.

Anticholinergic medications act to competitively antagonize acetylcholine at post-synaptic junctions. Therefore, vagal cholinergic-mediated bronchoconstriction of the large, central airways is inhibited, resulting in bronchodilation. The bronchodilatory effects of anticholinergics are additive with beta-agonists. Anticholinergics affect large, central airways, whereas beta-agonists affect smaller airways. Inhaled ipratropium bromide is an anticholinergic medication. Adding multiple high doses of ipratropium bromide to a selective short-acting beta-agonists (SABA) results in fewer hospital admissions, particularly in patients who have severe airflow obstruction. The use of ipratropium is recommended in the Emergency Department for moderate to severe exacerbations, but its continued use during hospitalization has not shown benefit.

Corticosteroids are highly affective and are one of the cornerstones of treatment in asthma exacerbations. Corticosteroids reduce inflammation and may restore beta-adrenergic responsiveness. Systemic corticosteroids decrease airway inflammation in moderate or severe exacerbations or for patients who fail to respond promptly and completely to SABA. Given early in the course of treatment, corticosteroids reduce the risk of hospital admissions. Common corticosteroids include prednisone, methylprednisolone, and prednisolone. Oral corticosteroids are recommended unless otherwise contraindicated.

Intravenous magnesium sulfate is an adjunctive therapy indicated in the management of acute, severe asthma. Magnesium sulfate leads to smooth muscle relaxation and bronchodilation; however, its usefulness in mild and moderate exacerbations has not been established.

Heliox is a mixture of helium and oxygen (usually 70:30). Heliox is less dense than inhaled air, generates less airway resistance by mechanism of increasing the tendency of laminar flow and decreasing the tendency of turbulent flow, thus requiring less mechanical energy to ventilate the lungs. The heliox mixture requires at least 70% helium for effect. So if the patient requires >30% oxygen, the heliox mixture cannot be used.

Mast cell modifiers (e.g., cromolyn), methylxanthines (e.g., theophylline), leukotriene inhibitors (i.e., montelukast, zafirlukast, zileuton) have no indication for use in the acute management of asthma.

A summary of the current recommendations for the management of acute asthma is shown in Table 1 [2].

Acute Asthma. Table 1 Management of acute asthma

Mild to moderate exacerbation (FEV1/PEFR $\geq$ 40%)	-Supplemental oxygen to achieve SaO$_2$ $\geq$ 90% - Short-acting beta-agonist (albuterol) - Oral corticosteroids if no immediate response to SABA or if recent corticosteroid use
Severe exacerbation (FEV1/PEFR < 40%)	- O$_2$, SABA, oral corticosteroids
	- Inhaled anticholinergic (ipratropium bromide)
	- Consider adjunctive therapy magnesium sulfate, heliox

Airway Management in Acute Asthma

When the clinician decides that respiratory failure is advanced or progressing despite therapy (imminent), intubation should be performed expeditiously before crisis ensues. Intubation should be performed by a clinician who has extensive experience in intubation and difficult airway management. An asthmatic in need of endotrachial intubation is with little physiologic reserve and at high risk of sustaining a rapid decline in oxygen saturation and blood pressure after receiving sedating medications and neuromuscular blocking agents. It is important to plan for and achieve intubation as early as possible once it has been determined that intubation is necessary. Rapid sequence intubation (RSI) is the preferred approach in such cases because it is the most rapid method for securing the airway with the highest likelihood of success. Pre-oxygenation can be performed with a bag valve mask if necessary. Small tidal volumes, high inspiratory flow rates, and prolonged expiratory phases should be utilized, mimicking the approach used during mechanical ventilation. Medications for RSI should be administered to the patient while they maintain the position of greatest comfort, which is generally sitting upright. The patient can be placed in the supine position to perform laryngoscopy and intubation after induction. Placement of a large endotracheal tube (8 or 9 mm in adults) is desirable to minimize airway resistance and facilitate aggressive pulmonary toilet.

Studies suggest that ketamine and propofol have bronchodilatory properties and thus are suitable induction agents for severe asthmatics. Barbiturates, such as thiopental, should be avoided because they can exacerbate bronchospasms through histamine release. Ketamine is a dissociated anesthetic with properties that provide benefits to severe asthma management. Ketamine acts directly as a smooth muscle dilator, indirectly by increasing circulation of catecholamines, inhibits vagal outflow, and does not cause histamine release. Propofol has bronchodilatory properties; however, it can result in hypotension. Intubated asthmatics should be deeply sedated and receive parenteral opioid analgesia with a non-histamine releasing opioid (e.g., fentanyl) in order to achieve complete relaxation and comfort for mechanical ventilation. Mechanical ventilation does not relieve airway obstruction; it merely eliminates the work of breathing and enables the patient to rest while the airflow obstruction is resolved.

Mechanical Ventilation in Acute Asthma

The potential complications of mechanical ventilation in an asthmatic include cardiovascular collapse and significant barotrauma. Bronchospasm, airway inflammation, edema, and mucus plugging that characterize asthma dramatically increases airflow obstruction, decreases expiratory flow, and prolongs the time needed to completely exhale prior to the onset of the next breath. When the expiratory time is insufficient, inadequate emptying between breaths causes progressive hyperinflation. Hyperinflation increases intrathoracic pressure, which increases pulmonary vascular resistance and decreases venous return. The net effect is reduced cardiac output which can lead to cardiovascular collapse and arrest. Barotrauma describes progressive hyperinflation causing overdistension and subsequent loss of the lungs structural integrity leading to interstitial emphysema or pneumothorax.

Special considerations must be made during mechanical ventilation of the severe asthmatic patients than would be typically provided to non-asthmatic patients due to this pathophysiology. During mechanical ventilation, the use of slower respiratory rates (e.g., 6–10 breaths/min), smaller tidal volumes (e.g., 6–8 mL/kg), shorter inspiratory time (e.g., adult flow rate 80–100 mL/min), and longer expiratory time (inspiratory to expiratory ratio 1:5) must be made [3]. Rapid inspiratory flow rate at a reduced respiratory frequency with adequate time for expiration decreases air-trapping, hyperinflation, and barotraumas, and is called permissive hypoventilation (hypercapnea). Patient-ventilator synchrony should also be maintained with adequate sedation.

Evaluation/Assessment

Fatal and near-fatal asthma exacerbations can occur sporadically and inexplicably, whether the baseline level of disease activity is mild, moderate, or severe. Therefore, any acute exacerbation of asthma may be a potentially fatal attack. Treatment should begin immediately following recognition of a moderate, severe, or life threatening exacerbation.

Initial assessment should include a brief history, brief physical examination, and for most patients, objective measures of lung function.

Patients typically present with the triad of chest tightness, cough, and wheezing. The purpose of the brief history is to determine the severity of the exacerbation as well as risk factors for death. Questions should include the time of onset and any potential causes of current exacerbations; severity of symptoms (especially compared with previous exacerbations) and response to any treatment given before admission to ED; all current medications and time of last dose; estimate of number of previous unscheduled office visits, ED visits, and hospitalization for asthma, particularly within the past year; any prior episodes of respiratory failure due to asthma (loss of consciousness, intubations, ICU admissions); other potentially complicating illness (especially pulmonary or cardiac disease). Risk factors for fatal and near-fatal asthma are listed in Table 2 [1].

The purpose of the initial brief physical examination is to assess severity and overall patient status. Special attention should be given to level of alertness, fluid status, presence of cyanosis, respiratory distress and wheezing. Wheezing is a common physical finding, but severity does not correlate with the degree of airway obstruction. The absence of wheezing may indicate critical airway obstruction, whereas increased wheezing may indicate a positive response to bronchodilator therapy. Drowsiness/agitation, paradoxical breathing, absence of wheezing or "silent chest" (representing absence of air movement), profound diaphoresis, inability to lay supine, bradycardia, or $PaCO_2$ >40 represents signs of impending respiratory arrest.

Objective measures, such as peak expiratory flow rates (PEFR) or forced expiratory volume in one second (FEV_1), should be obtained, if possible, with exception to cases of severe asthma or impending respiratory failure. For urgent or emergency care settings, severe exacerbations are indicated by PEFR/FEV_1 < 40% predicted. In these patients, adjuvant therapies should be considered.

Initial laboratory studies are not required in most patients, and if obtained, they should not delay initiation of treatment. Arterial blood gas (ABG) measurement may be reasonable in some patients who have suspected hypoventilation, severe distress, or FEV_1 or PEFR < 25% predicted after initial treatment. Respiratory drive is typically increased in asthma exacerbations, so a "normal"

Acute Asthma. Table 2 Risk factors for fatal and near-fatal asthma

Prior history of sudden severe exacerbations
Prior intubation for asthma
Prior admission for asthma to an intensive care unit (ICU)
Two or more hospitalizations for asthma in the past year
Three or more emergency care visits for asthma in the past year
Hospitalization or emergency care visit for asthma within the past month
Use of >2 SABA meter-dosed inhaler canisters per month
Current use or recent withdrawal from systemic corticosteroids
Difficulty perceiving asthma symptoms or severity
Comorbid disease, especially cardiac or chronic obstructive pulmonary disease
Psychiatric illness
Low socioeconomic status
Illicit drug abuse (especially inhaled cocaine and heroin)

PCO_2 indicates severe airflow obstruction and heightened risk of respiratory failure. Complete blood counts and chemistries are rarely helpful and may demonstrate a leukocytosis or transient electrolyte abnormities. A theophylline level should be sent to all patients currently taking theophylline. A beta-type-natriuretic peptide (BNP) level may help rule out cardiac asthma.

Chest radiography is not recommended for routine assessment, but should be obtained for patients suspected of a complicating cardiopulmonary process such as pneumonia, pneumothorax, or congestive heart failure (CHF).

An electrocardiogram (EKG) may be obtained in those with history of significant cardiovascular disease. If obtained, it may show a right-ventricular strain pattern which resolves with treatment. Older patients or those with profound hypoxia or those with impending respiratory failure may require continuous cardiac monitoring.

Disposition decisions are made on subjective and objective measures. The goal for discharge is FEV_1/PEFR $\geq 70\%$ predicted.

After-care

The long-term management of asthma focuses on reducing daily impairment and patient risk for fatal exacerbations. There are four essential components to asthma care: assessment and monitoring, patient education, control of factors contributing to asthma severity, and pharmacologic treatment.

Patients discharged from emergency care should be provided with a referral to follow-up asthma care in 1–4 weeks. Patients should be educated to monitor their symptoms, signs, and PEFR to recognize early deterioration. Inhaler techniques should be reviewed. Patients should be provided with a written action plan with current medications and specific instructions on early home management and when and how to seek emergency care. Instructions on how to control factors contributing to asthma severity and comorbid conditions should be given.

Recommended discharge medications should include short-acting beta-agonists (SABA), 3–10 days of burst oral corticosteroids, and consideration for initiation of inhaled corticosteroids.

A summary of discharge recommendations is listed in Table 3.

Prognosis

The prevalence of asthma symptoms and diagnosed asthma in the USA is among the highest in the world for both children and adults, reported to have increased 25–75% per decade during the period since 1960. The increase in hospital admission rates in the region reflects an increase in

Acute Asthma. Table 3 Summary checklist for hospital discharge

Review inhaler use technique
Follow-up visit
Peak flow meter
Action plan
Medications (SABA, oral corticosteroids, consider inhaled corticosteroids)

the prevalence of severe asthma. There has been an increase in the percentage of patients requiring intubation, even as the total number of hospital admissions for respiratory disease has decreased. The morbidity of asthma is considerable with approximately 40% of all children and adult with asthma having required hospitalization or emergency care treatment for asthma in the previous 12 months. Trends of asthma mortality in the USA contrast with those of most other Western countries in that there has been a progressive increase over the last two decades. Mortality rates are greatest in disadvantaged groups such as minorities and those with low socioeconomic status [4].

Despite concerns for increasing mortality, most patient survive acute asthma episodes.

Seventy to 80% of patients who present to emergency departments clear within 2 h of standard therapy. The relapse rate is approximately 7–15%, depending on how aggressive the patient is treated. However, the long-term mortality after a near-fatal event may be as high as 10% [5]. Patients with histories of previous ED visits and hospitalizations are at highest risk of relapse, regardless of management. Intubated patients are at the highest risk for mortality. These trends emphasize the importance of implementing education and management programs that specifically target high-risk groups.

References

1. National Asthma Education and Prevention Program (1997) Expert Panel Report Guidelines II: guidelines for the diagnosis and management of asthma. Publication 97-4051. National Institute of Health, Bethesda
2. National Asthma Education and Prevention Program (2007) Expert Panel Report Guidelines III: guidelines for the diagnosis and management of asthma. Publication 08-4051. National Institute of Health, Bethesda
3. Marik PE, Varon J, Fromm R Jr (2002) The management of acute severe asthma. J Emerg Med 23:257–268
4. Global Initiative for Asthma. Global Burden of Asthma. http://www.ginasthma.com/reportItem.asp?l1=2&l2=2&intId=94
5. McFadden ER Jr (2003) Acute severe asthma. Am J Respir Crit Care Med 168(7):740–759

Acute Bacterial Prostatitis

▶ Prostatitis

Acute Brain Dysfunction

▶ Septic Encephalopathy

Acute Brain Failure

▶ Encephalopathy and Delirium

Acute Calculous Cholecystitis

▶ Cholecystitis

Acute Cardiogenic Pulmonary Edema (ACPE)

▶ Heart Failure Syndromes, Treatment

Acute Care Surgery

ERNEST E. MOORE, CLAY COTHREN BURLEW
Department of Surgery, Denver Health Medical Center, University of Colorado Denver, Denver, CO, USA

Definition
Acute care surgery is a newly recognized surgical specialty in the USA that encompasses trauma surgery, surgical critical care, and emergency surgery [1].

Rationale
In the USA, trauma surgery has traditionally integrated surgical critical care to provide 24 h in hospital comprehensive patient management. To meet demands of the recent crisis in access to emergent surgical care [2], the discipline has been expanded to include emergency surgery; that is, broad-based general surgery to include urgent thoracic and vascular procedures. The fundamental goal is to provide emergent operative care for life or limb-threatening surgical problems within the first 24 h of hospitalization. Although considered a new specialty, in fact, this practice paradigm has existed in many urban safety-net hospitals in the USA serving as regional trauma centers [3]. However, the progressive fragmentation of general surgery, expanding knowledge and technical skills required, and limitations on residency work hours, has prompted the development of a formal fellowship to provide additional training. In sum, the rationale for the development of acute care surgery was based on the facts that (1) an increasing number of patients require emergent surgical care at a time of compromised access to such care, (2) the societal costs of maintaining a full registry of on-call specialists is prohibitive, and (3) trauma surgeons already provide 24 h in hospital patient care.

Scope of Practice
The American Association for the Surgery of Trauma (AAST) has implemented a fellowship to ensure the surgical expertise in managing acute surgical problems [4].

In addition to what has been considered trauma surgery (neck, thoracic, abdominal, and vascular procedures), the expanded capabilities include common emergent and urgent thoracic, abdominal, and vascular operations. In the process of defining this surgical training, consideration was given to selected neurosurgical and orthopedic trauma procedures. However, this option was not embraced by the respective national surgical societies and consequently has been de-emphasized.

Acute Care Surgery Fellowship
In the USA, prerequisite training is the completion of an Accreditation Council on Graduate Medical Education (ACGME) – Residency Review Committee (RRC) approved General Surgery Residency of 5-year duration. The fellowship consists of 2 years.

The first year is an ACGME-RRC-approved Surgical Critical Care Fellowship, during which the trainee may devote up to 25% of their time in direct operative care of critically ill patients. The second year focuses on emergency and elective surgical experience, and allows flexibility depending on the trainees' prior experience and future plans. In brief, the core rotations include:

Acute care surgery	4–6 months
Thoracic surgery	1–3 months
Vascular surgery	1–3 months
Hepatobiliary/pancreatic	1–3 months
Neurosurgery	1 month
Orthopedic surgery	1 month
Elective (burn, pediatric, endoscopy)	1–3 months

During this time, the trainee is expected to acquire operative management principles and technical procedural skills for a defined list of procedures, judged as essential or desirable [4].

Future Directions

The current training model of acute care surgery will continue to mature as the practice of acute care surgery evolves and patients' emergent needs become evident [5]. For example, selective angioembolization, endovascular stent placement, and CT-guided percutaneous sampling and drainage of torso fluid collections are logical additions to consider. The issue of selected emergent neurosurgical and orthopedic procedures warrants further deliberation.

References

1. The Committee to Develop the Reorganized Specialty of Trauma, Surgical Critical Care, and Emergency Surgery (2005) Acute care surgery – trauma, critical care, and emergency surgery. J Trauma 58:614–616
2. Division of Advocacy and Health Policy (2006) A growing crisis in patient access to emergency surgical care. Bull Am Coll Surg 91:8–20
3. Ciesla DJ, Moore EE, Moore JB et al (2005) The academic trauma center is a model for the future trauma and acute care surgeon. J Trauma 58:657–662
4. The Committee on Acute Care Surgery American Association for the Surgery of Trauma (2007) The acute care surgical curriculum. J Trauma 62:553–556
5. Representatives of the Participating Organizations in Congress (2009) Acute care congress on the future of emergency surgical care in the United States. J Trauma 67:1–7

Acute Cholecystitis

▶ Cholecystitis

Acute Coagulopathy of Trauma

▶ Coagulopathy

Acute Confusional State

▶ Encephalopathy and Delirium

Acute Coronary Syndrome: Risk Stratification

CHADWICK D. MILLER
Department of Emergency Medicine, Wake Forest University Baptist Medical Center School of Medicine, Winston-Salem, NC, USA

Synonyms

Prediction models

Definition

ACS Definition

Acute coronary syndrome (ACS) is comprised of two related entities: acute myocardial infarction (AMI) and unstable angina. Both entities are caused by an insufficient delivery of oxygen to cardiac myocytes. In myocardial infarction, a sustained disruption in the delivery of substrate leads to cellular death and necrosis. Unstable angina is typically an intermittent or incomplete disruption in cellular substrate delivery that by definition does not cause detectable amounts of cellular death. Unstable angina differs in definition from AMI in that no measurable myocardial necrosis, and therefore no elevated cardiac markers are present.

Risk Stratification

The concept of risk stratification is critical to the evaluation and treatment of ACS. Several levels of risk stratification are commonly used to determine prognosis and to direct treatment. The rationale for risk stratification is matching individual patients with diagnostic and treatment strategies most likely to provide a favorable outcome, deliver cost-effective care, and ideally both. Risk stratification tools commonly used in patients with ACS are listed in Table 1.

Evaluation and Assessment

Risk stratification of patients with ACS can be thought of in context of the clinical question to be answered. Common clinical questions arising in this population that are amendable to risk stratification are discussed below.

Acute Coronary Syndrome: Risk Stratification. Table 1 Components used in risk stratification of patients with NSTE ACS

Risk stratification component	Finding	Significance	Incorporated into risk stratification algorithm
ECG	ST-segment changes	Elevation: STEMI treatment Depression: highly specific for NSTE ACS	ACC/AHA guidelines GRACE TIMI NSTE ACS PURSUIT
Cardiac troponin	Elevated	Confirms MI; relates to prognosis and treatment	ACC/AHA guidelines GRACE TIMI NSTE ACS PURSUIT
Historical features	Multiple episodes in 24 h Typical versus atypical for ACS Use of aspirin	Typical symptoms, increased number, duration, or crescendo symptoms higher risk	ACC/AHA guidelines TIMI NSTE ACS PURSUIT
Physical exam findings of cardiac dysfunction	S3 JVD Killip classification	Suggests end-organ dysfunction and damage	ACC/AHA guidelines GRACE PURSUIT
Measures of hemodynamic or electrical instability	Arrhythmias, tachycardia, hypotension	Suggests end-organ dysfunction and damage	ACC/AHA guidelines GRACE PURSUIT
Demographic data and comorbid conditions	Age CAD risk factors Prior ACS Diabetes	Increases likelihood of complications/risk	ACC/AHA guidelines GRACE TIMI NSTE ACS PURSUIT

Purpose-driven risk stratification:

1. ST-segment elevation myocardial infarction (STEMI) versus non-ST-segment elevation (NSTE) acute coronary syndrome (ACS)
2. NSTE myocardial infarction (NSTEMI) versus unstable angina
3. Early invasive therapy
4. Advanced pharmacologic treatment

I. STEMI Versus NSTE ACS

The rapid diagnosis of STEMI is critically important to providing timely revascularization. The determination between STEMI and NSTE ACS is made solely on the basis of the electrocardiogram. ECG findings of ST-segment elevation >1 mV in two or more contiguous leads or a new left bundle branch block should prompt emergent treatment for ST-segment elevation myocardial infarction. Patients with these ECG findings, ongoing symptoms, and pain <12 h have complete coronary occlusion and emergent revascularization is indicated with either fibrinolytics or percutaneous coronary intervention (PCI). All patients with ST-segment elevation MI are relatively high-risk for adverse events.

The risk of mortality in STEMI can also be estimated based on ECG findings. ECG findings of anterior ST-segment elevation, left bundle branch blocks, or a large number of involved leads have an increased amount of myocardium at risk and therefore are associated with increased risk. Further, failure of ST-segment elevation to resolve after revascularization, or the development of Q waves represents additional high-risk ECG features.

II. NSTEMI Versus Unstable Angina

In patients with ACS but without ST-segment elevation, the differentiation between AMI and unstable angina is based on cardiac biomarkers. The most commonly used cardiac biomarkers are CK-MB and Troponin. These markers of cellular necrosis require cell breakdown and release into the circulation before they can be detected. With commonly available assays, this cycle requires a period of 6–8 h before detectable levels are found in the blood. Therefore, most patients undergo two or three serial cardiac markers at 3, 4, or 6 h intervals to detect patients with initially negative cardiac biomarkers that subsequently become positive.

III. Early Invasive Therapy

Early invasive therapy refers to cardiac catheterization and possible coronary revascularization early, typically in the first 24 h after presentation. Several clinical trials, meta-analyses, and guidelines support this practice as a means of improving outcomes among some patients. The alternative treatment approach, conservative therapy, involves pharmacologic therapy, stress testing, and selective angiography based upon stress test results. While an early invasive treatment pathway can be expected to increase angiography rates, it has also been shown to reduce mortality and be cost-effective among carefully selected patients.

The American College of Cardiology/American Heart Association (ACC/AHA) guidelines provide guidance for selecting patients with NSTE ACS for an early invasive strategy [1]. The class I recommendations include patients with refractory angina, hemodynamic or electrical instability, or increased risk for clinical events. Those at increased risk for clinical events include patients with elevated troponin, new ST-segment depression, signs or symptoms of heart failure, prior CABG, recent PCI (within 6 months), recurrent angina or ischemia at rest or with low-level activities, high-risk findings on noninvasive testing, reduced LV ejection fraction <40%, and a high thrombolysis in myocardial infarction (TIMI) or GRACE risk score.

IV. Advanced Pharmacologic Treatment

Basic treatment of patients with presumed or confirmed ACS includes aspirin, antithrombin therapy with either heparin or low molecular weight heparin, and consideration of anti-ischemic therapy. Treatment of ACS is complex and beyond the focus of this chapter; however, generalizations can be made regarding risk stratification and advanced pharmacologic therapy. As more drugs are added to a patient's treatment regimen, the risk of adverse events from treatment, such as bleeding, increases. In order for a patient to benefit from pharmacologic therapy, the risk reduction in adverse cardiac events resulting from adding a drug must outweigh the risk increase related to the treatment regimen. Therefore, patients at highest risk of cardiovascular adverse events have the most potential benefit from additional therapy. In contrast, patients with low risk of adverse events would be subjected to increased risk from therapy with little potential benefit. Two of the strongest predictors of risk for adverse events are elevated cardiac troponin and ST-segment deviation on the electrocardiogram. Patients with these features therefore stand to benefit the most from double (i.e., aspirin plus thienopyridine) or triple antiplatelet therapy (aspirin, thienopyridine, plus glycoprotein IIb/IIIa inhibition).

For a complete discussion of this topic, readers are referred to treatment guidelines from the ACC/AHA.

V. Risk Stratification Scoring Systems

Most scoring systems and decision rules are generally designed to provide prognostic information specific to patients with either STEMI or NSTE ACS. Therefore, these two are discussed separately. The GRACE risk score has prognostic value in both STEMI and NSTE ACS and is presented first. None of these risk scores are able to exclude ACS in ED patients with undifferentiated chest pain. Rather, they are derived and validated to provide treatment and prognostic guidance in patients with presumed ACS.

A. STEMI

Three risk stratification schemes for patients with STEMI are presented in this chapter, the GRACE risk score (discussed above), the TIMI risk score for STEMI, and the CADILLAC risk score.

GRACE

The GRACE risk score [2] is predictive of in-hospital mortality and is valid in patients with both STEMI and NSTE ACS. Elements of the GRACE risk score include age, Killip class, systolic blood pressure, heart rate, ST-segment deviation, cardiac arrest at presentation, serum creatinine, and elevated cardiac markers. A score is created based on the results for each component that is then converted into the risk for in-hospital mortality. An online calculator for the GRACE risk score is available at http://www.outcomes-umassmed.org/grace/ (accessed 7/15/2010).

TIMI for STEMI

The TIMI risk score for STEMI [3] has strong predictive value for mortality. The components include age, systolic blood pressure, heart rate, Killip class, anterior location of ST-segment elevation or left bundle branch block, diabetes, history of hypertension, history of angina, weight, and time to treatment. The decision aid yields a score from 0 to 14. A consistent increase in mortality is observed with increases in score, which is persistent across races and gender. Further, the TIMI risk score for STEMI is predictive of events occurring within the first 24 h, 1 month, 6 months, and 1 year. In-hospital mortality by TIMI risk score and the points for each component are noted in Fig. 1.

CADILLAC

The Controlled Abciximab and Device Investigation to Lower Late Angioplasty Complications (CADILLAC)

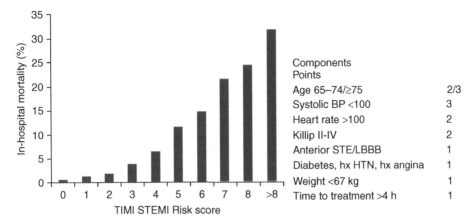

Components	Points
Age 65–74/≥75	2/3
Systolic BP <100	3
Heart rate >100	2
Killip II-IV	2
Anterior STE/LBBB	1
Diabetes, hx HTN, hx angina	1
Weight <67 kg	1
Time to treatment >4 h	1

Acute Coronary Syndrome: Risk Stratification. Figure 1 TIMI risk score for patients with STEMI

Acute Coronary Syndrome: Risk Stratification. Table 2
CADILLAC risk score

	Points
Baseline LV EF <40%	4
Renal insufficiency (creatinine clearance <60 ml/min)	3
Killip class 2 or 3	3
Final TIMI flow 0–2	2
Age >65 years	2
Anemia (hematocrit) (men <39%; women <36%)	2
Three vessel coronary disease	2

risk score [4] was derived to predict mortality at 30 days and 1 year based on clinical data and features at angiography among patients with STEMI. In contrast to GRACE or TIMI STEMI, the additional data obtained at angiography is incorporated and allows an additional level of risk stratification after intervention.

Components of the CADILLAC risk score include baseline left ventricular ejection fraction (LVEF) on angiography, renal insufficiency, Killip class, post-procedure TIMI flow grade, age, anemia, and three vessel disease (Table 2). These components are combined in an integer-based scoring system to create low risk (0–2), intermediate risk [3–5], and high-risk (≥6) categories. The 30-day mortality rate for low-risk patients is approximately 1%, 4% for intermediate risk, and 13% for high-risk.

Recommended Use of Scoring Systems in Patients with STEMI

Once STEMI is diagnosed, the immediate focus should be on emergent revascularization. In patients who may be questionable revascularization candidates, the TIMI STEMI or GRACE risk scores may assist clinicians in providing an estimate of the patient's risk for adverse cardiovascular outcomes. These risk scores may also be beneficial in patients who receive reperfusion with fibrinolytic agents and therefore do not have the necessary information to calculate risk using the CADILLAC risk score. After cardiac catheterization, the CADILLAC risk score can be used to integrate catheterization data with the clinical picture to provide a risk assessment.

B. NSTE ACS

Four risk scores are described in this chapter for use with patients with NSTE ACS. As demonstrated in Table 1, the risk stratification instruments have a large degree of overlap in their individual components. The risk strata obtained from using the framework in the ACC/AHA guidelines are linked to treatment recommendations and therefore this framework is commonly used. The GRACE, PURSUIT, and TIMI risk scores were derived to predict different outcomes at different time points. However, all three are useful in predicting with long-term outcomes.

ACC/AHA

The ACC/AHA guidelines [1] provide a framework for ascertaining the short-term risk for death or nonfatal MI among patients with presumed NSTE ACS. Features considered high-risk include:

Elevated cardiac biomarkers
ECG findings of ST-segment depression or new bundle
    branch block
Hemodynamic or electrical instability
End-organ dysfunction (pulmonary edema, rales, S3)
Advanced age (>75 years)

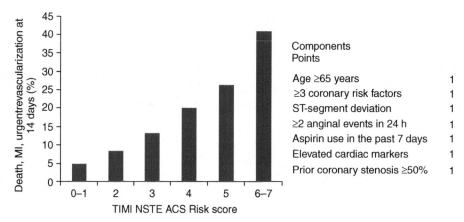

Components
Points

Age ≥65 years	1
≥3 coronary risk factors	1
ST-segment deviation	1
≥2 anginal events in 24 h	1
Aspirin use in the past 7 days	1
Elevated cardiac markers	1
Prior coronary stenosis ≥50%	1

Acute Coronary Syndrome: Risk Stratification. Figure 2 TIMI risk score for patients with NSTE ACS

Prolonged symptoms at rest (>20 min) or accelerating tempo of symptoms in the preceding 48 h

Based on this risk stratification system, all patients with biomarker proven MI are considered high-risk. Furthermore, all patients with STEMI should be considered high-risk. Finally, some patients with unstable angina will be considered high-risk. Risk categories using this system are linked to treatment guidelines published by the ACC/AHA with high-risk patients receiving more aggressive pharmacologic and interventional therapy.

TIMI Risk Score

The Thrombolysis in Myocardial Infarction (TIMI) risk score [5] for patients with NSTE ACS has been widely adopted. The scoring system consists of seven elements with each contributing one point. Elements include age ≥ 65 years, at least three risk factors for coronary artery disease (family history, hypertension, hypercholesterolemia, diabetes, current smoking), ST-segment deviation, two or more anginal events in the past 24 h, aspirin use in the past 7 days, and elevated cardiac markers. Mortality at 14 days increases with each increase in score ranging from approximately 5% among those with 0 or 1, to 41% among those with a TIMI risk score of 6 or 7 (Fig. 2).

The TIMI risk score has been extensively validated, has been shown to correlate with prognosis at 1 year, and also has utility in determining risk among ED patients with undifferentiated chest pain.

PURSUIT

The scoring system resulting from the PURSUIT trial [6] is unique in that it provides estimates for both 30-day mortality and the composite of 30-day mortality and reinfarction. Further, it provides separate estimates based

on whether the patient's diagnosis is unstable angina or myocardial infarction. Using the components of age, gender, Canadian cardiovascular society classification of angina, heart rate, systolic blood pressure, rales, ST-segment depression on the presenting ECG, a score is obtained ranging from 0 to 19. This score is then plotted on a curve to give an estimated event rate.

Recommended Use of Scoring Systems in Patients with NSTE ACS

As demonstrated in Table 1, the risk scoring systems for patients with NSTE ACS have a large degree of overlap in their components. It is not clear that one scoring system dominates or should be favored. Clinicians may choose to become familiar with and use one of these scoring systems. Alternatively, clinicians may choose to become familiar with the components that have the strongest predictive value, such as cardiac biomarkers, ECG findings, and hemodynamic status, and integrate this information into an unstructured clinical assessment.

References

1. Anderson JL, Adams CD, Antman EM et al. ACC/AHA (2007) Guidelines for the management of patients with unstable angina/non ST-elevation myocardial infarction. A report of the American College of Cardiology/American Heart Association Task Force on practice guidelines (writing committee to revise the 2002 guidelines for the management of patients with unstable angina/non ST-elevation myocardial infarction). Circulation 116(7):e148–304.
2. Granger CB, Goldberg RJ, Dabbous O et al (2003) Predictors of hospital mortality in the global registry of acute coronary events. Arch Intern Med 163:2345–2353
3. Morrow DA, Antman EM, Charlesworth A et al (2000) TIMI risk score for ST-elevation myocardial infarction: a convenient, bedside, clinical score for risk assessment at presentation: an intravenous nPA for treatment of infarcting myocardium early II trial substudy. Circulation 102:2031–2037

4. Halkin A, Singh M, Nikolsky E et al (2005) Prediction of mortality after primary percutaneous coronary intervention for acute myocardial infarction: the CADILLAC risk score. J Am Coll Cardiol 45:1397–1405

5. Antman EM, Cohen M, Bernink PJLM et al (2000) The TIMI risk score for unstable angina/non-st elevation MI: a method for prognostication and therapeutic decision making. J Am Med Assoc 284:835–842

6. Boersma E, Pieper KS, Steyerberg EW et al (2000) Predictors of outcome in patients with acute coronary syndromes without persistent st-segment elevation: results from an international trial of 9461 patients. Circulation 101:2557–2567

Acute Heart Failure

▶ Ventricular Dysfunction and Failure

Acute Heart Failure: Risk Stratification

Karina M. Soto-Ruiz[1,2], Joseph Varon[1,3], W. Frank Peacock[4]
[1]Dorrington Medical Associates, Houston, TX, USA
[2]School of Medicine, Universidad Autonoma de Baja California, Tijuana, Mexico
[3]The University of Texas Health Science Center at Houston, and The University of Texas Medical Branch at Galveston. Memorial Hermann Hospital, Texas Medical Center, Houston, TX, USA
[4]Department of Emergency Medicine, The Cleveland Clinic Cleveland Clinic Foundation, Cleveland, OH, USA

Synonyms

Acute pulmonary edema; Cardiogenic shock; Diastolic dysfunction; Heart failure; Left ventricular dysfunction; Systolic dysfunction

Definition

Heart failure is defined as the inability of the myocardium to provide sufficient cardiac output to meet the needs of the body. Heart failure may present with varying severity and require varying therapeutic interventions. Risk stratification is the performance of activities (e.g., laboratory and clinical testing) to determine a patient's need for acute intervention as well as short- or long-term prognosis.

Patients with heart failure are a large group that may benefit from risk stratification strategies.

Pre-existing Condition

Heart failure

Application

The ability to determine a patient's severity of illness at presentation would have great clinical utility. Unfortunately, no comprehensive model that is sufficiently accurate for clinical utility has been described. One model [1] has been prospectively validated to predict acute hospital mortality from data available within the first 10 min of presentation (age, systolic blood pressure, and ECG abnormalities). However, its validity for predicting morbidity, other acute sequelae, and its ability to identify low-risk patients that can be safely discharged home, is unknown. Thus physicians must use experience and clinical acumen when determining appropriate interventions and disposition decision in patients presenting with acute heart failure.

In acute HF, accurate volume status assessment is used to determine appropriate therapy. Errors in determining fluid status can result in unneeded or omitted therapy. Both types of errors are associated with increased mortality in the critically ill. Consequently, for early risk stratification, the physician must rely upon a number of individual objective parameters to provide guidance.

History and Physical Examination

The earliest data available at presentation for diagnosis and risk stratification is that obtained from the history and physical exam. When objectively evaluated, dyspnea on exertion, or the presence of edema have the highest sensitivity for circulatory congestion. Overall, the most specific symptoms suggesting circulatory congestion and a higher need of hospitalization are paroxysmal nocturnal dyspnea, orthopnea, and edema.

Other physical examination parameters have variable utility for diagnosis and increased short-term risk. Jugular venous distention (JVD) is associated with an elevated right atrial pressure, and the presence of either JVD or an S3 heart sound are independently associated with increased HF hospitalization, HF rehospitalization, and death from pump failure. If present, the S3 is highly specific for ventricular dysfunction and elevated left ventricular filling pressures. The S3 has the highest positive likelihood ratio (LR 11.0) for volume overload, but is not valuable as a negative predictor (LR 0.88). Finally, skin mottling, a function of poor peripheral perfusion from pump failure, is associated with a marked increase for in-hospital death, although its absence does not identify a patient at low risk.

Biomarkers

Objective measures of risk stratification have been described. The natriuretic peptides (NPs) of B-type natriuretic peptide (BNP), or its inactive precursor NTproBNP, can be used to differentiate patients with suspected heart failure from other causes of dyspnea and to assist in determining the severity of illness at presentation. NPs are produced by the myocardium in response to pressure or volume stress. When NP's are elevated (>500 pg/mL BNP or >900 pg/mL NTproBNP), the positive predictive value for a heart failure diagnosis is in the 90% range. These biomarkers also have high negative predictive values; when NP is low (<300 pg/mL NTproBNP or <100 pg/mL BNP), an alternative diagnosis should be considered. This then leaves a "gray zone" (300–900 pg/mL for NTproBNP, and 100–500 pg/mL for BNP), where additional testing is needed to determine the etiology of the clinical presentation.

It is important to consider non-heart failure causes of BNP alterations. Any myocardial stress (e.g., acute myocardial infarction or pulmonary embolism) may elevate natriuretic peptides, as can renal failure. In fact, some authors suggest that in the setting of moderate or severe renal failure, the reference range for abnormal BNP levels should be increased to 200 pg/mL. Alternatively, obesity may lower BNP levels, resulting in an inverse relationship between the NP level and body mass index. To correct for this phenomena, it is suggested that the BNP level should be doubled in patients with a body mass index >35, as a way of improving the sensitivity of a heart failure diagnosis. Ultimately, for accurate interpretation of an NP measurement, the clinical scenario must be considered.

The risk stratification value of NPs is their ability to identify heart failure patients at greater risk for short-term mortality. From the Acute Decompensated Heart Failure Registry (ADHERE), patients with a BNP >1,730 pg/mL at ED presentation had a 6% in-hospital mortality compared to those with a BNP level <430 pg/mL, whose in-hospital mortality rate was 2.2% [2]. Furthermore, patients with an elevated BNP were twice as likely to be admitted to the intensive care unit, and their hospital stay was prolonged by 1 day more than patients with lower levels.

ADHERE also identified that troponin provides prognostic data in patients with acute heart failure [3]. In this analysis, the authors reported a direct relationship between elevated troponin levels and in-hospital mortality. In patients with the highest quartile of troponin, the acute mortality rate was 6.3%, versus 1.7% in the lowest quartile. In addition, troponin positive patients required one half day longer in the intensive care unit and were hospitalized 1 day longer.

The results of NP and troponin testing can be combined to help risk stratification. In a separate ADHERE analysis [4], the combination of troponin and BNP assessment predicted acute mortality in patients arriving to the ED with acute heart failure. Patients with a positive troponin and BNP >840 pg/mL had an in-hospital mortality rate of 10.2%, compared to a mortality rate of approximately 4.5% when either one of BNP or troponin was elevated, and only 2.2% when neither was elevated.

These markers can also be used to identify patients who will benefit from interventions. Early diagnostic precision and time to treatment are considered clinically important in numerous conditions (e.g., acute coronary syndromes, hypoglycemia, and stroke); however, heart failure is not commonly considered in this group. In an analysis of nearly 15,000 heart failure patients hospitalized via the ED, mortality rates were stratified as a function of BNP quartile and time to intravenous loop diuretic administration [5]. In patients with a BNP <865 pg/mL, no time-dependent effect of loop diuretic dosing was found. However, if the initial BNP level was >865 pg/mL, a delay in diuretic administration was associated with increased mortality. In patients with a BNP level higher than 1,738 pg/mL, a delay in diuretic administration exceeding 5 h was associated with an increase in the acute in-hospital mortality from 5.1% to 7.3%.

A variety of additional tools are available for risk stratification in the acute care environment. In a study performing a classification and regression tree analysis of approximately 80,000 patients [6], the strongest predictor of in-hospital death was an elevated blood urea nitrogen (BUN). At presentation, if the BUN was >43 mg/dL, the mortality rate was about 9%, compared to only 2.7% in patients with a BUN below this. Additive to BUN, the second strongest predictor of acute mortality was the presenting systolic blood pressure (SBP). If the initial SBP was <115 mmHg, and the patient had an elevated BUN, in hospital mortality was approximately 15%, compared to only 2.1% in those with a SBP >115 mmHg. Finally, if the BUN was >43 mg/dL, the SBP below 115 mmHg, and the creatinine >2.75 mg/dL, the in-hospital mortality rate neared 22%.

Clearly, a number of acute mortality predictors for patients presenting with suspected acute heart failure exist. However for risk stratification, it is also valuable to identify patients at low risk for adverse outcomes. It is important to recognize that the absence of high-risk predictors does not identify low-risk patients. Although a much smaller data set, low-risk predictors have been identified to determine which patients can be managed in lower acuity environments. In one study of nearly 500 patients, a negative troponin and an initial SBP >160 mmHg identified a cohort that would be safely discharged within 24 h to survive and not require rehospitalization in the subsequent 30 days. A second study of 385 patients, found that a BUN below 30 mg/dL identified patients who could be successfully managed in a 24-h unit.

There are several implications in risk stratification of heart failure patients. As noted above, natriuretic peptides are helpful biomarkers for diagnosis and risk stratification. Furthermore, a positive troponin, BUN >43 mg/dL, SBP <115 mmHg, and creatinine >2.75 mg/dL, all contribute to the identification of patients presenting with acute heart failure at high risk for short-term mortality. Conversely, an SBP >160 mmHg, a negative troponin, and a BUN below 30 mg/dL identify patients with a low likelihood of short-term adverse events.

References

1. Selker HP, Griffith JL, D'Agostino RB (1994) A time-insensitive predictive instrument for acute hospital mortality due to congestive heart failure: development, testing, and use for comparing hospitals: a multicenter study. Med Care 32(10):1040–1052
2. Fonarow GC, Peacock WF, Phillips CO, Givertz MM, Lopatin M, ADHERE Scientific Advisory Committee and Investigators (2007) Admission B-type natriuretic peptide levels and in-hospital mortality in acute decompensated heart failure. J Am Coll Cardiol 49:1943–1950
3. Peacock WF IV, DeMarco T, Fonarow GC, DIercks D, Wynne J, Apple FS, For the ADHERE Investigators et al (2008) Cardiac troponin and outcome in acute heart failure. N Engl J Med 358:2117–2126
4. Fonarow G, Peacock WF, Horwich TB, Phillips CO, Givertz M, Lopatin M et al (2008) Usefulness of B-type natriuretic peptide and cardiac troponin levels to predict in-hospital mortality from ADHERE. Am J Cardiol 101:231–237
5. Maisel AS, Peacock WF, McMullin N, Jessie R, Fonarow GC, Wynne J, Mills RM (2008) Timing of immunoreactive B-type natriuretic peptide levels and treatment delay in acute decompensated heart failure. J Am Coll Cardiol 52:534–540
6. Fonarow GC, Adams KF Jr, Abraham WT, Yancy CW, Boscardin WJ, ADHERE scientific advisory committee study group, and Investigators (2005) Risk stratification for in-hospital mortality in acutely decompensated heart failure: classification and regression trees analysis. JAMA 293:572–580

Acute Intracerebral Hemorrhage

▶ Stroke, Blood Pressure Management

Acute Iron Poisoning

▶ Iron Overdose

Acute Ischemic Stroke

▶ Stroke, Blood Pressure Management

Acute Kidney Disease

▶ AKI, Concept of

Acute Kidney Diseases and Disorders (AKD)

▶ Decreased Estimated Glomerular Filtration Rate (eGFR): Interpretation in Acute and Chronic Kidney Disease

Acute Kidney Dysfunction

▶ AKI, Epidemiology of

Acute Kidney Failure

▶ AKI, Epidemiology of

Acute Kidney Injury (AKI)

▶ Acute Kidney Injury Biomarkers, Concept of
▶ ANP
▶ Decreased Estimated Glomerular Filtration Rate (eGFR): Interpretation in Acute and Chronic Kidney Disease

Acute Kidney Injury Biomarkers, Concept of

PRASAD DEVARAJAN
Department of Nephrology and Hypertension, Cincinnati Children's Hospital Medical Center University of Cincinnati, Cincinnati, OH, USA

Synonyms

Acute kidney injury (AKI); Acute renal failure; Structural biomarkers

Definition

Acute kidney injury (AKI) refers to a complex syndrome that comprises multiple causative factors and occurs in a variety of settings with varied clinical manifestations ranging from a minimal elevation in serum creatinine to anuric renal failure. AKI is characterized functionally by a rapid (within hours to days) decline in the glomerular filtration rate (GFR), and biochemically by the accumulation of nitrogenous wastes such as blood urea nitrogen and creatinine. The term AKI has largely replaced acute renal failure (ARF), the terminology historically used for this condition, since the latter designation overemphasizes the failure of kidney function and fails to account for the diverse spectrum of molecular, biochemical, and structural processes that characterize the AKI syndrome.

AKI is a common clinical condition, afflicting all ages in both hospital and community settings, and associated with potentially serious consequences and treatment options that are largely supportive in nature. The incidence of AKI in hospitalized subjects is estimated at a staggering 5–7%. The incidence is even higher in the intensive care unit (ICU) – about 25% – and carries an overall mortality rate of 50–80%. An increase in morbidity and mortality associated with AKI has been demonstrated in a wide variety of common clinical situations, including those exposed to radiocontrast dye, cardiopulmonary bypass, mechanical ventilation, sepsis, and other critical illnesses. In addition, AKI is a major risk factor for the development of nonrenal complications and it independently contributes to mortality.

AKI is largely asymptomatic, and establishing the diagnosis currently hinges on serial serum creatinine measurements. Unfortunately, serum creatinine is a delayed and unreliable indicator of AKI for a variety of reasons. First, even normal serum creatinine is influenced by several nonrenal factors such as age, gender, muscle mass, muscle metabolism, medications, hydration status, nutrition status, and tubular secretion. Second, a number of acute and chronic kidney conditions can exist with no increase in serum creatinine due to the concept of renal reserve – it is estimated that greater than 50% of kidney function must be lost before serum creatinine rises. Third, serum creatinine concentrations do not reflect the true decrease in glomerular filtration rate in the acute setting, since several hours to days must elapse before a new equilibrium between the presumably steady state production and the decreased excretion of creatinine is established. Fourth, an increase in serum creatinine represents a late indication of a functional change in glomerular filtration rate, which lags behind important structural changes that occur in the kidney during the early initiation and extension phases of AKI. Indeed, animal studies have identified several interventions that can prevent and/or treat AKI if instituted early in the disease course, well before the serum creatinine even begins to rise. The lack of early biomarkers has hampered our ability to translate these promising findings to human AKI. A troponin-like biomarker of AKI that is easily measured reflects early structural damage rather than late functional consequences, unaffected by other biological variables, and capable of both early detection and risk stratification would represent a tremendous advance in intensive care medicine.

In its simplest definition, a biomarker is anything that can be measured to extract information about a biologic state or process. The NIH Biomarkers Definitions Working Group has defined a biomarker as "A characteristic that is objectively measured and evaluated as an indicator of normal biological processes, pathogenic processes, or pharmacologic responses to a therapeutic intervention." In this chapter, we will review the general process for the discovery and validation of biomarkers, the characteristics of an ideal acute kidney injury biomarker, and the current status of novel AKI biomarkers.

Characteristics

The Process of Biomarker Discovery and Validation

The quest for biomarkers is as old as medicine itself. From the earliest days of diagnostic medicine in ancient Egypt, to the powerful discoveries of modern science, we have been searching for measurable biological cues that will allow us insight into the physiologic workings of the human organism. Biomarkers appear in every form. Body temperature, in the form of a fever, can signal infection. Blood pressure and cholesterol levels can predict cardiovascular risk. Tracking biomarkers such as height and weight can give clues to normal human growth and development. Such general biomarkers have been used for decades or even centuries and have remained powerful tools for assessing general biological activity. However, the era of personalized medicine is well upon us. Ushered in by the remarkable genomic and proteomic advances in our understanding of health and disease, personalized medicine promises a more precise determination of disease predisposition, diagnosis and prognosis, earlier preventive and therapeutic interventions, a more efficient drug development process, and a safer and more fiscally responsive approach to medicine. Biomarkers are the essential tools for the implementation of personalized medicine. The quest for the advancement of personalized medicine drives us further and further into the realm of molecular medicine to discover biomarkers with increasing sensitivity and specificity.

The biomarker development process has typically been divided into five phases, [1, 2] as shown in Table 1. The preclinical discovery phase requires high-quality, well-characterized tissue or body fluid samples from

Acute Kidney Injury Biomarkers, Concept of. Table 1
Phases of biomarker discovery, translation, and validation (Adapted from reference [2])

Phase	Terminology	Action steps
Phase 1	Preclinical discovery	• Discover biomarkers in tissues or body fluids • Confirm and prioritize promising candidates
Phase 2	Assay development	• Develop and optimize clinically useful assay • Test on existing samples of established disease
Phase 3	Retrospective study	• Test biomarker in completed clinical trial • Test if biomarker detects the disease early • Evaluate sensitivity, specificity, ROC
Phase 4	Prospective screening	• Use biomarker to screen population • Identify extent and characteristics of disease • Identify false referral rate
Phase 5	Disease control	• Determine impact of screening on reducing disease burden

carefully chosen animal or human models of the disease under investigation. In recent years, the ready availability of powerful tools to scan both the genome and the proteome of an organism have revolutionized and greatly accelerated biomarker discovery. Microarrays that can measure the entire complement of messenger RNA in a given sample type have yielded a number of promising biomarkers of kidney disease, and have also led to the discovery of novel disease mechanisms in many fields. This approach can be combined with other techniques, such as laser capture microdissection, to target specific areas of diseased tissue to give mechanistic clues not possible just a decade ago. A shortcoming of such transcriptomic profiling approaches is that one cannot directly measure biological fluids. Another problem with this approach is that ultimately messenger RNA does not always reflect protein levels or activity and must be further confirmed at the protein level prior to larger validation studies.

Proteomic approaches move a step beyond genomic studies and screen the actual proteins and peptides present in a sample. This approach allows one to go beyond simple translation of mRNA into protein, and allows a look into protein regulation, posttranslational modifications such as glycosylation and methylation, and even disease-specific fragmentation. There are a number of proteomic approaches including gel electrophoresis and modern mass spectrometry techniques such as matrix-assisted laser desorption ionization time of flight (MALDI-TOF) mass spectrometry and surface-enhanced laser desorption ionization time of flight (SELDI-TOF) mass spectrometry. These techniques are capable of identifying and quantifying proteins and peptides in exceedingly large numbers. The urinary proteome itself is quite large, with laboratories having identified over 1,500 proteins to date. The blood proteome is even larger, with over 3,000 nonredundant proteins identified in the plasma alone. Adding the proteome of the cellular component of blood will yield thousands more. To this end we have entered what has been termed an "open loop" or unbiased, approach to biomarker discovery. This is in stark contrast to the hypothesis driven approach of our past.

Desirable Characteristics of a Biomarker

What constitutes an ideal biomarker is highly dependent upon the disease under investigation. However, certain universal characteristics are important for any biomarker: (1) they should be noninvasive, easily measured, inexpensive, and produce rapid results; (2) they should be from readily available sources, such as blood or urine; (3) they should have a high sensitivity, allowing early detection, and no overlap in values between diseased patients and healthy controls; (4) they should have a high specificity, being greatly upregulated (or downregulated) specifically in the diseased samples and unaffected by comorbid conditions; (5) biomarker levels should vary rapidly in response to treatment; (6) biomarker levels should aid in risk stratification and possess prognostic value in terms of real outcomes; and (7) biomarkers should be biologically plausible and provide insight into the underlying disease mechanism [3, 4].

Of course, very few biomarkers will meet all of the characteristics of an ideal marker, but let us discuss these characteristics in a little more detail. First, a biomarker should be noninvasive. Regarding the source of biomarkers, the most readily available ones are urine and blood. These are substances obtained in the normal care of a patient, easily collected at the bedside, and associated with little to no health risks to the patient. Each source has desirable and negative characteristics. Urine is an excellent source of biomarkers produced in the kidney and thus may give better mechanistic insight into specific renal pathologies. Urine is less complex than serum and thus is easier to screen for potential biomarkers. Collection of urine is easy enough, and it can be readily employed in home testing kits. The handling of urine, however, greatly influences the stability of its proteins and measurements should be made immediately after collection or the urine should be promptly frozen at $-80°C$ to avoid degradation. Finally, urinary biomarker studies typically adjust for urine creatinine to account for differences in urine concentration due to hydration status and medications such as diuretics. However, the utility of urine creatinine in biomarker correction has been questioned due to its variable excretion throughout the day and its dependence on normal renal function. Serum or plasma can also be a good source of biomarkers and is even available in anuric patients. Serum is less prone to bacterial contamination than urine and is considered more stable. Serum biomarkers, however, are more likely to represent a systemic response to disease, rather than an organ response. There are exceptions, such as the troponins in cardiac disease. The real problem with serum as a source of biomarkers lies in the discovery phase. Serum has a wide range of protein concentrations across several orders of magnitude, with a small number of proteins (such as albumin) accounting for a large percentage of the volume.

The sensitivity and specificity of a biomarker go hand in hand. The receiver-operating characteristic (ROC) curve is a binary classification test, based on the sensitivity and specificity of a biomarker at certain cutoff points. ROC curves are often used to determine the clinical diagnostic value of a marker. The area under the ROC curve (AUC) is a common statistic derived from ROC curves. An AUC of 1.0 represents a perfect biomarker, while an AUC of 0.5 is a result that is no better than expected by chance. An AUC of 0.75 or greater is generally considered a good biomarker, while an AUC of 0.90 is considered an excellent biomarker. However, even a sensitive biomarker with what experimentally would be considered an excellent specificity of 90%, would still yield a false-positive rate of 10%, which may be unacceptably high for clinical use as a stand alone marker. As a result, the best approach clinically may be to find multiple biomarkers that can be combined as part of a panel to achieve even higher specificity. Lack of specificity and slow response to alterations in disease severity or treatment are primary reasons why serum creatinine is an unsatisfactory biomarker for renal disease, especially in AKI.

Characteristics of an Ideal AKI Biomarker

Many conventional markers of kidney function have suffered from a lack of specificity and poor standardized assays. The insensitivity of these measurements, such as casts and fractional secretion of sodium, make them poor candidates for the early detection of AKI. As mentioned, creatinine is an unreliable marker of acute changes in kidney function due to its slow response time and the fact that many variables can alter creatinine levels. Identification of early AKI biomarkers has been designated a top priority by the American Society of Nephrology and the concept of developing a new collection of tools for earlier diagnosis of disease states is a prominent feature in the National Institutes of Health road map or biomedical research.

Besides establishing the early diagnosis, biomarkers are needed for several other purposes in AKI [1–4]. Thus, biomarkers are needed for (a) pinpointing the location of primary injury (proximal tubule, distal tubule, interstitium, or vasculature); (b) determining the duration of kidney failure (AKI, chronic kidney disease, or "acute-on-chronic" kidney disease); (c) discerning AKI subtypes (prerenal, intrinsic renal, or postrenal); (d) identifying AKI etiologies (ischemia, toxins, sepsis, or a combination); (e) differentiating AKI from other forms of acute kidney disease (urinary tract infection, glomerulonephritis, or interstitial nephritis); (f) risk stratification and prognostication (duration and severity of AKI, need for renal replacement therapy, length of hospital stay, and mortality); (g) defining the course of AKI; and (i) monitoring the response to AKI interventions. Biomarkers are also desperately needed for use as surrogate endpoints in clinical trials evaluating potential therapeutics for AKI. Surrogate markers are precise measurements that can accurately correlate with a clinical endpoint. Surrogate endpoints can expedite clinical trials evaluating the safety and efficacy of new drug applications. If the intervention has the desired effect on the surrogate endpoint, then further evaluations are warranted to directly address the effect of the intervention on the appropriate clinical endpoint. This linking of the surrogate endpoint to the clinical endpoint is referred to as validation and is an essential step in the biomarker discovery process.

With respect to the desirable characteristics of AKI biomarkers, the most important remain those that are clinically applicable and can lead to early diagnosis and treatment of AKI. Other important properties of clinically relevant biomarkers of AKI are similar in concept to the properties of ideal biomarkers in general. Specific characteristics should include (a) measurements from noninvasive sources, such as blood or urine; (b) easy to perform either at bedside or in a standard clinical laboratory; (c) measurements should be reliable and have a rapid turnaround time; (d) they should be sensitive for early detection and have a wide dynamic range of values with cutoffs to allow for risk stratification; (e) they should be highly specific, and ideally allow for AKI subtype classification; and (f) they should be inexpensive to allow for broad global use.

The Current Status of Novel AKI Biomarkers

Not surprisingly, the pursuit of improved biomarkers for the early diagnosis of AKI and its outcomes is an area of intense contemporary research. For answers, we must turn to the kidney itself. Indeed, understanding the early stress response of the kidney to acute injuries has revealed a number of potential biomarkers. Many have successfully passed through the preclinical, assay development, and initial clinical testing stages of the biomarker development process. A number of biomarkers have now entered the prospective screening stage, facilitated by the development of commercial tools for their measurement on large populations across different laboratories. The most promising biomarkers being evaluated in humans are listed in Table 2, and their current status is briefly summarized below.

Acute Kidney Injury Biomarkers, Concept of. Table 2 Current status of novel urinary and plasma biomarkers for the early diagnosis of acute kidney injury

Biomarker name and source	Biomarker timing and accuracy	Cardiopulmonary bypass (CPB)	Contrast-induced nephropathy	Delayed graft function (DGF)	Critical care or emergency setting
Urine/plasma NGAL	Time post-insult	2 h post-CPB	2 h post-contrast	6 h posttransplant	Variable
	Time pre-AKI	2 days pre-AKI	1–2 days pre-AKI	2–3 days pre-DGF	2 days pre-AKI
	AUC-ROC	0.78	0.90	0.90	0.73
Urine IL-18	Time post-insult	12 h post-CPB	Not increased	6 h posttransplant	Variable
	Time pre-AKI	1–2 days pre-AKI		2–3 days pre-DGF	2 days pre-AKI
	AUC-ROC	0.75		0.90	0.73
Urine KIM-1	Time post-insult	12 h post-CPB	Not tested	Not tested	Not tested
	Time pre-AKI	1–2 days pre-AKI			
	AUC-ROC	0.78			
Urine L-FABP	Time post-insult	4 h post-CPB	6 h post-contrast	Not tested	Not tested
	Time pre-AKI	2 days pre-AKI	1–2 days pre-AKI		
	AUC-ROC	0.81	Not reported		
Plasma cystatin C	Time post-insult	6 h post-CPB	2–6 h post-contrast	Not tested	Variable
	Time pre-AKI	2 days pre-AKI	1–2 days pre-AKI		2 days pre-AKI
	AUC-ROC	0.62	Not reported		0.90

AUC-ROC, area under the receiver-operating characteristic curve, which is a measure of diagnostic accuracy
DGF, defined as dialysis requirement within the first week after transplant
Times shown are the earliest time points when biomarker concentrations become significantly increased from baseline

For the early prediction of AKI in various common clinical situations, a number of studies have now established neutrophil gelatinase-associated lipocalin (NGAL) as the most promising biomarker. A meta-analysis of published data has shown that early NGAL measurements can predict subsequent development of AKI, following temporally predictable injuries such as cardiac surgery, nephrotoxin administration, and kidney transplantation, and also in unselected populations such as critically ill subjects [5]. Both urine and plasma NGAL levels predict AKI with a very good to excellent diagnostic accuracy. Other emerging urinary biomarkers for the early diagnosis of AKI include interleukin-18 (IL-18), kidney injury molecule-1 (KIM-1), liver-type fatty acid binding protein (L-FABP), and the glutathione S-transferases. In the plasma, another promising AKI biomarker is cystatin C.

Biomarkers are also being examined for predicting the prognosis of AKI. Several publications have now demonstrated the utility of early urine and plasma NGAL measurements for predicting clinical outcomes of AKI, including duration and severity of AKI, length of hospital stay, dialysis requirement, and mortality. Positive correlations with AKI severity and mortality have also been reported in a limited number of studies for a number of other urinary (IL-18, KIM-1, N-acetyl-β-D-glucosaminidase, cystatin C) and plasma (cystatin C) biomarkers.

Summary

In addition to early diagnosis and prediction, it would be desirable to identify biomarkers capable of discerning AKI subtypes, identifying etiologies, predicting clinical outcomes, allowing for risk stratification, and monitoring the response to interventions. In order to obtain all of this desired information, a panel of validated biomarkers may be needed. The availability of a panel of AKI biomarkers could revolutionize renal and critical care.

References

1. Devarajan P (2007) Emerging biomarkers of acute kidney injury. Contrib Nephrol 156:203–212
2. Devarajan P (2007) Proteomics for biomarker discovery in acute kidney injury. Semin Nephrol 27:637–651
3. Parikh CR, Devarajan P (2008) New biomarkers of acute kidney injury. Crit Care Med 36(4 Suppl):159–165
4. Devarajan P (2008) Emerging urinary biomarkers in the diagnosis of acute kidney injury. Expert Opin Med Diagn 2(4):387–398
5. Haase M, Bellomo R, Devarajan P, Schlattmann P, Haase-Fielitz A, NGAL Meta-analysis Investigator Group (2009) Accuracy of neutrophil gelatinase-associated lipocalin (NGAL) in diagnosis and prognosis in acute kidney injury: a systematic review and meta-analysis. Am J Kidney Dis 54(6):1012–1024

Acute Kidney Injury During Pregnancy

Arun Jeyabalan
Department of Obstetrics, Gynecology, and Reproductive Sciences, University of Pittsburgh School of Medicine, Pittsburgh, PA, USA

Synonyms

Acute renal insufficiency in pregnancy; Pregnancy-related acute renal failure

Definition

Acute kidney injury (AKI) is broadly defined as an abrupt deterioration of renal function that results in retention of urea and nitrogenous waste products and in the dysregulation of fluid and electrolyte homeostasis [1]. Pregnancy-related AKI (PR-AKI), by definition, occurs during pregnancy, labor and delivery, and/or the postpartum period. There are two major categories of pregnancy-related AKI: (i) pregnancy-specific diagnoses and (ii) other etiologies relevant to women of childbearing age that may happen to coincide with pregnancy. Importantly, this condition poses a unique and important challenge as there are two patients to consider: the mother and her fetus.

Specific diagnostic criteria for AKI, even in the nonpregnant population, have been variable and often vague, thus clouding the existing literature and rendering the translation of research findings to bedside management challenging. To address this issue, the multidisciplinary AKI Network developed uniform standards for the diagnosis and staging of renal failure based on serum creatinine and urine output [2]. The proposed diagnostic criteria for AKI is an abrupt (within 48 h) reduction in kidney function defined as an absolute increase in serum creatinine of more than or equal to 0.3 mg/dL, a percentage increase in serum creatinine of more than or equal to 50% (1.5-fold from baseline), or a reduction in urine output (documented oliguria of less than 0.5 mL/kg per hour for more than 6 h). With pregnancy, the profound physiologic changes in the renal and cardiovascular systems must also be taken into account for proper diagnosis and management of AKI.

Renal Physiologic Changes in Pregnancy [3]

Anatomic changes occur as early as the first trimester including a marked increase in kidney size and volume primarily due to the increase in renal vascular volume and capacity of the collecting system. Dilation of the collecting system with hydronephrosis and hydroureter occurs in 80% of women by midpregnancy, likely due to the smooth muscle relaxation caused by progesterone and other hormones. Ureteral dilation is more dramatic on the right than the left secondary to external compression by the ovarian vascular plexus and the gravid uterus. Understanding these normal anatomic changes is important for the interpretation of renal imaging studies performed in the pregnant woman.

One of the most dramatic and early physiologic changes of pregnancy is the marked increase in renal blood flow that begins early in the first trimester. This increase is associated with reduced renal vascular resistance and increased maternal plasma volume and cardiac output. Progesterone, relaxin, and other luteal and placental hormones are likely responsible for the profound vasodilation and circulatory changes associated with pregnancy. Compared to the nonpregnant baseline, renal plasma flow increases by 50–85% over the course of pregnancy with a slight decrease at the end of gestation. An important consequence is a significant increase in glomerular filtration rate (GFR) of 40–65% above baseline. These changes have practical implications such as changes in normal laboratory parameters (Table 1). These include an increase in creatinine clearance by at least 25% over nonpregnant values as well as reduced serum concentrations of blood urea nitrogen and creatinine; thus, a serum creatinine of 0.9 mg/dL while considered normal in a nonpregnant adult, would be abnormal in a pregnant woman. The increased GFR also affects substrate handling, including an increase in proteinuria (up to 300 mg/dL) and often glucosuria. Despite this marked increase in GFR, the renal tubules function to preserve sodium balance and accomplish a net sodium retention of 500–900 mEq over the course of pregnancy. Water balance in maintained while plasma osmolality is reduced.

The kidney also plays an important role in acid–base homeostasis. The primary acid–base alteration during pregnancy is a respiratory alkalosis (pCO_2 is reduced by approximately 10 mmHg) secondary to increased minute ventilation. A compensatory metabolic acidosis occurs with decline in serum bicarbonate concentrations. While these adaptations are beneficial for the fetus by increasing the CO_2 gradient across the placenta to facilitate gas exchange, the maternal capacity to buffer acids is reduced. Understanding these acid–base changes is important in the management of pregnant women, particularly in the intensive care unit (ICU) setting.

Acute Kidney Injury During Pregnancy. Table 1 Normal laboratory parameters in pregnancy

Variable	Change compared to nonpregnant values	Approximate normal value in pregnancy
Serum creatinine	↓	0.5 mg/dL
Blood urea nitrogen (BUN)	↓	9.0 mg/dL
Creatinine clearance	↑	↑ ~25% above baseline
Uric acid	↓	2.0–3.0 mg/dL
Urinary protein excretion	Variable to ↑	Up to 300 mg/24 h
Sodium retention over pregnancy	↑	900–950 mEq
Plasma osmolality	↓	270 mOsm/kg H_2O
pCO_2	↓	27–32 mmHg
pH	↑	7.40–7.45
Serum bicarbonate	↓	18–20 mEq/L
Urinary glucose excretion	Variable to ↑	Variable

Treatment

Treatment principles of PR-AKI are as follows: (i) treat the underlying cause, (ii) prevent progression of renal damage, (iii) maintain supportive measures, and (iv) consider maternal health as primary while optimizing fetal well-being [3, 4]. A multidisciplinary team approach is recommended for the management of these complex patients including Maternal-Fetal medicine (high-risk obstetricians), critical care medicine, nephrology, and neonatology specialists. General management of PR-AKI will be discussed below. A detailed discussion of specific therapies based on diagnosis will follow in the next section.

Initial treatment should be directed at correcting the underlying causative factors and preventing progressive renal injury. As with the nonpregnant patient, the conventional approach of categorizing AKI etiology as prerenal, intrarenal, and postrenal provides a framework for guiding therapy in PR-AKI [1]. Prerenal AKI is a result of reduced renal perfusion. Hypovolemia (such as blood loss related to intra or postpartum hemorrhage, placental abruption, or placenta previa), hypotension (e.g., septic shock), or low cardiac output are common reasons for reduced perfusion of the kidneys and subsequent AKI.

If renal hypoperfusion is severe, prolonged or uncorrected, intrinsic renal damage or intrarenal AKI (e.g., acute tubular necrosis or cortical damage) may occur. Intrarenal AKI may also be caused by nephrotoxic drugs (e.g., aminoglycosides, nonsteroidal anti-inflammatory drugs) or immune-mediated damage (e.g., lupus nephritis) that may occur coincident with pregnancy. All nephrotoxic medication should be stopped to prevent further renal decline. Postrenal etiologies of AKI such as ureteral obstruction by the gravid or overdistended uterus or renal stones may be temporized by ureteral stents or percutaneous nephrostomy. If appropriate, delivery of the fetus will likely improve renal function.

By far, the most important tenet of PR-AKI management is improving and maintaining adequate renal perfusion to limit ongoing renal damage and reverse any pre-ischemic changes. This is generally done with intravenous administration of crystalloid or colloid solution, or in many obstetric situations of hemorrhage and disseminated intravascular coagulation, with packed red blood cells and other blood products as indicated. The rapidity of these interventions is guided by clinical status, pulmonary function, and urine output. In complicated cases, invasive hemodynamic assessments with central venous pressure monitoring with or without a pulmonary artery pressure catheter may be needed to guide management.

As with AKI in the nonpregnant individual, pharmacologic therapies for PR-AKI are secondary [3, 4]. The use of low-dose dopamine, believed to improve renal blood flow and clinical outcomes, is not supported by the current literature. Routine use of loop diuretics to prevent AKI during pregnancy is not recommended. An important pregnancy-specific consideration with vasoactive and diuretic medications includes the potential effect of reducing uterine blood flow and placental perfusion, thereby affecting fetal well-being.

Ongoing supportive care includes correcting the downstream effects of AKI such as hyperkalemia, metabolic acidosis, and anemia [3–5]. Hyperkalemia may be treated with polystyrene sulfonate (potassium-binding resin) or glucose/insulin during pregnancy. Metabolic acidosis may be acutely corrected using bicarbonate; however, the underlying cause should be treated. Furthermore, the physiologic respiratory alkalosis of pregnancy and compensatory decrease in plasma bicarbonate must be taken into account when addressing acid–base status in the pregnant woman. Anemia associated with PR-AKI is usually secondary to acute blood loss, hemolysis, and/or reduced hematopoiesis. In the acute setting, severe anemia is treated with red blood cell transfusion. Exogenous erythropoietin may be safely administered in pregnancy. Higher doses are usually needed to achieve a good response.

Renal replacement therapy (RRT, dialysis) should be considered if the previously mentioned measures are inadequate. The following general indications for RRT in pregnancy are similar to those in nonpregnant individuals: (i) volume overload, (ii) hyperkalemia refractory to medical management, (iii) metabolic acidosis, and/or (iv) symptomatic uremia (mental status changes, pericarditis, neuropathy). Both hemodialysis and peritoneal dialysis have been used successfully in pregnant women with chronic and end stage renal disease. Hemodialysis is more commonly used to achieve a rapid response in the acute setting. The precise type (intermittent versus continuous) as well as timing and thresholds for initiation of RRT in PR-AKI have not been determined. Experts recommend modification of RRT protocols during pregnancy including an increase in dialysis time and frequency, minimizing fluid shifts and hypotension, and maintaining serum urea <45–60 mg/dL [3]. For pregnancy-specific etiologies of AKI, dialysis is often temporary until renal function recovers.

With pregnancy there are two patients: the mother and her fetus. While maternal health comes first, fetal status must also be addressed. Adverse fetal and neonatal outcomes with AKI are most related to uteroplacental blood flow, which is highly dependent on maternal intravascular volume and cardiac function. Therefore, prompt volume resuscitation with intravenous fluids or blood/blood products is indicated. Safety of medications is also an important fetal consideration. For viable pregnancies (usually >24 weeks of gestation), fetal monitoring is recommended. Depending on the clinical situation, continuous or intermittent fetal heart rate monitoring or biophysical profile assessment by ultrasound can be used to evaluate fetal well-being. If preterm delivery is indicated, such as with preeclampsia for maternal benefit, antenatal glucocorticoids (betamethasone or dexamethasone) should be administered to reduce neonatal morbidity and mortality associated with prematurity. Neonatologists should be involved if delivery is being considered.

Evaluation and Assessment

Initial evaluation of the pregnant woman with AKI consists of a detailed history, physical examination, and laboratory assessment [3–5]. The primary cause of the AKI often becomes readily apparent based on clinical history; for example, with severe postpartum hemorrhage or placental abruption with preeclampsia. Serum creatinine is a key component of the diagnosis of AKI; of note, the normal range of serum creatinine is significantly lower in the pregnant patient (Table 1). Electrolytes, blood urea nitrogen, and complete blood count are useful as these factors can be primarily or secondarily affected by AKI. Urine electrolytes and microscopic evaluation may be helpful in differentiating between prerenal and intrarenal etiologies of AKI [1]. A functioning kidney with reduced perfusion responds by increasing sodium and water reabsorption with a concomitant reduction in urinary sodium excretion. This is reflected in the urine sodium concentration and fractional excretion of sodium ([(urine sodium × plasma creatinine)/(plasma sodium × urine creatinine)] × 100). Both would be low with prerenal etiologies, <20 mEq/L and <1%, respectively. With intrinsic causes, urine sodium and fractional excretion are expected to be higher, approximately >40 mEq/L and >2%, respectively. Lower urine osmolality with granular or cellular casts with white and red blood cells are also observed with intrarenal AKI. If postrenal causes of AKI are suspected, imaging of the urinary tract should be performed. Ultrasound is generally the first-line investigation for imaging of the urinary tract in pregnancy. Mild or moderate hydronephrosis, particularly on the right, is expected in pregnancy. Specialized serologic tests are used if the etiology of AKI is unclear and/or diagnoses not specific to pregnancy are being considered, such as lupus. Renal biopsy is rarely indicated during pregnancy, since an empiric diagnosis can be made with most cases of AKI and treatment instituted accordingly. Moreover, renal biopsy appears to be associated with increased morbidity during pregnancy. One possible exception is the sudden and unexplained deterioration of renal function before 28–30 weeks of gestation where iatrogenic preterm delivery may not be indicated and directed maternal therapy is likely to be beneficial. A multidisciplinary approach is recommended in making such decisions.

Specific Etiologies of PR-AKI

Pregnancy-specific etiologies of AKI can be categorized as disorders of hypertension and microangiopathy, volume depletion, infections, obstruction, and amniotic fluid embolism [3, 4].

Hypertensive and Microangiopathic Disorders Associated with Pregnancy

Preeclampsia and HELLP Syndrome

Preeclampsia is a common pregnancy-specific condition that affects 5–10% of all pregnancies. Diagnosis is based on new onset of hypertension and proteinuria after 20 weeks' gestation. With severe cases of preeclampsia,

maternal brain, lungs, kidney, liver, and platelets as well as fetal growth and well-being may be affected. Specific diagnostic criteria are presented in Table 2. HELLP syndrome is defined by the presence of hemolysis, elevated liver enzymes, and low platelets during the latter part of pregnancy. It is often considered to be a variant along the preeclampsia spectrum of disorders. Hypertension may or may not be present in HELLP syndrome.

Preeclampsia and related disorders are the most common cause of PR-AKI; however, the majority of women with preeclampsia do not develop AKI. It is estimated that AKI occurs in 1.5–2% of preeclamptic pregnancies. The incidence is higher with HELLP syndrome. The precise mechanisms by which preeclampsia predisposes to AKI are unclear, but may be a result of vascular dysfunction resulting in vasospasm and reduced renal perfusion. The major systemic features of preeclampsia are increased peripheral vascular resistance, endothelial dysfunction, vasospasm, activation of the coagulation and inflammatory cascades, platelet aggregation, resulting in ischemia, and multiorgan damage including AKI. Importantly, glomerular filtration rates and effective renal plasma flow are reduced by approximately 32% and 24% respectively compared to normal, third trimester pregnancy values. A superimposed insult such as obstetric hemorrhage or disseminated intravascular coagulation can lead to reduced intravascular volume and maternal AKI. Acute tubular necrosis is the most common pathology with preeclampsia-related AKI, with renal cortical necrosis observed in the most severe cases. Reported short-term RRT rates are reported to be 10–50% among these women with preeclampsia-associated AKI and maternal mortality rates of up to 10%.

Preeclampsia is a progressive disorder and the only effective treatment is delivery of the fetus and placenta. Mode of delivery (vaginal versus cesarean section) is dependent on clinical and obstetric factors. Supportive care to prevent progression of AKI is with IV fluid replacement and administration of blood and blood products as indicated. Beyond this, blood pressure control is important to prevent maternal cerebrovascular accidents. Intravenous magnesium sulfate is used to prevent seizures; circulating concentrations should be monitored with AKI given the risk of respiratory depression.

Acute Fatty Liver of Pregnancy

Acute fatty liver of pregnancy (AFLP) affects 1/5,000 to 1/10,000 pregnancies and is characterized by rapid progression of hepatic failure in late pregnancy. Clinical features include nausea, vomiting, malaise, abdominal pain, and less frequently, mental status changes. Diagnosis is

Acute Kidney Injury During Pregnancy. Table 2 Classification of hypertensive disorders of pregnancy

Mild preeclampsia	• New onset of sustained elevated blood pressure after 20 weeks' gestation in a previously normotensive woman ($\geq$140 mmHg systolic or $\geq$90 mmHg diastolic on at least two occasions 6 h apart) • Proteinuria of at least 1+ on a urine dipstick or $\geq$300 mg in a 24-h urine collection after 20 weeks
Severe preeclampsia (above criteria plus any of the items listed)	• Blood pressure $\geq$160 mmHg systolic or $\geq$110 mmHg diastolic • Urine protein excretion of at least 5 g in a 24-h collection • Neurologic disturbances (visual changes, headache, seizures, coma) • Pulmonary edema • Hepatic dysfunction (elevated liver transaminases or epigastric pain) • Renal compromise (oliguria or elevated serum creatinine concentration, $\geq$1.2 is considered abnormal in women with no history of renal disease) • Thrombocytopenia • Placental abruption, fetal growth restriction, or oligohydramnios (low amniotic fluid index)
Eclampsia	• Seizures in a preeclamptic women not be attributed to other causes
Superimposed preeclampsia (in women with chronic hypertension)	• Sudden and sustained increase in blood pressure with or without substantial increase in proteinuria • New onset proteinuria ($\geq$300 mg in a 24-h protein collection) in a woman with chronic hypertension and no proteinuria prior to 20 weeks of gestation[a] • Sudden increase in proteinuria or a sudden increase in blood pressure in a woman with previously well-controlled hypertension in a women with elevated blood pressure and proteinuria prior to 20 weeks of gestation[a] • Thrombocytopenia, abnormal liver enzymes, or a rapid worsening of renal function
HELLP syndrome	• Presence of *h*emolysis, *e*levated *l*iver enzymes, and *l*ow *p*latelets. This may or may not occur in the presence of hypertension and is often considered a variant of preeclampsia

[a]Precise diagnosis is often challenging and high clinical suspicion is warranted given the increase maternal and fetal/neonatal risks associated with superimposed preeclampsia

based on clinical presentation and moderately elevated liver transaminase enzymes, hyperbilirubinemia, elevated ammonia, coagulation abnormalities, and hypoglycemia. Low antithrombin III levels and modest elevations in creatinine are also observed. Features of preeclampsia may be coincident with acute fatty liver. Liver biopsy is rarely needed to make the diagnosis. There is an association between AFLP and an inherited defect in mitochondrial fatty acid oxidation, specifically a mutation in the long chain 3-hydroxyacyl coenzyme A dehydrogenase in the fetus and mother, which may account for a subset of cases.

The precise cause of AKI associated with acute fatty liver is not clear; fatty infiltration and/or hepatorenal syndrome have been proposed. Hemorrhage and disseminated intravascular coagulation, both of which are common with acute fatty liver of pregnancy, can accelerate

renal deterioration. Renal recovery is usually complete. Similar to preeclampsia, the cure is delivery with supportive care of the mother. Overall, recovery tends to be more protracted with AFLP and liver transplantation may be required in severe cases of hepatic failure.

Thrombotic Thrombocytopenic Purpura (TTP)/Hemolytic Uremic Syndrome (HUS)

Although these are not pregnancy-specific conditions, TTP and HUS often enter the differential diagnosis along with preeclampsia/HELLP syndrome and PR-AKI; therefore, we will briefly discuss their relevance in pregnancy. TTP/HUS is more common in women (70%) and during pregnancy (13%). Although mortality has decreased (range of 8–44%), long-term morbidity is significant. AKI is estimated to occur in two-thirds of patients, with a substantial proportion of women developing chronic renal insufficiency and hypertension. TTP and HUS are both characterized by microangiopathic hemolytic anemia, intravascular thrombi associated with consumption of platelets, thrombocytopenia, ischemia, and multiple organ involvement. TTP is conventionally described as a pentad of clinical findings: thrombocytopenia, hemolytic anemia, fever, neurologic abnormalities, and renal dysfunction. Features of HUS are similar except that renal dysfunction is more profound and neurologic problems are infrequent. Large multimers of von Willebrand's factor are found with TTP/HUS and recent evidence indicates the deficiency of a plasma protease, ADAMTS13, that cleaves these multimers.

When coincident with pregnancy, TTP/HUS can present very much like severe preeclampsia and/or HELLP syndrome. Proper diagnosis is important as treatments are different. Table 3 provides some general principles in differentiating between these conditions. With diseases along the preeclampsia spectrum, the proper treatment is delivery. On the other hand, timely institution of plasmapheresis is the primary treatment for TTP/HUS. Often the precise diagnosis is not made until after delivery, when preeclampsia, HELLP syndrome, and acute fatty liver of pregnancy would improve, while TTP/HUS does not. Glucocorticoids and aspirin are also treatment considerations with TTP/HUS. Supportive therapy and a multidisciplinary team approach are of key importance in the management of these patients.

Volume Depletion

Hemorrhage is the most common cause of volume depletion sufficient to cause AKI in pregnancy. Rarely, hyperemesis gravidarum may cause severe volume depletion that results in renal injury.

Obstetric hemorrhage can occur in any trimester, during the labor and delivery process, or postpartum. Uterine blood flow increases dramatically over the course of pregnancy approaching approximately 1,000 cc/min at full term; thus, obstetric hemorrhage can be massive and rapid. In the first and second trimesters, bleeding may be due to ectopic pregnancies or induced or spontaneous abortions. In the third trimester, placenta previa and placental abruption are common reasons for severe blood loss. Placenta previa refers to implantation of the placenta over the internal os of the cervix, rendering the woman at high risk for hemorrhage particularly with contractions and dilation of the cervix. Expectant management is an option for women with small amounts and self-limited vaginal bleeding; however, delivery by cesarean section is warranted for severe hemorrhage. Placental abruption refers to the separation of the placenta from the uterine wall. This can lead to fetal distress or death. In addition, a large or complete abruption is associated with substantial blood loss and disseminated intravascular coagulation, both risk factors for maternal AKI. Postpartum hemorrhage is most commonly caused by uterine atony which is the inability of the uterus to contract after delivery and stop bleeding from the vascular sinuses. Medical and

Acute Kidney Injury During Pregnancy. Table 3 Differential diagnosis of preeclampsia, acute fatty liver of pregnancy, TTP, and HUS[a]

	Preeclampsia/HELLP	Thrombotic thrombocytopenic purpura (TTP)	Hemolytic uremic syndrome (HUS)	Acute fatty liver of pregnancy
Onset	Usually third trimester	Median 23 weeks	Often postpartum	Close to term
Primary/unique clinical manifestation	Hypertension and proteinuria	Neurologic symptoms	Renal involvement	Nausea, vomiting, malaise
Purpura	Absent	Present	Absent	Absent
Fever	Absent	Present	Absent	Absent
Hemolysis	Mild	Severe	Severe	Mild
Platelets	Variable (normal or low)	Low	Variable (normal or low)	Variable (normal or low)
Coagulation studies	Variable	Normal	Normal	Prolonged abnormal
Hypoglycemia	Absent	Absent	Absent	Present
vWF multimers	Absent	Present	Present	Absent
Primary treatment	Delivery	Plasmapheresis	Plasmapheresis	Delivery

[a]The diagnosis may be confusing. Presence or absence of above features is not absolute, but may assist in the diagnosis. Precise diagnosis can often be made only after delivery. Preeclampsia, HELLP syndrome, and acute fatty liver of pregnancy resolve soon after delivery

conservative surgical therapies may be used to improve uterine tone and reduce blood loss; hysterectomy may be required for intractable bleeding. For any obstetric hemorrhage, aggressive initial and ongoing fluid resuscitation, replacement with blood and blood products, as well as correction of any coagulopathy are critical in preventing AKI and progressive renal damage.

Infection/Sepsis

Sepsis can lead to decreased renal perfusion secondary to hypotension and intravascular volume depletion as well as acute tubular necrosis. Pyelonephritis, chorioamnionitis (intrauterine infection), and pneumonia are the most common causes of sepsis during pregnancy. Pyelonephritis occurs in 1–2% of pregnant women with the increased risk attributed to the physiologic alterations including ureteral dilation secondary to smooth muscle relaxation, pressure on the ureters and bladder from the enlarging uterus, and possible increased susceptibility in pregnancy to endotoxin-mediated tissue damage. Pyelonephritis is also associated with a reduced glomerular filtration rate in pregnancy, which can compound the risk of AKI. The most common bacterial pathogen is E. coli. Other common pathogens are bowel commensals such as Klebsiella, Proteus, and enterococcal species. Significant maternal and fetal complications can occur with pyelonephritis warranting prompt diagnosis and treatment. Chorioamnionitis, an intrauterine infection involving the chorion and amniotic membranes, is quite common in pregnancy (0.5–10.5% of all deliveries); fortunately, bacteremia occurs in only 1–5% of these cases, with sepsis being even less common. Bacterial organisms ascending from the vagina, through the cervix, and into the uterus are the most common cause of infection. This is often a polymicrobial infection with common organisms being E. coli, group B streptococcus, Gardnerella species, peptostreptococcus, and anaerobes, to name a few. Globally, septic abortion is a major contributor to sepsis and AKI.

In general, treatment of sepsis consists of supportive measures including hydration, pressor support if needed, and antimicrobial therapy. Initial therapy with broad-spectrum antibiotics based on local and hospital microbiology and susceptibility information is recommended. Directed antibiotics based on culture and sensitivities may follow. For cases of chorioamnionitis and septic abortion, antibiotic penetration of the uterine cavity is inadequate and evacuation of the uterine contents is also necessary.

Obstruction

Although a rare cause of PR-AKI, the gravid uterus can cause urinary tract obstruction, particularly when overdistended as with polyhydramnios (high amniotic fluid volume), multiple gestation, or fibroids. Women with a solitary kidney, abnormal genitourinary tract, or prior urinary tract surgery are particularly susceptible to AKI related to obstruction. Nephrolithiasis may also cause obstruction and AKI. Ultrasound is used for initial evaluation but pyelogram and computed tomography (CT) scan may also be used for diagnosis and are generally safe in pregnancy. Treatment options include cystoscopy with retrograde ureteral stent placement or percutaeous nephrostomy. Delivery, as a treatment option, may be considered based on gestational age and response to other therapies.

Amniotic Fluid Embolism

Amniotic fluid embolism or "anaphylactoid syndrome of pregnancy" is a sudden and catastrophic pregnancy-specific event that can lead to AKI. Major features are abrupt and fulminant onset of respiratory failure, hypoxemia, cardiogenic shock, and disseminated intravascular coagulation. While the incidence is low at 7.7 per 100,000 births, the maternal mortality has been estimated to be 22%, with estimates in older studies of greater than 60%. Rapid resuscitation in the intensive care setting with respiratory and cardiovascular support, as well as intravascular volume resuscitation with correction of the coagulapathy can reduce multiorgan damage and mortality.

Other Causes of AKI Not Specific to Pregnancy

By far, pregnancy-specific causes of AKI, particularly during the third trimester, comprise the vast majority of PR-AKI. However, other causes of AKI coincident to pregnancy must be considered (discussed in detail elsewhere in this text and Refs. [4, 5]). Glomerulonephritis and autoimmune conditions such as systemic lupus erythematosus are particularly common in women of reproductive age. Differentiating between acute glomerulonephritis and preeclampsia may be particularly difficult in the late second and early third trimester. Some distinguishing features are summarized in Table 4.

Prognosis and After-care

Although overall maternal mortality associated with ICU admission is estimated to be 5–20%, maternal deaths related to AKI alone are rare. Overall, the prognosis for PR-AKI is good, with the majority undergoing complete or near complete renal recovery after the underlying cause of AKI is treated. Preexisting hypertension or renal disease are risk factors for requiring long-term RRT [3]. Women with residual renal insufficiency following AKI must be

Acute Kidney Injury During Pregnancy. Table 4 Features that may help differentiate preeclampsia and acute glomerulonephritis[a]

	Preeclampsia	Acute glomerulonephritis
Gestational age	Onset usually in the third trimester (by definition after 20 weeks')	Any
Hypertension	Present	Present
Systemic manifestations (may or may not be present)	• Neurologic (headache, scotomata, visual disturbances, seizures) • Hematologic (low platelets) • Hepatic involvement (elevated transaminases)	• Collagen-vascular disease (e.g., systemic lupus erythematosus with associated symptoms such as fatigue, arthralgias, rash, fevers) • Preceding infection (e.g., streptococcal infection)
Urine sediment	• Isolated proteinuria • Urine microscopy generally benign, may have findings of acute tubular necrosis (brown granular casts, renal tubular cells)	• Hematuria, RBC casts, oval fat bodies
Proteinuria	>300 mg/24 h (mild), >5 g/24 h (severe)	>2 g/24 h
Complement levels	Normal	↓
ANA	Normal	↑
Antistreptolysin-O titers	Normal	↑
Other autoantibodies	Generally normal	↑

[a]The diagnosis may be confusing. Presence or absence of above features is not absolute, but may assist in the diagnosis

followed closely with appropriate management of blood pressure and possibly renoprotective medications to prevent further decline of renal function.

Economics

Fortunately, the incidence of PR-AKI has declined to less than 1% of all pregnancies, largely attributable to the decline in illegal abortions and improved prenatal care and timely recognition and treatment of hypertensive disorders of pregnancy. The precise costs specifically related to PR-AKI are difficult to quantify as the renal injury is often a secondary outcome related to obstetric conditions such as preeclampsia or hemorrhage. The costs of neonatal care must also be considered.

References

1. Thadhani R, Pascual M, Bonventre JV (1996) Acute renal failure. N Engl J Med 334:1448–1460
2. Mehta RL, Kellum JA, Shah SV, Molitoris BA, Ronco C, Warnock DG, Levin A (2007) Acute kidney injury network. Acute injury network: report of an initiative to improve outcomes in acute kidney injury. Crit Care 11:R31
3. Jeyabalan A, Conrad KP (2010) Renal physiology and pathophysiology in pregnancy. In: Schrier RW (ed) Renal and electrolyte disorders, 7th edn. Lippincott Williams & Wilkins, Philadelphia, pp 418–474
4. Gammill HS, Jeyabalan A (2005) Acute renal failure in pregnancy. Crit Care Med 33(Suppl):S372–S384
5. Deering SH, Seiken GL (2004) Acute renal failure. In: Dildy GA III, Belfort MA, Saade GR, Phelan JP, Hankins GD, Clark SL (eds) Critical care obstetrics, 4th edn. Blackwell, Malden, pp 372–379

Acute Kidney Insufficiency

▶ AKI, Epidemiology of

Acute Myocardial Dysfunction

▶ Heart Failure Syndromes, Treatment

Acute Myocardial Infarction (MI)

▶ Coronary Syndromes, Acute

Acute Myocardial Inflammation

▶ Myocarditis and Acute Cardiomyopathies

Acute Pancreatitis

An inflammatory process of the pancreas, usually of sudden or rapid clinical onset, and typically presenting as upper abdominal pain with elevated levels of pancreatic enzymes in the blood.

Acute Phase Proteins

Are made by the liver during illness and infection to help the immune system.

Acute Pulmonary Edema

▶ Acute Heart Failure: Risk Stratification

Acute Pulmonary Embolism

▶ Pulmonary Embolism

Acute Quadriplegic Myopathy

▶ Mobility/Exercise, Early in ICU

Acute Radiation Syndrome

▶ Radiation Poisoning

Acute Renal Dysfunction

▶ AKI, Epidemiology of

Acute Renal Failure

▶ Acute Kidney Injury Biomarkers, Concept of
▶ AKI, Concept of
▶ AKI, Epidemiology of
▶ Kidney Injury, Acute

Acute Renal Failure of the Newborn

▶ AKI in the Newborn

Acute Renal Injury

▶ AKI, Epidemiology of

Acute Renal Insufficiency

▶ AKI, Epidemiology of

Acute Renal Insufficiency in Pregnancy

▶ Acute Kidney Injury During Pregnancy

Acute Respiratory Distress Syndrome (ARDS)

Acute lung injury of severe degree.

▶ Burns, Pneumonia

Acute Respiratory Distress Syndrome and Acute Lung Injury

JOAN R. BADIA
Unitat de Vigilancia Intensiva Respiratòria, Servei de Pneumologia, Institut Clínic del Tórax, IDIBAPS and CIBER de enfermedades respiratorias, Hospital Clínic de Barcelona, Barcelona, Spain

Synonyms

Adult respiratory distress syndrome; Diffuse alveolar damage; Respiratory distress syndrome; White lung

Definition

The acute respiratory distress syndrome (ARDS) was described in modern times by Ashbaugh et al. in 1967. They identified a series of 12 cases of a disorder characterized by sudden onset of tachypnea, diffuse pulmonary infiltrates on chest radiograph, devastating respiratory failure with hypoxemia, and decreased lung compliance. This syndrome is associated with a variety of precipitating factors, which cause lung injury by both direct and indirect mechanisms. Since its initial description ARDS has been recognized as a specific pathophysiological entity. However, patients with ARDS include a mixed population as regards clinical presentation, risk factors, and outcome.

In 1994 the results of a consensus conference by the American-European Consensus Committee (AECC) on ARDS were published [1]. This international expert panel defined ARDS as an entity associated with specific risk factors, that had a sudden onset and was characterized by hypoxemia [ratio of arterial partial pressure of oxygen to fraction of inspired oxygen (PaO_2/FIO_2) $\leq$ 200 mmHg] with bilateral infiltrates on chest radiograph in the absence of left atrial hypertension or clinical evidence of left heart failure (Table 1). In an attempt to identify early stages of the disease or less severe cases, the conference also defined the category of acute lung injury (ALI). This category included those patients meeting the abovementioned criteria but with a lower threshold of oxygenation impairment (PaO_2/FIO_2 $\leq$ 300 mmHg). The definition of the AECC was designed to be used in both clinical practice and research.

ARDS is a relevant health issue. It is a common condition that affects only the USA more than 100,000 patients per year, generating an estimation of more than a million days of hospital admission and occupation of beds in intensive care units (ICUs). The attributable mortality is also very high. In observational studies in unselected populations, the mortality rates are between 30% and 60%. In addition, those who survive often suffer a decline in health-related quality of life that can persist years after hospital discharge.

Acute Respiratory Distress Syndrome and Acute Lung Injury. **Table 1** AECC definition for ALI and ARDS

	Oxigenation[1]	Chest radiology	PWCP[2]
ALI	PaO_2/FIO_2 ratio $\leq$ 300 mmHg	Bilateral AD	$\leq$ 18 mmHg
ARDS	PaO_2/FIO_2 ratio $\leq$ 200 mmHg	Bilateral AD	$\leq$ 18 mmHg

ARDS and ALI have an acute onset and occur in the presence of risk factors. PCWP: pulmonary capillary wedge pressure.
[1]Oxigenation impairement is assessed regardless of the level of PEEP.
[2]Abscence of clinical data suggesting left heart failure as cause of the pulmonary infiltrates.

Characterization of ARDS

There is scientific evidence and general agreement on the fact that all patients with ARDS share a number of common features. First, ARDS occurs after exposure to known and well-established risk factors, and does not occur in their absence. ARDS is also a disease that presents with acute onset and is persistent over time. A key clinical feature is the presence of bilateral air space disease infiltrates on chest radiography. Figure 1 shows the radiography of a patient with ARDS. Finally, the severe disruption of gas exchange, with refractory hypoxemia, and decreased pulmonary compliance are also hallmarks of ARDS. The pathophysiology and the intimate mechanisms involved in the development of ARDS are extraordinarily complex and, to date, our understanding is still very incomplete. All these mechanisms are directly related to the initiation of an inflammatory cascade involving a wide variety of pathways, inflammatory cells, mediators, cytokines, chemokines, and the endothelium of the alveolar–capillary barrier and alveolar epithelium itself. This diversity has led some authors to consider the differentiation of ARDS in different pathologies, both in terms of triggering risk factors, type of injury on the lung (direct injury to the lung parenchyma or indirect injury), duration or clinical course of disease (early or late persistent), among others.

In its initial stage, ARDS is characterized by the presence of diffuse alveolar damage (DAD) involving both the epithelial layer and the vascular endothelium at the level of

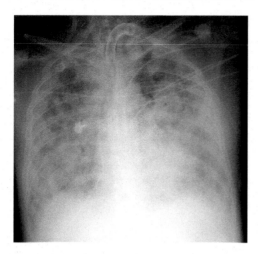 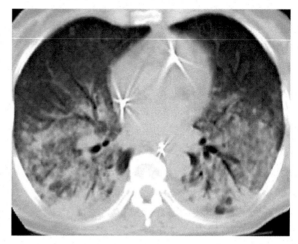

Acute Respiratory Distress Syndrome and Acute Lung Injury. Figure 1 Radiology in ARDS. The Chest radiography shows bilateral diffuse involvement with an air-space disease pattern. The computerized tomography of the thorax (right panel) shows that the infiltrates and consolidation predominate in dorsal regions of the lung, while anterior regions remain aerated

the alveolar–capillary membrane. The result is edema and alveolar flooding with fluid rich in proteins, inflammatory cells, and hemorrhagic material, leading to the formation of hyaline membranes and fibrosis. All these changes progress and result in the loss of barrier function and impairment of lung gas exchange. Knowledge about the mechanisms involved in the development of this highly specific lung injury is still limited. We do not have bio-chemical markers of inflammation, lung damage, or diffuse alveolar damage that may be helpful from the standpoint of clinical management of patients with ARDS. Moreover, in the vast majority of patients with ARDS it is not possible to obtain biopsies or lung tissue samples due to their critical condition. Thus, unlike what happens in other less acute and severe lung diseases, the identification of ARDS cannot be based on pathological examination. Therefore, the definition of ARDS is based on clinical observations and measures of changes in lung function, gas exchange, and mechanics caused by lung injury.

Risk Factors

As mentioned, the presence of specific risk factors as triggering events leading to the alveolar damage is a key element in the diagnosis of ARDS. The list of risk factors that have been associated with ARDS is extensive. Table 2 lists the most common of them. Sepsis has been one of the main risk factors associated with ARDS in different epidemiological studies. Approximately 30% of patients with

Acute Respiratory Distress Syndrome and Acute Lung Injury. Table 2 Risk factors for ALI and ARDS

Frequent	Less frequent
• Pneumonia	• Craneal trauma
• Bronchoaspiration	• Pulmonary contusion
• Sepsis	• Fat emboli
• Polytraumatism	• Toxic inhalation
• Multiple transfussion	• Substance abuse
	• Near drowning
	• Acute pancreatitis
	• Related to extracorporeal circulation
	• Pulmonay hemorrhage
	• Severe burns
	• Cardiopulmonary resucitation

severe sepsis or septic shock may develop ARDS or ALI. Viral and bacterial pneumonias are also a frequent cause for development of this complication. Polytraumatic patients with ARDS may develop a variety of mechanisms including direct trauma with pulmonary contusions, massive transfusions, or multiple bone fractures. In this subgroup of patients with ARDS the vital prognosis has improved notably in recent decades, coupled with advances in trauma care and general care of patients. Massive transfusion of blood products has also been identified as a risk factor for traumatic and nontraumatic patients. Some series have suggested that this may occur up to 25% of patients receiving 12 or more units of blood products. There is evidence that the incidence of ALI increases with storage time of transfused blood products. This type of transfusion-associated pulmonary injury is known as transfusion-related acute lung injury or TRALI (transfusion-related ALI). The patients with ARDS frequently have one or more of the risk factors described preceding the development of the syndrome. In the absence of risk factors differential diagnosis should be expanded and other causes of bilateral pulmonary infiltrates that may mimic ARDS have to be considered.

Diagnosis

The clinical expression in ARDS is related to the underlying cause and risk factors, the degree of the lung injury and the failure of other organs. The main signs and symptoms are those arising from respiratory failure. It is common to observe tachypnea, use of accessory muscles and increased work of breathing, and cyanoses among others. Arterial blood gases show severe arterial hypoxemia. The main pathophysiological mechanism of arterial hypoxemia in ARDS is the occurrence of shunt (pulmonary alveolar units well perfused but not ventilated). This is directly related to the occupation or consolidation of alveolar units by hyaline membranes and protein-rich fluid, together with collapse of dependent alveolar units. Simple chest radiography shows diffuse and bilateral alveolar infiltrates. Computed tomography of the chest demonstrates bilateral alveolar collapse and occupation predominantly of the dorsal regions of the lung, in dependent lower position on the supine patient [2]. Most patients require mechanical ventilation and characteristically show abnormal ventilatory mechanics, with a stiffer lung that is difficult to ventilate due to decreased lung compliance. Lung biopsy may be indicated in very much selected cases when the final diagnosis is unclear. However, because of the severity of respiratory failure it is not possible to consider the surgical procedure of the biopsy as a diagnostic method for most cases. At present the diagnosis is made when patients met the criteria described in the 1994 consensus definition of the AECC discussed earlier in this chapter. This definition is practical and has been used on a widespread basis. However, it has significant limitations that have been clearly demonstrated in recent years. One of the issues is the distinction between ALI and ARDS. The definition of ALI is intended to include patients with less severe forms of the same disease entity. The only difference between ALI and ARDS is the cutoff arbitrarily set oxygenation. However, the vast majority of patients with ALI progress and meet ARDS criteria

throughout its evolution, and on the other hand, other studies have shown a comparable mortality in cases of ARDS and ALI so this distinction is arguable. A second issue is the fact that the definition does not take into account the positive end expiratory pressure (PEEP) and dispenses with this in oxygenation criteria. PEEP is often used to recruit alveoli and open atelectatic lung units, improving gas exchange and oxygenation, and a direct impact on the relationship PaO_2/FIO_2 ratio. It is easy to understand whether a patient fulfilled ARDS criteria or not simply by varying the level of PEEP.

On the other hand rule out heart failure as underlying cause of pulmonary edema is not an easy task. Some studies question whether the use of pulmonary wedge pressure is the most effective method for this purpose.

Finally the reliability of radiographic criteria, bilateral infiltrates on frontal chest radiography, has been evaluated in several studies that show that the correlation between experts to identify ARDS is very moderate, with a suboptimal reliability between observers. One study compared the diagnostic performance of clinical parameters with autopsies on people who died and showed diffuse alveolar damage as a marker of ARDS. Diagnostic yield in sensitivity and specificity was not above 75% [3]. This study highlights the weaknesses of the definition and grouping of all patients who meet the definition of ARDS in the same category.

Treatment

The first step in treatment is always the identification and specific treatment, when possible, of the risk factor that triggers lung injury. This is particularly critical in the case of sepsis, where early treatment and control of the source of infection is essential to correct the systemic inflammatory response. The failure in this initial step perpetuates the inflammatory cascade and lung injury. Other than this a specific etiological treatment for acute lung injury and ARDS is not available. The most common cause of death in these patients is multiple organ dysfunction syndrome. Therefore, general supportive measures and organ failure treatment will be as important as the ventilatory support.

Mechanical Ventilation Strategy in ARDS

In ALI and ARDS support by noninvasive ventilation has been very inefficient. Thus, most patients will require intubation and conventional mechanical ventilation. Mechanical ventilation will be a key support measure to maintain respiratory function while lung damage resolves or improves. The current ventilatory strategy is based on two concepts: lung protection using a low tidal volume

(TV) and recruitment and stabilization of alveolar units using moderate levels of PEEP [4]. Conventionally, the use of a TV between 12 and 15 mL/kg of body weight has been considered the standard in mechanical ventilation. Subsequent studies have shown that the use of high TV induces overdistension and lung injury in healthy lungs and increases alveolar damage in patients with previous lung injury. In a lung with ARDS much airspace is collapsed or consolidated and mechanical ventilation overdistends the more preserved and aerated lung regions, aggravating lung injury, and inflammation. In simple terms, the lung-protective ventilation is based on ventilation with low TV to prevent alveolar overdistension of aerated areas. Moderate levels of PEEP are also applied to recruit alveoli and avoid cyclical collapse and reopening during the respiratory cycle. This strategy seeks to minimize induced lung injury, avoiding barotrauma (caused by high pressure in the respiratory system), the volutrauma (due to alveolar overdistention), and atelectrauma (due to instability associated with alveolar collapse and opening during mechanical ventilation). On the other hand there is some evidence suggesting that mechanical ventilation itself can induce an inflammatory response and promote systemic inflammation that may contribute to multiple organ dysfunction. Multiple randomized controlled trials have provided solid scientific evidence indicating that the use of lower tidal volume reduces mortality in patients with ARDS. The larger key studies are those carried out by a large collaborative research group that involves many hospitals in North America (ARDS Network). Data reported by these researchers and others are the basis of current recommendations for mechanical ventilation. The current state of the art for ventilation recommends the use of low TV (approximating 6 mL/kg of ideal body weight), and limiting airway pressure (plateau pressure or pressure after inspiratory pause as a measure of alveolar pressure below 30 cmH$_2$O). The modes of ventilation most commonly used are volume-controlled mode (CMV) or pressure (PCV). There are no studies to determine the superiority of either of these modes. Pressure is often used when mechanical alterations do not allow adequate alveolar ventilation and may improve removal of CO$_2$ and promote clinical stability in some cases. The use of PEEP is also a key element in mechanical ventilation in ARDS. The correct use of PEEP can recruit alveolar units and increase the proportion of ventilated lung to improve gas exchange. Moreover, PEEP also stabilizes the alveolar units to avoid the collapse and opening of the alveoli during the respiratory cycle which promotes more lung damage. There is no standardized approach to define the PEEP for each patient or a practical method to titrate. Several studies have helped to develop tables of PEEP adjustment based on the requirements of FiO$_2$ and level of PEEP and may be helpful in clinical practice, though, are based only on oxygenation parameters and do not take into account variables of respiratory mechanics.

Recruitment maneuvers have been proposed to achieve the opening of collapsed alveoli. Involve the application of high pressures in the air for a short period of time. It has been shown that these maneuvers improve oxygenation only transiently and do not seem to have greater advantages than the application of moderate PEEP continuously. Its routine use is not indicated and should be considered on an individual basis.

Hemodynamic Monitoring and Fluid Therapy

Hemodynamic monitoring using a pulmonary artery catheter does not get better results than conventional monitoring and is associated with increased incidence of complications. Therefore, the routine use of pulmonary artery catheter is not necessary. A fluid balance neutral or mildly negative is associated with a shorter duration of mechanical ventilation and stay in intensive care, although not to a significant reduction in mortality. International recommendations advice restriction of the entry of fluids and avoidance of a positive fluid balance when possible.

Other Rescue Therapies and Interventions

Prone Position

Placing patients with ARDS and ALI in the prone position can improve oxygenation and respiratory mechanics in approximately two thirds of the patients. The mechanisms involved include increased lung volume by recruiting the dorsal lung regions, redistribution of perfusion to ventilated areas and obtaining a more homogeneous distribution of ventilation. The outcome is best if applied early in the course of the disease (<48 h) and prolonged (most of the day initially). Several trials have currently failed to demonstrate an improvement in survival with this strategy and it should be considered an adjunctive measure. It is contraindicated in some situations such as pregnancy, head trauma or intracranial hypertension, pelvic or spinal fractures, hypotension, and hemodynamic instability.

Corticosteroids

The use of corticosteroids for the treatment of ARDS has been a controversial issue. It is an appealing possibility treatment as ARDS is primarily an inflammatory disease of the lung. Since the early 1990s several studies have focused on the use of steroids in ARDS, with often conflicting results. A recent large randomized controlled trial showed an improvement in oxygenation and lung compliance improved with corticosteroids. However, there was no difference in mortality at 60 days and a higher incidence of neuromyopathy was observed in the treatment arm of the study. Shorter series has shown a possible benefit in early administration of corticosteroids, but the level of evidence provided does not endorse the systematic indication at this time.

Ventilation with High Frequency Oscillation (HFOV)

The use of high frequency ventilation has been proposed as a ventilatory modality in this situation. High frequency ventilation (jet or oscillation) leads to high mean pressures that promite alveolar recruitment, while maintaining very low tidal volume s(1–3 mL/kg), avoiding overdistention of alveolar units. Several trials have shown that high-frequency oscillation ventilation achieves these goals, and can be used safely. However, increased survival with HFOV has not been demonstrated. Further controlled studies are in progress and more information needs to be obtained to support the systematic use of this strategy.

Others

Numerous other procedures and treatments have been studied and can improve specific physiological parameters, but have failed to improve survival or other relevant outcome measures. Examples of these are extracorporeal membrane oxygenation devices (ECMO). Studies with conventional ECMO in adults show a possible benefit, although trials have been performed only in highly selected subgroups of patients and in specialized centers. There are no randomized trials in adults regarding the use of more simple devices without external pump. These systems allow the removal of CO_2 and could be considered as a salvage procedure in patients with extreme hypercapnia, or as an adjuvant method to use extremely low tidal volumes. Experience with these devices is limited and indications should always be individualized in selected cases. Nitric oxide has also been tested in ARDS. The inhalatory administration of this gas with selective vasodilator effect on the pulmonary circulation improves PaO_2 in some patients but has not shown any effect on survival. The use of pulmonary surfactant in adults, liquid ventilation with perfluorocarbons, nonsteroidal anti-inflammatory drugs, ketoconazole, antioxidants, Almitrine, or inhaled prostacyclin has not demonstrated any efficacy in ARDS.

Prognosis

The ARDS mortality rate varies largely depending on the patient's age and the presence of associated organ dysfunction. In recent years, the overall impression of the intensive care community has been that associated mortality was actually decreasing due to improved general care, better mechanical ventilation practices, and increased awareness of the disease. Some recent studies have systematically evaluated the evolution of ARDS mortality over time suggests that this mortality has not really decreased as expected [5]. These data show a significantly lower mortality in highly selected patients included in randomized studies, compared with mortality in prospective case series without exclusion criteria. The current figures for expected mortality could be about 40% in the general population of patients with ARDS and 30–40% in selected patients included in RCTs. Among patients who survive lung function is recovered almost completely in 6–12 months but neuropsychiatric disorders and neuromuscular impairment are common sequelae in this group of critically ill patients [6].

References

1. Bernard GR, Reines HD, Brigham KL et al (1994) The American European consensus conference on ARDS: definitions, mechanisms, relevant outcomes and clinical trials coordination. Am J Resp Crit Care Med 149:818
2. Gattinoni L, Caironi P, Pelosi P, Goodman LR (2001) What has computed tomography taught us about the acute respiratory distress syndrome? Am J Respir Crit Care Med 164:1701
3. Esteban A, Fernandez-Segoviano P, Frutos-Vivar F et al (2004) Comparison of clinical criteria for the acute respiratory distress syndrome with autopsy findings. Ann Intern Med 141:440
4. Investigators ARDSnet (2000) Ventilation with lower tidal volumes as compared with traditional tidal volumes for acute lung injury and the acute respiratory distress syndrome. N Engl J Med 342 (1301):2000
5. Phua J, Badia JR, Adhikari NK et al (2009) Has mortality from acute respiratory distress syndrome decreased over time? A systematic review. Am J Respir Crit Care Med 179:220–7
6. Herridge MS, Cheung AM, Tansey CM et al (2003) One-year outcomes of the survivors of acute respiratory distress syndrome. N Engl J Med 348:683

Acute Respiratory Failure

▶ Acute Respiratory Failure, Mechanisms of

Acute Respiratory Failure, Mechanisms of

JOSÉ A. LORENTE, NICOLÁS NIN
CIBER de Enfermedades Respiratorias, Hospital Universitario de Getafe, Universidad Europea de Madrid, Madrid, Spain

Synonyms

Acute respiratory failure; Acute respiratory insufficiency

Definition

Acute respiratory failure (ARF) is diagnosed when the patient is unable to ventilate (maintain P_aCO_2 within the normal range) or to adequately oxygenate the blood (maintain P_aO_2 within the normal range).

Clinical presentation of ARF usually fits into one of four categories. Acute hypoxemic respiratory failure (or type I) causes hypoxemia mainly because of increased shunt fraction (Q_s/Q_t). Acute ventilatory respiratory failure (or type II) is characterized by hypoventilation and hypercarbia. Perioperative acute respiratory failure is caused by a number of factors including the formation of atelectasis due to reduced functional residual capacity, fluid overload, bronchospasm, or retained airway secretions (type III). Acute respiratory failure in hypoperfusion states is characterized by decreased mixed venous O_2 saturation ($S_{mv}O_2$) due to low cardiac output, hypovolemia, and increased oxygen consumption by respiratory muscles (type IV).

Ventilatory requirements are relative to the metabolic demand of the patient. In addition, ventilatory function depends on neuromuscular function. Thus, patients may have respiratory failure with normal lungs (i.e., inability to eliminate CO_2 in situations of increased CO_2 production, muscle weakness, or respiratory depression). Also, acute respiratory failure in hypoperfusion states is often characterized by normal intrinsic lung function.

Characteristics

Mechanisms of Hypoxemia

The five mechanisms of hypoxemia are: (i) low alveolar partial pressure of oxygen (P_AO_2), (ii) ventilation/perfusion (V/Q) mismatch, (iii) increased shunt fraction, (iv) diffusion abnormality, and (v) low mixed venous oxygen saturation ($S_{mv}O_2$). Differential diagnosis of the different causes of hypoxemia is of great clinical relevance to help diagnose the underlying condition and anticipate response to treatment (Table 1).

Low P_AO_2

Low P_AO_2 can be due to decreased FiO_2 (high altitude) or to hypoventilation (decreased P_ACO_2). The alveolar gas equation dictates

$$P_AO_2 = FiO_2(P_B - PH_2O_v) - P_aCO_2/R \qquad (1)$$

Where

P_AO_2 is alveolar PO_2, FiO_2 is fraction of inspired oxygen, P_B is barometric pressure (760 mmHg at sea level), PH_2O_v is the pressure of water vapor, and R is the respiratory quotient (R = 0.8). Thus, during hypoventilation for a given increase in P_ACO_2, P_AO_2 decreases, and consequently P_aO_2 decreases.

V/Q Mismatch

It is the most common cause of hypoxemia in ARF. V/Q mismatch occurs in conditions in which ventilated areas are poorly perfused (increased V/Q ratio), or certain areas normally perfused are poorly ventilated (decreased V/Q

Acute Respiratory Failure, Mechanisms of. Table 1 Mechanisms of hypoxemia

Mechanism of hypoxemia	A-a gradient	Response to increase in FiO_2	Common causes
Low P_AO_2			
– Decreased FiO_2	Normal	Yes	High altitude
– Hypoventilation	Normal	Yes	Narcotic overdose
V/Q mismatch	High	Yes	COPD
Shunt (Qs/Qt)	High	No	Pulmonary edema
Diffusion abnormality	High	No	Pulmonary fibrosis
Low $S_{mv}O_2$	High	No	Heart failure

P_AO_2: alveolar PO_2; A-a gradient: difference $P_AO_2-P_aO_2$; Qs/Qt: fraction of shunted blood flow relative to total blood flow; $S_{mv}O_2$: mixed venous oxygen saturation; COPD: chronic obstructive pulmonary disease

ratio, i.e., bronchospasm). The extreme abnormalities of V/Q mismatch are represented by shunt (perfused areas not ventilated at all, V/Q = 0) and dead space ventilation (ventilated areas not perfused at all, V/Q = ∞).

More than one mechanism may determine hypoxemia in a given condition. For instance, in COPD, V/Q mismatch may be the main determinant of hypoxemia, whilst the decreased P_AO_2 (due to increased P_ACO_2 because of respiratory center depression) will also contribute.

Shunt (Qs/Qt)

This may be intracardiac (as in right-to-left shunt) or intrapulmonary. Any condition resulting in occupation of the alveolar space (edema, pus, or blood) will result in increased shunt fraction.

The measurement of shunt fraction requires that the patient is breathing air at a FiO_2 of 100%. Any "shunt" measured with lower FiO_2 may represent venous admixture due to V/Q mismatch (areas with low V/Q). Hypoxemia due to low V/Q ratio will respond to increased FiO_2, and therefore is not a true shunt. Only hypoxemia due to true shunt (V/Q = 0) will not respond to increased FiO_2.

Diffusion Abnormality

It is not usually the cause of hypoxemia, unless the capillary blood transit time is shortened, as seen in high cardiac output states and tachycardia.

Low $S_{mv}O_2$

Pulmonary arterial blood becomes fully oxygenated in its pulmonary capillary transit regardless of its saturation ($S_{mv}VO_2$) (except under conditions of impaired capillary diffusion and decreased transit time). However, if alveoli are flooded, mixed venous blood is not adequately oxygenated. Under these circumstances, oxygenation becomes dependent on $S_{mv}O_2$.

Blood passing through functional alveoli, will increase its oxygen saturation to nearly 100% regardless of $S_{mv}O_2$. However, blood passing through nonfunctional alveoli will not increase its oxygen saturation. This non-oxygenated blood will mix with the fully oxygenated blood, and their combination will result in a given S_aO_2. Thus oxygen saturation of blood traversing nonfunctional alveoli equals $S_{mv}O_2$. The higher this value, the higher the saturation of venous blood once it has mixed with fully oxygenated blood.

$S_{mv}O_2$ can be boosted by increasing oxygen delivery or by decreasing oxygen consumption. This is the mechanism by which muscle paralysis, control of hyperthermia, fluid challenge, or inotropic drugs can improve gas exchange in

conditions characterized by increased shunt fraction such as the Acute Respiratory Distress Syndrome (ARDS).

Mechanisms of Hypercapnia

Ventilatory or hypecapnic respiratory failure occurs in situations in which the patient is unable to eliminate the CO_2 produced. Then P_aCO_2 rises and respiratory acidosis (high P_aCO_2, low pH) ensues.

In steady-state conditions, the rate of production of CO_2 equals the rate of CO_2 elimination. CO_2 elimination depends on alveolar ventilation (the amount of air coming in and out from the alveolar space each breath, V_AO_2) and on P_ACO_2. Since CO_2 readily diffuses cell membranes, and PCO_2 of inspired room air is zero, $P_ACO_2 = P_aCO_2$. Thus

$$VCO_2 = V_A * P_aCO_2 * K$$

where K = 0.86. Total tidal volume (V_T) in each breath is the sum of the air participating in gas exchange (alveolar air, V_A) and that not participating in gas exchange (dead space, both anatomic and physiologic, V_D). Thus

$$V_T = V_A + V_D$$

And therefore,

$$V_A = V_T - V_D,$$

and

$$VCO_2 = (V_T - V_D) * P_aCO_2 * K$$

Thus,

$$P_aCO_2 = VCO_2/(V_T - V_D) * K \qquad (2)$$

This equation helps understand the different causes of hypercapnia: (i) increased CO_2 production, (ii) decreased tidal volume, and (iii) increased dead space ventilation.

Hypoxemic Respiratory Failure

The major pathophysiological derangement in this type of respiratory failure is increased shunt fraction. Alveolar flooding explains that large alveolar units are excessively perfused for their degree of ventilation. Alveoli can be occupied by edema, pus, or blood. Thus pulmonary edema, pneumonia, and pulmonary hemorrhage are common causes of hypoxemic respiratory failure. Edema in the alveoli can be formed by increased capillary hydrostatic pressure (hydrostatic or cardiogenic pulmonary edema) or by increased capillary permeability (hyperpermeability or noncardiogenic edema, as it happens in ARDS).

The pressure respiratory muscles have to generate to distend the lungs are increased in these conditions. The negative pressure required for lung distention depends on (i) the resistive pressure (P_r), which is determined by airway resistance (R) and inspiratory flow rate (V_i) ($P_r = V_i * R$); (ii) the respiratory elastic recoil pressure (P_{el}), determined by the change in lung volume (ΔV) and lung elastance (E) ($P_{el} = \Delta V * E$). As elastance in increased, a greater P_{el} has to be generated, resulting in greater work of breathing and greater risk of muscle fatigue.

Therefore, these patients often require mechanical ventilation and high mean airway pressures to expand the lungs and maintain oxygenation.

Hypercapnic Respiratory Failure

Hypercapnic respiratory failure is a condition in which ventilation is insufficient to maintain normal P_aCO_2 for the level of CO_2 production (VCO_2). Hypercapnia is synonymous with alveolar hypoventilation. Causes of hypercapnia include increased CO_2 production, decreased tidal volume ventilation, and increased dead space ventilation. One of these three mechanisms explains hypercapnia in the different causes listed below. Decreased V_T is the cause of hypercapnia in decreased neuromuscular capacity (CNS, nerve, or muscle dysfunction). Increased VCO_2 or increased dead space ventilation are the cause of hypercapnia in conditions associated with increased ventilatory load.

Treatment goals in these patients differ from hypoxemic respiratory failure. In hypercapnic ventilatory failure treatment is directed to increase alveolar ventilation. If respiratory drive or muscle strength are decreased, mechanical ventilation is required to sustain ventilation until the cause has been treated. Hypoxemia is not a problem as it responds easily to increased FiO_2.

Patients with increased mechanical load (increased airway resistance) may also need mechanical ventilation as the increased ΔP required to sustain ventilation ($P_r = V_i * R$, see above) may lead to muscle fatigue.

Decreased Neuromuscular Capacity

Impairment in the neuromuscular component of respiration is seen in conditions characterized by decreased respiratory center output, muscle weakness, and muscle fatigue. Neuromuscular dysfunction leads to decreased V_T and therefore increased P_aCO_2 (see Eq. 2).

Decreased Respiratory Center Output

Decreased respiratory center output is characterized by decreased respiratory drive and normal muscle strength generation. Conditions associated with decreased respiratory center output include sedative overdose, hypothyroidism, metabolic alkalosis, semistarvation, and central alveolar hypoventilation (idiopathic – i.e., primary alveolar hypoventilation or Ondines′ curse-, or secondary to neurologic lesions such as trauma, infection, infarction, Shy-Drager syndrome, demyelination, and obesity hypoventilation syndrome). Severe hypercapnia depresses the CNS and decreases respiratory center output, aggravating hypercapnia, and in turn further depressing the respiratory center.

Respiratory Muscle Weakness

Respiratory muscle weakness is seen in chronic conditions such as a number of neuromuscular disorders (stroke, amyotrophic lateral sclerosis, spinal cord injuries, poliomyelitis, Guillain-Barré syndrome, neuropathies due to intoxication –arsenic, thallium-, acute intermittent porphyria, myasthenia gravis, acid maltase deficiency, muscular dystrophies), as well as in malnutrition, endocrine disturbances (hypo and hyperthyroidism, acromegaly), acidosis, renal failure, cancer, denervation, diabetes mellitus, and AIDS.

A number of acute conditions in the critically ill patient are associated with respiratory muscle weakness and may compromise ventilation, including trauma and burns, ventilator-associated muscle dysfunction, critical illness polyneuropathy, acid base disturbances, and decreased oxygen delivery.

Hyperinflation may comprise ventilation. In hyperinflation the inspiratory muscles work at unfavorable position of the length–tension relationship. The diaphragm is flattened and there is less zone of apposition, resulting in less effective contraction and less thoracic cage expansion. Also, the elastic recoil of the thoracic cage increases, as inspiratory muscles must work not only against the elastic recoil of the lung but also against the elastic recoil of the thoracic cage. Hyperinflation occurs in COPD (where it contributes to ventilatory failure), asthma, bronchiolitis, cystic fibrosis, and lymphangioleiomyomatosis. Other acute conditions such as pneumonia, ARDS, and chest trauma also present hyperinflation.

Respiratory Muscle Fatigue

Respiratory muscle fatigue occurs in conditions of an increased respiratory load applied over a long time. It may occur in acute bronchoconstriction, obesity, and during weaning from mechanical ventilation.

Increased Ventilatory Load

Increased ventilatory load may cause hypoventilation because of all three mechanisms: decreased V_T (mechanical load), increased VCO_2, and increased dead space ventilation.

In conditions of increased ventilatory load, normally operating compensatory mechanisms correct the hypercapnia. Thus hypercapnia cannot be explained solely based on these mechanisms and other causes must be sought to explain the increased P_aCO_2.

Increased Mechanical Load

Increased airway resistance, dynamic elastance, and intrinsic PEEP all contribute to increased respiratory load in patients with ARF. These changes are seen in rapid shallow breathing and in upper airway obstruction.

Increased Ventilatory Requirements

Increased ventilatory requirements occur in conditions associated with increased CO_2 production or increased dead space ventilation.

Increased CO_2 Production is seen in sepsis, trauma, burns, fever, drugs such as salicylates, and increased lipid utilization (which increases RQ).

Increased Dead Space Ventilation

Increased dead space ventilation occurs in patients with V/Q mismatch and areas of high V/Q ratio. Dead space in this context (also called physiologic dead space) refers to the sum of anatomic dead space (airway normally not participating in gas exchange, that is, the airway from the nose and mouth to bronchioles) and alveolar dead space (alveoli that receive little or no blood flow, with high V/Q ratio).

However, increased dead space ventilation does not cause hypercapnia by itself, as the normal response to increased P_aCO_2 is to increase minute ventilation to augment V_A and therefore keep P_aCO_2 within a normal range. Only those patients unable to increase alveolar ventilation will develop hypercapnia.

Increased dead space ventilation occurs in COPD, ARDS, and other lung diseases, most notably pulmonary thromboembolism.

Postoperative Acute Respiratory Failure

It is practical to identify this type of respiratory failure, although there is no single pathophysiological mechanism involved. Postoperative patients may have pain, fluid overload, respiratory depression because of sedative administration, increased intra-abdominal pressure, and muscle wasting. All these factors will lead to reduced FRC, increased alveolar closing volume, and lung collapse. Muscle fatigue and respiratory depression will result in alveolar hypoventilation. The end result will be both hypoxemic and ventilatory respiratory failure.

Acute Respiratory Failure in Shock

Patients in severe shock often present with respiratory failure requiring mechanical ventilation. Many factors

explain respiratory failure under these conditions. Patients with cardiogenic shock may have increased work of breathing due to pulmonary edema, low muscle flow resulting in impaired inspiratory muscle contraction, and low $S_{mv}O_2$ because of low cardiac output. In sepsis, V/Q mismatch, increased respiratory load (increased CO_2 production), increased respiratory drive, noncardiogenic pulmonary edema, and muscle dysfunction induced by endotoxin, cytokines, acidosis, electrolyte abnormalities, or drugs, all contribute to respiratory failure. Thus patients with shock require mechanical ventilation even though the lungs appear normal, until all underlying factors have been corrected.

Diagnosis

Hypoxemia

In airflow obstruction, alveolar occupation or interstitial disease, hypoxemia develops because large alveolar units are excessively perfused for their degree of ventilation (low V/Q ratio, increased venous admixture). Hypoxemia will respond to increased FiO_2 unless V/Q = 0 (true shunt).

In any of the listed causes of hypoxemia with impaired gas exchange (increased $P(A-a)O_2$) V_A is reduced because there are large numbers of alveoli poorly perfused causing increased dead space ventilation (increased V_D/V_T). However, hypercapnia does not ensue because total minute volume (V_E) increases to maintain a normal P_aCO_2. This is why these patients have to augment their respiratory rate to increase minute ventilation. A normal or high P_aCO_2 is an ominous clinical sign indicating muscle fatigue and the impending necessity of mechanical ventilation.

Thus, isolated impairment in gas exchange (in which A-a gradient is high) from any of the listed causes is not associated with hypercapnia. However, in conditions characterized by impairment in gas exchange, the magnitude of neuromuscular weakness or respiratory load that causes hypercapnia is less than that in the absence of abnormalities in gas exchange. These conditions favoring hypercapnia are usually characterized by V/Q mismatch, and total minute ventilation (V_T) is high despite a decreased alveolar ventilation.

Hypercapnia

In ventilatory ARF, hypercapnia is associated with mild hypoxemia, as P_AO_2 decreases for any increase in P_aCO_2 (see alveolar gas equation). In these cases, the alveolar–arterial PO_2 gradient ($P(A-a)O_2$) is normal, and hypoxemia is corrected by increasing the FiO_2.

Acute Respiratory Failure, Mechanisms of. Table 2 Differential diagnosis of hypercapnia

Normal P(A-a)O_2: alveolar hypoventilation with normal gas exchange
Normal muscle strength
Decreased respiratory drive
Increased mechanical load
Increased ventilatory load
Decreased muscle strength
Respiratory muscle weakness
Respiratory muscle fatigue
High P(A-a)O_2: alveolar hypoventilation with abnormal gas exchange
Airway disease (i.e., COPD)
Interstitial disease (i.e., pulmonary fibrosis)
Alveolar disease (i.e., ARDS)

Thus during hypercapnia the measurement of a normal P(A-a)O_2 is required to diagnose a nonpulmonary disorder (Table 2). These disorders are always characterized by low V_T. As a consequence, they are often associated with microatelectasis, retention of secretions and pneumonia, resulting in V/Q mismatch and a high P(A-a)O_2. Thus a high P(A-a)O_2 does not rule out a nonpulmonary cause of hypercapnia.

The diagnosis of hypercapnic ARF is based on the demonstration of an increased P_aCO_2 in arterial blood gases. However, many patients have chronic respiratory failure and an already high baseline P_aCO_2. To determine if the hypercapnia is chronic or acute (acute-on-chronic respiratory failure) the magnitude of the increase in serum bicarbonate has to be assessed.

As indicated above, among the different causes of hypercapnia, respiratory muscle weakness and fatigue are characterized by decreased muscle strength whereas decreased respiratory drive and increased mechanical or ventilator load have preserved muscle function.

References

1. Weinberger SE, Schwartzstein RM, Weiss JW (1989) Hypercapnia. N Engl J Med 321:1223–1231
2. Laghi F, Tobin M (2003) Disorders of the respiratory muscles. Am J Resp Crit Care Med 168:10–48
3. Manthous CA (2006) ARDS redux. Clin Pulm Med 13:121–127
4. Berger KI, Goldring RM, Rapoport DM (2009) Obesity hypoventilation syndrome. Semin Respir Crit Care Med 30:253–261
5. O'Donnell DE, Parker CM (2006) COPD exacerbations. 3: Pathophysiology. Thorax 61:354–361
6. Calverley PM (2003) Respiratory failure in chronic obstructive pulmonary disease. Eur Respir J Suppl 47:26s–30s

Acute Respiratory Insufficiency

▶ Acute Respiratory Failure, Mechanisms of

Acute Salicylate Toxicity

▶ Salicylate Overdose

Acute Severe Asthma

▶ Acute Asthma

Acute Toxic-Metabolic Encephalopathy

▶ Encephalopathy and Delirium

Acute Tubular Necrosis (ATN)

▶ AKI, Concept of
▶ Kidney Injury, Acute

Adenosine 2A Agonists in Acute Kidney Injury

RAMSEY J. DAHER, MARK D. OKUSA
Division of Nephrology and the Center for Immunity, Inflammation and Regenerative Medicine, University of Virginia Health System, Charlottesville, VA, USA

Trade Names
None

Class and Category
Anti-inflammation

Indications

None yet

Dosage

Not determined yet

Preparation/Composition

Not determined yet

Contraindications

Not determined yet

Adverse Reactions

Hypotension with high doses

Drug Interactions

Not determined yet

Mechanisms of Action

Pathogenesis of Acute Kidney Injury. Classically, acute kidney injury (AKI) due to ischemia results from unfavorable changes in renal blood flow as a consequence of vasospasm, alterations in ultrafiltration coefficient, tubular obstruction and/or back leak. Much progress has been made in defining mechanisms that contribute to ischemic AKI. The molecular responses that occur after reperfusion are likely maladaptive and lead to endothelial and epithelial cell injury. The reduction of renal blood flow causes an activation of bone marrow–derived immune cells, endothelial cells, and epithelial cells, and initiates a decline in GFR. Leukocytes then adhere to the endothelial cells, which leads to ▶ inflammation and extension of cellular injury (extension phase). In the early phase, ischemia and/or reperfusion initiate changes in vascular endothelial cells, tubular epithelial cells, and resident renal dendritic cells (DCs) that cause the loss of immune system homeostasis in the kidney [1]. As a result, leukocytes are attracted to and are activated within the post-ischemic kidney, potentiating the direct damage inflicted on kidney parenchymal cells by ischemia/reperfusion (IR). Compared to the early/innate response to kidney IR, less is known about the late phase of I/R injury (IRI) that necessitates the activation of the adaptive immune response. The late or adaptive immune response to specific antigens (from pathogens or dead endogenous cells) occurs over the course of several days and includes DC maturation and antigen presentation and CD4$^+$ and CD8$^+$ T lymphocyte proliferation and activation. Reparative processes likely involve participation of alternatively activated M2 macrophages, DCs, regulatory T (Treg) cells, and bone marrow–derived stem cells.

Adenosine 2A receptors. Adenosine is a nucleoside whose extracellular concentrations vary from 300 to 1,200 nM. Normally, the adenosine concentration in kidney is less than 1 µM; however, within 2 min of renal ischemia, adenosine concentration increases sixfold and its metabolite hypoxanthine increases 300-fold (see [2]).

Four subtypes of adenosine receptors have been cloned: A_1, A_{2A}, A_{2B}, and A_3 [1, 2]. Adenosine receptors are G-protein-coupled receptors and have seven transmembrane-spanning domains, an extracellular amino terminus, cytoplasmic carboxy terminus, and a third intracellular loop that is important in binding G-proteins. The human adenosine receptors share an overall identity of 30% at the amino acid level; the transmembrane domains of these four receptors are 45% shared. A_{2A} adenosine receptors stimulate adenylyl cyclase and increase the production of cyclic AMP by coupling to stimulatory G proteins (G_s) or to G(olf) in tissues in which G(olf) is expressed as the primary stimulatory G-protein. Serine/threonine protein phosphatase, mitogen-activated protein kinase (MAP kinase), protein kinase C, and phospholipase D might also participate in mediating the effects of A_{2A} receptor activation [2].

The functional characterization of the A_{2A} adenosine receptor has been aided by the development of selective pharmacological agents, a monoclonal antibody, molecular cloning of A_{2A} receptors, and generation of the A_{2A} receptor knockout mouse (as reviewed in [1, 2]). CGS21680 and ATL146 ester (e) [3] are selective A_{2A} agonists that have been used principally to examine the effect of A_{2A} receptor activation. The selectivity of ATL146e is due to substitutions at the C2 and 5' positions. Radioligandbinding studies indicate that ATL146e has a higher affinity for A_{2A} receptors than CGS21680 [4]. Additional characterization of the A_{2A} receptor has been aided by specific A_{2A} receptor antagonists, such as ZM241385 (refer to [3]).

Localization of adenosine A_{2A} receptors. A_{2A} receptors are expressed in both renal and nonrenal tissues. A_{2A} receptor mRNA has been detected in the outer medullary descending vasa recta as well as the glomerulus. Immunohistochemistry has also located A_{2A} receptors in cortical collecting duct of kidneys. Functional data indicate that A_{2A} receptor activation is involved in the control of glomerular filtration rate and causes vasodilatation of the descending vasa recta following preconstriction with angiotensin II. Additionally, afferent and efferent arteriolar vasodilatation in response to adenosine is blocked by the adenosine A_{2A} antagonist KF-17837. These results suggest that A_{2A} receptors modulate renal hemodynamics and could serve as important therapeutic targets. In nonrenal tissue, A_{2A} receptors are abundantly expressed in the brain (especially in caudate putamen), in hematopoietic tissues/cells including spleen, thymus, leukocytes, and platelets and, to a lesser extent, in heart, lung, and blood vessels. A_{2A} receptors are also expressed in many of the bone marrow–derived leukocytes such as neutrophils, lymphocytes, monocytes, mast cells, and basophils. Thus the expression of A_{2A} receptors in multiple tissues suggests a heterogeneous role in regulating important homeostatic cellular functions.

A_2 receptor activation blocks inflammation. Adenosine accumulates during ischemia in many different tissues. Although activation of A_{2B} and A_3 receptors mediate a proinflammatory response, activation of A_1 and A_{2A} receptors reduces inflammation and tissue injury. The expression of A_{2A} receptors on inflammatory cells allows adenosine to regulate inflammation. Thus, while infection or reperfusion injury activates the inflammatory process, activation of A_{2A} receptors attenuate inflammation and reduce injury. The proinflammatory process is necessary during infection and contributes to the successful eradication of pathogens. However, prolonged and unregulated inflammation that can occur following IR or infections may irreversibly damage tissue. During IRI, endogenous adenosine accumulates in response to hypoxia and probably has a crucial role in terminating an overactive immune system. This mechanism of adenosine-mediated dampening of inflammation is not unique to the kidney and has been seen in hepatic injury. Renal IRI is also more pronounced in A_{2A} receptor knockout mice compared with wild-type mice (as summarized in [1]). These data indicate that activation of A_{2A} receptors by endogenous adenosine functions to attenuate inflammation and tissue injury.

In vitro studies have generated insight into the mechanism by which A_{2A} receptor agonists block inflammation (as reviewed [1]). The abundant expression of A_{2A} receptors on immune cells is central to abrogating the inflammatory response. For example, adenosine works on activated neutrophils to decrease the levels of superoxide anion and hydrogen peroxide, both of which contribute to the inflammatory response. These anti-inflammatory effects of adenosine are A_{2A} receptor-mediated, as A_{2A} agonists such as CGS21680 and ATL146e attenuated the oxidative burst and release of superoxide anion from activated neutrophils. A_{2A} receptor agonists also block neutrophil adhesion to endothelial cells by inhibiting expression of $\alpha4\beta1$ integrin very late antigen (VLA)-4, which is normally present in activated neutrophils. Release of the proinflammatory cytokines TNF-α and IL-12 by macrophages is blocked by A_{2A} agonists; an effect that can be reversed via small interfering RNA to A_{2A} receptors.

The ▶ humoral immune response is delayed in comparison to the ▶ innate immune response initiated by the inflammatory cells discussed above. Antigen-specific signaling requires several interactions between the T cell and the antigen presenting cell (APC). The T cell receptor interacts with the MHC and antigenic peptide on the APCs, while costimulation may come from CD28 on T cells interacting with CD80 and CD86 proteins on the APC. T cell activation is associated with enhanced secretion of IFN-γ and IL-2 and expression of IL-2 receptor α chain (CD25), an effect that is blocked by A_{2A} agonists. TCR-mediated activation of T cells is associated with increased expression of A_{2A} receptor mRNA, which may indicate potential regulatory mechanisms for curtailment of activation events. Given the marked reduction of IFN-γ and IL-2 following A_{2A} receptor stimulation, A_{2A} agonists seem to target T_H1 cytokines.

A_{2A} receptors are involved in several mechanisms relating to acute kidney injury, which makes these proteins a prime target for treatment. Early studies showed that a systemic infusion of adenosine was actually detrimental to kidney function, as it led to vasoconstriction and a decrease in GFR (as reviewed [1, 2]). However, those effects were likely due to the activation of A_1 receptors. The discovery of A_{2A} receptor-specific compounds has shown that activation of A_{2A} receptors is protective in injury-reperfusion studies. Since the initial observation that A_{2A} receptor activation ameliorates renal IRI in rat kidneys [2], significant advances have been made in characterizing the mechanism and target of action. ATL146e markedly reduced damaging effects by ~70% when infusion was initiated prior to, or at the time of, IRI. Using the A_{2A} agonist DWH-145e (later renamed ATL146e) in rats attenuated IR, an effect reversed with ZM241385, a selective A_{2A} antagonist [2]. Tissue protection with the optimally effective dose of A_{2A} agonist (1–10 ng/kg/min) (as summarized in [1, 2]) was not due to any change in systemic blood pressure [4]. Protective effects of A_{2A} agonists have also been detected during IR of the heart, lung, and spinal cord, and in inflammatory bowel disease and sepsis (as reviewed [2]). These studies suggest that A_{2A} agonists may be useful in blocking common injury pathways in a wide variety of disorders.

Both in vivo and in vitro data suggest that A_{2A} agonists exert their protective effects through direct action on hematopoietic, endothelial cells or proximal tubule cells (as reviewed in [1]). Furthermore, this protective effect of adenosine A_{2A} receptor activation is mediated by increases in cAMP, as revealed by renal IRI studies with rolipram (a phosphodiesterase IV inhibitor) and ATL146e. Infusion of either drug alone reduced renal injury in a dose-dependent manner. Rolipram and ATL146e reduced myeloperoxidase activity, an enzyme marker of neutrophils, by 60% and 70%, respectively. However, the co-infusion of both compounds led to a reduction in plasma creatinine by 90% as well as a further decrease in MPO activity that was greater than either compound alone [1]. ATL146e's protective mechanisms were at least in part mediated through neutrophils. Using ATL146e caused a 70% reduction in neutrophil accumulation in kidney post-IRI as compared with vehicle-treated mice. Using high-resolution microscopy combined with flow cytometry, it was demonstrated that A_{2A} agonists reduce transmigration of neutrophils from the intravascular space to the interstitium and produce a decrease in vascular permeability. Additionally, the enhanced expression of the ▶ adhesion molecules P-selectin and ICAM-1 following IRI was reduced with A_{2A} agonists. This observation was consistent with the idea that A_{2A} agonists limit IRI due to an inhibitory effect on neutrophil adhesion.

Given the ubiquitous expression of A_{2A}Rs, the precise target of A_{2A} agonist action in mediating tissue protection in vivo was not known. In order to determine the target of action of A_{2A} receptor agonists, chimeric mice were generated by irradiating wild-type mice and repopulating their bone marrow with marrow from A_{2A} receptor knockout mice [5]. Therefore, these chimeric mice had a full complement of A_{2A} receptors in all tissues that normally express the proteins except bone marrow–derived cells. The protective effect of A_{2A} receptor agonists following ischemia reperfusion was absent from these chimeric animals, in contrast to the control group in which wild-type marrow was used to reconstitute the marrow of irradiated wild-type mice. These findings indicated that the primary target of A_{2A} receptor agonists is bone marrow–derived cells. Further studies demonstrated that activation of A_{2A} receptors expressed on CD4 cells and not macrophages mediated tissue protection [1].

Extracellular adenosine acts on A_{2A} receptors, which can raise cAMP, resulting in an inhibition of T-cell receptor triggered activation. Additional, T cells are likely inhibited by hypoxia inducible transcription factor 1α (▶ HIF-1α) through activation of the cAMP response element (CRE) and the hypoxia response element (HRE). These mechanisms work in concert to inhibit activated T-effector cells in damaged tissues.

Clinical applications. Currently A_{2A} agonists are not marketed for use in humans for the prevention or treatment of AKI in humans. There are minimal side effects associated with the A_{2A} agonist ATL146e due to its short half life (minutes) with the exception of transient hypotension in rats following bolus iv administration of ATL146e at dose levels of 3.5 and 6.9 µg/kg. However at doses that block inflammation (1–10 ng/kg/min used in IR studies), there were no hemodynamic effects. ATL146e is currently in phase III clinical trials for use in pharmacologic stress myocardial perfusion imaging and may find use as an alternative to dipyridamole or adenosine. Thus, future studies should be directed to humans in the treatment and prevention of AKI by A_{2A} agonists.

Conclusion

A broad-based anti-inflammatory strategy against AKI is an attractive therapeutic option. A_{2A} receptor agonists act proximally to disrupt the cascade of inflammation that occurs following reperfusion injury and might be a lead candidate for clinical trials.

References

1. Li L, Okusa MD (2006) Blocking the Immune respone in ischemic acute kidney injury: the role of adenosine 2A agonists. Nat Clin Pract Nephrol 2:432–444
2. Okusa MD (2002) A2A adenosine receptor: A novel therapeutic target in renal disease. Am J Physiol 282:F10–F18
3. Rieger JM, Brown ML, Sullivan GW, Linden J, Macdonald TL (2001) Design, synthesis, and evaluation of novel adenosine A2A receptor agonists. J Med Chem 44:531–539
4. Okusa MD, Linden J, Macdonald T, Huang L (1999) Selective A2A-adenosine receptor activation during reperfusion reduces ischemia-reperfusion injury in rat kidney. Am J Physiol 277:F404–F412
5. Day Y-J, Huang L, McDuffie MJ, Rosin DL, Ye H, Chen JF et al (2003) Renal protection from ischemia mediated by A2A adenosine receptors on bone marrow-derived cells. J Clin Invest 112 (6):883–891

Adhesion Molecules

Proteins located on the cell surface that mediate binding with other cells or with the extracellular matrix in the process called cell adhesion.

Adrenal Conditions, Hypercortisolism/ Hyperaldosteronism

RUI P. MORENO
Unidade de Cuidados Intensivos Polivalente, Hospital de Santo António dos Capuchos, Centro Hospitalar de Lisboa Central, E.P.E, Lisbon, Portugal

Introduction

The adrenal glands (also known as suprarenal glands) are two triangular-shaped endocrine glands that are located in the retroperiteneum, on top of the kidneys, one on each side. They main physiological task is the production and release of stress-related hormones. Each adrenal gland is separated into two distinct structures, the adrenal cortex and the adrenal medulla, both of which produce hormones. The cortex, that surrounds the medulla, mainly produces glucocorticosteroids (including cortisol), mineralocorticosteroids (aldosterone), and androgens (such as testosterone), under the regulation hormones produced by the pituitary gland and hypothalamus, as well as by the rennin-angiotensin-aldosterone system; the medulla mainly produces catecholamines, adrenaline (or epinephrine) and noradrenaline (norepinephrine), under control from the sympathetic system (and in a less extension by the cortisol released by the adrenal cortex).

The normal response during times of stress, as occurs during any critical illness, is an increased function of the adrenal cortex and of the adrenal medulla. The hormones produced by the adrenal cortex (e.g., glucocorticoids and aldosterone) are crucial in driving the physiological adaptation to illness in order to maintain the homeostasis. However, as for almost any other hormones, an inappropriate – sometimes fatal – increase in adrenal function could lead to major changes in fluid and electrolyte balance, in energy metabolism, and in immune function.

Hypercortisolism

The condition of hyperadrenocorticism is a disorder characterized by increased circulating levels of glucocorticoids (primarily cortisol). Usually an easily recognizable disorder, it may arise in clinical practice from three causes:

- An excess production by the pituitary gland of adrenocorticotropic hormone or corticotrophin (ACTH)
- An excess production of cortisol originating in the adrenal gland
- An iatrogenic administration or factitious ingestion of excessive doses of exogenously administered glucocorticoids

The description by Harvey Cushing of the disease included the existence of truncal obesity, hypertension, fatigability and weakness, amenorrhea, hirsutism, purplish abdominal striae, edema, glucosuria, osteoporosis, and a tumor of the pituitary gland. Two forms of the disease are usually considered: those in which the hyperproduction of cortisol is secondary to an hyperproduction of ACTH by the pituitary gland, with bilateral adrenal hyperplasia, the so-called *Cushing's Disease*; and those, in which the clinical manifestations result from the chronic exposure to excess glucocorticoids, independently from the source, the so-called *Cushing's Syndrome*. In these cases, the disease may be due to the ectopic overproduction of ACTH (from other tumors, most commonly the oat cell–type lung cancer, but also thymus, pancreas, ovary, and thyroid cancers), those in which the overproduction of cortisol is primary due to adrenal cancer (about 20–25% of the cases) or by the exogenous administration of ingestion of excessive doses of exogenously administered glucocorticoids [1]. The Cushing's syndrome is rarely an admitting diagnosis to critical care (except in the rare cases in which the syndrome presentation is due to severe hypokallemic alkalosis and glucose intolerance), but life-threatening infections, diabetes, and a high mortality rate in surgeries are all associated with chronic severe hypercortisolism.

The positive diagnosis of Cushing's Syndrome requires the biologically demonstration of chronic hypercortisolism, usually using 24-h urinary cortisol, urinary 17-hydroxysteroids (17-OHS), late-evening plasma or salivary cortisol, or the dexamethasone suppression test (either the short midnight 1 mg test or the classical 48-h-low-dose classical test). Characteristically, despite being sometimes very difficult to measure adequately in the ICU, the following laboratory findings are seen:

- Elevation in urinary free cortisol (usually greater than 150 µg/24 h).
- Loss of diurnal rhythm of plasma ACTH and cortisol (very difficult to access in the patient with critical illness due to the loss in circadian rhythm); evening cortisol levels are greater than 10 µg/dL; excretion of urinary 17-OHS also loses its daily rhythm.

- Loss of ACTH suppressibility by physiologic doses of dexamethasone (1 mg at midnight does not prevent the morning increase > 10 µg/dL or 0.5 mg every 6 h of dexamethasone for 48 h starting at 6 am). Urinary 18-OHS and 17-KS levels fall to less than 50% of control levels. This test can be complemented by the administration of Corticotropin-releasing hormone (CRH) as IV bolus at a dose of 1 µg/kg body weight and plasma cortisol and ACTH levels accessed at −15, −10, −5, and 0 min before administration and then at 5, 15, 30, 45, and 60 post CRF administration.

These exams are complemented by the determination of the plasma levels of ACTH and by imaging exams targeting the pituitary and the adrenal glands. Once excluded the exogenous chronic administration of glucocorticosteroids, a suppressed ACTH plasma levels indicate an adrenal cause to the syndrome either malign or benign; a measurable or increase ACTH plasma levels indicate usually a pituitary tumor (Cushing's Disease) or an ectopic production of ACTG of malignant origin. In rare cases, where the biological and imaging diagnosis are uncertain, sampling the ACTH plasma in the inferior petrosal sinus may be necessary.

Care should be taken to distinguish the true Cushing's syndrome from pseudo-Cushing states, usually with mild hypercortisolism, that include active alcoholism and withdrawal from ethanol intoxication, stressful situations, renal failure, anorexia and bulimia nervosa, the depressed phase of affective disorders, primary glucocorticoid receptor resistance, and severe obesity. In these cases, the dexamethasone-CRH test seems to be more accurate than the classical tests [2].

Given the high morbidity and mortality associated with the Cushing's syndrome, treatment should be initiated as soon as possible, targeting the correction of the adrenal oversecretion and the ablation and/or destruction of the tumor. The optimal treatment option is still surgical, and consists in the remotion of the responsible tumor, ideally with preservation of the anterior pituitary function, complemented sometimes by radiotherapy or in the surgical removal of the adrenal gland involved. The medical treatment of the condition is still not optimal due to the high rate of failure and secondary effects, and it can be done with medical treatments directed at the pituitary gland (with the PPAR-γ rosiglitazone, the dopamine agonist cabergoline, the new somatostatin analogue SOM-239 or with temozolomide, all experimental or with inconsistent results) or directed at the at the adrenal gland

(with Op'DDD, that specifically destroys the adrenal cortex; with inhibitors of cortisol synthesis such as metyrapone or ketoconazole; with glucocorticoid antagonists such as mifepristone). In some cases, total bilateral adrenalectomy has been used to suppress the steroidogenesis process. Also, in the intensive care setting, the only inhibitor of the steroidogenesis available in IV formulation, the sedative etomidate, has been used in the acute preparation of the patient intolerant to the other available therapies before the surgical removal of the tumor [3].

Hyperaldosteronism

The primary hyperaldosteronism is a syndrome of hypertension and hypokalemia that is responsible for 6–13% of the cases of hypertension in some referenced populations of the adult patients [4].

Although much more rare in the ICU that hypercortisolism, it should be suspected in patients with admission to ICU for management of troublesome hypertension, refractory or difficult to control hypokalemia, rapidly progressive heart failure, and various dysrhythmias. Suspicion of the diagnosis should always arise when these manifestations occur, particularly when hypokalemia is refractory to potassium supplementation. Without timely diagnosis and treatment, these patients will succumb to lethal dysrhythmias.

The etiology of the syndrome is in about 70% of the patients unilateral adenoma, in 20–30% idiopathic bilateral hyperplasia or, rarely, adrenocortical carcinoma.

The diagnosis can usually be made, measuring the aldosterone and rennin levels at 8 am (after overnight recumbence) and 4 h later (after the patient being upright for 4 h). These measurements should only be made when the patient on a diet that provides at least 100 mEq of NaCl a day after correction of the hypokalemia. Caution should be used when measuring the aldosterone/rennin ratio (ARR) to diagnose primary hyperaldoteronism and all drugs know to affect it stopped (e.g., beta-adrenergic blockers, nonsteroidal anti-inflammatory agents), diuretics (including potassium-sparing diuretics), dihydropyridine calcium channel antagonists, and angiotensin converting enzyme inhibitors and renin inhibitors, contraceptives and progesterone. Other factors might interfere with the test, such as age over 65, method of blood collection, renal function, and phase of the menstrual cycle in women [5]. There exists a certain variability among laboratories in the interpretation of the ratio among different groups, with cutoffs of the ARR as different as 20 and 100 being considered as positives (with plasma aldosterone expressed as ng/dL and plasma rennin as ng/mL/h). In doubt, the fludrocortisone test can be used as the confirmatory test [6].

Since surgically correctable forms of primary aldosteronism are characterized by unilateral aldosterone hypersecretion and renin suppression, it is important to diagnose and locate an aldosterone-producing adenoma (also known as Conn's adenoma and aldosteronoma), primary unilateral adrenal hyperplasia, and rare cases of aldosterone-producing adrenocortical carcinoma. In these forms, unilateral adrenalectomy can cure aldosterone excess and hypokalemia, but not necessarily hypertension. Once the diagnosis is confirmed, adrenal imaging methods should be performed for all patients. If surgery is considered, taking into consideration the clinical context and the desire of the patient, bilateral adrenal vein sampling may eventually be performed to detect whether or not aldosterone hypersecretion is unilateral because even the CT scan will miss 50% of the adenomas and incorrectly lateralize the adenoma in occasional cases [6].

The differential diagnosis of hypokalemic hypertension with low renin includes mineralocorticoid excess, with the mineralocorticoid being cortisol or 11-deoxycorticosterone, apparent mineralocorticoid excess, pseudohypermineralocorticoidism in Liddle syndrome or exposure to glycyrrhizic acid [4].

Prognosis is usually good if the tumor can be removed, with the majority of patients recovering significantly from the renal lesions of the hypertension, even when albuminuria is already present [7]. Patients with a raised ratio then undergo confirmatory suppression tests.

References

1. Bertagna X, Guignat L, Groussin L, Bertherat J (2009) Cushing's disease. Best Pract Res Clin Endocrinol Metab 23:607–623
2. Yanovski JA, Cutler GB Jr, Chrousos GP, Nieman LK (1993) Corticotropin-releasing hormone stimulation following low-Dose dexamethasone administration. A new test to distinguish Cushing's syndrome from pseudo-Cushing's states. JAMA 269:2232–2238
3. Dabbagh A, Sa'adat N, Heidari Z (2009) Etomidate Infusion in the critical care setting for suppressing the acute phase of Cushing's syndrome. Anesth Analg 108:238–239
4. Amar L, Plouin P-F, Steichen O (2010) Aldosterone-producing adenoma and other surgically correctable forms of primary hyperaldosteronism. Orphanet J Rare Dis 5:9
5. Stowasser M, Taylor PJ, Pimenta E, Al-Asaly Ahmed AH, Gordon RD (2010) Laboratory investigation of primary aldosteronism. Clin Biochem Rev 31:39–56
6. Rayner BL (2002) Screening and diagnosis of primary aldosteronism. Cardiovasc J SA 13:166–170
7. Sechi LA, Novello M, Lapenna R, Baroselli S, Nadalini E, Colussi GL, Catena C (2006) Long-term renal outcomes in patients with primary aldosteronism. JAMA 295:2638–2645

Adrenal Conditions, Insufficiency/Failure

DJILLALI ANNANE
General ICU, Raymond Poincaré Hospital (APHP), University of Versailles SQY, Garches, France

Synonyms

Adrenal failure; Adrenocortical insufficiency; Corticosteroid insufficiency; Critical illness related corticosteroid insufficiency; Relative adrenal insufficiency

Definition

Adrenal insufficiency is a condition in which cortisol synthesis, delivery, and/or uptake by tissues is compromised. It is classified into primary adrenal insufficiency when the adrenocortical cells are damaged or cortisol metabolism is altered and secondary adrenal insufficiency when corticotrophin releasing hormone or adrenocorticotrophin hormone synthesizing hypothalamic or pituitary cells are damaged. In primary adrenal insufficiency, impaired mineralocorticoid synthesis is common. Secondary adrenal insufficiency may be associated with failure of other pituitary axes in particular of the thyroid and gonad axes.

The term "critical illness related corticosteroid insufficiency" (CIRCI) has been recently introduced to replace the term "relative adrenal insufficiency" [1]. It is characterized by a situation of insufficient cellular corticosteroids activity for the severity of patient's illness, i.e., for the intensity of the systemic inflammatory response.

Treatment

Symptomatic Treatment

One of the main complications of adrenal insufficiency is hypovolemia and salt wasting. Thus, immediate fluid and sodium replacement are required. In addition, intravenous vasopressor therapy should be titrated to restore systolic blood pressure and tissue perfusion.

Hormone Replacement Therapy

Mechanisms of Action of Corticosteroids

Glucocorticoids cross freely the cells membrane to interact with a specific glucocorticoid receptor in the cytosol [2]. Activation of the glucocorticoid-glucocorticoid receptor complex triggers conformational changes with dissociation from other proteins (particularly shedding from heat shock proteins) and dimerization, allowing the translocation of the complex to the nucleus and interaction with general transcription factors, adapter proteins, and various co-activators, resulting in transrepression (indirect genomic effects) and transactivation (direct genomic effects) properties. Glucocorticoids also interact with membrane sites inducing non-genomic effects.

Genomic Effects

The glucocorticoid-glucocorticoid receptor complex directly activates or represses target genes by binding to hormone responsive elements in promoter or enhancer regions and by binding to other DNA sequence-specific activators. Glucocorticoids transactivated genes for chemokines, cytokines, complement family members, and innate immune-related genes, including scavenger and Toll-like receptors. They also transrepressed adaptive immune-related genes, and may simultaneously transactivate and repress inflammatory T-helper subsets and apoptosis-related gene clusters. The interaction between glucocorticoids, NF-kB, and activator protein-1 represents the main glucocorticoid-induced, DNA-independent mode of transrepression. In addition, the induction of IkB-alpha by glucocorticoids further inhibits NF-kB-dependent gene transcription. Glucocorticoids may also regulate inflammatory mediators by acting at the post-transcriptional level, on mRNA or on proteins.

Non-genomic Effects

Non-genomic effects may be nonspecific or specific. Nonspecific effects include direct membrane effects of glucocorticoids in the hypothalamic synaptosomes controlling the negative feedback loop, rapid restoration of the sympathetic modulation of cardiac and vessels activity, and potentiation of exogenous catecholamines action. Specific non-genomic effects include interaction between the glucocorticoid-glucocorticoid receptor complex and p38 mitogen-activated protein kinase, interaction between membrane binding sites for glucocorticoids and mitochondrial membrane potential, and nonnuclear activation of phosphatidylinositol 3-kinase and of protein kinase Akt.

Main Effects of Corticosteroids

Metabolic Effects

Corticosteroids increase blood glucose concentration by inducing insulin resistance at the level of skeletal muscles and adipocytes, liver neoglucogenesis, and glycogenolysis. Thereby, corticosteroids divert glucose toward insulin-independent tissues such as neurons and inflammatory cells. They also enhance lipolysis and proteolysis, providing amino acids for neoglucogenesis.

Immune Effects

Corticosteroids increase neutrophils count by releasing bone-marrow polymorphonuclear cells and by inhibiting neutrophils migration and apoptosis. They promote apoptosis of eosinophils and basophils and improve opsonization and the activity of scavenger systems. They suppress the synthesis and release of inflammatory mediators such as cytokines, nitric oxide, prostaglandins, and leukotrienes.

Corticosteroids block dendrite cell maturation, interfere with antigens presenting cells, and prevent differentiation of CD4+ T cells into T-helper (Th) 1 lymphocytes by blocking the IL-12 secretion monocytes/macrophages and dendritic cell. They promote Th2 recruitment by increasing IL-10 secretion acting in synergy with IL-4. Thus, Corticosteroids induce a shift from cellular toward humoral immune response.

Cardiovascular Effects

Corticosteroids interact with cardiac and vessels smooth muscles, maintaining vascular tone, endothelium integrity, capillary permeability, and myocardial inotropic activity. Corticosteroids act in synergy with norepinephrine and angiotensin II. Immediate corticosteroids effects on the cardiovascular system are likely non-genomic resulting from direct intra-cellular calcium mobilization, or activation of endothelial nitric oxide synthase via the P38 mitogen-activate protein kinase or the phosphatidylinositol 3-kinase/protein kinase system.

Observed Clinical Effects During Critical Illness

In various critical illnesses, including sepsis, acute respiratory distress syndrome, trauma, postoperative patients, corticosteroids reduced clinical and biological symptoms of exaggerated systemic inflammatory response, reduced the need for vasopressor therapy or mechanical ventilation, prevented the development of organ dysfunction and fasten the resolution of established organ failures, shortened length of stay and may improve survival [1].

Practical Use of Corticosteroids

Intravenous administration of hydrocortisone is the gold standard for the treatment of adrenal insufficiency. Critical illness related corticosteroid insufficiency should be treated with 200–300 mg of hydrocortisone given as intravenous bolus of 50 mg q6 or 100 mg q8, or as a continuous infusion of about 10 mg/h. The duration of treatment may be adapted to specific conditions and logically hydrocortisone therapy should be given as long as symptoms of CIRCI are present. In septic shock, hydrocortisone therapy should be given for 5–7 days at full dose and may or may not be tapered off over 3–6 days [1, 3]. In acute lung injury, corticosteroids may be given for up to 4 weeks. Administration of fludrocortisone is optional and requires advice from an endocrinologist.

Tolerance

Corticosteroids dramatically increased blood glucose to levels that may affect patients' morbidity and mortality. Therefore, during corticosteroid therapy it is paramount that blood glucose levels are maintained lower than 150 mg/dL by the means of continuous insulin therapy. Corticosteroids with mineralocorticoid activity may cause hypernatremia, hypokalemia, and metabolic alkalosis. Therefore, a close monitoring of serum electrolytes levels and acid–base equilibrium is mandatory in corticosteroid-treated intensive care unit patients. Corticosteroids replacement therapy may not increase the risk of hospital-acquired infections in critically ill patients. However, this treatment may blunt the febrile response to infection and interferes with white cells count and inflammatory parameters. Then, corticosteroids replacement therapy may mask the acquisition of a new infection. Physicians need to systematically screen for lung superinfection with daily chest X-ray and lung cultures twice weekly, for blood stream infection with blood cultures twice weekly, for urinary tract infection with cultures twice weekly, as well as screening for any other potential new site of infection. Indeed, corticosteroids, early enteral nutrition, and stress ulcer prophylaxis should be carefully considered to prevent gastrointestinal bleeding [1, 3].

Evaluation/Assessment

Risk Factors for Adrenal Insufficiency in the Intensive Care Unit

Systemic Inflammatory Response Syndrome

Various critical illnesses may be associated with adrenal insufficiency. In fact, any condition that is characterized by an exaggerated systemic inflammatory response likely is associated with CIRCI [1]. Sepsis is probably the most common cause of adrenal insufficiency in the intensive care unit. Sepsis-induced pro-inflammatory mediators activate the hypothalamic-pituitary-adrenal axis via multiple pathways including afferent fibers of noradrenergic and vagus nerves, and circum ventricular organs [2]. In sepsis, the accumulation of pro-inflammatory mediators

interferes at all levels of the hypothalamic-pituitary-adrenal axis to decrease cortisol synthesis. In turn, the resulting adrenal insufficiency favors the accumulation of pro-inflammatory mediators in a vicious circle. Sepsis may also result in low levels of cortisol binding globulin and albumin, with increasing circulating free cortisol levels. However, the cortisol cannot be appropriately delivered to inflamed tissues without its specific carrier. Other mechanisms of tissue resistance to corticosteroids may include down regulation of the glucocorticoid receptor alpha or decrease in its affinity for cortisol, and over expression of the 11 beta hydroxysteroid dehydrogenase.

Shock, Kidney Failure, and Coagulation Disorders

The adrenal glands are characterized by limited venous drainage and thus the increased arterial flow during critical illness results in prompt enlargement of the glands subsequently exposing them to hemorrhage and necrosis. Cardiovascular or renal failure, bacteremia, coagulation disorders, and the use of anticoagulant drugs are the main risk factors for adrenal hemorrhage and necrosis.

Drugs

A number of drugs may alter cortisol production and metabolism [1, 2]. In brief, previous treatment with glucocorticoids even topical form of the drug may induce a prolong suppression of the hypothalamic-pituitary-adrenal axis. Several drugs that are commonly used in the intensive care unit may also inhibit cortisol synthesis. They may include sedatives, particularly etomidate (specific inhibitor of the 11-β-hydroxylase), or antibiotics, particularly antifungal drugs.

Clinical Diagnosis

Common clinical symptoms of adrenal insufficiency like fever, abdominal pain, vomiting, hypotension, or altered consciousness are very common and nonspecific signs in intensive care unit patients. However, intensive care unit physicians should consider adrenal insufficiency in patients with hypotension poorly responsive to fluid replacement or vasopressor therapy, with sustained signs of overt organ inflammation (e.g., persistent acute respiratory distress syndrome), or with difficulties to be weaned from life-supportive therapies.

Laboratory Investigations

Nonspecific Laboratory Tests

Hypoglycemia, hyponatremia, hyperkalemia, and increased eosinophils count are commonly found in adrenal insufficiency and should alert intensive care unit physicians. However, these abnormalities are nonspecific and insufficient to decide for hormone replacement therapy.

Specific Laboratory Tests

Although there is no definite test for the diagnosis of adrenal insufficiency in critically ill patients, in practice, physicians should rely on the standard short corticotrophin test [1]. The insulin tolerance test cannot be used in the intensive care unit. Firstly, this test is cumbersome and requests trained physicians and nurses. Secondly, insulin resistance is very common in critical illness, thus, lowering the reliability of the insulin tolerance test, and increasing the risk of severe hypoglycaemia given the on/off response type. The overnight metyrapone test is also cumbersome and dangerous for a routine use in critically ill patients. This test relies on evaluation of increase in plasma concentrations of corticotrophin and 11B deoxycortisol after metyrapone-induced fall in cortisol levels. It is unlikely that corticotrophin and 11 B deoxycortisol could be measured in a timely fashion. In addition, metyrapone by blocking cortisol synthesis may rapidly worsen patient's hemodynamic status and may precipitate death. The standard high dose corticotrophin remains the most practical test for the diagnosis of adrenal insufficiency during critical illness. It consists in measuring cortisol before and 30 and 60 minutes after following an intravenous bolus of 250 μg of ACTH. It is considered that a basal cortisol level lower than 10 μg/dL or a post corticotrophin increment in cortisol <9 μg/dL is suggestive of CIRCI [1, 4]. In patients with low albumin levels, total cortisol levels are less reliable and because free cortisol levels could not be obtained in a timely fashion, the diagnosis of adrenal insufficiency in these patients may remain problematic. Determination of salivary concentrations of free cortisol is not ready for routine use in the intensive care unit. Finally, computed tomography scan can help demonstrate damage to the adrenal glands.

After-care

In most cases of CIRCI, patients recover a normal adrenal function after recovery from their critical illness [1, 2]. In rare cases of irreversible anatomic damages to the hypothalamic-pituitary-adrenal axis, patients remain dependent of hormonal replacement therapy. In practice, patients should be weaned off corticosteroids a priori being discharged from the intensive care unit. If the cessation of treatment is associated with rebound in signs of systemic inflammatory response, new onset of shock or respiratory failure, intensive care physicians should seek for advices from an endocrinologist to rule out or to optimize the treatment of a persistent adrenal failure.

Prognosis

In animals, removal of the adrenal cortex increased dramatically endotoxin-related mortality whereas destruction of the medulla with intact cortex has no effect on mortality. It is known for almost a century that bilateral necrosis of the adrenals precipitated death in patients with severe infection. Numerous observations have convincingly shown that chemical adrenalectomy (e.g., with prolonged infusion of etomidate) increased mortality in critically ill patients. Critically ill patients with CIRCI are more likely dependent of vasopressor therapy and mechanical ventilation hospital mortality reaching 60% [1, 4].

References

1. Marik PE, Pastores SM, Annane D, Meduri GU, Sprung CL, Arlt W, Keh D, Briegel J, Beishuizen A, Dimopoulou I, Tsagarakis S, Singer M, Chrousos GP, Zaloga G, Bokhari F, Vogeser M (2008) Recommendations for the diagnosis and management of corticosteroid insufficiency in critical ill adult patients: consensus statements from an international task force by the American College of Critical Care Medicine. Crit Care Med 36(6):1937–1949
2. Prigent H, Maxime V, Annane D (2004) Science review: mechanisms of impaired adrenal function in sepsis and molecular actions of glucocorticoids. Crit Care 8:243–252
3. Annane D, Bellissant E, Bollaert PE et al (2009) Corticosteroids in the treatment of severe sepsis and septic shock in adults: a systematic review. JAMA 301:2362–2375
4. Annane D, Maxime V, Ibrahim F, Alvarez JC, Abe E, Boudou P (2006) Diagnosis of adrenal insufficiency in severe sepsis and septic shock. Am J Respir Crit Care Med 174:1319–1326

Adrenal Failure

▶ Adrenal Conditions, Insufficiency/Failure

ß-Adrenergic Antagonist Toxicity

BRENNA M. FARMER
Division of Emergency Medicine, Weill Cornell Medical Center, New York, NY, USA

Synonyms

ß-Blocker toxicity

Definition

ß-adrenergic agonism occurs with stimulation of the ß-receptor. The ß1 receptor is mainly located in the heart and results in increased heart rate (tachycardia) when stimulated. Medications that stimulate ß1-receptors are used to increase chronotropy and inotropy in the heart. The ß2-receptor is located in the vasculature and lungs. Its stimulation results in vasodilatation and bronchodilation. Medications that stimulate ß2-receptors are used to treat conditions associated with bronchoconstriction such as asthma or chronic obstructive pulmonary disease. Agonism of ß3-receptors is rarely discussed for medical conditions. ß-agonists like albuterol are used to move potassium into cells when hyperkalemia is present.

ß-adrenergic antagonists are medications used to treat and or manage several medical conditions including: hypertension, coronary artery disease, congestive heart failure, atrial fibrillation, migraines, and other chronic headaches. They are used to control heart rate and blood pressure. These medications include: atenolol, carvedilol, esmolol, labetolol, metoprolol, and propanolol as well as many others. These medications are often discussed as being selective for β1-receptors (such as atenolol, esmolol, or metoprolol) versus having no selectivity (such as propanolol). Carvedilol and labetolol also have some α-1 receptor antagonist effects.

ß-adrenergic antagonist toxicity is a spectrum of signs and symptoms that can include: depressed mental status or coma, bradycardia and/or conduction delays, hypotension, seizures, hypoglycemia, hyperkalemia, metabolic acidosis from lactate production, and multisystem organ failure due to poor perfusion [1]. Toxicity occurs after intentional overdose or therapeutic misadventures.

Some ß-receptor antagonists have varying effects on the sodium channel. These antagonists are known as "membrane-stabilizing" ß-blockers and include propanolol, oxprenolol, acebutolol, and others. Their toxicity profile may include specific toxicities associated with sodium channel blocking effects. Specific effects include widening of the QRS on the electrocardiogram and ventricular dysrhythmias.

Treatment

All patients presenting with ß-adrenergic antagonist toxicity should be managed as a critically ill patient. They should have their airway, breathing, and circulation assessed. The airway should be secured with endotracheal intubation and mechanical ventilation as clinically indicated. Supplemental oxygen should be administered to all patients at risk for poor perfusion from ß-adrenergic antagonist toxicity. All patients should have intravenous access secured, preferably with two large-bore peripheral intravenous lines (either 14 or 16 gauge) to allow for rapid fluid resuscitation if necessary. Patients with hypotension should receive initial intravenous fluid resuscitation with isotonic fluid (normal saline or lactated Ringers). All patients should have an electrocardiogram performed to evaluate for bradycardia, other dysrhythmias, and conduction abnormalities. They should be connected to telemetry and have continuous heart rate and blood pressure monitoring to assess for development of dysrhythmias, hypotension, and deterioration.

The next step in managing these patients is to consider gastrointestinal decontamination. For patients with a normal mental status who are protecting their airway, activated charcoal (1g/kg) should be given orally. For patients with endotracheal tubes, a nasogastric (NG) tube should be placed and activated charcoal (1 g/kg) should be administered through the NG tube. The administration of activated charcoal is to try to decrease the amount of ß-adrenergic antagonist absorbed into the blood stream from the gastrointestinal tract. If a sustained release, controlled release, extended release, or other long-term release product was ingested, whole bowel irrigation with polyethylene glycol with electrolyte solution (PEG ELS) can be initiated through an NG tube to try to increase the gastrointestinal transit of the ß-adrenergic antagonist and thereby, hopefully, decreasing the absorption into the blood stream. For severely poisoned patients with recent ingestions, orogastric lavage with a large-bore tube (Ewald tube) may be considered as a form of decontamination. For unstable patients, resuscitative measures should supersede gastrointestinal decontamination. Once stabilized, these critically ill patients may benefit from gastrointestinal decontamination.

For patients presenting with bradycardia advanced cardiac life support measures should be initiated. As a first-line agent, atropine can be given. It acts to stimulate the vagus nerve and thereby increase inotropy and chronotropy. When patients do not respond to this therapy, calcium salts should be considered.

Calcium salts (gluconate, if given peripherally due to it being less irritating on the vein; chloride, if a central venous catheter is in place) increase chronotropy and inotropy. They bypass the antagonized ß-receptor to stimulate release of calcium from the sarcoplasmic reticulum to affect excitation-contraction coupling, provide necessary substrate for generation of action potentials from the sinoatrial node, and aid in the maintenance of vascular tone [2]. Calcium gluconate delivers one-third the milliequivalents of calcium compared to calcium chloride. This difference must be a consideration when using calcium gluconate.

Glucagon

Glucagon is a hormone synthesized in the pancreatic α cells and is generally considered a first-line agent (or antidote) for ß-adrenergic antagonist toxicity. It directly stimulates the G-protein on the blocked ß-adrenergic receptor complex. It bypasses the blocked ß-receptor and allows activation of the adenylate cyclase pathway to increase cyclic AMP intracellularly. This increase in cyclic AMP results in excitation-contraction coupling through release of calcium from the sarcoplasmic reticulum. Thereby, glucagon increases inotropy and chronotropy on a ß-adrenergic antagonized heart. Peripherally, it also increases the amount of glucose available for cardiac myocytes and vascular smooth muscle cells to use as an energy source. Recommended doses range from 3 to 10 mg as intravenous boluses and from 3 to 10 mg/h when given as infusions. Infusion rates are set at the milligram rate that a patient responds to (i.e., if a patient improves with a 5 mg bolus dose, an infusion rate of 5 mg/h glucagon should be given) [2]. The major adverse effects from glucagon are nausea and vomiting. Symptomatic control with an antiemetic may be necessary.

Insulin-Euglycemia Therapy

This therapy, sometimes described as hyperinsulin-euglycemia therapy or HIET, is used in patients refractory to the above measures. It is often used in combination with other discussed therapies. Insulin is secreted by the pancreatic β-islet cells to allow for the utilization of glucose as a cellular energy source. During times of stress, the heart shifts from using free fatty acids to glucose for metabolic function. In multiple canine models and case reports, HIET has shown improvement in cardiac function with increased contractility and blood pressure. Insulin is usually given as a 1 unit/kg intravenous bolus followed by an infusion at 0.5 unit/kg/h, which is titrated by 0.5 unit/kg upward as needed. It usually takes 30–60 min to see any effect from this therapy. To maintain euglycemia in these patients, a dextrose infusion is also often initiated to maintain the patient's serum glucose between 100 and 250 mg/dL [2]. Patients must also have their serum potassium monitored as insulin causes potassium to shift into the cells. Supplementation may be required to keep serum potassium at near normal or normal concentration. When patients are titrated off HIET, potassium concentrations usually return to normal.

Adrenergic Agonists: Vasopressors

Dopamine, norepinephrine, and or epinephrine may be required if a patient has refractory hypotension despite the above measures. These agents increase heart rate by increasing inotropy. They increase blood pressure by increasing chronotropy and peripheral vasoconstriction. Echocardiography or invasive cardiac monitoring may aid in the choice of a particular vasopressor. Often, these agents are used in conjunction with the above measures. Vasopressin is rarely used or mentioned in the literature for ß-adrenergic antagonist toxicity. Use of any vasopressor may increase the risk for gut or extremity ischemia as a result of severe peripheral ischemia due to the amount needed to keep the heart rate and blood pressure at desirable ranges, particularly if used alone.

Intravenous Lipid Emulsion

Intravenous lipid emulsion therapy has been introduced as a "last resort" therapy for patients' toxic from lipid soluble drugs/toxins. This antidote was first introduced for bupivacaine and local anesthetic toxicity, but has been studied for calcium channel antagonists, lipid soluble ß-antagonists, and numerous other lipid soluble toxins with resulting cardiac toxicity. Use of this therapy is generally reserved for those patients not responding to the above therapies or who deteriorate to cardiac arrest despite the above measures. There are two basic theories as to why this intervention may work for lipid soluble ß antagonist toxicity (such as from propanolol). The first theory suggests that the lipid emulsion creates a lipid compartment in the blood to draw the lipid soluble drug off the ß-receptor and sequesters it so that it cannot interact with the receptor to cause toxicity. The second theory suggests that the lipid provides energy in the form of free fatty acids to the cardiac myocyte to improve heart function. Several animal experiments and case reports supporting the use of this therapy can be found on the web site www.lipidrescue.org. The recommended dose is a bolus injection of 1.5 mL/kg of 20% intravenous fat emulsion, followed by an infusion of 0.25 mL/kg/min over 30–60 min. The initial bolus may be repeated 1–2 times if asystole persists and the infusion may be titrated upward if blood pressure remains low (www.lipidrescue.org).

Sodium Bicarbonate

Sodium bicarbonate as an intravenous bolus of 1–2 mEq/kg may benefit patients experiencing a widened QRS, ventricular dysrhythmias, or severe hypotension from the membrane-stabilizing ß-adrenergic antagonists. If this therapy is used, patients should have their serum potassium monitored as sodium bicarbonate can induce hypokalemia. Patients should also be monitored on telemetry if this therapy is used, as hypokalemia can increase the risk of torsades de pointes.

Extraordinary Measures and Hemodialysis

In patients severely poisoned from ß-adrenergic antagonist ingestion, the above therapies may not improve their condition. These patients may require extraordinary measures such as an intra-aortic balloon pump or extracorporeal mechanical oxygen until the drug is metabolized (out of the body) and toxicity resolves. Atenolol, sotalol, and nadolol are water-soluble and may be removed by hemodialysis. Case reports are available supporting the use of these measures.

Evaluation/Assessment

All patients presenting with possible or potential for ß-adrenergic antagonist toxicity should have their vital signs monitored. An intravenous catheter should be placed and laboratories for whole blood counts, electrolytes, renal function, lactate, liver function, and troponin sent for analysis. These studies will allow for evaluation of systemic hypoperfusion from toxicity. An electrocardiogram should be obtained as a screen for cardiac dysrhythmias including bradycardia or conduction abnormalities. Sinus bradycardia and first-degree heart block are common in patients who develop symptoms from their ß-blocker exposure [3]. An observation period of 6 h is recommended for patients who have ingested a regular release ß-receptor antagonist. If the patient maintains normal vital signs, mental status, and physical examination, he/she may be medically cleared for evaluation by psychiatry. A 24-h observation period is recommended for any patient ingesting any sustained-, extended-, or controlled-release product as these products may cause delayed toxicity. All symptomatic patients should be monitored in a unit with intensive care capabilities.

Epidemiology

ß-adrenergic antagonist exposures are reported to poison control centers every day. In the 2008 National Poison Data System report, there were 21,282 cases mentioning ß blockers with 9,787 exposures to ß-blockers. Out of the 1,315 deaths related to a poisoning, six deaths were deemed due to a ß-blocker (as a single agent). ß-adrenergic antagonists exposures involved 54 cases with major effects while 653 cases resulted in moderate effects (based on the NPDS categories) [4]. Propanolol, metoprolol, atenolol, labetolol, and the generic label of

"ß-blocker" were among the ß-adrenergic receptor antagonists mentioned in those cases resulting in fatalities and or major or moderate effects [4]. A study done evaluating 11 years of reports to the NPDS from 1985 to 1995 revealed 52,156 ß-blocker exposures with 164 cases resulting in death [5]. Propanolol was the most commonly implicated ß-blockers in fatal cases [5].

Prognosis

The prognosis of these patients depends on their underlying comorbidities, amount ingested, time to recognition and treatment of ingestion, response to therapy, and availability of intensive care.

References

1. Heath A (1984) ß-adrenoceptor blocker toxicity: clinical features and therapy. Am J Emerg Med 2:518–525
2. Kerns W II (2007) Management of ß-adrenergic blocker and calcium channel antagonist toxicity. Emerg Med Clin N Am 25:309–331
3. Love JN, Enlow B, Howell JM et al (2002) Electrocardiographic changes associated with ß blocker toxicity. Acad Emerg Med 40:603–610
4. Bronstein AC, Spyker DA, Cantilena LR et al (2009) 2008 Annual report of the American Association of Poison Control Centers' National Poison Data System (NPDS): 26th Annual Report. Clin Toxicol 47:911–1084
5. Love JN, Litovitz TL, Howell JM et al (1997) Characterization of fatal ß blocker ingestion: A review of the American Association of Poison Control Centers data from 1985 to 1995. J Toxicol Clin Toxicol 35:353–359

Adrenocortical Insufficiency

▶ Adrenal Conditions, Insufficiency/Failure

Adsorption

CLAUDIO RONCO[1], ZACCARIA RICCI[2]
[1]Department of Nephrology, St. Bortolo Hospital, Vicenza, Italy
[2]Department of Pediatric Cardiac Surgery, Bambino Gesù Children's Hospital, Rome, Italy

Synonyms

Flow distribution; Hemoperfusion; Isotherm; Mass separation; Sorbents; Synthetic polymers; Zeolites

Definition

The possibility of removing solutes from blood in order to obtain blood purification by means of the physical-chemical principle of adsorption.

Pre-existing Condition

Both the characteristics of some solutes that make their removal difficult, and the limited efficiency of some dialysis membranes, have spurred a significant interest in the use of further mechanisms of solute removal such as adsorption [1]. Materials with high capacity of adsorption (sorbents) have been utilized for about 50 years in extracorporeal blood treatments. The evolution in knowledge and clinical use of sorbents can be summarized in Table 1.

The analysis of the molecular structure of a sorbent as well as the study of the chemical–physical mechanisms involved in the process of adsorption are fascinating and may contribute to understand the potential for clinical application [2].

Application

Basic Principles

The mixing of chemicals to form a mixture is a spontaneous, natural process accompanied by an increase in entropy or randomness. The inverse process of separation of that mixture into its constituent species is not a spontaneous process and requires an expenditure of energy. If the mixture comes as two or more immiscible

Adsorption. Table 1 Development of sorbents in extracorporeal blood therapies

1850 First inorganic allumosilicates (zeolites) used to exchange NH4 & Ca
1910 Water softeners using zeolites display instability in presence of mineral acids
1935 Adams and Holmes synthetize the first organic polymer ion exchange resin
1950 Application of synthetic porous polymers (styrene or acrylic acid based) (Spherical beeds: trade names of Amberlyte, Duolite, Dowex, Ionac and Purolite)
1960 Manipulation of physical-chemical characteristics (commercial use)
1970 Application in blood purification techniques such as hemoperfusion
1980–2000 Improved design and coating for better hemocompatibility of adsorbent materials
2000 and beyond: Search for new sorbent materials and new possibilities of application

phases we can use gravity, pressure, or electrical fields, but if it exists in a single homogeneous phase different processes must be applied such as:

- Separation by phase addition or creation (distillation, crystallization, desublimation)
- Separation by barrier (reverse osmosis, dialysis, microfiltration, ultrafiltration)
- Separation by solid agent (adsorption, chromatography, ion exchange)
- Separation by external field or gradient (electrodialysis, electrophoresis)

In clinical settings, blood purification techniques mostly rely on the second and the third group of processes [3]. While, however, diffusion and convection are mostly used for membrane filtration processes, adsorption is generally employed in blood detoxification techniques such as hemoperfusion. Diffusion may be limited by the diffusion coefficients of the molecules or by other factors such as temperature, surface area, and distance. Convection on the other hand is mostly limited by the sieving properties of the membrane and the flux of solvent obtained in response to a positive pressure gradient. When these processes are inadequate to remove the wanted molecules from patient's blood, the use of adsorbents may become the alternative pathway for blood purification. Hemoperfusion is in fact a technique in which patient's blood is circulated through a unit containing a sorbent material. Blood purification is obtained by absorption of molecules on to the sorbent particles. Sorbents can be synthetic or natural. In the past, problems related to hemoperfusion were mostly due to the incompatibility of the biomaterial used as a sorbent. In fact, the first sessions of hemoperfusion were accompanied by chills, fever, cutaneous rush, thrombocytopenia, leucopenia, and Aluminum load.

Today, these reactions are prevented in two ways: (a) separating plasma from red cells and circulating only the separated plasma through the sorbent bed; (b) making the sorbent bio or hemocompatible by coating the particles with specific biomaterials.

If the use of sorbents is quite justified in poisoning or acute intoxications, is there a rationale for the use of sorbents in chronic or acute blood purification techniques? The efficiency of membrane separation processes in hemodialysis is limited by membrane permeability. To overcome this problem, high flux membranes have been introduced. However, the efficiency for solutes of middle-high molecular weight is limited by the low diffusion coefficients of those solutes. A further improvement has come with hemodiafiltration and even better with on-line hemodiafiltration where the high rate of ultrafiltration increases significantly middle-high solute clearance. Nevertheless, the possible selectivity of adsorptive processes, and the possibility of placing the sorbent in direct contact with blood may be seen as a further step toward increasing the efficiency of the blood purification process.

The sorbent however must be hemocompatible and adequately coated, size-dependent nonselective adsorption may cause unwanted losses and a completely different kinetics for middle-large molecules could be expected in comparison to that commonly observed in hemodialysis.

To make an adequate adsorbent therapy one needs an effective and safe sorbent material, an adequately designed sorbent cartridge and finally an optimal utilization of the available surface of the sorbent [1].

Sorbent Materials and Structure

Sorbents can be found in nature as raw materials or they can be synthetically produced in the laboratory.

Natural sorbents such as Zeolites (Alumino silicates) are inorganic porous polymers with porosity deriving from their crystal structure (today they can be synthetically modified to control the structure of the internal pore system). Other typical sorbents such as porous carbons, are cellulose-derived organic polymers prepared by controlled thermal oxidation (Fig. 1).

Synthetic sorbents are constituted by different polymers of synthetic origin. Almost all polymerizable monomers can be built up into large molecules via a multitude of reactions. Difunctional monomers tend to aggregate in linear polymeric structures while high functional monomers tend to polymerize in cross linked structures. Divinylbenzene is generally used as a potent crosslinker (Fig. 2). They can also exist in forms of granules or fibers that are functionalized with specific substances (Fig. 3).

Sorbents exist in granules, spheres, cylindrical pellets, flakes, and powder. They are solid particles with single particle diameter between 50 µm and 1.2 cm. Surface area to volume ratio is extremely high in sorbent particles with a surface area varying from 300 to 1,200 m^2/g. They can also be defined as (a) macroporous = pore size > 500 Å (50 nm), (b) mesoporous = pore size 20–500 Å, and (c) microporous = pore size < 20 Å.

The surface to volume ratio is enormous and it is generally described by the following equation:

$$S/V = \pi d_p L \left(\pi d^2_p L / 4 \right) = 4 d_p \qquad (1)$$

where d_p = pore diameter and L = pore length. If ε_p = fractional particle porosity and ρ_p = particle density the specific surface area per unit of mass S_g is

$$S_g = 4 \varepsilon_p / \rho_p d_p \qquad (2)$$

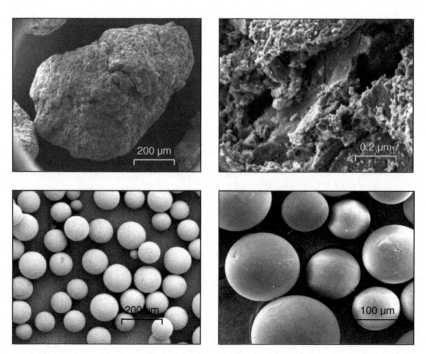

Adsorption. Figure 1 Scanning electron microscopic view of a natural sorbent (uncoated charcoal) at different magnifications (*top panels*) and of a synthetic polymer in granules (*bottom panels*)

Sorbents

Natural   Synthetic

Zeolites (alumino silicates)   Almost all polymerizable monomers
  Inorganic porous polymers   can be built up into large molecules
  with porosity deriving from their   via a multitude of reactions
  crystal structure (today synthetically
  made to control the structure of the   Difunctional monomers
  internal pore system)
                                           Linear

Porous carbons   High functional monomers
  Cellulose-derivedorganic
  polymers prepared by controlled   Cross
  thermal oxidation   linked

                                          Divinylbenzene (potent crosslinker)

Adsorption. Figure 2 Description of sorbent characteristics and distinction between ▶ natural and synthetic sorbents

A   Styrene + divinylbenzene   Three-dimensional polymeric network

B

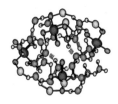

Copolymeric particles   Polyamyde fiber   Polystirenic a-chloro
(styrene +   functionalized with   acetoamydomethylate
divinylbenzene   DEAE   functionalzed with
crosslinked)   (diethylamminoethyl-)   PMXB

Adsorption. Figure 3 Panel A (*top*): In most synthetic sorbents, styrene is crosslinked by divinylbenzene forming solid gels
in spherical or granular form (40 mm–1.2 cm). The characteristics are peculiar: Ionic functional groups attached, Typical moisture
content (w. saturated) 40–65 wt%, Particle density = 1–1.5 g/cm^3 (water swollen), Bulk density = 0.5–1 g/cm^3 when packed in
beds, Fractional bed porosity = 0.3–0.4. **Panel B** (*bottom*): other forms of synthetic sorbents can be generated beyond the
mixture styrene-divinylbenzene (left); adsorbent materials can also be represented by polymeric substrates possibly
functionalized with specific chemical substances such as polyamyde fibers functionalyzed with DEAE (Diethylamminoethyl-)
(center) and Polystirenic a-chloroacetoamydo-methylate functionalzed with polymixin-B

To make an example, if $\varepsilon_p = 0.5$ and ρ_p is 1 g/cm^3 = 1 × 106 g/m^3 and $d_p = 20$ Å (20 × 10^{-10} m), then $S_g = 1,000$ m^2/g. In other words, 1 g of sorbent material provides a potential surface for adsorption of 1,000 m^2. In reality we will see that not all the surface is utilized and many factors contribute to the fraction of surface utilized for adsorption in different conditions.

Requirements for a Sorbent

A suitable sorbent material must have high selectivity/affinity to enable sharp separation and high capacity to minimize the amount of sorbent employed to make a commercial product. The sorbent should have favorable kinetics and transport properties for rapid sorption of the target solutes, chemical and thermal stability, low solubility in the contacting fluid, and mechanical strength to prevent crushing or erosion.

In a sorbent cartridge for clinical purposes, the material must have free flowing tendency for ease filling and emptying of the packed bed, high resistance to fouling for long adsorption life, maximal biocompatibility with no tendency to promote undesirable chemical reactions or side effects. Finally the sorbent must be cost effective and the possibility of regeneration should be explored for possible multiple uses. Unwanted losses of hormones, proteins, and drugs must be identified and addressed as potential side effects. Adequate anticoagulation should also be scheduled to prevent clotting or platelet losses.

Mechanism of Adsorption of Solutes in Porous Media

For the adsorption of a solute onto the porous surface of an adsorbent, the following steps are required: (a) External (interphase) mass transfer of the solute from the bulk fluid by convection through a thin film or boundary layer, to the outer surface of the sorbent; (b) Internal (intraphase) mass transfer of the solute by pore diffusion from the outer surface of the adsorbent to the inner surface of the internal porous structure; (c) Surface diffusion along the porous surface; (d) adsorption of the solute onto the porous surface (Fig. 4). The adsorption mechanism involves physical-chemical forces of different nature and provide the basis for the final kinetics of solute removal.

The interphase is a crucial aspect since it permits to bring the solution and the molecules to be removed in contact with the sorbent. When sorbents are contained in a cartridge, it is quintessential that a uniform flow of the bulk solution (it can be ultrafiltrate, plasma, or whole blood) is achieved inside the unit. For example, in the case of sorbent granules, the most uniform flow profile can be obtained when beds are packed carefully with spherical particles of equal size.

Packing densities between 40% and 60% are considered optimal to prevent channeling of the flow and thus, loss of efficiency.

To perform an effective sorbent therapy it is important to ensure that blood flow is equally distributed within the packed sorbent particles so that all the sorbent material is

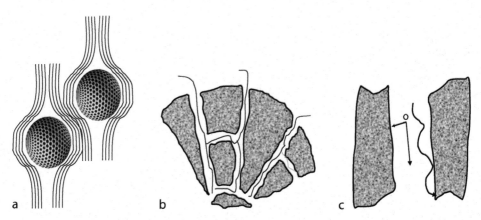

Adsorption. Figure 4 Mechanisms of mass transport from the bulk solution to the sorbent surface: (**a**) External (interphase) mass transfer of the solute from the bulk fluid by convection through a thin film or boundary layer, to the outer surface of the sorbent. (**b**) Internal (intraphase) mass transfer of the solute by pore diffusion from the outer surface of the adsorbent to the inner surface of the internal porous structure. (**c**) Surface diffusion along the porous surface and adsorption of the solute onto the porous surface

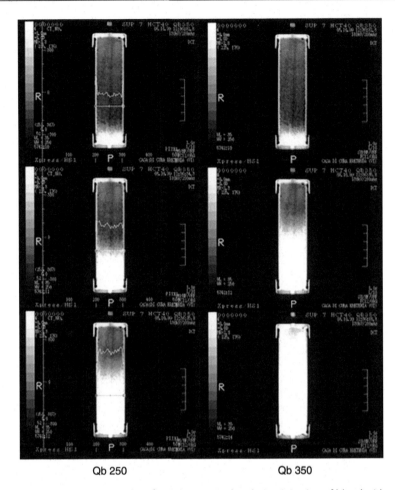

Qb 250   Qb 350

Adsorption. Figure 5 Computerized tomography of a sorbent cartridge during injection of blood with contrast medium to study the flow distribution within the packed sorbent bed

adequately and effectively utilized (Fig. 5). The flow distribution inside the cartridge of sorbent is one of the main issues concerning the performance and the reliability of the device. Any type of channeling phenomenon may affect the quantity of solute adsorbed per unit of sorbent and influences the saturation of the unit. Since blood is a non-Newtonian fluid, one must carry out an accurate analysis of the flow distribution taking into consideration different conditions of flows and blood viscosity. The flow distribution in packed beds can be theoretically modeled using equations of physical chemistry and transport. The structure of the packing is usually complex, and the resulting flow pattern is complicated. There are tortuous paths through the interstitial space of the bed, which consists of channels (pores) of various diameters. In well-packed beds the diversity of channel diameters and velocities in the individual channels is small. Then the packed bed can be approximated as a bundle of tortuous

capillary tubes. In practice, some wide-diameter channels and gaps in the packing structure may be present and the local flow velocity is relatively low. This may result in the undesirable phenomenon of channeling of the flow which may facilitate clotting.

The internal mass transfer or intraphase can be seen as a convective transport of the solute through the structure of the sorbent. This once again depends on the packing density, the differential pressure, and the permeability coefficient of the particle. Very seldom this is fully optimized and the sorbent is generally utilized only in minimal part due to insufficient permeation of the bulk solution in the structure of the particle (Fig. 6).

Finally, the physical-chemical mechanisms regulating molecular surface adsorption are multiple: once the molecule is brought to the surface of the sorbent, different ▶ chemical and physical forces are involved such as Van der Waals forces generated by the interaction between

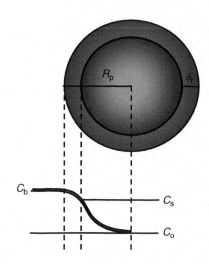

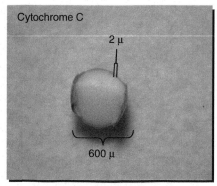

Surface penetration depends on
surface shear rate, coating,
hydration, and molecular
diffusion coefficient

Adsorption. Figure 6 The intraphase or internal mass transfer is described by the difference between the concentration of a solute in the blood (C_b) and the concentration in different internal zones of the sorbent particle (from C_s at the surface to Co in the innermost zone). On the right side a practical example with cytochrome C in a sorbent particle (Image courtesy of Dr. Winchester)

electrons of one molecule and the nucleus of another molecule; these are weak and generally reversible. Ionic bonds are generated by electrostatic attraction between positively charged and negatively charged ions; these are typical of exchange ion resins. Hydrophobic bonds are also present and generated by the hydrophobic affinity of the sorbent and the solute molecules (Fig. 7).

Efficiency of Adsorption

Porous polymers can be designed and constructed with varying internal surface selectivity and varying pore sizes so that molecules can be separated from each other based upon size, geometry, and individual binding properties.

To make a selective or partially selective process of adsorption, one needs to know the properties of the molecules to be separated or removed. If the information is lacking the properties of the molecules under analysis can be ascertained by combining a number of available analytical measurements to develop an understanding of the molecular distinctives or by trial and error through adsorption isotherms (Fig. 8).

When a liquid mixture is brought into contact with a microporous solid, adsorption of certain components in the mixture takes place on the internal surface of the solid. The maximum extent of adsorption occurs when equilibrium is reached. No theory for predicting adsorption curves is universally embraced. Instead, laboratory experiments must be performed at fixed temperature

(Separation processes are energy intensive and affecting entropy) for each liquid mixture and adsorbent to provide data for plotting curves called *adsorption isotherms*. Adsorption isotherms can be used to determine the amount of adsorbent required to remove a given amount of solute from the solvent.

Another measure of the efficiency of the unit is obtained by using marker molecules to determine the so-called mass transfer zone. The mass transfer zone is the portion of the cartridge length that goes from a fully saturated sorbent to a completely unsaturated condition. In Fig. 9, different possibilities are described to define the characteristics of the unit. Mass transfer zone determination also helps to define the design of the unit and the expected time of efficiency before saturation.

Biocompatibility of Sorbents

The biocompatibility of a system utilizing sorbents for extracorporeal therapies should be studied considering different aspects. First of all the sorbent must be resistant and must have a structure that prevent delivery of micro particles or fragments of the material. To further prevent dissemination of small particles in the body, cartridges are provided with a screen that allows free passage of blood but retains particles or their fragments (Fig. 10). A derivate measure of biocompatibility in this sense is given by the behavior of the end-to-end pressure drop in the unit throughout the treatment. Fouling of the screens due to

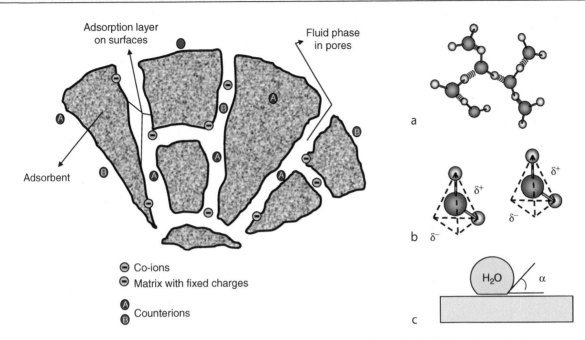

Adsorption. Figure 7 Physical-chemical mechanisms regulating molecular surface adsorption: Once the molecule is brought to the surface of the sorbent, different chemical and physical forces play the final role including (**a**) Van der Waals forces generated by the interaction between electrons of one molecule and the nucleus of another molecule (weak and generally reversible). (**b**) Ionic bonds generated by electrostatic attraction between positively charged and negatively charged ions. (Typical of exchange ion resins). (**c**) Hydrophobic bonds, generated by the hydrophobic affinity of the sorbent and the solute molecules

cell or albumin trapping may result in increased resistance to flow and thus in increased pressure drop inside the cartridge. The second aspect is the intrinsic structure of the sorbent material; if the material goes in direct contact with blood, then it must be hemocompatible, i.e., it must not cause unwanted reactions (from complement activation to cytokine release), leucopenia, thrombocytopenia, or adsorption of albumin beyond a certain limit. All these effects can be partially prevented by coating the surface of the granules or the fibers with a biocompatible material such as polysulfone. In this case however, the coating may render the sorbent less efficient because the intraphase component of the transport may be negatively affected. To avoid this inconvenience, some techniques include a plasma separation process so that cells do not enter in contact with the sorbent, the plasma is circulated through the sorbent bed, and finally blood is reconstituted after an extracorporeal single pass treatment.

Rationale for the Use of Adsorption in Clinical Settings

Is there a rationale for the use of sorbents in acute critical illness and kidney injury? The question has already been posed for chronic patients and the answers are multiple: Assuming there is a humoral disorder that is dependent on circulating molecules and the final target of a therapy is to remove them, the process of adsorption seems to offer some specific benefits. There is a limited efficiency of membrane separation processes (HD-HF) both due to molecule- and membrane-dependent factors. In this case an extra mechanism of solute removal beyond diffusion and convection may provide extra efficiency. There is a possible selectivity or size exclusion adsorptive process so that specific substances can be removed from the circulation and finally, there is in some cases the possibility of placing the sorbent in direct contact with blood facilitating the adsorption process. On the other hand, one must face the limitations imposed by the use of sorbents including the fact that sorbent must be hemocompatible or adequately coated to prevent reactions, size-dependent nonselective adsorption may cause unwanted losses, and finally sorbents might alter the requirement for heparin in the extracorporeal circuit. Nevertheless, the use of sorbents in clinical practice may offer some interesting advantages and some of them have already become evident.

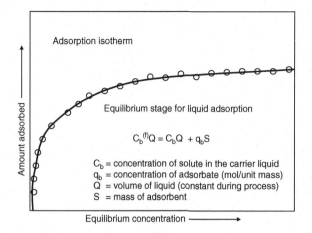

Adsorption. Figure 8 Typical example of an adsorption isotherm

Typical modalities for the utilization of sorbents in extracorporeal therapies are represented in Fig. 11. These techniques have been applied to the management of both acute and chronic renal failure [4].

Hemoperfusion (HP)

Classically, hemoperfusion has been described as a technique in which the sorbent was placed in direct contact with blood in an extracorporeal circulation. Hemoperfusion has the advantage of a much simpler circuit, but it requires a very biocompatible sorbent because of the direct contact with blood and with blood cells in particular. Charcoal has a high adsorbing capacity especially for low molecular weight waste products that accumulate during kidney or liver failure. Its use in hemoperfusion however requires a coating of the sorbent

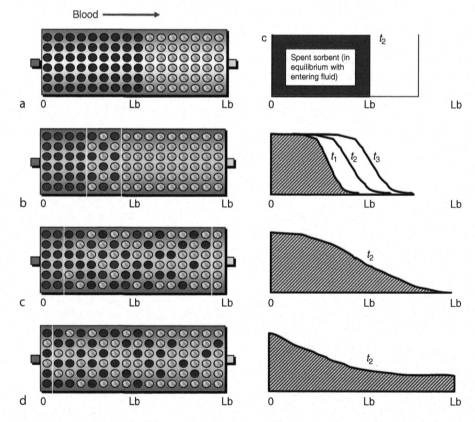

Adsorption. Figure 9 Evaluation of unit efficiency by determination of mass transfer zones: for this test a colored marker molecule is generally utilized. Configuration (**a**) the mass transfer zone is near 0 and this is the Ideal Stoichiometric front for a fixed bed adsorption. (**b**) Uneven concentration front builds mass transfer zones but the dimension of each mass transfer zone at each time is lower than 1/3 of the length of the unit (*L*). (**c**) The mass transfer zone occupies the entire length of the unit; in this condition, the flow-through condition is obtained immediately after the beginning of the treatment. (**d**) The mass transfer zone is larger than the length of the unit (MTZ > Lb); this condition describes a poor design, the presence of channeling phenomena or a poorly efficient sorbent material and leads to typical breakthrough conditions

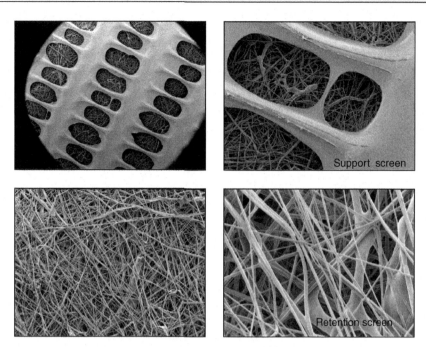

Adsorption. **Figure 10** Screens are used in cartridges to prevent dissemination of sorbent particles and fragments into the circulation (*top panels* depict support screens, *bottom panels* depicts retention screens) (Images courtesy of Prof. Ghezzi)

surface to make it biocompatible. Coated charcoal, although biocompatible, has a remarkably reduced adsorptive capacity due to the cut-off of the coating material. More recently, synthetic polymers have been introduced with remarkable capacity for adsorption. The size selectivity is only offered by the size of the pores on the surface of the granular elements and not by the material itself. In spite of this, specific advantages have been experimentally demonstrated in removing poisons, cytokines, or even endotoxins. For the specific types of hemoperfusion we suggest to read the relevant chapters in this book.

Hemoperfusion Coupled with Hemodialysis (HPHD)

Sorbents have also been used in conjunction with hemodialysis (Hemoperfusion-hemodialysis = HPHD). In this case the sorbent unit is placed in series with the dialyzer, just before it. The reason why it is always placed before is that the dialyzer adjust for temperature or other abnormalities induced by the sorbent (e.g., acidosis). In this setting, the sorbents are hemocompatible and they are mostly utilized in the attempt to remove molecules such as beta-2 microglobulin that are poorly removed by dialysis.

Another approach consists on the use of sorbents in "uncoated" form. These however cannot be placed in direct contact with whole blood and they are used for the treatment on-line of the ultrafiltrate or the plasmafiltrate.

Double Chamber Hemodiafiltration (HFR)

In these system, plasma water is separated from whole blood and, after passing through the sorbent, it is reinfused into the blood circuit reconstituting whole blood structure. This technique has mostly been used in chronic dialysis as a particular form of hemodiafiltration.

Coupled Plasmafiltration Adsorption (CPFA)

Continuous plasmafiltration adsorption is a modality of blood purification in which plasma is separated from whole blood and circulated in a sorbent cartridge. After the sorbent unit, plasma is returned to the blood circuit and the whole blood undergoes hemofiltration or hemodialysis. The rationale consists in the attempt to achieve adequate removal of molecules that are not removed by other hemofiltration or hemodialysis techniques. The advantage is to exclude the blood cells from contact with the sorbent and to reinfuse endogenous plasma after nonselective simultaneous removal of different sepsis-associated mediators without the need of donor plasma. The main issue is concerning the sparing effect on endogenous plasma as compared to potential unwanted losses of autologous plasma compounds.

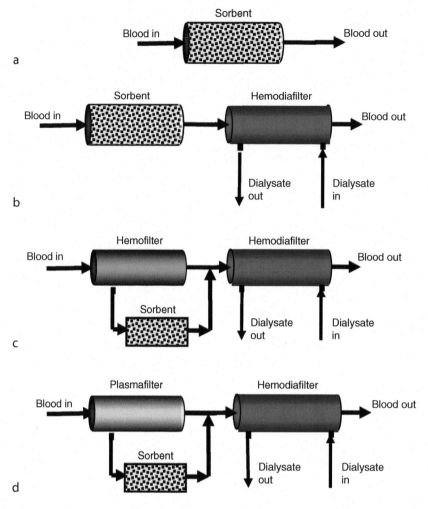

Adsorption. Figure 11 Possible modes of application of sorbents: (**a**) Hemoperfusion (HP). (**b**) The sorbent unit is placed in series before the hemodialyzer (hemoperfusion-hemodialysis HPHD). (**c**) The sorbent unit is placed on-line in the ultrafiltrate produced from a hemofilter. The hemofilter is placed in series with the hemodialyzer. The system is used for on-line hemodiafiltration in chronic patients and it is defined Paired Filtration Dialysis with sorbent (HFR). (**d**) The sorbent unit is placed on-line in the plasmafiltrate produced from a plasmafilter. The plasmafilter is placed in series with the hemodiafilter. The system is used for critically ill patients with septic shock and it is defined Coupled Plasmafiltration Adsorption (CPFA)

This technique has mostly been used in septic patients showing specific advantages of blood purification, restoration of hemodynamics, and immunomodulation (see specific chapter in this book).

In another technique using uncoated sorbents (Detoxification plasmafiltration, DTPF HemoCleanse, Inc., West Lafayette, IN), a hemodiabsorption mechanism is associated with a push-pull plasmafiltration system (a suspension of powdered sorbents surrounding 0.5 μm plasma filter membranes). Bidirectional plasma flow (at 80–100 mL/min) across the plasmafiltration membrane provides direct contact between plasma proteins and powdered

sorbents, as well as clearance of cytokines (tumor necrosis factor-α, interleukin-1β, and interleukin-6).

A major criticism may be risen concerning the removal of beneficial substances or drugs by the mechanism of adsorption. We assessed the different adsorptive properties of a hydrophobic resin for the most-commonly used antibiotics. Except for Vancomycin, where a modest removal can be observed, the levels of other antibiotics such as Tobramycin or Amikacin tend to remain stable over time.

Efficiency and adequacy of treatment, known milestones in the extracorporeal treatment for chronic renal failure, are now reconsidered in critical care nephrology. The complex scenario of sepsis must not be underestimated. Notwithstanding, 20 years or so after the first descriptions, we all face a disease with an ever increasing incidence and unacceptably high mortality. Innovative techniques address the importance of dedicated extracorporeal systems for sespis where acute renal failure is just one of the pathologic complications.

This wider approach to the concept of blood purification opens new perspectives in a revisited strategy for the application of extracorporeal treatments.

Sorbents in Sepsis

The cellular and humoral response of the host to bacterial invasion results in a series of symptoms and organ derangements which are mediated by the presence of chemical mediators.

Continuous renal replacement therapies (CRRT) have gained increased popularity for their ability to insure the removal of excess fluid and waste products in septic patients with acute kidney injury. However, removal rates and clearances of the different proinflammatory cytokines (IL-1, TNF) and lipid mediators (PAF) are hindered by poor membrane passage.

Innovative approaches: include high volume hemofiltration and the use of superpermeable membranes. The latter are still under investigation for the possible excessive leakage of albumin. Plasmafiltration techniques have shown an increase in TNF clearance by 2 orders of magnitude and have demonstrated some improved survival in septic animals. However plasmapheresis is hardly considerable as a CRRT.

The combined requirements of a continuous renal replacement therapy with high sieving capacity and possible selective removal of sepsis-associated mediators, seem to find an answer in the application of sorbents. The most interesting experience with sorbents in sepsis has been done with CPFA. CPFA has been utilized with the rationale of reinfusing endogenous plasma after nonselective simultaneous removal of different sepsis-associated mediators without the need of donor plasma.

In vitro studies demonstrated that removal rates of cytokines were different according to varying sorbents tested. More importantly, when tested at different linear velocities, their efficiencies in removing cytokines were far away above the mass of individual cytokines calculated on the basis of the highest levels detected in the plasma of septic patients.

In animal studies coupled plasmafiltration adsorption resulted in a significant ($p = 0.0041$) survival (85%) at 72 h with respect to rabbits injected with lipopolysaccharide,

but not treated with coupled plasmafiltration adsorption [5]. It must be emphasized that the overall net effect on survival could be due to the removal not only of the TNF or PAF, but also to many other mediators not monitored in the study.

In a prospective randomized cross-over trial aimed at comparing clinical and biological effects of coupled plasmafiltration adsorption versus continuous venovenous hemofiltration (CVVH) in critically ill septic patients significant improvement were observed after 10 h of CPFA. Despite the fact that all patients had relatively low plasma concentrations of cytokines (TNF-α, IL.1β), the sorbent adsorbed almost 100% of the cytokines in the plasmafiltrate. In all patients, starting the treatment, the in vitro TNF production of circulating monocytes to exogenous lipopolysaccharide was remarkably impaired in relation to monocytes from healthy subjects. When the same patient was studied after 5- and 10-h treatment with CPFA, the ability of monocytes to produce TNF-α was restored in the range seen for normal monocytes. Coincubation experiments with a monoclonal antibody directed against IL-10 could abrogate (60%) monocyte unresponsiveness. In CVVH, abrogation of monocyte unresponsivess was only partial as compared to CPFA and significantly delayed (after 10-h treatment). At the hemodynamic level, all patients (APACHE score > 20) showed increased peripheral vascular resistances that allowed a significant reduction in the dose of vasopressor drugs at 5 h and remained steadily low after 10-h treatment. The reduction of vasopressor drugs was not observed during CVVH. These data suggest the possibility that CPFA may insure better hemodynamics in highly unstable patients than CVVH. Since the CPFA may be modular to conventional CVVH, the system may ensure a fluid and salt balance together with an enhanced blood purification.

In the concept of using extracorporeal therapies for sepsis, there has been a widespread tendency to remove "bad factors" rather than to attempt to bring about a restoration of balance of physiological factors. Often, too much emphasis has been placed on individual markers. The results obtained with CPFA suggest that treatments should focus more carefully on a "balancing hypothesis" trying to restore a correct equilibrium between immunological suppression and activation.

The results obtained in clinical practice were in fact the basis to formulate the "peak concentration hypothesis" and to offer a possible explanation of the beneficial effects of sorbents in septic patients. The unselective but continuous removal of the peak concentrations of both pro and antiinflammatory mediators may in fact lead to a kind of immunomodulation with partial restoration of the immunohomeostasis.

The rationale for exposing the plasma to the sorbent in a plasma filtration system is to exclude the blood cells from contact with the sorbent and to reinfuse endogenous plasma after nonselective simultaneous removal of different sepsis-associated mediators without the need of donor plasma. The main issue is concerning the sparing effect on endogenous plasma as compared to potential unwanted losses of autologous plasma compounds.

The major advantages can be summarized in a restoration of cell responsiveness to exogenous LPS, improvement of the pathological apoptosis detected in sepsis, improved HLA-DR expression as a measure of the immunoresponse of the patient, improved phagocytosis capacity, and finally increased systemic vascular resistances and significant reduction of the dose of norepinephrine required to maintain a stable hemodynamics in patients. Since CPFA may be modular to conventional CVVH, the two modalities can be carried out in series. The system may ensure a fluid and salt balance together with enhanced blood purification for various molecules and a combined effect on immunomodulation.

In order to underline the growing importance and developments of sorbents applied to blood purification, we should also consider the new polystirene-based fiber to which polymixin-B (Pmx-B) is covalently bound: whole blood of septic endotoxemic patients is circulated for some hours through the cartridge, obtaining a removal of endotoxin, selectively affine to Pmx-B. This technique is matter of a specific chapter in this book.

Finally we should say that new sorbent materials are also appearing on the scene and soon they will be available for clinical trials.

References

1. Ronco C, Bordoni V, Levin NW (2002) Adsorbents: from basic structure to clinical application. Contrib Nephrol 137:158–164
2. Ronco C, Brendolan A, Winchester JF, Golds E, Clemmer J, Polaschegg HD, Muller TE, La Greca G, Levin N (2001) First clinical experience with an adjunctive hemoperfusion device designed specifically to remove β_2-microglobulin in hemodialysis. Blood Purif 19:260–263
3. Tetta C, Cavaillon JM, Camusi G, Lonneman G, Brendolan A, Ronco C (1998) Continuous plasma filtration coupled with sorbents. Kidney Int 53(suppl 66):S186–S189
4. Ronco C, Brendolan A, Dan M, Piccinni P, Bellomo R, De Nitti C, Inguaggiato P, Tetta C (2000) Adsorption in sepsis. Kidney Int 58 (suppl 76):S148–S155
5. Tetta C, Gianotti L, Cavaillon JM, Wratten ML, Fini M, Braga M, Bisagni P, Giavaresi G, Bolzani R, Giardino R (2000) Coupled plasma filtration adsorption in a rabbit model of endotoxic shock. Crit Care Med 28:1526–1533

Adult Respiratory Distress Syndrome

▶ Acute Respiratory Distress Syndrome and Acute Lung Injury

Advanced Cardiac Life Support (ACLS)

Refers to the protocolized medical care provided to patients suffering from severe cardiovascular compromise or cardiac arrest due to tachydysrhythmia, such as ventricular fibrillation, bradydysrhythmia, asystole, or pulseless electrical activity (PEA). ACLS is based on algorithms developed by the American Heart Association (AHA); these algorithms dictate pharmacotherapy, cardiac pacing, electrical cardioversion and defibrillation, and immediate procedural interventions for reversible causes of cardiac arrest, such as needle chest decompression for tension pneumothorax.

Advanced Hemodynamic Monitoring

A method for the management of high-risk surgical and critically ill patients beyond physical examination and conventional monitoring of vital signs.

Advanced Trauma Life Support

JAMEEL ALI
Division of General Surgery, St. Michael's Hospital
University of Toronto, Toronto, ON, Canada

Definition

The Advanced Trauma Life Support (ATLS®) program has become the standard of trauma resuscitation internationally. To date, the program has been introduced into 64 countries with over one million physicians trained internationally and over 50% from outside North America.

Another 15 countries have indicated interest in having this program [1].

Characteristics

Because many trauma victims present with multiple injuries and immediate definitive anatomical diagnosis is not possible, the ATLS® initial approach to resuscitation is based on the identification and recognition of degrees of life threat caused by the injuries rather than the specific diagnosis of the injury. This has led to a prioritization of care related to the degree of life threat which in turn is related to the time required before irreversible damage or death occurs following injuries. This approach to trauma resuscitation includes three phases: the Primary Survey, Secondary Survey, and Definitive Care.

During the primary survey, the approach is physiologic and not based on identification of specific injuries but on the effect of these injuries on the ability to sustain life.

The secondary survey is a sequential head-to-toe anatomical approach to identify specific injuries which themselves may not be immediately life threatening but could, in time, cause death or significant morbidity.

The third phase is termed the Definitive care phase and this incorporates management techniques aimed at definitively treating specific injuries such as the fixation of fractures etc.

The ATLS® program also identifies "adjuncts" to the primary and secondary surveys. These adjuncts facilitate the application of the principles of resuscitation.

The Primary Survey

The stages of the primary survey are delineated by the letters of the alphabet: A, B, C, D, and E as follows: A – Airway with Cervical spine control; B – Breathing; C – Circulation; D-neurologic Disability; E – complete Exposure of the patient.

This order of priority in the primary survey is based on the degree of life threat related to the time element. For instance, although bleeding in C for circulation can result in organ damage and death, if both airway and circulatory problems coexist, irreversible damage or death occurs more rapidly from the airway problem than from the abnormality in C or circulation. It is important to recognize that abnormalities in A – Airway may occur as a result of a primary airway injury or severe shock or other abnormalities such as severe head injury. However, it does not matter initially which one of these injuries produces the airway problem because the approach to the airway would be the same that is clearing and securing the airway. It should be recognized that in instances where multiple care givers are available for managing the patient, simultaneous

management of the airway, breathing, and circulatory abnormalities could occur. However, in that setting it is crucial to have one person designated as "team leader" to coordinate the management of the patient so that the overall management follows the sequence of the degree of life threat posed by the different physiologic derangements resulting from the injury. Another important concept is that the primary survey and resuscitation are conducted simultaneously.

Adjuncts to Resuscitation

Protective equipment (gown, mask, eye shield, gloves, boots, etc.) need to be worn by all personnel caring for the trauma patient. Level I warmer (or other warming device) should be immediately available for infusing warm fluids and the room temperature should also be high to protect from hypothermia. EKG monitoring, arterial blood gas, pulse-oximetry, CO_2 detector, FAST (Focused Abdominal Sonogram for Trauma), as well as x-ray capabilities for conducting a chest x-ray and x-ray of the pelvis should be available. A lateral cervical spine x-ray with open odontoid view is practiced in many institutions but most trauma centers use the CT scan for radiologic assessment of the spine.

Another adjunct to the assessment and management of the patient is an orogastric tube inserted to decompress the stomach and also to assess for possible upper gastrointestinal hemorrhage. Although the nasogastric route is easier for gastric intubation, this route should be avoided especially when a basal skull fracture is suspected.

Airway with C-Spine Control (C – Denotes Cervical)

Whenever airway intervention is contemplated it is essential to consider the risk of cervical spine injury and protect the spine accordingly by maintaining the spine in the neutral position with a ▶ C-collar. C-spine control should be maintained as a preventive measure during resuscitation. Definitive diagnosis of a C-spine injury is made later.

Recognizing that the commonest cause of obstruction of the airway in the trauma patient is posterior displacement of the tongue in the pharynx, simple maneuvers such as jaw thrust, chin lift together with removal and suctioning of foreign bodies, and secretions would allow the insertion of an oropharyngeal airway with bag valve mask ventilation in order to provide oxygenation. Once the oxygenation has been improved by this maneuver, if the patient is still unable to maintain a patent airway, then attempts should be made to secure the airway in a definitive manner (the ▶ definitive airway is defined as a cuffed tube in the trachea – note that the tube does not need to be cuffed in the infant). The definitive airway is secured usually by nonsurgical means failing which the surgical airway option should be chosen. Although in some instances the naso-tracheal route is chosen, it is generally considered more appropriate to use the oro-tracheal route especially if there is concern about a possible basal skull fracture in the patient. Prior to endotracheal intubation, the patient should be preoxygenated and if the patient is combative consideration should be given to using intravenous sedatives and/or short acting paralyzing agents to facilitate the intubation process. Although the laryngeal mask airway (LMA) is used in many centers it is not uniformly recognized as a definitive airway because of its ease of dislodgement. Other techniques such as introducing the endotracheal tube over a bronchoscope or using the gum-elastic bougie are very useful in securing the airway in a patient with anatomical or mechanical abnormalities.

Patients with evidence of inhalation injuries such as facial burns, hoarseness, carbonaceous sputum, etc., should be considered for early intubation prior to the development of expected airway edema which would make the procedure much more difficult.

Failure to secure the airway by these measures warrants consideration of a surgical airway. The method of choice in adults is the surgical cricothyroidotomy. The needle cricothyroidotomy is preferred in infants. The needle cricothyroidotomy provides oxygenation support for period of 30–40 min but after this time hypercapnea results and the tube should therefore be replaced by a tracheostomy in the operating room if the airway problem has not resolved. Before attaching the intubated patient to positive pressure ventilation one should quickly determine whether there is presence of a simple pneumothorax by clinical examination or quick chest x-ray since positive pressure ventilation could result in the conversion of a simple pneumothorax to a life-threatening tension pneumothorax. In most instances there is clear evidence that a simple pneumothorax is not present and once the patient is intubated mechanical ventilation is instituted with 100% oxygen. The position of the endotracheal tube is ascertained by clinical examination, the detection of CO_2 in the expired gas, and a chest x-ray.

B –Breathing

A quick physical examination would tell whether there is tachypnea, asymmetric chest wall movement, a sucking chest wound, dullness to percussion or hyper-resonance with decreased air entry. The hypotensive patient with hyper-resonance on one side of the chest, particularly with elevated jugular venous pressure should be treated by prompt needle decompression of the pleural space and if this confirms the presence of tension pneumothorax the maneuver should be followed by insertion of large bore (32 French) chest tube in the fourth or fifth intercostal space just anterior to the mid-axillary line and the tube is connected to the underwater seal apparatus. Whenever a chest tube is placed, physical examination and a chest x-ray should be conducted to confirm proper location of the tube.

The other major breathing threat to life in the primary survey is the presence of an open pneumothorax which presents with an audible sound of air entering the pleural space and an open wound in the chest wall. The larger the chest wall opening relative to the size of the main stem bronchus the more rapid the deterioration in the patient. Because of the opening to the atmosphere, during spontaneous ventilation the patient is unable to generate a negative pleural pressure which is required for the expansion of the lung. Accumulation of air in the pleural space with compression of the lung results in the same hemodynamic and ventilatory abnormalities found in the tension pneumothorax. Recognition of this abnormality requires prompt occlusion of the opening followed by chest tube insertion. When the opening is very large, intubation and positive pressure ventilation will temporarily correct the hemodynamic and ventilatory compromise until surgical closure of the defect.

C-Circulation

Circulatory abnormality resulting in hypoperfusion in the trauma patient is considered hemorrhagic until proven otherwise. The overall approach to the circulation in the trauma patient, therefore, consists of (1) the search for a source of hemorrhage, (2) stopping the hemorrhage, and (3) reestablishing blood volume through large bore (14–16 gauge) venous access. At the time of the venous access, blood should be taken for cross and type as well as CBC and toxicology screen.

Identifying the Source of Hemorrhage and Principles of Management

The source of the hemorrhage should be considered as either external or internal and begins with a look for an external source by complete assessment of the trunk, extremities, head, and the back of the patient while log rolling. At the time of log rolling a rectal examination should be done to determine whether there is any evidence of neurologic injury as well as whether there is a high riding prostate in the male to suggest a possibility of a urethral injury prior to inserting a foley catheter for monitoring urine output. In the presence of a major pelvic fracture and blood at the urethral meatus or a high riding or boggy prostate on the digital rectal examination, a urethrogram should be conducted to assess the integrity of the urethra and if the urethra is intact the foley catheter is inserted. Otherwise urologic consultation is sought before decompressing or intubating the bladder by other means. The spine board should be removed after the ▶ log roll and in-line immobilization should be maintained by having the patient on a flat firm surface with a C-collar and neck bolsters in place. Thereafter, the spine board should only be used for transferring the patient in order to prevent ducubitus ulceration which is a major form of morbidity in severely injured patients.

Any external source of hemorrhage should be controlled by direct digital pressure and application of pressure bandages to stop the hemorrhage temporarily until definitive care could be provided.

The search for an internal source of hemorrhage begins with a physical examination of the chest followed by a chest x-ray. These two methods should allow identification of the chest as a source of hemorrhage. Even a small hemothorax should be treated in the trauma situation with chest tube insertion which allows the decompression of the pleural space as well as monitoring of the volume and rate of blood loss. Most patients with traumatic hemothorax do not require thoracotomy to control the bleeding because the source of the bleeding is usually parenchymal and stops spontaneously particularly on lung reexpansion with chest tube insertion. However, massive hemothorax which is generally regarded as a volume of at least 1,500 cc with continued bleeding is an indication for thoracotomy for controlling the hemorrhage. The hemorrhage in massive hemothorax usually arises from a systemic source such as an intercostal artery, internal mammary artery, or a major intrathoracic vascular structure.

The abdomen is assessed clinically for distention, bruising and if the patient is alert, signs of tenderness or guarding but the mainstay of assessing the abdomen for bleeding in the emergency setting is sonography (FAST-focused assessment sonogram in trauma). If the patient is in shock and there is a penetrating mechanism most of these patients require laparotomy. On the other hand a blunt mechanism with hypotension warrants a short trial of fluid administration looking for hemodynamic improvement. Failure to obtain a good hemodynamic response prompts laporotomy. In the primary survey, assessment of the abdomen is aimed at determining whether or not laparotomy is required, the chief indications for laparotomy being significant continuing hemorrhage especially in a penetrating mechanism, presence of signs of perforation or in some cases penetration of the peritoneum (relative indication).

The pelvis is next assessed by a combination of physical examination and pelvic x-rays. If a pelvic fracture is diagnosed, restriction of the expansion of the pelvic volume is accomplished by the application of pelvic binders or temporary bed sheet and more definitively application of an external fixator. In addition to volume resuscitation, if there is failure to respond, consideration needs to be given to angio embolization. Pre-peritoneal packing has been reported to be beneficial in controlling the pelvic hemorrhage and this is becoming a frequent early option for controlling major hemorrhage from pelvic fractures [2].

Although bleeding from the scalp in a young child could account for hypovolemic shock, in the adult head injured patient, hypotension is not usually due to the head injury and another source of the hypotension should be sought.

One of the triggers for suggesting hypoperfusion in the trauma patient is the presence of hypotension. However, it should be recognized that the blood pressure could be maintained, especially in young adults at the expense of perfusion. The systolic blood pressure is the product of stroke volume and peripheral vascular resistance and when stroke volume is diminished from loss of circulating blood volume the peripheral vascular resistance through the release of catecholamines could maintain the blood pressure at normal or even at higher than normal levels. Indeed, in the classification of hemorrhagic shock in the trauma patient where Class I is considered to be up to 15% of the total blood volume, Class II up to 30% and Class III 40% of total blood volume it is only after the Class III has been reached or almost 2 L of blood in an adult will hypotension occur. In assessing for blood loss in the trauma patient, a drop in blood pressure is, therefore, a very late sign and one should assess for signs of hypoperfusion such as tachycardia, cool extremities, and increased base deficit, rather than relying on blood pressure measurement alone.

Nonhemorrhagic Sources of Hypoperfusion

Apart from volume loss, nonhemorrhagic sources of hypotension or hypoperfusion in the trauma patient should be considered. The main entities are tension pneumothorax, cardiac tamponade, and neurogenic shock. Although septic shock can occur in the trauma patient it is usually a late presentation. When traumatic septic shock occurs, treatment consists of fluid resuscitation, antimicrobials, and removal of the septic focus while maintaining cardiorespiratory dynamics.

Both tension pneumothorax and cardiac tamponade differ from hypovolemic shock by presenting with distended neck veins. Hypovolemia, tension pneumothorax, and cardiac tamponade all have in common tachycardia, hypotension, narrowed pulse pressure, and evidence of peripheral vasoconstriction. The differentiating feature is, therefore, the presence of flat nondistended neck veins in the hypolovemic patient. The major differentiating features between a tension pneumothorax and cardiac tamponade are the hyper resonance and decreased breath sounds on the side of the tension pneumothorax. The finding of hemopericardium on FAST examination in the presence of hypotension indicates cardiac tamponade as the diagnosis. If, in spite of physical examination, there is still doubt about whether the hypotension is due to cardiac tamponade or tension pneumothorax, the patient should be treated with needle decompression of the pleural space and that should release the tension pneumothorax as well as give the diagnosis which should be followed by insertion of a chest tube. The diagnosis of tension pneumothorax should be clinical and not radiologic.

Cardiac tamponade in the trauma patient should be treated initially by pericardiocentesis or pericardial window followed by emergency room thoracotomy if the patient is severely hemodynamically compromised. Ideally, the patient should be taken to the operating room for repair of the cardiac wound.

Neurogenic shock differs from other forms of shock in the trauma patient by having warm extremities and a widened pulse pressure. There is usually a lack of tachycardia unless the cardiac sympathetics are preserved. The neurogenic shock results from a disruption of the sympathetic nervous system leading to the vasodilatation, hypotension, and relative bradycardia. The initial treatment of the patient in neurogenic shock is volume infusion because of the relative hypovolemia resulting from an expanded vascular space. Occasionally, atropine for severe bradycardia or alpha agonists for severe hypotension is necessary.

Apart from identifying and stopping hemorrhage in the trauma patient volume resuscitation is required and this necessitates the establishment of large bore [14–16 gauge] venous access. The approach is to first attempt peripheral venous access in the antecubital veins and failing this promptly going to central venous access through the femoral, subclavian, or internal jugular routes. In many centers the establishment of central venous access is facilitated under ultrasound guidance. Although it is also possible to use the intra-osseous route in adults, in most instances it is not necessary. However, in infants and young children the intra-osseous route is more frequently applied when there is failure to gain venous access on at least two attempts in the vasoconstricted patient.

Volume infusion should be followed by monitoring the patient for an appropriate response. Rapid infusion of warm crystalloids is first instituted and if there is major blood loss, warmed cross matched blood should be administered. If there is not enough time to obtain this then type-specific or emergency group O blood should be administered. With massive infusions, consideration should be given to early administration of platelets, fresh frozen plasma, and cryoprecipitate and in special circumstances recombinant factor VIIa. The usual initial dose of crystalloids is 1–2 L for adults and 20 mL/kg for pediatric patients and this is given as rapidly as possible. The patient response is monitored by urinary output, evidence of correction of base deficit, as well as return to normal hemodynamics. The patient who usually has less than 20% blood volume loss and usually does not require surgical intervention or blood administration may be classified as a rapid responder. The transient responder may have moderate ongoing bleeding up to 40% as demonstrated by a transient improvement in hemodynamics. These patients may or may not require blood as well as crystalloid, and consideration needs to be given to possible surgical intervention. The minimal or nonresponder continues to have abnormal hemodynamics in spite of rapid volume infusion and these patients may have either massive blood loss over 40% of total blood volume or the hemodynamic abnormality may not be due to blood loss at all. If hemorrhage is the cause, these patients require immediate blood transfusion and usually surgical intervention.

D – Neurologic Disability

Initial assessment of the head injured patient requires determination of the Glasgow Coma Scale (GCS) score, pupillary response, and any lateralizing signs. This mini neurologic examination provides a baseline for detecting improvement or deterioration.

The mainstay of initial treatment of the patient with head injury is the prevention of ▶ secondary brain injury by maintaining adequate oxygenation and perfusion. Oxygenation would require an adequate airway and patients with a GCS score of eight or less will require mechanical ventilation with endotracheal intubation because of the inability to spontaneously maintain the airway. Adequate perfusion requires appropriate venous access and isotonic fluid administration.

Prevention of secondary brain injury not only requires maintenance of perfusion and oxygenation but also control of intracranial pressure by maneuvers such as temporary hyperventilation (PCO_2 30–35) and decompression of an expanding hematoma. CT scan is also a very important tool in assessing and guiding management of these patients to prevent secondary brain injury. In the presence of seizures, anticonvulsant therapy is required and failure to maintain seizure-free activity warrants consideration for endotracheal intubation and mechanical ventilation with paralysis.

The Cushing response to head trauma results in an elevation in mean arterial blood pressure that counteracts an increase in intracranial pressure so that the cerebral perfusion pressure is maintained. It is therefore inappropriate to try to decrease the systemic blood pressure in these patients since this is a compensatory mechanism to maintain cerebral perfusion pressure.

Oxygenation, ventilation, volume infusion, monitoring of the GCS, and frequent CT scan are, therefore, key elements in the assessment and management of the head-injured patient as well as craniotomy for evacuation of mass lesions.

E – Exposure

Complete examination of the trauma patient is essential in order to avoid missing injuries particularly posteriorly. In order to accomplish this the patient is log-rolled, with one person maintaining stability of the cervical spine, two persons maintaining the thoracic and lumbar spine, another one supporting the extremities while one person examines the back for signs of bleeding or deformity or evidence of spine injury. Once the examination is complete the patient should be promptly covered with warm blankets in order to maintain normothermia. As mentioned earlier, prevention of hypothermia also involves the administration of warmed fluid in a warm environment.

Secondary Survey

The secondary survey is a head-to-toe anatomical assessment of the patient for injuries that are not immediately life-threatening but if left unattended could produce a later life threat and certainly could produce major morbidity. It is a systematic approach and it is conducted only after the primary survey is completed. Indeed, in many patients, the secondary survey is not completed until the patient has been to the operating room to control hemorrhage or evacuate an intracranial hematoma.

During the secondary survey the scalp and head and neck area are examined in detail for any evidence of injury. There is now an opportunity to reexamine the chest by inspection, percussion, palpation, and auscultation to reassess the position of the tubes, the drainage of chest tubes and the reassessment of the abdomen including sometimes a second FAST. Examination of all extremities is conducted including power, tone, sensation and reflexes, and assessing for possible ligamentous injuries and other minor fractures. In the trauma patient, x-rays should be performed liberally if there is any suggestion of injury to the joint or bony areas. However, these assessments should not delay the primary survey and resuscitation and should not delay the transfer of the patient who requires a higher level of care than is provided at the receiving institution.

During the secondary survey a detailed assessment of the musculoskeletal system should be undertaken and a close look for such entities as the compartment syndrome especially in patients who are unconscious or who have been in shock or have had massive fluid resuscitation. When clinical assessment is not sufficient to establish the diagnosis of compartment syndrome, compartment pressure should be measured and prompt fasciotomy conducted to preserve neurovascular integrity and muscle viability.

During the secondary survey, if there is any clinical suspicion of spine injury appropriate imaging should be conducted. In most instances this requires CT scan imaging and if there is an abnormality of the spine then the entire spine should be assessed radiologically since a fracture in one area of the spine is associated with a noncontiguous fracture in another area of the spine in 10% of cases. In most severely injured patients CT scan of the entire spine is conducted.

Because physical findings and hemodynamic status could change very quickly, reevaluation is a common theme during all phases, especially during primary survey and secondary survey.

Definitive Care Phase

The definitive care phase of management of the trauma patient takes place only after the primary and secondary surveys have been completed, and involves treatment of specific fractures, investigation of findings such as hematuria without major hemodynamic sequelae, the treatment of facial fractures, ligamentous injury, and other non-life-threatening injuries.

Special Considerations

Although the priorities of management as outlined in the ATLS® program are the same for all trauma patients, there are anatomic and physiologic differences peculiar to four groups that is the pediatric patient, the pregnant patient, the elderly, and the conditioned athlete that warrant special consideration. Following are some highlights of these differences which impact on presentation and management of trauma in these populations.

Children

Trauma is the leading cause of death in this age group and there is a vigorous physiologic response initially but precipitous deterioration when the compensatory mechanisms have been overwhelmed. The child is particularly prone to develop hypothermia and failure to recognize the shortness of the trachea could result in right main stem-bronchus intubation. The presentations of head, chest, and musculoskeletal injuries including fracture patterns are also different. Hemodynamic parameters such as heart rate, blood pressure, urine output are age dependent and the doses of drugs, size of tubes all warrant special attention in this age group. The ▶ Broselow™ Pediatric Emergency Tape (Armstrong Medical Industries Inc.) is a helpful adjunct in managing these patients.

Pregnancy

In pregnancy, there are two patients – the fetus and the mother. The best treatment for the fetus is appropriate resuscitation of the mother. Hypotension in the late trimester may be associated with compression of the vena cava by the gravid uterus and this supine hypotension could be improved by manually displacing the uterus or if there is no sign of spine injury turning the patient to the left lateral position. In the Rh-negative mother with trauma one should be conscious of the possibility of iso-immunization and Rh-immune globulin (Rhogam) should be administered even with minimal injury, since as small a volume of .01 mL of Rh-positive blood during feto-maternal hemorrhage will sensitize 70% of Rh-negative mothers.

The Elderly

The elderly patient has diminished physiologic reserve and decompensates much earlier for the same level of insult. Frequently there are associated comorbidities that would affect presentation and outcome as well as medications such as anticoagulants and beta blockers which could compound presentation and management of these patients. Outcome on the elderly patient sustaining trauma therefore depends on early aggressive therapy.

The Athlete

The well-conditioned athlete could present with very misleading hemodynamics. The heart rate is frequently lower than normal. The absence of tachycardia should not be regarded as a reliable indicator of normovolemia in assessing and managing these patients.

Transfer to Definitive Care

Throughout the course of management of the trauma patient, a major consideration is whether or not the patient requires transfer to a higher level of care. The transfer decision is based on the patient's needs as well as the resources and capabilities of the treating institution. Whenever the patient's needs exceed the institutional resources then consideration should be given to transfer and this should be done as early as possible after resuscitation has been achieved. The transfer process should not be delayed for diagnostic tests that would not affect the management at the primary institution. Communication between physicians and selection of the most appropriate mode of transport are essential. Transfer should not be to the nearest institution but more importantly to the nearest appropriate institution that is capable of meeting the needs of the patient.

Advanced Trauma Life Support. Table 1 Mortality pre and post ATLS

Mortality among all trauma patients		
	Total Patients	Dead
Pre-ATLS	413	279
Post-ATLS	400	134
There was a twofold decrease in overall mortality after ATLS. Mortality: Pre = 2 × post-ATLS.		
ISS Category and Mortality		
ISS	Mortality Pre (%)	Mortality Post (%)	Odds Ratio
LE 24	47.9	16.7	4.5
25–40	91.0	71.0	1.2
41 +	100	100	
Post-ATLS trauma mortality improved for all ISS categories except for those exceeding ISS of 40.			

Impact of the ATLS Program

The above outline of the Advanced Trauma Life Support approach to trauma care was designed to improve the level of care provided to trauma victims. The program has been adopted throughout the world but has it made a difference in the management of trauma patients? Knowledge base assessed by MCQ examinations have shown immediate improvement in the post-ATLS trained physicians compared to their pre-ATLS performance. Within 6 months there has been significant attrition of this cognitive skill, the attrition being greater in physicians who treat less than 50 major trauma cases per year. Although there is attrition of clinical resuscitation skills as measured by an organized approach to the trauma patient and adherence to priorities, this attrition is not as severe. The principles of trauma management taught in the ATLS program seem to prevail with time at a higher level than the cognitive element. Again, physicians practicing in institutions where they see more than 50 trauma patients per year performed better as far as clinical skills are concerned. This was also borne out by testing performance in simulated trauma patient situations using Objective Structured Clinical Examination (OSCE) methodology.

Advanced Trauma Life Support. Table 2 Percentage of mortality of blunt and penetrating injuries

	Blunt (%)	Penetrating (%)
Pre-ATLS	76.7	19.7
Post-ATLS	46.2	6.3

Trauma patient outcome improved for both penetrating and blunt injuries post-ATLS

A study in the developing country of Trinidad and Tobago of trauma patient outcome shows that pre-ATLS mortality was twice as high for the same injury severity as post-ATLS mortality and this was so for both penetrating and blunt trauma [3] (Tables 1 and 2). It was further demonstrated that when comparing institutions that had the ATLS course the resuscitative procedures were more commonly instituted after the ATLS course was administered than previously [4] (Fig. 1).

One of the other results or outcome of the ATLS course is the spawning of other training courses in trauma such as the Pre-hospital Trauma Life Support program which has been shown to improve trauma outcome further following its introduction after the ATLS program.

Conclusion

The Advanced Trauma Life Support program was instituted after a recognized need for improving trauma care and it has now become the international standard for resuscitation of trauma patients. The approach of dividing the care into phases of primary survey with adjuncts and resuscitation, secondary survey with adjuncts and reevaluation, definitive care and transfer is a very simple and easily applied approach. This program has been shown to improve trauma resuscitation knowledge, improvement in trauma skills, as well as improvement in trauma patient outcome.

References

1. Ali J (2008) Program: historical perspectives and future directions. Fraser Gurd lecture. J Trauma 64(5):1149–1158
2. Cothren CC, Osborn PM, Moore EE, Morgan SJ et al (2007) Preperitoneal pelvic packing for hemodynamically unstable pelvic fractures: a paradigm shift. J Trauma 62(4):834–838

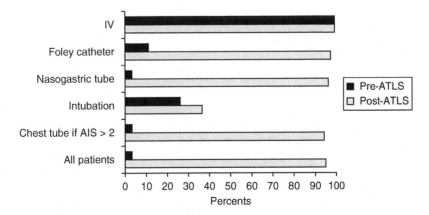

Advanced Trauma Life Support. Figure 1 Percentage of procedures administered in the emergency department. Less than 10% of the procedures were instituted in the emergency department before ATLS compared with over 90% after ATLS

3. Ali J, Adam R, Butler AK et al (1993) Trauma outcome improves following the Advanced Trauma Life support [ATLS] program in a developing country. J Trauma 34:890–899
4. Ali J, Adam R, Stedman M et al (1994) Advanced Trauma Life Support Program increases emergency room application of trauma resuscitative procedures in a developing country. J Trauma 36(3):391–394

Advanced Trauma Life Support (ATLS)

Advanced trauma life support (ATLS) is defined and standardized by the American College of Surgeons (ACS) and refers to specific medical care needed to adequately assess and resuscitate trauma patients. This includes recognition of the severity of injury, determining appropriate level of care, providing the correct IV fluid and blood products to trauma patients, and initial stabilization of life- or limb-threatening injuries.

Aerosolized Antibiotics

RICHARD D. BRANSON, BRYCE R. H. ROBINSON
Division of Trauma and Critical Care, University of Cincinnati, Cincinnati, OH, USA

Synonyms
Antibiotics via the respiratory tract; Inhalational antibiotics

Definition
Inhaled antibiotics entail the delivery of antimicrobial therapy directly to the respiratory tract by an aerosolized format.

Pre-existing Condition
Antibiotic therapy delivered directly to the infected airways has been a goal of clinicians for over 50 years. Such systems allow for the direct interaction of pharmaceuticals to diseased airways avoiding complications associated with systemic delivery approaches (enteral and parenteral). The rate of use of such products has escalated over the last several years due to increasing technological advances. The introduction of jet and ultrasonic nebulizers in addition to the advent of dry powder delivery devices allows for a more efficient method as compared to historical atomizers. Such devices now allow for the lower airways to be targeted, broadening the anatomical distribution of drug. The use of escalation can also be attributable to gains in the development of specialized aerosolized formulations of existing drugs by the pharmaceutical industry.

Cystic Fibrosis
Work with aerosolized antibiotics emerged from chronic care delivered to those with cystic fibrosis (CF). The majority of those with CF have airways that are colonized by gram-negative organisms, specifically *Pseudomonas aeruginosa*. Treatment of acute exacerbation in these patients becomes complicated in that aminoglycosides are often the preferred agent though have a great deal of difficulty penetrating into the sputum when intravenous (IV) preparations are used. To reach an appropriate concentration in the sputum, toxic levels are often required. Repeated courses of lower dosed IV antibiotics led to the anticipated development of drug resistance. To combat this phenomenon, inhaled antibiotic therapy for CF has been focused on the delivery of these agents as suppressive therapy between periods of acute attacks [1]. However, the use of inhaled antibiotics for acute respiratory exacerbations in CF patients may offer little benefit over IV therapy though such therapy may be beneficial in non-CF populations with chronic bronchiectasis and tracheobronchitis [2, 3].

Mechanical Ventilation
Critically ill or injured patients often require mechanical ventilation in an intensive care unit (ICU) during the course of their illness. Mechanical ventilation predisposes these patients to airway colonization to gram-negative organisms or *Staplococcus aureus*. Because of heavy antibiotic use within ICUs, multidrug resistant organisms are emerging as part of this colonization. Mechanical ventilation is a significant risk factor for the development of ventilator-associated pneumonia (VAP) with virulent and/or resistant organisms.

The microbiologic patterns of ICU pneumonias often require the delivery of high tissue concentrations of drug or the use of pharmaceuticals with otherwise objectionable side effects due to the presence of these bacteria. IV antibiotics often have poor penetration into lung parenchyma limiting effectiveness against these difficult pneumonias. To achieve the necessary tissue concentrations with the use of IV aminoglycosides, the risk of ototoxicity and nephrotoxicity are well described. The use of polymyxins is increasing because of continued emergences of multidrug resistant pneumonias though frustration surrounds their use because of the known side effects of nephrotoxicity, neuromuscular blockade, and neurotoxicity.

Inhaled antibiotic therapy in the ICU has been shown to deliver high concentrations of antibiotics directly to the endobrochial tree to minimize the effects of systemic use or when multidrug resistant patterns mandate such therapy. The use of aerosolized aminoglycosides allows for sputum concentrations to be 10–50 times greater than serum levels with equivalent IV dosing. Low systemic concentrations of drug are reported when inhaled delivery is utilized alleviating concerns over parenteral complications. Clinical success has been reported with the use of inhaled antibiotics with traditional systemic choices for both VAP with *Pseudomonas*, *Acinetobacter*, and multidrug resistant ICU pneumonias. Further work is emerging that the use of monotherapy inhaled antibiotics may be a safe and effective alternative to combination systemic therapy for VAP [4]. Nonetheless, the use of inhaled antibiotics for the prophylaxis of pneumonia in mechanically ventilated patients is neither effective nor supported at this time.

Application

Instruments: At present there are no metered dose inhalers for aerosolized antibiotic delivery. In spontaneously breathing subjects an updraft nebulizer is commonly used. However, in order to protect the caregiver and reduce the antibiotic freely floating in the air, filters are used to trap the antibiotic aerosol. Similarly in the ventilator circuit an updraft nebulizer or vibrating mesh nebulizer is used. The advantage of the vibrating mesh nebulizer is that it coordinates aerosol delivery with inspiration and does not impact ventilator performance. When used with a ventilator, a filter must be placed proximal to the exhaled monitoring port to protect the sensors. The filter is typically placed prior to the initiation of aerosolization and removed when the therapy is complete. Failure to change the filter will result in increased resistance and elevated airway pressures (Figs. 1 and 2).

Schedule: Aerosolized tobramyacin and other aminoglycosides are commonly delivered every 8 h. Aerosolized colistin is typically given every 12 h.

Access: Aerosol can be delivered via a mouthpiece and updraft nebulizer and requires 10–12 min to complete the treatment. In a mechanically ventilated patient, the nebulizer is placed in the circuit in the inspiratory limb. Using an updraft nebulizer will require 10–12 min. The vibrating mesh nebulizer will require much longer as medication is only aerosolized during inspiration.

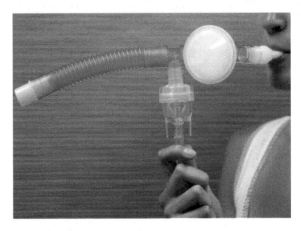

Aerosolized Antibiotics. Figure 1 Updraft nebulizer with expiratory filter for delivery of aerosolized antibiotics

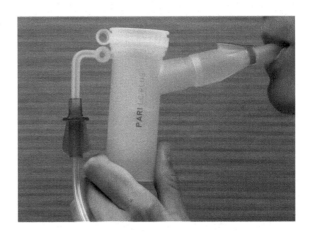

Aerosolized Antibiotics. Figure 2 Pari nebulizer often used for delivery of tobramycin aerosol

Monitoring: The most common side effect of aerosolized antibiotics is bronchospasm. This may be alleviated by pretreatment with a bronchodilator. Auscultation is the most important tool for detection of wheezing. In ventilated patients, changes in peak inspiratory pressure and peak inspiratory flow may suggest increased airway resistance.

Complications

Limitations for the use of inhaled antibiotics do exist. The effects of mucus plugging, excessive secretions, and consolidation on drug delivery are still unclear. Well-established literature as to the systemic exposure that one may see is still uncertain as more antibiotics are delivered in an aerosolized form. Concern still exists over the potential increase of multidrug resistant bacteria if antibiotic instillations were to become airborne repetitively in an clinical environment. Large prospective trials are needed to clarify the above concerns but also to objectively define beneficial populations for its use. Nonetheless, inhaled antibiotics continue to progress at a rapid pace as an encouraging option in the treatment of significant pulmonary infections. A potential technical issue revolves around the effects of the drugs on the expired side of the ventilator. Filters can be placed in line to protect the volume- and pressure-monitoring transducers, but must be changed to prevent increased resistance or occlusion. When filters are not used, heated sensors evaporate the diluents leaving the residue of the drug on the sensor and altering function.

References

1. Langton Hewer SC, Smyth AR (2009) Antibiotic strategies for eradicating Pseudomonas aeruginosa in people with cystic fibrosis. Cochrane Database Syst Rev 7:CD004197
2. O'Riordan TG (2000) Inhaled antimicrobial therapy: from cystic fibrosis to the flu. Respir Care 45:836–845
3. Bilton D, Henig N, Morrissey B, Gotfried M (2006) Addition of inhaled tobramycin to ciprofloxacin for acute exacerbations of Pseudomonas aeruginosa infections in adult bronchiectasis. Chest 130:1503–1510
4. Falagas ME, Agrafiotis M, Athanassa A, Siempos II (2008) Administration of antibiotics via the respiratory tract as monotherapy for pneumonia. Expert Rev Anti Infect Ther 6:447–452

Afterload

Lara Wijayasiri[1], Andrew Rhodes[2], Maurizio Cecconi[2]
[1]Department of Anaesthesia, St. George's Hospital, London, UK
[2]Department of Intensive Care, St. George's Hospital, London, UK

Synonyms

Pulmonary vascular resistance; Systemic vascular resistance

Definition

In the simplest of terms, afterload can be thought of as the load or resistance against which the heart has to work in order to eject a given volume of blood. However, this definition fails to reflect the various parameters that affect afterload and therefore a more in-depth definition is required. Based on LaPlace's law ($T = (P \times r)/2$, where T = tension, P = intraventricular pressure, and r = intraventricular radius), afterload can be defined as the stress within the ventricular wall that develops during systolic ejection. Note that the terms "tension" and "stress" are interchangeable as tension is equal to wall stress (S) multiplied by wall thickness (h). Hence, LaPlace's law can also be written as $S = (P \times r)/2\ h$. This principle highlights the dependence of afterload on ventricular radius and wall thickness. At a given pressure, afterload is increased with an increase in intraventricular radius (dilatation) and is reduced by an increase in ventricular wall thickness (e.g., concentric hypertrophy).

Characteristics

Factors increasing left ventricular afterload:

- Valvular obstruction – for example, aortic stenosis
- Increased systemic vascular resistance (SVR)
- Decreased aortic compliance
- Increased left intraventricular volume

Factors increasing right ventricular afterload:

- Valvular obstruction – for example, pulmonary valve stenosis
- Increased pulmonary vascular resistance (PVR)
- Increased right ventricular volume

An acute increase in afterload shifts the Frank–Starling curve (length–tension relationship) down and to the right. As afterload increases, the velocity of myocardial shortening decreases (based on force–velocity relationship) and therefore during a finite period of systole, less blood gets ejected resulting in a reduced stroke volume and an increased end-diastolic volume. This leads to a secondary increase in ventricular end-diastolic volume (preload) as venous return is added to the increased end-systolic volume. Therefore, during the next contraction, stroke volume is increased due to the Frank–Starling mechanism. This intrinsic ability of the heart to restore stroke volume towards normal in the context of an acute increase in afterload is known as the Anrep effect [1, 2].

Measurement of Afterload

SVR and PVR are commonly used as clinical indices of left and right ventricular afterload, respectively, and therefore factors affecting these are crucial determinants of ventricular afterload. Vascular resistance refers to the forces that oppose or "resist" the flow of blood within a vascular bed. The two main components of vascular resistance are:

- Flow component – refers to the frictional opposition of blood flow through the vessels of which blood viscosity is a major determinant – the greater the viscosity, the higher the vascular resistance
- Reactive component – refers to vascular compliance and inertia of the ejected blood and is dependent on the pulsatile nature of the pressure waveform – the lower the compliance, the higher the vascular resistance

Factors Affecting SVR

- Vessel diameter – Hagen–Poiseuille law states that resistance is inversely related to the fourth power of the radius ($R \propto 1/r^4$), which means that halving the radius of a vessel increases the resistance to blood flow 16-fold. Vasoconstriction, especially of smaller arterioles (e.g., due to α_1 adrenoceptor agonists, sympathetic nervous system activation, circulating catecholamines, angiotensin II, vasopressin, and hypothermia) increases SVR. Vasodilatation (e.g., due to β_2 adrenoceptor agonists, lactic acid, hydrogen ions, nitric oxide, hyperthermia, and sepsis) decreases SVR [2–4].
- Compliance of the systemic circulation.
- Blood viscosity and hematocrit.

Factors Affecting PVR

- Vessel diameter – vasoconstriction (e.g., due to hypoxia, acidosis, hypercapnia, and histamine) increases PVR, while vasodilatation (e.g., due to nitric oxide, prostacyclin, and sildenafil) reduces PVR.
- Positive pressure ventilation increases PVR.
- Disease states – left to right cardiac shunts, mitral stenosis, pulmonary fibrosis, pulmonary emboli, obstructive sleep apnea, and high altitude all increase PVR with the risk of developing pulmonary hypertension.
- Compliance of the pulmonary circulation.
- Blood viscosity and hematocrit.

However, both SVR and PVR cannot be measured directly and instead they are derived using the principle of Ohm's law, which relates cardiac output, pressure, and resistance ($V = I \times R$, where V = voltage, now representing pressure, I = current, now representing flow or cardiac output and R = resistance).

$$SVR \ (dyne.s/cm^5) = 80 \times (MAP - RAP)/CO$$

where, MAP = mean arterial pressure (mmHg) RAP = right atrial pressure (mmHg) CO = cardiac output (l/min)

Normal values for SVR range from 800 to 1200 dyne.s/cm^5. However, it is typically quoted as SVR index (SVRI) in order to standardize values to body surface area. Normal values for SVRI range from 1900 to 2400 dyne.$s/cm^5/m^2$.

$$PVR \ (dyne.s/cm^5) = 80 \times (PAP - PAOP)/CO$$

where, PAP = pulmonary artery pressure (mmHg) PAOP = pulmonary artery occlusion pressure (mmHg)

Typical values for PVR lie below 250 dyne.s/cm^5. Again these are typically quoted as PVR index (PVRI), which range from 255 to 285 dyne.$s/cm^5/m^2$.

Limitations of SVR and PVR

The major limitation of using SVR and PVR data are that they are derived values. The equations used to calculate these parameters do not take into consideration the effects of viscosity, pulsatile flow, and/or pressure changes that occur in the various vascular beds. Furthermore, these equations assume a linear relationship between flow and pressure, which in reality does not exist. Therefore, these derived values are prone to error and should be used judiciously by those who understand the associated flaws and pitfalls of the data.

References

1. Norton JM (2001) Toward consistent definitions for preload and afterload. Adv Physiol Educ 25(1–4):53–61
2. Klabunde RE (2005) Cardiovascular physiology concepts, 1st edn. Lippincott Williams & Wilkins, Philadelphia, pp 72–75
3. Mebazaa A, Gheorghiade M, Zannad FM et al (2008) Acute heart failure, 1st edn. Springer Verlag, London, pp 44–45
4. Parrillo JE, Dellinger RP (2008) Critical care medicine: principles of diagnosis and management in the adult, 3rd edn. Mosby Elsevier, Philadelphia, pp 39–52

AH

Absolute humidity. It is the mass of water vapor held in a given volume of gas at a particular temperature.

AIDS

Acquired immunodeficiency syndrome – the syndrome caused by HIV that occurs when defined opportunistic infections occur as a result of progressive immune damage.

Air Embolus

▶ Bronchovenous Air Embolism

Air Hunger

▶ Dyspnea: Differential Diagnosis

Airborne Transmission

This refers to disease transmission, where droplet nuclei (resulting from evaporated droplets) or dust particles containing microorganisms can remain suspended in the air for long periods of time, allowing organisms to enter the upper and lower respiratory tracts. Organisms transmitted in this manner must be capable of surviving for a long period of time outside the body and must be resistant to drying. This differs from droplet transmission, in that droplets are too large to be airborne for long periods of time, and quickly settle out of air. A well-fitted N95 mask may provide protection against airborne transmission.

Airflow Obstruction

▶ Decompensated Chronic Obstructive Pulmonary Disease

Airway Assessment

▶ Airway Management

Airway Control

▶ Tracheal Intubation in Acute Procedures

Airway Management

STUART F. REYNOLDS, PETER G. BRINDLEY
Division of Critical Care Medicine, University of Alberta Hospitals, Edmonton, AB, Canada

Synonyms

Airway assessment; Airway pharmacology; Bag-valve-mask ventilation; Difficult airway; Endotracheal intubation; Rapid sequence intubation

Definition

Airway management involves ensuring airway patency, protecting the lungs from aspiration (airway protection), and aiding oxygenation and ventilation. It is one of the most common and most urgent invasive procedures in the intensive care unit (ICU). It is, therefore, also an obligatory skill for intensive care physicians. Comprehensive airway management requires knowledge, procedural dexterity, and judgment in each of the following areas: preparation, airway assessment, basic maneuvers, laryngoscopy, endotracheal intubation (ETI), pharmacology, and post-intubation care.

Pre-existing Condition

Common indications for tracheal intubation include decreased level of consciousness (LOC), a threat to airway patency (whether from bulbar dysfunction, trauma, aspiration, or airway edema from inhalational injury, infection, or angioedema), and/or cardiac or pulmonary dysfunction (such that the patient cannot adequately oxygenate or ventilate). However, the commonest reasons for intubation differ if we compare the ICU, emergency room (ER), and operating room (OR). Typically, endotracheal intubation facilitates the provision of general anesthetic for surgical procedure. In the ER, central nervous system (CNS) dysfunction leads to intubation more often than in the ICU, whereas, pulmonary and/or cardiac dysfunction leads to intubation more commonly in the ICU.

Indications

Ventilation enables gas exchange; whereby blood receives oxygen and expels carbon dioxide. Aberrant blood gas values are often used to initiate an ICU consult regarding whether airway management is required. This approach does identify patients in peril, but in reality, is physiologically simplistic. Therefore, intensivists need an understanding of hypoxemia (low partial pressure of arterial oxygen), hypoxia (low cellular oxygen, usually identified by lactic acidemia), and acute hypercapnia/hypercarbia (usually identified by decreased blood pH or increased $PaCO_2$). While a comprehensive review is beyond our scope, a basic understanding is required to guide airway management.

Hypoxemia includes rare causes such as low barometric pressure, hypoventilation, low fractional inspired oxygen, low venous oxygen, or diffusion abnormalities. However, the vast majority of cases are due to imbalance between lung perfusion (Q) and ventilation (V). This is known as V/Q mismatching, and has a spectrum ranging from pathologic shunt, all Q but no V, to dead space, all V but no Q. Pathologic shunts can be secondary to pulmonary parenchymal disease (water, pus, cells, or blood in the alveolar space), pulmonary vascular disease (pulmonary arteriovenous malformations, or physiologic shunting in the case of end-stage liver disease), or extrapulmonary causes (whether from right-to-left intracardiac shunts, or venous-to-arterial systemic shunts). In reality, the diseased alveolar-capillary interface exhibits heterogeneity as shunt and dead space often coexist. However, these two extremes can be distinguished – both therapeutically and diagnostically – because oxygen therapy will *not* improve the hypoxemia from shunt, but will from dead space and V/Q mismatch.

Hypercapnia (increased $paCO_2$) results from inadequate ventilation relative to production. Dead space, from disorders such as obstructive lung disease and pulmonary embolus, can therefore cause elevated arterial carbon dioxide in those with inadequate ventilatory drive. However, most awake patients mitigate this through hyperventilation, and therefore more often present as hypoxemia. While conditions such as malignant hyperthermia, fever, and sympathetic excess can also cause hypercapnia due to excess carbon dioxide production, this is also rare in the ICU. What this means is that ICU hypercarbia is usually due to either decreased minute ventilation (whether from sedation, central nervous system dysfunction, or neuromuscular compromise) or the aforementioned pathologic dead space. In short, a systematic approach is required to determine if it is time to supplement or control respiratory efforts. It is also needed to understand the cause and ameliorate the problem.

Application

Preparation

It has been argued that "failing to prepare means preparing to fail." As such, the skilled physician understands that airway management requires preparation, situational awareness, and sufficient skills to coordinate all resources (both equipment and personnel). Control of the evolving crisis is vital, but is not the focus of this review. However, in this vein, the mnemonic "**Y BAG PEOPLE**" does provide a useful construct for preparation [1]. It stands for **Y**ankauer suction; **B**VM; **A**ccess vein; **G**et your team ready; **P**osition the patient; **E**ndotracheal tubes (and check cuffs); **O**ropharyngeal Airway; **P**harmacy (prepare drugs); **L**aryngoscope – variety of blades and confirm the light is working; and **E**valuate for a difficult airway. When verbalized, this mnemonic also reminds physicians not to provide positive pressure ventilation to patients who are meeting their gas exchange needs with spontaneous efforts. This reminder may seem trite, but it is common during crises to see spontaneously breathing patient receiving bag-valve-mask ventilation. In this setting, positive pressure insufflates the stomach thereby increasing the chance of emesis and aspiration. Obviously, if the patient is not meeting gas exchange needs then 100% oxygen and BVM should be expedited.

Airway Assessment

The difficult airway is defined by anatomic, historical, and clinical factors that increase the likelihood of being unable to oxygenate, unable to ventilate, and/or unable to intubate. The incidence of difficult tracheal intubation (DTI): defined as the need for more than three intubation attempts or attempts at intubation that last >10 min in patients undergoing anesthesia, is typically reported between 1% and 3%. The incidence of a difficult intubation in ICU patients is as high as 20%. The difference is related primarily to patient and situational factors, not the physician's specialty [2].

Significant research has provided clues, albeit imperfect, as to which patients will be more difficult. As such an airway assessment is beneficial. However, these models were typically developed for anesthetists working with patients in the OR. Given the acuity of critical illness, it is hardly surprising that most models have not been validated to the ICU or ER. Regardless, the presence of risk factors is useful as it encourages the clinician to redouble efforts to ensure that alternative strategies are readily available, and that help is nearby.

The Mallampati classification is widely promoted for patients undergoing elective intubation. In short, a cooperative, awake patient sits upright, and, without phonating, protrudes his/her tongue. The physician analyzes how much of the posterior pharynx and uvula can be visualized. There is a four-point grading system, from best to worst. Reasonable correlation exists between class I/II and easy laryngoscopy, while class III/IV is suggestive of difficulty. Obviously, though, this is of limited use for emergency intubations in the ICU. However, similar information may be obtained and proximal airway obstruction may be ruled out by visualizing the oropharynx with a tongue blade. As well, the intensivist can perform a rapid airway assessment and assess a patient's interincisor distance (three finger breadths or mouth opening greater than 3 cm- and ideally greater than 5 cm- suggests adequate room for insertion and rotation of the laryngoscope blade) (Fig. 1) and thyromental distance (three finger breadths or a span of greater than 6 cm suggests that the glottis opening is likely to be in a good position to be visualized; and not in an excessively anterior position) (Fig. 2). Furthermore the Intensivist can also perform a mandibular protrusion test (the ability to cover the upper lip with the lower incisors).

Large observational studies have reviewed historical and physical characteristics of OR patients [3, 4]. The goal was to determine predictors and incidence of both difficult and impossible mask ventilation. They concluded rates of 1.4% for difficult mask ventilation (DMV) and 0.16% for impossible mask ventilation. The terrifying combination of difficult or impossible ventilation *as well as* difficult intubation occurred 0.37% of the time. The independent predictors of difficult mask ventilation (DMV) included: obesity, presence of a beard, Mallampati III or IV, age >57, limited jaw protrusion, and a history of snoring. The independent predictors of impossible mask ventilation were: history of neck irradiation, sleep apnea, and either a beard or Mallampati III/IV visualization. Risk factors for the combination of difficult or impossible mask ventilation and difficult intubation included: Mallampati III/IV, abnormal cervical spine, thick obese neck, thyromental distance <6 cm, mouth opening <3 cm, limited mandibular protrusion, snoring, sleep apnea, and obesity (Fig. 3). Additional risk factors for a difficult airway include limitations in spinal movement (e.g., rheumatoid or osteoarthritis, spondyloarthropathies, trauma, even severe diabetes) or macroglossia (e.g., in hypothyroidism and Down's Syndrome).

Our practice is to briefly obtain a history of previous difficult intubation, neck irradiation, neck pathology, or snoring. As well, during preparation we assess the patients interincisor distance, thyromental distance, and if the patient can cooperate we perform a mandibular protrusion test. We inspect the oropharynx. We also note the presence of obesity (Fig. 4). If any historical factors are present or physical assessment abnormal we ensure that adjuncts or a difficult airway cart is available.

Basic Maneuvers

Positioning

The optimal position for intubation attempts has been summarized as the "sniffing position" or "sniff the morning air position." While several authors have argued that novices fail to understand what is implied by this analogy, it is intended to communicate neck flexion at the lower cervical spine, extension at the upper cervical spine, and positioning the ears at level with the sternum (Fig. 5). This position should not be attempted in patients with suspected spinal trauma or pathology. Fortunately, there is also evidence suggesting that simple neck extension alone is as effective as the "sniffing position" in nontrauma patients undergoing endotracheal intubation in the OR. Recumbence may be also difficult in many ICU patients, whether from obesity, pulmonary edema, or ascites. In these patients meticulous attention to head position and use of semi-fowler's, reverse Trendelenburg, or ramp-up position will assist

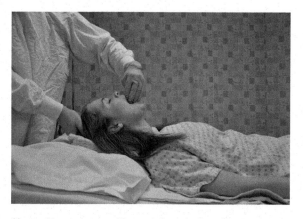

Airway Management. Figure 1 Inter-incisor distance

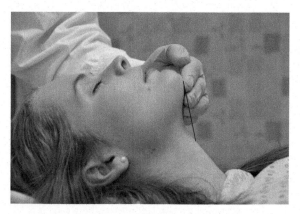

Airway Management. Figure 2 Thyro-mental distance: >6 cm suggests adequate laryngoscopic view

Risk Factors	DMV*	IMV**	DMV/IMV and DTI
Historical			
Sleep Apnea	♦	♦	♦
Snoring	♦	♦	♦
Neck Irradiation		♦	□
Physical			
Obesity	♦	♦	♦
Thick Neck	♦	♦	♦
Edendulous dentition	♦		
Thyromental distance < 6 cm	♦	♦	♦
Mouth Opening < 3 cm	♦		♦
Limited MPT^Φ	♦		♦
Beard	♦	♦	□

* Difficult Mask Ventilation ** Impossible Mask Ventilation
Φ Mandibular Protrusion Test
Modified from Kheterpal, S, Martin, L, Shanks, A et al. Prediction and Outcomes of Impossible Mask Ventilation: A Review of 50,000 Anesthetics. Anesthesiology 2009; 110:891–897

Airway Management. Figure 3 Risk factors for DMV and DTI

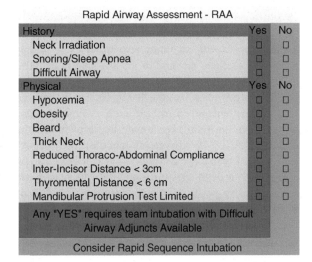

Rapid Airway Assessment - RAA

History	Yes	No
Neck Irradiation	□	□
Snoring/Sleep Apnea	□	□
Difficult Airway	□	□
Physical	**Yes**	**No**
Hypoxemia	□	□
Obesity	□	□
Beard	□	□
Thick Neck	□	□
Reduced Thoraco-Abdominal Compliance	□	□
Inter-Incisor Distance < 3cm	□	□
Thyromental Distance < 6 cm	□	□
Mandibular Protrusion Test Limited	□	□

Any "YES" requires team intubation with Difficult Airway Adjuncts Available

Consider Rapid Sequence Intubation

Airway Management. Figure 4 Rapid airway assessment

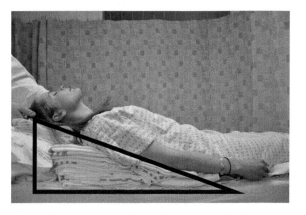

Airway Management. Figure 5 Sniffing position. Note the patients ears are at the level of the sternum, the lower cervical spine is flexed; and the upper cervical spine is extended

preoxygenation, BVM, laryngoscopy, and intubation (Fig. 6).

Airway Patency

Discussions of ICU airway management often emphasize laryngoscopy and special adjuncts to intubation. It is paramount to emphasize that intensivists first need to be experts in maintaining airway patency, oxygenation, and ventilation with a bag-valve-mask (BVM). Airways in critically ill patients may be obstructed for a multitude of reasons (oral secretions, blood, vomit, trauma, redundant oropharyngeal tissue secondary to edema or adiposity, and above all from inadequate oropharyngeal muscular tone). Obstruction may manifest as stridor, or increased

Airway Management. Figure 6 Ramp up position

respiratory effort, tracheal tug, paradoxical chest abdominal movements, or worsening hypoxemia. If unresolved this can deteriorate to bradycardia and cardiac arrest. As part of airway assessment, the intensivist should rapidly identify and remedy obstruction by suctioning and clearing the oropharynx. If the airway remains compromised, a head-tilt-chin-lift or jaw thrust maneuver often helps. If the patient has suspected or identified spinal pathology the chin-lift should be avoided, but the jaw thrust still utilized to open and maintain the airway. These maneuvers work by increasing the distance between the soft palate and posterior tongue – the most common area of obstruction.

If the airway remains obstructed despite a clear oropharyngeal space and a head-tilt-chin-lift or jaw thrust maneuver, the cause of obstruction may be more distal. It may also be the result of laryngospasm which usually responds to simple maneuvers such as gentle suctioning, cessation of airway stimulation, and repositioning by chin-lift or jaw thrust and gentle BVM. If cricoid pressure is being applied then easing up may help. Adjuncts to the above measures include oropharyngeal airways (OPA) (Fig. 7) and nasopharyngeal airways (NPA) (Fig. 8). The OPA is a noxious stimulus thus should be utilized in patients that are either adequately sedated or are unconscious; otherwise it may promote emesis and aspiration. NPAs are somewhat easier for patients to tolerate; but topicalization of the nasal mucosa with local anesthetic and vasoconstrictors is recommended in awake patients. Use of the NPA is contraindicated in patients with signs of basal skull fracture or with severe facial trauma. In rare instances, both an OPA and NPA are required. If these adjuncts are not adequate the next considerations are to directly visualize for an obstruction with direct laryngoscopy or fiberoptically. If no obstruction is readily apparent insert a rescue device such as a laryngeal mask airway (L.M.A.) to assist oxygenation and ventilation. Meanwhile preparations should be underway for a surgical airway if the patient is not able to be ventilated or oxygenated.

Preoxygenation and BVM Ventilation (BVM)

Both preoxygenation and BVM ventilation can be difficult in the critically ill. Preoxygenation, or alveolar denitrogenation, is ideally achieved through the provision of 100% oxygen via face-mask or BVM to the patient for at least 5 min. The goal is to replace alveolar nitrogen with oxygen thereby creating a reservoir of oxygen to prevent hypoxemia during subsequent intubation. This may be challenging in critically ill patients because of concurrent cardiopulmonary pathology, or if patients have low functional residual capacity due to obesity, abdominal pathology or preexisting lung derecruitment. Of note, even transient hypoxia in patients with ARDS has been associated with neurocognitive deficits; thus every opportunity should be taken to maintain adequate oxygenation.

In patients with an intact respiratory drive that is providing adequate rate and depth of respiration, 100% oxygen can be delivered via a high flow oxygen mask, non-rebreather mask, or the BMV device. In patients that are spontaneously breathing but have limited effort, oxygenation and ventilation should be augmentation by squeezing the BVM. Preoxygenation of the acutely hypoxemic patient with an intact respiratory drive can also be augmented through the provision of 100% oxygen via a non-invasive positive pressure circuit (e.g., CPAP or Bipap), or via a BVM with a tight seal and a PEEP valve. Regardless, the clinician must look, listen, and feel to assess whether the patient is being adequately oxygenated (and ventilated). He/she should *look* for chest expansion,

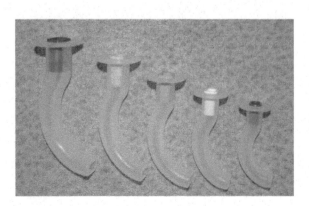

Airway Management. Figure 7 Oropharyngeal airways

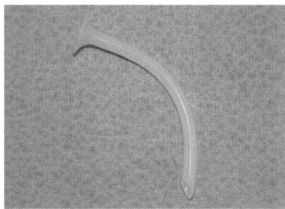

Airway Management. Figure 8 Nasopharyngeal airway

filling of the reservoir bag of the BVM, improving pulse oximeter reading, and improvement in color. He/she should *listen* for any hiss indicative of a poor seal, and for a pulse oximeter tone indicative of an adequate saturation. He/she should *feel* the compliance of the self-inflating bag, or leaking air against one's hand from poorly sealed mask. If inadequate ventilation is identified, despite assurance of an open airway, then two-person BVM should be performed.

Laryngoscopy and Tracheal Intubation

Laryngoscopy and tracheal intubation is the standard-of-care for the emergency airway. Clinicians should be prepared to use alternate airway devices or procedures (e.g., fiber-optic modalities – flexible bronchoscope, GlideScope™, and the surgical airway). As such, the patient should be optimally positioned and preoxygenated (as discussed above). Dentures, which improve the seal obtained during BVM, should be removed for intubation. Cricoid pressure may decrease the likelihood of aspiration but may worsen glottic view. In contrast, external laryngeal manipulation (also known as a BURP maneuver: backward, upward, rightward pressure on the thyroid cartilage) typically improves glottic view, but does not protect against aspiration.

A variety of laryngoscopes are available. The Macintosh blade is curved in order to conform to the shape of the tongue and so that its blade tip can be placed in the vallecula. As the blade tip is lifted, pressure on the hyoepiglottic ligament helps lift the epiglottis, thereby exposing the underlying glottic opening. A size 3 Macintosh blade is appropriate for the majority of adult patients, although for those with long necks, a Macintosh 4 may be needed. Straight laryngoscopy blades such as the Miller, Phillips, or Wisconsin also displace the tongue to the left but unlike the Macintosh they directly elevate the epiglottis. Often used as the blades of choice in pediatric patients, they can also be useful in the adult patient with an "anterior" larynx, small mandible, large tongue, or prominent incisors. Cadaveric studies suggest that the Miller blade produces less movement of an unstable cervical vertebra – thus may be the blade of choice in multitrauma patients. The McCoy blade has the shape of the Macintosh, but also features a levering distal tip to lift the hyoepiglottic ligament.

The laryngoscope handle should be held in the left hand and close to the blade, and the head approximately level with the intubator's xiphisternum. Following Macintosh blade insertion, the clinician's right hand can be placed under the patient's occiput. With this hand lifting the head, additional lower neck flexion and head extension can be performed. The blade should be inserted to the right of the tongue. This should occur slowly and deliberately, to enable time to identify anatomy at the blade tip. By "looking-as-you-go," clinicians avoid placing the blade too far. After the epiglottis is identified, the blade tip is advanced into the vallecula. The blade tip is then centered, by moving it to the left, and an additional lift applied along the longitudinal axis of the laryngoscope. The handle should be lifted – not levered – at an angle no more than 30° to the floor. If a chosen blade it too short to successfully contact the hyoepiglottic ligament at the junction of the tongue base and epiglottis, the epiglottis may not move out of the way. Too long a blade can occasionally trap and push back the epiglottis, creating a worse glottic view. Curved blades can also be used to directly elevate the epiglottis in the same way as a straight blade, but failure to engage the hyoepiglottic ligament is a common reason for novices to be unsuccessful.

The prepared endotracheal tube, with lubricated stylet inserted, should then be passed by an assistant to the clinician's open right hand. This cooperative approach avoids interrupting direct visualization of the cords. The best ways to confirm a properly placed tube is to watch it go through the cords. Other signs include end-tidal carbon dioxide ($ETCO_2$) detection, auscultation of air entry to the hemithoraces at the midaxillary line, and normalization of oxygen saturation. Esophageal detection devices neither confirm tracheal placement of the endotracheal tube nor detect esophageal placement, and thus should not be used. Once positioned, the tube is held with one hand, the laryngoscope removed, and the cuff inflated with 5–10 ml of air.

Post-intubation Care

The clinician should now shift focus to post-intubation care and monitoring of complications. The endotracheal must be secured to prevent displacement. The level at which to secure the endotracheal tube is determined both clinically and radiographically. Generally, securing the endotracheal tube at 24 cm for men and 22 cm for women will result in the endotracheal tube resting 2–5 cm above the carina. It is important to remember that the distance traveled by the endotracheal tube between full neck flexion to full neck extension can be 10 cm. Thus excessive neck movement may result in an unforeseen extubation or mainstem bronchus intubation. Various commercial devices are available to secure the endotracheal tube; but in most circumstances use of cloth tape is sufficient. In cases of facial trauma or burns, the endotracheal may need to be secured with a silk tie to a tooth.

Post-intubation hypoxemia and/or hypotension are not uncommon in the critically ill patient. Thus a systematic approach to each should be applied. In the face of hypoxemia – the mnemonic **CODE** provides a construct to quickly identify and respond to common causes of post-intubation hypoxemia. The clinician should assess for **C**ollapse: whether from pneumothorax or atelectasis. Pneumothorax, either tension or simple may result because of intubation and the provision of positive pressure; identified by noting unequal auscultation, asymmetrical chest movement, and resonance on percussion; and remedied via the placement of 14 G needle in the second intercostals space or formal tube thoracostomy. Atelectasis may occur during intubation, particularly in situations where there is cephalad deflection of the diaphragm (obesity, ascites, etc.) or aspiration of gastric contents. Atelectasis is identified via auscultation and radiographic changes, and remedied through the provision of positive end expiratory pressure (PEEP) or bronchoscopy. **O**bstruction of the endotracheal tube secondary to aspirated contents, secretions, or a kink is suggested by the inability to pass a suction catheter down the endotracheal tube. Removing the obstruction may require additional suctioning or bronchoscopy, or reintubation. **D**isplacement, resulting in extubation can be identified by noting a continuous endotracheal cuff leak, or a reduction of ETCO2. Displacement resulting in mainstem bronchus intubation can be detected by noting unilateral breath sounds during auscultation. **E**quipment failure should be sought by following the oxygen supply from the patient to source; and ensuring all connection are secure and the patient is receiving 100% oxygen. Patients should be removed from mechanical ventilator and provided 100% oxygen via the bag-valve device.

Post-intubation hypotension is usually multifactorial, and most commonly associated with the provision of positive pressure ventilation combined with hypovolemia and induction medications. The best treatment for this complication is prevention by identifying patients at risk of hypotension – particularly hypovolemic and hemodynamically compromised patients. During the preparation phase of intubation, hypovolemic patients should receive boluses of isotonic crystalloid in anticipation of hypotension; in addition, strong consideration should be given to starting either vasopressors or inotropes in patients with septic shock or cardiac dysfunction, prior to induction. Although these are the most common causes of hypotension, the clinician must rule out tension pneumothorax as a cause of vascular collapse during intubation or immediately after intubation.

Airway Pharmacology

Airway management in the critically ill requires expertise with airway pharmacology. It also requires an understanding of how pharmacokinetics can change in the critically ill, thereby making the physiologic effects of drugs less predictable [5]. The first practical tip is that physicians should, therefore, guard against overzealous drug administration. This can result from a simple stress-induced desire to rapidly sedate the patient. It can also result from failure to compensate for slower circulatory drug delivery, or decreased drug metabolism, or from a failure to appreciate the patient's deceased hemodynamic reserve. As such, it is useful to emphasize that you can always give more, but you cannot take it away once given. The second tip is that proper drug selection may mean balancing competing goals: preserving hemodynamic stability, but achieving patient compliance, and attenuating the physiologic consequences of airway manipulation (see below). The goal is to increase chance of successful intubation, but decrease the risk of complications (such as aspiration, and hemodynamic collapse). Regardless, for these reasons, experts in airway management are also experts in airway pharmacology.

Physiology of Airway Management

The human homunculus reveals tremendous amount of the somatosensory cortex devoted to the oropharynx and larynx. In other words, these areas are richly innervated with sensory fibers, and stimulation can result in pain, agitation, and physiologic reflexes. Stimulation of reflexes intended to protect the airway, such as the gag, can result in emesis and aspiration. Airway stimulation, from both laryngoscopy and endotracheal tube insertion, can also cause sympathetic discharge. This "pressor response" can cause tachycardia and hypertension which can exacerbate ongoing myocardial ischemia, dysrhythmias, hypertension, or cerebral edema. Excessive stimulation of the cholinergic portion of the autonomic nervous system can cause bronchorrhea, bronchoconstriction, and bradycardia (the so-called cholingergic response). Thus airway stimulation can increase intracranial pressure and worsen ischemia. Therefore, patients unlikely to tolerate adverse physiologic consequences of laryngoscopy and tracheal intubation (e.g., those with myocardial or cerebral ischemia, elevated intracranial pressure, dissecting aneurysm, hypertensive crisis, asthma, or COPD, to name but a few) will typically benefit from a preinduction agent. These agents include opioids, local anesthetics, beta-adrenergic antagonists, and nondepolarizing neuromuscular blockers (NMBA), each of which are summarized in table form, and discussed below.

Specific Agents

Opioids are central to airway management because of their analgesic and sedative properties. Fentanyl, a synthetic opioid, is commonly used. It has 50–100 times the affinity for μ receptor, and increased lipid solubility compared to morphine. This results in an agent that is very potent with a rapid onset and short duration. Fentanyl effectively blunts the hypertensive response to airway stimulation, although with marginal effects on tachycardia. Other synthetic opioids such as remifentanil, sufentanil, and alfentanil are more effective at blunting both the hypertensive and tachycardic response to intubation. However, caution is advised when using opioids in circulatory shock, as they can block the compensatory sympathetic response to the extent that cardiovascular collapse can ensue. In addition, when administered rapidly in a large dose, these synthetic opioids can be associated with chest wall rigidity and masseter spasm, thereby further complicating oxygenation, ventilation, and intubation. This idiosyncratic reaction is variably responsive to naloxone, and often requires neuromuscular blockade (see below).

Lidocaine, an amide local anesthetic (and class 1B anti-arrhythmic drug), is commonly used to diminish the "pressor response," reduce airway reactivity, mitigate intracranial hypertension, and decrease the incidence of dysrhythmias during intubation. It is used more often in North America than Europe. Regardless, to be most effective, lidocaine should be administered intravenously, 3 minutes prior to laryngoscopy, and at a dose of 1.5 mg/kg. Occasionally awake laryngoscopy and intubation is required. Effective blunting of laryngeal and cholinergic reflexes can be accomplished through topical application of aerosolized lidocaine via a DeVilbiss Atomizer or nebulizer; and the gag reflex may be attenuated by placing lidocaine ointment or spray to the posterior third of the tongue.

Esmolol is a rapid onset, short-acting, cardio-selective beta-adrenergic receptor site antagonist that effectively diminishes the tachycardic response to intubation. However, esmolol can have an unpredictable effect upon the hypertensive response. A combination of esmolol (2 mg/kg) and fentanyl (2 μg/kg) may have a synergistic effect for reducing both the tachycardia and hypertension associated with tracheal intubation and laryngeal manipulation. Caution is recommended in patients likely to be hypovolemic, as they may have become reliant upon the compensatory tachycardia to maintain cardiac output and blood pressure.

Some rapid sequence induction protocols (Fig. 9) are combined with a preinduction dose of nondepolarizing NMBA. This is typically given to patients with suspected raised intracranial or intraocular pressure, for whom succinylcholine administration is planned. This is because succinylcholine use is associated with fasciculations. These can increase intracranial or intraocular pressure, and elevate serum potassium – a particular risk in crush injuries, head injury, stroke, and preexisting neuromuscular disease. A low "defasciculating dose" (one tenth of the intubation dose) of a nondepolarizing NMBA, such as rocuronium, will minimize fasciculations and therefore attenuate adverse effects. A low dose of nondepolarizing NMBA in the brief preinduction interval, given just before sedating induction drugs, does not cause paralysis that conscious patients would otherwise find dysphoric.

Induction/Sedative-Hypnotic Medications

Induction anesthetic agents facilitate intubation by inducing unconsciousness. Clinicians and researchers have suggested, the ideal induction agent for an ICU patient would have a rapid onset of action, short duration of action, analgesic properties, minimal drug interactions, metabolism and excretion that is independent of renal or hepatic function, minimal depression of hemodynamics or respiratory drive, and would maintain cerebral perfusion pressure. It should not be surprising that no single agent yet exists. As with all ICU treatment, agents must be tailored to specific patient needs. Numerous medications are available, but we shall focus on those most useful in ICU. The patient's individual clinical status will determine if the induction agent should be administered by rapid bolus, used as part of a rapid sequence induction protocol (Fig. 9) or be slowly titrated. All induction agents can suppress the myocardium; thus hypotension or shock can result. As a result, unless precluded by patient acuity, it is advisable to first ensure adequate venous access and to provide intravenous fluid boluses and/or vasoactive agents prior to the induction agent. This is intended to reduce the likelihood of post induction hypotension and shock.

Etomidate, an imidazole derivative, has rapid onset of action, short duration, relative cardiac stability, and is associated with reduced cerebral oxygen demands: all of which suggest it would be attractive for induction. Indeed, this drug has been a cornerstone of ER inductions in the United States. However, growing literature has reported adrenal suppression and even death. This was believed to only occur with continuous infusion of etomidate. However, evidence has now shown that even a single dose can cause adrenal suppression, and the use in patients with severe sepsis/septic shock is associated with higher mortality. Thus in patients requiring intubation because of severe sepsis or septic shock, etomidate should not be used, especially as alternative agents are available. However, in

Select Critical Conditions and Associated Steps for Airway Management

Time (min)	RSI Step	Severe Sepsis & Septic Shock	Hypoxic Respiratory Failure (ARDS, Pulmonary Edema, Obesity) - Stable CVS	Hypoxic Respiratory Failure (ARDS, CHF, Obesity) - unstable CVS	Asthma/COPD	Isolated Head Trauma or Brain Injury - CVS stable	Polytrauma with Brain Injury	Poly trauma	Coma/Altered Mental Status, Status Epilepticus - Stable CVS	Shock - compensated (Non-septic)	Hypertensive Crisis, Acute ischemia - heart, brain	Uncompensate Shock
−5	**Preparation & Preoxygenation**											
	Y-BAG-PEOPLE	✓	✓	✓	✓	✓	✓	✓	✓	✓	✓	✓
	100% NRB or via BVM	✓	✓	✓	✓	✓	✓	✓	✓	✓	✓	✓
	Special Considerations											
	NIV or BVM with PEEP		✓	✓								
	Ramp up or Reverse Trendelenberg Position		✓	✓								
	Large Bore IV access or CVC	✓		✓								
	Fluid Bolus	✓		✓	✓					✓		✓
	Vasopressors/Inotropes	✓		✓						✓		✓
	Bronchodilators				✓							
−3	**Pre-medication**											
	Lidocaine 1.5 mg/kg IV OR				✓	✓	✓		✓		✓	
	Fentanyl 3 mcg/kg over 2 min					✓	✓		✓		✓	
0	**Induction Options**											
	INDUCTION AGENT OPTIONS – Use only one. Consider Dose Reduction if Risk of Hypotension											
	Propofol 1–2 mg/kg	x	✓	x		✓	x	x	✓	x	✓	x
	Ketamine 1–2 mg/kg	✓	✓	✓	✓	✓	✓	✓	✓	✓	x	x
	Etomidate 0.2–0.3 mg/kg	x	✓	✓		✓	✓	✓	✓	✓	✓	x ✓
	Scopalamine 0.6 mg IVP		✓	✓								
	Paralysis											
	Succinylcholine 1.5 mg/kg or Rocuronium 1.0 mg/kg	✓	✓	✓	✓	✓	✓	✓	✓	✓	✓	✓
	Special Considerations											
	NMBA Contraindicated											
	Remifentanyl with Propofol		✓			✓			✓			
+1	**Intubation**											
	Laryngoscopy and Tracheal Intubation	✓	✓	✓	✓	✓	✓	✓	✓	✓	✓	✓
	In-line cervical neck stabilization					✓	✓	✓	Consider if suspect secondary to trauma			
	Special Maneoevers											
	BURP Maneuver (Unable to Visualize Glottic Opening)	✓	✓	✓	✓	✓	✓	✓	✓	✓	✓	✓
1+	**Confirmation**											
	Auscultate gastric then bilateral axillae	✓	✓	✓	✓	✓	✓	✓	✓	✓	✓	✓
	ETCO2 Detection	✓	✓	✓	✓	✓	✓	✓	✓	✓	✓	✓
	Secure ETT	✓	✓	✓	✓	✓	✓	✓	✓	✓	✓	✓

Airway Management. Figure 9 Adjuncts and steps for RSI

patients that are hypotensive because of hypovolemia, multitrauma, or cardiac dysfunction, etomidate may be suitable. Other adverse effects include nausea, vomiting, and myoclonic movements. The latter is not of consequence if an NMBA is co-administered.

Ketamine, a phencyclidine derivative, is unique as an induction agent as it causes a dissociative anesthesia, rather than hypnosis. It has potent analgesia, and sympathomimetic effects, but minimal effects on spontaneous respiration or airway protection. It selectively inhibits the cortex and thalamus, while stimulating the limbic system. It also causes functional disorganization of the neural pathways running between the cortex, thalamus, and limbic system. This means the patient often does not appear to be anesthetized and can swallow and open eyes, but does not process information such as pain or memories. Regardless, it is frequently given with an amnestic, such as midazolam to prevent an emergence reaction. Ketamine causes direct bronchial smooth muscle relaxation, and subsequent bronchodilation. It can also increase oral-pharyngeal and laryngeal secretions, and in very rare instances laryngospasm. Premedication with glycopyrrolate (0.005 mg/kg, or 250–500 mcg) may attenuate secretions but is usually not required. Due to the sympathomimetic effects it can augment blood pressure and heart rate. However, because it can increase myocardial oxygen demands and worsen supply–demand imbalance, caution is advised in patients with ongoing cardiac ischemia and hypertensive crisis. Paradoxically, ketamine can also cause *hypotension* due to direct myocardial suppression in patients in an uncompensated shock state. Furthermore, traditionally at least, ketamine was contraindicated in brain injury because of augmentation of cerebral blood flow and resultant increase in intracranial pressure. This dogma needs to be challenged, particularly in the trauma patient where head injury and shock coincide [4]. After all, in brain injury, the goal is to ensure adequate supply to the ischemic penumbra, in order to minimize further injury. Cerebral autoregulation normally maintains cerebral blow flow (CBF), but is deranged by brain injury. Thus CBF becomes proportional to cerebral perfusion pressure. Ketamine either increases or has a neutral response on cerebral perfusion pressure, and reduces cerebral oxygen consumption. Thus, ketamine is probably a rationale induction agent in the brain-injured patient considering its cerebral DO_2/VO_2 profile.

Propofol is a lipid-soluble drug that induces hypnosis in a single arm-brain circulation time. It is favored due to rapid onset and rapid recovery. However, it has no analgesic activity, and is therefore typically given with fentanyl. Propofol reduces ICP, and reduces the cerebral metabolic demands. At induction doses it induces apnea, and profound muscular relaxation. In fact, when given in conjunction with the semi-synthetic opioids it produces intubation conditions similar to an NMBA. Like ketamine, propofol causes direct bronchodilation. However, propofol use as an ICU induction agent is limited because its negative inotropic and vasodilatory properties can result in hypotension. This is particularly pronounced in patients with hypovolemia or poor left-ventricular function. These effects can be attenuated through concomitant intravenous fluid boluses, or ephedrine administration (0.15 mg/kg IV). As a result, propofol use should be targeted to hemodynamically stable patients requiring intubation for altered mental status, isolated head injury, status epilepticus, asthma, or isolated respiratory failure. Anaphylaxis can occur in patients with egg or soy allergies.

The short-acting benzodiazepine, midazolam (versed®), is commonly administered in the ICU either as a bolus (2.5–5.0 mg IV) for procedural sedation, or as an infusion (0–10 mg/h) to facilitate mechanical ventilation. The relatively slow onset of action makes midazolam unsuitable for rapid sequence intubation. However, its potent anxiolytic properties may facilitate awake intubation if used in conjunction with intravenous opioid and topical local anesthetic.

Some ICU patients, particularly those with uncompensated shock, will not tolerate even small doses of induction agents. As a result, Scopolamine (0.4–0.6 mg IV bolus) can be considered. It is a potent amnesic, that when given prior to neuromuscular blockade reduces the likelihood of patient recall of the event, and has minimal hemodynamic consequences.

Neuromuscular blocking agents (NMBA) facilitate intubation by causing brief paralysis of skeletal muscle. There are two classes of NMBA: depolarizing and nondepolarizing. Depolarizing agents activate the acetylcholine receptor whereas nondepolarizing agents competitively inhibit the acetylcholine receptor. NMBAs have no direct effect on blood pressure or cardiac output, though agents such as pancuronium can cause vagolysis and tachycardia. Neither class of NMBA should be utilized routinely in the setting of a predictable difficult airway.

Succinylcholine, a depolarizing NMBA, is a dimer of acetylcholine molecules that binds to the acetylcholine receptor in a biphasic manner. It first opens sodium channels and causes a brief depolarization of the cellular membrane – noted clinically as muscular fasciculations. Subsequently acetylcholine-medicated synaptic transmission is prevented through occupation of the acetylcholine receptor. Succinylcholine is enzymatically degraded in the liver and in plasma via pseudocholinesterases.

Due to its rapidity of onset (30–60 s), and short duration (5–15 min), succinylcholine is the most commonly administered muscle relaxant. Effective ventilation typically returns after 8–10 min. Major complications include hyperkalemia, bradycardia, and malignant hypothermia. Most deaths, secondary to succinylcholine-induced hyperkalemia, involved children with previously undiagnosed myopathies. Adult patients, intubated using succinylcholine, generally experience a modest change in serum potassium. The hyperkalemic effect is pronounced in chronic or subacute, neuromuscular conditions, cerebrovascular accidents, and burn and crush injuries. Regardless, if a patient's EKG is demonstrating changes attributable to hyperkalemia, succinylcholine is contraindicated.

Absolute contraindications to succinylcholine include a personal or familial history of malignant hyperthermia. Patients who experience masseter-spasm upon induction with either thiopental or fentanyl are at increased risk of developing malignant hyperthermia from succinylcholine. Chronic neuromuscular diseases, chronic central nervous system injury, or myopathies result in upregulation of acetylcholine receptors and thus an exaggerated hyperkalemic response after administration of succinylcholine. Deficiencies of plasma pseudocholinesterase will result in prolonged paralysis; thus it is a contraindication to the use of succinylcholine. Many anesthesiologists will use succinylcholine within the first 24 h after an extensive burn or acute CNS injury that denervates muscle (i.e., a spinal injury), but avoid its use thereafter. Succinylcholine-associated dysrhythmias are mediated by postganglionic muscarinic receptors and preganglionic sympathetic receptors. Bradydysrhythmias are most commonly observed, but there are rare reports of asystole and ventricular tachyarrhythmias. Most instances occur in pediatric patients or in adults after the use of multiple doses of succinylcholine. Dysrhythmias may be prevented in adults by premedicating with a vagolytic dose of atropine (0.4 mg IV), prior to repeating succinylcholine.

Succinylcholine may cause an increase in intragastric pressure, presumably because of drug-induced fasciculations. However aspiration usually does not result, because of a coincident increase in tone of the esophageal sphincter. Succinylcholine increases both intraocular and intracranial pressure, but these effects are transient and clinically insignificant.

Traditionally, 1.5 mg/kg of succinylcholine is administered for intubation because a lower dose may relax the central laryngeal muscles before the peripheral musculature. This laryngeal relaxation could both promote aspiration due to glottic incompetence while also complicating intubation because masseter function may remain intact.

Nondepolarizing NMBAs provide an alternative to succinylcholine for either paralytic-assisted intubation or rapid sequence intubation. Rocuronium, an aminosteroid drug, has a relatively rapid onset of action (1–2 min) and intermediate duration of action (45–70 min). A recent systematic review compared succinylcholine versus rocuronium (0.6 mg/kg) and concluded succinylcholine produced superior intubation conditions when rigorous standards were used to define "excellent" conditions. The two agents had similar efficacy when "adequate" intubation conditions were established. No differences were found, however, if propofol was used for induction, or if the dose of rocuronium was increased to 1.0 mg/kg. However, use of this higher dose of rocuronium prolongs the duration of paralysis.

Reversal of nondepolarizing blocking NMBA can be accelerated using acetylcholinesterase inhibitors, such as neostigmine or edrophonium, concomitantly with vagolytic drugs i.e., glycopyrrolate or atropine. The only absolute contraindication to rocuronium is an allergy to aminosteroid NMBA. However, great caution should be taken to select appropriate patients for nondepolarizing NMBA because of their long duration of action. As such, practitioners should be wary when facing the potentially difficult airway. After all, if the patient cannot be successfully intubated, then there is a risk of dangerous hypoxemia and acidosis unless an airway and BMV can be maintained for the prolonged period of drug-induced paralysis (45–70 min).

In recent years, the selective relaxant binding agent (SRBA) Sugammadex has been approved for use in some European countries. Sugammadex is modified of cyclodextrin that encapsulates rocuronium molecules resulting in fast reversal of paralysis. Sugammadex is not dependent upon the use of acetylcholinesterase inhibitors; thus autonomic instability is negated. Sugammadex also reverses vecuronium-induced neuromuscular paralysis.

References

1. Reynolds SF, Heffner J (2005) Airway management of the critically ill patient: rapid-sequence intubation. Chest 127:1397–1412
2. Jaber S, Amraoui J, Lefrant JY et al (2006) Clinical practice and risk factors for immediate complications of endotracheal intubation in the intensive care unit: a prospective, multiple-center study. Crit Care Med 34(9):2355–2361
3. Kheterpal S, Han R, Tremper K et al (2006) Incidence and predictors of difficult and impossible mask ventilation. Anesthesiology 105:885–891

4. Kheterpal S, Martin L, Shanks A et al (2009) Prediction and out-
    comes of impossible mask ventilation: a review of 50,000 anesthetics.
    Anesthesiology 110:891–897
5. Boucher B, Wood G, Swanson J (2006) Pharmacokinetic changes in
    critical illness. Crit Care Clin 22:255–271

Airway Pharmacology

▶ Airway Management

Airway Protection

▶ Tracheal Intubation in Acute Procedures

AIS 2005 Military

The AIS 2005 Military was developed to more accurately
describe commonly seen multi-mechanistic combat injuries such as soft-tissue fragment wounds; high velocity
penetration; blast injuries (mutilating or non-mutilating),
and/or bilateral and multiple injuries that result from
improvised explosive devices (IEDs, which account for
65-76% of combat injuries). The AIS 2005-Military
codes were derived by identifying each combat injury
that is more severe than the corresponding civilian injury,
and increasing the AIS code by one or two increments of
severity to reflect the increased risk of injury or morbidity
in a military setting.

AKD/AKI, Approach to the Patient with

JOHN A. KELLUM, NATTACHAI SRISAWAT
Department of Critical Care Medicine, University of
Pittsburgh School of Medicine, Pittsburgh, PA, USA

Cause of AKI

Once a diagnosis of AKI has been established, it is important to stratify the patient's condition by etiology. AKI can
be caused by insults that can be broadly divided into three
categories: prerenal, renal (intrinsic), and postrenal. This
stratification is important because current recommended
therapeutic models are tailored to these types of insults.
However, the categories are overly simplistic and, particularly with respect to prerenal insults, the line between
purely functional changes and parenchymal injury can be
very blurry [1].

Prerenal mechanisms of AKI see detail in ▶ prerenal
azotemia. Table 1 summarizes prerenal causes of AKI.

Postrenal mechanisms of AKI can be divided by anatomy into intrarenal (intratubular) obstruction and
extrarenal obstruction, which result from obstruction of
the urinary collecting system. While extrarenal obstruction can be further divided into upper (the level of ureter
or renal pelvis) and lower urinary tract (the level of bladder or urethra). Of note, upper urinary tract obstruction,
unless bilateral, may not manifest as AKI since the ipsilateral kidney, if normally functioning, can usually maintain
overall function. Table 1 summarizes common postrenal
causes of AKI (intrarenal and extrarenal).

Intrinsic mechanisms of AKI can be categorized by
anatomy: tubular (acute tubular necrosis, ATN), interstitial (acute interstitial nephritis, AIN), glomerular (acute
glomerulonephritis, AGN), and vascular (acute renal vascular disorder). Table 1 summarizes cause of intrinsic
causes of AKI.

– *Acute tubular necrosis (ATN)* results from prolonged
   exposure to ischemia, or from direct toxin damage
   (nephrotoxic). The natural history of "self-limited"
   ATN is a steady rise in sCr (injury stage), followed by
   stabilization (plateau stage), and an eventual decline in
   those measures (recovery stage) during 7–21 days. The
   typical urine finding in ATN is "muddy brown cast"
   which is a coarse granular casts containing necrotic
   tubular epithelial cells. However, this finding is neither
   sensitive nor specific for ATN. Impaired tubular
   reabsorptive function (FE Na >1) is also a common
   finding of ATN.
– *Acute interstitial nephritis (AIN)* see detail in ▶ interstitial nephritis.
– *Acute glomerulonephritis (AGN) and rapidly progressive
   glomerulonephritis (RPGN)* comprise a spectrum of
   glomerular diseases that may present as AKI, or may
   present with progressive decline in renal function over
   days to weeks (subacute kidney injury). The hallmark
   finding from phase contrast microscopic examination
   of the urine is dysmorphic red blood cells and red
   blood cell casts. Decreasing serum complement levels

AKD/AKI, Approach to the Patient with. Table 1 Causes of AKI

1. Prerenal Mechanisms
Decreased effective extracellular fluid volume
– Extracellular fluid loss: burns, diarrhea, vomiting, diuretics, salt-wasting renal disease, primary adrenal insufficiency
– Extracellular fluid sequestration: pancreatitis, burns, crush injury, nephrotic syndrome, malnutrition, advanced liver disease
Decreased cardiac output
Myocardial dysfunction: myocardial infarction, arrhythmias, cardiomyopathies, severe cor pulmonale
Cardiac tamponade
Peripheral vasodilatation
Drugs: antihypertensive agents
Sepsis
Miscellaneous: adrenal insufficiency, hypomagnesemia, hypercapnia, hypoxemia
Severe renal vasoconstriction
Sepsis
Drugs: NSAIDs, alpha-adrenergic agonists
Hepatorenal syndrome
Mechanical occlusion of renal arteries
Thrombotic occlusion
Miscellaneous (emboli, trauma)
2. Intrinsic Mechanisms
Renal vascular disorders
Vasculitis, Malignant hypertension, Scleroderma, Thrombotic thrombocytopenic purpura, Hemolytic-Uremic syndrome,
Disseminated Intravascular Coagulation, Mechanical renal artery occlusion, Renal vein thrombosis
Acute glomerulonephritis
Postinfectious glomerulonephritis (post-streptococcal glomerulonephritis)
Membranoproliferative glomerulonephritis
Rapidly progressive glomerulonephritis
Lupus nephritis
Acute interstitial nephritis (AIN)
Drugs: Penicillins, sulfonamides, rifampicin, cimetidine, captopril, allopurinol, NSAIDs
Infections: Leptospirosis
Infiltrative disease: Sarcoidosis, Leukemia, Lymphoma
Connective tissue disease
Acute tubular necrosis (ATN)

AKD/AKI, Approach to the Patient with. Table 1 (Continued)

Renal ischemia (prolonged prerenal AKI)
Nephrotoxins (aminoglycosides, radiocontrast agents, amphotericin B
Pigmenturia (myoglobulinuria, hemoglobulinuria)
3. Postrenal AKI
Intrarenal (Intratubular)
Crystal deposition: uric acid (rhabdomyolysis), calcium oxalic acid (ethylene glycol intoxication), methotrexate, acyclovir, triamterene, sulfonamide
Protein deposition: light chains, myoglobin, hemoglobin
Extrarenal
Ureteral, Pelvic
– Intrinsic lesion: tumor, stone, blood clot, fungal ball
– Extrinsic lesion: retroperitoneal and pelvic malignancy, fibrosis, ligation
Bladder: stone, blood clot, tumor, neurogenic, prostatic, prostate (hypertrophy, malignancy)
Urethral: stricture, phimosis

are seen in various disorders: (Systemic Lupus Erythemotosus, post-Streptococcal (post infectious) glomerulonephritis, Shunt nephritis, Subacute bacterial endocarditis, membranoproliferative glomerulonephritis, Cryoglobulinemia) – the mnemonics 4SMC can be used to recall these disorders. Other serologies such as markers for hepatitis B and C virus, antinuclear antibodie, anti-neutrophil cytoplasmic antibodies, anti-glomerular basement membrane antibodies, anti-HIV, and anti-streptococcal antibodies, may also be helpful in making a diagnosis.

– *Acute renal vascular disorders associated with AKI* can be divided into large-vessel and small-vessel disease. The large-vessel includes renal artery thromboembolism, and renal vein thrombosis. The common finding of large-vessel disease is renal infarction, usually presenting with flank pain, hematuria, and elevated serum lactate dehydrogenase. As with upper urinary tract obstruction, unilateral disease may not manifest as a decline in renal function if the remaining kidney is healthy. Small-vessel disease may result from ateroembolization of cholesterol crystal, hemolytic-uremic syndrome, thrombotic thrombocytopenic purpura, scleroderma renal crises, and disseminated intravascular coagulation.

Diagnostic Approach of the Patient Who Has AKI

The diagnostic approach of patient who is suspect of AKI can be divided into five steps (Fig. 1):

Step 1: Rule out Conditions with High BUN, sCr without Decreasing of GFR (Pseudoazotemia)

There are many factors which may cause an increased BUN and sCr without decreasing glomerular filtration rate (GFR). The production rate of urea and creatinine is an important contributor to BUN (hypercatabolic state, increased protein intake, infusion of amino acid, gastro-intestinal bleeding, corticosterioid administration, tetracycline), and sCr (rhabdomyolysis). Moreover, decreased tubular secretion of creatinine by drugs such as cimetidine, trimethoprim (with, or without sulfamethoxazole) can also cause a mild increase in creatinine.

Step 2: Differentiate between Acute or Chronic Kidney Disease (CKD)

The next step for a patient who has true decline in GFR is exclusion of chronic kidney disease (CKD) by history, physical examination, and laboratory investigation.

History

History of signs or symptoms associated with renal disease such as nocturia (may reflect loss of concentrating ability), edema, hematuria, persistent elevations of BUN, and sCr (if applicable) for more than 3 months should be sought. A family history of polycystic kidney disease should also be checked.

Physical Examination

Unfortunately, there are no specific signs to differentiate between AKI and CKD, but anemia, dry skin, and chronic hypertension point toward CKD.

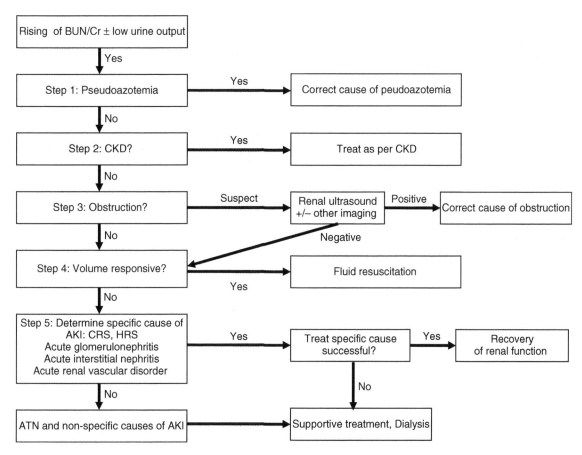

AKD/AKI, Approach to the Patient with. Figure 1 Flow chart of diagnostic approach and treatment of AKI patients

Laboratory Investigation

Plain KUB and renal ultrasonography are important diagnostic tools for differentiation of CKD. Patient who have CKD will have small-sized kidneys (usually less than 8.5 cm) and increase echogenicity of renal parenchyma. However, there are some causes of CKD that do not have small-size kidney such as diabetic nephropathy, adult polycystic kidney disease, HIV-associated nephropathy (HIVAN), infiltrative disease (lymphoma), obstructive uropathy, and xanthogranulomatous pyelonephritis.

Step 3: Exclude of Urinary Tract Obstruction

The clinical presentation of urinary tract obstruction varies with the location, duration, and degree of obstruction. Thus, a thorough history and physical examination are key factors in patient evaluation.

History

Upper urinary tract obstruction can manifest as flank pain, and/or referred pain to groin. Nausea and vomiting are also common and usually occur when obstruction is acute. Lower urinary tract obstruction (bladder, urethra) can manifest as voiding dysfunction such as urgency, frequency, nocturia, incontinence, decreased stream, hesitancy, postvoid dribbling, and a sensation of inadequate emptying. Suprapubic pain or a palpable bladder indicates urinary retention. Infection may be present, and patients may experience dysuria. Hematuria may be present with or without infection.

Physical Examination

Digital rectal examination can reveal prostatic enlargement, decreased rectal tone, or prostatitis. Urethral stricture often requires cystoscopy for diagnosis. Meatal stenosis is usually apparent on physical examination. Patients with urethral stricture may report a history of trauma, instrumentation, or sexually transmitted disease. They may also experience a split urinary stream. In women, the presence of uterine or bladder prolapse can be visualized on a pelvic examination. A urethral diverticulum can also be palpated on pelvic examination.

Laboratory Investigation

Plain KUB for radio-opaque stones and renal ultrasonography (CT scan if needed) for diagnosed hydronephrosis are important diagnostic tests for urinary tract obstruction.

Step 4: Exclude Reversible Prerenal Causes of AKI

After excluding obstruction, the next step is the differentiation between volume responsive and unresponsive AKI.

In a patient who has true volume depletion, the diagnosis of prerenal azotemia is usually not difficult. Intravascular volume depletion may be manifested by hypotension, orthostatic hypotension, flat neck veins, poor skin turgor, and dry oral mucosa. Urine sediment is without casts or cellular elements, and the urine is concentrated (specific gravity >1.015; urine osmolality >350 mOsm/kg) with a low urine sodium concentration (<20 mmol/L). The fractional excretion of sodium (FENa), is usually <1%.

$$FENa = \frac{[(urine\ sodium\ x\ plasma\ creatinine)/}{(plasma\ sodium\ x\ urine\ creatinine)] \times 100}$$

However, none of the above indices have sufficient sensitivity or specificity to be used as definitive tests for prerenal azotemia. Moreover, the concomitant use of diuretics may decrease the utility of urine sodium measurements. In the setting of diuretic use, the fractional excretion of urea (FE urea) has been advocated as an alternative to FENa. In patients who have prerenal azotemia, the fractional excretion of urea is usually less than 35%, compared with normal values of more than 60% (Table 2) [2]. Unfortunately FEurea has only marginally better test characteristics compared to FENa. Finally, all any of these tests provide is a measure of intact tubular function. If tubular function is intact, it does not rule out the presence of intrinsic AKI in a variety of settings (e.g., sepsis, rhabdomyolysis) and if tubular function is disrupted it does not preclude concomitant volume depletion or low renal perfusion. A more useful paradigm may be the concept of volume responsive AKI in which AKI can

AKD/AKI, Approach to the Patient with. Table 2 Interpretation fractional excretion of sodium (FE Na)

1. FE Na <1%
– Prerenal azotemia
– Severe renal vasoconstriction: hepatorenal syndrome, NSAIDs, Disease of afferent arteriole (TTP, scleroderma), sepsis, early phase of myoglobinuric renal failure, radiocontrast induced nephropathy
– Early obstructive uropathy
2. FE Na >2%
– Acute tubular necrosis
– Non-reabsorbable anion: bicarbonate, glucose, mannitol
– Mineralocorticoid deficiency
– Late obstructive uropathy
– Chronic kidney disease
– Diuretic use

be attenuated by volume resuscitation vs. established AKI that is no longer helped by fluid. Indeed the continued administration of fluid a patient with volume *unresponsive* AKI can only cause harm.

Step 5: Investigate the Specific Cause of AKI

To differentiate between the various causes of AKI requires a careful clinical history and physical examination. Urine microscopy also may provide useful clues to diagnosis. The presence of dysmorphic RBCs, and RBC casts are strongly suggestive AGN. The presence of WBC casts and eosinophiluria suggests the diagnosis of AIN. When the diagnosis remains uncertain, especially if there is suspicion of AGN or AIN, a kidney biopsy may be needed. Prerenal causes of AKI including volume depletion, cardiorenal and hepatorenal syndromes, and renal vascular disease are all treated very differently and should be distinguished.

In summary, AKI is a commonly encountered syndrome in the hospital, especially the ICU. The diagnosis of the specific cause of AKI is stilled based on careful attention to patient history, thorough physical examination, aided by urinary microscopy and urinary indices.

References

1. Kellum JA (2008) Acute kidney injury. Crit Care Med 36:S141–S145
2. Carvounis CP, Nisar S, Guro-Razuman S (2002) Significance of the fractional excretion of urea in the differential diagnosis of acute renal failure. Kidney Int 62(6):2223–2229

AKI in the Newborn

Patrick D. Brophy, Michelle Baack
Department of Pediatrics, University of Iowa Children's Hospital, Carver College of Medicine, Iowa City, IA, USA

Synonyms

Acute renal failure of the newborn; Neonatal acute kidney injury; Neonatal acute renal failure

Definition

Although guidelines have been developed and validated for defining acute kidney injury (AKI) in adults and children, no such criteria have been established for the neonatal population. Defining AKI in the newborn is complex and requires consideration of normal renal maturation as well as maternal creatinine. Typically AKI is diagnosed by an elevated serum creatinine (SCr), decreased glomerular filtration rate (GFR), and/or a reduction in the kidney's ability to regulate salt and water homeostasis. In 2004, a working definition of AKI, called RIFLE (risk, injury, failure, and loss and end stage renal disease) was developed and implemented for adults (www.ADQI.net) (Table 1). A modified pediatric RIFLE classification was proposed in 2007, which accounts for lower baseline SCr levels in children (Table 1). A second working definition of AKI was proposed by the Acute Kidney Injury Network (AKIN), a collaborative group of investigators

AKI in the Newborn. Table 1 Working RIFLE (risk, injury, failure, and loss and end stage renal disease) definitions for acute kidney injury (AKI) classifications in adults and children (Adapted from Askenazi, et al. 2009)

RIFLE		Ped RIFLE		
Class	Serum Cr or GFR	Class	eCrCl	Urine output
Risk	SCr increase by 150% OR GFR decreased by 25%	Risk	CrCl decreased by 25%	<0.5 mL/kg/h × 8 h
Injury	SCr increase by 200% OR GFR decreased by 50%	Injury	eCrCl decreased by 50%	<0.5mL/kg/h × 16 h
Fail	SCr increase by 300% or is >4.0mg/dL OR GFR decreased by 75%	Fail	eCrCl decreased by 75% or <35 mL/min per 1.73 m² BSA	<0.3 mL/kg/h × 24 h or anuric for 12 h
Loss	Failure >4 weeks	Loss	Failure >4 weeks	
ESRD	Failure >3 months	ESRD	Failure >3 months	

from all major critical care and nephrology societies. To date, there is no specific classification system to define AKI in neonates due to the complexity of the maturing kidney [1].

Using adult/pediatric AKI classifications for neonates (birth to 28 days post birth) is problematic for many reasons. Newborn kidney function is considerably different than that of a mature adult kidney in both glomerular and tubular functions. Nephrogenesis is not complete until approximately 34–36 weeks gestation, and thereafter, renal function gradually matures to adult function. At birth, GFR is very low and urine flow rates less than 1 mL/kg/h may initially be appropriate and not harmful. In fact, initial voiding might be delayed until 24 h of life in some normal term infants. Furthermore, nearly half of the cases of neonatal AKI are nonoliguric in nature. Serum creatinine (SCr) levels are initially a reflection of maternal levels and thereafter vary based on muscle mass, hydration status, chronological age, and gestational age (GA). Also, medications and bilirubin may effect SCr measurements if performed by the Jaffe's reaction instead of other enzymatic analyses. Newborns undergo a 10–15% postnatal loss of extracellular water accompanied by sodium loss. This sodium loss is more pronounced in premature infants who have immature tubules. Additionally, in premature infants SCr is even higher than term infants due to a physiologically normal but relatively low GFR and increased tubular reabsorption of creatinine across leaky tubules. Therefore, initially after birth, elevated SCr, low GFR/urine output, or impairment in concentrating ability of the neonatal kidney are not necessarily of clinical significance in all but the most extreme circumstances. However, SCr levels and urine output that do not normalize with kidney maturation are indicative of renal injury. Normal kidney maturation must be understood and accounted for so adjustments for age and prematurity can be considered while determining a renal injury state in an infant [1].

Physiology

Two major physiologic processes concurrently active in the maturing kidney include adapting glomerular and tubular functions. Normative data have now been reported for infants of different gestational ages. Glomerular function can best be assessed by serial measurements of serum creatinine (SCr) and creatinine clearance (CrCl), while tubular function is estimated by fractional excretion of sodium (FeNa). Both progress as the kidney matures from neonatal function to adult function [2].

Glomerular Physiology

Normal glomerular function progresses in direct correlation with postnatal age but gestational age is the key factor determining rate of maturation. After birth, the immature kidney must rapidly increase filtration despite minimal renal blood flow due to a relatively low mean arterial blood pressure and high intrarenal vascular resistance. Additionally, mean arterial blood pressure correlates with gestational age. Therefore, as expected, preterm infants with lower renal blood flow and more immature kidneys have a lower CrCl than term infants and it takes a longer time to attain adult glomerular function. GFR (mL/min $\times$ 1.73 m^2) may be as low as 10 in the 28-week preterm infant during the first week of life whereas it can be double that in a term (40 weeks) infant over the same period. Serum creatinine at birth, in infants of all gestational ages, is a reflection of the mother's SCr level and is a poor marker of kidney function in the neonate. SCr may increase over the first 36–96 h of life then gradually decrease as postnatal mean blood pressure increases and renal vascular resistance falls particularly in preterm infants [2]. In term infants, SCr reaches a stable average neonatal level of 0.4 mg/dL by 1–2 weeks of age. However in preterm infants, SCr may continue to increase to a peak at 4 days of age and then decline to stable values by 3–8 weeks of life. Overall, glomerular function, as measured by CrCl and SCr, increases progressively in all neonates and the rate of increase correlates positively to the gestational age. See Table 2 for further information on GFR in healthy preterm infants. Anoxia, sepsis, acidosis, or exposure to nephrotoxic medications further decrease renal perfusion and may adversely affect the immature neonatal glomerular function leading to AKI [3].

Tubular Physiology

The second important physiologic process in the maturing kidney is tubular function. Tubular function, as measured by fractional excretion of sodium (FeNa), progressively improves with postnatal age from initial values that correlate to gestational age [2]. Infants may need this increased sodium loss to maintain sodium balance until extracellular fluid reduction, which is normal after birth, is complete. Premature infants have a higher FeNa at birth, up to 5% compared to 1% in adults and 3% in term infants. Additionally, preterm infants have a slower rate of tubular maturation [3]. This may be protective for the development of hypernatremia initially but ultimately accounts for a higher sodium requirement among very premature infants after the first week of age. A positive sodium balance in the neonate is a prerequisite for growth

AKI in the Newborn. Table 2 The evolution of glomerulo-filtration rate in preterm infants as renal development occurs ex utero (Adapted from Askenazi, et al. 2009)

Age	Inulin clearance/GFR (mL/min/1.73 m²)
Preterm infants	
1–3 days	14.0 ± 5
1–7 days	18.7 ± 5.5
4–8 days	44.3 ± 9.3
3–13 days	47.8 ± 10.7
1.5–4 months	67.4 ± 16.6
Term infants	
1–3 days	20.8 ± 5.0
4–14 days	36.8 ± 7.2
1–3 months	85.3 ± 35.1
4–6 months	87.4 ± 22.3
7–12 months	96.2 ± 12.2
1–2 years	105.2 ± 17.3

and development, and at postnatal weeks 4–6, there is avid incorporation of sodium into the tissues, which exaggerates the late hyponatremia often seen in premature infants. For these reasons, serum sodium levels and FeNa alone cannot be used as a marker for AKI.

At this time, the best way to define AKI in the neonate is to consider the developmental phases that infants go through and the immediate post-uterine environment while evaluating traditional clinical and laboratory markers of renal function in an infant. Several clinical studies in at-risk neonatal populations further define neonatal AKI based on plasma creatinine concentrations that increase or remain consistently elevated after their presumed maternal influence has subsided. Practically speaking, spot creatinine values are not as valuable as serial measurements. Additionally, SCr is a late marker of kidney function and levels may not change until 25–50% of kidney function has already been lost. Multiple studies on the use of novel urine and serum biomarkers to identify kidney injury early in the course of illness are ongoing and very promising. In the near future, levels of neutrophil gelatinase-associated lipocalin (NGAL), interleukin-18 (IL-18), or kidney injury molecule-1 (KIM-1) may be utilized to identify AKI hours after an insult, allowing intervention early in the process [1]. Unfortunately, these biomarkers are not readily available or standardized for the neonate at this time. Therefore, clinically based criteria in addition to knowledge about maturational changes of the kidney should be used to identify AKI in the newborn.

Treatment

The primary focus of management of AKI in the newborn should be directed at the initiating event. Precisely defining and addressing the factors leading up to AKI may lead to a rapid reversal of kidney dysfunction in neonatal patients with prerenal causes. Prerenal factors such as hypotension, hypovolemia, hypoxia, and acidosis should be rapidly corrected. The acuity of correction is guided by the degree of cardiovascular instability and the presence or absence of shock. Adequate ventilation and hydration are essential for proper management of AKI in this period. It is imperative to realize that insensible water losses in the term infant and very low birth weight infants can be significant in the first week of life and congenital abdominal wall or spinal defects may exacerbate this. Minimizing insensible loss is beneficial. When indicated, treatment of sepsis, heart failure or adrenal crisis is essential. Fluid deficits should be initially corrected with 20 mL/kg of isotonic saline solution in a goal-directed fashion. Subsequent fluid challenges are based on initial response in terms of restoring effective circulating volume and blood pressure as well as renal response in the form of urine output. If indicated and tolerated, the use of IV thiazide and furosemide as well as maintenance of oncotic intravascular pressure (with albumin) may reestablish urine output. If subsequent diuresis is not noted in the next few hours, other causes of intrinsic AKI must be suspected and evaluated [4]. In the hypotensive infant with prerenal AKI that is not responsive to fluid resuscitation, dopamine administration (followed by additional vasopressors as needed) may support blood pressure by improving renal blood flow. Treatment of obstructive AKI involves assuring adequate drainage of the urinary tract. Bladder catheterization is imperative in infants with bladder outlet obstruction including posterior urethral valves and neurogenic bladder. Intrinsic AKI should also aim at eliminating inciting causes especially nephrotoxic drugs when possible.

Complications associated with AKI may include acidosis, hyperkalemia, hypocalcemia, and hyponatremia. Each of these complications must be addressed in order to provide adequate restoration of internal homeostasis. Volume and fluid overload has been associated with increased mortality and should also be addressed. Patients with anasarca have a reduction of tissue perfusion, and even if they are making urine, their kidneys are unable to maintain fluid and solute removal adequately enough to maintain nominal fluid balance. This is a form of AKI and aggressive therapy in order to promote diuresis and reduce fluid overload is indicated in such patients.

Renal Replacement Therapy in the Neonatal Acute Kidney Injury Patient

Neonates with AKI, like other children, may require the utilization of renal replacement therapy as a bridge until renal injury improves. This may also be utilized for longer-term therapy if the acute injury progresses to chronic renal insufficiency or end stage renal disease. Renal replacement therapy (RRT) includes peritoneal dialysis, hemodialysis, or hemofiltration.

Peritoneal dialysis has been a preferred modality for infants. As a general rule, it is easy to perform and does not require anticoagulation. Low volume peritoneal dialysis (5–10 mL/kg) through a Tenckhoff catheter generally has minimal impact on the hemodynamic status of the neonate and provides effective control of uremia, fluid, and solute exchange. Disadvantages include slower correction of metabolic parameters and increased risk of peritonitis. Recent abdominal surgery, ostomies, massive organomegaly, or intra-abdominal masses are contraindications to peritoneal dialysis. Long-term peritoneal dialysis has been effectively used in very low birth weight infants [5].

When peritoneal dialysis is not an option, clinicians may opt for hemodialysis. However, this can place the infants, particularly critically ill ones, at significant risk for hypotension due to large extracorporeal blood volume shifts. Because of this, the utilization of continuous renal replacement therapy has become increasingly popular. In both cases, vascular access and anticoagulation are required. Continuous venovenous hemofiltration (CVVH), continuous venovenous hemodialysis (CVVHD), or continuous venovenous hemodiafiltration (CVVH-DF) provide optimal fluid removal without rapid shifts in hemodynamics or solutes. These treatment approaches seem to be reasonably tolerated in infants who are critically ill [5]. It should be noted that these therapies may be technically challenging and although improvement in outcomes have been realized in the past few years the mortality rate remains significant. Ultimately, choice of RRT is based on patient characteristics, physician choice, institutional experience, and equipment availability.

Evaluation/Assessment

Once AKI is suspected, finding the primary etiology is important for further classification and treatment of the disease. There are three major classes of AKI: prerenal, intrinsic, and obstructive AKI. Table 3 defines the more common causes of these diseases.

Prerenal AKI

Prerenal failure is the most common cause of AKI in the neonatal intensive care unit (NICU). In the immediate period after birth, mean arterial blood pressure is low, leading to a low GFR. Additional stresses from systemic hypotension, hypovolemia, hypoxia, or acidosis lead to inadequate perfusion and prerenal AKI. These can be seen from perinatal asphyxia, blood loss, sepsis, cardiac anomalies, UAC thrombosis, or abdominal compartment syndrome from closure of abdominal wall defects for instance. Although an elevated FeNa is typically used to differentiate prerenal from intrinsic causes of AKI in children and adults, high sodium losses in the immature kidney make this more challenging. Normal FeNa at 29–30 weeks gestational age (GA) is 6% and infants over 31 weeks GA is 3%. Additionally, infants less than 32 weeks GA have very elevated FeNa in the first 5 days of age. A FeNa less than 3% in a term infant may indicate prerenal AKI but this must be adjusted for preterm infants, especially in the first few days of life. FeNa more than 3% in a term infant is more suggestive of intrinsic AKI [4]. In prerenal AKI, restoring renal perfusion early in the course of disease may lead to resolution without renal sequelae. Further insult from medications that inhibit the kidney's ability to compensate during this time of hypoperfusion can lead to acute tubular necrosis and intrinsic renal damage.

Intrinsic and Postrenal AKI

Other types of AKI in the neonate include intrinsic or obstructive causes. Intrinsic AKI implies damage or congenital dysfunction of the kidney itself, whereas obstructive AKI is postrenal and caused by abnormalities in the drainage system of the urinary tract. Ultrasonography is noninvasive, inexpensive, and a simple measure that is mandatory in assessing AKI in the neonate. It is very helpful in diagnosing obstructive nephropathy. If indicated by ultrasound, obstructive AKI should urgently be treated with catheterization or other measures to relieve obstruction and prevent further renal damage. Intrinsic AKI should be considered if FeNa is high as described above and there is no other immediately treatable causes identified by renal ultrasound [4]. Drugs commonly used in the NICU can interfere with the kidney's intrinsic ability to compensate for poor perfusion or be directly toxic to the kidney. Common insulting agents include indomethacin, theophylline, aminoglycosides, vancomycin or amphotericin B, and dosage adjustments or alternative therapy should be considered in infants with AKI.

In any infant with AKI monitoring, clinical and laboratory tests during the course are essential. Effective

AKI in the Newborn. Table 3 Etiology and classification of neonatal AKI

Prerenal AKI	Intrinsic AKI	Obstructive AKI
Decreased intravascular volume –Twin–twin or fetal–maternal transfusion –Perinatal hemorrhage/placental abruption –Placental insufficiency, i.e., severe oligohydramnios, IUGR –Hemolytic disease –Dehydration –Increased insensible water loss, i.e., ELBW, GI losses, gastroschisis/omphalocele, Diabetes insipidus	*Kidney disease* –Acute tubular necrosis, i.e., hypoxia/ischemia, drugs, IV contrast or endogenous toxins (rhabdomyolysis) –Interstitial nephritis, i.e., drug induced or idiopathic –Polycystic kidney disease –Renal dysplasia or hypoplasia –Renal agenesis –Renal tubular dysgenesis –Congenital nephrotic syndrome	*Obstructive uropathies* –Ureteropelvic junction obstruction –Severe vesicoureteral reflux –Posterior urethral valves –Bladder outlet obstruction or neurogenic bladder dysfunction
Shock, hypotension, acidosis, or hypoxemia –Perinatal asphyxia –RDS/PPHN –Sepsis –Necrotizing enterocolitis –DIC –Cardiac tamponade/CHF –ECMO or cardiopulmonary bypass –Adrenal insufficiency	*Nephrotoxic Drugs* –ACE inhibitors –Aminoglycosides –Amphotericin B –Antiepileptics –Indomethacin/NSAIDs –Theophylline	
Renal artery obstruction –Vascular thrombosis –Umbilical catheters –Abdominal compartment syndrome, i.e., closure of congenital abdominal wall defects		

circulating volume should be assessed by following vital signs, physical exam, urine output, central venous pressure, and renal perfusion monitoring (with near infrared spectroscopy). Serial SCr, blood urea nitrogen (BUN), electrolytes, blood gas, and FeNa levels should be followed in the initial stages of neonatal AKI. Additionally, a complete blood count including platelets, urinalysis, calcium, phosphorous, and magnesium should also be considered in AKI that does not resolve with initial interventions. Renal ultrasound should be performed for all infants with AKI to rule out obstructive nephropathy.

After-care

At the present time, recommendations for aftercare are unclear because the long-term outcomes secondary to neonatal AKI are not well defined. However, many clinicians are now developing AKI follow-up clinics in order to monitor such patients and provide early therapy should chronic kidney disease (CKD) develop. There is certainly mounting evidence that damage to the developing

nephron mass in the neonatal or perinatal period can lead to the development of subsequent chronic kidney disease. Late onset development of CKD typically manifests as proteinuria and hypertension followed by an elevated Blood Urea Nitrogen (BUN) and SCr [5]. The economic impact of this remains to be determined. It is likely higher than recognized and increasing with the increasing numbers of surviving premature infants. Newborns with AKI need lifelong monitoring of their renal function, blood pressure, and urinalysis.

Prognosis Epidemiology and Outcomes

Determining the exact incidence and outcome of infants with AKI is also limited by the difficulty defining AKI and separating out comorbidities. Unfortunately, most available data are based on small, single-center studies that usually focus on a subset of the neonatal population. Published studies estimate the incidence of AKI in critically ill neonates is between 8% and 24%. It is certainly higher in at-risk categories. Infants with severe asphyxia have a 66% occurrence rate of AKI, and 56% of infants with a 5-min APGAR score of ≤ 6 have AKI. In one prospective study, term infants with sepsis had a 26% incidence of AKI [1].

At present, studies suggest that infants with AKI have a higher mortality rate both during and after hospitalization. Prognosis of neonatal AKI is highly dependent on the underlying etiology. Infants with nonoliguric AKI had excellent survival rates, but infants with oliguric or anuric AKI had a mortality rate range of 25–78%. Cause of death was seldom solely from renal disease but more often from comorbidities [4]. At present, patients who require the use of renal replacement therapy have a significant risk of mortality in the first year of life. Infants receiving prolonged RRT for kidney damage alone have approximately 50% increase in mortality in the first year of life. If patients have associated comorbidities including lung disease, cardiac disease, or other, their mortality rate rises logarithmically. Overlapping factors associated with high mortality include multiorgan failure, hypotension, hemodynamic instability, or the need for pressors, mechanical ventilation, or dialysis.

In addition to an increase in mortality, infants with AKI have other short-term morbidities. It should be evident that fluid and electrolyte disturbance and worsening renal disease can occur. New evidence also suggests that a systemic inflammatory response may occur, worsening other neonatal disease states. Infants with lung disease have an increased propensity for worsening respiratory status if they develop AKI. Not only can oliguric AKI lead to pulmonary edema secondary to volume overload, but it may also increase serum levels of neutrophil counts, cytokines, and free radical levels that may be associated with increased inflammation in the lung [1].

Neonatal AKI may also lead to progressive renal injury and CKD. Although most infants with prerenal AKI rarely have long-term renal insufficiency, 88% of infants with congenital uropathies and AKI develop CKD [4]. Furthermore, over 50% of children have at least one sign of CKD, 3–5 years after the initial event [1]. As the definition of neonatal AKI evolves, more outcome studies will be important to further understand the epidemiology of kidney injury.

With the advent of improved biomarkers for defining neonatal AKI such as NGAL, IL-18, and KIM-1, improved diagnosis should develop over the next several years. These novel biomarkers should help clinicians employ therapeutic interventions earlier in the course of AKI, when reversal without sequelae is more likely. Additionally, understanding epidemiology and outcomes will ensue. Long-term studies are required in order to fully appreciate the prognostic significance of neonatal AKI and its impact on resource management and health care costs.

References

1. Askenazi DJ, Ambalavanan N et al (2009) Acute kidney injury in critically ill newborns: what do we know? What do we need to learn? Pediatr Nephrol 24(2):265–274
2. Gallini F, Maggio L et al (2000) Progression of renal function in preterm neonates with gestational age < or = 32 weeks. Pediatr Nephrol 15(1–2):119–124
3. Drukker A, Guignard JP (2002) Renal aspects of the term and preterm infant: a selective update. Curr Opin Pediatr 14(2):175–182
4. Gouyon JB, Guignard JP (2000) Management of acute renal failure in newborns. Pediatr Nephrol 14(10–11):1037–1044
5. Andreoli SP (2004) Acute renal failure in the newborn. Semin Perinatol 28(2):112–123

AKI, Concept of

John A. Kellum, Nattachai Srisawat
Department of Critical Care Medicine, University of Pittsburgh School of Medicine, Pittsburgh, PA, USA

Synonyms

Acute kidney disease; Acute renal failure; Acute tubular necrosis (ATN)

Terminology

Acute kidney injury (AKI) is a common clinical syndrome defined as a sudden onset of reduced kidney function resulting in the retention of nitrogenous waste products, dysregulation of extracellular volume and electrolytes. However, before 2004, this clinical syndrome lacked uniform terminology and definitions. This state of varying definitions gave rise to wide range of incidence estimates for acute renal failure from 1% to 25% of ICU patients and lead to mortality rate estimates from 15% to 60%. Evidence from recent studies has demonstrated that even minimal increases in serum creatinine are associated with a dramatic impact on the risk for mortality. For this reason, the term acute renal failure, which was first introduced by Homer W. Smith in 1951 in a chapter of his textbook "The kidney-structure and function in health and disease" was replaced by that of acute kidney injury (AKI), as defined by RIFLE criteria and AKI staging (see below). Importantly, AKI is not synonymous with acute renal failure, but rather incorporates the entire spectrum of the syndrome from minor changes in renal function to

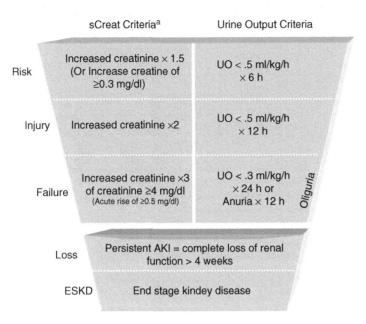

AKI, Concept of. Figure 1 Demonstration of the RIFLE criteria for AKI (used With Permission [1]). sCreat = serum creatinine concentration; UO = urine output; GFR = glomerular filtration rate; ARF = acute renal failure. [a]All serum creatinine references are based on changes from baseline values. The Risk criteria includes the modifications recommended by AKIN [2]

requirement for renal replacement therapy. Figure 1 summarizes the historical milestone of AKI.

RIFLE and AKIN Staging

In 2004, the Acute Dialysis Quality Initiative (ADQI) group developed the RIFLE system through a broad consensus of the experts [1]. The aim of this classification was to standardize the definition of AKI. The characteristics of this system are summarized in Fig. 1. The acronym RIFLE stands for the increasing severity classes Risk, Injury, and Failure, and the two outcome classes Loss and End-Stage Kidney Disease. The three severity grades are defined on the basis of the changes in serum creatinine or urine output where the worst of each criterion is used. Also, two outcome criteria (Loss and End-Stage Kidney Disease), are defined by the duration of loss of kidney function, 4 weeks and 3 months, respectively. As of early 2010, RIFLE has been validated in more than 550,000 patients around the world, and the original article describing these criteria has been accessed more than 150,000 times.

In 2007, the AKI network (AKIN), a multidisciplinary, international group proposed some small modifications to the RIFLE criteria [2]. These modifications can be summarized as follows (Fig. 1): (a) broadening of the "Risk" category of RIFLE to include an increase in serum creatinine of at least 0.3 mg/dl even if this does not reach the 50% threshold, (b) setting a 48 h window on the

documentation of AKI using the 0.3 mg/dl cutoff, and (c) categorizing patients as "Failure" if they are treated with renal replacement therapy regardless of what their serum creatinine or urine output is at the point of initiation. AKIN also proposed that stages 1, 2, and 3 be used instead of R, I, and F. These differences between ADQI-RIFLE and AKIN Stages might therefore appear quite modest, but indeed, that was precisely the intent. Figure 2 shows a conceptual model of AKI developed by AKIN for the purpose of furthering research in this field.

How to Classify RIFLE Criteria and AKIN Staging

Figure 3 summarizes a series of case examples of how to classify RIFLE criteria. Case 1 is an example of how the AKIN modification can provide for earlier recognition of AKI (D3 versus D5). Furthermore, had creatinine peaked at 1.4, the case would have been "missed" by the original RIFLE threshold of 50%. However, application of the AKIN criteria requires that creatinine be measured. If for example, creatinine was not measured on D1 or D2, the diagnosis of AKI could not be made until D6. Therefore when data are limited, using a baseline creatinine allows for the diagnosis of AKI earlier. By contrast, case 2 would have been diagnosed and classified the same according to either set of criteria. Case 3 is another example of the limitation of the AKIN criteria. If we restrict to a 48-h

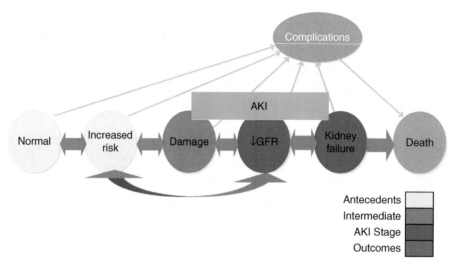

AKI, Concept of. Figure 2 Acute Kidney Injury conceptual model developed by AKIN (the Acute Kidney Injury Network) at the Vancouver Summit 2006 (www.akinet.org)

Admission day

Pt No.	sCr D1	sCr D2	sCr D3	sCr D4	sCr D5	sCr D6	sCr D7	Comments
1	1.0	1.1	**1.3**	1.4	1.5	**2.1**	1.5	- AKI is reached on D3 (by AKIN) and Max stage = 2 on D6 (2x compared to baseline)
2	1.0	1.1	1.1	1.3	**1.5**	1.4	1.2	-AKI is reached on D5 (both methods) and Max stage = 1
3	1.0	1.1	1.2	1.3	1.4	**1.5**	1.6	-AKI is reached on D6 (by RIFLE) and Max stage = 1 on D6 (<2x compared to baseline)
4	1.0	1.1	**1.3**	1.4	1.5	**2.5** and start RRT	2.0	-AKI is reached on D3 (by AKIN) and Stage 3 is reached on D6 (start of RRT)
5	**2.0**	1.8	1.6	1.5	1.3	1.0	1.0	-AKI is reached on D1 (by RIFLE compared to a known or estimated baseline). Stage 2 is already present on D1. Note that baseline of 1.0 is also confirmed at D6

In these examples, all patients have baseline serum creatinine = 1.0 mg/dl

AKI, Concept of. Figure 3 Classification of AKI patients by RIFLE criteria and AKIN staging

time window rule, we cannot diagnose AKI by serum creatinine because within no 48-h time window did the serum creatinine increase by 0.3 mg/dl or more, even though the serum creatinine increased more than 50% from baseline. ADQI also included Glomerular filtration rate (GFR) in the original RIFLE criteria but with the understanding that it would only be used as a rough "guide" since few patients will have GFR measured and

a non-steady-state GFR is of limited value in any case. GFR was therefore eliminated in the AKIN modification. Case 4 is the example of using RRT criteria regardless of serum creatinine to classify AKIN staging. Finally, case 5 shows a case of community-acquired AKI where the peak creatinine occurs at (or prior to admission). Here the patient can be diagnosed with AKI if the baseline of 1.0 mg/dl is known or estimated (e.g., using MDRD equation). Note that even if a baseline is unavailable, the creatinine of 1.0 on D6 and after, confirms that this is (was) a case of AKI.

Thus, subtle but important differences between AKIN and RIFLE criteria emerge when applied across patients. However, there are several caveats. First, the urine output criteria is the same for both AKIN and RIFLE and many patients will be diagnosed by this criterion before creatinine changes manifest. Second, in clinical practice, as opposed to retrospective database studies, clinicians are free to obtain additional and more frequent measures of creatinine. Indeed, for high risk patients, measuring creatinine every 12 or even every 8 h might be appropriate. It should also be stressed that quantifying and recording urine output is an extremely important and underutilized biomarker of AKI.

Another recommendation from ADQI was how to handle the absence of a baseline serum creatinine. The ADQI group recommended using the MDRD equation to back-estimate a baseline serum creatinine using a low normal value for GFR (75 ml/min/m^2). This approach was first operationalized by Hoste et al. who used the lowest of the following as the baseline when no baseline was available: hospital admission creatinine; ICU admission creatinine; MDRD estimated creatinine [3]. By using the lowest of these three, the authors ensured that a subject admitted with a low creatinine would have that information included (and thus a higher maximum RIFLE class if the creatinine increased) while a subject admitted with a high creatinine and no history of CKD would be classified based on a change from a theoretical baseline estimated from MDRD.

AKI, as defined by the RIFLE criteria and AKIN staging, is now recognized as an important ICU syndrome along side other ICU syndromes such as ALI/ARDS consensus criteria and the consensus definitions for SIRS/sepsis/severe sepsis and septic shock.

References

1. Bellomo R, Ronco C, Kellum JA, Mehta RL, Palevsky P (2004) Acute renal failure – definition, outcome measures, animal models, fluid therapy and information technology needs: the second international consensus conference of the Acute Dialysis Quality Initiative (ADQI) Group. Crit Care 8(4):R204–R212, Acute Dialysis Quality Initiative workgroup
2. Molitoris BA, Levin A, Warnock DG, Joannidis M, Mehta RL, Kellum JA et al (2007) Improving outcomes of acute kidney injury: report of an initiative. Nat Clin Pract Nephrol 3(8):439–442, Acute Kidney Injury Network working group
3. Hoste EA, Clermont G, Kersten A, Venkataraman R, Angus DC, De Bacquer D et al (2006) RIFLE criteria for acute kidney injury are associated with hospital mortality in critically ill patients: a cohort analysis. Crit Care 10(3):R73

AKI, Epidemiology of

Eric A. J. Hoste
Department of Internal Medicine, Ghent University Hospital, Ghent, Belgium

Synonyms
Acute kidney dysfunction; Acute kidney failure; Acute kidney insufficiency; Acute renal dysfunction; Acute renal failure; Acute renal injury; Acute renal insufficiency

Definition
Acute renal failure (ARF) was in the past the general term for the condition described now as acute kidney injury (AKI). At present, it is used by some authors to define AKI patients who are treated with renal replacement therapy (RRT), in other words, the most severe stage of AKI.

AKI is defined by a generic definition as an abrupt and sustained decrease in renal function resulting in retention of nitrogenous (urea and creatinine) and nonnitrogenous waste products [1]. Although this definition adequately describes the condition of AKI, it leaves much room for interpretation. What is the exact definition for the crucial words abrupt, sustained, and decrease of renal function? A more precise and practical definition for AKI is offered by the Risk Injury Failure Loss and End stage renal disease (RIFLE) classification for AKI (Table 1) [2]. This classification defines three increasing severity grades of AKI (R, I, and F) based upon an increase of serum creatinine or a decrease of urine output. It also consists of two outcome stages (L and E). This classification is increasingly used in clinical studies since its publication. The RIFLE classification was adopted in a modified form by the Acute Kidney Injury Network (AKIN), a consortium that units all major international critical care and nephrological societies, as the AKI diagnostic and classification system [3]. The modifications that were introduced were considered details and not essential for the RIFLE classification system. The first modification was renaming of the three severity grades R, I, and F, into stage 1, 2, and 3. This renaming is done for consistency with the staging system for chronic kidney disease. Second, AKI patients who were treated with RRT were classified as stage 3, as they obviously represent the most severe form of AKI, irrespective of serum creatinine increase or duration of oliguria. Third, in RIFLE the change of serum creatinine was defined relative to a baseline creatinine. In the AKI system, AKI is defined on a documented increase of serum creatinine during a 48-h period. The 48-h time frame was introduced to

AKI, Epidemiology of. Table 1 Acute kidney injury (AKI) defined by the risk injury failure loss and end stage renal disease (RIFLE) classification and the modifications by the acute kidney injury diagnostic and classification system

	Creatinine criteria	Urine output criteria
Risk or stage 1	↑ ≥ 0.3 mg/dL or ≥150% and <200% compared to baseline	<0.5 mL/kg for 6 h
Injury or stage 2	≥200% and <300% compared to baseline	<0.5 mL/kg for 12 h
Failure or stage 3	≥300%, or > 4.0 mg/dL and increase > 0.5 mg/dL	<0.3 mL/kg for 24 h or anuria for 12 h
	RRT	

exclude clinically less significant periods of prerenal azotemia. Fourth, an absolute increase of serum creatinine of 0.3 mg/dL or greater was also defined as AKI stage 1. This is based upon literature that small absolute increases of serum creatinine also have important implications to outcome [4, 5].

Data on the epidemiology of AKI according to the AKI diagnostic and staging system is still limited. Initial studies confirmed that these modifications were not essentially changing the strength of the RIFLE classification [6–8]. However, a more recent study demonstrates that there are important differences in the populations described by both definitions of AKI [9].

Characteristics

Classification of AKI

On Etiology

AKI is typically a multifactorial disease. Intensive care unit (ICU) patients typically develop this disease as a consequence of several factors, and several insults. AKI is also a heterogeneous disease; there are several possible underlying disease states that may lead to the clinical syndrome of AKI. AKI is classically classified according to the underlying etiology of AKI as prerenal, intrinsic renal, and postrenal. According to this classification, only intrinsic AKI is true kidney disease, and prerenal and postrenal AKI are a consequence of disease in other organ systems, i.e., decreased kidney perfusion (prerenal disease) and diseases leading to obstruction of the urine outflow tract (postrenal). When postrenal and prenal disease status exist for longer periods, this may lead to acute tubular necrosis, one of the causes of intrinsic AKI. Prerenal and renal causes of AKI are most common in ICU patients, accounting for over 95% of AKI cases.

Common causes that may lead to decreased arterial perfusion of the kidney and prerenal AKI in ICU patients are all types of shock, decompensated congestive heart failure, liver cirrhosis, and medication induced decreased glomerular perfusion such as after administration of non-steroidal anti-inflammatory drugs, and angiotensin-converting enzyme inhibitors. Postrenal failure may be caused by, e.g., prostate hypertrophy, or by tumor masses obstructing the ureters. Intrinsic renal failure can be the consequence of disease of the renal vasculature (e.g., vasculitis in systemic disease), glomeruli (acute glomerulonephritis), interstitial cells (acute interstitial nephritis, secondary to, e.g., betalactam antibiotics), or the tubules (acute tubular necrosis secondary to toxins agents such as aminoglycosides, or ischemic secondary to prolonged periods of prerenal failure).

Community and Hospital Acquired

In parallel to infectious disease states, one can also classify AKI as community acquired, and nosocomial, either hospital acquired or ICU acquired [10, 11]. Nosocomial AKI is more often caused by multiple factors and multiple insults and occurs in patients with multiple organ dysfunction syndrome. An example may be a patient with abdominal infection who develops septic shock, undergoes surgery, and is treated with nephrotoxic aminoglycosides. Ten days after the initial insult, the patient has recurrent fever and undergoes a contrast enhanced CT scan to rule out an abdominal abscess.

Epidemiology

The incidence rate of AKI depends on the definition and the characteristics of the population taken for study. The population incidence of AKI defined by the RIFLE classification has been estimated in a Scottish region as 2,147 patients per million inhabitants per year (pmp/year) [12]. In ICU settings, the incidence of AKI defined by the RIFLE classification varies between 10% in ICU's with patients with low severity grade and 67%, in a US tertiary care referral center specialized in organ transplantation [13, 14]. In a general ICU, the incidence is probably between 35% and 50% [6, 9, 15, 16].

When AKI is defined as treatment with RRT (AKI-RRT), the population incidence varies between 80 and

270 pmp/year, comparable to the incidence of acute lung injury/acute respiratory distress syndrome (ARDS) in the USA [16–19]. On average 5% of ICU patients will be treated with RRT [20, 21].

The incidence of AKI is steadily increasing between 3% and 11% per year [18, 22–26]. This reported increase may in part be caused by reporting bias. Some of the data are from large ICD-9 based databases that are also used for billing purposes [18, 24]. Also, increased awareness that small increases of serum creatinine are important may have led to increased reporting of AKI. However, when the same definition for AKI was used for a 20-year period, as in the Australian New Zealand ICU database, the incidence of AKI also increased over the study period [23]. Factors that may explain this are the older patient population admitted to modern western ICUs, increased initial survival of severely ill patients as a consequence of advances in ICU care, and the admission of patients with severe comorbidity who were denied ICU care in the past, such as patients with hematologic malignancies.

Outcome

Patients with AKI have an increased mortality. This effect is present in different settings and in both the less severe stages of AKI, and in the most severe stages.

Less severe AKI is associated with increased risk for mortality even after correction for other covariates. This is demonstrated in contrast-associated AKI, defined as a 25% increase of serum creatinine or an absolute increase of 0.5 mg/dL [27]. After cardiac surgery, when serum creatinine increased between 0 and 0.5 mg/dL [4, 28]. And, in a hospital wide cohort, when serum creatinine increased with of 0.3 mg/dL or 25% [5]. Also, AKI defined by the different RIFLE classes was associated with mortality, in different ICU settings [13, 14, 29, 30].

ICU patients with AKI who are treated with RRT carry a mortality between 50% and 60% [20, 31]. As in less severe AKI, also severe AKI has an independent effect on mortality [32, 33].

Several sources report a decreasing trend of mortality of AKI patients treated with RRT. This may be attributed by improved treatment strategies (renal and nonrenal) for these severely ill patients [18, 23, 34]. However, also changes in case mix, and criteria for initiation of RRT may have influenced this.

In surviving patients, recovery of kidney function is an important endpoint. Up to 18% of patients are discharged from the hospital with permanent need for RRT or end stage kidney disease (ESKD). Also, patients who are discharged from the hospital without need for RRT, have an increased risk for developing ESKD, and for mortality

in the 5 years following hospital discharge [35, 36]. Especially, patients who had chronic kidney disease before ICU admission are at increased risk for developing ESKD [37].

Symptoms of AKI encompass the effects of failing of the different functions of the kidneys. Volume overload is one of the important symptoms that lead to increased morbidity such as decreased wound healing, intraabdominal hypertension, and pulmonary edema [38]. This is important, because common dogma is that volume therapy may prevent or treat prerenal and renal forms of AKI. The fact that restricted fluid therapy may even be beneficial for kidney function was demonstrated in ARDS patients, in whom this strategy resulted in a near significant trend for less RRT [39]. Volume overload is even an independent factor that contributes to the increased mortality in AKI patients [40]. Other untoward symptoms are electrolyte abnormalities such as hyperkalemia and hyponatremia and acidosis that can be found in 40–60% of patients with severe AKI, before start of RRT [41]. Infection may be one of the other leading causes of mortality in AKI patients. Similar to data in chronic dialysis patients, AKI patients also experience an increased incidence of infection [42–44]. This in itself may explain mortality, but also antimicrobial treatment of infections in ICU patients with AKI may play a role in this. Data on antibiotic prescription in patients with decreased kidney function are most based on data in patients with chronic kidney disease. In ICU patients with AKI, distribution volume may be importantly increased, which makes that in many cases the proposed reduction of antibiotic dose leads to insufficient antibiotic dosing and inadequate therapy. Also, RRT may vary in so many details (blood flow, dialysis flow, predilution, postdilution, membrane, duration of therapy, etc.) that proposed antibiotic dosing strategies for RRT are not necessarily comparable to the specific RRT technique you are using.

A final factor that may explain increased morbidity and mortality of AKI is that AKI is probably an important motor of other organ dysfunctions. An example for this may be the so-called organ cross talk between kidneys and lungs. Animal experimental data demonstrated that after AKI, the lungs will develop gene activation of inflammatory mediators, change in aquaporins and sodium cannels, infiltration with neutrophils, and albumin-rich exsudate, leading to a clinical syndrome of ARDS [45–48].

References

1. Lameire N, Van Biesen W, Vanholder R (2005) Acute renal failure. Lancet 365:417–430
2. Bellomo R, Ronco C, Kellum JA, Mehta RL, Palevsky P, Acute Dialysis Quality Initiative w (2004) Acute renal failure – definition, outcome

measures, animal models, fluid therapy and information technology needs: the Second International Consensus Conference of the Acute Dialysis Quality Initiative (ADQI) Group. Crit Care (London, England) 8:R204–R212

3. Mehta RL, Kellum JA, Shah SV, Molitoris BA, Ronco C, Warnock DG, Levin A (2007) Acute Kidney Injury Network (AKIN): report of an initiative to improve outcomes in acute kidney injury. Crit care (London, England) 11:R31

4. Lassnigg A, Schmidlin D, Mouhieddine M, Bachmann LM, Druml W, Bauer P, Hiesmayr M (2004) Minimal changes of serum creatinine predict prognosis in patients after cardiothoracic surgery: a prospective cohort study. J Am Soc Nephrol 15:1597–1605

5. Chertow GM, Burdick E, Honour M, Bonventre JV, Bates DW (2005) Acute kidney injury, mortality, length of stay, and costs in hospitalized patients. J Am Soc Nephrol 16:3365–3370

6. Bagshaw SM, George C, Bellomo R, for the ADMC (2008) A comparison of the RIFLE and AKIN criteria for acute kidney injury in critically ill patients. Nephrol Dial Transplant 23:1569–1574

7. Lopes JA, Fernandes P, Jorge S, Goncalves S, Alvarez A, Costa ESZ, Franca C, Prata MM (2008) Acute kidney injury in intensive care unit patients: a comparison between the RIFLE and the Acute Kidney Injury Network classifications. Crit Care (London, England) 12:R110

8. Kellum JA (2008) Defining and classifying AKI: one set of criteria. Nephrol Dial Transplant 23:1471–1472

9. Joannidis M, Metnitz B, Bauer P, Schusterschitz N, Moreno R, Druml W, Metnitz PG (2009) Acute kidney injury in critically ill patients classified by AKIN versus RIFLE using the SAPS 3 database. Intensive Care Med 35:1692–1702

10. Hsu CY, McCulloch CE, Fan D, Ordonez JD, Chertow GM, Go AS (2007) Community-based incidence of acute renal failure. Kidney Int 72:208–212

11. Liano F, Pascual J (1996) Epidemiology of acute renal failure: a prospective, multicenter, community-based study. Madrid Acute Renal Failure Study Group. Kidney Int 50:811–818

12. Ali T, Khan I, Simpson W, Prescott G, Townend J, Smith W, MacLeod A (2007) Incidence and outcomes in acute kidney injury: a comprehensive population-based study. J Am Soc Nephrol 18:1292–1298

13. Cruz D, Bolgan I, Perazella M, Bonelli M, de Cal M, Corradi V, Polanco N, Ocampo C, Nalesso F, Ronco C (2007) North East Italian prospective hospital renal outcome survey on acute kidney injury (NEiPHROS-AKI): targetting the problem with the RIFLE criteria. CJASN 2:418–425

14. Hoste EA, Clermont G, Kersten A, Venkataraman R, Angus DC, De Bacquer D, Kellum JA (2006) RIFLE criteria for acute kidney injury are associated with hospital mortality in critically ill patients: a cohort analysis. Crit Care 10:R73

15. Ostermann M, Chang RW (2007) Acute kidney injury in the intensive care unit according to RIFLE. Crit Care Med 35:1837–1843

16. Hoste EAJ, De Corte W (2007) The epidemiology of acute kidney injury in the ICU. Acta Clin Belg 62:314–317

17. Korkeila M, Ruokonen E, Takala J (2000) Costs of care, long-term prognosis and quality of life in patients requiring renal replacement therapy during intensive care. Intensive Care Med 26:1824–1831

18. Waikar SS, Curhan GC, Wald R, McCarthy EP, Chertow GM (2006) Declining mortality in patients with acute renal failure, 1988 to 2002. J Am Soc Nephrol 17:1143–1150

19. Goss CH, Brower RG, Hudson LD, Rubenfeld GD (2003) Incidence of acute lung injury in the United States. Crit Care Med 31:1607–1611

20. Uchino S, Kellum JA, Bellomo R, Doig GS, Morimatsu H, Morgera S, Schetz M, Tan I, Bouman C, Macedo E, Gibney N, Tolwani A, Ronco C (2005) Acute renal failure in critically ill patients: a multinational, multicenter study. JAMA 294:813–818

21. Metnitz PG, Krenn CG, Steltzer H, Lang T, Ploder J, Lenz K, Le Gall JR, Druml W (2002) Effect of acute renal failure requiring renal replacement therapy on outcome in critically ill patients. Crit Care Med 30:2051–2058

22. Swaminathan M, Shaw AD, Phillips-Bute BG, McGugan-Clark PL, Archer LE, Talbert S, Milano CA, Patel UD, Stafford-Smith M (2007) Trends in acute renal failure associated with coronary artery bypass graft surgery in the United States. Crit Care Med 35:2286–2291

23. Bagshaw SM, George C, Bellomo R (2007) Changes in the incidence and outcome for early acute kidney injury in a cohort of Australian intensive care units. Crit Care (London, England) 11:R68

24. Xue JL, Daniels F, Star RA, Kimmel PL, Eggers PW, Molitoris BA, Himmelfarb J, Collins AJ (2006) Incidence and mortality of acute renal failure in Medicare beneficiaries, 1992 to 2001. J Am Soc Nephrol 17:1135–1142

25. Hou S, Bushinsky D, Wish J, Cohen J, Harrington J (1983) Hospital-acquired renal insuffciency: a prospective study. Am J Med 74:243–248

26. Nash K, Hafeez A, Hou S (2002) Hospital-acquired renal insufficiency. Am J Kidney Dis 39:930–936

27. Levy EM, Viscoli CM, Horwitz RI (1996) The effect of acute renal failure on mortality. A cohort analysis. JAMA 275:1489–1494

28. Lassnigg A, Schmid ER, Hiesmayr M, Falk C, Druml W, Bauer P, Schmidlin D (2008) Impact of minimal increases in serum creatinine on outcome in patients after cardiothoracic surgery: do we have to revise current definitions of acute renal failure? Crit Care Med 36:1129–1137

29. Uchino S, Bellomo R, Goldsmith D, Bates S, Ronco C (2006) An assessment of the RIFLE criteria for acute renal failure in hospitalized patients. Crit Care Med 34:1913–1917

30. Kuitunen A, Vento A, Suojaranta-Ylinen R, Pettila V (2006) Acute renal failure after cardiac surgery: evaluation of the RIFLE classification. Ann Thorac Surg 81:542–546

31. The VA/NIH Acute Renal Failure Trial Network (2008) Intensity of renal support in critically ill patients with acute kidney injury. N Engl J Med 359:7–20

32. Chertow GM, Levy EM, Hammermeister KM, Grover F, Daley J (1998) Independent association between acute renal failure and mortality following cardiac surgery. Am J Med 104:343–348

33. Hoste EA, Lameire NH, Vanholder RC, Benoit DD, Decruyenaere JM, Colardyn FA (2003) Acute renal failure in patients with sepsis in a surgical ICU: predictive factors, incidence, comorbidity, and outcome. J Am Soc Nephrol 14:1022–1030

34. Desegher A, Reynvoet E, Blot S, De Waele J, Claus S, Hoste E (2006) Outcome of patients treated with renal replacement therapy for acute kidney injury. Crit Care 10:P296

35. C-y H, Chertow GM, McCulloch CE, Fan D, Ordonez JD, Go AS (2009) Nonrecovery of kidney function and death after acute on chronic renal failure. Clin J Am Soc Nephrol 4:891–898

36. Schiffl H, Fischer R (2008) Five-year outcomes of severe acute kidney injury requiring renal replacement therapy. Nephrol Dial Transplant 23:2235–2241

37. Ishani A, Xue JL, Himmelfarb J, Eggers PW, Kimmel PL, Molitoris BA, Collins AJ (2009) Acute kidney injury increases risk of ESRD among elderly. J Am Soc Nephrol 20:223–228

38. Dalfino L, Tullo L, Donadio I, Malcangi V, Brienza N (2008) Intra-abdominal hypertension and acute renal failure in critically ill patients. Intensive Care Med 34:707–713
39. Wiedemann HP, Wheeler AP, Bernard GR, Thompson BT, Hayden D, deBoisblanc B, Connors AF Jr, Hite RD, Harabin AL (2006) Comparison of two fluid-management strategies in acute lung injury. N Engl J Med 354:2564–2575
40. Payen D, de Pont A, Sakr Y, Spies C, Reinhart K, Vincent J, the Sepsis Occurrence in Acutely Ill Patients I (2008) A positive fluid balance is associated with a worse outcome in patients with acute renal failure. Crit Care 12:R74
41. Uchino S, Bellomo R, Ronco C (2001) Intermittent versus continuous renal replacement therapy in the ICU: impact on electrolyte and acid- base balance. Intensive Care Med 27:1037–1043
42. Hoste EA, Blot SI, Lameire NH, Vanholder RC, De Bacquer D, Colardyn FA (2004) Effect of nosocomial bloodstream infection on the outcome of critically ill patients with acute renal failure treated with renal replacement therapy. J Am Soc Nephrol 15:454–462
43. Reynvoet E, Vandijck DM, Blot SI, Dhondt AW, De Waele JJ, Claus S, Buyle FM, Vanholder RC, Hoste EA (2009) Epidemiology of infection in critically ill patients with acute renal failure. Crit Care Med 37:2203–2209
44. Thakar CV, Yared JP, Worley S, Cotman K, Paganini EP (2003) Renal dysfunction and serious infections after open-heart surgery. Kidney Int 64:239–246
45. Hassoun HT, Grigoryev DN, Lie ML, Liu M, Cheadle C, Tuder RM, Rabb H (2007) Ischemic acute kidney injury induces a distant organ functional and genomic response distinguishable from bilateral nephrectomy. Am J Physiol Renal Physiol 293:F30–F40
46. Rabb H, Wang Z, Nemoto T, Hotchkiss J, Yokota N, Soleimani M (2003) Acute renal failure leads to dysregulation of lung salt and water channels. Kidney Int 63:600–606
47. Kim DJ, Park SH, Sheen MR, Jeon US, Kim SW, Koh ES, Woo SK (2006) Comparison of experimental lung injury from acute renal failure with injury due to sepsis. Respiration 73:815–824
48. Hoke TS, Douglas IS, Klein CL, He Z, Fang W, Thurman JM, Tao Y, Dursun B, Voelkel NF, Edelstein CL, Faubel S (2007) Acute renal failure after bilateral nephrectomy is associated with cytokine-mediated pulmonary injury. J Am Soc Nephrol 18:155–164

Alanyl-Glutamine Dipeptide

▶ Glutamine

Alcohol Intoxication

▶ Ethanol Intoxication

Alkaline Phosphatase

▶ Tubular Enzymuria

Allergic Interstitial Nephritis

▶ Interstitial Nephritis, Acute

Allergic Shock

▶ Anaphylactic Shock

"All-in-One" Solutions

"All-in-one" PN solutions, also called "ternary" PN solutions, contain protein, carbohydrate, lipid, trace elements, vitamins, water, and electrolytes altogether in the same solution. "All-in-one" PN solutions have replaced the separated administration of macronutrients. The "all-in-one" solutions allow obtaining a lower and constant load of glucose and lipid substrates, reducing the risk of overfeeding.

ALP

▶ Tubular Enzymuria

Alpha-1-Microglobulin

▶ Serum and Urinary Low Molecular Weight Proteins

Alterations in Coagulation in Acute Renal Failure

▶ Bleeding and Hemostasis in Acute Renal Failure

Altered Mental Status

▶ Encephalopathy and Delirium

Alternative Airways

EDWARD T. DICKINSON
Department of Emergency Medicine, Hospital of the
University of Pennsylvania Ground Ravdin, Philadelphia,
PA, USA

Introduction

Modern medical dogma states that definitive emergency airway control requires that a cuffed tube be placed in the trachea by means of either an orotracheal, nasotracheal, or surgical airway approach. In the vast majority of cases, this task is accomplished by the placement of an oral endotracheal tube under direct visualization of the vocal cords with a laryngoscope. However, in an increasing number of emergency situations, non-definitive advanced airway devices are being used to temporize the airway to allow for effective ventilation when placement of an endotracheal tube is either impossible or impractical. Collectively, these non-endotracheal devices are referred to as *alternative airways (AAs)*.

Historical Perspective

Supraglottic and esophageal obturator alternative airways (AAs) have been available for over 3 decades. The earliest marketed AAs were esophageal obturator airways that were rigid tubes blindly inserted into the esophagus. The esophageal obturator airway (EOA) and a later version that allowed for gastric decompression via the airway (EGTA) first came into use almost 4 decades ago. This first generation of AA devices were designed as primary airway control devices and marketed for use by less-trained rescuers (such as prehospital emergency medical services (EMS) providers) for rapid insertion in respiratory and cardiac arrest patients in the out-of-hospital setting.

In subsequent years, technical advancements in AA design and the acceptance of AAs as "rescue airways" for physicians, in situations where endotracheal intubation is either not possible due to patient anatomy or lack of operator expertise, has greatly expanded the use of these devices in both prehospital and hospital emergencies. Indeed, the 2010 American Heart Association's evidenced-based guidelines for advanced cardiac life-support acute resuscitation gives AA devices equal footing with endotracheal intubation as equivalently recommended means of securing the airway of patients in cardiac arrest [1]. Although the endotracheal intubation remains the most definitive way of securing the airway, the direct laryngoscopy necessary for intubation has proven to be a more difficult and time-consuming procedure than the blind insertion of an AA [2]. In the setting of cardiac arrest, where the length of interruption of chest compressions has been shown to be inversely proportional to survival, the prolonged interruption of chest compression demonstrated with endotracheal intubation attempts in some studies is deemed unacceptable. In this setting, it is felt the speed benefits of AA insertion outweigh its lack of definitiveness. Thus, both AA insertion and endotracheal intubation modalities are equally weighted in the AHA cardiac arrest guidelines.

Clinical Use of Alternative Airway Devices

The decision when to utilize an AA rather than an endotracheal tube for emergency airway control is based on various considerations, including clinical situation, patient anatomy, and the expertise of the medical personnel. In the prehospital setting, the AA may be the only advanced airway device the provider is authorized to use in a given emergency medical services (EMS) system. Alternatively, in some systems when paramedics are allowed to perform endotracheal intubation, protocol may dictate that an alternative airway be placed after two failed attempts at conventional endotracheal intubation.

In emergency situations in hospital-based emergency and critical care medicine, AAs are most often deployed in situations when clinicians are unable to successfully perform endotracheal intubation. In this role, the alternative airway is considered a "rescue airway" that allows effective ventilation to critically ill or cardiac arrest patients. In light of the recent AHA guidelines, it is likely AAs will gain an increased primary airway role during in-hospital cardiac arrests.

All alternative airways have commonalities in their clinical use. No airway device is perfect. The ideal AA should have the following attributes:

1. When properly placed, allows for effective ventilation of the patient.
2. The design is simple enough that it allows for adequate skill retention so that the clinician can effectively use the device despite the fact that it might only be used in a rare emergency situation.
3. Design allows for rapid insertion.
4. The design accommodates the potential subsequent placement of an endotracheal tube with minimal risk to the patient.

Perhaps the two most clinically significant commonalities of all alternative airway devices are that all these devices are largely restricted to use in the unconscious patient, and that AAs are designed for short-term use only. If the patient will continue to require ongoing airway control, then the AA will need to be replaced by a definitive airway, most commonly an orally placed endotracheal tube.

Each alternative airway device has a specific technique for the controlled transition of the AA to an endotracheal tube. Regardless of the device being used, it is essential that the transition occurs in as controlled a fashion as possible, minimizing the risk of complications such as hypoxia and aspiration that can occur during airway change over. Certain caveats for the transition of an alternative airway device to an endotracheal are applicable to all these devices. First and foremost, the decision to simply "yank" the AA and then try to perform endotracheal intubation is ill advised *unless* patient assessment shows that the alternative airway is not providing adequate ventilation. Patients who have had an AA placed as a "rescue airway" after failed intubation attempts may present with iatrogenic airway challenges in addition to any preexisting anatomic challenge the patient may have. Often these, patients have sustained some degree of upper airway trauma from laryngoscope manipulations as well gastric distension, with resultant vomiting from excessive bag-valve-mask ventilation prior to the airway placement. The clinical reality is that if the AA is providing adequate ventilation, then the conversion to a definitive airway should be conducted in a calm, well-planned, and methodical fashion. Key generic steps in the conversion of the AA to an endotracheal tube include the following:

If the alternative airway has the capacity to allow the passage of a gastric tube (the Combitube® and King Airway LTS-D™ for example), then the stomach should be fully decompressed and suctioned prior to any conversion procedure.
The patient should be pre-oxygenated with 100% oxygen.
Continuous ECG, end-tidal CO_2, and pulse ox monitoring should be in place.
Appropriate equipment for the procedure (endotracheal tube introducer, laryngoscope, etc.) should be assembled and tested.
The clinician with the most expertise in alternative airways should direct the procedure.
A physician with expertise and equipment for the establishment of a surgical airway should be present at bedside in case the airway proves to be unobtainable by any means.
If during a conversion attempt hypoxia develops, then the alternative airway can be again used to provide ventilation prior to another attempt at endotracheal intubation.

Alternative Airway Designs

Although there are numerous designs and brands of alternative airways currently available, they can be broadly categorized as either esophageal-seated or supraglottic-seated airways [3].

Esophageal-Seated Airways

The earliest alternative airways devices widely marketed were of the esophageal-seated type. The Esophageal Obturator Airway (EOA) and later variation that allowed for gastric decompression, the Esophageal Gastric Tube Airway (EGTA), were initially marked for use by prehospital personnel and used as a primary device to secure the airway in the unconscious unresponsive patients. The device has two parts: a rigid tube approximately 14 in. long with a higher pressure balloon at the distal tip and a face mask that attaches to the proximal end of the tube. After blind insertion, the EOA/EGTA is designed to be inserted into the esophagus where the obturating balloon is inflated which then allows pulmonary ventilation by channeling air into the pharynx when the face mask is ventilated. The device requires an excellent mask seal in order to be effective. The device never gained significant traction as an in-hospital device and to this day remains largely relinquished to prehospital care use in certain regions.

Conversion of the EOA/EGTA to an oral endotracheal tube is best accomplished by separating the face mask from the esophageal tube and performing direct laryngoscopy around the tube. If an EGTA is to be converted, gastric decompression prior to the removal of the esophageal tube is recommended. If oxygen desaturation or other difficulty is encountered during endotracheal intubation attempts, simply reattach the mask to the EOA/EGTA tube and ventilate the patient while preparing for another attempt at intubation.

The two key limitations of the EOA design is that it is ineffective without an excellent mask seal, and that although the majority of the time the tube does come to rest in the esophagus as designed, it is equally ineffective if the tube is placed in the trachea. Subsequent generations of esophageal-seated AA devices have taken into account these significant limitations of the relatively simple EOA design. First, none of the newer devices have a facemask, and thus do not rely on operator-dependent mask seal for effective ventilation. Second, in case the tube is blindly inserted into the trachea, a secondary ventilation lumen that allows direct endotracheal ventilation is incorporated into the newer esophageal-seated AA designs.

The resultant generation of esophageal-seated AAs is broadly referred to as *multi-lumen, multi-port airways*. Examples include Combitube®, the PTL®, and the Rusch

Easytube® airways. All these devices are still blindly inserted and designed to have their long tubes come to rest in the esophagus. Once placed, a distal balloon is inflated to block the esophagus in the same fashion as their ancestral EOA. However, to obviate the need for a face mask seal, these AAs utilize a second large balloon attached to the mid-tube that when inflated fills the patient's pharynx. With the esophagus obturated by the distal balloon and the potential for air to escape from the mouth or nose blocked by the pharyngeal balloon, ventilation is accomplished via ventilation ports on the shaft of the tube between the two balloons. When both balloons inflated, ventilation is directed into the trachea and lungs because all other means of gas egress are blocked.

Clinical experience and limited published data have shown that in approximately 10% of multi-lumen, multi-port-airway insertions, the tube comes to rest in the trachea. These AA devices are designed to accommodate this possibility by the addition of an endotracheal tube incorporated as a second ventilation lumen. The tracheal ventilation lumen is identified by a second 15 mm ventilation port adapter on the airway.

If as designed, the multi-lumen, multi-port esophageal-seated AA device is blindly placed in the esophagus, then conversion to an oral endotracheal tube is best accomplished by deflating the proximal pharyngeal balloon and intubating the trachea under direct visualization around the esophageal tube. Alternatively, if the airway is found to be inserted into the trachea, the patient de facto already has a definitive airway. In this situation, there are two options: the AA can be left in place and the patient ventilated via the endotracheal lumen with the proximal balloon deflated, or the AA can be converted to a conventional endotracheal tube by use of a tube changer or similar device.

The most recent variant of the esophageal-seated airway is the King Airway™. This device is notably shorter than the multi-lumen, multi-port airways but utilizes the same dual balloon system allowing ventilation to be directed into the trachea and lungs because all other means of gas egress are blocked. The King airway™ is specifically designed to be too short in length to allow endotracheal placement. Thus, it does not have an endotracheal ventilation port or lumen. To assure proper tube length, the King Airway™ comes in five different sizes from pediatric to large adult. Tube-length sizing makes the King Airway™ unique among esophageal-seated airways in that it can be used in pediatric patients.

Conversion of the King Airway™ to an oral endotracheal tube is best accomplished by insertion of either an endotracheal tube introducer (aka Bougie™) or an Aintree® intubation catheter mounted over a fiberoptic

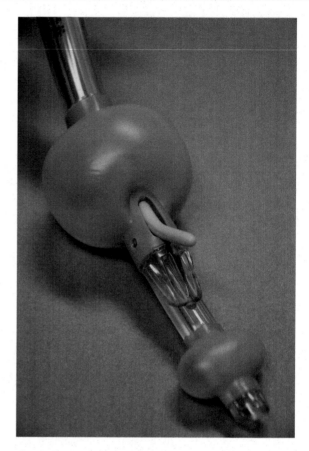

Alternative Airways. Figure 1 Endotracheal Tube Introducer emerging from King™ Airway conversion ramp

bronchoscope down the conversion ramp of the device (Fig. 1). Once a device is passed through the airway's ramp into the trachea, the King™ can be withdrawn over the device and an endotracheal tube is then inserted over the device that then acts like a tube changer.

Supraglottic-Seated Airways

Supraglottic-seated airways are the second major class of alternative airways. Following blind insertion, these airways allow effective ventilation by forming a snug seal around the laryngeal inlet with the soft "mask" on the distal portion of the device. The archetype of this airway class is the Laryngeal Mask Airway (LMA). There are many commercial variants of the LMA-type supraglottic airway currently available. These AA devices include the I-Gel®, the intubating LMA, and the LMA-Unique™. Because it is essential that the mask be properly sized to fit around the laryngeal inlet, these devices come in various sizes from pediatrics patients up through adults.

The LMA and its variants have traditionally been used for brief elective operative procedures in patients with

2. Wang HE et al (2009) Interruptions in cardiopulmonary resuscitation from paramedic endotracheal intubation. Ann Emerg Med 54:645–652
3. Levitan RM (2004) The Airway Cam guide to intubation and practical emergency airway management. Airway Cam Technologies, Wayne, PA

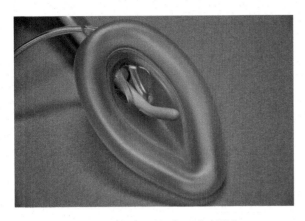

Alternative Airways. Figure 2 Endotracheal Tube Introducer emerging from LMA (Source: Both photos by Ed Dickinson, M.D. Photo use permission granted)

empty stomachs. The use of laryngeal mask devices in emergency patients with full stomachs is generally considered to be problematic due to the risk of aspiration if vomiting occurs.

The conversion of supraglottic airways to an endotracheal tube is generally accomplished by passing an endotracheal tube, an endotracheal tube introducer (Fig. 2) or a fiberoptic intubating bronchoscope directly down the lumen of the device. If intubation difficulties (including hypoxia) are encountered during conversion to an endotracheal tube, attempts should be discontinued and the patient re-ventilated through the supraglotic airway's lumen prior to subsequent attempts.

Summary

Alternative airway devices are becoming increasingly ubiquitous in emergency and critical care medicine. Whether their role is as a rapidly inserted primary airway device or as a "rescue" airway in cases of failed attempts at conventional endotracheal intubation, it is essential that the practitioner be thoroughly versed in the use of the AA device and in their practice environment. Consideration of what defines the practice environment must also include those airways used by the local prehospital personnel local who transport critically ill patients to the hospital. To assure safe and effective utilization of these devices, the clinician must know how insert, assess placement, ventilate, remove, and secure a definitive airway around the device.

References

1. Field JM, Hazinski F, Sayre MR et al (2010) Executive summary: 2010 American Heart Association guidelines for cardiopulmonary resuscitation and emergency cardiovascular care. Circulation 122: S640–S656

Alveolar Echinococcosis (AE)

▶ Echinococcosis, Alveolar

Alveolar Hydatid Disease

▶ Echinococcosis, Alveolar

Amb-d

Amphotericin B deoxycholate.

American College of Surgeons Resources Document

ALEXANDER L. COLONNA, J. WAYNE MEREDITH
Wake Forest University Baptist, Medical Center,
Medical Center Boulevarde, Winston-Salem, NC, USA

Synonyms

Resources for the Optimal Care of the Injured Patient (2006); *Optimal Hospital Resources for Care of the Injured Patient* (1976)

Definition

Published by the American College of Surgeons Committee on Trauma (ACS-COT), the resources document establishes guidelines for care of the injured patient. The ACS-COT was founded in 1922 by Charles L. Scudder, MD, FACS and focuses on improving the care of the injured patient, believing that trauma is a surgical disease demanding surgical leadership [1].

Characteristics

History

Trauma as a disease was most likely the first to be treated by early man, as its sequelae are often easily visible in the form of wounds and fractures. As civilizations evolved and expanded, so did human conflicts. War became more common and the need to care for the wounded increased. The earliest medical records from ancient Egypt described the treatment of traumatic wounds as does early literature like Homer's *Iliad*. The Romans had special quarters for the care of sick or wounded soldiers called *valetudinaria*. Great advancements in trauma care continued to be made through the Middle Ages, the Renaissance, and the Industrial Revolution closely coinciding with the major wars of these eras. Hand in hand with the increase in basic scientific knowledge and operative technique was the realization that the development of trauma systems, especially during the Korean and Vietnam wars, was an integral part of improving outcomes [2].

The first civilian trauma center was created in Birmingham, England in 1941. The first two trauma centers in the USA were opened in San Francisco and Chicago in 1966. Maryland then developed a statewide trauma system, followed by Illinois in 1971 which created the first trauma system legislature. Germany developed a nationwide trauma system in the 1970s that significantly decreased traffic accident mortality. In 1976 the ACS-COT developed guidelines for the care of trauma patients and published it as *Optimal Hospital Resources for the Care of the Injured Patient*. This document has undergone several revisions until reaching the latest version published in 2006 as *Resources for the Optimal Care of the Injured Patient*. It underwent a clear change from describing optimal hospital resources to describing optimal care given available resources forcing the development of a full trauma system, not solely trauma centers, realizing that no single facility can provide all care to all patients at all times.

The resources document describes the ideal *inclusive trauma system* comprised of prevention, access, acute hospital care, rehabilitation, and research. It describes a network of definitive care facilities differing in resource depth, Levels I to IV. The guidelines also describe in detail prehospital and interhospital care, clinical functions of the various specialties involved in trauma care, posthospital care, process improvement and research, and finally the verification process. The overall goal is to better define what resources are necessary to provide the best care for the injured patient, using evidence-based recommendations when available [3].

Trauma Systems

The goal of a trauma system is to reduce the burden of injury to individuals and society. As such, this requires a group of related injury-oriented facilities, personnel, and organizational entities operating in a coordinated fashion within a defined geographic region. To achieve this goal the ACS has developed recommendations and provided a system of trauma center verification. Trauma should be approached as a public health problem, requiring a public health model in which the core functions of assessment, policy development, and assurance are implemented. A successful trauma system also participates in community outreach to prevent trauma. Primary prevention includes programs directed toward decreasing the incidence of trauma (e.g., minimum drinking age, gun control laws), secondary prevention policies to decrease the severity of the trauma once it occurs (e.g., seatbelt and helmet laws), and tertiary prevention measures to improve the outcomes of trauma patients (e.g., process improvement, compliance).

The basic components of a trauma system can be broken down into two major sections, administrative and clinical. The administrative components include leadership, system development, legislation, and finances. The clinical component includes injury prevention, human resources, prehospital care, definitive care facilities, information systems, evaluation, all hazards preparedness, and research. Trauma systems also have a special obligation to participate in disaster preparation and management. Disaster planning requires a cooperative multidisciplinary effort by local medical resources; police and fire departments; local, regional, and national governments; and industry.

Prehospital and Interhospital Care

Prehospital stabilization and emergency transportation systems were enhanced from lessons learned in military conflicts. Initial management of the injured patient at the scene of injury consists of assessment, extrication, initiation of resuscitation and stabilization, and rapid transport to the closest appropriate facility. The protocols that guide this care should be established by trauma health care providers as a team to establish continuity of care and consistency of protocols throughout the trauma system. Essential components of resuscitation should be limited to airway management, hemorrhage control, stabilization of fractures, and immobilization of the spine.

As patients are being readied for transport they must be triaged to the appropriate facility. A priority has been given to reducing undertriage, with acceptance of resulting overtriage, since undertriage can result in preventable morbidity and mortality from delays in reaching definitive care. An overtriage rate of 25–50% is acceptable while keeping the undertriage rate to 1–5%. The trauma system's performance improvement program should carefully monitor the triage criteria to achieve these goals.

Trauma systems facilitate the transfer of patients between the initial stabilizing facility and the receiving facility that has access to definitive or specialized care that a patient requires. Written agreements and transfer plans are essential in order to have these protocols in place before the acute patient need arises. Physician to physician contact is essential to complete the transfer of a patient based solely on the patient's needs. Also there should be well-established protocols outlining injuries or patterns of injury that should be transferred to a higher level of care. However, injured patients who are hemodynamically unstable may undergo appropriate operative control of life-threatening hemorrhage prior to transfer to a higher level of care if there is a qualified surgeon and operating room resources available.

Trauma Centers

In order to become a trauma center a hospital must have the commitment of the staff and management in order to allocate the necessary resources and provide the specialty care necessary for injured patients. A trauma center must have nine elements in place. These are: hospital organization, medical staff support, the trauma program, the trauma medical director, the trauma resuscitation team, the trauma program manager, the trauma service, the trauma registrar, and the trauma performance improvement and safety program. Specific guidelines are provided in the resource document describing the makeup of these elements and the regular upkeep of these elements with written commitments.

The trauma medical director is a board-certified surgeon who provides leadership for the entire trauma program. The resuscitation team is a multidisciplinary group that responds to trauma codes. A trauma center must also have a trauma service that provides structure for the care of the injured patient. The trauma program manager and registrar provide administrative and research assistance to maintain the development, implementation, and evaluation of the trauma program. A multidisciplinary peer review committee is also necessary for performance improvement.

In order to assure that the right patient gets to the right facility at the right time, the ACS resources document describes the various trauma center levels and their roles in the trauma system. These levels range from I to IV, with one center of the highest available level serving as the lead center for the region. Ideally this would be a Level I trauma center, serving as a regional resource and usually situated in a large city or population dense area, that manages a large number of severely injured patients (Injury Severity Score >16). A Level I trauma center has 24 hour in-house availability of an attending surgeon or a postgraduate year four or five resident. A surgically directed critical care service, resident education, trauma research program, injury prevention and control, and community outreach are all also deemed essential for a Level I trauma center.

The Level II trauma center has many of the same criteria as the Level I center, although it may function as an adjunct to the Level I center in population dense areas. In rural areas a Level II center may be the lead institution of the regional trauma system. Level II trauma centers aspire to the same standards as Level I centers, but are not required to have graduate medical education, research capabilities, or specific volume requirements [4]. The key aspect of the Level II trauma center is close cooperation between higher and lower level centers in order to properly triage patients.

The last level of fully functional trauma care is the Level III center. These hospitals serve smaller rural areas or urban communities that may not have immediate access to higher levels of care. These trauma centers have the capability to initially manage the majority of trauma patients and have transfer agreements with Level I and II centers. They are expected to have surgical leadership, a trauma director, a trauma team, and a performance improvement system. The Level IV center is generally located in a rural area and supplements care in a larger system by recognizing injuries, initiating resuscitation, and transferring patients to a higher level of care. The Level III and IV centers may be the lead center of a rural trauma system.

Rural trauma centers and systems must be developed to mitigate the specific challenges of the area. Optimal care of a patient can be delayed or limited by geography, weather, distances, or resources. The low-volume nature of rural trauma puts extra pressure on providers to maintain their skill sets. Also integral to a rural trauma center and system is a trauma registry that can track patients and a robust performance improvement (PI) process that can continuously evaluate the best use of limited resources to maximize the benefit to the local population. Level III or even IV centers may be the lead facility in isolated areas, and it is incumbent for these centers to have established transfer protocols as part of an inclusive trauma system.

Clinical Functions

General surgery is the foundation of the trauma center. Ideally the trauma director is board-certified, has demonstrated an interest and leadership of trauma care, and serves as the "captain" of the resuscitation team. Certification in and the teaching of Advanced Trauma Life Support (ATLS) is required. The day-to-day care of patients on the trauma service and the response to new trauma admissions can be closely integrated within a general surgery residency program. In Level I and II centers the general surgeon is dedicated to the trauma center while on duty and must have a documented backup call schedule. The general surgeon must participate in multidisciplinary PI in all trauma center levels. Level I and II trauma center directors must participate in regional and national trauma organizations and maintain adequate continuing medical education (CME).

Emergency medicine physicians are integral to a functioning trauma center. Level I, II, and III centers must have an emergency department (ED) director that is board-certified. There must also be an appropriate level of staffing commiserate with the trauma center level at all times in the ED. The emergency physician must be involved with the care of trauma patients, participate in PI, and maintain CME. ATLS certification of the ED physician is optimal.

Neurosurgery should be available to care for severe traumatic brain and spinal cord injury promptly and continuously. They must participate in the ED evaluation or be continuously available for neurotrauma, per the hospitals protocols in Level I and II centers. Level III centers may not have neurosurgical coverage and thus need established transfer protocols with higher level centers. As with the other specialties, neurosurgeons must participate regularly in the care of neurotrauma, participate in PI, and maintain current trauma-related CME.

Over half of trauma patients that are admitted have an orthopedic injury. However, patients with isolated simple fractures do not necessitate a trauma evaluation. Multiply injured patients require very close interaction with the trauma service and orthopedics. There are three kinds of orthopedic trauma patients. The first has isolated closed musculoskeletal injury and can be managed by ED physicians and orthopedists alone. The second has fractures of multiple long bone or joints and requires trauma team evaluation to ensure that associated injuries are not missed. Once resuscitated these patients should have early aggressive fracture stabilization. The third kind of patient has multiple fractures of long bones, joints, and/or spine with associated injuries of other organ systems. These patients mandate a high level of care by the trauma

team working closely with orthopedics and other necessary specialties like otolaryngology, plastic surgery, and ophthalmology. In Level I and II centers an orthopedist must be available continuously for ED evaluation. There must also be associated ancillary services, operating room staff, and operating room (OR) availability. A Level I trauma center must have an orthopedic trauma tram and director with dedicated call and backup call schedules. Integration with an orthopedics residency is highly desirable. A Level II trauma center must also have an orthopedic trauma team. A Level III trauma center may have 24 h orthopedic availability or it must have established transfer protocols with higher level centers. Again, the orthopedist must participate in PI, regular clinical care of trauma, and CME. Rehabilitation, physical therapy, and pain management service protocols are also recommended.

Collaborative clinical services such as anesthesiology, OR staff, postanesthesia care unit, radiology, critical care, laboratory, respiratory therapy, hemodialysis are necessary for the multidisciplinary care of the severely injured patient. Level I and II trauma centers must have anesthesia attendings available 24 h a day. Level III trauma centers are not required to have in-house anesthesiologists, but anesthesia services must be promptly available when needed. Level I trauma centers must have an operating room and staff available continuously. Level II and III trauma centers must have these resources promptly available. The requirements are similar for radiology and ancillary services based on the level of the trauma center.

Burn Care and Pediatric Trauma recommendations are also included in the resources document. Burn center referral criteria are specific and include: partial-thickness burns greater than 10% of the total body surface area; burns involving the face, hands, feet, genitalia, perineum, or major joints; full thickness burns; electrical burns, including lightning; chemical burns; inhalation injury; burns in patients with multiple medical comorbidities; burned multitrauma patients; and burned children. The development of a functioning burn system parallels the development of trauma systems. The pediatric trauma system requires similar overall commitments and organization as well. Pediatric surgery involvement within a dedicated children's hospital is optimal. The resource document specifies the additional need for board certification by the pediatric surgeon, neurosurgeon, and orthopedist. A pediatric trauma center must also have a pediatric trauma service, participate in PI, educate and perform outreach with the community.

The National Organ Transplantation Act of 1984 and the 1986 Omnibus Budget Reconciliation Act established the United Network for Organ Sharing and requires hospitals to notify family members of the option to donate. The hospital's trauma program plays a major role in identifying potential organ donors since 75% of organs come from deceased donors and of these cadaveric transplants 40% are trauma patients. A trauma center must collaborate with an organ procurement organization (OPO) to identify potential organ donors early and assist in discussing organ donation with the family. Complete and irreversible loss of function of the brain and brainstem is the definition of brain death set by the Uniform Determination of Death Act. Once brain death has been declared the patients care should be optimized to maintain perfusion of potential organs, ideally by the surgical critical care section of the trauma service.

Posthospital Care and Outreach

Rehabilitation starts at day one of hospitalization as the goal of trauma care is to return the patient to preinjury status. A multidisciplinary rehabilitation team should evaluate patients as early in their hospitalization as possible. Physical therapy is best started well in advance of neurological or orthopedic recovery to minimize the effects of prolonged immobilization. There are multiple rehabilitation assessments including the Functional Independence Measure, the Short Form-36, and the Quality of Well Being Index that can assist in quantifying a patient's recovery potential. Part of the rehabilitation from traumatic injury includes awareness of posttraumatic stress disorder (PTSD) since the prevalence of PTSD has been estimated at about 5–10% of the American population. Trauma patients may require different kinds of specialized rehabilitation based upon their injury pattern and age such as spine injury, brain injury, or orthopedic injury, and geriatric or pediatric. These different groups of patients do best at facilities with resources specifically directed at these injury patterns. Rehabilitation needs in the critical care arena should not be overlooked. Level I and II centers must have physical therapy, occupational therapy, and speech therapy available in the ICU.

Trauma centers have a responsibility to engage in community outreach and education. Outreach takes the form of public education, injury prevention programs, professional education, and making resources available to the community. Public education serves multiple roles of raising awareness of injury prevention and prompt utilization of care as life saving. First aid and CPR courses teach basic management to the layperson that can save lives. Professional education like the ATLS course and residency programs teaches the next generation of trauma professionals and help those already engaged in the care of

the injured patient both obtain certification and maintain skills already acquired.

Injury prevention programs are perhaps the best and sometimes only way to reduce the impact of trauma on a community. Evidence-based efforts like violence awareness programs, alcohol education/intervention, and injury surveillance have been shown to decrease trauma rates. There are three levels of injury prevention: primary, secondary, and tertiary based on the timing of the intervention. Developing an injury prevention program includes selecting a target injury, acquiring and analyzing data, developing an intervention, formulating a plan, implementation, and evaluating and revising the program.

Research and Education

Level I trauma centers must demonstrate research and scholarly activities. The resources document outlines specific publication requirements. There must be a research infrastructure in place to facilitate productive scholarly activity, which makes it no coincidence that most Level I trauma centers are in academic medical centers. An essential tool for this research is the trauma registry. This registry must link to the National Trauma Data Bank (NTDB) and be managed by a dedicated trauma registrar. The data in the hospitals registry can be used for PI, public health outreach, injury prevention, trauma systems outcomes measurement, resource utilization, and research. With all of these various uses, the trauma registry is one of the most important tools in the trauma center's armamentarium.

In addition to the research and scholarship activities based on the trauma registry, trauma centers are encouraged to participate in residency programs. The leadership of the trauma program, especially at Level I centers, must also participate in national meetings such the American Association for the Surgery of Trauma (AAST), the Eastern Association for the Surgery of Trauma (EAST), and the Western Trauma Association (WTA).

Performance Improvement

The performance improvement and patient safety (PIPS) section of the resources document describes a robust system for monitoring, evaluating, and improving the performance of a trauma program. Using filters that select cases to evaluate from the trauma registry for multidisciplinary peer review, the PIPS program aims to improve the care of the injured patient. An effective program has authority and accountability, a well defined organizational structure, objectively defined standards to determine quality of care, and explicit definitions of outcomes derived from relevant standards. All trauma centers must document a functioning PIPS program that has administrative accountability, assesses trauma privileges for providers, and implements corrective actions.

Trauma Center Consultation and Verification

The resources document provides the standards by which trauma centers can be measured. The purpose of trauma center verification is to assess whether a potential trauma center meets the guidelines published by the ACS-COT. The designation of a trauma center must be made in the context of a trauma system; the verification process compliments this and allows for independent oversight of standards. The ACS does not designate trauma centers itself; it verifies that properly designated centers have the resources outlined in the document available. The designation of trauma facilities is a geopolitical process by which empowered entities, governmental or otherwise, are authorized to do so. Research has been published that shows a trauma center can improve its outcomes by simply participating in trauma center verification. The verification team will closely examine the trauma center and will either grant or deny verification, but will also identify areas of excellence and areas that need improvement to comply with the guidelines [5].

References

1. American College of Surgeons Committee on Trauma (2006) Resources for the optimal care of the injured patient. American College of Surgeons, Chicago, IL
2. Pruitt B, Pruitt J (2008) History of trauma care. In: Moore E, Feliciano D, Mattox K (eds) Trauma. McGraw-Hill, New York, pp 3–23
3. Trunkey D (2008) The development of trauma systems. In: Asensio J, Trunkey D (eds) Current therapy of trauma and surgical critical care. Mosby Elsevier, Philadelphia, PA, pp 1–4
4. Trunkey D (2008) Trauma care and trauma systems: past present and future. In: Flint L, Meredith JW et al (eds) Trauma contemporary principles and therapy. Lippincott Williams & Wilkins, Philadelphia, PA, pp 3–38
5. Ehrlich PF et al (2002) American college of surgeons, committee on trauma verification review: does it really make a difference? J Trauma 53(5):811–816

An Emergency Medical Technician (EMT)

Is a member of the health-care team who provides care to patients ranging from basic life support (BLS) to advanced life support (ALS), depending on the level of training. EMT personnel usually practice in the pre-hospital setting, but may also work in emergency departments, intensive care units, clinics, or other locations.

Anaerobic Infections

ALI EL-SOLH
Medical Research, VA Western New York Healthcare System, Buffalo, NY, USA

Synonyms

Abscess; Empyema

Definition

Anaerobic bacteria refer to microorganisms that fail to grow on an agar surface in the presence of 10% CO_2 in air (18% oxygen). Bacteria are classified as microaerophilic if they grow anaerobically or under 10% CO_2 in air. Facultative bacteria can grow in both the presence and absence of air [1].

Epidemiology and Pathogenesis

Non-sporulating anaerobes exist normally in the crevices of the skin, in the nose, mouth, throat, intestine, and vagina. Differences in oxygen tension, pH, and ability of these bacteria to adhere to epithelial surfaces account for the diversity of anaerobic flora within the body. The majority of non-sporulating anaerobic infections stem from indigenous flora. Despite the identification of more than hundreds of anaerobic species, relatively few of them are commonly responsible for human infection. The second source of anaerobic infection originates from the introduction of spores into a normally sterile site. Spore-producing anaerobes live in the soil and water, and are generally more difficult to eradicate. Once they gain access to a human host via an open wound or minor incision, the exosporium triggers spore germination culminating in bacterial replication.

The outcome of an anaerobic infection depends on the balance between the bacterial load, the virulence of the infecting organisms, and the host defense mechanisms. Infection results when an anatomical barrier is disrupted by trauma, surgery, or underlying disease whereby these organisms gain access to the usually sterile body sites. Host conditions that interfere with blood supply or delivery of oxygen lower the oxidation-reduction potential and favor the growth of anaerobic bacteria. Predisposing illnesses like vascular disease, diabetes mellitus, immunosuppression, and splenectomy interfere with phagocytosis and intracellular killing, promoting a suitable milieu for bacterial proliferation. Depending on the characteristics of the anaerobic genus, three virulence factors have been implicated in the pathogenesis of anaerobic infection:

the production of toxins and exoenzymes, the ability to adhere to host tissues, and the nature of the polysaccharide surface constituents. Toxins are responsible for the majority of observed clinical syndromes caused after anaerobic infections, such as paralytic syndromes produced by *Clostridium tetani* and *C. botulinum* neurotoxins; diarrhea induced by *C. difficile* toxins A and B; and enterotoxemia due to *C. perfringes* enterotoxin. These toxins act either on the cell membrane or on specific targets in the cytosol whereby they inhibit enzymatic reactions or block functional receptors.

The exact incidence of anaerobic infections in critically ill patients is unavailable. Difficulties in obtaining adequate cultures free of contamination by aerobic bacteria or normal flora and the lack of reliable transport and culture media have long underestimated the frequency of anaerobic infections in intensive care units. However, these infections are encountered frequently in oral, surgical, and obstetric gynecological specialties.

Treatment
Principles that guide the treatment of anaerobic infections in critically ill patients:

1. Modification of the environment that promotes the proliferation of anaerobic organisms by performing debridement of necrotic tissues, drainage of pus collection, and release of trapped gas in order to improve blood circulation and tissue oxygenation
2. Monitoring the expansion and the spread of the underlying infection into healthy tissues
3. Knowledge of the nature and spectrum of microbial agents specific to the site of the infection
4. Awareness of the susceptibility profile of local pathogens
5. Optimization of the pharmacokinetic and pharmacodynamic properties of antimicrobial agents at the infection site
6. Proven efficacy and acceptable side effects

Anaerobic Infections of the Central Nervous System Infection
Anaerobic bacteria can cause various intracranial infections, including intracranial abscesses, subdural empyema, and meningitis. The main access of anaerobes to the CNS is by contiguous spread from adjacent structures (skull, ear, sinuses). The true incidence of anaerobic meningitis in critically ill patients is unknown because anaerobic cultures of the CNS are rarely performed. The predominant anaerobes are Gram-negative bacilli (including *Bacteroides fragilis* and *Fusobacterium* species).

Anaerobic meningitis is predominantly monomicrobial, but mixed anaerobic–aerobic infection can occur in the presence of ventricular peritoneal shunt or dermal sinus tract infection. Principles of treatment are based on eliminating the associated foci of infection and antimicrobial therapy. Adequate cerebrospinal fluid penetration is critical to sterilization of the meningeal space and satisfactory outcome. Hence, cefoxitin and clindamycin should be not be used if anaerobic bacteria is suspected.

Intracranial abscesses include brain abscess, subdural, and extradural empyema. The most common predisposing factors are congenital cardiac disease, systemic arteriovenous shunts, chronic otitis media, sinusitis, and penetrating trauma. Knowledge of the primary site of infection can be useful in determining the etiology and microbial therapy of the brain abscess. Anaerobic Gram-negative bacilli (*Prevotella, Porphyromonas,* and *Bacteroides*) are commonly recovered in association with ear and sinus infections, while Gram-positive cocci (especially *Peptostreptococci* species) are more prevalent in association with oral or congenital heart disease. Because *Bacteroides fragilis* group and some strains of *Prevotella* species, *Porphyromonas* species, and *Fusobacterium* species are penicillin resistant, empiric therapy should include active agents that can penetrate the blood–brain barrier. These include metronidazole, chloramphenicol, ticarcillin plus clavulanic acid, imipenem, and meropenem. Caution should be used however in administering carbapenems and various beta-lactam antibiotics because high doses of these agents may be associated with seizure activity.

Anaerobic Infections of the Head, Mouth, and Neck

Acute Sinusitis
In critically ill patients, paranasal sinusitis is an important cause of occult fever and can lead to severe complications such as meningitis, pneumonia, and sepsis. In contrast to community-acquired chronic sinusitis where anaerobes account for more than 90% of isolates, organisms implicated in nosocomial sinusitis are frequently those responsible for other hospital acquired infections [2]. In the rare instances where acute sinusitis is associated with dental infections of the upper premolars or molars, anaerobic organisms predominates the microbial spectrum. The most common anaerobes isolated are *Peptostreptococcus* species, *Fusobacterium* species, and pigmented *Prevotella* and *Porphyromonas* species. Most strains of *Prevotella* and *Fusobacterium* were considered susceptible to penicillin. However, penicillin-resistant strains have emerged in

the last two decades. Successful therapy of sinusitis in critically ill patients requires broad spectrum coverage with a β-lactam/β-lactamase inhibitor, second- or third-generation cephalosporins (cefdinir, cefuroxime-axetil, and cefpodoxime proxetil), or respiratory fluoroquinolones that possess anaerobic activity. Macrolides, trimethropim-sulfamethoxazole, and clindamycin are less effective because of growing bacterial resistance and may be considered for patients with antimicrobial allergy. The recommended duration is at least 14 days, although no controlled studies have established the duration of therapy sufficient to control the infection in this setting.

Deep Neck Space Infections

Severe deep neck space infections (DNIs), sometimes resulting in descending mediastinitis, are potential complications of odontogenic infections. Overall, DNIs are significantly less common today than in the pre-antibiotic era but are often underestimated. In pre-antibiotic era, 70% of DNIs arose from tonsillitis or pharyngitis, while nowadays poor dental hygiene and intravenous drug abuse have become the most common nonsurgical causes of DNI in adults, followed by foreign body ingestion and infections of unknown origin. The submandibular space is the most frequently encountered location for both single-space and multi-space odontogenic infections, followed by the buccal and parapharyngeal space. DNIs most frequently are polymicrobial processes with *Streptococcus* and *Staphylococcus* species as well as anaerobes playing the major pathogenic role. *Actinomyces* species account for 3–4% of such cases in nonsurgical patients. Life-threatening forms of DNI infections that are frequently encountered in intensive care setting include Ludwig's angina and Lemierre's syndrome [3].

Ludwig's Angina

Ludwig's angina is a rapidly spreading cellulitis of the floor of the mouth involving the sublingual, submandibular, and submental spaces. It is characterized by a brawny, hard induration of the floor of the oral cavity with tongue elevation and airway compromise. The clinical presentation consists of malaise, dysphagia, bilateral cervical swelling, neck tenderness, dysphonia, elevation and swelling of the tongue, pain in the floor of the mouth, sore throat, restricted neck movement, and stridor suggestive of impending airway obstruction.

The infection has usually an odontogenic cause pointing to a decayed mandibular molar tooth. The roots of these teeth extend inferiorly to the mandibular insertion of the mylohyoid muscle. Abscesses of these molars are believed to erode and perforate into the mandible and then expand into the submandibular space. Once the submandibular space is penetrated, infection of this region ensues. Other less common causes include submandibular sialoadenitis, mandibular fractures, or trauma resulting from intubation or after bronchoscopy.

Ludwig's angina has been reported in patients with history of alcoholism, diabetes mellitus, aplastic anemia, and immunodeficiency disorders, although the majority of those presenting with the disease have no prior comorbid conditions. A mixed flora of aerobic and anaerobic microbes, including streptococcal species, *S. aureus*, *Borrelia vincentii*, *Fusobacterium*, and *Bacteroides* species, is implicated in most cases. *Eikenella corrodens* is becoming a more frequently cultured facultative anaerobic pathogen with significant clinical implication because this organism tends to be resistant to clindamycin.

Management is directed toward securing a patent airway, providing systemic antibiotic therapy, and instituting early surgical decompression of the sublingual, submental, and submandibular spaces. Thirty-five percent will require an airway control in the form of either endotracheal intubation or tracheotomy. Blind nasotracheal intubation is contraindicated, and rapid sequence induction for orotracheal intubation is controversial given the potential difficulties in obtaining adequate laryngoscopic visualization. Cricothyroidotomy is considered the preferred method in the acute period given that low tracheostomy carries the potential risk of spreading the infection to the mediastinum. Administration of an immediate dose of 10–20 mg of dexamethasone followed by 4–6 mg every 6 h for 48 h provides initial chemical decompression by decreasing edema and cellulitis. Antibiotic therapy consists of a combination of β-lactamase–resistant penicillin in combination with metronidazole. For those patients allergic to penicillin, a quinolone can be used instead. If indicated, surgical decompression and drainage are performed with removal of all offending teeth in the first 24–48 h. Mortality ranges from 0% to 8.5% and occurs secondary to pneumonia, sepsis, empyema, and respiratory obstruction.

Lemierre's Syndrome

The syndrome refers to an acute pharyngeal infection with the anaerobe *Fusobacterium necrophorum*, a Gram-negative rod that normally inhabits the oropharynx. The classic presentation of Lemierre's syndrome involves a previously healthy adolescent or young adult who develops anaerobic septicemia 3–5 days after primary oropharyngeal, tonsillar, or peritonsillar infection that initially may not be clinically impressive. The infection usually begins with a sore throat, followed by fever, septicemia, thrombosis, and metastatic abscesses that also can affect the spleen, liver, joints, bones, and soft tissues. Purulent thrombophlebitis of the internal jugular vein can lead to pulmonary and other distant emboli. The responsible bacteria produce a lipopolysaccharide endotoxin with strong biologic activity, as well as a leukocidin and hemolysin, assisting in destruction of white and red blood cells. Hemagglutinin production augments the fulminant nature of the disease, causing platelet aggregation and septic thrombus formation.

Confirmation of Lemierre's syndrome is provided by demonstration of *F. necrophorum* on blood culture. Treatment of Lemierre's syndrome is high-dose parenteral antibiotics directed against anaerobes. Resistance data available for *Fusobacterium* species in general indicate that up to 41% in the United States are beta-lactamase positive. Antibiotic coverage should include agents such as clindamycin, metronidazole, or beta-lactam antibiotic combinations with a beta-lactamase inhibitor, such as ampicillin-sulbactam or ticarcillin-clavulanate, until sensitivity testing can be performed on bacterial isolates (clindamycin, metronidazole, chloramphenicol, imipenem, or cefodizime). Most cases with favorable outcomes have been treated for 6 weeks or longer. Ligation of the infected internal jugular vein is reserved for refractory disease with ongoing emboli or sepsis. Heparin use is controversial but may be considered for refractory cases as well.

Pleuropulmonary Anaerobic Infections

Aspiration of oropharyngeal contents is by far the most important risk factor for the development anaerobic pulmonary infections. Dysphagia caused by esophageal lesions, neurologic impairment as a result of seizures, cerebrovascular accidents, or altered consciousness secondary to sedatives or alcohol intoxication are invariably present on admission. Other conditions that would harbor anaerobic infections include conditions that interfere with clearance of aspirated materials such as foreign bodies and neoplasm.

The incidence of anaerobic pleuropulmonary infections in critically ill patients is not known due to the stringent requirements for recovery of anaerobic organisms. Furthermore, the polymicrobial nature of these infections makes more likely that the pathogenesis of pneumonia is attributed to coexisting aerobic microorganisms. Data about microbiological etiology of severe community-acquired anaerobic lung infection are derived mostly from small case series of patients who were diagnosed with aspiration pneumonia, lung abscesses, and

pleural empyema. The most commonly encountered anaerobes were pigmented *Prevotella* species, nonpigmented *Prevotella* species, *Fusobacterium nucleatum*, *Peptostreptococcus* species, and *Bacteroides melaninogenicus*. Other unusual anaerobes include *B. fragilis*, *Eubacterium* species, *Lactobacillus* species, *Propionibaterium* species, and *Capnocytophaga* species. In two large studies, the average number of anaerobic strains per case reviewed was between 2.4 and 3.2. Twelve percent of specimens had only one anaerobe isolated. The recovery rate ranged from 16% to 100% depending on the diagnostic techniques used.

The role of anaerobic bacteria in the pathogenesis of ventilator associated pneumonia (VAP) remains undetermined. Isolation of anaerobic pathogens requires specific collection techniques, transportation conditions, and culture media which are difficult to achieve during samplings of the lower respiratory tract on high inspiratory fraction of oxygen. Clinical investigations that included the first episode of bacteriologically documented VAP have reported a wide range of anaerobic organisms recovery, ranging from 0% to 23% [4]. The main strains isolated were *Prevotella melaninogenica* (36%), *Fusobacterium nucleatum* (17%), and *Veillonella paravula* (12%). The probability of recovering anaerobic bacteria was increased in orotracheally intubated patients and patients in whom pneumonia occurred during the 5 days after ICU admission.

Anaerobic lung infections in critically ill patients have a variety of clinical presentations depending on underlying risk factors, the type, and the volume of fluid aspirated. No single clinical feature is diagnostic of the underlying disease. Early in the process, focal areas of pneumonitis are observed on chest radiographs which can progress with time to dense segmental infiltration with numerous small cavitations. These may coalesce to form a lung cavity that is undistinguishable from a tuberculosis cavity or a cavitating bronchogenic carcinoma. The cavitation of a lung abscess however is characterized by a thick wall with surrounding infiltrate localized in the gravity-dependent area of the lung. An air-fluid level is typically observed.

The routine use of bronchoscopy in the diagnosis and management of anaerobic lung infection is controversial. Antimicrobials are the main stay of therapy in the early stage of anaerobic pneumonia. In the presence of identifiable risk factors and a compatible diagnostic chest radiograph showing disease in the dependent regions of the lung, a diagnostic procedure may not be required. A similar approach may be applicable for suspected anaerobic lung abscess if the diagnosis is supported by clinical and radiologic presentation, and the patient is showing signs of clinical improvement. However, diagnostic bronchoscopy may be indicated to rule out the presence of tuberculosis or atypical pathogens responsible for cavitary lung lesions. *Legionella micdadei, Mycobacterium fortuitum, Streptococcus mitis*, and *Eikenella corrodens* have all been reported as the causative agents of lung abscess. In immunocompromised patients, the list of pathogens may include *Corynebacterium equi, Rhodococcus equi, Pneumocystis jiroveci*, and *Salmonella* species. Bronchoscopy is also advocated for patients with delayed resolution and those who fail to respond to antimicrobial therapy. A history of limited sputum expectoration in patient with suspected anaerobic lung abscess may warrant a bronchoscopy due to the possibility of endobronchial lesion. Findings suggestive of neoplasm include also lack of a risk factor for anaerobic infection, lack of constitutional symptoms, a white blood count less than 11×10^9/L, and absence of an infiltrate surrounding the abscess. Careful consideration should be given for a large abscess cavity (>6–8 cm in diameter) prior to performing a bronchoscopy because of the potential evacuation of the abscess contents into the bronchial tree.

A dreadful sequelae of anaerobic lung infections is the formation of bronchopulmonary fistula complicated with an empyema. At times, it may be difficult to differentiate between cavitary lung abscess and empyema on plain radiograph due to close proximity of the parenchymal lesion to the pleural space. A computed tomographic (CT) scan of the chest can be helpful in making this distinction. A lung abscess has the characteristics of an irregular wall width, a blurred outer margin, an oval or round shape with minimal distortion to the adjacent lung. In contrast, an empyema appears more to have a uniform wall width, a lenticular shape, and an obtuse chest-wall angle. The adjacent pulmonary parenchyma is usually compressed.

The type of approach to a patient who may have an anaerobic lung infection depends on the extent of disease on presentation. As with most bacterial infections, proper identification and treatment of underlying causative agents is paramount for a satisfactory outcome. Antibiotic resistance among anaerobic bacteria has been on the rise. Penicillins used to be the standard treatment for anaerobic pleuropulmonary infections. In the 1980s, two therapeutic trials showed superiority of clindamycin to penicillins in reducing the failure rates and shortening the time for elimination of putrid sputum. Clindamycin appears also to enhance phagocyte killing. Hence, the most recent guidelines for the management of pneumonia with suspected anaerobic bacteria recommend clindamycin as the first line agent. More recent studies show that β-lactam/β-lactamase inhibitor combinations are also effective. The use of metronidazole as monotherapy with anaerobic lung infection is discouraged in view of the high therapeutic failure (43%) that has been linked to metronidazole-resistant microaerophilic and aerobic streptococci. If metronidazole is to be used, it is advisable to combine it with another drug such as penicillin. Erythromycin and other macrolides such as azithromycin and clarithromycin have good activity against anaerobes but have relatively poor activity against *Fusobacterium*. Other drugs such as cefoxitin, imipenem, meropenem, tigecycline, and moxifloxacin have adequate anaerobic coverage, but their use in treating anaerobic lung infections has not been examined in large randomized trials.

Clinicians should be aware of infections caused by *Eikenella corrodens*, a slow-growing, nonmotile, facultative anaerobic, Gram-negative bacillus which is commensal of the oral cavity, intestinal, and genital tracts. The most common clinical sources of this organism are human bite wounds, head and neck infections, and respiratory tract infections. The organism is uniformly resistant to clindamycin and metronidazole. When suspected, the addition of β-lactam/β-lactamase inhibitor, penicillin, or a quinolone should be entertained.

The duration of therapy in critically ill patients with anaerobic lung infection must be tailored to the clinical presentation and microbiological infection. Antibiotic therapy is usually recommended for 7–10 days for uncomplicated cases, whereas 4–8 weeks may be required for complex cases involving necrotizing pneumonia, lung abscesses, or empyema. Longer therapy has been advocated until the pulmonary infiltrate has cleared or there is only a small stable residual lesion.

Intra-abdominal and Pelvic Anaerobic Infections

In critically ill patients, intra-abdominal and pelvic anaerobic infections run the gamut from minor problems that respond to systemic antibiotics to life-threatening catastrophes. Intraperitoneal, retroperitoneal, and visceral anaerobic infections occur generally as complication of appendicitis, cholecystitis, diverticulitis, pelvic inflammatory disease, tubo-ovarian infection, surgery, or trauma. The polymicrobial nature of abdominal and pelvic abscesses is apparent in the majority of patients, where the number of isolates in an infectious site varies between two and six. The average number of isolates is five in intra-abdominal infection (3.0 anaerobes and 2.0 aerobes) per specimen and four in pelvic infections (2.8 anaerobes and 1.2 aerobes) per specimen.

The microbiology of intra-abdominal abscesses that develop following perforation of viscera is made up of the gastrointestinal flora at the level of the perforation. The predominant anaerobic bacteria are *B. fragilis*, *Peptostreptococcus* species, and *Clostridium* species, whereas the most commonly isolated aerobic and facultative bacteria are Enterobacteriaceae and Group D *Enterococcus* species. A similar pattern also exists in the microbiology of pelvic, vulvo-vaginal, and prostatic abscesses, which originate from the rectal and cervical flora. The predominant anaerobic bacteria are *P. bivia*, *P. disiens*, and *Peptostreptococcus*, whereas the common aerobic and facultative bacteria include Enterobacteriaceae, *N. gonorrhoeae*, and Group B streptococci. In cases of septic abortion and uterine gas gangrene, *Clostridium* species should be included also in the list of microbial etiology.

Early diagnosis of intra-abdominal or pelvic infection is paramount in preventing progression from bacterial contamination to abscess formation. The treatment of these infections is based on source control which focuses on three principles: drainage, debridement, and restoration of anatomy and function. No single- or multiple-antimicrobial regimen has been consistently shown to be superior or inferior for community-acquired intra-abdominal infection. Metronidazole, clindamycin, a carbapenem (i.e., imipenem), cefoxitin, or β-lactam/β-lactamase inhibitor are the drugs of choice. Metronidazole is also a very potent amoebicide. An aminoglycoside, a quinolone (in adults), or a third-generation cephalosporin should be added if Gram-negative enteric bacteria are present. Because susceptibility profiles for *Bacteroides fragilis* isolates often show significant resistance to clindamycin, cefotetan, cefoxitin, and quinolones, these drugs should not be used alone empirically in contexts in which these organisms are likely to be encountered. Antimicrobial agents, especially when used without surgical drainage, should be given for at least 6–8 weeks. A shorter course, of 4–6 weeks, may be used when good surgical drainage has been achieved.

Skin and Soft Tissue Infections

Anaerobic infections of the skin and soft tissue develop in areas contaminated by the indigenous flora following penetrating foreign body, trauma, ischemia, or surgery. Necrotizing fasciitis and anaerobic gangrenous cellulitis dominate the majority of cases seen in intensive care units. These infections are usually polymicrobial in nature. A mean of 4.8 bacterial species are isolated with a roughly 3:2 ratio of anaerobes to aerobes. The predominant anaerobes are *Clostridium* species, *Peptostreptococcus* species, *Prevotella* species, *B. fragilis* group, and *Porphyroonas*

species. Early symptoms resemble those of cellulitis, but progressive skin changes such as skin ulceration, bullae formation, necrotic eschars, and fluid draining from the site can occur rapidly as the infection progresses. Sepsis and organ failure can develop before the skin changes are recognized. Although X-rays show occasionally gas in tissues, CT or MRI studies are needed to delineate the extent of the infection. Surgical exploration, extensive incisions, and deep probing beyond the involved areas of necrosis are often necessary to determine the extent of muscle involvement. Frequent surgical debridement and drainage of fluid collection may be necessary till granulation tissue is established. Antimicrobial therapy for mixed aerobic and anaerobic bacteria is indicated when polymicrobial infection is suspected. Cefoxitin, tigecycline, carabapenems, beta-lactam/beta-lactamase inhibitors, clindamycin, or metronidazole alone or in combination are all effective agents against anaerobic skin and soft tissue infections. When used in conjunction with surgery and antibiotics, hyperbaric oxygen therapy enhances wound healing and may reduce morbidity by reducing the rate of amputation.

Anaerobic Bacteremia

Anaerobic bacteremia has been gradually decreasing over the past few years because of empirical treatment with antibiotics and surgical prophylaxis against anaerobes. Anaerobic bacteremia that is considered to be clinically significant accounts for <4% of anaerobic blood cultures. The gastrointestinal tract accounts for half of anaerobic bacteremias followed by the female genital tract (20%) and soft tissue infections (8%). Intestinal obstruction, diabetes mellitus, undrained abscess, recent gastrintestinal and obstetric gynecologic surgery, use of cytotoxic or steroids, and malignant neoplasms are among the recognized risk factors [5]. Dental and oral surgery can also predispose to anaerobic bacteremia particularly in the setting of subacute endocarditis.

Anaerobic Gram-negative bacilli represent about 75% of anaerobic bacteremia, mostly of the *Bacteroides* group. Many of these cases are polymicrobial in nature and originate predominantly from infections below the diaphragm. *Bacteriodes fragilis* is the most common blood isolate recovered from these patients. Anaerobic bacteremia due to non-sporulating, Gram-positive bacilli include members of the genera *Actinomyces*, *Bifidobacterium*, *Eggerthella*, *Eubacterium*, *Lactobacillus*, and *Propionibacterium*. Almost all patients with these clinically significant bacteremias have underlying diseases, with gastrointestinal tract disease and malignancy being the most common. Other species responsible for anaerobic bacteremia include *Peptostreptococcus* species, *Clostridium* species, and *Fusobacterium* species.

The mortality associated with an anaerobic bloodstream infection is high. *Bacteroides* bacteremia has been associated with a mortality rate of up to 50% depending on the species recovered (*B. thetaiotaomicron* > *B. distasonis* > *B. fragilis*). Lower death rates have been documented in patients who have undergone surgical interventions.

References

1. Kasper DL (1991) Infections due to mixed anaerobic organisms. In: Wilson JD, Braunwald E, Isselbacher KJ, Petersdorf RG, Martin JB, Fauci AS, Root RK (eds) Harrison's principles of internal medicine, 12th edn. McGraw-Hill, New York, pp 584–590
2. Brook I (2008) Anaerobic infections: diagnosis and management. Informa Healthcare, New York
3. Ramadan H, El Solh A (2004) Update on otolaryngology in critical care. Am J Respir Crit Care Med 169:1273–1277
4. Chastre J, Fagon JY (2002) Ventilator-associated pneumonia. Am J Respir Crit Care Med 165:867–903
5. Salonen J, Eerola E, Meurman O (1998) Clinical significance and outcome of anaerobic bacteremia. Clin Infect Dis 26:1413–1417

Analgesia

▶ Pain Management

Anaphylactic Shock

BRIAN H. ROWE
Department of Emergency Medicine, University of Alberta, Edmonton, AB, Canada

Synonyms

Allergic shock; Anaphylaxis

Definition

Anaphylaxis is a medical emergency that requires immediate diagnosis and treatment in order to avoid life-threatening consequences. Definitions of anaphylaxis have conflicted over the years; however, recent clarity has emerged based on consensus symposia. In simple terms, "*anaphylaxis* is a serious allergic reaction that is rapid in onset and may cause death" [1]. More detailed revisions of the definition [1] for health professionals using clinical criteria suggest that anaphylaxis is highly likely when any one of the following three criteria occurs:

1. Acute onset of an illness (minutes to several hours) with involvement of the skin and/or mucosal tissue (e.g., hives/urticaria, pruritus, flushing, swollen lips, tongue, or uvula) associated with *at least one* of the following:
   (a) Respiratory compromise (e.g., dyspnea, wheeze, and/or stridor)
   (b) Reduced blood pressure
   (c) Associated symptoms of organ dysfunction (e.g., hypotonia, syncope, and incontinence)
2. Two or more of the following that occur rapidly after exposure to a likely allergen for that patient (minutes to several hours):
   (a) Involvement of the skin and/or mucosal tissue
   (b) Respiratory compromise
   (c) Reduced blood pressure or associated symptoms
   (d) Persistent gastrointestinal symptoms (e.g., cramps, vomiting)
3. Anaphylaxis should be suspected when patients are exposed to a known allergen and develop hypotension.

Most patients with anaphylaxis demonstrate "hypersensitivity," which implies an inappropriate immune response to generally harmless antigens; anaphylactic shock represent the most dramatic and severe form of immediate hypersensitivity. Anaphylaxis occurs as part of a clinical continuum. It is critical to remember that it can begin with relatively minor symptoms and rapidly progress to a life-threatening respiratory and cardiovascular reaction.

The causes of anaphylaxis are many and varied. Foods (especially nuts and shellfish), medications (especially antibiotics), insect stings, and allergen immunotherapy injections are the most common provoking factors for anaphylaxis; however, any agent capable of producing a sudden degranulation of mast cells or basophils can induce anaphylaxis. For the most part, anaphylaxis arises from the activation of mast cells and basophils through a mechanism involving cross-linking of IgE and aggregation of the high-affinity receptors for IgE. Upon activation, mast cells and/or basophils quickly release preformed mediators from secretory granules, including histamine, which sets up further inflammation cascade effects.

The majority of anaphylaxis patients arrive to an emergency department setting, and those with anaphylaxis often present via ambulance. How common is anaphylaxis in the allergic population? Research suggests that physicians under-diagnose anaphylaxis, which leads to significant under-estimation of the prevalence of anaphylaxis. For example, in one study of ED visits for food allergies, 51% were defined by the authors as meeting criteria for anaphylaxis. The same authors examined ED presentations of insect allergies and found 31% met the criteria for anaphylaxis. It is likely that many cases of anaphylaxis are both under-recognized and under-treated; however, anaphylactic shock is likely not misdiagnosed because of its severity at presentation.

Given the mechanisms described above, it is not surprising that severe acute asthma and anaphylaxis can coexist. Since there is considerable overlap between these two syndromes their treatment also overlaps and it is important to recognize this. This article will focus on the pathophysiology, clinical features and management of anaphylaxis, and anaphylactic shock.

Treatment

Clinical Presentation: Anaphylaxis is the most severe life-threatening form of a systemic allergic reaction, often involving respiratory or cardiovascular compromise. The initial clinical signs of systemic allergic reactions include diffuse urticaria and angioedema. These major symptoms are in most cases accompanied by any of the following: abdominal pain or cramping, nausea, vomiting, diarrhea, bronchospasm, rhinorrhea, conjunctivitis, dysrhythmias, and/or hypotension. The clinician should be aware that even mild, localized urticaria can progress to full anaphylaxis, and even to death.

The "classic" presentation of anaphylaxis begins with pruritis, cutaneous flushing, and urticaria. These symptoms are followed by a sense of fullness in the throat, anxiety, a sensation of chest tightness, shortness of breath, and lightheadedness. As the cascade progresses, decreased level of consciousness, respiratory distress, and circulatory collapse may ensue. In its severest form, loss of consciousness and cardiorespiratory arrest may result. A complaint of a "lump in the throat" and hoarseness heralds life-threatening laryngeal edema in a patient with symptoms of anaphylaxis.

The diagnosis of anaphylaxis and anaphylactic shock are made clinically. There are no particular drug tests that will aid the clinician in this diagnosis. Some have advocated the use of tryptase measures; however, this test is largely unavailable or the results arrive after the patient's condition has improved. In general, for patients with severe reactions and in those with underlying cardiovascular disease, cardiac monitoring is important,

particularly when adrenergic agonists are used in treatment. Monitoring using pulse oximetry is also useful.

Priority Treatment: Anaphylaxis, as defined by airway compromise or hypotension, is obviously a true medical emergency and must be rapidly assessed and treated. With *suspected* anaphylaxis, the single most important step in treatment is the rapid administration of epinephrine. Moreover, with this rapid administration, many of the secondary measures discussed below may not be necessary.

Airway: Patients should be given sufficient oxygen to maintain arterial oxygen saturation greater than 90%. Securing the airway is always the first priority. The airway should be examined for signs and symptoms of angioedema (e.g., uvula edema or "hydrops," audible stridor, respiratory distress, hypoxia). If angioedema is producing respiratory distress, intubation should be considered an early intervention, since delay may result in complete airway obstruction secondary to progression of angioedema.

Most patients with anaphylaxis will not require intubation or assisted ventilation, especially if severe cases are recognized early and managed aggressively. In the event of airway compromise, the use of high flow oxygen, or even noninvasive ventilation would be considered risky practice. The key intervention is airway control through intubation and the safest approach possible is required. Intubation should ideally be performed by someone with knowledge of airway techniques and the potential complications associated with intubation and positive pressure mechanical ventilation.

A variety of approaches to securing the airway are available; however, an approach including a rapid sequence intubation (RSI) protocol is recommended. For example, a common approach in patients with airway disease is proposed by the Canadian Thoracic Society and seems reasonable: intravenous induction with ketamine (1.5 mg/kg) or propofol (2–2.5 mg/kg) followed by paralysis with intravenous succinylcholine (1.5 mg/kg) or rocuronium (0.6–1.2 mg/kg). Other therapeutic options are available, and clinicians should become comfortable with one and use it in this situation.

Adrenaline/Epinephrine: Epinephrine is a mixed alpha (α_1) and beta (β_2) receptor agent; the α_1 receptor activation reduces mucosal edema, membrane leakage, and treats hypotension while the β_2 receptor activation provides bronchodilation and controls mediator release [2]. Epinephrine is the drug of choice and the first drug that should be administered in acute anaphylaxis; however, evidence suggests that it is underused. Studies suggest that the use of epinephrine is lower than second line therapies such as corticosteroids and antihistamines in treatment of all allergic reactions including anaphylaxis [3]. Moreover, the 12-year trend in the USA shows a statistically significant decline in epinephrine use and use in only 50% of the cases defined as anaphylaxis [3]. Finally, epinephrine is often dosed suboptimally to treat anaphylaxis, and is under-prescribed for potential future self-administration. Experts believe that most of the reasons proposed to withhold its clinical use are flawed, and that the therapeutic benefits of epinephrine exceed the risk when given in appropriate (e.g., intramuscular) doses. These results are concerning and suggest that clinicians who treat anaphylaxis and anaphylactic shock need to be aggressive with this agent.

For less severe symptoms, intramuscular epinephrine can be administered [2]. The dose is epinephrine 0.3–0.5 mg (0.3–0.5 mL of the 1:1,000 dilution) repeated every 5–10 min according to response or relapse. Intramuscular dosing provides higher, more consistent, and more rapid peak blood epinephrine levels than subcutaneous administration, and should now be the treatment of choice for adults and children [4]. Moreover, injections into the thigh are more effective at achieving peak blood levels than are injections into the deltoid area. If the patient is refractory to treatment despite repeated intramuscular epinephrine, then an epinephrine infusion should be instituted. Caution is warranted in patients taking β-blockers, because epinephrine use may result in severe hypertension secondary to unopposed β-adrenergic stimulation.

Volume Expansion: When hypotension or shock are present, it is generally thought to be the result of distributive shock and responds to fluid resuscitation. Patients should receive a saline bolus of 1–2 L (10–20 ml/kg repeated as needed) concurrently with the epinephrine treatment. There is currently insufficient evidence to suggest that albumen or hypertonic saline should replace saline as the crystalloid of choice.

Vasopressor Agents: In patients with signs of cardiovascular compromise or collapse, epinephrine may be delivered intravenously. Initially, epinephrine 100 µg (0.1 mg) IV should be given as a 1:100,000 dilution. If the patient is refractory to the initial bolus, then an epinephrine infusion can be started, by placing epinephrine 1 mg (1.0 mL of the 1:1,000 dilution) in 500 mL of saline and administering at a rate of 1–4 µg/min (0.5–2 mL/min), titrating to effect.

While some clinicians may be hesitant to give intravenous epinephrine because of its side effects (e.g., tachycardia, arrhythmia, tremor), it should be stressed that the initial adult dose is very dilute, is given over 5–10 min, and can be stopped immediately if arrhythmias or chest pain occur. If epinephrine is ineffective, other vasopressor agents with alpha-adrenergic activity (e.g., norepinephrine or dopamine) may be reasonable alternatives.

Adjunctive Treatment: In addition to the priority treatments described above, there are other treatments that may benefit patents with anaphylaxis and anaphylactic shock. It is important to note that given the life-threatening nature of this condition, the evidence for many of these treatments is based on consensus and expert opinion.

Corticosteroids: All patients with anaphylaxis should receive systemic corticosteroids. These agents depress the immune and inflammatory response and are responsible for a myriad of effects that may be beneficial in anaphylaxis including influencing protein metabolism, membrane stabilization, and inhibiting the release of further immune and inflammatory mediators. Intravenous methyl-prednisolone (80–125 mg) or hydrocortisone (250–500 mg) are equally appropriate. Methyl-prednisolone produces less fluid retention than hydrocortisone and is preferred for elderly patients and for those patients in whom fluid retention would be problematic (e.g., renal and cardiac impairment). Increasing use of corticosteroids has been observed in US emergency departments [3]. Finally, the use of very high dose systemic corticosteroids is likely unnecessary as available evidence suggests limited additional benefits with this approach.

Antihistamines: All patients with anaphylaxis should receive intravenous histamine-1 (H_1) blockers, such as diphenhydramine (25–50 mg); however, evidence suggests this is not always the case [3]. Because the histamine-2 (H_2) blockers are effective in shock refractory to epinephrine, fluids, steroids, and H_1 blockers, it is recommended that H_2 antihistamines be considered as well in the intensive care setting [5].

If considered, H_2 blockers such as ranitidine and cimetidine may be used in anaphylaxis. Cimetidine should not be used for patients who are elderly (side effects), with multiple comorbidities (interference with metabolism of many drugs), have renal or hepatic impairment, or whose anaphylaxis is complicated by β-blocker use (prolongs metabolism of β-blockers and may prolong anaphylactic state). After the initial intravenous dose of steroids and antihistamines, the patient may be switched to oral medication.

Antiasthmatic/Bronchospasm Therapy: If bronchospasm is present, either as an exacerbation of asthma or de novo bronchospasm related to histamine release, a selective bronchodilator, such as intermittent or continuous nebulized albuterol/salbutamol, should be instituted. For severe bronchospasm refractory to the above-mentioned treatments, other treatments such as anticholinergics and magnesium sulfate can be added. Anticholinergic agents should be added to nebulized albuterol (ipratropium bromide 250–500 µg/dose) in severe acute bronchospasm every 20 min for an hour and every 4 h afterwards. Magnesium sulfate improves pulmonary functions and reduces admissions when administered in severe acute asthma. It is inexpensive and free of major side effects when used in single doses of magnesium sulfate 2 g intravenously over 20–30 min in adults. Bronchodilator and stimulant agents should be used with caution (lower dose and slower rate) in elderly patients.

Intravenous aminophylline and β-agonists have no role to play in the early management of acute bronchospasm because their benefits are marginal, as compared to other agents, and their side-effect profiles are impressive. There are no data yet on the role of leukotriene receptor antagonists in the treatment of anaphylaxis.

Glucagon: Concurrent use of β-blockers by the patient is a risk factor for severe prolonged anaphylaxis. For patients taking β-blockers with hypotension refractory to fluids and epinephrine, intravenous glucagon should be used in a dose of 1 mg every 5 min until hypotension resolves, followed by an infusion of 5–15 µg/min.

Evaluation/Assessment

Effectiveness: In the vast majority of patients, signs and symptoms begin suddenly, often within 60 min of allergen exposure. In general, the faster the onset of symptoms, the more severe the reaction, as evidenced by the fact that one-half of anaphylactic fatalities occur within the first hour. After the initial signs and symptoms have abated, patients are at risk for a recurrence of symptoms. The exact incidence of this biphasic phenomenon is unclear, although it has been reported in 3–20% of patients.

Most patients with anaphylaxis do not need more than a single dose of epinephrine, and response is relatively immediate. Additional treatments including corticosteroids, fluids and antihistamines are often also provided; however, other agents are not needed in all cases of anaphylaxis [3]. It is unusual not to observe a response to this therapeutic approach. Overall, approximately 4% of allergic presentations require hospitalization and death from anaphylaxis early in the course or in the prehospital setting.

Complications of Treatment: In general, anaphylactic shock is reversible and patients make excellent recoveries. The complications associated with anaphylactic shock can be divided into those arising from airway interventions, those related to monitoring, those from the associated bronchospasm or asthma, and those related to underlying cardiac disease.

Airway complications generally arise from the process of intubation. The local airway complications can be as minor as post-extubation hoarseness and sore throat. The more severe airway complications include failure to secure the airway resulting in the need for a cricothyroidotomy. Overall, these complications can be mitigated by early consideration of airway control through intubation, use of the highest level of expertise, and the use of RSI techniques.

Well-known issues relating to monitoring of patients in an intensive care setting with central venous access include pneumothorax, bleeding, nerve injury, arterial puncture, arrhythmia, and infection. Morbidity and mortality statistics are dependent on the expertise of the individual performing the procedure and are likely decreasing with the increasing use of bedside ultrasound.

There are many reports of serious pulmonary complications when asthma and bronchospasm occur with anaphylaxis. Once intubated, barotrauma can occur and pneumothorax can result. The operator may influence the severity of these complications by adjusting the volume, rate, and end-tidal pressures during ventilation; however, careful monitoring should mitigate these problems.

Some of the mediators released in anaphylactic shock have a direct effect on myocardial tissue. In patients with preexisting heart disease, hypotension and hypoxia may be partially due to ischemic myocardial dysfunction. Since epinephrine is still required for most patients, clinicians need to be aware of this potential toxicity in adults and those with known cardiac disease. If pulmonary congestion occurs, clinicians must monitor fluid resuscitation carefully.

Economics: The "cost" of anaphylaxis and anaphylactic shock is difficult to determine, since there are few reports in the literature. The majority of the treatments for anaphylaxis are inexpensive and most patients are discharged, so the costs are generally low; however, when cases are severe and the airway is compromised, the incremental hospital cost of care for these patients is high. The societal costs of anaphylaxis are also unknown; however, the lost years of productive life resulting from the death of a young person from anaphylactic shock and cardiorespiratory collapse is large. With the increasing presence of allergies in the developed world, it is likely that the societal burden of anaphylaxis will increase. Furthermore, these costs do not take into account the post-anaphylaxis care of patients following referrals for allergy testing, consultations, immunotherapy, and future ED and physician visits. Finally, the costs to patients and families of patients with anaphylaxis are unclear.

After-care

All unstable patients with anaphylaxis refractory to treatment or where airway interventions were required should be admitted to the intensive care unit. Patients who receive epinephrine should be observed; however, the timing of observation is based on experience rather than clear evidence. Observation for at least several hours after the end of treatment appears routine. If patients remain symptom free after appropriate treatment following 4 h of observation, the patient can be safely discharged home. Estimates on the occurrence of late recurrence reactions vary, yet they are thought to be rare; however, prolonged observation periods should be considered in patients with a past history of severe reaction and those using β-blockers. Other factors to consider in discharge planning include distance from medical care, whether the patient lives alone, significant comorbidity (including but not limited to asthma), and age.

A prescription and clear instructions on the use of an epinephrine autoinjector (usually one each for home, work, and vehicle) should be provided to patients with anaphylaxis when the risk of another reaction is judged to be substantial. Patients who have suffered an anaphylaxis episode should also be discharged with a prescription for a short course of systemic corticosteroids and antihistamines. Finally, to prevent future events, patients discharged with anaphylaxis and anaphylactic shock should leave with a referral to an allergist (where possible), an appointment for allergy testing, educational information (including encouragement to wear personal identification of this condition), and appropriate follow-up.

Prognosis

The short-term prognosis of patients with anaphylactic shock and anaphylaxis is usually very good; complete recovery is expected. Short-term prognosis is largely dependent on the underlying cause, the early use epinephrine, the timing of advanced interventions, and patient comorbidities. For most patients, response to therapy is lifesaving and rapid; the majority of patients are discharged without any sequelae. The long-term prognosis for patients with anaphylactic shock and anaphylaxis varies, since reexposure without adequate preventive strategies in place may lead to a catastrophic outcome. Long-term prognosis is largely dependent on identifying and avoiding the underlying trigger(s), the availability of an epinephrine autoinjector at future events, and patient education on avoidance and early treatment.

References

1. Sampson HA, Munoz-Furlong A, Bock SA, Schmitt C, Bass R, Chowdhury BA, Decker WW, Furlong TJ, Galli SJ, Golden DB, Gruchalla RS, Harlor AD Jr, Hepner DL, Howarth M, Kaplan AP, Levy JH, Lewis LM, Lieberman PL, Metcalfe DD, Murphy R, Pollart SM, Pumphrey RS, Rosenwasser LJ, Simons FE, Wood JP, Camargo CA Jr (2005) Symposium on the definition and management of anaphylaxis: summary report. J Allergy Clin Immunol 115(3):584–591
2. Simons FE (2008) Emergency treatment of anaphylaxis. Brit Med J 336(7654):1141–1142
3. Gaeta TJ, Clark S, Pelletier AJ, Camargo CA (2007) National study of US emergency department visits for acute allergic reactions, 1993 to 2004. Ann Allergy Asthma Immunol 98(4):360–365
4. Simons FE, Gu X, Simons KJ (2001) Epinephrine absorption in adults: intramuscular versus subcutaneous injection. J Allergy Clin Immunol 108(5):871–873
5. Winbery SL, Lieberman PL (2002) Histamine and antihistamines in anaphylaxis. Clin Allergy Immunol 17:287–317

Anaphylaxis

Anaphylaxis is an acute multisystem life-threatening Type I of hypersensitivity reaction.

▶ Anaphylactic Shock

Anatomic Resection

▶ Hepatic Lobectomy

Anemia Management

HOWARD L. CORWIN
Departments of Medicine and Anesthesiology, Dartmouth–Hitchcock Medical Center, Lebanon, NH, USA

Anemia is common in critically ill patients. On ICU admission, two-thirds patients have a hemoglobin concentration less than 12 g/dL and by ICU day 3 almost 95% of patients still in the ICU are anemic. The anemia observed in these critically ill patients persists throughout the duration of their ICU and hospital stay. As a consequence of the anemia, critically ill patients receive a large number of RBC transfusions. Observational studies conducted in Europe and the USA have noted that RBC transfusions were administered to approximately 40–45% of all critically ill patients admitted to the ICU and to over 50% of trauma patients. On average, critically ill patients receive almost 5 units of RBCs during their ICU stay. This has remained constant over the past 2 decades despite the intense scrutiny of transfusion practice in general and transfusion practice in the ICU in particular. Over 80% of patients are still anemic at the time of ICU discharge and 10–15% of these patients are transfused post ICU discharge. Anemia of the critically ill persists long after ICU discharge and may persist longer than 6 months in over 50% of patients [1].

Etiology of Anemia

Active bleeding, while important, is only responsible for a small portion of the anemia observed in critical illness. Only about 25% of RBC transfusions are given in the ICU for active bleeding. On the other hand, phlebotomy is a major factor contributing to anemia and the need for blood transfusions in the critically ill patient. In the past, ICU patients have been reported to be phlebotomized as much as 65 ml per day, while more recently, phlebotomy losses of 40 ml per day were still noted in ICU patients. However, it is now becoming clear that the view of anemia in the critically ill as simply the result of excessive phlebotomy by "Medical Vampires" is not completely accurate. Red blood cell production in critically ill patients is not normal and decreased RBC production is also important in the development and maintenance of the anemia observed in the critically ill [1].

Over 90% of ICU patients have low serum iron (Fe), total iron binding capacity (TIBC), and Fe/TIBC ratio, but have a normal or, more usually, an elevated serum ferritin level. On the other hand, nutritional deficiencies are uncommon. At the same time, serum erythropoietin levels are only mildly elevated, with little evidence of reticulocyte response to endogenous erythropoietin. Erythropoietin levels in the critically ill are mildly elevated when compared to adults without anemia; however, erythropoietin levels are significantly lower when compared to patients with iron-deficiency anemia, despite similar hematocrits. The blunted erythropoietin response observed in the critically ill appears to result from inhibition of the erythropoietin gene

by inflammatory mediators. These same inflammatory cytokines directly inhibit RBC production by the bone marrow and may produce the distinct abnormalities of iron metabolism. An inappropriately low erythropoietin response to anemia persists for as long as 6 months following ICU discharge. Patients who are slow to recover from their anemia tend to have evidence of ongoing inflammation. In summary, anemia of critical illness therefore is a distinct clinical entity characterized by blunted erythropoietin production and abnormalities in iron metabolism similar to what is commonly referred to as the anemia of chronic disease [2].

Consequences of Anemia

As a consequence of anemia O_2-carrying capacity is decreased; however, tissue oxygenation is preserved at hemoglobin levels well below 10.0 g/dL. Following the development of anemia, adaptive changes include a shift in the oxyhemoglobin dissociation curve as well as hemodynamic and microcirculatory alterations. As a consequence more O_2 can be released to the tissues at a given pO_2; offsetting the effect of reduced O_2-carrying capacity of the blood. At the same time, O_2 delivery to vital organs is preserved through increased cardiac output and central and regional reflexes redistribute organ blood flow [1, 3].

There is good evidence that low levels of hemoglobin can be tolerated in healthy subjects. Hematocrits of 10–20% have been shown to be well tolerated in animal and human studies. These studies as well as data from the Jehovah's Witness population clearly demonstrate that hemoglobin concentrations falling significantly below the "10/30" threshold can be tolerated by individuals who are not critically ill. Whether this is also applicable to critically ill patients is less clear. While the presence and degree of anemia has been observed to be associated with worse clinical outcomes in almost all critically ill populations which have been studied; the precise role, if any, that anemia plays in the observed increase in morbidity and mortality is unknown. However, these observations in large part have driven the efforts to prevent and/or correct anemia in the critically ill [1, 3].

Management of Anemia

Reduction of blood loss. The approach to acute blood loss is directed toward control of the bleeding source, correction of coagulation abnormalities, and antithrombolytic agents. However, more important for the majority of critically ill patients is phlebotomy blood loss. It has been repeatedly demonstrated that reducing phlebotomy blood loss is associated with less RBC transfusion. Several techniques have been employed to achieve the goal of phlebotomy reduction including minimizing discard blood loss (e.g., closed sampling techniques) and use of small volume blood sample tubes. As important, although less well studied, is the reduction of unnecessary laboratory studies, e.g., elimination of standing blood draw orders.

Red blood cell transfusion. Red blood cell transfusions are commonly utilized in patients with anemia in an attempt to increase oxygen delivery to the tissues and in turn improve tissue oxygenation. The rationale for this therapeutic approach is that an increase in hemoglobin will increase the oxygen-carrying capacity of blood and thus provide more oxygen delivery to delivery-dependent tissue. Historically, RBC transfusions have been viewed as a safe and effective means of improving oxygen delivery to tissues. However, over the last 25 years transfusion practice has come under intense scrutiny. Initially, concerns related to the risks of transfusion-related infection drove the process. Today advances in transfusion medicine have greatly decreased the risk of viral transmission during RBC transfusion; however, other newly identified risks of RBC transfusion (i.e., immunomodulation, age of blood, TRALI) now drive the examination of RBC transfusion practice. The new appreciation of RBC transfusion risks has in led to a more critical examination of RBC transfusion benefits. In view of the prevalence of anemia and the resulting large number of RBC transfusions, these issues are particularly important in the critically ill patient population [3].

The best evidence available regarding the efficacy of RBC transfusion in critically ill patients comes from a randomized controlled trial conducted by the Canadian Critical Care Trials Group (TRICC Trial) [4]. In this study, a liberal transfusion strategy (hemoglobin 10.0–12.0 g/dL, with a transfusion trigger of 10.0 g/dL) was compared to a restrictive transfusion strategy (hemoglobin 7.0–9.0 g/dL, with a transfusion trigger of 7.0 g/dL) in a general medical and surgical critical care population. The TRICC Trial documented an overall nonsignificant trend toward decreased 30-day mortality in the restrictive group, however there was a significant decrease in mortality in the restrictive group among patients who were less acutely ill (APACHE II scores less than 20) and among patients who were less than 55 years of age. The TRICC Trial, in combination with observational studies of critically ill patients demonstrating worse clinical outcomes associated with RBC transfusion, have raised questions regarding the validity of the historic assumption that RBC transfusions are beneficial for critically ill patients with anemia. To date, there are no convincing data to support the routine use of RBC transfusion to treat anemia in hemodynamically stable critically ill patients

without evidence of acute bleeding. In fact, the data available suggests that RBC transfusions are associated with worse clinical outcomes [5].

In the absence of acute bleeding, hemoglobin levels of 7.0–9.0 g/dL are well tolerated by most critically ill patients and that a transfusion threshold of 7.0 g/dL is appropriate. There is still controversy as to the appropriate transfusion threshold for critically ill patients with acute ischemic cardiac disease. A transfusion trigger of between 8.0 g/L and 10.0 g/dL would seem reasonable for patients with acute coronary syndromes until further evidence becomes available [3].

Erythropoietin. A major feature of the anemia of critical illness is a failure of circulating erythropoietin concentrations to increase appropriately in response to the reduction in hemoglobin levels. These observations have suggested that treatment with pharmacological doses of erythropoietin (epoetin alpha) might decrease exposure to allogeneic blood in critically ill patients by increasing erythropoiesis thus resulting in a higher hemoglobin, a more rapid return to a normal hemoglobin, and in turn a reduced need for RBC transfusions.

The above rationale led to several randomized trials in critically ill patients, which demonstrated a reduction in RBC transfusion with epoetin alpha treatment in critically ill patients in the ICU as well as critically patients discharged to long-term care facilities. However, a more recent large randomized trial of epoetin alpha treatment in critically ill patients did not demonstrate a decrease in RBC transfusion, although hemoglobin concentration did increase. The absence of transfusion benefit in this more recent trial likely reflected a change in transfusion practice as compared to the earlier studies. Of note, although there was no transfusion reduction observed, there was a significant reduction in mortality in trauma patients who received epoetin alpha treatment [6].

Given that the mortality benefit observed in trauma patients occurred in the absence of a reduction in RBC transfusion, the likely explanation for the mortality improvement is related to non-hematopoietic effects of epoetin alpha. Erythropoietin has actions aside from stimulating the bone marrow to produce mature erythrocytes. Erythropoietin acts as a cytokine with antiapoptotic activity. In this latter role, erythropoietin has been demonstrated in preclinical and small clinical studies to protect cells from hypoxemia/ischemia. Multiple tissues express erythropoietin and the erythropoietin receptor, in response to stress and mediate local stress responses. These "non-hematopoetic" activities of erythropoietin in protecting cells suggest a role for erythropoietin in the critically ill. Apoptosis is important in the pathogenesis of many critical illnesses such as sepsis and multiorgan failure. Similar mechanisms may possibly be involved in mediating injury in trauma patients. Further preclinical and clinical studies will be necessary to establish the mechanism responsible for the epoetin alpha effects.

An important additional observation was a significant increase in thrombotic events noted with epoetin alpha treatment. In a *post hoc* analysis, the increase in thrombotic events was not observed in epoetin alpha patients receiving heparin (prophylactic or therapeutic).

Recommendations for Anemia Management in the Critically Ill

In summary, based on the available data in the critically ill several recommendations can be made:

1. Given the well-documented risks associated with RBC transfusion and the absence of clear evidence for efficacy of RBC transfusion in critically ill patients, in the absence of acute bleeding or acute ischemic cardiac disease, a transfusion threshold of 7.0 g/dL is appropriate for most critically ill patients.

2. A transfusion threshold between 8.0 and 10.0 g/dL is appropriate for patients with acute coronary syndromes until further evidence becomes available.

3. Epoetin alpha administration will increase the hemoglobin concentration in critically ill patients; however, it does not result in a reduction in RBC transfusion in the critically ill if a conservative transfusion threshold is used. Therefore, in the acute setting treatment with epoetin, alpha is of little benefit with the possible exception of patients admitted to the ICU following trauma. In view of the increase in risk of thrombotic events any patients receiving epoetin alpha in the ICU should receive prophylactic anticoagulation if possible.

4. Efforts should be directed toward minimizing phlebotomy blood loss via limiting laboratory testing and phlebotomy blood volume.

References

1. Corwin HL, Hebert PC (eds) (2004) Blood transfusion in the critically Ill, Critical care clinics, Vol 20 2. WB Saunders, Philadelphia
2. Corwin H, Krantz S (2000) Anemia in the critically ill: "Acute" anemia of chronic disease. Crit Care Med 28:3098–3099
3. Hebert P, Timon A, Corwin HL (2007) Controversies in blood transfusion in the critically ill. Chest 131:1583–1590
4. Hebert PC, Wells G, Blajchman MA, Marshall J, Martin C, Pagliarello G et al (1999) A multicenter, randomized, controlled clinical trial of transfusion requirements in critical care. Transfusion requirements in critical care investigators, canadian critical care trials group. New Engl J Med 340:409–417
5. Marik PE, Corwin HL (2008) Efficacy of RBC transfusion in the critically ill: A systematic review of the literature. Crit Care Med 36:2667–2674
6. Corwin HL (2007) Erythropoietin in the critically ill: Forest and trees. Can Med Assoc J 177:747–749

Anesthesia, Local

JOEL M. BARTFIELD
Department of Emergency Medicine, Albany Medical College, Albany, NY, USA

Definition

Local anesthesia is being defined as the administration of anesthetics though administration at the site of an injury or prior to performing a painful procedure. Local anesthetics are typically either amide or ester "caine" anesthetics and are most often administered by injection.

Introduction

Emergency physicians commonly provide local anesthesia to patients requiring laceration repair and anesthesia for bedside procedures. Most typically, local anesthetics are given by injection. Our goal should always be to provide safe and effective anesthesia utilizing techniques which minimize pain of administration. This chapter will review techniques to minimize pain of infiltration followed by a general overview of local anesthetics including alternatives to traditional agents.

Minimizing Pain of Injection

One simple way to minimize patient anxiety is to conduct anesthesia preparation including withdrawing anesthetics and needle and syringe preparation out of the eyesight of the patient. Pain of local anesthetic infiltration is influence by several factors. These include the type of anesthetic, needle size, pH and temperature of the solution, and speed and depth of injection [1]. The best studied technique for minimizing pain is buffering. Local anesthetics are marketed in slightly acidic solutions in order to increase their shelf life. Since they are weak bases they are largely ionized in acidic solutions. It is the unionized base form of the anesthetic which is thought to cross nerve cell membranes and provide anesthesia. Several studies have shown that buffering solutions to approximately physiologic pH decreases the pain of infiltration presumably by increasing the amount of unionized base form [2]. Buffering is accomplished by adding sodium bicarbonate (1 meq/ml) to anesthetic in approximately a 10:1 dilution (10 ml of anesthetic to 1 ml of sodium bicarbonate). This can be accomplished by adding 2 ml of sodium bicarbonate to a 20-ml vial of anesthetic. Buffered lidocaine can be used for up to 1 week after preparation with no clinical change in efficacy [3].

Warming local anesthetics has been inconsistently shown to reduce pain of infiltration. However, pain has been consistently shown to decrease by slow infiltration and subcutaneous injection as opposed to intradermal injection [1]. Pain of infiltration can also be decreased by infiltration from within the wound rather through intact skin. Pretreatment of wounds with topical tetracaine and other combination topical anesthetics minimize the pain associated with anesthetic infiltration.

Local Anesthesia Without Injection

A number of different combinations of agents have been studied as topical anesthetics thus completely obviating the need for needle infiltration. TAC, a combination of tetracaine (0.5%), adrenaline (1:2,000), and cocaine (11.8%) was the first combination to be studied and introduced into clinical practice. Although shown to be moderately effective, the potential toxicity associated cocaine has lead TAC to be replaced by agents and combinations of agents.

Topical 5% lidocaine with epinephrine and lidocaine, adrenaline, and tetracaine (LET) have both compared favorably to TAC. EMLA™ cream, a eutectic mixture of lidocaine and prilocaine, has been used successfully as an anesthetic on intact skin prior to invasive procedures such as phlebotomy, intravenous insertion, and lumbar puncture. Both EMLA™ and LET have been shown to reduce the pain of infiltration of local anesthetics.

Local anesthetics can be "infiltrated" into skin without use of a needle. Two ways this can be accomplished include jet injection or iontophoresis. Jet injection involves the use of a device which essentially sprays material at high pressure (200 PSI) into the skin. The technique is limited by the fact that only small amounts (0.1 ml) of anesthetic can be infiltrated.

Iontophoresis takes advantage of the fact that anesthetics exist in solution as salts of weak bases and therefore are positively charged. By exposing anesthetic solutions to an electrical field they can be forced into the skin. The technique has been studied in volunteers and prior to intravenous catheter placed in pediatric patients. Limitations include the need for specialized equipment and time delay required for administration.

Dosage Considerations

Local anesthetics have dosage-related toxicities. While a weight-based (mg/kg) dosing is useful in pediatric patients, in adult patients, the maximum safe dosages is generally expressed in absolute terms. It is important to note that maximum safe doses are for subcutaneous or intradermal injections. If anesthetics are accidentally injected intravascularly, toxicity can be expected at a much lower dose. The maximum safe amount of plain lidocaine in an adult patient is 300 mg or 30 cc of a 1% solution (since a 1% solution contains 1,000 mg/100 ml or 10 mg/ml). Maximum dosages for commonly used local anesthetics are provided in Table 1.

The practitioner has several options if volumes approaching maximum dosages are anticipated. These include: selection of a less toxic agent, dilution of the agent, providing anesthesia as a nerve or field block which often requires less volume than simple local anesthesia, and the addition of epinephrine. The vasoconstrictive properties of epinephrine increase the amount of local anesthetic which can be injected by decreasing systemic absorption. Epinephrine-containing solutions are commercially available for some anesthetics such as lidocaine;

Anesthesia, Local. Table 1 Maximum safe dosages for selected anesthetics

Generic name	Trade name	Classification	Adult dosage	Pediatric dosage
Lidocaine	Xylocaine	Amide	300 mg	4 mg/kg
Lidocaine w/epi[a] epinephrine	Xylocaine w/epi[a]	Amide	500 mg	7 mg/kg
Bupivacaine	Marcaine	Amide	175 mg	1.5 mg/kg
Bupivacaine w/epi[a]	Marcaine w/epi[a]	Amide	225 mg	3 mg/kg
Procaine	Novocain	Ester	500 mg	7 mg/kg
Procaine w/epi[a]	Novocain w/epi[a]	Ester	600 mg	9 mg/kg

[a]epi = epinephrine

otherwise epinephrine can be added in approximately a 1:100,000 dilution. While a more bloodless field is provided by the use of epinephrine, it also has several disadvantages including the theoretical increase risk of infection, limitations in use in parts of the body with end-arteriolar circulation, and increase pain of infiltration.

Alternatives to Commonly used Local Anesthetics

Local anesthetics are generally of the "caine" family. The two classifications of these agents are amide and esters. Amides and esters differ in their metabolism. Esters (of which procaine (Novocaine™) is the prototype) were the first to be developed. They are metabolized in plasma by pseudocholinesterases. Amides such as lidocaine are metabolized by the liver. Since esters have a relatively high incidence of allergic reactions, amides are most often utilized.

True anaphylaxis to local anesthetics, particularly amides, is extremely rare. Even patients who report an allergy to lidocaine are rarely found to be truly allergic by skin testing. However, if a patient claims to be allergic to lidocaine, it is obviously incumbent on the treating physician to avoid the use of lidocaine unless a true allergy can be reasonably excluded.

The first step in evaluating a patient who states that he/she is "allergic" to local anesthetics is to define the true nature of the previous reaction. A detailed history may reveal that a reported "allergic reaction" was really a vasovagal reaction related to the procedure being performed. If a true "allergic reaction" cannot be excluded, choosing an alternative class anesthetic would be reasonable. For instance, if a patient had a known allergy to lidocaine, an amide anesthetic, an ester anesthetic such as tetracaine could be used safely. Unfortunately patients are often unable to identify which specific anesthetic caused a previous allergic reaction. Even in situations when an allergy to lidocaine, per se is identified, it is more likely that the allergy is to methylparaben, the preservative used in multi-dose vials, rather than to lidocaine itself. Ester anesthetics would not be a good choice for a patient with a methylparaben allergy since they are degraded to para-amino benzoic acid (PABA), a chemical which is closely related to methylparaben. Single dose lidocaine (lidocaine used for IV use) contains no preservatives and would therefore be a reasonable alternative to multi-dose lidocine if it was possible to determine that an individual patient was allergic to methylparaben rather than lidocaine itself. However, it is often impossible to make this distinction without performing skin testing which is impractical in the acute setting. Alternatives to traditional "caine" anesthetics have therefore been sought.

The antihistamine diphenhydramine (Benadryl™) has been shown to be an effective local anesthetic. Its chemical structure is closely related to local anesthetics but different enough that it does not share antigencity with local anesthetics. Although a 1% solution of diphenhydramine provides anesthesia comparable to 1% lidocaine, the solution is considerably more painful to administer than lidocaine. Diphendramine, 0.5%, is less painful but unfortunately also less effective. Buffering diphenhydramine with sodium bicarbonate was not found to decrease its pain of infiltration. Other properties

Anesthesia, Local. Table 2 Comparison of types of anesthesia

	Advantages	Disadvantages
Topical	Painless	• Not always reliable, (works best on face)
		• Danger of absorption if used on mucus membranes
		• Cannot be used on areas with end-arteriolar circulation
Local	• Ease of technique	• May require high volumes of anesthetic
	• Reliability	• May be excessively painful in certain locations (tips of extremities, palms, soles)
Nerve/field blocks	• Does not distort anatomy	• Only useful for certain locations
	• Requires lower volume of anesthetic	• Not as reliable as local

which make diphenhydramine an unattractive alternative to caine anesthetics are side effects which include sedation, local irritation, erythema, vesicle formation, tissue necrosis and prolonged anesthesia. Given these disadvantages of diphenhydramine, other non-"caine" anesthetics have been sought for patients who are allergic to lidocaine.

Benzyl alcohol (as found as a preservative in multidose normal saline) has been shown to have local anesthetic properties. Its pain of administration compares favorably to lidocaine; however its short duration of action (a few minutes) limits its utility. The addition of epinephrine, 1:100,000 increases the duration of activity of benzyl alcohol. Although the duration of action is still somewhat shorter than lidocaine, benzyl alcohol with epinephrine is a viable alternative to patients with caine anesthetic allergies [4]. Benzyl alcohol with epinephrine 1:100,000 can be prepared by making a 1:100 dilution of epinephrine, 1:1,000, with multi-dose normal saline that contains 0.9% benzyl alcohol.

Local Versus Regional Anesthesia

Anesthesia for laceration repair and other common bedside procedures is generally accomplished by local infiltration. Local infiltration has the advantages of being easy to perform; and is reliable and safe providing proper technique is utilized and toxicity is not exceeded. Direct infiltration of local anesthetics, particularly those containing epinephrine, also has the advantage of providing hemostasis.

Local anesthesia has several noteworthy disadvantages. Infiltration of anesthetics in and around wounds distorts anatomy and can make subsequent repair of lacerations more difficult. As compared to nerve blocks, local anesthesia often requires larger volumes of anesthetic. Additionally, local infiltration requires multiple injections. Table 2 summarizes advantages and disadvantages nerve blocks, topical, and local anesthesia.

Nerve blocks will be discussed in the chapter on regional anesthesia.

References

1. Arndt KA, Burton C, Noe JM (1983) Minimizing the pain of local anesthesia. Plast Reconstr Surg 72:676–679
2. Bartfield JM et al (1990) Buffered versus plain lidocaine as a local anesthetic for simple laceration repair. Ann Emerg Med 19:1387–1389
3. Bartfield JM et al (1992) Buffered lidocaine as a local anesthetic: An investigation of shelf life. Ann Emerg Med 21:16–19
4. Bartfield JM, May-Wheeling HE, Raccio-Robak N, Lai S-Y (1999) Benzyl alcohol with epinephrine as an alternative local anesthetic to lidocaine with epinephrine. Acad Emerg Med 6:496

Anesthesia, Regional

JOEL M. BARTFIELD
Department of Emergency Medicine, Albany Medical College, Albany, NY, USA

Definition

For purposes of this chapter, regional anesthesia is being defined as the injection of an anesthetic other than a local injection directly into a wound, laceration, or body part for which local anesthesia is desired. Regional anesthesia can be divided into two main types, field blocks and nerve blocks.

Characteristics

Field Blocks

Field blocks provide anesthesia by infiltration of an anesthetic in the skin surrounding the area of interest. The technique is relatively easy to accomplish and generally provides reliable anesthesia without disrupting anatomy. However, field blocks can only be used in certain areas of the body with appropriate sensory innervation and anatomy. Common areas that can be anesthetized by field blocks include the forehead, ear, and nose. A disadvantage of field blocks is that they often require a large volume of anesthetics as compared to nerve blocks, or sometimes even local anesthesia.

Nerve Blocks

Nerve blocks provide regional anesthesia by anesthetizing single nerves or groups of nerves that supply sensory innervation to particular areas of the body. Like field blocks, nerve blocks have the advantage of providing anesthesia without distorting anatomy. Unlike field blocks, nerve blocks generally require a relatively small volume of anesthetic and can often be performed through a single injection. Nerve blocks in certain areas of the body are relatively easy to perform and master. This chapter will focus on some general principles of nerve blocks and then on specific blocks which are clinically useful and commonly performed. These include digital nerve blocks and blocks involving nerves supplying sensation to the hand, foot, and face.

General Principals

The practitioner should be mindful of several general principals when performing nerve blocks.

1. A good working knowledge of anatomy is essential in order to successfully perform nerve blocks. Care should be taken to identify landmarks.

2. It is essential to utilize proper antiseptic technique particularly when deep injections are being administered.
3. Prior to performing a block, patients should be told that they might feel paresthesias during the procedure. If paresthesias are elicited (indicating that the needle is very close to the target nerve), the needle should be withdrawn slightly and then the anesthetic should be injected.
4. Since vascular structures tend to run close to nerves, it is important to always aspirate prior to injecting.
5. An adequate amount of anesthetic should be injected in the area of the nerve.
6. After infiltration, if possible the area should be gently massaged (to help to diffuse the anesthetic into the nerve being blocked).
7. It may take several minutes for nerve blocks to take effect.
8. If a block has been unsuccessful, the block can be reattempted or local anesthesia can be administered (remembering not to exceed the maximum allowable amount of local anesthetic).

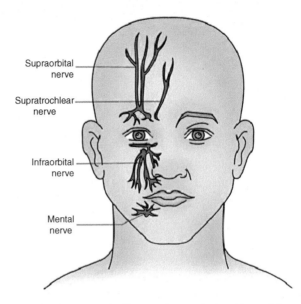

Anesthesia, Regional. Figure 1 Anatomical positions of three branches of the trigeminal nerve

Specific Nerve Blocks

Facial Nerve Blocks
Nerve blocks offer distinct advantages over local anesthesia for the management of facial injuries. In the case of lacerations (assuming the location lends itself to a nerve block) complete anesthesia can be achieved without distorting the edges of the laceration. The trigeminal nerve supplies sensation to the face. All three branches of this nerve, the supraorbital, infraorbital, and mental nerves, are easily blocked. The three nerves exit from foramina that fall along a line that connects the medial aspect of the pupil with the corner of the mouth (Fig. 1).

Supraorbital and Supratrochlear Nerves
The supraorbital nerve supplies sensation to most of the forehead. The area near the bridge of the nose is supplied by the supratrochlear nerve. The supraorbital nerve exits at the supraorbital foramen and the supratrochlear nerve exits 5–10 mm medial to it. The supraorbital foramen is easily palpated as a notch in the medial one third of the superior orbital rim. Both nerves can be blocked by superficial injection at this easily identifiable location.

Infraorbital Nerve
The infraorbital nerve supplies sensation to the medial aspect of the mid-face including the upper lip. The nerve exits through the infraorbital foramen. The foramen is easily palpated just below the inferior border of the orbit

along the line previously described. The infraorbital nerve can be blocked either by injection through intact skin or through buccal mucosa (author's preferred method). Injection thorough the buccal mucosa has been shown to be less painful and more reliable [1]. The nerve is blocked by inserting a ¾ inch needle to the hub into the buccal-mucosal sulcus opposite the upper canine and palpating the foramen as the anesthetic is slowly injected. Care must be taken to introduce the needle along the surface of the maxilla in order to avoid puncturing the globe and the outer surface of the face.

Mental Nerve
The mental nerve supplies sensation to the superior chin and lower lip. This nerve exits through the mental foramen. This notch is easily identified along the previously described line in the lateral chin. Similar to the infraorbital nerve, there are two approaches to blocking the mental nerve, transcutaneous or intraoral (author's preferred method) injection. The latter technique was shown to be more reliable and less painful in a study involving ten volunteers [2]. The block is accomplished by inserting a ¾ inch needle to the hub into the buccal-mucosal fold opposite the lower canine and palpating the foramen as the anesthetic is slowly injected.

Digital Nerve Block
There are two sets (palmar and dorsal) of digital nerves, which each run along the lateral aspect of the digit. For the

middle three fingers, the palmar nerves supply most of the sensation to the fingertip. Therefore only the palmar nerve needs to be blocked for the middle three fingers. In order to provide good anesthesia for the first and fifth digit, the dorsal nerves have to be blocked in addition to the palmar nerves. The digital arteries run in close proximity to the digital nerves. Since these arteries supply end arterial circulation to the finger and toe tips, care must be taken to avoid injury to them and anesthetics with epinephrine should be avoided for digital nerve blocks.

Buffered lidocaine has been shown to be less painful to administer for digital nerve blocks then plain lidocaine [3]. There are several acceptable techniques for performing digital nerve blocks. The nerve can be blocked either at the metacarpophalangeal (MCP) joint or metatarsopahalangeal (MTP) joint or anywhere along its course. Digital blocks can be performed by introducing the needle through the dorsal or ventral surface of the digit. MCP and MTP blocks are best performed by injecting between the digits on either side of the digit being blocked. MCP and MTP blocks are easy to learn; however, one study involving 30 volunteers, found MCP blocks to be less reliable (23% failure rate versus 3% failure rate) and to have a slower onset (6.35 min versus 2.82 min) compared to conventional digital blocks [4].

Nerve Blocks of the Hand

A thorough knowledge of sensory innervation is important when planning for nerve blocks in the hand. Figure 2 demonstrates the typical sensory innervation of the hand. It is important to remember that there is some individual variation and therefore multiple blocks may be required. Since local infiltration into the hand, particularly into the thick palmar skin can be particularly painful, nerve blocks are particularly useful.

Ulnar Nerve Block

The ulnar nerve can be blocked at the wrist or the elbow. The wrist is preferable since the nerve can be easily damaged at the elbow due to its superficial location and close proximity to boney structures. The nerve lies between the flexor carpi ulnaris tendon and the ulnar artery at the wrist. It can be blocked either by introducing the needle between these two structures or by introducing the needle underneath the flexor carpi ulnaris tendon at the ulnar aspect of the wrist (author's preferred method). With either technique care should be taken to avoid injection into the ulnar artery by aspirating prior to injection. A total of 5–7 cc of agent is injected to achieve anesthesia. The ulnar nerve can also be blocked at the elbow by infiltrating small amounts of anesthesia in proximity to the nerve that runs in the groove

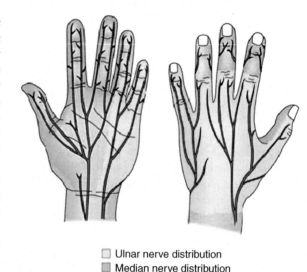

☐ Ulnar nerve distribution
▨ Median nerve distribution
☐ Radial nerve distribution

Anesthesia, Regional. Figure 2 Sensory distribution of the nerves supplying the hand

between the medial epicondyle of the humerus and the olecranon of the ulna.

Median Nerve Block

The median nerve is located between the palmaris longus and the flexor carpi radialis tendons. The palmaris longus can be located by having the patient oppose the thumb and fifth finger and flex the wrist against resistance. This tendon is congenitally absent approximately 20% the time. In these instances, the nerve can be found approximately 1 cm ulnar to the flexor carpi radialis. The median nerve is blocked by puncturing the flexor retinaculum between the two wrist creases at the location of the nerve and injecting 5–8 cc of agent at this site.

Radial Nerve

The radial nerve follows the radial artery and then fans out dorsally distal to the wrist. The nerve is blocked by injecting into the anatomic snuff box and laying a 6–8 cm wheel of anesthetic as a field block across the dorsal portion of the radial aspect of the wrist.

Nerve Blocks of the Ankle

Ankle blocks are more difficult to accomplish than the other blocks discussed in this chapter. Familiarity with these blocks can be very useful, however, since local anesthesia to the sole of the foot is both difficult to accomplish and painful to administer due to skin thickness. Five different nerve blocks at the ankle can be utilized to

Superficial peroneal distribution

Sural nerve distribution

Deep personal distribution

Posterior tribial nerve distribution

Anesthesia, Regional. Figure 3 Sensory distribution of the nerves supplying the foot

provide anesthesia to the foot. Multiple blocks are often employed since sensory innervation is somewhat variable. The sole of the foot is supplied by the tibial nerve (which branches into the medial and lateral plantar nerve) and the sural nerve (Fig. 3). The most lateral aspect of the dorsum of the foot is supplied by the sural nerve with the remainder supplied by the superficial and deep peroneal nerves and the saphenous nerve (Fig. 3).

Tibial Nerve (Medial and Lateral Plantar Nerves) Block
The tibial nerve is located in close proximity to the tibia between the medial malleolus and the Achilles' tendon. This nerve is blocked by injecting 5 cc of anesthetic agent between the posterior tibial artery and the Achilles' tendon just posterior to the medial malleolus. The block is easiest to perform with the patient in the prone position with the foot in slight dorsiflexion.

Sural Nerve Block
The sural nerve is located between the lateral malleolus and the Achilles' tendon. The sural nerve is relatively superficial as compared to the tibial nerve, and therefore requires a more superficial injection. The sural nerve can be blocked by injecting 5 cc of anesthetic superficially in

a fan-like distribution just lateral to the Achilles' tendon at the top of the lateral malleolus.

Superficial Peroneal, Deep Peroneal, and Saphenous Nerve Blocks
All three of these nerves should be blocked in order to provide adequate anesthesia to the dorsum of the foot. With the patient in a supine position, the skin is punctured between the extensor hallucis longus and anterior tibial tendons at a point parallel to the superior aspect of the medial malleolus. The deep peroneal nerve is blocked by a deep injection between the two tendons, while the other two nerves are blocked by superficial injections. The needle is then withdrawn and redirected subcutaneously toward the lateral malleolus to block the superficial peroneal nerve and then medially to block the saphenous nerve. A total of 15 cc of agent will usually be required to block all three nerves.

References
1. Lynch MT et al (1994) Comparison of intraoral and percutaneous approaches for infraorbital nerve block. Acad Emerg Med 1:514–519
2. Syverud SA et al (1994) A comparative study of the percutaneous versus intraoral technique for mental nerve block. Acad Emerg Med 1:509–513
3. Bartfield JM, Ford DT, Homer PJ (1993) Buffered versus plain lidocaine for digital nerve blocks. Ann Emerg Med 22:216–219
4. Knoop K, Trott A, Syverud S (1994) Comparison of digital versus metacarpal blocks for repair of finger injuries. Ann Emerg Med 23:1296–1300

Angio Embolization

▶ Angioembolization, Hepatic

Angioembolization, Hepatic

THOMAS M. SCALEA
Shock Trauma Center, University of Maryland School of Medicine, Baltimore, MD, USA

Synonyms
Angio embolization; Liver embolization

Definition
Angiography is a radiographic technique that allows imaging of vascular beds, allowing the identification of vascular

injuries or lesions. When using this technique for the liver, the arteries imaged are the aorta, the common and proper hepatic arteries and the left and right hepatic arteries with their branches. Embolization involves occluding vascular lesions or injuries utilizing one of a variety of occlusion materials. The technique is described below. The liver has a dual blood supply, and nutrient flow enters the liver via both the hepatic artery and the portal vein. Imaging of the portal venous circulation, while possible, is technically much more difficult than imaging the hepatic arterial circulation. In addition, portal venous pressures are much lower than that seen in the hepatic artery. Thus, injuries only rarely become symptomatic and require embolization. On these rare occasions, the portal vein is generally accessed from the superior vena cava. A guidewire must then be placed into the liver substance and bridged from the hepatic venous circulation, into the portal venous circulation, similarly to performing a transjugular intrahepatic portosystemic shunt. The guidewire can then be advanced to the level necessary in the portal vein and the injury can be stented or embolized.

Indications

Angiographic embolization has become a mainstay in the treatment of hepatic pathology. While the technique can be used for a number of disease states, it is probably most often used to extend the nonoperative therapy following blunt trauma. Angiography has the ability to diagnose vascular lesions deep in the hepatic parenchyma. These are not visible at the time of open surgical exploration. Embolization can achieve hemostasis without the need for laparotomy and/or the major blood loss that usually accompanies major hepatic repair or resection [1, 2].

There are no clear guidelines for angiography and subsequent embolization following hepatic trauma. There are, however, some generally accepted guidelines. The higher the grade of hepatic injury, the more likely the patient is to fail simple observation. Thus, these higher grade injuries likely come with an increased incidence of intrahepatic vascular injury that could therefore benefit from embolization. Certainly, patients with pseudoaneurysms or other vascular abnormalities seen on CT scan are good candidates for angiographic embolization (Fig. 1–3). Some patients developed delayed complications such as hemobilia, following nonoperative management of high grade liver injuries. Even if a vascular abnormality is not seen on CT scan, diagnostic angiography should come with a high yield, and embolization should be curative. Finally, some would advocate diagnostic angiography for patients at particular risk such as those with penetrating injury through the midportion of the

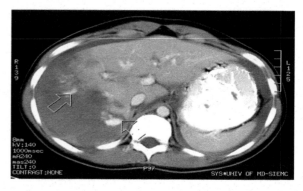

Angioembolization, Hepatic. Figure 1 The 16-year-old female presented after a high-speed vehicular crash. CT scan shows a number of large vascular injuries deep in the substance of the liver

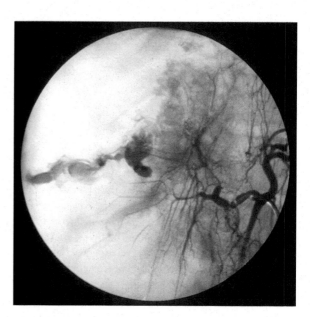

Angioembolization, Hepatic. Figure 2 Diagnostic angiography reveals four very large vascular injuries

liver. There are no good data supporting hepatic angiography for any of these indications, yet these are common indications for its use.

Angiographic embolization has gained wide popularity as part of a multidisciplinary strategy when using damage control following severe either blunt or penetrating trauma [3]. Damage control involves an abbreviated initial laparotomy, utilizing packing for adjunctive hemostasis. The patient is then resuscitated in the Intensive Care Unit and non-lifesaving surgical procedures are deferred until the patient is more stable. Arguably, severe liver

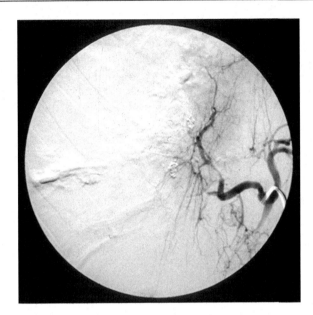

Angioembolization, Hepatic. Figure 3 These were all successfully occluded using stainless steel coils

injury is the most common indication for damage control. In that scenario, major hepatic bleeding is controlled at the time of initial operation. Perihepatic packing can be life-saving in helping to tamponade nonsurgical bleeding. These patients often have vascular injuries that have been temporized. Thus, early postoperative angiographic embolization can be key to obtain final hemostasis and prevent rebleeding at the time of unpacking.

Technique
Patients with large vascular injuries can sometimes have them identified at the time of a flush aortogram. More commonly, patients undergo selective hepatic artery angiography in order to identify the number and location of vascular injuries that can be treated with embolization. Several techniques of embolization exist, each with its advantages and disadvantages.

Highly selective embolization is usually accomplished with a combination of small stainless steel coils and gel foam. Utilizing this technique, a small guidewire is inserted to the level of the vascular injury. The injury can then be selectively occluded. If there are a number of injuries located adjacent to each other, coils can be deposited just distal to each of these injuries. The catheter can then be pulled back and the area flooded with gel foam. This allows for embolization of all of the injuries but prevents distal migration of the embolization material.

Maneuvering the wire out peripherally in the liver can be problematic in patients in shock with accompanying vasospasm. Tight packing may also produce vasospasm, potentially limiting the angiographer's ability to access peripheral vascular injuries. In this case, more proximal embolization can be used. Depositing coils more proximally decreases the pressure head to the area of injury. Spontaneous hemostasis can occur. This technique, of course, renders a much larger portion of the liver potentially ischemic. In addition, if collateral flow maintains hemorrhage from the injured blood vessel, the angiographic window is now closed. Occasionally, the coils can be placed very proximally such as embolizing the entire right or left hepatic arteries. Similar to hepatic artery ligation, this usually results in good hemostasis.

Blind gel foam embolization has the advantage of being one among the simplest of techniques. In this case, gel foam is cut to the desired size and then blindly delivered into the right or left hepatic artery. The gel foam particles travel into the hepatic parenchyma, carried by liver blood flow, until they reach the blood vessels that match their size. Blind gel foam embolization can be quite effective, particularly in people with a large number of injuries in one lobe of the liver. This technique can be particularly effective in patients who are hemodynamically quite labile, as it can be performed rapidly. Because the particles travel distally, this can cause substantial hepatic necrosis.

Complications
While hepatic angioembolization can be lifesaving, it does come with a significant rate of complications [4]. Certainly all patients are at risk for any of the complications reparable to the angiogram such as femoral artery injury, acute renal failure from contrast nephropathy, and/or inadvertant placement of a coil. The most common hepatic complication after angioembolization is major hepatic necrosis. We have recently described this as occurring in 20% of patients who undergo angioembolization for high grade liver injury [5]. The reason for this high rate is unclear. As the liver has dual blood supply, one would imagine that flow through the portal vein would be sufficient to maintain hepatic viability after angiographic embolization. It may be that many of these patients have concomitant portal venous injury adjacent to their hepatic artery injury. In addition, perihepatic packing and/or hematoma within the hepatic parenchymal may produce a local compartment syndrome, impeding flow through the portal vein.

Major hepatic necrosis is most often treated with either multiple hepatic debridements or formal hepatic lobectomy. We have had good success with both techniques. While a 20% incidence of major complications seems high, it is also important to remember that many of these patients in the past died of hemorrhage. We now simply consider this as part of the progression of damage control. While hepatic lobectomy is certainly an operative procedure of magnitude, it should be able to be accomplished successfully once the patient is stabilized. Based on our recent experience, we now perform lobectomy early, after major hepatic necrosis has been identified.

Conclusion

Hepatic angioembolization has the ability to be lifesaving, particularly following major hepatic injury. Absolute indications have not been clearly described and will vary from institution to institution based on local expertise and interests. Hepatic embolization can be used in stable patients with particular injury subsets, but is probably most often used as part of a damage control philosophy. There is a substantial complication rate of angioembolization, which often requires hepatic lobectomy.

References

1. Hagiwara A, Murata A, Matsuda T, Matsuda H, Shimazaki S (1992) The efficacy and limitations of transarterial embolization for severe hepatic injury. J Trauma 52:1091–1096
2. Wahl WL, Ahrns KS, Brandt MM, Franklin GA, Taheri PA (2002) The need for early angiographic embolization in blunt liver injuries. J Trauma 52:1097–1101
3. Johnson JW, Gracias VH, Gupta R et al (2002) Hepatic angiography in patients undergoing damage control laparotomy. J Trauma 52:1102–1106
4. Mohr AM, Lavery RF, Barone A et al (2003) Angiographic embolization for liver injuries: low mortality, high morbidity. J Trauma 55:1077–1082
5. Dabbs DN, Stein DM, Scalea TM (2009) Major hepatic necrosis: a common complication after angioembolization for treatment of high-grade liver injuries. J Trauma 66:621–629

Angioembolization, Splenic

Kareem R. AbdelFattah, Joseph P. Minei
Division of Burns, Trauma, and Critical Care, Department of Surgery, UT-Southwestern Medical Center, Dallas, TX, USA

Synonyms

Splenic Angiography; Splenic Arteriography with Embolization; Splenic Embolization

Definition

Splenic angioembolization (SAE) is the process of utilizing vascular interventional techniques to manage injury to or, occasionally, diseases of the spleen. In trauma, this technique is an adjunctive maneuver in the nonoperative management (NOM) of the hemodynamically stable patient with splenic injuries. The process includes angiography, which utilizes catheter-based techniques to deliver radio-opaque contrast material into blood vessels for visualization of the vascular anatomy, followed by possible intervention with embolization. Splenic embolization refers to occlusion of the splenic artery or its branches using various materials.

Pre-existing Condition

Splenic injuries are one of the most common reasons for laparotomy after blunt abdominal trauma, however the majority of patients experiencing splenic trauma will be managed nonoperatively (NOM). Splenic embolization is most commonly used for the patient who has experienced blunt trauma resulting in injury to the spleen. Although it has been applied in other areas of medicine, such as the treatment of some chronic spleen disorders, it is used with much more frequency in the trauma setting. Mortality rates of patients with splenic injury in the early part of the twentieth century approached nearly 100%. It was not until reports of fatal infections in children after splenectomy led practitioners to attempt NOM that a more conservative treatment model became standard. Reports of splenic embolization in blunt injury were first reported in the 1980s, and became common during the 1990s. Now, the procedure has been used to treat splenic injuries in patients who exhibit ongoing blood loss but maintain hemodynamic stability, and has been considered in those patients with CT scan findings that portend a failure of a conservative approach. Those findings include contrast extravasation, pseudoaneurysms, arteriovenous fistulas, or significant hemoperitoneum.

Patient Selection

Although splenic embolization has been used for nearly 20 years, there still remains controversy regarding optimal patient selection, as the role of splenic embolization has not fully evolved in current trauma care. Trauma centers should have a basic algorithm in place which, depending on local expertise and standards of practice, will outline the management of the patient with blunt abdominal trauma with an identified injury to the spleen (Fig. 1). The basic principles of surgery and trauma should be followed in determining which patients would benefit most from splenic angioembolization. Hemodynamically unstable patients are best served in the operating room, and patients that are hemodynamically stable, despite the degree of injury, may be given a trial of nonoperative management. It is this latter group from which the

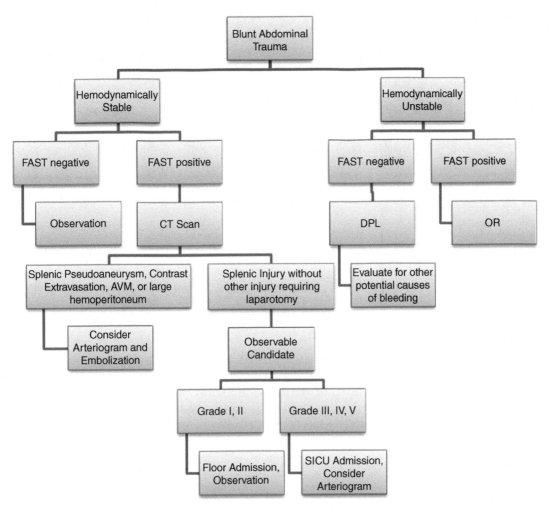

Angioembolization, Splenic. Figure 1 Sample algorithm for blunt abdominal trauma with splenic injury. *FAST* Focused Abdominal Sonography in Trauma, *DPL* Diagnostic Peritoneal Lavage, *OR* Operating Room, *SICU* Surgical Intensive Care Unit

majority of patients considered for angiographic intervention should be selected.

Patients that suffer blunt abdominal trauma who are stable, in whom there is concern for intra-abdominal injury, should undergo abdominal CT scanning with IV contrast (Fig. 2a). Oral contrast administration is not necessary due to time constraints in the trauma setting. Modern CT scanners are fast and reliable in determining the presence of intra-abdominal injuries, and can be of great use in the diagnosis of splenic injuries in the stable patient. The identification of active contrast extravasation, pseudoaneurysm, arteriovenous fistula, large amounts of hemoperitoneum, or a high grade of injury (Table 1) are all findings in which literature has supported the use of angiography and possible embolization secondary to the reportedly high incidence of failure of NOM. Using these

as the basis for selective criteria, approximately 8–15% of patients will become candidates for the use of splenic angioembolization.

Application

A failure rate of 10% can be expected in the nonoperative management of splenic injuries [2]. Generally, higher-grade injuries will result in a higher rate of failure. The objective of splenic angioembolization is to reduce the failure rate of nonsurgical management, and studies have shown NOM success rates between 75% and 100% when observation is combined with selective use of SAE [3, 4]. Patients who have undergone embolization but exhibit ongoing bleeding may be candidates for a repeat procedure as long as hemodynamic stability is maintained.

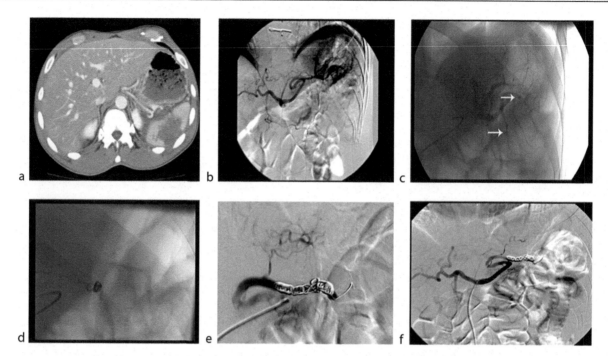

Angioembolization, Splenic. Figure 2 CT scan (**a**) and angiography (**b**, **c**) demonstrating a Grade IV Spleen Injury with active extravasation. This patient was a hemodynamically stable 43-year-old male who suffered an aggravated assault and was noted to have the injury on CT scan. He required multiple metal coils placed in the splenic artery (**d**–**f**) to stop extravasation from two locations. The patient underwent repeat CT scan 5 days later for abdominal pain, and a small low-density area was seen, thought to be an area of infarction. No further intervention was required, and the patient was discharged in good condition

Angioembolization, Splenic. Angioembolization, Splenic. Table 1 AAST grading scale for splenic injuries (1994 Revision) [1]

Grade	Injury description
I	Subcapsular hematoma of less than 10% of surface area; capsular tear of less than 1 cm in depth
II	Subcapsular hematoma of 10–50% of surface area. Intraparenchymal hematoma of less than 5 cm in diameter; laceration of 1–3 cm in depth and not involving trabecular vessels
III	Subcapsular hematoma of greater than 50% of surface area or expanding and ruptured subcapsular or parenchymal hematoma; intraparenchymal hematoma of greater than 5 cm or expanding; laceration of greater than 3 cm in depth or involving trabecular vessels
IV	Laceration involving segmental or hilar vessels with devascularization of more than 25% of the spleen
V	Shattered spleen or hilar vascular injury

Splenic angioembolization is directed at the splenic artery and its branches. The procedure begins by performance of nonselective angiography of the aorta in order to visualize the origin of the splenic artery. While this is usually a branch of the celiac axis, variations exist and must be accounted for. Once this is complete and the splenic artery has been selected, the interventionist's goal is to control hemorrhage.

Technique

Splenic angioembolization requires catheterization of the arterial system, most commonly via femoral artery access. Depending on access issues and anatomy, the brachial artery can be used as an alternative site for access. Once the femoral artery has been identified on ultrasound, it can be accessed using an 18-gauge needle, or in some cases, a micropuncture technique. The Seldinger technique is used to place a catheter over a wire once access is achieved. A 5- to 6-French introducer sheath is most commonly placed at the start of the procedure; however, the use of micro-catheters is required for many interventions, especially if subsegmental arterial branches are to be accessed. Selective angiography of the spleen via the splenic artery is obtained in order to determine the extent of the injury (Fig. 2b, c). A radio-opaque dye is injected into the catheter once the splenic artery has been accessed in order to visualize the injury. Once the vessel suspected to be feeding the injury is identified, a variety of materials may be used to complete embolization. Metallic coils (Fig. 2d–f) and gelfoam (Fig. 3d) are the most commonly used agents; however, other substances have included sodium tetradecyl sulfate, cyanoacrylate, polyvinyl alcohol (PVA), microspheres, and vascular plugs. Many of these materials do not embolize the vessel primarily; rather, they promote thrombosis at the site of placement. Therefore, it is important to be aware of the patient's coagulation profile, and those patients who develop coagulopathy may not be able to benefit from these procedures. The notable exception to this is gelfoam, which acts to physically clot the vessel. Gelfoam is a water-insoluble, pliable material which acts

as a hemostatic agent in many settings, although it is known to be absorbed over time, which can later lead to recanalization of an injured vessel.

Depending on the location and extent of bleeding, the interventionist must decide whether to embolize proximally (e.g., the main splenic artery), or to perform selective embolization of small branches of the splenic artery which are feeding the injury in question. No studies have compared the effectiveness or complication rates between these approaches. In either approach, embolization is effective secondary to the decrease in splenic blood pressure which allows for hemostasis at the site of injury. Again, the patient's coagulation status becomes important for this process. The most obvious advantage to proximal embolization over distal is procedure time, which depending on other injuries may be critical in the injured patient.

The success rate for splenic angioembolization ranges from 83% to 92%. Failure is usually defined as the continuation of hemorrhage, or other complications such as

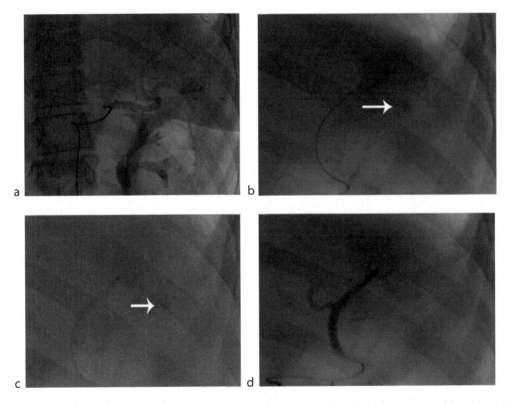

a

b

c

d

Angioembolization, Splenic. Figure 3 Angiography (**a–c**) and gelfoam embolization (**d**) of a 39-year-old female involved in an MVC. Contrast extravasation was noted on CT scan and confirmed on angiography. A third-order branch of the splenic artery was selected using a microcatheter setup, and gelfoam used for embolization with resultant decrease of blood flow to the area

infarction or infection. The failure rates of splenic angioembolization may depend on the substance used in the vessel, although this is controversial. Some studies have shown no differences between different embolization materials, whereas others show significant differences in failure rates between, for example, permanent embolization with metal coils versus gelfoam, which has the potential for recanalization of the vessel. It should be noted that the finding of intraperitoneal air following angioembolization is not an absolute indication for mandatory splenectomy.

Complications

Although significant developments have changed the procedure since its first use, it still entails a number of important complications that practitioners should consider. A complication rate of 20–30% can be expected with the use of the technique [5]. Major complications include ongoing bleeding, splenic infarction, splenic abscess, coil migration, and contrast-induced nephropathy. In several series, the rate of ongoing bleeding is between 40% and 60%. Most of these reports do not describe whether bleeding was from the original identified bleed or a secondary location; however, at least one study reported rebleeding to occur in 11% of patients and missed injuries to be identified in 3% [3]. The rate of splenic infarction has been reported in up to 60% of patients treated with proximal embolization, and as high as 100% in patients treated with distal embolization. These patients are generally asymptomatic and do not require intervention. Splenic abscesses occur in approximately 5% of patients, presenting usually with fever, abdominal pain, and occasionally splenomegaly. Patients will often present with high WBC counts, and will have non-enhancing low-density lesions. Most of these patients can be managed with percutaneous drainage. Complications related to the vascular access portion of the case must also be considered, including hematoma at the site of puncture as well as infection risks if the catheter is left in place.

Post-Procedure Considerations

All patients who undergo surgical splenectomy receive the *Haemophilus influenza* vaccine (Hib vaccine or PRP vaccine), pneumococcus vaccine (Prevnar), and meningococcal vaccine, as they incur a small but dangerous risk of overwhelming postsplenectomy sepsis. While splenic embolization likely does not result in the same immunologic disadvantages as splenectomy [6], some centers will vaccinate patients undergoing the procedure in which the indication was a high-grade injury. It should be noted that even with proximal splenic artery embolization, the spleen will retain perfusion through collateral branches including the short gastric arteries. Distal embolization will usually result in a significant portion of the spleen retaining its primary blood supply. Still, there is a risk of splenic infarction following the procedure, which may have a delayed presentation.

References

1. Moore EE et al (1995) Organ injury scaling: spleen and liver (1994 Revision). J Trauma 38:323
2. Peitzman AB, Heil B, Rivera L et al (2000) Blunt splenic injury in adults: Multi-institutional Study of the Eastern Association for the surgery of trauma. J Trauma 49(2):177–187, discussion 187–179
3. Haan JM, Biffl W, Knudson MM et al (2004) Splenic embolization revisited: a multicenter review. J Trauma 56(3):542–547
4. Sclafani SJ, Shaftan GW, Scalea TM et al (1995) Nonoperative salvage of computed tomography-diagnosed splenic injuries: utilization of angiography for triage and embolization for hemostasis. J Trauma 39(5):818–825, discussion 826–817
5. Ekeh AP, McCarthy MC, Woods RJ, Haley E (2005) Complications arising from splenic embolization after blunt splenic trauma. Am J Surg 189(3):335–339
6. Tominaga GT, Simon FJ Jr, Dandan IS et al (2009) Immunologic function after splenic embolization, is there a difference? J Trauma 67(2):289–295

Angiography with Therapeutic Embolization

▶ Musculoskeletal Trauma, Pelvic Angioembolization

Angiotensin II

▶ Renal Blood Flow Regulation

Animal Bite Wounds

▶ Bite Injuries

Anoxic Hypoxia

▶ Arterial Hypoxemia

ANP

PATRICK T. MURRAY
School of Medicine and Medical Science, University
College Dublin, Dublin, Ireland

Synonyms

Acute kidney injury (AKI); Atrial natriuretic factor (ANF);
Atrial natriuretic hormone (ANH); Atrial natriuretic pep-
tide (ANP); Atriopeptin; Auriculin; Natriuretic peptides;
Hypertension

Trade Names

Anaritide, Carperitide

Definition

The term "natriuretic peptide" refers to a peptide that
induces natriuresis (the urinary excretion of sodium).
Several endogenous peptides are produced, stored, and
released in the heart in response to myocardial
stretch. Once released, a natriuretic peptide binds to its
receptors in the kidney and blood vessels, and promotes
salt excretion (which lowers blood volume) and blood
vessel relaxation (which lowers BP). This endocrine
mechanism links the heart and kidney in maintaining
a fine balance of electrolytes, body fluid, and blood pressure [1]. ANP was first discovered in 1981 by a team led
by de Bold et al.; after it was observed that injection of
atrial tissue extracts into rats caused copious natriuresis.
The mammalian natriuretic peptide family has three
structurally related members, namely atrial natriuretic
peptide or factor (ANP or ANF), brain or B-type natriuretic peptide (BNP), and C-type natriuretic peptide
(CNP). Urodilatin (URO) is a natriuretic peptide that
has been isolated in human urine. It is derived from the
same precursor as ANP but its post-translational modification is dissimilar. Urodilatin exerts similar diuretic and
natriuretic actions to those as ANP. Dendroaspis natriuretic peptide (DNP) was isolated from the venom of
Dendroaspis augusticeps (the green mamba snake) and
its function in humans is not fully understood. This
article will focus on the structure, synthesis, secretion,
pharmacological actions, safety, and clinical effects of
ANP. BNP is discussed in detail in the succeeding chapter. ANP and synthetic analogs of ANP (anaritide and
carperitide) have been investigated as potential therapies
for the treatment of acute kidney injury (AKI) and
other diseases.

Structure, Synthesis, and Secretion

Biologically active ANP is a 28-amino acid peptide. All
natriuretic peptides share structural similarities in a
17-amino acid core ring and a cysteine bridge. Natriuretic
peptides are synthesized as preprohormones. ANP is
derived from a preproANP molecule containing 151
amino acids. PreproANP is a single copy gene called
NPPA and is located on the short arm of chromosome 1
at location 1p36.21. *NPPA* accounts for 1–3% of all
messenger RNA (mRNA) in the cardiac atria. The
preproANP molecule contains a 25-amino acid signal
peptide that permits post-translational modification and
processing into the proANP molecule. Removal of the
signal peptide forms a 126-amino acid proANP molecule.
ProANP is stored within atrial granules and released by
exocytotic fusion of granule with the plasma membrane.
Simultaneously, a specific protease, corin, cleaves proANP
into biologically active ANP and an N-terminal fragment
that enter the circulation. Corin is a transmembrane
cardiac serine protease and is highly expressed on the
extracellular surface of atrial cardiomyocytes. Atrial tissues
derived from corin knockout mice contain proANP but no
ANP and are indeed hypertensive and have cardiac hypertrophy. Several single nucleotide polymorphisms within
the NPPA and corin-coding regions have been identified
and are linked to hypertension. One of them (−C664G) is
located in the promoter region of the ANP gene, *NPPA*.
The −C664G allele in humans was associated with low
plasma ANP levels, high blood pressure, and left ventricular hypertrophy. To date, a number of SNPs in the human
corin gene have been identified. Two non-synonymous
SNPs (T555I/Q568P) in a minor corin allele have been
found to be more common in African Americans than
Caucasians and are associated with an increased risk for
hypertension and an enhanced cardiac hypertrophic
response to high blood pressure. Patients with this allele
had a greater left ventricular mass than that in control
patients with wild-type alleles but similar systolic blood
pressure. The finding of corin variants in African Americans suggests a potential role of corin in hypertension in
human and encourages more research to identify new
corin mutations that may cause essential hypertension [2].

The major site of ANP production is the human atrial
myocardium, with greater production from the right
atrium than the left. ANP mRNA is detectable in the
ventricular myocardial cells but is only 1–2% that of the
atria. The major stimulus for ANP secretion by atrial
myocyte is stretch, volume overload, and conditions that
increase cardiac preload and/or afterload, such as congestive heart failure (CHF). Other stimuli include primary
aldosteronism, the syndrome of inappropriate secretion of

antidiuretic hormone, and volume overload associated with renal failure and valvular heart disease. Uncomplicated essential hypertension does not increase the production of ANP; however, in the presence of congestive cardiac failure, ANP levels rise. Atrial tachycardia can increase ANP secretion in the absence of an elevation of atrial pressures. Multiple pharmacological agents can increase ANP secretion and include alpha and beta agonists, cholinergic agents, phorbol esters, calcium ionophores, and endothelin.

Mechanism of Action

Natriuretic peptides mediate their physiological effects through activation of three different cell surface receptors named natriuretic peptide receptor (NPR)-A, NPR-B, and NPR-C. ANP preferentially binds NPR-A and NPR-C. ANP has a higher affinity for NPR-A and NPR-C than that of BNP. NPR-B is only weakly sensitive to ANP and BNP. NPR-A and NPR-B are single transmembrane-spanning proteins coupled to cyclic guanylate monophosphate (cGMP)-dependent signaling cascades. NPR-C, also known as clearance receptor, is a single transmembrane-spanning receptor that is devoid of guanylyl cyclase activity. NPR-C contains a very short 37-amino acid cytoplasmic tail that bears no homology to the cytoplasmic domains of the other two natriuretic peptide receptors. Activation of NPR-C couples through Gi protein-mediated inhibition of adenylate cyclase. All three natriuretic peptides bind to this receptor in the order of ANP > CNP > BNP. Binding of peptides to NPR-C leads to internalization and lysosomal degradation of the peptide.

NPR-A is most abundant in large blood vessels, kidney, heart, adrenals, and to a lesser extent in brain. NPR-B appears to be localized solely to neuronally derived tissue such as brain, pituitary, and adrenal medulla. NPR-C is the most widely and abundantly expressed natriuretic peptide receptor and is located in several tissues, including vascular endothelium, kidney, heart, adrenal gland, and smooth muscle.

Clearance of ANP

ANP has a short half-life of 1–3 min and high total body clearance. Clearance of ANP involves two main pathways and the relative clinical significance of each mechanism versus another remains controversial [3]. The first important mechanism involves the aforementioned clearance receptor, NPR-C. Peptide-NPR-C complex endocytose within target cells where lysosomes degrade peptide. Unoccupied NPR-C returns to plasma membrane to sequester further peptide ligands. NPR-C knockout mice are characterized, in part, by prolonged half-life of exogenous ANP. NPR-C knockout mice have a reduced ability to clear exogenous ANP and are hypotensive.

Another important mechanism of clearance of ANP involves proteolytic cleavage in the circulation. A circulating metallopeptidase known as neutral endopeptidase 24.11 (NEP 24.11) hydrolyses the natriuretic peptides. NEP 24.11 is widely distributed on the surface of endothelial cells, smooth muscle cells, cardiac myocytes, fibroblasts, and the brush border membranes of the renal proximal tubules. NEP inhibitors increase the half-life of ANP both in vivo and in vitro, however, NEP knockout mice do not exhibit increased natriuretic peptide function. Renal clearance of ANP has been described, but plays a minor role in the elimination of ANP from the circulation.

Dosage

There have been multiple clinical trials involving the experimental use of ANP and its synthetic analogs. In these trials, doses of synthetic human ANP ranged from 0.01 to 0.1 µg/kg/min. Infusions durations varied from 3 h to 5 days. In general, low-dose ANP is well tolerated with adverse events reported only at the higher doses. Anaritide infusions range from 0.05 to 0.20 µg/kg/min. Urodilatin has been infused at a rate of 20–40 ng/kg/min for 7 h to 6 days.

Adverse Reactions

The hemodynamic effects of natriuretic peptides have been widely investigated in both healthy volunteers and in patients with various cardiavascular conditions. ANP and its synthetic analogs are generally well tolerated. Hypotension is the most commonly encountered adverse event. In a 6-year prospective open label registry of 3,777 patients with acute heart failure treated with carperitide, the incidence of adverse events was 16.9%, the most frequent being hypotension (9.5%), which resolved spontaneously in 96% of patients. Other documented adverse events of ANP include disturbances of renal function (3.2%), serum electrolyte disturbances (3.0%), and liver function derangement (2.8%) [4].

In one meta-analysis, involving 1,861 participants, low-dose ANP was not associated with any significant adverse events, including hypotension. The incidence rates of hypotension, arrhythmias (premature ventricular contractions and ventricular tachycardia), and change in serum creatinine were increased in the ANP treatment group when compared with the control group when high-dose ANP was used. In contrast, the incidence of hypotension and other adverse events were eliminated when low doses of ANP or analog were used [5].

Physiologic Effects of ANP

The spectrum of bioactivities for ANP and its analogs continues to be illustrated in both human clinical investigations and animal disease models. ANP mediates physiological effects ranging from diuresis, a reduction in blood volume and therefore a reduction in cardiac output and systemic blood pressure. Renal sodium reabsorption is reduced and the overall effect of ANP on the body is to counter increases in blood pressure and volume caused by the renin–angiotensin system. Other physiological effects of ANP range from effects on lipolysis, endochondral ossification, and inhibition of cardiac hypertrophy and remodeling.

Renal Effects

ANP increases glomerular hydrostatic pressure by dilating afferent arterioles while constricting efferent arterioles and relaxes glomerular mesangial cells. This effect increases glomerular filtration rate (GFR), resulting in greater delivery of sodium and water to the tubules for excretion. The hormone blocks the tubular reabsorption of sodium and chloride. ANP promotes vasorelaxation, increases endothelial permeability, causes antagonism of the renin–angiotensin system by inhibition of renin secretion, reduces aldosterone secretion by the adrenal cortex, redistributes renal medullary blood flow, disrupts tubuloglomerular feedback, and reverses endothelin-induced vasoconstriction. The overall physiological effect of ANP is to drive diuresis and natriuresis and promote hemoconcentration. ANP has been shown to improve renal function by increasing glomerular filtration and urinary output. The clinical utility of ANP and its analogs in the prevention and treatment of AKI is discussed in more detail below.

Vascular Effects

ANP relaxes vascular smooth muscle cells in arterioles and venules and thereby lowers systemic blood pressure and cardiac output. Secondary effects of ANP on blood pressure may also be achieved through natriuresis and diuresis and other aforementioned renal effects. These effects on blood pressure control are mediated via activation of the NPR-A receptor and elevation of vascular smooth muscle cGMP. ANP null mice or mice lacking NPR-A receptor have elevated systolic blood pressure, whereas ANP overexpression results in hypotension. The hypertension in ANP null mice is sensitive to high dietary salts,

indicating that ANP may play a role in regulating response to salt in vivo.

Effects on Cardiac Hypertrophy and Remodeling

It is not surprising that the natriuretic peptide system, with actions that decrease blood pressure and blood volume, would also have antihypertrophic properties. However, there is an increasing body of evidence to suggest that ANP and more specifically NPR-A plays a local growth inhibitory role in cardiac hypertrophy. Mice lacking NPR-A have marked cardiac hypertrophy and chamber dilation disproportionate to their increased blood pressure suggesting the NPR-A system moderates the cardiac response to hypertrophic stimuli. Transgenic overexpression of ANP causes a decrease in heart weight and prevents right ventricular hypertrophy induced by pulmonary hypertension. In vitro, ANP inhibits norepinephrine, angiotensin II, and endothelin-1 induced hypertrophy in rat cardiac myocytes via a cGMP-dependent pathway. Mice lacking BNP do not display increased cardiac hypertrophy, although they do develop cardiac fibrosis, suggesting a role for role for BNP in cardiac remodeling.

Effects on Lipolysis

The natriuretic peptide system seems to play an important role in lipid metabolism, possibly affecting the pathophysiology of obesity and obesity-related disorders, such hypertension. Intravenous ANP infusion is followed by plasma NEFA and glycerol concentration increase (reflecting lipid mobilization). Human fat cell lipolysis was, until recently, thought to be mediated exclusively by a cAMP-dependent protein kinase (PKA)-regulated pathway under the control of catecholamines and insulin. ANP mediates lipolysis in human fat cells via the NPR-A through a cGMP-dependent protein kinase (PKG) signaling pathway independent of cAMP production and PKA activity. Reduced plasma levels of natriuretic peptides have been reported in obese patients especially those with hypertension. Further studies, however, are needed to completely establish the mechanisms involved in ANP-induced lipolysis and true clinical relevance of this new pathway.

Application

The two most widely studied synthetic analogs of ANP are anaritide and carperitide. Anaritide is a synthetic 25-amino acid peptide lacking the first three amino-terminal residues and has similar activities to the mature

28-amino acid peptide. Carperitide is a synthetic 28-amino acid peptide.

Initial studies using ANP and its synthetic analogs in healthy human subjects have demonstrated natriuretic, diuretic, hemoconcentration, and blood pressure lowering effects. However, the hemodynamic and renal effects of ANP in congestive heart failure (CHF) patients have been rather disappointing, with only modest effects on sodium excretion and changes in urine volume. There appears to be a marked attenuation of the renal and hemoconcentrating responses to ANP in CHF patients. Although initially considered to be a state of ANP deficiency, it has become evident that plasma levels of ANP are frequently elevated in patients with CHF and positively correlated with the severity of cardiac failure, such that the highest reported concentrations of ANP in the circulation are found in CHF. In patients and dogs with CHF, ANP is a weak counter regulatory hormone, insufficient to overcome the substantial systemic and regional vasoconstriction mediated by the SNS, RAAS, and AVP. However, despite the blunted renal response to ANP in CHF, elimination of this peptide by antibody blockade or antagonism of NPR-A further decreases sodium excretion and urine flow. Furthermore, blockade of the natriuretic system in CHF removes the inhibitory effect of ANP on the actions of angiotensin II. Therefore, the increase in natriuretic peptides is still considered an important adaptive or compensatory mechanism aimed at reducing peripheral vascular resistance and maintaining effective blood volume regulation in overt CHF.

The renal hyporesponsiveness to ANP and its analogs in CHF patients has not been well delineated, but potential explanations include downregulation of natriuretic peptide receptors in the kidney, increased activity of NEP, reduced production or increased degradation of cGMP, increased renal sympathetic activity, or hyperaldosteronism and reduced distal sodium delivery.

In the USA, anaritide or carperitide is currently not licensed for use in CHF. Nevertheless, in 1995, caperitide was launched in Japan for use in congestive cardiac failure. The clinical utility of carperitide as a first-line agent in the treatment of acute decompensated cardiac failure was demonstrated in a prospective observational study (COMPASS study). Of 1,832 patients enrolled in this uncontrolled study, 1,254 patients (83.2%) had symptomatic recovery in the acute phase of acute decompensated heart failure using carperitide monotherapy [4].

Multiple clinical trials exploring the therapeutic potential of ANP or one of its synthetic analogs in the prevention or treatment of AKI have been conducted [5]. Many of these studies showed conflicting results, which may be explained in part by the different doses of ANP (high versus low), clinical setting (medical versus surgical), type of analog used, and whether AKI was established or not (treatment versus prevention).

In a pilot study, anaritide increased creatinine clearance and reduced the need for renal replacement therapy in patients with established acute renal failure, without improving overall patient survival [6]. This small pilot study was performed subsequently led to two large randomized, placebo-controlled trials [7, 8], in which anaritide ultimately failed to improve the overall rate of dialysis-free survival in hospitalized patients with established AKI of various etiologies. However, preplanned subgroup analysis of the initial large trial in patients with acute tubular necrosis by Allgren and colleagues found that anaritide did improve dialysis-free survival in patients with oliguria (27% in anaritide treatment group, 8% in the placebo group) [7]. Conversely, in patients with nonoliguric AKI, anaritide apparently worsened dialysis-free survival (59% in placebo group, 48% in anaritide treatment group). It was also found that the incidence of hypotesion was higher in the patients who did not have oliguria than those who did. This finding raised the possibility that anaritide therapy may have resulted in decreased renal perfusion and further ischemic injury in the patients without oliguria, thus worsening renal function. This hypothesis was further tested in another prospective trial, restricted to patients with acute tubular necrosis and oliguria, performed by Lewis and colleagues [8]. In this randomized, double blind, placebo-controlled trial, 222 patients with oliguric acute renal failure were randomized to treatment with a 24-h infusion of anaride (0.2 μg/kg/min) or placebo. The dialysis-free survival in the Anaritide group was 21% group and 15% in the placebo group ($P = 0.22$). Thus, there was no beneficial effect of Anaritide on dialysis-free survival in patients with oliguric acute renal failure. Of note, a significantly greater proportion (95%) of patients in Anaritide treatment group developed hypotension (systolic blood pressure of less than 90 mmHg) compared to the placebo group (55%) [8]. Taken together, these relatively large trials confirmed that dose-dependent hypotension caused by Anaritide limits its clinical utility, even in oliguric patients, and should be avoided in future AKI trials.

In a small randomized controlled pilot study by Sward et al. 2004, high-risk patients undergoing cardiopulmonary bypass who developed rise in serum creatinine >50% from baseline and circulatory shock requiring inotropes were randomized to low-dose recombinant human ANP (50 ng/kg/min) or placebo [9]. Human ANP significantly enhanced creatinine clearance in contrast to placebo: 21% of patients in the hANP group compared with 47% in the placebo group needed dialysis within 21 days (hazard ratio 0.28; $p = 0.009$). Thus, it appears that the use of low-dose ANP early in the course of AKI may be more beneficial than prior approaches.

Similarly, in a prophylaxis trial, Mitaka et al. 2008 randomized 40 patients undergoing open abdominal aortic aneurysm repair to either human ANP (0.01–0.05 μg/kg/min) or placebo for 48 h, beginning immediately before cross-clamp [10]. Serum concentrations of creatinine and blood urea nitrogen were significantly lower and urine volume and creatinine clearance were significantly higher in the hANP group than in the placebo group. In addition, urinary NAG/creatinine ratio was also significantly lower in the hANP group than in the placebo group. The patients in this study were administered low-dose hANP at 0.01–0.05 μg/kg/min and the infusion was commenced during the operation and continued for 48 h. Overall, these results indicate that intraoperative and postoperative infusion of hANP at a low dose (0.01–0.05 μg/kg/min for 48 h) preserved renal function in patients undergoing abdominal aortic aneurysm repair. This study raises the potential role for prophylactic hANP infusion to improve perioperative renal function and outcomes in patients undergoing aortic occlusive surgery [10].

It is difficult to make any definitive statement about the role of ANP and its analogs in AKI. The randomized controlled trials discussed above have shown inconsistent effects for renal endpoints. In 2008, a comprehensive meta-analysis of current literature concerning ANP in adults with or at risk for AKI [5]. Many of the earlier clinical trials were underpowered and excluded for lack of randomization or a control group. The meta-analysis finally identified 19 eligible studies that included 1,861 participants. The authors pooled analysis of 11 prevention trials and 8 treatment trials of AKI. For the prevention of AKI, ANP used in low doses was well tolerated and may be associated with some improvement in clinical outcomes (requirement of renal replacement therapy, lengths of ICU stay, and hospitalization). Beneficial effects were most prominent in the post-cardiac surgery setting. Overall, however, ANP therapy (particularly in high doses) for established AKI, was not associated with any significant clinical benefits, and was associated with hypotension and other adverse effects [5].

In summary, further high-quality studies are required to make a definitive statement regarding the efficacy and effectiveness of ANP in the management of AKI. Particular attention must be paid to the selection and perhaps titration of the dose of ANP used to minimize adverse effects and maximize beneficial effects on renal perfusion and function in AKI. Further large clinical studies are needed to investigate the apparent beneficial effects of ANP on renal function in perioperative patients undergoing cardiovascular surgery and in other settings.

References

1. Potter RP, Yoder AR, Flora DR et al (2009) Natriuretic peptides: their structures, receptors, physiologica functions and therapeutic applications. Handb Exp Pharmacol 191:341–366
2. Zhou Y, Jiang J, Cui Y et al (2009) Corin, atrial natriuretic peptide and hypertension. Nephrol Dial Transplant 24:1071–1073
3. Candace LYW, Burnett JC (2007) Natriuretic peptides and therapeutic applications. Heart Fail Rev 12:131–142
4. Nomura F, Kurobe N, Mori Y et al (2008) Multicenter prospective investigation on efficacy and safety of carperitide as a first-line drug for acute heart failure syndrome with preserved blood pressure COMPASS: carperitide effects observed through monitoring dyspnea in acute decompensated heart failure study. Circ J 72(11):1777–1786
5. Nigwekar SU, Navaneethan SD, Parikh CR et al (2009) Atrial natriuretic peptide for management of acute kidney injury: a systematic review and meta-analysis. J Am Soc Nephrol 4(2):261–272
6. Rahman SN, Kim GE, Mathew AS, Goldberg CA, Allgren R, Schrier RW, Conger JD (1994) Effects of atrial natriuretic peptide in clinical acute renal failure. Kidney Int 45(6):1731–1738
7. Allgren RL, Marbury TC, Rahman SN et al (1997) Anaritide in acute tubular necrosis. New Engl J Med 336:828–834
8. Lewis J, Salem MM, Chertow GM et al (2000) Atrial natriuretic factor in oliguric acute renal failure. Anaritide acute renal failure study group. Am J Kidney Dis 36:767–774
9. Sward K, Valsson F, Odencrants P et al (2004) Recombinant human atrial natriuretic peptide in ischemic acute renal failure: a randomized placebo-controlled trial. Crit Care Med 32:1310–1315
10. Mitaka C, Kudo T, Jibiki M et al (2008) Effects of human atrial natriuretic peptide on renal function in patients undergoing abdominal aortic aneurysm repair. Crit Care Med 36(3):745–751

Anterior Scalene Syndrome

▶ Thoracic Outlet

Anterior Spinal Cord Syndrome

▶ Spinal Cord Injury Syndromes

Anthozoa

▶ Jellyfish Envenomation

Anthrax

CAITLIN W. HICKS[1,2], PETER Q. EICHACKER[3]
[1]Cleveland Clinic Lerner College of Medicine, Cleveland, OH, USA
[2]Howard Hughes Medical Institute–National Institutes of Health Research Scholar, National Institutes of Health, Bethesda, MD, USA
[3]Critical Care Medicine Department, Clinical Center, National Institutes of Health, Bethesda, MD, USA

Synonyms

Anthrax pneumonia; Bacillus anthracis infection; Ragpicker's disease; Ragsorter's disease; Woolsorter's disease; Woolsorter's pneumonia

Definition

Anthrax infection is caused by *Bacillus anthracis*, a large, gram-positive bacterium that exists in either a dormant spore or actively replicating vegetative rod form. The spore is found in soil around the world although active disease is more common in warmer and wetter locations. Infection occurs most commonly in herbivore mammals, either domestic or wild (e.g., cattle, sheep, goats, camels, antelopes, and other herbivores) that ingest spores during grazing.

Anthrax infection in humans is caused when *B. anthracis* spores enter the body through the skin, are ingested by eating contaminated meat, or are inhaled, resulting in cutaneous, gastrointestinal, or inhalational anthrax, respectively [1]. Human infections normally result from contact with contaminated animals or animal products; there are no known cases of human-to-human transmission [2]. For cutaneous and gastrointestinal anthrax, low-level germination occurs when endospores reach a primary site in the subcutaneous layer or gastrointestinal mucosa, respectively, leading to local edema and necrosis. Remaining endospores are phagocytosed by local macrophages, which migrate to regional lymph node. Vegetative anthrax bacilli grow in the lymph node, creating regional hemorrhagic lymphadenitis. Bacteria then spread through the blood and lymph, proliferate and produce high levels of exotoxin that appear largely responsible for organ injury and eventual death. In a small number of cases, systemic anthrax can lead to meningeal involvement by means of lymphatic or hematogenous spread [3]. For inhalational anthrax, endospores enter alveolar spaces where they are phagocytosed by macrophages and transported to mediastinal lymph nodes.

Vegetative forms develop, replicate, and again cause hemorrhagic lymphadenitis. While this mediastinal lymph node involvement serves as a source of systemic bacterial spread and toxin production, it also produces lymphatic obstruction, parenchymal edema, and pleural effusions. Death results from septicemia, toxemia, or pulmonary complications as a result of the action of exotoxin secreted by anthrax bacilli [2].

Two virulence factors, a capsule and toxin production, play a primary role in the pathogenesis of anthrax infection. The capsule consists of poly D-glutamic acid and contributes to pathogenicity by enabling the vegetative bacterial form to evade the host-immune defenses (i.e., it is antiphagocytic) and provoke septicemia. The bacteria also produces three proteins (protective antigen (PA), lethal factor (LF), and edema factor (EF)) that makeup the bacteria's two exotoxins: lethal toxin (LeTx) and edema toxin (ETX). These toxins are binary or A-B type toxins. Protective antigen is the B component that initiates cell binding and uptake of either of the two toxigenic or A components, LF and EF. Lethal factor is a zinc metalloprotease that inactivates mitogen-activated protein kinase kinase and causes lysis of macrophages in vitro [4]. While LF has been demonstrated to inhibit important host cell functions (e.g., innate and adaptive immunity and apoptosis) how it contributes to death associated with LeTx is unclear [5]. Edema factor is a calmodulin-dependent adenyl cyclase that increases cellular cAMP concentration and impairs host defenses, including inhibition of phagocytosis [4]. It causes edema when injected subcutaneously into experimental animals.

The relative ease with which anthrax can be grown in the laboratory and spread environmentally, along with its virulence, has made it a potential weapon of bioterrorism [5]. It is also worth noting that a new syndrome of anthrax associated with soft tissue infection is just now coming to light based on a recent outbreak in the United Kingdom [16].

Treatment

Active Infection

Treatment of anthrax must be considered in the context of those patients with likely or diagnosed active disease and of those who have potentially been exposed but do not yet demonstrate clinical symptoms. Of those patients with diagnosed active disease, treatment recommendations differ depending on which stage of the disease is present (i.e., stage 1 (mild disease) versus stage 2 (disease with shock and respiratory failure)). For patients affected with stage 1 active inhalational anthrax, the CDC recommends IV treatment with ciprofloxacin or doxycycline and one or two additional antimicrobials [6]. Initial therapy may be altered based on the clinical course of the patient; one or two oral antimicrobials may be adequate as the patient improves. IV and oral antimicrobial treatment should be continued for a period of no less than 60 days. The treatment regimens for stage 1 gastrointestinal or oropharyngeal anthrax are the same as those recommended for stage 1 inhalational anthrax [6].

For patients affected with stage 2 active inhalational anthrax, IV ciprofloxacin is recommended over doxycycline as the primary antimicrobial agent unless ciprofloxacin use is contraindicated [7]. This is mainly because fluoroquinolones are bactericidal whereas tetracyclines are bacteriostatic. Ciprofloxacin is also favored over doxycycline because meningeal involvement is likely in systemic anthrax cases, and CNS penetration of ciprofloxacin in the presence of meningeal inflammation is much higher than the poor CNS penetration of doxycycline. In addition to ciprofloxacin, at least 1 or more additional agents with adequate CNS penetration and in vitro activity against B. anthracis (e.g., ampicillin or penicillin, meropenem, rifampin, or vancomycin) should be used in the treatment of systemic cases of anthrax regardless of clinical suspicion of meningeal involvement. Clindamycin is strongly recommended for inclusion in the antimicrobial regimen because of its potential ability to inhibit protein synthesis, which may reduce exotoxin production [7]. As with stage 1 disease, patients affected with stage 2 inhalational anthrax should follow a 60-day course of antimicrobial therapy, with adjustment of the regimen to treatment with oral antimicrobials based on the clinical course of the disease in the patient [6]. The treatment regimens for stage 2 gastrointestinal or oropharyngeal anthrax are the same as those recommended for stage 2 inhalational anthrax [6].

Patients affected with localized or uncomplicated cases of naturally acquired cutaneous anthrax should be treated with oral ciprofloxacin or doxycycline for 60 days [6]; previous guidelines have suggested treating cutaneous anthrax for 7–10 days, but 60 days is now recommended given the likelihood of exposure to aerosolized B. anthracis [8]. Oral amoxicillin is an option for completion of therapy following clinical improvement, since penicillin has been shown to render cutaneous anthrax lesions culture-negative within 24 h, and has long been the treatment of choice in many parts of the world [7]. For severe cases of cutaneous anthrax with signs of systemic involvement, extensive edema, or lesions on the head or neck, IV therapy using a multidrug approach is recommended [6].

Aside from antimicrobial therapy, there are a number of adjunctive interventions that may be applicable for treating active anthrax disease. These include postexposure administration of anthrax vaccine to accelerate active immunity to the bacteria or its toxin, agents designed to directly inhibit anthrax toxins, and thoracentesis to improve respiratory mechanics and remove a potential reservoir of anthrax toxin.

Anthrax vaccine adsorbed, AVA (BioThrax; BioPort Corporation, Lansing, MI, USA), is an aluminum hydroxide–precipitated preparation of PA from attenuated, nonencapsulated B. anthracis cultures of the Sterne strain that has been used in the USA. The current UK-licensed anthrax vaccine (anthrax vaccine precipitated, AVP) produced by the Health Protection Agency (HPA; Porton Down, UK) is similarly composed of alum-precipitated PA from the Sterne strain of B. anthracis, along with a much smaller amount of LF.

Researchers are becoming increasingly aware of the importance of toxin production in the pathogenesis of anthrax, leading to an increasing interest in developing immunoglobulin-based therapies directed at these bacterial components. In the USA, two preparations have received considerable attention and have actually been purchased or contracted for by federal agencies. One is an immunoglobulin preparation derived from individuals previously vaccinated with AVA vaccine, known as anthrax immune globulin (AIG) (Emergent BioSolutions Inc., Rockville, MD, USA). Treatment with this preparation in two recent cases of life-threatening inhalational anthrax infection was associated with a successful outcome in one, although not the other. There is presently a supply of this antibody available from the CDC under an Investigational New Drug protocol for the treatment of patients with confirmed life-threatening anthrax. The second preparation receiving recent attention is a human monoclonal antibody generated against recombinant PA, raxibacumab (ABthrax) and produced by Human Genome Sciences (HGS; Rockville, MD, USA). Administration of raxibacumab has been shown to be safe in uninfected humans. In April 2009, HGS completed the delivery of 20,000 doses of Raxibacumab to the US Strategic National Stockpile. In July 2009, HGS received a second order for 45,000 doses of raxibacumab from the US Government, to be delivered over a period of 3 years beginning near the end of 2009.

In addition to AVA based and raxibacumab, there are other antibody-based preparations directed at PA, LF, and EF that have been proposed as potential anthrax treatments and are now under study. Finally, there are a variety of non-antibody-based therapies designed to inhibit anthrax toxin function that have shown promise in in vitro and in vivo studies but which are too extensive to review here [5].

Several lines of evidence suggest that continued chest drainage or intermittent thoracentesis may be important in the management of inhalational anthrax cases. This intervention appeared effective in patients during the 2001 inhalational anthrax outbreak and in the more recent 2006 case. In this latter case, analysis of serial samples showed high pleural fluid lethal toxin levels, and the case's positive outcome has been attributed to a combination of improved mechanical effects on respiration from fluid drainage as well a reduction in lethal toxin levels. Evaluation of the treatment of inhalational anthrax cases from 1900 to 2005 has also suggested that pleural fluid drainage may be associated with decreased mortality [3].

Glucocorticoids have also been considered as possible adjunctive therapy for patients with serious systemic illness due to inhalation anthrax, including anthrax patients with meningoencephalitis and patients with extensive edema involving the head and neck. A retrospective review of 70 cases of anthrax meningoencephalitis from 1966 to 2002 reported a 14% decrease in overall mortality among patients treated with glucocorticoids as an adjunct to antimicrobial therapy, though it is not possible to draw conclusions from such a small study. It has also been shown that at very low concentrations, LeTx represses glucocorticoid receptor transactivation in both a cellular system and animal model, further suggesting that glucocorticoids may have therapeutic value in anthrax patients. However in this latter study, treatment with dexamethasone treatment was not beneficial in toxin-challenged animals.

Patients presenting with anthrax infection and shock should be treated aggressively with the same type of hemodynamic support utilized for septic shock due to other types of bacterial infection [9]. It must be noted, however, that it is currently unknown how the vascular effects of LeTx and ETx might alter responsiveness to conventional hemodynamic support [5]. Recent research suggests that during anthrax infection and shock, both conventional hemodynamic support and toxin-directed agents may be necessary for optimal outcome.

Postexposure Prophylaxis

Historically, penicillin has been the preferred treatment for anthrax since most naturally occurring B. anthracis strains are sensitive to it [9]. However, penicillin resistance has been found in some naturally occurring strains possibly due to the low antibiotic levels achieved in pulmonary secretions, tissues, and alveolar macrophages with oral agents. Based on this observation, participants at

a recent CDC conference on anthrax postexposure prophylaxis (PEP) recommended treatment with ciprofloxacin or doxycycline as equivalent first-line antimicrobial agents [7].

In addition to the recommendation for 60 days of oral antimicrobial therapy as PEP following potential inhalation exposure to aerosolized B. anthracis, the CDC also calls for treatment with a 3-dose series of AVA administered at time zero, 2 weeks, and 4 weeks. In order to maximize the benefits of the vaccine, it should be offered within 10 days of exposure. In 2008, the CDC's Advisory Committee on Immunization Practices (ACIP) recommended the use of AVA for both pregnant and lactating women exposed to aerosolized B. anthracis spores, as well as the consideration of vaccine use among children exposed to B. anthracis spores.

Preexposure Prophylaxis

The AVA has been licensed by the FDA since 1970 for the preexposure prophylaxis against inhalational anthrax in persons at risk of acquiring the disease occupationally, including members of the US armed forces, woolen mill workers, laboratory workers, and veterinarians [10]. The vaccine can be administered to healthy individuals aged 18–65 years, and has a dosage schedule that requires vaccination subcutaneously at 0, 2, and 4 weeks and 6, 12, and 18 months. Yearly boosters are given to maintain immunity [11].

Evaluation/Assessment

The determination of individual patient exposure to B. anthracis on the basis of environmental testing is complex due to the uncertain specificity and sensitivity of rapid field tests and the difficulty of assessing individual risks of exposure. In 2001, the CDC developed interim case definitions for anthrax. A confirmed case was defined as a clinically compatible one that was laboratory confirmed by the isolation of B. anthracis from the patient, or by laboratory evidence based on at least two supportive tests employing nonculture detection methods [12]. B. anthracis can be isolated from numerous clinical samples, including blood, skin lesion exudates, cerebrospinal fluid (CSF), pleural fluid, sputum, and feces. In systemic infections, organisms can easily be cultured from the blood if the sample is collected prior to antimicrobial therapy. Anthrax should immediately be considered if Gram's stain of specimens reveals high concentrations of gram-positive bacilli growing in chains.

Because of the infection's rapid progression, clinical or laboratory suspicion of anthrax should be followed by expeditious testing of clinical samples and early initiation of antibiotic therapy. Isolates suspected to be *B. anthracis* should be sent to a Laboratory Response Network (LRN) reference laboratory for identification and characterization and local or state health departments should be notified. While most clinical laboratories do not have the experience or facilities required to identify *B. anthracis*, LRN laboratories have the testing capability for the specific and rapid identification of the bacteria. These tests include susceptibility to gamma phage lysis, an LRN real-time PCR assay, a direct fluorescent assay (DFA), and a time-resolved fluorescent assay (TRF) for specific detection of *B. anthracis* antigens. A commercially available immunochromatographic test, the Redline Alert (Tetracore, Inc.), which tests nonhemolytic Bacillus isolates cultured on sheep blood agar, has also been approved by the US Food and Drug Administration (FDA) for the presumptive identification of *B. anthracis* isolates.

Patients with inhalational anthrax that has progressed are typically found to have mediastinal adenopathy and hemorrhagic pleural effusions [3]. Anthrax infection is unusual in that mediastinal changes can be detected relatively early in the course of infection by chest radiography, although similar findings may be found with *Histoplasma capsulatum* [2].

Effectiveness

B. anthracis is highly susceptible to a variety of antimicrobial agents including penicillin, chloramphenicol, tetracycline, erythromycin, streptomycin, and fluoroquinolones. It is not susceptible to cephalosporins or trimethoprim-sulfamethoxazole and these agents should not be used for treatment of active disease. If taken, antibiotics are effective at preventing people in the incubation stage or early disease stage from proceeding to later stages, but generally do not prevent people in the intermediate or fulminant stages from disease progression or death.

Data from animal studies provides evidence that postexposure vaccination with AVA can shorten the duration of antibiotic prophylaxis required to protect against inhalational anthrax, and may impact public health management of a bioterrorism event. Infected individuals presenting with symptomatic inhalational anthrax who are treated, recover, and seroconvert may not require 60 days of antibiotic therapy, as recommended by the current guidelines, although additional research is warranted.

Tolerance

Historically, penicillin has been the preferred treatment for anthrax since most naturally occurring *B. anthracis* strains are sensitive to it [9]. However, penicillin resistance

has been found in some naturally occurring strains possibly due to the low antibiotic levels achieved in pulmonary secretions, tissues, and alveolar macrophages with oral agents. Based on this observation, participants at a recent CDC conference on anthrax postexposure prophylaxis (PEP) recommended treatment with ciprofloxacin and doxycycline as equivalent first-line antimicrobial agents [7].

Studies on the safety of four lots of the AVA, involving approximately 16,000 doses administered to approximately 7,000 participants were submitted by the Centers for Disease Control and Prevention, in support of licensure of the vaccine [13]. Mild reactions (e.g., erythema ≤ 3 cm) were reported in up to 20% of recipients, but more moderate (>3 cm to <12 cm) and severe (≥ 12 cm) reactions occurred in less than 3% and 1% of cases, respectively. Systemic reactions, reported in four individuals ($<0.06\%$), consisted of fever, chills, nausea, and general body aches, and were transient. Therefore the risks associated with anthrax immunization are much less than those associated with no intervention, indicating that vaccination should be strongly considered in populations at high risk of disease.

Pharmacoeconomics

Public health planners are uncertain how the anthrax vaccine should be used as part of a comprehensive strategy for addressing the bioterrorism threats posed by *B. anthracis*. There is a great deal of debate as to whether the general population should be immunized against *B. anthracis*, or whether the vaccine should only be used as a postexposure prophylaxis. In an effort to solve this debate, a number of theoretical models have been created that analyze cost effectiveness and overall mortality that would result from preexposure vaccination versus postexposure vaccination versus no vaccination. In general, postexposure vaccination along with appropriate antibiotic therapy has been found to be the most cost-effective response compared with other strategies [14]. However, the validity of these findings depends on many factors, including the safety and efficacy of prolonged antibiotic prophylaxis, adherence to antibiotic regimens, the time delay before postexposure antibiotic prophylaxis is initiated, and vaccine characteristics such as efficacy, safety, and time to achieve immunity.

In addition, these models make assumptions that there would be adequate supplies of antibiotics and anthrax vaccine available, and that all exposed persons needing postexposure prophylaxis could be identified. In reality, these assumptions may not prove reasonable, and thus disease prevention rates may be overestimated.

This is particularly true in the event of a large bioterrorism attack.

After-care

Patients with an alleged exposure to anthrax should be started on antibiotic treatment and a schedule of AVA immunization as recommended by the CDC, and instructed to follow up with their primary care physician if they experience new and/or rapidly worsening dry cough, difficulty breathing, fever, chills, weakness (typically severe and beginning 1–2 days after exposure), or a new skin ulcer with a black center surrounded by swelling (typically appearing on the hands, feet, face, or neck and beginning within days to 1 week after exposure).

There are no data to suggest that patient-to-patient transmission or person-to-person transmission of anthrax occurs. Therefore while standard barrier precautions are recommended for all hospitalized anthrax patients, the use of barrier precautions are not indicated and there is no need to immunize or provide PEP to healthcare workers or household contacts. However, contact isolation precautions should be used for patients with draining cutaneous anthrax lesions. Human and animal remains infected with *B. anthracis* should be cremated rather than buried to prevent any further spread of disease [9].

Prognosis

Cutaneous anthrax has accounted for 95% of all anthrax infections in the USA [15]. While the course of cutaneous anthrax is often self-limited, antibiotic treatment is recommended to decrease the likelihood of systemic disease. Without antibiotic therapy, mortality due to malignant edema (characterized by severe edema, induration, multiple bullae, and symptoms of shock) has been reported to be as high as 20%. With appropriate antibiotic treatment, death due to cutaneous anthrax is rare [15].

While the cutaneous form of anthrax is typically diagnosed early and therefore treated relatively easily, the gastrointestinal and inhalational forms are much more insidious, with early symptoms that are mild and similar to gastroenteritis or an upper respiratory tract infection. As a result, early diagnosis of these forms of anthrax is difficult and the disease can abruptly develop into a systemic form resistant to treatment and rapidly fatal. The mortality rate with gastrointestinal anthrax can approach 100% [2]. Morbidity is due to blood loss, fluid and electrolyte imbalances, and subsequent shock. Death results from intestinal perforation or anthrax toxemia. In the rare case in which a patient does survive, most symptoms subside in 10–14 days.

In the twentieth-century series of US cases on anthrax infection, the mortality rate of occupationally acquired inhalational anthrax was 89%, but the majority of these cases occurred before the development of critical care units and, in most cases, before the advent of antibiotics. However, the mortality rate in patients in the 2001 US outbreak who had developed shock was still very high. Up to half of patients with inhalational anthrax develop hemorrhagic meningitis with concomitant meningismus, delirium, and obtundation. In these cases, cyanosis and hypotension progress rapidly, with death occurring within hours [9].

References

1. Holty JE, Kim RY, Bravata DM (2006) Anthrax: a systematic review of atypical presentations. Ann Emerg Med 48(2):200–211
2. Dixon TC, Meselson M, Guillemin J et al (1999) Anthrax. N Engl J Med 341(11):815–826
3. Holty JE, Bravata DM, Liu H et al (2006) Systematic review: a century of inhalational anthrax cases from 1900 to 2005. Ann Intern Med 144 (4):270–280
4. Bradley KA, Mogridge J, Mourez M et al (2001) Identification of the cellular receptor for anthrax toxin. Nature 414(6860):225–229
5. Sherer K, Li Y, Cui X et al (2007) Lethal and edema toxins in the pathogenesis of *Bacillus anthracis* septic shock: implications for therapy. Am J Respir Crit Care Med 175(3):211–221
6. Centers for Disease Control and Prevention (2001) Update: investigation of bioterrorism-related anthrax and interim guidelines for exposure management and antimicrobial therapy, October 2001. JAMA 286(18):2226–2232
7. Stern EJ, Uhde KB, Shadomy SV et al (2008) Conference report on public health and clinical guidelines for anthrax. Emerg Infect Dis 14 (4):07–0969
8. Inglesby TV, Henderson DA, Bartlett JG et al (1999) Anthrax as a biological weapon: medical and public health management. Working group on civilian biodefense. JAMA 281 (18):1735–1745
9. Inglesby TV, O'Toole T, Henderson DA et al (2002) Anthrax as a biological weapon, 2002: updated recommendations for management. JAMA 287(17):2236–2252
10. Bartlett JG, Inglesby TV Jr, Borio L (2002) Management of anthrax. Clin Infect Dis 35(7):851–858
11. Friedlander AM, Pittman PR, Parker GW (1999) Anthrax vaccine: evidence for safety and efficacy against inhalational anthrax. JAMA 282(22):2104–2106
12. Centers for Disease Control and Prevention (CDC) (2001) Update: investigation of anthrax associated with intentional exposure and interim public health guidelines, October 2001. MMWR 50 (41):889–893
13. National Institutes of Health, Office of Public Health Preparedness, Centers for Disease Control and Prevention (2001) Optimizing post-exposure prevention of inhalation anthrax: issues and options. National Academy of Sciences, Washington, DC
14. Brookmeyer R, Johnson E, Bollinger R (2004) Public health vaccination policies for containing an anthrax outbreak. Nature 432 (7019):901–904
15. Tutrone WD, Scheinfeld NS, Weinberg JM (2002) Cutaneous anthrax: a concise review. Cutis 69(1):27–33
16. Booth MG, Hood J, Brooks TJ et al (2010) Anthrax infection in drug users. Lancet 375:1345–1346

Anthrax Pneumonia

▶ Anthrax

Anti-arrhythmic Therapy

S. Uddin[1], Susanna Price[2]
[1]Department of Intensive Care, King's College Hospital, London, UK
[2]Department of Intensive Care, Royal Brompton Hospital, London, UK

Definition

The term "arrhythmia" is derived from the Greek a-, loss + rhythmos, rhythm – meaning loss of rhythm and is used to describe any cardiac rhythm associated with abnormal myocardial contraction. These include:

- Tachyarrhythmias – greater than 100 bpm (adults)
- Bradyarrhythmias – less than 60 bpm (adults)
- Irregular rhythms – fibrillation, flutter, premature/ectopic contractions

Antiarrhythmic therapy is used to correct or control any pathological arrhythmias. Common pathological arrhythmias in the ICU are shown below:

Atrial fibrillation (AF)	Chapter X
Atrial flutter	Chapter Y
AV reentrant tachycardias	Chapter Y
AV node reentrant tachycardias	Chapter Y
Ventricular fibrillation (VF)	Chapter Z
Ventricular tachycardia (VT)	Chapter Z

Characteristics

Arrhythmias may be asymptomatic or an incidental finding when cardiac monitoring is in use, and may be demonstrated by an abrupt change in heart rate and/or blood pressure. In critically ill patients the incidence of arrhythmias is approximately 10% [1], with atrial dysrhythmias, in particular AF occurring more commonly in postoperative patients. The incidence of AF is up to 60% after cardiac surgery for valve disease and revascularisation [2]. Ventricular dysrhythmias are more commonly encountered in mixed medical and surgical critical care units with over a third associated with primary cardiac pathology. Whether these rhythm disturbances are clinically relevant or result in adverse outcomes is not entirely clear in the general medical ICU population; however post-cardiac surgery they are associated with increased morbidity and possibly mortality [3, 4]. Thus, the need for routine anti arrhythmic therapy is similarly unclear, however current clinical experience would suggest that any arrhythmia associated with hemodynamic instability or adverse clinical signs, requires urgent assessment and treatment – see Fig. 1. In the presence of cardiac arrest, patients should be managed according to the current ALS guidelines [5, 6].

It must be remembered that on occasion the arrhythmia may be part of an appropriate physiological response, for example, tachycardia in response to hypovolemia or sepsis, and first-line management therefore should be targeted at treating reversible and precipitating factors (Table 1). Similarly, a heart rate that would normally be considered within the normal range might be inappropriately slow for a critically ill patient, and be considered as a relative bradycardia. In all cases, associated risk factor for arrhythmia should be sought and corrected where possible (see relevant chapters). Specific antiarrhythmic therapy is only indicated if there is continued hemodynamic/cardiovascular disturbance despite correction of reversible factors (see table), or when a particularly pressing indication for restoration of normal sinus rhythm exists (e.g., in patients with a stenotic cardiac lesion, those with complex congenital heart disease, or patients with severely impaired ventricular function).

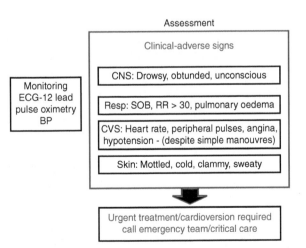

Anti-arrhythmic Therapy. Figure 1 Assessment algorithm for arrhythmia on the ICU. *ECG* electrocardiogram, *BP* blood pressure, *O₂* oxygen, *CNS* central nervous system, *RESP* respiratory system, *SOB* short of breath, *RR* respiratory rate, *CVS* cardiovascular system

Anti-arrhythmic Therapy. Table 1 Factors potentially contributing to arrhythmia on the ICU

Factor	Cause	Common clinical examples
Electrolytes	K$^+$, Mg^{++}, glucose, acidosis	Post surgery, bowel obstruction
Volume status	Hypovolemia or hypervolemia	Resuscitation, diarrhea, sepsis
Myocardial ischemia	Perfusion- revascularisation, mechanical support (IABP)	Prolonged arrhythmia in pre existing heart failure
	Hypoxia (hypercarbia)	Pneumonia
Temperature	Hypothermia or hyperthermia	Drowning
		Post-cardiac surgery
Pacemaker failure	Lead fracture	Post-cardiac surgery
	Antiarrhythmic drugs	
	Pacing generator failure	
↑Sympathetic drive	Pain, agitation	ICU admission
		Surgery
		Pain
		Anxiety

K$^+$ potassium ion, *Mg^{++}* magnesium ion, *IABP* intra-aortic balloon pump, *ICU* intensive care unit

Antiarrhythmic therapy can be divided into electrical or pharmacological methods, the selection of which depends upon the urgency for treatment, the arrhythmia, and the underlying cause. Electrical methods include defibrillation for VF (cardioversion for VT), cardioversion, overdrive/underdrive pacing, pacemaker implantation, and/or ablation.

Electrical Antiarrhythmic Therapy

Cardioversion is the delivery of energy that is synchronized to the QRS complex. Defibrillation is nonsynchronized delivery of energy, for example, the shock is delivered randomly during the cardiac cycle. Electrical cardioversion/defibrillation should generally be considered as first-line treatment in the management of unstable patients with cardiac arrhythmias [6] (Fig. 1). When considering the energy required, several factors are relevant including type of defibrillator, size of patient, recent cardiac/thoracic surgery, duration of arrhythmia, and type of arrhythmia. Modern biphasic defibrillators can successfully terminate arrhythmias at lower energies than older monophasic defibrillators. There is also emerging evidence that escalating energies on successive shocks may not be necessary when using biphasic defibrillators [7]. Complications of cardioversion/defibrillation include worsening arrhythmia, embolization, myocardial dysfunction, myocardial necrosis, hypotension, pulmonary edema, and skin erythema/burns. Cardioversion may be used for the treatment of atrial and ventricular tachycardia (see Chapters Table 2).

Anti-arrhythmic Therapy. Table 2 Indications for cardioversion/defibrillation

Treatment	Indication
DC cardioversion	Sustained monomorphic VT
	Fast AF, SVT with CVS compromise
Defibrillation	Ventricular fibrillation
Ablation	AVRT
	AV nodal reentrant tachycardia
	Atrial tachycardia
	Atrial flutter
	Idiopathic ventricular tachycardia
	Bundle branch entrant tachycardia

DC cardioversion, direct current cardioversion, *VT* ventricular tachycardia, *Fast AF* atrial fibrillation with a rapid ventricular response rate, *SVT* supraventricular tachycardia, *CVS* cardiovascular system, *AVRT* atrioventricular reentry tachycardia, *AV* atrioventricular

With increasing numbers of patients with heart failure undergoing treatment with device therapy (implantation of cardioverter-defibrillators), intensivists must be aware of their presence. These devices can detect tachyarrhythmias, and when appropriately programmed terminate using either anti-tachycardia pacing and/or cardioversion/defibrillation. Inhibition of these devices using a magnet should usually be avoided if at all possible. If a patient with an implanted defibrillator or pacemaker has undergone external defibrillation/cardioversion, device interrogation is indicated.

On occasion, recurrent tachycardias may be treated by the electrophysiologists using ablation in the cardiac catheter laboratories. Ablative therapy involves destruction or modulation of abnormal electrical conduction pathways within the heart using high-frequency alternating currents. Cardiac ablation has progressed over the last decade with the technical developments including saline cooling and radiofrequency ablation (RFA). RFA is now indicated as first-line therapy for several dysrhythmias both atrial and ventricular. Although not contraindicated, there is limited evidence in critically ill patients. Even when indicated, intermediate stabilization with drug therapy may be required as ablation services may not be immediately feasible or available. Where recurrent tachyarrhythmias occur in a critically ill patient that might be potentially amenable to ablation, discussion with an electrophysiologist is warranted.

Pacing involves electrical stimulation to the cardiac muscle either ventricular or atrial (or both) to cause electrical depolarization and thus cardiac contraction. It may be temporary or permanent. Pacing nomenclature with the devices as generally encountered on the ICU is relatively simple (A – atrium, V – ventricle, D – dual, I – inhibit). The three-letter code relates to the chamber being paced, the chamber being sensed, and the potential action of the device (either pace or inhibit). An example is DVI pacing (paces the atrium and ventricle, senses only the ventricle, and inhibits output from the pacing generator if an R wave is sensed). Pacemakers can be used to treat bradyarrhythmias, to allow safe control of tachyarrhythmias with drug therapy (by avoiding the risk of excessive bradycardia), or to terminate reentrant tachycardias using overdrive pacing. Additional uses of pacing post-cardiothoracic surgery in patients with heart failure facilitate mechanisms to increase cardiac output by echo-guided optimization of atrioventricular and/or ventricular-ventricular delay. The indications for pacing in bradycardia and tachycardia are discussed in the relevant chapters.

Pharmacological Antiarrhythmic Therapy

Pharmacological therapy may be used to treat arrhythmias (either alone or in conjunction with electrical therapy). Drugs are generally classified using the Vaughn Williams classification, with the exception of Digoxin (Table 2). This classification is based upon the mechanism of the effect on the cardiac action potential (Fig. 2). Other antiarrhythmic drugs that fall outside the Vaughn Williams classification include Atropine, Isoprenaline, Magnesium, and Glycopyrollate (Table 3).

The assessment and treatment of individual arrhythmias on the ICU are discussed in detail in the relevant chapters in this encyclopedia. Several issues in critically ill patients with rhythm disturbances warrant specific mention, however.

Areas for Special Consideration

Rate Versus Rhythm Control in AF

There is ongoing debate as to whether (in the hemodynamically stable patient) the aim of antiarrhythmic therapy should be to correct rhythm or control rate in this arrhythmia. A recent Cochrane review summarized the

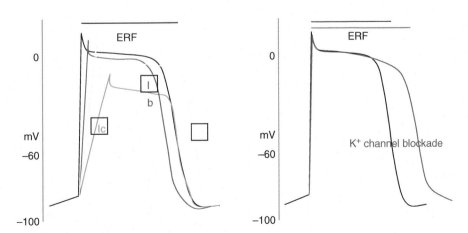

Anti-arrhythmic Therapy. Figure 2 Diagram showing the cardiac action potentials and the site of action of antiarrhythmic agents shown in Table 2. *X-axis* time, *y-axis* voltage, *mV* millivolts, *ERF* effective refractory period, *K⁺* potassium ions

Anti-arrhythmic Therapy. Table 3 Vaughn Williams Classification of antiarrhythmic drugs (see Fig. 2 for action potential)

V-W class			
I	Sodium channel blockade	Reduce phase 0 slope and peak of action potential	
	Ia	↓↓ Phase 0 slope	Quinidine
		↑ AP duration	Procainamide
		↑ Effective refractory period	Disopyramide
	Ib	↓ Phase 0 slope	Lidocaine
		↓ AP duration	Mexilitine
		↓ Effective refractory period	Phenytoin
	Ic	↓↓↓ Phase 0 slope	Flecainide
		↔ AP duration	Propafenone
		↔ Effective refractory period	
II	Beta blockade	↓ SAN automaticity	Atenolol
		↓ Heart rate and conduction	Metoprolol
			Sotalol
III	Potassium channel blockade	Delay repolarisation (phase 3)	Amiodarone
		↑ AP duration	Bretylium
		↑ Effective refractory period	Sotalol
IV	Calcium channel blockade	Block L-type calcium channels	Amlodipine
		Most effective at SA and AV	Nifedipine
		Nodes	Verapamil
		↓ Heart rate and conduction	Diltiazem

V-W class Vaughn Williams class, *AP* action potential, *SAN* sinoatrial node

AFFIRM, PIAF trials and found that rate control was as effective as rhythm control in chronic AF [8–10]. Of note, these studies were conducted in noncritically ill patient populations. Critically ill postoperative patients may have a number of reversible precipitating factors which when addressed may result in an increased successful cardioversion rate. The success of conversion to sinus rhythm is related to the duration of AF. Thus, in critically ill patients with new onset AF, cardioversion (either electrical or pharmacological) may be more readily achieved. Further, as this group of patients often have concomitant cardiac dysfunction and low cardiac output states, restoration of sinus rhythm and atrial kick may be key to improving the clinical state of the patient (Chapter X).

Anticoagulation and Risk of Embolization

Before attempted conversion to sinus rhythm is considered (either electrically or pharmacologically) is the need

for anticoagulation, as cardioversion is associated with pulmonary or systemic embolization. This is more likely without prior anticoagulation in patients with AF > 48 h, rheumatic heart disease, severe left ventricular dysfunction, or other structural heart disease associated with intracardiac thrombus formation. The incidence of thromboembolic complications varies, but in a large nonrandomized series that included 437 patients, embolism occurred in 5.3% of non-anticoagulated patients compared to 0.8% of those receiving anticoagulation [11]. The risk of embolic complications can be reduced if trans-oesophageal echo (TOE) is performed prior to cardioversion to establish absence of preexisting thrombus. However, the risk of embolization continues for several weeks even after restoration of sinus rhythm due to delayed return of normal atrial activity from atrial stunning. The current recommendation is to anticoagulate patients with chronic AF for 3–4 weeks prior and for at least 4 weeks following elective cardioversion. The recommendations for critically ill patients are less clear being dependant on coexisting clinical risks [12].

Antiarrhythmic Therapy in Congenital Heart Disease

Anti-arrhythmic therapy in adult patients with congenital heart disease warrants special mention. These patients must not be regarded the same as those with structurally normal hearts, as what is relatively benign rhythm disturbance in a normal heart can result in rapid and catastrophic hemodynamic instability. Expert advice should always be sought with respect to all aspects of treatment. Supraventricular arrhythmias are very common in this population of patients with loss of sinus rhythm being one of the most common indications for hospital admission. Atrial fibrillation and flutter are frequent for those who had had no operative repair of their malformation [13]. In patients with univentricular circulation and/or a systemic right ventricle, atrial arrhythmias should be regarded as malignant, and cardioversion (electrical or pharmacological) should be performed as soon as possible after presentation. For all congenital patients, special consideration should be given to:

- Effects of anaesthesia/sedation on the circulation (the most senior anesthetist possible should be used) as hemodynamic instability may rapidly follow induction of anesthesia.
- Anticoagulation may be suboptimal prior to cardioversion: where urgent cardioversion is indicated (vide supra) intravenous heparin should be administered.
- TOE should be considered for all the usual indications, and in those with significant chamber enlargement.
- Post-cardioversion bradycardia/asystole: consideration must always be given to how the patient could be paced if this complication occurs. Some patients (i.e., total cavo-pulmonary connection (TCPC), left atrial isomerism) there may be no direct connection between the venous return and the ventricle.

References

1. Reinelt P, Karth GD, Geppert A, Heinz G (2001) Incidence and type of cardiac arrhythmias in critically ill patients: a single center experience in a medical-cardiological ICU. Intensive Care Med 27 (9):1466–1473
2. Maisel WH, Rawn JD, Stevenson WG (2001) Atrial fibrillation after cardiac surgery. Ann Intern Med 135:1061
3. Almassi GH, Schowalter T, Nicolosi AC, Aggarwal A, Moritz TE, Henderson WG et al (1997) Atrial fibrillation after cardiac surgery: a major morbid event? Ann Surg 226(4):501–511, discussion 11–13
4. Brathwaite D, Weissman C (1998) The new onset of atrial arrhythmias following major noncardiothoracic surgery is associated with increased mortality. Chest 114(2):462–468
5. Blomstrom-Lundqvist C, Scheinman MM, Aliot EM et al (2003) ACC/AHA/ESC guidelines for the management of patients with supraventricular arrhythmias. Eur Heart J 24:1857–1897
6. Nolan J, Deakin C, Soar J et al (2005) European Resuscitation Council Guidelines 2005. Resuscitation 67:S39–S86
7. Schneider T, Martens PR, Paschen H et al (2000) Multicenter, randomized, controlled trial of 150-J biphasic shocks compared with 200- to 360-J monophasic shocks in the resuscitation of out-of-hospital cardiac arrest victims. Optimized Response to Cardiac Arrest (ORCA) Investigators. Circulation 102:1780–1787
8. Crystal E, Garfinkle MS, Connolly SS, Ginger TT, Sleik K, Yusuf SS (2004) Interventions for preventing post-operative atrial fibrillation in patients undergoing heart surgery. Cochrane Database Syst Rev 4:CD003611
9. Wyse DG, Waldo AL, DiMarco JP, Domanski MJ, Rosenberg Y, Schron EB et al (2002) A comparison of rate control and rhythm control in patients with atrial fibrillation. N Engl J Med 347 (23):1825–1833
10. Hohnloser SH, Kuck KH, Lilienthal J (2000) Rhythm or rate control in atrial fibrillation – pharmacological Intervention in Atrial Fibrillation (PIAF): a randomised trial. Lancet 356(9244):1789–1794
11. Bjerkelund CJ, Orning OM (1969) The efficacy of anticoagulant therapy in preventing embolism related to D.C. electrical conversion of atrial fibrillation. Am J Cardiol 23:208
12. The Management of Atrial Fibrillation. NICE clinical guidelines. http://www.nice.org.uk/Guidance/CG36NICE guidelines
13. ACC/AHA/ESC guidelines for the management of patients with supraventricular arrhythmias (2003) Eur Heart J 24:1857–1897

Antibiotic Tolerance

This in vitro phenomenon is observed when bacteria are inhibited by low concentrations of an antimicrobial agent but are killed at much higher concentrations (MBC/MIC-ratio≥1/32).

Antibiotic-Associated Diarrhea

▶ Clostridium Difficile-Associated Diarrhea

Antibiotics via the Respiratory Tract

▶ Aerosolized Antibiotics

Antibiotics: Resistance Mechanisms and Clinical Relevance

Joseph P. Lynch, III
Division of Pulmonary, Critical Care Medicine, Allergy, and Clinical Immunology, The David Geffen School of Medicine at UCLA, Los Angeles, CA, USA

Antimicrobial resistance continues to escalate globally and is associated with heightened mortality and morbidity [1]. Clones of multidrug resistant (MDR) bacteria have disseminated globally, and in some cases, infections are essentially untreatable with existing antimicrobial agents [1, 2]. Antimicrobial resistance is particularly problematic in the intensive care unit (ICU) [1]. Ventilator-associated pneumonia (VAP) and other infections acquired in the ICU (e.g., catheter- or device-associated infections, skin/soft tissue infections (SSTI), wound infections, urinary tract infections (UTIs), blood stream infections (BSI)) are often caused by opportunistic bacteria with an array of antibiotic resistance mechanisms. The most important factors predisposing to antibiotic resistance in hospitals include prior use of antimicrobials, prolonged hospitalization or residence in an ICU, prolonged mechanical ventilation (MV), need for invasive devices, and severity and acuity of illness.

Mechanisms of Antibiotic Resistance

Mechanisms responsible for antibiotic resistance include enzymatic inactivation or modification of antibiotics; alteration in the bacterial target site(s); permeability barriers to influx of antibiotics; active efflux pumps (that extrude antibiotics from bacterial cells) [1]. Mutations conferring resistance typically increase over time; the rate of increase may be amplified by selection pressure from antibiotic use. Over the past 2–3 decades, resistance rates to a variety of antibiotics have escalated dramatically within the USA and globally. Clonal spread of resistant organisms between hospitals, geographic regions, and continents has fueled the explosive rise in resistance [1]. Selection pressure from antibiotic use amplifies and perpetuates resistant clones. Antimicrobial resistance rates are highest in ICUs, because of the debilitated state of patients, prolonged hospital stays, comorbidities, and liberal use of antibiotics.

Prevention of Resistance

Judicious use of antibiotics and aggressive infection-control measures are essential to minimize spread of antimicrobial resistance [1, 2]. In hospital settings, several strategies to curtail or reduce emergence of resistance include restriction of certain antibiotic classes, initial empiric combination therapy, directed (pathogen-specific) therapy, shortening duration of therapy, rotating antibiotics, computer-assisted antibiotic management, vigilant infection-control policies, and patient cohorting. These strategies are sometimes, but not consistently, effective in curtailing epidemics of antibiotic-resistant organisms. Awareness of local resistance patterns and prior antibiotic exposure (among individual patients) are essential to guide empirical antibiotic therapy. When a causative agent is identified, therapy should be "de-escalated." Tailoring (narrowing) antibiotic therapy for proven pathogens, and shortening duration of antibiotic therapy, may limit the selection pressure driving resistance (in both hospital and community settings).

Empirical Choice of Antibiotic

Selecting the best antibiotic regimen requires an awareness of local susceptibility patterns within the institution, the ICU, and prior antibiotic exposure among individual patients. Exposure to antibiotics is an independent risk factor for emergence of antimicrobial resistance. For empirical treatment, a careful antibiotic history should be obtained. Ideally, if patients have received a particular class of antibiotics within 30 days, that antibiotic class should *not* be used.

Gram-Positive Cocci

Antibiotic resistance in Gram-positive pathogens has increased at an alarming rate over the past 2 decades. The problem is most apparent in hospitals (particularly in ICUs). In the following section, we discuss methicillin-resistant staphylococci (both coagulase-positive and -negative) and vancomycin-resistant *Enterococcus faecium* (VREF), Gram-positive organisms that are endemic in most hospitals in the USA and worldwide.

Staphylococcus aureus

Staphylococcus aureus (*S. aureus*) is the leading cause of nosocomial infections in the USA and globally (accounting for >20% of VAP, 15% of BSI, and >30% of SSTI) [3]. Intravascular catheters are the major cause of BSI due to *S. aureus*.

Prevalence and Epidemiology of MRSA

Currently, most *S. aureus* isolates in hospitals are methicillin-resistant (MRSA). Further, MRSA is endemic in many long-term care facilities (LTCF) and in individuals with specific risk factors (e.g., comorbidity, human immunodeficiency virus (HIV) infection, injection drug abusers, and prior hospitalization). Additionally, in the mid-1990s, community-acquired (CA)-MRSA emerged as a cause of serious infections, even in healthy individuals with no risk factors [3]. These CA-MRSA strains are genetically distinct from strains traditionally detected in health-care institutions (e.g., hospital and LTCF). Most isolates of CA-MRSA are derived from a single clone (USA300 clone). This clone contains virulence factors (including Panton–Valentine leukocidin (PVL) gene) that markedly increase morbidity and mortality [3]. CA-MRSA predominantly cause SSTI (often with necrosis and abscess formation) but may cause invasive disease including BSI, necrotizing pneumonia, empyema, and endocarditis [3]. The USA300 clone is endemic in the USA and is gaining ground in the rest of the world [3].

Risk Factors for Colonization or Infection with MRSA

Risk factors for colonization and infection with MRSA include prior or prolonged antibiotic therapy, hospital source, residence in ICU or LTCF, presence of indwelling catheters, dialysis, surgical wounds, corticosteroids, diabetes mellitus, neurosurgery, and exposure to patients colonized or infected with MRSA. Colonization of the nasopharynx, skin, or surgical wounds is associated with an increased risk for MRSA infections. CA-MRSA may infect previously healthy individuals; outbreaks of CA-MRSA infections have been noted in closed populations (e.g., children in day-care centers, military recruits, athletes, prison inmates, gay males, and native Americans) [3].

Nosocomial infections caused by MRSA have been associated with increased mortality rates, hospital length of stay (LOS), and costs compared with MSSA. This heightened mortality likely reflects host and demographic factors (e.g., comorbidities) and/or differences in efficacy of therapy rather than intrinsic differences in the virulence of the organism.

Mechanisms of Antibiotic Resistance

Methicillin resistance is mediated by the chromosomal gene, *mec*A, which alters penicillin-binding protein-2a (PBP2a) and confers resistance to all β-lactam antibiotics (including carbapenems). Most strains of hospital-acquired MRSA are resistant to multiple non-β-lactam antibiotic classes (e.g., macrolides, aminoglycosides (AGs), fluoroquinolones (FQs), sulfonamides, tetracyclines, etc.). The prevalence of nosocomial MRSA increased dramatically within the last 3 decades, via dissemination of a few dominant "epidemic" clones, some of which are MDR [3].

Treatment of Nosocomial MRSA

Vancomycin is the cornerstone of therapy for MRSA. However, anti-staphylococcal penicillins or cefazolin remain the drugs of choice for MSSA. Importantly, vancomycin is *less* effective than β-lactam antibiotics against serious infections due to MSSA. MRSA isolates are almost universally susceptible to vancomycin, linezolid, daptomycin, quinupristin/dalfopristin (Q/D), and tigecycline. Resistance to vancomycin (a glycopeptide) is rare. Linezolid and Q/D remain active against glycopeptide-resistant strains (>99% susceptibility). Risk factors for resistance to linezolid include indwelling prosthetic devices and prolonged therapy with linezolid. Although vancomycin is most often used to treat MRSA, optimal therapy for serious MRSA infections has not been established. Vancomycin is not bactericidal, lacks activity against organisms growing in biofilm, and penetrates poorly into the lung. Combining vancomycin with a second antibiotic (e.g., rifampin, gentamicin, linezolid, clindamycin, etc.) has not been shown to improve outcomes over vancomycin alone, and may increase toxicities [4]. The addition of clindamycin or linezolid may antagonize the anti-staphylococcal activity of vancomycin [4]. Linezolid achieves better intrapulmonary deposition than vancomycin, but clinical superiority for MRSA pneumonia has not been proven. Daptomycin is at least as effective as vancomycin for bacteremias and endocarditis [5], but should not be used for pneumonia since daptomycin is inactivated by surfactant.

Treatment of Community-Acquired MRSA

Most CA-MRSA remain susceptible to trimethoprim/sulfamethoxazole (T/S) or tetracyclines. In recent years, CA-MRSA (USA300 isolates) acquired additional mechanisms of resistance to macrolides (mediated by [*msr*(A)]), clindamycin [*erm*(A) and *erm*(C)], tetracycline [*tet*(K) and *tet* (M)], mupirocon (*mupA*)), and FQs [3]. Further, USA300 isolates displaying reduced susceptibility to vancomycin, daptomycin, and T/S have been detected. Thus, USA300 is rapidly acquiring MDR, much like

USA100 (the most commonly isolated strain of MRSA in the USA in nosocomial settings) [3].

Coagulase-Negative Staphylococci (CNS)

Coagulase-negative staphylococci (i.e., *S. epidermidis*, *S. saprophyticus*, *S. haemolyticus*) are important causes of catheter-related infections, BSI, and SSTI in the ICU. In the USA, CNS account for >30% of nosocomial BSI.

Risk Factors for Colonization or Infection with CNS

Patients with indwelling medical devices (e.g., central venous catheters, neurosurgical shunts, prosthetic heart valves, artificial joints), are at greatest risk for infections due to CNS. Prior receipt of β-lactam antibiotics is a risk factor for colonization or infection with methicillin-resistant CNS.

Mechanism of Antimicrobial Resistance

Methicillin resistance in CNS is caused by the same *mec*A gene found in MRSA. Currently, >75% of nosocomial isolates of CNS in the USA are resistant to methicillin.

Therapy

Vancomycin is the drug of choice for infections due to CNS. Although rare, some strains of *S. epidermidis* and *S. haemolyticus* have acquired high-level resistance to glycopeptides (i.e., vancomyin and teicoplanin). Agents with excellent activity against CNS include linezolid, tigecyline, Q/D, and daptomycin [6].

Enterococci

Enterococci (predominantly *E. faecium* and *E. fecalis*) are important causes of UTI, BSI, and device-associated wound infections in ICU patients. During the 1990s, enterococci became the second leading cause of infection among hospitalized patients in the USA. Importantly, vancomycin-resistant enterococci (VRE), initially described in Europe in 1986, have disseminated globally [1].

Risk Factors for Colonization or Infection with VRE

Risk factors for colonization or infection with VRE include previous antibiotic exposure (particularly to vancomycin, cephalosporins (CEPHs), or agents with anaerobic activity), enteral feeding, exposure to patients with VRE or contaminated environmental sources, prolonged hospital stay, severe debilitation, immunosuppression, malignancy, organ transplant recipients, chronic renal or hepatic failure, trauma, and residence in ICUs or LTCFs. Colonization with VRE precedes infections; colonization

can persist for extended periods (sometimes >1 year). The most important mechanism of spread is via carriage on the hands of caregivers. Transmission from colonized individuals may lead to endemic and epidemic spread of VRE in hospitals or LTCRs. VRE can survive for up to 7 days on environmental surfaces. Infection-control measures are critical to limit the spread of VRE in hospitals.

Mechanisms of Antimicrobial Resistance

Antimicrobial resistance among enterococci escalated dramatically over the past 2 decades [1]. Enterococci are *intrinsically* resistant to many antimicrobial agents including CEPHs, penicillins (PCNs), T/S, clindamycin, FQs, and low-dose AGs. *Acquired* resistance emerged to high-dose β-lactams, AGs, glycopeptides, macrolides, tetracyclines, and other antibiotic classes. In 1979, high-level resistance to gentamicin (due to AQ-modifying enzymes) was noted. In the 1980s, resistance to β-lactam antibiotics due to mutations in penicillin-binding proteins (PBPs), β-lactamase production, or a combination of mechanisms followed. In 1986, VRE was reported in Europe. Vancomycin resistance is mediated by small genetic elements (transposons) (*van*A through *van*F). Within a decade of the sentinel report, the incidence of VRE skyrocketed globally. By 2002, >35% of clinical isolates of *E. faecium* in ICUs in the USA were resistant to vancomycin.

Therapy

For *susceptible* strains of enterococci, ampicillin is indicated. For serious infections, ampicillin should be *combined with* an AG to achieve synergy. However, when *high-grade* AG resistance is noted, synergy will not occur. For ampicillin-resistant strains, vancomycin is the drug of choice. Agents with excellent in vitro activity (>99%) against enterococci (including VRE) include linezolid, Q/D, daptomycin, and tigecycline [6].

Gram-Negative Bacteria

Gram-negative bacteria (GNB) accounted for 65–80% of VAP, 70% of ICU-acquired UTIs, 34–56% of ICU-acquired surgical-site infections, and 24–33% of ICU-acquired BSIs in the USA from 1986 to 2003 [7, 8]. Over the past 2 decades, resistance among GNB increased sharply [1, 2]. Resistance of *K. pneumoniae* to third-generation CEPHs increased from <3% in the late 1980s to >20% in the early 1990s, subsequently plateauing at 15–20% [8]. The percentage of *Acinetobacter* isolates resistant to third-generation CEPHs increased from 25% in 1986 to almost 70% in 2003 [7]. Because of space constraints, we will discuss only a few GNB of particular importance in the ICU including extended-spectrum β-lactamase (ESBL)-producing *Enterobacteriaceae*, *Pseudomonas aeruginosa*, and *Acinetobacter* spp.

Enterobacteriaceae

Bacteria within the family Enterobacteriacea (which include *Enterobacter* spp, *K. pneumoniae*, *Escherichia coli*, *Proteus* spp, *S. marcescens*, and *Citrobacter* spp) are important nososomial pathogens. Within the past decade, resistance to β-lactam antibiotics and carbapenems (CPs) among *Enterobacteriaceae* increased substantially [2].

Extended-Spectrum β-Lactamases (ESBLs)

Extended-spectrum β-lactamases (ESBLs), encoded on plasmids, were first recognized among *K. pneumoniae* in Europe in the early 1980s, and spread rapidly worldwide [1]. The plasmid is transferable to other *Enterobacteriaceae* (e.g., *E. coli*, *Proteus* spp, *Serratia marcescens*). ESBLs confer resistance to third-generation CEPHs, extended-spectrum PCNs, and aztreonam. ESBL-producing strains typically remain susceptible to CPs, but CP resistance is increasing [9]. By the mid-1990s, 9–14% of isolates of *K. pneumoniae* in US hospitals expressed ESBLs, with higher rates at some centers. Rates of ESBL-producing organisms vary widely in different geographic regions and from institution to institution [2]. Additional resistance determinants to non-β lactam antibiotics (e.g., FQs, AGs, tetracyclines, and T/S) emerged, leading to MDR [10].

Risk Factors for Infection or Colonization with ESBLs

Risk factors associated with infection or colonization with ESBLs include prior use of antimicrobials, residence in an ICU, indwelling devices, increased severity of illness, prolonged hospital stay, emergency intra-abdominal surgery, LTCF stay, and MV [10]. Clonal dissemination has been noted within and between hospitals, associated with endemic and epidemic outbreaks. Ominously, CA-ESBL-producing *Enterobacteriaceae* have been noted in adults with no recent contact with health-care facilities [10].

Treatment

Carbapenems are the preferred therapy for serious infections due to ESBLs. However, widespread use of CPs for "empiric" use can lead to resistance [9]. Resistance to CPs may emerge due to hyperproduction of plasmid-mediated ampC/β-lactamase, loss of porin proteins, or carbapenemases. Cefepime is active against most ESBLs, but activity decreases as the inoculum increases; this "innoculum effect" is dose dependent and may compromise efficacy of cefepime in serious infections. For susceptible strains, FQs may be used, but resistance rates to FQs have skyrocketed [10]. Outbreaks of ESBL in nosocomial settings may be curtailed by restricting the use of broad-spectrum CEPHs (particularly ceftazidime). Switching to CPs or β-lactam/β-lactamase inhibitors may curtail outbreaks, but long-term use may drive resistance.

Non-fermenting Gram-Negative Pathogens

Pseudomonas aeruginosa

Pseudomonas aeruginosa (PA), an aerobic Gram-negative rod, is the leading cause of VAP (16–43%), and may cause SSTI, UTI, BSI, and wound infections.

Risk Factors for Colonization or Infection with PA

P. aeruginosa primarily colonizes or infects patients with specific or nonspecific impairments in host defenses (e.g., immunosuppression, burns, neutropenia, organ transplant recipients, need for MV; bronchiectasis; COPD). Colonization with PA increases with length of hospitalization and severity of illness, and may lead to invasive infections. In normal hosts, invasive infections may occur when there is disruption of normal skin or mucous membranes, or insertion of urinary or intravascular catheters or endotracheal tubes. Risk factors for pseudomonas VAP include acute respiratory distress syndrome (ARDS), "late onset" (>4 days) pneumonia, prior receipt of antibiotics, and prolonged MV (>6 days) [11]. *P. aeruginosa* is ubiquitous in hospital environments, and may thrive in sinks, food, plants, and on environmental surfaces. Outbreaks of nosocomial PA infections have been linked to contaminated environmental sources or cross-infection from colonized patients or health-care workers.

Mechanisms of Antimicrobial Resistance

P. aeruginosa is *intrinsically* resistant to many antibiotics (via constitutive expression of AmpC β-lactamase and efflux pumps) and can *acquire* resistance to antibiotics by diverse mechanisms including enzymes (e.g., carbapenemases, AG-modifying enzymes, DNA gyrase), active efflux pumps, and porin protein alterations (affecting permeability) [12]. Combinations of resistance mechanisms (e.g., efflux, impermeability, and production of inactivating enzymes) may lead to MDR. Most MDR-PA remain susceptible to polymyxins (e.g., colistimethate sodium), but some isolates are resistant to all antibiotics [12]. Importantly, PA forms biofilms that constitute sanctuary sites for bacterial replication and may compromise efficacy of antibiotics.

Treatment

Optimal therapy for serious infections due to PA is not well defined, as randomized therapeutic trials are lacking. Mortality associated with *P. aeruginosa* VAP is high (>40%) which in part reflects the debilitated state of patients infected with this organism. Clinical failure rates, persistence of the organism, and relapse rates are high, even with appropriate therapy [11].

The most active agents (>75% activity) against PA are AGs (particularly amikacin), CPs, piperacillin/tazobactam, cefepime, and ceftazidime [11]. Among the FQs, ciprofloxacin and levofloxacin have the best antipseudomonal activity, but rates of resistance to these agents exceed 30%. Unfortunately, CP-resistant and MDR strains have emerged. For CP-resistant or MDR strains, sulbactam and the polymyxins may retain activity.

Antimicrobial resistance among PA develops rapidly under selection pressure [11]. Many experts recommend treating serious PA infections with two agents to which the organism is susceptible. *Theoretically*, combining agents may achieve synergy and limit the emergence of resistance. However, clinical data supporting the superiority of combination therapy are lacking. For serious infections due to PA, we advise initial therapy with an antipseudomonal β-lactam (or CP) *combined with* an AG or FQ. For pseudomonas VAP, therapy should be continued for 15 days, since shorter duration of therapy (e.g., 8 days) was associated with higher relapse rates. Treatment of MDR-PA is difficult. Combinations of β-lactams, FQs, and AGs may achieve synergy, even when strains are resistant to the individual antibiotics. Polymyxin E (colistin) may be effective against MDR-PA [11]. Nebullized tobramycin or colistin have been tried for VAP due to MDR-PA [11], but have not yet been shown to improve clinical outcomes.

Acinetobacter baumannii

Bacteria within the genus *Acinetobacter* (principally *A. baumannii*) are aerobic Gram-negative coccobacilli that cause opportunistic infections in critically ill or debilitated patients [13]. *Acinetobacter* spp account for 8% of VAP and 2% of nosocomial BSI in the USA; rates are higher in subtropical regions [13]. Mortality rates with BSI or VAP due to *Acinetobacter* spp are high (30–75%); these high mortality rates in part reflect comorbidities and severity of illness.

Risk Factors for Colonization or Infection with *Acinetobacter* spp

Infections due to *Acinetobacter* spp are more common in the summer season (in temperate climates) and in subtropical regions [13]. *Acinetobacter* spp were implicated in SSTI sustained during disasters in warm climates (e.g., tsunamis, earthquakes, military wounds, bombings) [13]. *Acinetobacter* spp is an important cause of BSI and SSTI in wounded military personnel in Iraq and Afghanistan [13]. *Acinetobacter* spp have assumed increasing importance as nosocomial pathogens over the past 2 decades. In the USA, rates of VAP due to *Acinetobacter* spp increased from 1986 to 2003 whereas no increase was observed for any other GNB [8].

Risk factors for acquisition of *Acinetobacter* species include invasive procedures or devices, prolonged ICU stay, MV, enteral feedings, and recent use of broad-spectrum antibiotics. In critically ill patients, *Acinetobacter* spp may colonize the gastrointestinal tract, skin, and respiratory tract, and may be a precursor of infection. *Acinetobacter* spp are ubiquitous in the environment, and may survive for prolonged periods on wet or dry surfaces [13]. Contaminated environmental sources and transmission via medical personnel may cause outbreaks of nosocomial infections. Dissemination of a limited number of clones may cause endemic and epidemic spread within hospitals. Outbreaks have ceased following aggressive infection-control measures and modification of antibiotic use (particularly restricting CP and broad-spectrum antibiotics) [1].

Mechanisms of Antimicrobial Resistance

Nosocomial *Acinetobacter* spp are often resistant to CEPHs, penicillins, FQs, and AGs. Susceptibility rates are highly variable in various regions/countries and hospitals [2]. All *A. baumannii* strains produce AmpC β-lactamases encoded in chromosomes that confer low-level resistance to CEPHs. High-grade resistance to all β-lactams (except CPs) may occur due to hyperproduction of AmpC β-lactamases, alterations in PBPs, reduced permeability (due to altered porin proteins), efflux pumps, and plasmids [13]. The activity of FQs, AGs, and tetracyclines against *A. baumannii* (AB) is variable. Carbapenems are the preferred agents to treat AB, but CP resistance may develop via several mechanisms including plasmid-mediated serine and metallo-β-lactamases (carbapenemases), decreased outer membrane permeability, and altered PBPs [13]. In the USA, CP resistance among *A. baumannii* increased from 9% in 1995 to 40% in 2004 [13]. Within the past decade, epidemics of infections due to CP-resistant AB clones were noted in the USA, Latin America, Europe, and Asia [2]. CP-resistant strains are usually MDR but sulbactam, the polymyxins, and tigecycline (the first of the glycylglycines) often remain active against MDR-AB [13]. Ominously, strains of *Acinetobacter* resistant to *all* antimicrobials have emerged.

Treatment of MDR *A. baumannii*

Although data are limited, I recommend two active agents for serious infections due to *Acinetobacter* spp. For SSTI or surgical-site infections, debridement is an essential part of therapy. For initial, *empiric* antibiotic therapy, CP may be combined with an AG. Provided isolates are susceptible, ticarcillin/clavulanate, piperacillin/tazobactam, ceftazidime, FQs, or tigecycline may be used. For CP-resistant AB, ampicillin/sulbactam (due to the sulbactam component) may be effective therapy. Colistin (polymyxin E) may be used to treat strains resistant to *all* commonly used antibiotics. Colistin can be administered IV or via nebulization. Despite good in vitro activity, colistin may be less effective in vivo (particularly for pneumonia). Favorable responses were cited with tigecycline (alone or in combination with colistin) in some patients with MDR-AB. Hospital outbreaks of *Acinetobacter* infections may reflect environmental contamination. Removal or disinfection and sterilization of contaminated equipment (e.g., ventilator or nebulizer tubing) or fomites may eliminate the problem [13]. Even MDR-AB strains usually remain susceptible to disinfectants and antiseptics [13].

Summary

Antimicrobial resistance in ICUs is an escalating problem, with devastating consequences on morbidity, mortality, and health-care costs. Strategies to limit resistance in the ICU must be multifaceted. Initial empirical treatment should be aggressive, taking into account antibiotic susceptibility profiles within the ICU or institution. Following identification of an organism(s), therapy should be de-escalated (pathogen-directed). Attention to pharmacokinetics (PK), pharmacodynamics (PD), appropriate antibiotic, dose, and duration are essential. When endemic or epidemic spread of antibiotic-resistant bacteria occurs, aggressive infection-control efforts (including cohorting, isolation, hygiene measures), in tandem with elimination or restriction of certain antibiotic classes, may be required [1, 2].

References

1. Hawkey PM (2008) The growing burden of antimicrobial resistance. J Antimicrob Chemother 62(Suppl 1):i1–i9
2. Livermore DM (2009) Has the era of untreatable infections arrived? J Antimicrob Chemother 64(Suppl 1):i29–i36
3. Tenover FC, Goering RV (2009) Methicillin-resistant Staphylococcus aureus strain USA300: origin and epidemiology. J Antimicrob Chemother 64(3):441–446
4. Deresinski S (2009) Vancomycin in combination with other antibiotics for the treatment of serious methicillin-resistant Staphylococcus aureus infections. Clin Infect Dis 49(7):1072–1079
5. Bhavnani SM, Prakhya A, Hammel JP, Ambrose PG (2009) Cost-Effectiveness of daptomycin versus vancomycin and gentamicin for patients with methicillin-resistant Staphylococcus aureus bacteremia and/or endocarditis. Clin Infect Dis 49(5):691–698
6. Erlandson KM, Sun J, Iwen PC, Rupp ME (2008) Impact of the more-potent antibiotics quinupristin-dalfopristin and linezolid on outcome measure of patients with vancomycin-resistant Enterococcus bacteremia. Clin Infect Dis 46(1):30–36
7. Rahal JJ (2009) Antimicrobial resistance among and therapeutic options against gram-negative pathogens. Clin Infect Dis 49(Suppl 1): S4–S10
8. Gaynes R, Edwards JR (2005) Overview of nosocomial infections caused by gram-negative bacilli. Clin Infect Dis 41(6):848–854
9. Kochar S, Sheard T, Sharma R, Hui A, Tolentino E, Allen G, Landman D, Bratu S, Augenbraun M, Quale J (2009) Success of an infection control program to reduce the spread of carbapenem-resistant Klebsiella pneumoniae. Infect Control Hosp Epidemiol 30(5):447–452
10. Ben-Ami R, Rodriguez-Bano J, Arslan H, Pitout JD, Quentin C, Calbo ES, Azap OK, Arpin C, Pascual A, Livermore DM, Garau J, Carmeli Y (2009) A multinational survey of risk factors for infection with extended-spectrum beta-lactamase-producing enterobacteriaceae in nonhospitalized patients. Clin Infect Dis 49(5):682–690
11. El Solh AA, Alhajhusain A (2009) Update on the treatment of Pseudomonas aeruginosa pneumonia. J Antimicrob Chemother 64(2): 229–238
12. Strateva T, Yordanov D (2009) Pseudomonas aeruginosa – a phenomenon of bacterial resistance. J Med Microbiol 58(Pt 9):1133–1148
13. Munoz-Price LS, Weinstein RA (2008) Acinetobacter infection. N Engl J Med 358(12):1271–1281

Anticoagulant Medication

▶ Anticoagulation Reversal in the ED

Anticoagulation in Extracorporeal Circuits (CVVH, ECMO)

ANNE-CORNÉLIE J. M. DE PONT
Academisch Medisch Centrum, Academisch Ziekenhuis bij de Universiteit van Amsterdam, Amsterdam, The Netherlands

Synonyms

Prevention of thrombosis in systems processing the blood outside the body

Definition

Anticoagulation in extracorporeal circuits aims at the prevention of thrombosis in systems processing the blood outside the body, such as extracorporeal membrane oxygenation, hemodialysis, hemofiltration, and plasmapheresis.

Pre-existing Condition

In the intensive care unit, a variety of conditions may require the use of extracorporeal techniques. Extracorporeal membrane oxygenation may be used in patients with severe cardiopulmonary failure, renal failure is treated by means of hemodialysis or hemofiltration, and in case of liver failure the molecular adsorbent recirculating system may be used. Finally, plasma exchange is being used for specific indications such as thrombotic thrombocytopenic purpura and the Guillain–Barré syndrome.

During the use of extracorporeal techniques, the occurrence of circuit thrombosis is a major problem: it reduces treatment efficacy, leads to blood loss for the patient, and increases workload and costs. Several studies have addressed the pathophysiology of circuit thrombosis, but the exact mechanism by which it occurs, has not yet been elucidated. Multiple factors may play a role: activation of the contact system and the tissue factor pathway, activation of leukocytes and platelets, but also factors related to the extracorporeal treatment itself, such as turbulent flow, repeated stasis of blood, hemoconcentration, and blood-air contact [1, 2].

Application

If anticoagulation is needed to prevent the occurrence of circuit thrombosis, the choice can be made for either systemic or regional anticoagulation. The choice for either of these strategies depends on the presence of an indication for systemic anticoagulation, the bleeding risk, and the probability of side effects of the anticoagulant used.

Systemic Anticoagulation

The choice of an anticoagulant for the prevention of thrombosis in the extracorporeal circuit depends on several issues, such as experience with the drug, its pharmacokinetic and pharmacodynamic properties, the likelihood of adverse events, and the costs of the drug and its monitoring. Unfractionated heparin is the drug most frequently used to prevent thrombosis in extracorporeal circuits. Other drugs used are low molecular weight heparins, direct thrombin inhibitors, and factor Xa inhibitors.

Unfractionated Heparin

Unfractionated heparin is a highly sulfated mucopolysaccharide, heterogeneous with respect to molecular size, anticoagulant activity, and pharmacokinetics. Its anticoagulant effect is mediated by the binding to antithrombin, an endogenous inhibitor of various activated clotting factors. The heparin molecule binds to antithrombin through a high affinity pentasaccharide sequence, thereby converting antithrombin from a slow to a rapid inhibitor. Small heparin chains containing the pentasaccharide sequence only catalyze factor Xa inhibition by activating antithrombin, whereas heparin chains of sufficient length to bridge antithrombin to thrombin also exert thrombin inhibition [3].

Heparin also binds to other plasma proteins, which reduces its anticoagulant activity. Proteins binding heparin include factor VIII and fibrinogen, acute phase proteins often elevated in critically ill patients. This explains why the response to heparin among critically ill patients is individually different.

Heparin is cleared from the circulation by two mechanisms: cellular binding and renal elimination. Binding to endothelial cell receptors and macrophages leads to rapid internalization and depolymerization, whereas renal elimination is a much slower process.

Treatment with heparin carries the risks of both drug resistance and bleeding. Drug resistance is associated with antithrombin deficiency, increased heparin clearance, and elevations in heparin binding proteins including the acute phase proteins factor VIII and fibrinogen. The risk of heparin-associated bleeding increases with the dose. Monitoring of the extent of anticoagulation is usually performed through the augmented partial thromboplastin time (APTT). In critically ill patients, however, elevated levels of factor VIII may shorten the APTT without diminishing the antithrombotic effect of heparin [3]. In these cases, monitoring through an anti-Xa assay is recommended, since the result of this assay more closely mirrors the antithrombotic effect of heparin.

The use of unfractionated heparin has several advantages: its half-life is relatively short (0.5–3 h), it is easily reversible with protamine, the experience with unfractionated heparin is large, and it is cheap. However, both drug resistance and bleeding are common and unfractionated heparin carries a 1–5% risk of heparin-induced thrombocytopenia (HIT).

Low Molecular Weight Heparins

Low molecular weight heparins have several advantages compared with unfractionated heparin: their pharmacokinetics are more predictable, obviating the need of anti-Xa monitoring during continuous dosing, and the incidence of HIT is much lower (0.5–1%). However, low molecular weight heparins have a longer half-life (2–4 h), they are not fully reversible with protamine, and they are more expensive than unfractionated heparin.

Heparin-Induced Thrombocytopenia (HIT)

Heparin-induced thrombocytopenia (HIT) occurs when heparin forms a complex with platelet factor (PF)4, a protein derived from the platelet granule. The heparin-PF4 complex induces antibodies causing platelet activation and aggregation. This may lead to a procoagulant state carrying the risk of major arterial and venous thromboembolism [4]. Although HIT is uncommon (less than 1% of the ICU patients with thrombocytopenia actually have HIT), it may represent a serious danger to the patient, therefore timely diagnosis is important. HIT is a clinicopathological syndrome and its diagnosis is based on both clinical signs and serological tests. Clinical signs include a typical fall in platelet count within one week after the first heparin challenge, the presence of arterial or venous thrombosis, skin lesion at the heparin injection site, and anaphylactic reactions after the injection of heparin. Serological tests demonstrating the presence of antibodies to the heparin-PF4 complex are the enzyme linked immunosorbent assay (ELISA) and the serotonin release assay (SRA). When the two tests are combined, a sensitivity of nearly 100% can be reached. However, antibody testing is not always directly available. To facilitate the diagnosis, a scoring system has been developed, the so-called 4Ts-test (Table 1). In this test, four items each score 0–2 points, summarizing to a maximum of 8. A score of 6–8 indicates high probability of HIT, 4–5 intermediate, and 0–3 low probability.

Anticoagulants for Patients with HIT

In case of high probability of HIT, all heparins must be stopped and a different anticoagulant strategy must be chosen. There are two classes of anticoagulants suitable for the treatment of patients with HIT: direct thrombin inhibitors and factor Xa inhibitors [4].

Direct Thrombin Inhibitors

Direct thrombin inhibitors selectively block the activity of thrombin, preventing the conversion of fibrinogen to fibrin and thus thrombus formation. The most frequently used drugs in this class are lepirudin, bivalirudin, and argatroban. These agents have in common that their anticoagulant effect is not reversible. However, the agents differ in the way they are metabolized and eliminated, which has a consequence for their half-lives and their use in clinical practice (Table 2). Since extracorporeal circuits are most often used to treat acute kidney injury, argatroban is most suitable for the use in this setting, because of its nonrenal elimination and the relatively large experience with the drug. Lepirudin commonly elicits antibody generation, which leads to the formation of large lepirudin-antibody complexes. Since these complexes cannot readily be eliminated by extracorporeal circulation, this leads to a prolonged half-life and an increased risk of bleeding. Therefore, the use of lepirudin during extracorporeal treatment is strongly recommended against.

Anticoagulation in Extracorporeal Circuits (CVVH, ECMO). Table 1 Probability of heparin-induced thrombocytopenia: the 4Ts test

	Points (0, 1, or 2 for each of four categories: maximum score = 8)		
	2	1	0
Thrombocytopenia	>50% platelet decrease to a nadir ≥20	30–50% platelet decrease, or nadir 10–19, or >50% decrease secondary to surgery	<30% platelet decrease or nadir <10
Timing of onset of platelet decrease[a]	Days 5–10 or ≤1 day with recent heparin (past 30 days)	>day 10 or timing unclear or <1 day with recent heparin (past 31–100 days)	<day 4 (no recent heparin)
Thrombosis or other sequelae	Proven new thrombosis, skin necrosis, or acute systemic reaction after intravenous heparin	Progressive or recurrent thrombosis, erythematous skin lesions, suspected thrombosis	None
Other causes of platelet decrease	None evident	Possible	Definite

[a]First day of heparin exposure considered day 0
Pretest probability score: 6–8 indicates high, 4–5 intermediate, 0–3 low

Factor Xa Inhibitors

Factor Xa inhibitors are divided into indirect inhibitors, which prevent factor Xa activity through its natural inhibitor antithrombin, and direct inhibitors, which block factor Xa activity by binding to its catalytic subunit independently of antithrombin. The indirect factor Xa inhibitors danaparoid and fondaparinux can be considered for treatment or prevention of HIT associated thrombosis [4]. Similarly to direct thrombin inhibitors the anticoagulant effect of danaparoid and fondaparinux is not reversible. Moreover, both drugs have a long half-life (ranging from 17 to 24 h) and are cleared predominantly by the kidney, making them less suitable for patients with renal failure (Table 2). However, when carefully dosed and monitored through anti-Xa effect, danaparoid and fondaparinux can be used as anticoagulants in extracorporeal circuits.

Regional Anticoagulation

The term regional anticoagulation refers to the titration of an anticoagulant into the blood entering the processing device, with reversal of the anticoagulant effect after the device. Regional anticoagulation can be performed with heparin and protamine or with sodium citrate and calcium. The advantage of regional anticoagulation is that it restricts anticoagulation to the extracorporeal circuit, lowering the patient's risk of bleeding.

Anticoagulation in Extracorporeal Circuits (CVVH, ECMO).
Table 2 Properties of anticoagulants suitable for the treatment of patients with heparin-induced thrombocytopenia

Anticoagulant	Properties
Direct thrombin inhibitors	
Argatroban	Hepatobiliary elimination Half-life 40–50 min
Bivalirudin	Metabolism renal (20%) and enzymatical (80%) Half-life 25 min
Lepirudin	Renal elimination Half-life 80 min 40–60% antibody formation
Factor Xa inhibitors	
Danaparoid	Renal elimination Half-life 24 h Potential cross-reactivity with PF4
Fondaparinux	Renal elimination Half-life 17–20 h

Heparin and Protamine

Regional heparinization is technically complicated, since it is difficult to determine how much protamine is needed to neutralize the effect of heparin. After the heparin-protamine complex has been taken up and metabolized by the reticuloendothelial system, heparin and protamine are released into the circulation again, complicating the dosing schedule. Moreover, protamine infusion is associated with systemic hypotension and pulmonary hypertension, activation of inflammatory mediators, and platelet dysfunction [5].

Sodium Citrate and Calcium

In recent years, regional anticoagulation of hemofiltration circuits with sodium citrate and calcium has gained large interest. If an algorithm is used, the technique is easy to perform, and it has been demonstrated to be superior to systemic anticoagulation with heparin with respect to filter survival. Moreover, bleeding complications and transfusion requirements are significantly lower during regional anticoagulation with citrate than during systemic anticoagulation with heparin [5].

When regional anticoagulation with citrate is applied, citrate not only acts as an anticoagulant, but also as a buffer. Sodium citrate is infused into the blood entering the hemofilter and a buffer-free substitution fluid with calcium is infused into the blood leaving the filter. Part of the sodium citrate is filtered into the ultrafiltrate, whereas another part enters the systemic circulation and is metabolized to bicarbonate by the liver and skeletal muscles. Therefore, the maintenance of a normal blood pH depends both on the amount of sodium citrate infused and the ability of the patient to metabolize the citrate to bicarbonate. If the amount of citrate infused is too low, the production of bicarbonate will be too low and a normal anion gap (AG) acidosis will ensue.

During hemofiltration, cells and proteins accumulate on the filter membrane, making it less permeable for the sodium citrate infused. When this occurs, a larger proportion of sodium citrate will be entering the systemic circulation. The metabolization of this larger proportion of citrate to bicarbonate may cause metabolic alkalosis. On the other hand, if the patient is unable to metabolize the larger proportion of citrate, this will cause a high anion gap metabolic acidosis, because citrate is converted to citric acid, an acid not accounted for in the anion gap equation (AG = [Na$^+$] − ([Cl$^-$] + [NaHCO3$^-$])). Therefore, both metabolic alkalosis and metabolic acidosis may be caused by citrate intoxication. Another clue to diagnose citrate intoxication is the calcium ratio (Ca/iCa), that is

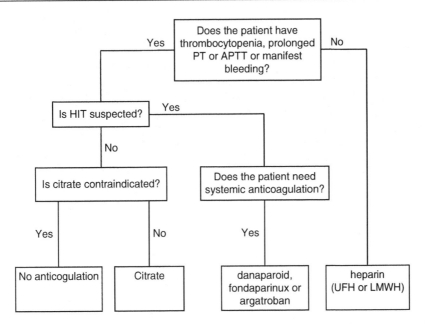

Anticoagulation in Extracorporeal Circuits (CVVH, ECMO). Figure 1 Algorithm for the choice of an anticoagulant during extracorporeal treatment. PT: prothrombin time; APTT: augmented partial thromboplastin time; HIT: heparin-induced thrombocytopenia

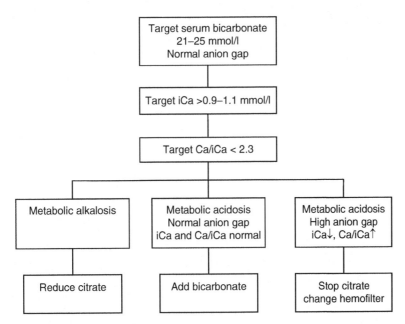

Anticoagulation in Extracorporeal Circuits (CVVH, ECMO). Figure 2 Algorithm for the management of regional anticoagulation with citrate during extracorporeal treatment. iCa: ionized calcium

the total calcium concentration divided by the ionized calcium concentration. Normally, the ratio between total and ionized calcium is below 2.1. In case of citrate intoxication, however, the excess citrate binds calcium, making the ionized calcium concentration decrease, whereas the bound calcium concentration increases. Therefore, the calcium ratio will increase to levels above the cutoff range of 2.1–2.5 [2].

Use of Algorithms

The choice for an anticoagulant strategy during extracorporeal treatments can be facilitated by the use of an algorithm. Use of an algorithm ensures that all factors possibly influencing the effect of a certain anticoagulant are taken into account. In this way, the risk of adverse events may be reduced. Examples of algorithms for the choice of an anticoagulant technique during hemofiltration and for the application of regional anticoagulation with citrate are shown in Figs. 1 and 2.

References

1. Despotis GJ, Avidan MS, Hogue CW Jr (2001) Mechanisms and attenuation of hemostatic activation during extracorporeal circulation. Ann Thor Surg 72:S1821–S1831
2. Joannidis M (2007) Oudemans-van Straaten HM. Clinical review: patency of the circuit in continuous renal replacement therapy. Crit Care 11:218
3. Hirsh J, Bauer KA, Donati MB et al (2008) Parenteral anticoagulants. Chest 133:141S–159S
4. Warkentin TE, Greinacher A, Koster A et al (2008) Treatment and prevention of heparin-induced thrombocytopenia: American College of Chest Physicians evidence-based clinical practice guidelines (8th edition). Chest 133:340–380
5. Oudemans-van Straaten HM, Wester JP, de Pont AC et al (2006) Anticoagulant strategies in continuous renal replacement therapy: can the choice be evidence-based? Intensive Care Med 32:188–202

Anticoagulation Reversal in the ED

TYLER W. BARRETT, BRETT F. BECHTEL
Department of Emergency Medicine, Vanderbilt University Oxford House, Nashville, TN, USA

Synonyms

Anticoagulant medication; Heparin; Vitamin K antagonists; Warfarin

Definition

Anticoagulation refers to the process of impeding the coagulation of blood. Anticoagulation reversal entails treatments to restore a patient's blood coagulation pathways to normal or near normal levels.

Characteristics

Anticoagulants are a class of medications that interfere with various steps of the coagulation process. Vitamin K Antagonists (VKA) include warfarin, acenocoumarol,

fluinidone, and phenprocoumon and function by inhibiting the regeneration of vitamin K. Vitamin K is an essential cofactor in the synthesis of coagulation factors II, VII, IX, X, and inhibitors protein C, protein S, and protein Z [1–3]. Warfarin is the most common anticoagulant in the USA and has a half-life of 40 h, which impacts reversal strategies [2, 3].

Unfractionated heparin (UFH) is a short acting drug with a half-life of 60–120 min. UFH binds to antithrombin resulting in the inhibition of the coagulation cascade [2]. Low-molecular weight heparin (LMWH) predominantly inhibits factor Xa and has a half-life of 3–12 h resulting in less frequent dosing intervals [2]. Additional selective anticoagulants include direct thrombin inhibitors (lepirudin, bivalirudin, and argatroban) and a selective factor Xa inhibitor (fondaparinux) [4]. Antiplatelet agents include aspirin, clopidrogrel, and ticlodipine. Aspirin irreversibly blocks the platelet enzyme cyclooxygenase resulting in inhibition of platelet aggregation for the 10-day life of the platelet. Clopidogrel and ticlodipine inhibit adenosine diphosphate-induced platelet aggregation and have half-lives of 8–12 h.

Major bleeding episodes include intracranial or retroperitoneal hemorrhages and bleeding events that result in death, hospitalization, or transfusion [1, 3, 4]. Major gastrointestinal and urinary tract bleeding events occur in 1–4% of patients per year treated with VKA [1]. The incidence of intracranial hemorrhage among VKA users is less common with reported annual event rates of 0.25–1% [1, 5]. The American College of Chest Physicians defines minor bleeding as reported episodes that do not require additional testing, referrals, or visits [3].

The primary risk factors for anticoagulation-induced bleeding complications include intensity of anticoagulant effect (i.e., higher goal international normalized ratio (INR) have increased bleeding rates), length of anticoagulant therapy, patient characteristics (age, genetic predisposition, comorbid conditions), and concomitant use of medications that also interfere with blood coagulation [4, 5].

Indications for Reversing Anticoagulation

Rapid reversal is essential when patients are experiencing life-threatening bleeding such as intracranial and gastrointestinal hemorrhage, hemorrhagic shock, or have a need for an emergent surgical procedure [2, 4, 5]. Physicians should also consider reversal when bleeding occurs in the deep muscles, retro-orbital spaces, or within joints. Additional indications for considering the risk and benefits of reversal include treatment of open long bone fractures and management of septic shock [1]. The treatment for life-threatening bleeding requires that the INR be rapidly normalized. The decision to reverse a patient's anticoagulated state should also include consideration of the potential thrombogenic risk while not therapeutically anticoagulated [1]. Patients with mechanical heart valves, especially mitral valves, are at increased risk for thromboembolism with rates as high as 4% per year or 0.02% per day when not anticoagulated [1]. Individuals with atrial fibrillation, prior ischemic stroke or transient ischemic attack, or cardiomyopathy with reduced ejection fraction are also at increased risk for thromboembolism [4, 5].

Treatment Options for Reversing Vitamin K Antagonist Anticoagulation

The American College of Chest Physicians' guidelines provide clear, detailed pathways for treating patients with elevated INRs [3]. The guidelines include detailed management of patients with supratherapeutic INR in the absence of bleeding. These guidelines are summarized in Table 1. Treatment options for reversing VKA include: cessation of anticoagulant, vitamin K replacement, fresh frozen plasma (FFP) transfusion, prothrombin complex concentrates (PCC), and recombinant factor VIIa [1–5].

Vitamin K can be administered parenterally or orally. The subcutaneous administration of vitamin K is not recommended due to the unpredictable absorption and response [5]. The injectable form may also be given orally when vitamin K pills are unavailable [2]. Intravenous administration of vitamin K has been associated with anaphylactoid reactions with a reported rate of 3 per 10,000 doses [5]. Many of these episodes occurred with older formulations that contained polyethoxylated castor oil. The modern micelle formulation is thought to have a lower risk of anaphylactoid reactivity [2, 5]. Doses for vitamin K range from 1 to 10 mg depending on INR level and seriousness of bleeding. Vitamin K's full effect does not occur until 12–24 h following administration due to the time needed for hepatic synthesis of new clotting factors [1]. Therefore, vitamin K replacement alone is not sufficient for reversal in the setting of life-threatening bleeding.

FFP contains all vitamin K dependent coagulation factors. Transfusion of FFP is the most commonly used treatment for VKA reversal in North America despite multiple small observational studies reporting the longer time required for INR correction compared to PCC [1, 3]. FFP is administered as a blood-group specific product. The usual dose of FFP administered for emergent reversal is 15 ml/kg of body weight equaling a typical FFP volume of 1,500–2,000 mL. A lower 5–8 ml/kg dose may be

Anticoagulation Reversal in the ED. Table 1 The American College of Chest Physicians' recommendations for managing elevated INRs or bleeding in patients taking VKAs [3]

INR	Asymptomatic or minor bleeding	Major bleeding at any elevated INR level	
If INR above therapeutic range but <5	1. Lower or omit next dose of VKA. Monitor INR and resume at same or lower dose when INR is therapeutic. Consider vitamin K 1–2.5 mg, if needed, for increased bleeding risk.	1. Hold VKA therapy.	
		2. All patients with major bleeding should receive vitamin K 10 mg by slow IV infusion. May repeat dose every 12 h.	
INR ≥5 but ≤9	1. Hold next 1–2 doses of VKA. Monitor INR and resume at same or lower dose when INR is therapeutic. May consider vitamin K 1–2.5 mg orally if increased bleeding risk. If more rapid reversal needed (i.e., urgent procedure), vitamin K 5 mg dose may be given for expected INR reduction within 24 h.	*If potentially life-threatening hemorrhage or need for emergent surgery, the goal is to rapidly normalize the INR. Proceed with the following:*	
		3a. Administer fresh frozen plasma (10–15 mL/kg). Smaller dose of 5–8 mL/kg might be sufficient for reversal of therapeutic INR	
		or	
INR ≥9	1. Hold VKA therapy. Give vitamin K 2.5–5 mg orally for expected substantial INR reduction within 24–48 h. Monitor INR and resume at appropriately adjusted dose when INR is therapeutic. Use additional vitamin K if needed.	3b. Prothrombin complex concentrate (25–100 U/kg)	
		or	
		3c. Recombinant Factor VIIa (10–90 ug/kg)	
		4. Repeat Steps 2 and 3a–c, if necessary, to stop hemorrhage and normalize INR	

Definitions: Major bleeding is defined as life-threatening bleeding that requires treatment, hospitalization, or transfusion [3]. Minor bleeding as reported episodes that do not require additional testing, referrals, or visits [3].

sufficient in urgent reversal of therapeutic INR levels [3]. FFP has a number of limitations that must be considered when emergent reversal is needed. Firstly, frozen plasma must be thawed prior to transfusion. Secondly, the required high volume of FFP can be problematic for elderly patients or individuals with heart or renal failure. FFP is also associated with transfusion-related acute lung injury (TRALI). TRALI occurs more often after FFP transfusion than any other blood product component [1, 5].

PCC provides an alternative to FFP. The aforementioned limitations for FFP limit its utility in many of the patient populations who are most likely to be taking VKA (i.e., elderly, heart failure). PCC was originally approved to treat hemophilia B but its role in reversing anticoagulation has been actively studied. PCC contains approximately 25 times higher concentration of the Vitamin K dependent clotting factors than are present

in FFP [2]. PCC does not require ABO blood type compatibility. Many PCC formulations undergo viral inactivation processes to reduce the risk of viral transmission [1]. The most recent PCC formulations often include anticoagulants (i.e., Proteins C, S, Z and antithrombin III) to decrease the risk of thromboembolic complications [1]. The higher concentration of coagulation factors in PCC results in a significantly smaller required volume for reversal (60 ml of PCC is equivalent to 2 L of FFP) [1]. The recommended PCC dose ranges from 25 to 100 U/kg depending on product used and desired level of reversal [1, 4]. Studies comparing speed of INR correction between FFP and PCC have reported faster INR normalization with mean post-treatment INR of 1.3 within 15 min of completing the PCC infusion compared to a post-treatment INR of 2.3 in 12 patients receiving 4 units of FFP [1]. This is due in part to faster PCC

Anticoagulation Reversal in the ED. Table 2 Reversal options for common anticoagulants (Adapted from tables within referenced articles [1, 4])

Anticoagulant	Minor bleeding	Major bleeding
Unfractionated heparin (UFH)	1. Consider stopping UFH based on indication for treatment and bleeding risk. 2. Close observation.	1. Slow IV infusion of protamine 1 mg/100 U of UFH given in past 4 h. (Keep dose <100 mg over 2 h to reduce risk of hypotension and bradycardia.) 2. Titrate additional doses to bleeding status. Monitor hemodynamics and aPTT.
Low-molecular weight heparin (LMWH)	1. Consider stopping LMWH based on indication for treatment and bleeding risk. 2. Close observation.	1. Slow IV infusion of protamine 1 mg per 1 mg of LMWH given in past 8 h. Decrease dose to 0.5 mg of protamine for every 1 mg LMWH given between 8 and 12 h prior to event (keep dose <100 mg over 2 h). 2. Titrate additional doses to bleeding status. Monitor hemodynamics, aPTT, and INR.
Antiplatelet agents (aspirin, clopidogrel, and ticlodipine)	1. Consider stopping drug based on indication for treatment and bleeding risk. 2. Close observation.	1. Platelet transfusion to increase platelet level by 20,000–50,000.
Direct thrombin inhibitors (lepirudin, bivalirudin, and argatroban)	1. Consider stopping drug based on indication for treatment and bleeding risk. 2. Close observation. 3. No approved treatment.	1. No approved treatment. 2. Desmopressin acetate 0.3 µg/kg in normal saline IV over 15 min. 3. Transfuse ≥10 units of cryoprecipitate. 4. Monitor INR, aPTT, thrombin times.
Pentasaccharide (fondaparinux)	1. Consider stopping drug based on indication for treatment and bleeding risk. 2. Close observation. 3. No approved treatment.	1. No approved treatment. 2. In life-threatening bleeding, consider recombinant factor VIIa (10–90 ug/kg). 3. Monitor INR, aPTT, thrombin-generation times.

Definitions: Major bleeding is defined as life-threatening bleeding that requires treatment, hospitalization, or transfusion [3]. Minor bleeding as reported episodes that do not require additional testing, referrals, or visits [3]. aPTT=activated partial thromboplastin time

preparation (does not require thawing) and infusion (smaller volume) [1].

Recombinant factor VIIa has been evaluated as a treatment for VKA in small case series and been found to have generally favorable results [2]. Recombinant factor VIIa has a half-life of 2.8 h and thrombosis rates of up to 7% have been reported [2, 4]. Future clinical trials are needed to determine the value of recombinant factor VIIa in emergent VKA reversal.

Reversing Unfractionated Heparin and Low-Molecular Weight Heparin

The short half-life of unfractionated heparin (UFH) results in approximately 3 h of anticoagulation [2]. Conservative treatment for minor bleeding episodes might be observation and close monitoring of bleeding and hemodynamics (Table 2). In situations of life-threatening bleeding requiring immediate correction, protamine may be administered. Protamine, a mixture of peptides extracted from fish sperm cell nuclei, is administered intravenously and binds to UFH forming a stable inactive salt [2]. Protamine is dosed based on the amount of UFH administered within the previous 4 h with 1 mg of protamine able to neutralize 100 units of UFH [2, 4]. Protamine should not be given faster than 50 mg per 10 min due to risk of histamine release with associated hypotension, bradycardia, and bronchoconstriction [2]. There is no proven treatment for reversing low-molecular weight heparin [4]. Protamine will neutralize LMWH's antithrombin effect (approximately 60% of its total anticoagulation effect) but does not completely reverse the Factor Xa inhibition [2, 4]. When presented with a patient with life-threatening bleeding taking enoxaparin or dalteparin within the last 8 h, consider administering 1 mg of protamine per 1 mg of enoxaparin or 1 mg of protamine per 100 units of dalteparin [4]. If bleeding continues, a second dose of protamine 0.5 mg per 1 mg enoxaparin or 100 U dalteparin should be administered [4].

Direct Thrombin Inhibitors

There are no accepted treatments for reversing direct thrombin inhibitors [4]. Recombinant factor VIIa, PCC, and deamino-D-arginine vasopressin (DDAVP) have been studied as possible treatment options but none are currently approved [4]. DDAVP promotes the release of Factor VIII and von Willebrand factor from plasma endothelium resulting in increased hemostasis [4].

Selective Factor Xa Inhibitors

Fondaparinux, a pentasaccharide anticoagulant, binds to antithrombin inhibiting its affinity to bind Factor Xa [4].

There are no specific antidotes for this drug class [4]. FFP, PCC, and protamine administration do not adequately reverse the medication's anticoagulant effect [4]. Small studies have suggested that recombinant factor VIIa might partially reverse the pentasaccharide's effect but definitive studies are still needed [4].

Antiplatelet Agents

Aspirin irreversibly inhibits platelet aggregation for the life of the platelet, typically 10 days. No specific antidote treats aspirin's effects. Patients with life-threatening bleeding who are on chronic aspirin therapy require platelet transfusions. The goal should be to raise the affected individual's platelet level by 20,000–50,000. The longer elimination times for clopidogrel and ticlodipine make reversal more challenging. Unlike aspirin that is eliminated rather quickly, clopidogrel and ticlodipine remain and may potentially inhibit newly transfused platelets.

References

1. Vigué B (2009) Bench-to-bedside review: Optimising emergency reversal of vitamin K antagonists in severe haemorrhage - from theory to practice. Crit Care 13(2):209
2. Schulman S, Bijsterveld NR (2007) Anticoagulants and their reversal. Transfus Med Rev 21(1):37–48
3. Ansell J, Hirsh J, Hylek E, Jacobson A, Crowther M, Palareti G (2008) American College of Chest Physicians. Pharmacology and management of the vitamin K antagonists: American College of Chest Physicians Evidence-Based Clinical Practice Guidelines (8th Edition). Chest 133(6 Suppl):160S–198S
4. Crowther MA, Warkentin TE (2008) Bleeding risk and the management of bleeding complications in patients undergoing anticoagulant therapy: focus on new anticoagulant agents. Blood 111(10):4871–4879
5. Makris M, van Veen JJ, Maclean R (2010) Warfarin anticoagulation reversal: management of the asymptomatic and bleeding patient. J Thromb Thrombolysis 29(2):171–181

Antidiuretic Hormone (ADH)

► Vasopressin

Anti-glomerular Basement Membrane (GBM) Disease

► Pulmonary-Renal Syndrome

Antimicrobial Administration in Critical Infections

DAVID F. GAIESKI[1], MUNISH GOYAL[2]
[1]Department of Emergency Medicine, Hospital of the University of Pennsylvania, Philadelphia, PA, USA
[2]Department of Emergency Medicine, Washington Hospital Center, Washington, DC, USA

Synonyms

Early administration of antibiotics; Empiric antibiotics; Time to antibiotics

Definition

A management strategy for patients with infection and evidence of tissue hypoperfusion that incorporates appropriate antimicrobial administration into the proximal phase of resuscitation.

Characteristics

▶ Except on few occasions, the patient appears to die from the body's response to infection rather than from . . . the infection itself. (Sir William Osler, Evolution of Modern Medicine, 1904)

Introduction

While not all infections require antimicrobials, some bacterial, viral, and fungal infections require antimicrobial therapy to eradicate the causative agent and prevent further progression of disease. If left untreated, the body may mount an inflammatory response to an infectious agent as a form of self-defense. This response to infection is known as sepsis and exists on a continuum of severity. When an infectious agent causes tissue hypoperfusion, rapid administration of antimicrobials becomes crucial.

If the septic patient is left untreated, organ dysfunction may develop. This is known as severe sepsis and is accompanied by a marked increase in mortality. Septic shock occurs when inadequate systolic blood pressure (SBP) or mean arterial pressure (MAP) persists despite adequate restoration of intravascular volume. Recently the concept of cryptic septic shock has added another category to the sepsis continuum. Patients with cryptic septic shock have elevated or normal SBP or MAP accompanied by elevated serum lactate levels as a marker of significant tissue level hypoperfusion. The addition of this category recognizes that the central component of shock is not a specific level of blood pressure but rather inadequate oxygen delivery to meet tissue level oxygen demands.

As sepsis progresses along this severity continuum, at some point it becomes a time sensitive disease where inflammation is rapidly progressing, immunomodulatory dysfunction begins, and reversible organ dysfunction becomes irreversible organ injury.

Timing of Antimicrobial Administration

Administration of appropriate antimicrobials to patients with progressive infections is central to halting disease escalation. What is less clear is where along the continuum the rapidity of administration of these antimicrobials becomes central to efficacy. Put another way, early on in the infectious process (e.g., a developing pneumonia), a delay of hours in administering antibiotics may have no impact on outcome. On the other hand, when that pneumonia has progressed to septic shock, administration of appropriate antibiotics rapidly takes precedence such that a small delay may have significant impact on the chances of survival. Aggressiveness of antibiotic timing must be balanced with appropriateness of antibiotic use. We are not suggesting a cavalier approach to administration of antibiotics – clinicians must clearly differentiate which infections require antimicrobial therapy for eradication and deliver these agents in an appropriately timely fashion.

In a retrospective analysis, Fine et al. [1] demonstrated that hospitalized Medicare patients with pneumonia who had antibiotics administered within 8 h of admission had lower 30-day mortality than those receiving the antibiotics at greater than 8 h. Similarly, also using patients in a Medicare database, Houck et al. [2] found that for patients who had not received prehospital antibiotics, administration of the first dose of antibiotics within 4 hours of admission was associated with a lower 30-day mortality rate. The accuracy of these findings and the extent to which they are primarily driven by the importance of early antibiotics in critically ill patients have not been resolved.

Further insight into the impact of antimicrobials on disease progression comes from animal experiments including Kumar et al.'s murine model of septic shock [3]. In this model, intraperitoneal implantation of a gelatin-coated *Escherichia coli* capsule was employed. Over the next 6–15 h, a stereotypical pattern of inflammation, organ dysfunction, increasing serum lactate levels, and emerging hypotension develops if the animals remain untreated. Kumar and his colleagues demonstrated that this pattern of progression was reversible with administration of appropriate antimicrobials until the animals reached a tipping point, occurring between 12 and 15 h after intraperitoneal implantation, coincident with increasing lactate levels and the onset of sustained hypotension. The MAP in septic mice began to differ from sham mice and baseline values within 9 h of implantation. In mice receiving antimicrobials 12 versus 15 h after implantation, the 96-hour survival rate was 80% and 13.3%, respectively. Eighteen hours after implantation, administration of appropriate antimicrobials had no impact on mortality, as all of these mice, as well as controls, were dead at 96 h.

Kumar also performed a retrospective analysis of a large database of ICU patients with septic shock, examining the relationship between the duration of time from the onset of hypotension to the initiation of appropriate antimicrobials and survival [4]. They found a stepwise decrease in survival with antimicrobial delays such that if patients with septic shock received appropriate antimicrobials in the first hour after onset of hypotension, mortality was 20%, but if appropriate antimicrobials were delayed to the sixth hour, mortality exceeded 60%. On average, each hour's delay to appropriate antimicrobial initiation was associated with a 7.6% decrease in survival. Extensive details about the adequacy of hemodynamic resuscitation in these patients are not available. However, in multivariate analysis controlling for intravenous fluid resuscitation, vasopressor use, APACHE II score, and double coverage of the causative agent, time to appropriate antimicrobial was most strongly associated with survival.

As the idea of a whole bundle of sepsis care has emerged and been embraced by the Surviving Sepsis Campaign (SSC), early antimicrobial administration has been accompanied by hemodynamic optimization, also known as early goal-directed therapy (EGDT), ventilator management strategies to prevent acute lung injury, glucose management strategies, and other aspects of critical care. The SSC based their recommendations on the data from Kumar's retrospective trial and one other trial, which demonstrated that a delay of greater than 12 h in administering empiric antifungal coverage in febrile oncology patients with candidemia resulted in increased mortality. They recommended that appropriate antimicrobial therapy be administered within 1 h of recognition of severe sepsis or septic shock. The competing demands of initial resuscitation, along with the crowding seen in many EDs, make this a difficult task to achieve in most instances.

A couple of investigators have studied the relationship between early antimicrobial administration and outcomes in patients with severe sepsis or septic shock who were managed using an algorithmic resuscitation strategy. Varpula et al. [5] studied the impact of early treatment guidelines, including early antibiotic administration and early hemodynamic optimization, on outcomes in patients with severe sepsis and septic shock in Finland. In

a cohort of 92 patients, they found that a "delayed start to antibiotics was the most significant individual early treatment variable resulting in increased mortality." Significantly reduced mortality was noted in patients in whom antibiotic therapy was initiated less than 3 h after presentation. However, only 53% of the patients received antibiotics within 3 h and specific screening and resuscitation goals specified by EGDT (assessment of lactate, CVP, MAP, $ScvO_2$) were only addressed in a minority of patients. Gaieski et al. [6] investigated the relationship between time from triage to appropriate antimicrobials and time from qualification for EGDT to appropriate antimicrobials in a cohort of 261 patients treated with EGDT for severe sepsis or septic shock. All patients had their EGDT goals addressed and optimization attempted during the first 6 h after presentation to the ED. The median time from triage to first antimicrobial administration was 119 min and the median time from qualification for EGDT to antimicrobials was 42 min. Mortality was decreased when time from triage to administration of appropriate antimicrobials occurred in less than 1 h (<1 h, 19.5% versus >1 h, 33.2%). Similar mortality reduction was seen when time from qualification for EGDT to administration of appropriate antimicrobials was less than 1 h (<1 h, 25.0% versus >1 h, 38.5%). These results remained when analyzed for cryptic septic shock versus hypotensive septic shock and in multivariate analysis examining intravenous fluid volume, age, and APACHE II score.

When patients with sepsis reach the tipping point of the development of severe sepsis with tissue hypoperfusion manifested as increased serum lactate level or persistent hypotension, early appropriate antimicrobial administration takes on increasing importance. In these patients, appropriate antimicrobials should be started within 1 h of recognition of shock. Further studies are needed to better understand timing of antimicrobial administration in less severe disease and in different infectious processes (meningitis, pneumonia, pyelonephritis).

Emergency and intensive care health providers should develop protocols to optimize antibiotic administration. These protocols should include bundles of antimicrobials based upon suspected source, suspected organism, up-to-date local antibiograms, administration time, and cost. Once antimicrobials are selected, these medications should be placed in the ED and ICU to minimize delays. If multiple antimicrobials will be administered, those that can be rapidly administered should be given first. A multidisciplinary quality assurance program is important to track compliance with antimicrobial choice and timeliness.

This review supports the current international guidelines recommending early administration of appropriate antimicrobials in patients with severe sepsis and septic shock.

References

1. Fine MJ et al (1997) A prediction rule to identify low-risk patients with community-acquired pneumonia. New Eng J Med 336(4):243–250
2. Houck PM et al (2004) Timing of antibiotic administration and outcomes for medicare patients hospitalized with community-acquired pneumonia. Arch Int Med 164(6):637–644
3. Kumar A et al (2006) The duration of hypotension before the initiation of antibiotic treatment is a critical determinant of survival in a murine model of *Escherichia coli* septic shock: association with serum lactate and inflammatory cytokine levels. J Infect Dis 193:251–258
4. Kumar A et al (2006) Duration of hypotension before initiation of effective antimicrobial therapy is the critical determinant of survival in human septic shock. Crit Care Med 34(6):1589–1596
5. Varpula M et al (2007) Community-acquired septic shock: early management and outcome in a nationwide study in Finland. Acta Anaesthesiol Scand 51(10):1320–1326
6. Gaieski DF (2010) Impact of time to antibiotics on survival in patients with severe sepsis or septic shock in whom early goal-directed therapy was initiated in the emergency department. Crit Care Med 38(4):1045–1053

Antioxidants, Clinical Importance

METTE M. BERGER, LUCAS LIAUDET
Adult Intensive Care Medicine Service and Burn Center, CHUV (University Hospital), Lausanne, Switzerland

Synonyms

Free radical scavenger

Characteristics

Reactive Oxygen and Reactive Nitrogen Species

The presence of free radicals in biological materials was first identified by Commoner in 1954. A further major step in the field was the recognition, by Furchgott and Zawadzki, that the vascular endothelium releases a chemical factor relaxing the vascular smooth muscle, which was soon identified by Ignarro as the free radical nitric oxide (NO·). Since then, free radicals have been recognized both as fundamental molecular devices essential to normal cell physiology, as well as potent cytotoxic species involved in virtually every human disease [1].

Free radicals are molecules or fragments of molecules containing one or more unpaired electrons in their molecular orbitals, which make the basis of their strong chemical reactivity. Indeed, the stabilization of the unpaired electron(s) requires the abstraction of one or more electrons to neighboring molecules. Such ability is shared by some non-radical species with a highly positive redox potential, including hydrogen peroxide or peroxinitrite (see below) [2]. Collectively, such radical and non-radical species are termed oxidants. These belong to two major families, namely, the reactive oxygen species (ROS) and the reactive nitrogen species (RNS).

ROS are oxygen-centered, and their parent molecule is the superoxide anion radical (O_2^-, the superscripted dot representing the unpaired electron). Reaction of O_2^- with other molecules (either directly or indirectly through enzyme or metal catalysis, such as iron-catalyzed Fenton reaction) yields secondary ROS, including the hydroxyl radical OH· and hydrogen peroxide (H_2O_2, non-radical). The main sources of O_2^- are the mitochondria and various enzyme systems. Under physiological conditions, about 2% of electrons entering the mitochondrial respiratory chain "leak" directly to oxygen, mainly at the ubiquinone binding sites of Complex I and Complex III, resulting in the one electron reduction of oxygen, forming O_2^-. Thus, O_2^- is a byproduct of normal cell respiration, which does not accumulate due to rapid detoxification by the mitochondrial superoxide dismutase (see below). This process becomes however significant under conditions of cell hypoxia and mitochondrial damage, which increase electron leak.

The major enzymatic sources of O_2^- are xanthine oxidoreductase (XOR) and nicotinamide adenine dinucleotide phosphate (NADPH) oxidase (NOX). XOR is a ubiquitous molybdene flavoprotein normally working as a xanthine deshydrogenase (XDH) involved in purine catabolism, converting xanthine and hypoxanthine into uric acid. Under certain circumstances (such as tissue ischemia), XDH is converted into xanthine oxidase (XO), which generates significant amounts of O_2^- during purine catabolism. NOX is an enzyme complex mainly present in leukocytes, but also found in endothelial and vascular smooth muscle cells. It is formed from five major subunits ($p40^{phox}$, $p47^{phox}$, $p67^{phox}$, $p22^{phox}$, and $gp91^{phox}$), assembled on a membrane-bound vesicle upon cell activation, which fuses with the plasma membrane to release O_2^-. Although of a much lesser importance, additional enzymes with an NADPH oxidase function may also generate O_2^- under certain conditions (not detailed here due to space limitation), including nitric oxide synthase, cytochrome p450 and cyclo-oxygenase.

RNS are nitrogen-centered species, whose parent molecule is NO. The major sources of NO˙ production are the NO synthases (NOS), which convert L-arginine into L-citrulline and NO˙ via a five-electron oxidative reaction. Three NOS isoforms exist, namely, neuronal (type I), inducible (type II), and endothelial (type III). All three use NADPH and molecular oxygen as cosubstrates, and contain similar prosthetic groups and cofactors. Under physiological conditions, NO˙ produced in low concentration acts as a messenger and cytoprotective (antioxidant) device, by interacting directly with transition metals and other free radicals, and by promoting the S-nitrosylation of cysteine residues (SNO) within proteins, thereby modulating their biological activity. Alternatively, in conditions favoring higher fluxes of NO˙ and simultaneously promoting the generation of O_2^- (for instance, circulatory shock or systemic inflammation), the chemistry of NO˙ is redirected toward indirect effects, related to the formation of higher nitrogen oxides, most significantly peroxynitrite ($ONOO^-$). The latter is a highly reactive non-radical oxidant formed from the diffusion-limited reaction of NO with O_2^- (rate constant k between 6.6 and 19 $\times$ $10^9\,M^{-1}\,s^{-1}$). In addition to promote oxidative reactions, peroxynitrite also introduces a particular modification of tyrosine residues within proteins, termed nitration (adjunction of a $- NO_2$ group within the aromatic ring of tyrosine). Nitration results from a radical attack of the tyrosine residue by the nitrogen dioxide radical (NO_{2}˙), which is mainly formed following the reaction of peroxynitrite with CO_2, yielding the radicals CO_3^- (carbonate) and NO_2.

Antioxidant Defense Mechanisms

Antioxidants are substances able to compete, at low concentrations, with other oxidizable substrates, thereby inhibiting (or delaying) their oxidation. Two main categories of antioxidants occur in biological systems, namely, enzymatic and nonenzymatic. The major antioxidant enzymes are represented by superoxide dismutase (SOD), catalase, and the selenoproteins glutathione peroxidase and thioredoxin reductase. SOD enzymes are ubiquitous metalloproteins, classified according to their localization and the metal present at their active site (MnSOD present in mitochondria, and Cu-Zn SOD present in the cytosol and the extracellular milieu). SODs catalyze the dismutation of O_2^- (1).

$$2O_2^- + 2H^+ \rightarrow O_2 + H_2O_2 \quad (1)$$

Catalase, a ubiquitous homotetrameric protein especially concentrated in the liver and erythrocytes, decomposes hydrogen peroxide into water (2).

$$2H_2O_2 \rightarrow 2H_2O + O_2 \quad (2)$$

All selenoproteins contain selenocysteine [3]: the glutathione peroxidase family (GPX: $n = 6$), the thioredoxin reductases (TRXR, $n = 3$), and selenoproteins H, N, and P are essential for the redox homeostasis; some further selenoproteins are probably also involved in redox mechanisms. The GPXs reduce hydrogen peroxide into water by oxidizing reduced glutathione (3), the latter being reduced back by glutathione reductase in the glutathione cycle (4)

$$H_2O_2 + GSH \rightarrow 2H_2O + GSSG \quad (3)$$

$$GSSG + NADPH + H^+ \rightarrow 2GSH + NADP^+ \quad (4)$$

The thioredoxin reductases, located in the cytosol and in the mitochondria, reduce oxidized thioredoxins (TRs), which themselves reduce disulphide bridges in oxidized proteins, using two redox active cysteine-bound thiols (5, 6)

$$TR - SH + prot - SS \rightarrow TR - SS + prot -SH(\text{action of TRs}) \quad (5)$$

$$TR - SS + NADPH + H^+ \rightarrow TR - SH + NADP^+ \quad (6)$$
$$(\text{action of TRXRs})$$

The glutharedoxins are additional members of the TR superfamily. They use cysteine-bound thiols to reduce disulphide bridges and they are reduced back nonenzymatically by reduced glutathione. Finally, the peroxiredoxins (PRXs) represent a recently identified group of essential antioxidant proteins. PRXs use a redox active cysteine to directly scavenge H_2O_2. They appear to play a critical role in antioxidant defenses within the mitochondria, which do not possess catalase.

Among the nonenzymatic antioxidants, reduced glutathione (GSH) plays the most important role. GSH is a tripeptide formed by the amino acids Glu-Cys-Gly. It is abundantly present in all cell compartments, at concentrations of about 5–10 mM. The thiol (–SH) group of cysteine supports the biological antioxidant activity of GSH, by serving as an electron donor. GSH is used as a cofactor for GPX. It can also directly scavenge various free radicals, such as OH˙ (hydroxyl) and O˙ (singlet oxygen), and allows the regeneration of other antioxidants, including vitamin C and vitamin E. Oxidized glutathione (GSSG) is reduced back by the activity of the enzyme glutathione reductase. Additional nonenzymatic antioxidants are represented by α-tocopherol (vitamin E), ascorbate (vitamin C), β-carotene, and flavonoids. Furthermore, most free amino acids, although relatively weak antioxidants, represent quantitatively important free radicals scavengers due to their high intracellular concentrations.

Targets and Cytotoxic Pathways Elicited by ROS and RNS

When the generation of ROS-RNS exceed endogenous antioxidant defenses, redox homeostasis can no more be maintained, resulting in a state of oxidative stress. Other terms used to describe such imbalance are nitrosative stress (excess NO˙ production) and nitroxidative stress (excess peroxynitrite generation).

ROS and RNS initiate lipid peroxidation by abstracting a hydrogen atom from polyunsaturated fatty acids (PUFA), resulting in the formation of lipid hydroperoxyradicals, conjugated dienes and aldehydes, which can attack neighboring PUFAs, generating additional radicals that propagate the free radical reaction and the degeneration of membrane lipids, causing membrane permeability and fluidity changes with significant biological consequences.

ROS-RNS also damage proteins by oxidizing thiols, iron/sulfur centers, and zinc fingers. As mentioned earlier, tyrosine nitration is a specific alteration promoted by peroxynitrite within proteins, whereas enhanced S-nitrosylation occurs in states of nitrosative stress. These various alterations may result into a gain or loss of function, or an enhanced degradation of the modified proteins, including ionic pumps, metabolic enzymes, structural proteins, and signaling proteins. A major group of proteins particularly vulnerable to inactivation by oxidants are those involved in mitochondrial electron transport, including NADH:ubiquinone oxidoreductase (Complex I), cytochrome oxidase (Complex IV), and ATP synthase (Complex V). Such inactivation may precipitate bioenergetic failure, leading to cell dysfunction and eventually cell death. Another critical consequence of protein oxidation/nitration is altered cell signaling. While subtle changes of cellular redox state is a key mechanism of cellular homeostasis (redox signaling), enhanced ROS-RNS formation may promote long lasting and pathological alterations of cell signaling. Disturbed signaling relies on the modification of cell receptors (e.g., growth factor receptors), protein kinases (e.g., MAP kinases), protein phosphatases, and transcription factors (e.g., NF-κB, AP-1, and HIF-1).

Another key target of oxidants is DNA. Free radicals damage nucleobases, especially guanine due to its low redox potential, resulting in the formation of 8-oxoguanine. Oxidants further attack the sugar phosphate backbone of DNA by abstracting a hydrogen atom from the deoxyribose moiety, opening the sugar ring and generating DNA strand breaks. Importantly, such DNA strand breaks are sensed by the nuclear enzyme poly(ADP-ribose) polymerase (PARP), leading to its activation and the consumption of its substrate, nicotinamide adenine dinucleotide (NAD^+). Excessive activation of PARP in conditions of intense oxidative stress therefore results in NAD shortage and in the breakdown of ATP production. It is assumed that PARP activation therefore largely contributes to the development of so-called cytopathic hypoxia.

Antioxidant Status During Critical Illness

Critically ill patients, whatever the etiology of their disease, are characterized by increased production of oxygen or NO derived free radicals. Although oxidative stress is part of the normal defense mechanisms, it may become deleterious in the critically ill patient, when escaping endogenous control, and several critical conditions including ARDS and sepsis are either caused, worsened, or maintained by increased ROS production [4]. A central paradigm of organ dysfunction has been shown to be impaired oxygen utilization (cytopathic hypoxia) with overwhelming oxidative stress and impaired phosphorylation and ATP depletion at the mitochondrial level [5].

A large proportion of endogenous antioxidant defenses is ensured by vitamins and trace elements with antioxidant functions. Several analytical methods have been used for research for assessment of oxidative stress and antioxidants in blood, cells, and tissues, but these methods can generally not be used in clinical settings, where the analysis in the circulating compartments remains the only possibility despite its limitations [6]. Indeed the blood/plasma concentrations only reflect the flow between compartments and not real status. Nevertheless, low plasma concentrations of, for example, selenium have been shown to be associated with low activity of the selenium-dependent enzymes such as the glutathione peroxidase (GPX) family. This relation between low concentration and low activity has also been shown to be true for other antioxidant micronutrients.

The circulating concentrations of most trace elements (particularly Fe, Se, Zn), of their carrier proteins and water soluble vitamins decrease during the acute phase response and its systemic extension (SIRS). The trace elements and vitamins are redistributed via cytokine-mediated mechanisms to organs, tissues, and cells with increased activity during inflammation such as the liver, spleen, kidney, and the reticulo-endothelial system. Low plasma levels of antioxidant micronutrients have been repeatedly shown during critical illness, in association with evidence of peroxidative damage (increased malondialdehyde production etc.), or low antioxidant enzyme activity. Nevertheless, the low plasma concentrations observed in the ICU have many causes. In addition to the SIRS-mediated redistribution of micronutrients from the circulating compartment to tissues and organs, acute losses through biological fluids (exudates, drains, effluents form continuous renal replacement, other digestive losses), or dilution due to resuscitation fluids and insufficient intakes contribute heavily too. The compartmental depletion of endogenous AOX defenses results in a disturbance in the prooxidant-antioxidant balance in favor of the former resulting in cell damage and disease.

Several micronutrients, including selenium, limit the release of NFκB caused by increased ROS, thereby limiting the extension of the inflammatory response. It has been hypothesized that the redistribution of trace elements occurring during the acute phase response may therefore be deleterious if prolonged, due to the depletion of the circulating compartment's AOXs.

Further, critically ill patients frequently have preadmission suboptimal or deficient status: an important part of the population is indeed exposed to the risk of micronutrient deficiency caused, for example, by changes in eating habits in Western countries, but also the lower food concentration of micronutrients. The most common deficits involve vitamin C (hypovitaminosis present in 47% of hospitalized patients), vitamin B1 (present in 20% of hospital and ICU admissions), selenium and zinc (10–20% of the population does not consume RDA requirements), all involved in antioxidant and immune defenses. Should we bother about this abnormal prehospital or ICU admission status? Animal models show that pre-event status negatively impacts on outcome: pre-burn selenium deficiency is associated with increased baseline lipid peroxidation, not reversible by Se supplementation; in models of sepsis, preexisting zinc deficiency worsens organ damage. These negative consequences may well be true to humans.

Antioxidant Supplementation Candidates

Among micronutrients, selenium appears as the most potent AOX agent in clinical settings, followed by zinc, vitamins C, E, and β-carotene [4]. Other compounds, generally present in food, do have AOX properties, such as urea, glucose, bilirubin, proteins, vitamin C, vitamin E, carotenoids, melatonin, coenzyme Q, lipoic acid, the n-3 polyunsaturated fatty acids, eicosapentaenoic (EPA) and docosahexaenoic (DHA) acids, and glutamine (see specific § for w-3 PUFA and glutamine). They are present in human plasma, and are candidates for therapeutic use, but this review will focus on the nutritional components. Due to their clinical availability, known mechanisms of action and presumed safety, as well as to the possibility of systemic supplementation under control of circulating levels, AOX research in critical illness has focused mainly on four micronutrients: vitamins C and E, selenium and zinc, in combination (or not) with other agents.

Intervention strategies may be (1) preventive, maintaining or restoring the normal antioxidant capacity, or (2) "therapeutic," that is, delivering antioxidant nutrient supplements in conditions caused or worsened by oxidative stress, as is the case in critical illness. Therapeutic targets may be the endothelium, the mitochondria, or the circulating compartment. The aim of the intervention can be substrate provision, cofactor provision, or membrane stabilization.

Trials in Critically Ill Patients

A selection of high quality trials is summarized in Table 1. The use of supra-nutritional pharmacological doses has been associated with clinical benefits in several critical care conditions such as major burns, trauma, and severe sepsis, that is, in conditions with an important inflammatory response. The benefits have included reduction of fluid resuscitation requirements and improved wound healing in burns, reduction of organ dysfunction, shortening of ICU stay, of hospital stay, reduction of mortality in other categories, as well as several biological benefits that did not all translate to clinical effects. Alleged mechanisms include mainly antioxidant activity of the micronutrients, but other mechanisms should be kept in mind particularly regarding zinc, which is involved in the intermediary metabolism and most steps of immune defense.

Conclusions

The multiple insults inflicted to biomolecules by oxidants result in significant cytotoxicity, ranging from subtle derangements of specialized cellular functions to apoptosis or even necrosis in case of overt oxidative damage. As such, oxidants and free radicals are considered plausible culprits in the cardiovascular failure, organ dysfunction, and inflammatory changes that occur in critically ill patients. This makes the basis for the development of efficient antioxidant and free radical scavenging therapies.

Among micronutrients, selenium appears as the most potent antioxidant agent in critical care settings, followed by zinc, vitamin C, and vitamin E. The published supplementation trials show that antioxidant micronutrient

Antioxidants, Clinical Importance. Table 1 Selection of antioxidant micronutrient trials in critically ill patients, by publication year

Trial/year	N patients/ diagnosis	Study design	Dose/duration	Outcome/comments
Young et al., J Neurotrauma 1996;13:25	68 Patients with closed brain injury	PRCBT	Zinc 20 mg/day for 2 weeks followed by 12 mg (enteral)	Improved neurological outcome
Berger et al., Am J Clin Nutr 1998	21 Patients with major burns	PRCBT	Cu 3 mg, Se 350 mcg, Zn 35 mg for 8 days, IV	Reduction of IL-6 levels, lipid peroxidation, infectious complications, and normalized length of ICU stay in trace element group
Angstwurm et al., Crit Care Med, 1999; 27:1807	42 Patients with severe SIRS, mainly due to pneumonia	PRCBT	Selenium supplements for 9 days, IV	Significant reduction of acute renal failure with 3 (14%) vs 9 (43%) patients; $P < 0.035$; and a nonsignificant reduction of mortality in selenium group
Porter et al., Am Surg, 1999; 65:478	18 Major trauma patients	PRCBT	N-acetylcysteine, selenium, and vitamins C and E for 7 days	Reduction of infectious complications (8 vs 18) and fewer organ dysfunctions (0 vs 9) in intervention group
Tanaka et al., Arch Surg, 2000;135:326	37 Patients with major burns	Before and after	Vitamin C 66 mg/kg per hour for 24 h, IV	30% Reduction of fluid resuscitation volume, improved PaO2/FiO2 ratio, reduction of length mechanical ventilation in vitamin C group
				Hypothesis: capillary permeability normalization through a NO mediated endothelial mechanism
Berger et al., Nutritonal Research 2001; 21:42	32 Critically ill trauma patients	PRCBT	Selenium 500 µg IV, 150 mg vitamin E enteral	Normalization of thyroid function (triiodothyronine, and thyroxin concentrations), with improved antioxidant status in the supplemented patients
Nathens et al., Ann Surg, 2002; 236:814	595 Including 542 trauma	PRCBT	3 g ascorbic acid, 3 g tocopherol during the ICU stay or 28 days	Reduction of relative risk of pulmonary morbidity was 0.81 (95% confidence interval 0.60–1.1), and multiple organ failure 0.43 (95% confidence interval 0.19–0.96) shortened ICU length of stay
Brooks et al., Lancet, 2004; 363:1683	270 Children with pneumonia	PRCBT	Zinc 20 mg/day (oral)	Reduced duration of severe pneumonia, and of hospital stay
Angstwurm et al., Crit Care Med, 2006;35:118	249 Patients with severe SIRS, sepsis, and septic shock	PRCBT	Selenium 1,000 µg/day for 14 days IV	8-day mortality rate was significantly reduced to 42.4% compared with 56.7%
Berger et al., Crit Care 2006; 10:R153	41 Patients with major burns	PRCBT	Cu 3 mg, Se 350 mcg, Zn 35 mg IV for 8–14 days depending on burn size	65% reduction of nosocomial pneumonia
				Substitution rather than supplementation : Doses were calculated to compensate for the exudative losses

Antithyroid Peroxidase Antibodies. Table 1 (Continued)

Trial/year	N patients/ diagnosis	Study design	Dose/duration	Outcome/comments
Heyland et al., JPEN, 2007; 31:109	58 Critically ill ventilated patients	Prospective, open-label, dose-escalating clinical trial	Glutamine, Selenium, Zinc combinations by IV and enteral route	Normalization of oxidative parameters and a reduction in the blood cell mitochondrial DNA/nuclear DNA ratio, that is, a reduction of oxidative damage
Forceville et al., Crit Care. 2007; 11:R73	60 Patients with severe septic shock	PRCBT	Selenium 4 mg on first day, 1,000 ug/day on the 9 next days	No effect: no obvious toxicity but trends to prolonged ventilation and more respiratory complications in the selenium group
				Ceiling effect > 750–1,000 mcg/day?
Berger et al., Crit Care, 2008; 12:R101	200 Including 77 trauma	PRCBT	Se 270 mcg, Zn 30 mg, vitamin C 1.1 g, vitamin B1 100 mg for 5 days, IV	Reduction of inflammatory response (CRP)
				Shortening of hospital stay in surviving AOX trauma patients (-10 days: $p = 0.045$)
Collier et al., JPEN, 2008; 32:384	4,294 Critically ill trauma	Before and after	Vitamin C 1 g, vitamin E 1,000 UI, and selenium 200 mcg for 7 days	28% Relative risk reduction in mortality and a significant reduction in both hospital and ICU length of stay
Barbosa et al., JBCR, 2009; 30:859	32 Children with major burns	PRCBT	Vitamin E, vitamin C, and zinc	Decreased malondialdehyde plasma levels and reduced wound healing time
Andrews et al., BMJ, 2011; 342:d1442	505 Critically ill patients	PRCBT Factorial design	Selenium 500 mcg Glutamine 20 g	Insufficient doses and duration of supplementation Less infections with selenium for $\geq$5 days (OR:0.53)

IV intravenous, *PRCBT* prospective randomized + placebo controlled + double blinded

supplementation has very few side effects, limited costs, and potential clinical beneficial effects on critical illness. The most successful trials until now have included selenium in doses 300–1,000 mcg/day. The optimal doses and combinations of antioxidants are still to be determined. Indeed, if levels of oxidative stress are increased and probably deleterious when prolonged, it is still uncertain to which levels we should reduce them. If circulating levels of antioxidant micronutrients are inadequately low, which levels should supplementation achieve for optimal antioxidant defenses and adequate balance between them and oxidative stress? An ongoing large size trial combining selenium and glutamine (REducing Deaths due to OXidative Stress = REDOXS) should provide some of the answers.

References

1. Dröge W (2002) Free radicals in the physiological control of cell function. Physiol Rev 82(1):47–95
2. Pacher P, Beckman JS, Liaudet L (2007) Nitric oxide and peroxynitrite in health and disease. Physiol Rev 87(1):315–424
3. Reeves MA, Hoffmann PR (2009) The human selenoproteome: recent insights into functions and regulation. Cell Mol Life Sci 66(15):2457–2478
4. Berger MM, Chiolero RL (2007) Antioxidant supplementation in sepsis and systemic inflammatory response syndrome. Crit Care Med 35(9 Suppl):S584–S590
5. Dare AJ, Phillips AR, Hickey AJ et al (2009) A systematic review of experimental treatments for mitochondrial dysfunction in sepsis and multiple organ dysfunction syndrome. Free Radic Biol Med 47(11):1517–1525
6. Berger MM (2009) Vitamin C requirements in parenteral nutrition. Gastroenterology 137(5 Suppl):S70–S78

Antithyroid Peroxidase Antibodies

In autoimmune thyroid disease, proteins that mistakenly try to attack the thyroid peroxidase (TPO) enzymes that help the thyroid gland make hormone.

Antivenom

Antivenom is a biological product used in the management of poisonous bites and stings. Antivenom is produced by injecting a small amount of the target venom into an animal. The animal will develop an immune response to the venom, producing antibodies against the venom's active molecule. The antivenom can then be harvested for use.

Anuria

► Oliguria in Children
► Oliguria, Clinical Significance
► Oliguria, Investigation and Management

Anxiolytics

► Sedative-Hypnotic

Aortic Counterpulsation

PASCAL VRANCKX[1], MARCO VALGIMIGLI[2], P. W. SERRUYS[3]
[1]Medical Director Cardiac ITU, Hartcentrum Hasselt, Hasselt, Belgium
[2]Director of the Cath. Laboratory, University of Ferrara, Cardiovascular Institute, Arcispedale S. Anna Hospital, Ferrara, Italy
[3]Director of the Department of Interventional Cardiology Thoraxcenter, Erasmus Medical Centre, GD, Rotterdam, The Netherlands

Synonyms

Intra-aortic balloon counterpulsation; Intra-aortic balloon pumping; Intra-aortic balloon support

Definition

The intra-aortic balloon pump (IABP) is currently the most widely used of all circulatory assist devices; its action is based on the concept of *counterpulsation* with the assumption that the reduction in end-diastolic pressure improves left ventricular (LV) function. Counterpulsation improves LV performance by favorably influencing myocardial oxygen balance. It increases myocardial oxygen supply by diastolic augmentation of coronary perfusion and decreases myocardial oxygen requirements through a reduction in the afterload component of cardiac work [1] (Fig. 1).

The indications and applications for IABP have come a long way since the early days of counterpulsation. After almost four decades of use, IABP has become a mature technology. It is the most common method of mechanical cardiac assistance in acute cardiology today.

Pre-existing Condition

Acute Myocardial Infarction

The potential indications for IAB support in patients with ST-segment-elevation myocardial infarction include

- Management of acute heart failure and cardiogenic shock attributable to LV myocardial pump failure in the setting of ST-segment-elevation ACS in the contemporary reperfusion era
- Management of acute heart failure and cardiogenic shock attributable to mechanical complications (e.g., functional and/or structural mitral insufficiency, ventricular septum defect) in the setting of ST-segment-elevation ACS
- High-risk acute myocardial infarction patients, with or without hemodynamic compromise, to rest the heart, reduce the infarct size, and improve clinical outcome

Early, brisk, and sustained reperfusion significantly improves survival after acute myocardial infarction (MI). Primary percutaneous coronary intervention (PCI) in patients with evolving ST-segment-elevation ACS decreases infarct size and the rates of recurrent ischemia, reinfarction, and stroke, and improves survival, as compared with pharmacologic reperfusion therapy. Despite a high rate of patency obtained through primary PCI, myocardial recovery is often suboptimal, and mortality, especially in high-risk patients, such as those with anterior myocardial infarction and acute heart failure is still considerable. Recovery of myocardial performance following successful revascularization of the infarct-related artery may require several days. During this period, many patients succumb to low cardiac output. IAB support is the method of choice for mechanical assistance, since IABP can result in significant improvement of LV performance and initial hemodynamics [2]. Although recent guidelines supported the use of IABP counterpulsation as the method of first choice for mechanical assistance in cardiogenic shock, the efficacy of routine IABP use adjunctive to primary percutaneous coronary

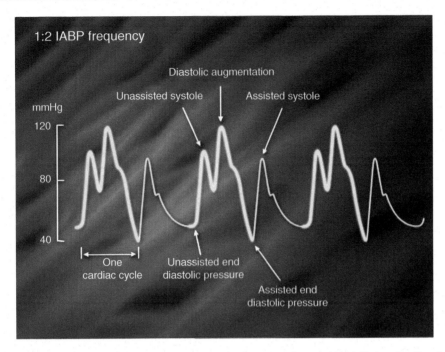

Aortic Counterpulsation. Figure 1 IABP pressure curve, 1:2 ratio of assist. With proper IAB inflation, the dicrotic notch assumes a V-shaped morphology. With proper deflation, the balloon-assisted end-diastolic pressure is lower than the nonassisted end-diastolic pressure; the assisted systole is lower or at least equal to unassisted systole (Reproduced with permission from MAQUET Cardiovascular)

intervention in cardiogenic shock was recently questioned [3]. IABP is incapable of supporting a patient with complete hemodynamic collapse. Also, a prophylactic IABP strategy after primary PTCA in hemodynamically stable high-risk patients with AMI does not decrease the rates of infarct-related artery reocclusion or reinfarction, promote myocardial recovery, or improve overall clinical outcome.

Myocardial necrosis is a time-dependent phenomenon following coronary occlusion. A critically important goal of reperfusion is to restore flow to the infarct-related artery as quickly and as completely as possible, but the ultimate goal of reperfusion in ST-segment-elevation ACS is to reduce myocardial damage and to improve myocardial perfusion in the risk area. Yet, despite flow restoration in epicardial coronary arteries, limited reperfusion at the tissue level due to microvascular obstruction has been documented, and is also known as the "no-reflow phenomenon." This progressive process, which evolves mainly within the first 48 h after reperfusion, may significantly contribute to myocardial infarction extension. Ischemic time is a major independent driver of the probability microvascular dysfunction. This suggests that there might be a therapeutic window for intervention to limit myocardial infarction (extension). Controlled,

randomized studies of early, preferentially, pre(re)perfusion intra-aortic counterpulsation in small animal models of acute MI and subsequent reperfusion have demonstrated improved myocardial perfusion, reduction in microvascular obstruction, and accelerated rate of LV functional recovery. Prolonged and efficient mechanical unloading of the myocardium during ischemia and reperfusion reduced LV pressure work and myocardial oxygen consumption, and proved beneficial for ventricular function, even after late reperfusion. This concept is currently under investigation in high-risk MI patients.

High-Risk Angioplasty

With increasing operator experience and refinement of angioplasty hardware and technique and adjunctive pharmacological treatment, the morphologic and the clinical profile of patients acceptable for coronary angioplasty has widened considerable. PCI is now considered in many high-risk subgroups in which mechanical revascularization was previously contraindicated. At all times, the benefits of a specific PCI procedure should be weighed against the risks involved, taking into account alternative treatment strategies. IABP is suggested to act as a stabilizing measure or to prevent catheterization laboratory events.

Prophylactic IABP may prevent intraprocedural events in high-risk patients with severe depression of the LV ejection fraction (EF ≤ 30%) and/or specific anatomical features (e.g., unprotected left main coronary artery disease). Prophylactic aortic counterpulsation proved superior to provisional ("standby") among patients with low ejection fraction in reducing death, periprocedural MI, stroke, and urgent CABG (0% versus 17%, p 0.001). However, these are still small series of patients, and the decision to proceed with aortic counterpulsation before high-risk PCI still remains a judgment call and should be considered on a case-by-case basis, mainly because of the lack of solid evidence.

Cardiac Surgery

In the early phase, IABP use by cardiothoracic surgeons was when difficulties arose weaning patients off cardiopulmonary bypass following CABG. Early implantation of an intra-aortic balloon pump (IABP) together with pharmacological support leads to the successful weaning from cardiopulmonary bypass in 70–90% of all patients, with hemodynamic recovery and successful explantation of the IABP in 60–70% of the patients [4]. Response to treatment may already be assessed after 60 min, using simple clinical parameters. Nonresponders may need to upgrade to more sophisticated extracorporeal cardiopulmonary assist [5, 6]. Preoperative prophylactic IAB counterpulsation insertion is advocated to reduce surgical mortality in elective or emergency high-risk patients because it provides better hemodynamic stability and coronary perfusion and minimizes low-output syndrome and organ dysfunction. Short-term perioperative "pulsatile" perfusion, implementing aortic counterpulsation, may provide a theoretical advantage of improvement of organ perfusion, due to a reduction of vasoconstrictive reflexes, an optimized oxygen consumption, and a reduction of acidosis. There is expanding evidence supporting prophylactic IABP insertion in high-risk patients preparing for CABG, namely those with critical coronary anatomy (including left main disease) and/or severe LV dysfunction and/or (non) ST-segment-elevation ACS. However, the randomized evidence is from a number of small trials, with a high proportion of unstable patients recruited at a single institution. The assessment of perioperative IABP efficacy still will require a randomized trial.

Heart Transplantation

The IABP has also been used as a bridge to transplant in patients with severe cardiomyopathy. Transplant rejection may be another indication for aortic counterpulsation, as unloading the left ventricle and increasing perfusion of the right ventricle could possibly improve outcomes.

Children

There is class IIa grade C evidence for IABP use in hemodynamically unstable children. However, the use of the IABP in children has been limited, partly because of technical difficulties, although appropriate equipment has been developed. Physiologic differences including greater compliance of the pediatric aorta, the large bronchial vessel in cyanotic diseases, and the higher heart rates in children make augmentation difficult to achieve.

Refractory Tachycardia and Ventricular Irritability

Several anecdotal reports have cited the cessation of arrhythmias after the initiation of aortic counterpulsation, especially ventricular tachycardia and ventricular fibrillation. ACC/AHA guidelines give a class IIa recommendation for IABP therapy in patients with severe malignant arrhythmias that are driven by underlying cardiac ischemia and are refractory to medical therapy.

The IABP is one of the most versatile support devices used in the management of patients suffering from the complications of acute cardiovascular disease. The relative ease and speed at which this device can be applied among patients with a rapidly deteriorating hemodynamic picture have led to its use as a first-line intervention among critically unstable patients. Interventional cardiologists are now the predominant users of this device in practice; the value of the IABP has been established among cardiothoracic surgeons. With this improved risk-benefit ratio, the IABP may probably be applied in other clinical situations to enhance patient outcomes. Indications of interest are

- Preoperative insertion in high-risk noncardiac surgical patients
- Severe sepsis and septic shock

Application

The balloon is positioned in the proximal descending aorta. The balloon is inflated in diastole concurrently with closure of the aortic valve and is held in inflation until onset of the next ventricular systole. The balloon is then rapidly deflated. The inflation of the balloon displaces blood in the aorta (by an amount equal to the volume of the balloon) toward the coronary tree, thereby increasing (augmenting) coronary perfusion pressure and blood flow (Fig. 1). The collapse of the balloon creates a reduction in impedance of the left ventricular ejection,

Aortic Counterpulsation. **Table 1** Conditions interfering
with the hemodynamic effects of IAB pumping

Position of the balloon in the aorta
Heart rate and rhythm
Size and volume of the balloon
Compliance of the aorta (aortic pressure volume relation)

and decreased afterload, and consequently reduces left
ventricular work. The hemodynamic effects of IAB
pumping are dependent on several factors (Table 1). For
decades, the ability to increase distal coronary blood
beyond severe coronary obstruction stenosis with IABP
have been debated. However, in early work, coronary
hemodynamics and flow measurements might have been
adversely affected by impeding distal coronary flow as the
Doppler guide wire passed beyond the stenosis. However,
when assessed totally noninvasive by currently available
transthoracic Doppler echocardiography, IAB support
produced significant distal flow enhancement even in
patients with critical proximal stenosis.

The Clinical System for Intra-Aortic Balloon Pumping

Our IABC cardiac assistance system consists of a catheter
and a balloon inserted mostly through a femoral
arteriotomy into the thoracic aorta. Over the last several
decades, there has been a dramatic improvement in the
technology and refined percutaneous insertion techniques.
These advancements have lowered major complication
rates associated with IABP rates to the low single digits.

Patient Instrumentation

IA Balloon Insertion

"Pre-warned is pre-armed." A complete vascular physical
examination should be performed prior to IABP insertion. It should include the palpation of all lower extremity
pulses, as well as auscultation of the lower abdomen and
the femoral arteries.

The femoral artery is *cannulated* providing a modified
Seldinger technique. Strategies aimed at reducing femoral
artery access site complications, such as use of fluoroscopy
and vascular echography to guide femoral artery access,
have been introduced and implemented into practice. An
angiogram of the iliofemoral bed may allow to identify
significant peripheral vascular disease. Prophylactic percutaneous angioplasty with or without the use of vascular
stents can be considered. A Teflon-coated guide wire is

advanced through the lumen. The needle is removed and
a step dilator is passed over the wire to predilate the
subcutaneous tissue and the arterial cannulation.

Figure 2 illustrates the correct *positioning* of the IAB
catheter. The IAB mounted on a catheter is inserted
into the descending aorta mostly percutaneously
through a femoral artery in the leg. The balloon is
positioned with the tip just distal to the left subclavian
artery (be sure you feel the radial pulse in the left arm:
the tip of the balloon is not occluding the left subclavian inflow). The intra-aortic balloon is inflated with
helium, an inert gas that is easily absorbed into the
bloodstream in case of accidental balloon rupture. Its
low molecular weight enables very quick pendeling of
the gas, allowing the pump system to support high and
irregular heart rates.

IA Balloon Removal

The tubing should not be placed to negative pressure to
avoid stiffening of the balloon in preparation for removal.
The balloon and sheath, if used, should be slowly removed
as a unit and pressure applied distally to allow blood flow
from the arterial access site for a few seconds. This maneuver clears clots that may have formed at the insertion site
to flow out of the artery. Manual pressure or a mechanical/
pneumatic hemostasis device can then be applied slightly
above the insertion site until hemostasis is achieved. The
distal pulses should be checked regularly and the patient
kept supine for at least 6 h to reduce possible bleeding
complications.

Balloon Construction

IAB catheter technology has evolved over time. Different
sizes are currently available, allowing to tailor balloon size
to patient length (Fig. 3). Smaller catheter diameter sizes
and the option for sheathless insertion should improve
distal limb blood flow and further contribute to
a reduction of vascular complications, especially in
patients with heavy arterial calcification, ileofemoral disease, or obesity. IAB catheters available today may integrate innovative fiber-optic technology as mentioned
already. The introduction of Durathane balloon membranes may offer improved abrasion and fatigue resistance
and reduced insertion force, and should allow for immediate inflation at start-up.

The Console

In order for the IAB pump to perform its function of
cardiac assistance, the timing of balloon inflation and
deflation must be extremely accurate and responsive to

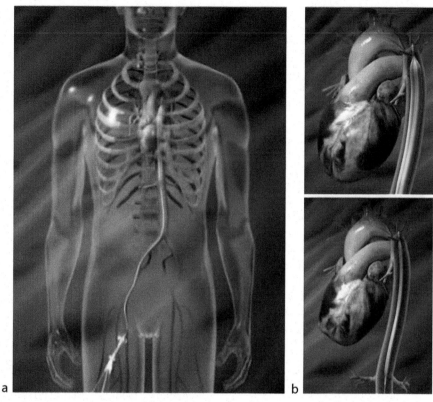

a   b

Aortic Counterpulsation. Figure 2 Proper positioning of the IAB catheter in the descending aorta: balloon inflation/deflation. Diagrammatic representation of IABP inflation and deflation and its effects on blood flow as timed by the cardiac cycle. (**a**) During diastole, the IABP is inflated, increasing diastolic pressure thus augmenting flow not only into the coronary arteries but also into the great vessels and the renal arteries. (**b**) During systole, the IABP is deflated, creating a void where the inflated balloon was, and thus increasing forward flow into the aorta and to the periphery (Reproduced with permission from MAQUET Cardiovascular)

changes in heart rate. When inflated, the balloon is timed in concert with the mechanical cardiac cycle to inflate at the start of diastole, augmenting diastolic pressure, which increases coronary perfusion and oxygen delivery to the myocardium. It is timed to deflate just before the start of systole.

IABP hemodynamic effects are dependent on the appropriate balloon catheter size and timing of inflation and deflation during diastole. The pumping chamber, activated by helium, is usually synchronized with the heart by signals from the electrocardiogram, or the central aortic pressure transducer. The implementation of fiber-optic pressure signal transmission to a patient monitor results in a faster time to therapy and faster signal acquisition. IABP triggering can also be set according to AV pacing or internal triggering. Timing errors typically produce characteristic pressure waveform changes that can easily be recognized. Early recognition is crucial as errors

can be potentially life threatening or lead to ineffective cardiovascular support.

Extreme tachycardia and/or cardiac arrhythmias may affect the efficiency of the IAB counterpulsation. Recently introduced, more sophisticated timing and trigger source automation allow the pump to react quickly, even in the presence of rate and rhythm changes. Efforts should be made to suppress cardiac arrhythmias while the patient is on IAB support. Pressure trigger is not recommended in atrial fibrillation.

Anticoagulation

Few studies have investigated the need for intravenous anticoagulation in the setting of IABP use. Industry guidelines do not require anticoagulation especially when the IABP is being used at a 1:1 ratio. However, it is reasonable to recommend appropriate intravenous anticoagulation in patients without contraindications and when IAB

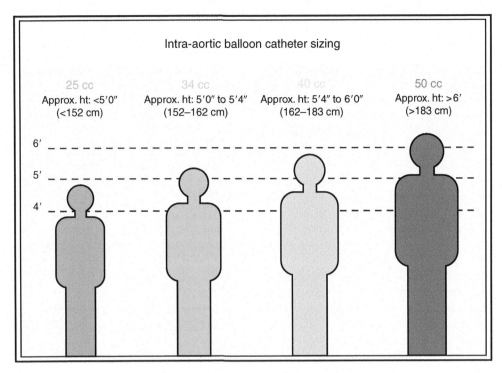

Aortic Counterpulsation. Figure 3 Intra-aortic balloon catheter reference guide (Reproduced with permission from MAQUET Cardiovascular)

support is planned for greater than 24 h and/or in lower assist ratios.

Contraindications

Absolute contraindications for IAB pump use include severe aortic valve insufficiency and (acute) aortic dissection. The presence of an aortic aneurysm, severe iliofemoral vascular disease, and history of aortic surgery are relative contraindications. In these situations, best clinical judgment should guide decision making on whether or not to utilize the IABP.

Complications

An international prospective registry – the Benchmark Counterpulsation Outcomes Registry – followed outcomes in over 22,000 subjects treated with an IABP for a range of indications [7]. The principle complications associated with IAB support are (Table 2)

- Trauma to the arterial wall occurring while inserting and advancing the guide wire or balloon (laceration, dissection, wall hematoma)
- Limb ischemia (mostly disappears with catheter removal)

Aortic Counterpulsation. Table 2 Investigator reported events in the Benchmark Counterpulsation Outcomes Registry

Severe access site-related bleeding	1.4%
Vascular injury	0.7%
Major limb injury	0.5%
Amputation	0.1%
Bowel, renal, and spinal cord infarcts	0.1%
Infection	0.1%
Stroke	0.1%
Venous thrombosis	0.1%
Death	0.05%

- Dislodged thrombus or atherosclerotic plaque with distal embolization
- Hematologic complications: damage to blood cells (thrombocytopenia, red blood cell hemolysis) and heparin-induced thrombocytopenia
- Renal dysfunction
- Infection
- Access site bleeding and retroperitoneal hematoma
- Balloon leak/rupture

Despite the demonstrable technologic advances, vascular complications remain the major risk. The prevalence of PAD ranges up to 12% in patients with CAD; most are asymptomatic. PAD relates to access complications, including bleeding, following transfemoral vascular procedures for symptomatic CAD. Major bleeding after percutaneous coronary intervention (PCI) has been linked with increased morbidity and mortality. Implementation of routine Doppler ultrasound techniques to detect vascular blood flow is advocated.

Elective IABP insertion may be linked with CIN through various mechanisms: (1) as a marker of significant hemodynamic disturbances during PCI; (2) as a marker of very severe atherosclerotic disease without hypotension; (3) as a source of atheroemboli to the renal circulation during insertion, pulsation, or removal; (4) as a partial occlusion of the renal blood flow if it is positioned too low (i.e., in the abdominal instead of the descending thoracic aorta); and (5) as a marker of increased vascular complications and post-PCI hypotension.

IAB Support in Specific Conditions

Cardiac Arrest

When defibrillating a patient, the operator should stand clear of the pump. During chest compression or cardiocerebral resuscitation, the use of ECG or arterial pressure trigger is advocated to allow synchronization of the assist to the rate and rhythm of chest compressions.

Transport/Portable Operation

During a portable operation, the console is powered by a rechargeable battery. Prior to transport, the battery should be fully charged (*Note*: a reduction in run time may be expected over a battery's life due to age, storage temperature, and discharge depth. A spare battery pack or [external] AC power should be provided in case of long distance transport). Check for sufficient helium supply (*Note*: this is of particular importance during air transport as the balloon will refill repeatedly). Ensure the helium cylinder yoke handle is tight. The console should be tightly "docked" during transport.

References

1. Williams DO, Korr KS, Gewirtz H et al (1982) The effect of intraaortic balloon counterpulsation on regional myocardial blood flow and oxygen consumption in the presence of coronary artery stenosis in patients with unstable angina. Circulation 66:593–597
2. DeWood MA, Notske RN, Hensley GR, Shields JP, O'Grady WP, Spores J, Goldman M, Ganji JH (1980) Intraaortic balloon counterpulsation with and without reperfusion for myocardial infarction shock. Circulation 61:1105–1112
3. Cheng JM, den Uil CA, Hoeks SE, van der Ent M, Jewbali LSD, van Domburg RT, Serruys PW (2009) Percutaneous left ventricular assist devices vs. intra-aortic balloon counterpulsation for treatment of cardiogenic shock: a meta-analysis of controlled trials. Eur Heart J 30:2102–2108. First published on 8 July 2009, doi:10.1093/eurheartj/ehp292
4. Pennington DG, Swartz M, Codd JE et al (1983) Intra-aortic balloon pumping in cardiac surgical patients: a nine year experience. Ann Thorac Surg 36:125–131
5. Hausmann H, Potapov EV, Koster A et al (2002) Prognosis after the implantation of an intra-aortic balloon pump in cardiac surgery calculated with a new score. Circulation 106:I-203–I-206
6. Davies AR, Bellomo R, Raman JS, Gutteridge GA, Buxton BF (2001) High lactate predicts the failure of intraaortic balloon pumping after cardiac surgery. Ann Thorac Surg 71:1415–1420
7. Cohen M, Urban P, Christenson JT et al (2003) Intra-aortic balloon counterpulsation in US and non-US centres: results of the Benchmark Registry. Eur Heart J 24(19):1763–1770

Aortic Dissection

Ian Loftus
St. George's Healthcare NHS Trust, London, UK

Synonyms

Aortic syndrome; Aortic ulcer; Intramural hematoma

Definition

Acute dissection results from sudden tear of the intima and separation of the layers within the aortic wall. This results in the longitudinal and spiralling flow of pulsatile blood between the inner and outer layers of the tunica media propagating the extent of dissection with the variable formation of both true and false lumina. Dynamic obstruction of the true lumen by the expanding false lumen can result in organ or limb ischemia.

Acute Aortic Syndrome

Related to aortic dissections, penetrating aortic ulcers and intramural hematomas occur in a more elderly hypertensive population in whom women predominate. Grouped together, the three pathologies comprise the **acute aortic syndrome** and are representative of degenerative changes encountered in the atherosclerotic aortic wall. In comparison to acute aortic dissection, visceral and limb ischemia do not appear to be a prevalent feature of either penetrating ulcers or intramural hematomas. Clinical presentation is often indistinguishable from acute aortic dissection and can only be made radiologically.

Penetrating ulcers are typically localized to the thoracic descending aorta but may arise in the abdominal aorta. Localized ulceration of the aortic wall is thought to arise from rupture of atheromatous plaque breaching the internal elastic lamina. This is associated with disruption of the tunica media with parietal aortic hematoma and has the potential for dissection, embolization, pseudoaneurysm formation, and free rupture.

Intramural hematoma is defined by the presence of a localized collection of blood within the tunica media of the aorta, most likely as a result of hemorrhage from the adventitial vasa vasorum, in the absence of an initial intimal tear. A significant proportion develops into dissections.

Clinical Features and Diagnosis

Dissections of the aorta can occur throughout its length. A patient's symptoms and signs may evolve reflecting underlying temporal hemodynamic changes. The classical descriptive pain of aortic dissection is sudden ripping, severe, migratory pain which may radiate anteriorly to the neck (in ascending arch dissections) or between the shoulder blades (descending aorta). This is usually associated with high blood pressure. Chest X-ray may reveal a widened mediastinum. However, up to a fifth of patients have minimal or no reported symptoms indicative of dissection. Spontaneous thrombosis or enlargement of false lumina together with the presence or absence of spontaneous fenestrations of the intimal flap will ultimately dictate vascular compromise and/or infarction of end-organs, presenting with mesenteric or renal ischemia or vascular compromise to the lower limbs.

The clinical diagnosis of aortic dissection is made in only two thirds of patients at initial presentation and in a third of patients, diagnosis will only be determined at postmortem. The inadvertent treatment of these patients with antithrombotic therapy (for presumed acute coronary syndrome) is associated with hemorrhagic complications and increases in-hospital mortality significantly.

Risk Factors for Acute Aortic Dissection

Systemic hypertension is the most common predisposing factor for aortic dissection and is found in up to three quarters of patients presenting with aortic dissections. Increased ventricular contractility and systolic hypertension exacerbate adverse hemodynamic forces acting upon a contracting heart and relatively mobile aortic arch and tethered descending thoracic aorta.

Following the initiation of intimal tearing, these predisposing mechanical and anatomical factors act together to increase the size of the intimal tear and blood flow through the false lumen.

Other predisposing factors include atherosclerosis, connective tissue disorders predisposing to medial aortic necrosis such as Marfan's and Ehlos Danlos syndromes, familial aneurysm syndromes, aortic coarctation and anomalies of the aortic valve or arch, the presence of a biscupid aortic valve, vascular inflammatory disorders, pregnancy, trauma, primary aldosteronism, iatrogenic injuries, methamphetamine abuse and chronic cocaine use.

Classification

The two most commonly used classification systems for thoracic dissections are the Debakey and Stanford systems, of which the Stanford classification is most frequently used.

The Stanford classification separates dissections of the thoracic aorta into those which involve the ascending aorta – **type A** (with or without involvement of the descending thoracic aorta see Fig. 1), and those that solely involve the descending thoracic aorta – **type B** (Fig. 2).

The Debakey classification categorizes dissections into three types:

- **Type I** – a tear in the ascending aorta with the dissection flap extending for a variable length into the arch of the aorta or beyond
- **Type II** – a dissection restricted wholly to the ascending aorta
- **Type III** – a dissection restricted to the descending thoracic aorta, sparing both the ascending aorta and arch

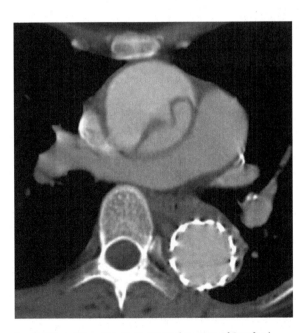

Aortic Dissection. Figure 1 CT axial section of Stanford type A involving aortic arch with true and false lumina, and descending thoracic stent in situ

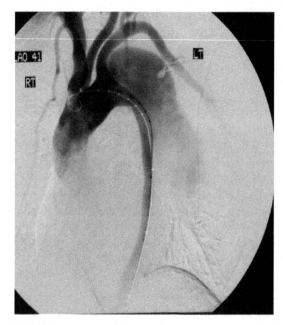

Aortic Dissection. Figure 2 Arch aortogram of a type B dissection demonstrating true luminal collapse and extraluminal expansion of false lumen

Dissections of the aorta can be further classified into those which are **acute** when the clinical diagnosis is made within 2 weeks following the onset of symptoms and **chronic** dissections when the diagnosis is made after this time point. This is to an extent a rather arbitrary classification and should not always dictate treatment.

Treatment, Evaluation, and Assessment

Imaging

Contrast-enhanced computer tomography and magnetic resonance imaging has superseded aortography as the gold standard first line imaging, allowing for rapid diagnosis. This provides clear delineation of the entire aorta, and assessment of lumen size, thrombus volume, and aortic wall calcification. Three-dimensional reconstruction of the enhanced aorta allows for accurate quantification of intramural hematoma and the location of major aortic branches allowing planning of surgical or endovascular repair.

Blood Pressure Control

Unlike Stanford type A dissections, in which emergency replacement of the aortic arch is mandated, the management of acute and chronic Stanford type B dissections remains controversial.

Immediate blood pressure control is mandatory in all patients with aortic dissection to prevent further progression of the dissection flap. Evidence of end-organ ischemia may dictate urgent operative intervention but medical stabilization is still essential and should usually be within a critical care setting with invasive blood pressure monitoring.

Commonly used antihypertensive regimens include titrated intravenous beta blockade with labetolol or propanolol to maintain a systolic pressure between 100 and 120 mmHg. Sotalol in patients with atrial fibrillation may also be used, with adjustment for impaired renal clearance.

In those patients in whom β-blockade is contraindicated, Clonidine is a centrally acting agent which may be administered by slow i.v. infusion in doses of up to 1.5 mg/24 h. This can be combined with short-acting vasodilators such as dihydralazine in typical doses of 100–150 mg/day. In some instances, refractory hypertensive crises may be aborted with the judicious use of sodium nitroprusside to reduce peripheral vascular resistance and left ventricular preload, in doses of 0.2–10 μg/kg/min.

Once stabilized, conversion of i.v. therapy to oral antihypertensive agents is desirable. Long-term blood pressure control is essential if the patient is otherwise treated conservatively to prevent further propagation of the dissection and aortic dilatation.

Surgical and Endovascular Considerations for Repair of Aortic Dissections

Acute type A dissection should be managed surgically by a cardio-thoracic team, preferably with an aortic interest. Surgery involves aortic root repair and entails a significant risk of mortality and morbidity. A proportion of patients are deemed unsuitable for intervention and the prognosis is poor.

Current consensus suggest that emergent surgical intervention for acute complicated type B aortic dissections be indicated by aortic rupture, rapid aortic expansion, retrograde aortic dissection, visceral and limb ischemia, neurological deficit, or intractable pain.

Open surgical replacement of the diseased aorta has been traditionally performed through a left posterolateral thoracotomy with prosthetic graft replacement of the descending thoracic aorta, in conjunction with single lung ventilation, full heparinization, cardiopulmonary bypass, profound hypothermia, cerebrospinal fluid drainage, and circulatory arrest in an attempt to minimize morbidity particularly in reference to stroke and paraplegia rates. The concomitant morbidity associated with thoracotomy remains significant, particularly in patients who often have coexistent cardiac failure, chronic obstructive lung disease, and renal insufficiency. Mortality reported in available surgical series may well be subject to publication bias, retrospective data collection, nonrepresentative population selection, and by the inherent natural selection of patients surviving transfer to high volume tertiary vascular referral centers. Nonetheless, data from the IRAD database suggests an improving but significant mortality rate for emergent complicated type B dissections over the last 5 years, with contemporary reported in-hospital mortality rates of 17% [1, 2].

A paradigm shift in the surgical management of these patients began in the late 1990s with the reporting of patients being treated with custom-designed covered stents. Studies demonstrated the feasibility and technical success in endovascular sealing of the proximal intimal entry tear in patients with type B thoracic dissections. Covering the intimal tear was associated with near or complete thrombosis of the false lumen in 80–100% of patients at subsequent follow-up. In keeping with the known natural history of complicated type B dissections and outcome data from the IRAD registry, patients with aortic branch vessel ischemia or occlusions fared worse following endoluminal stent deployment as compared to uncomplicated cases with no branch vessel involvement, with reported 30 day mortality of 17%. Of interest, sealing the primary entry tear resulted in revascularization of the true lumens of affected ischemic branch vessels without the need for further fenestrations, visceral revascularization or laparotomy.

The subsequent rapid advance in stent graft design has led to a steady increase in the number of patients with acute aortic syndromes treated using endovascular techniques, and has led to endovascular enthusiasts advocating an expansion to the indications and applications to include uncomplicated chronic type B dissections. Repair can be performed with percutaneous or open approach to a single femoral artery, preferably under general anesthetic, and insertion of a variety of commercially available stent grafts to the thoracic aorta under radiological control (Fig. 3). In acute dissections, the priority is to close the entry tear, and generally long lengths of aorta do not need to be covered. In chronic dissections often longer lengths of aorta need to be covered and consideration should be given to the prophylactic placement of a spinal drain.

Blood pressure should be controlled up to the deployment of the stent and in deploying within the arch the systolic pressure should be below 100 mmHg at this point. Having covered the tear the blood pressure can be permitted to rise. This is important if long lengths of aorta are covered, to prevent spinal malperfusion. There is a

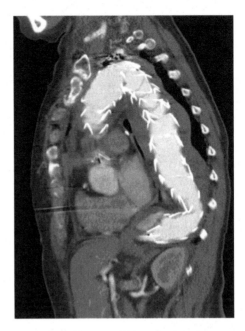

Aortic Dissection. Figure 3 CT in sagittal section demonstrating endovascular stent graft placed proximally across the aortic arch with endograft extensions deployed in descending thoracic aorta

significant risk of paraplegia from endovascular and open thoracic aortic repair. Driving the spinal perfusion pressure by controlled hypertension and spinal drainage reduces the risk and should be maintained in those most at risk for 3 days postoperatively.

The possibility of combining covered stents with uncovered bare metal branch vessel stenting in the abdominal aorta, and endoluminal aortic fenestrations has obviated the need for open surgical intervention and aortic cross clamping, thereby minimizing surgical trauma and blood loss with avoidance of a thoracotomy. Furthermore, patients historically deemed unfit to withstand traditional open surgical repair of the thoracoabdominal aorta could well be managed with a combined open mesenteric revascularization with subsequent endovascular grafting of the thoracoabdominal aorta. Endovascular options for type A dissections are at present limited but developments in stent graft technology make this an interesting challenge for the future.

After-care

Early postoperative care should involve careful blood pressure control and prevention of paraplegia. The mean arterial pressure should be kept above 100 mmHg for the first 3 days and in selected patients where spinal cord ischemia is deemed high risk (long length of aorta covered, previous aortic surgery, continues sedation, and ventilation after surgery), a spinal drain should be kept in situ for 3 days. The pressure should be maintained at 10 cmH$_2$O, with a maximum drainage of 30 mL/h. The drain can subsequently be clamped for 24 h prior to removal and unclamped should neurology develop.

Following endovascular repair, all patients should continue to receive adequate blood pressure management and should enter into CT-scan surveillance programs to monitor the condition of the rest of the aorta and the position of the stent graft. Most center recommend yearly CT scan for at least the first 5 years.

Type B dissections treated conservatively also need long-term surveillance of the aorta. The follow-up protocol should be determined on a patient by patient basis but initially CT scans may be required fairly regularly eventually dropping to yearly.

Prognosis

Acute dissection is the most common life threatening condition of the aorta affecting 5–30 per million people per year. Left untreated, the majority of patients with dissections involving the ascending aorta will die within days of an acute episode.

Patients presenting with descending thoracic aortic dissections seem to fare better, with one in ten patients ultimately dying before leaving hospital. Ultimately, these patients are at risk of aortic rupture with nearly 20% of these patients requiring some form of surgical or endovascular intervention.

Judicious medical, surgical, and endovascular management of this condition aims to reduce propagation of the dissection plane and concomitant branch vessel compromise, halt aortic expansion, and prevent fatal aortic rupture.

Early recognition of these disease entities in conjunction with urgent and pertinent management is the key to a successful outcome in these patients.

The mortality risk is highest in the first 48 h with a plateau in cumulative mortality at 14 days. Over half of the patients presenting the Stanford type A dissection die within 2 days without emergent surgery as a result of aortic rupture and acute aortic valvular regurgitation. Survival after urgent surgical intervention approaches 75%. Of those who do survive surgical repair, 90% are still alive for 3 years. There is no role for conservative management except in the most moribund patient with an unsalvageable premorbid history or in those patients who have refused surgery.

The presence of persistent pain indicative of progressing dissection, refractory systemic hypertension, distal organ ischemia, and aortic expansion or rupture occurs in up to a fifth of type B dissections. These so-called **complicated** Type B dissections require emergent surgical or endovascular intervention, in spite of which historical series suggest that up to a third will ultimately die. Independent predictive risk factors for in-hospital mortality in these patients are the absence of chest or back pain at presentation, female gender, the presence of acute limb, or visceral ischemia, in-hospital hypotension or shock, a widened mediastinum, the detection of periaortic hematoma, aneurysmal aortic dilatation of greater than 6 cm, altered consciousness, acute renal failure, and the need for life saving surgery. The actuarial survival rate for patients with a type B dissection, who do leave hospital, however approaches 71%, 60%, 35%, and 17% at 1, 5, 10, and 15 years following discharge [3].

Chronic complications following aortic dissections are related to the persistence of a blood flow through a patent false lumen with resultant aortic expansion and attendant risk of rupture. A fifth of all patients treated conservatively continue to have a patent false lumen without evidence of thrombosis, with only a minority of demonstrating evidence of spontaneous healing. It is estimated that 20–40% of the patients who survive the acute phase of will develop significant aneurysmal dilatation of the descending thoracic or thoracoabdominal aorta. Previous studies have estimated that in the absence of postoperative false lumen thrombosis, aortic expansion continues at a variable rate up to 4 mm/year. The risk of rupture is reported to be greater in women than in men and once the aorta reaches 6 cm or greater is estimated to be 30%. Despite this, there is probably no indication at present to intervene for asymptomatic acute type B dissections.

Regarding endovascular repair, the European collaborators registry/Eurostar registry has yet to provide outcome data beyond 1 year, and has yet to provide conclusive evidence that late aortic rupture is not a cause for concern following endovascular repair despite little evidence of aortic expansion or endoleak [4]. The Talent Thoracic Retrospective Registry demonstrated in-patient mortality of less than 5%, but a small proportion (1.5%) of patients continued to have a pressurized false lumen despite stenting, which ultimately caused death upon rupture [5]. Up to 3% of patients suffered device failure, in terms of either migration of the stent graft, failure of graft fabric integrity, or modular disconnection and a third of all patients required either surgical or a second endovascular procedure by 5 years.

Eggebrecht et al. reported on the outcome of 609 patients from 39 observational series that had undergone endovascular stent-graft placement in aortic dissection.

Sixty percent of these patients underwent emergent endovascular repair. Early procedural failure or surgical conversion occurred in 4% with a further 6% of patients requiring additional endovascular intervention. In three quarters of the patients, thrombosis of the false lumen was achieved but 3% of patients still died of aortic rupture within 2 years. Major complication rates still occurred in18% of cases, with an associated in-patient mortality of 6% and combined procedural stroke and paraplegic rate of 4%. Kaplan Meier estimates of survival rates demonstrated a significant survival advantage in favor of patients treated for chronic dissections as opposed to acute dissections (3.2% ± 1.4% versus 9.8% ± 2.2%) associated with a 50% reduction in in-hospital complications (9.1% ± 2.3% versus 21.7% ± 2.8%). Overall survival rates were reported to be 93.3% ± 1.4% at 30 days, 89.9% ± 1.7% at 1 year and 88.8% ± 1.9% at 2 years which compares favorably to outcome data reported by the IRAD registry of an 11% in-hospital mortality rate in medically treated patients and 31.4% mortality rate in surgically treated patients.

The rapid acceptance of endovascular techniques has yet to be met with well designed multicenter randomized controlled trials for endovascular versus open surgical repair. There is no available data on long-term benefit of stenting over open surgery with regard to prevention of late aortic expansion and rupture. Widespread application has been further tempered by the current lack of American FDA approval for the use of commercially available thoracic endografts for thoracic dissections.

In summary, type A dissections require immediate open surgical repair in specialist units. Complicated acute type B dissections should be considered for endovascular treatment, which is technically feasible with an acceptable operative morbidity and mortality in comparison to open surgical aortic replacement. Patients require intensive scrutiny during longer-term follow-up to exclude stent failure, migration, infection, and modular disconnection.

References

1. Tsai TT, Fattori R, Trimarchi S, Isselbacher E, Myrmel T, Evangelista A et al (2006) Long-term survival in patients presenting with type B acute aortic dissection: insights from the International Registry of Acute Aortic Dissection. Circulation 114(21):2226–2231
2. Eggebrecht H, Nienaber CA, Neuhauser M, Baumgart D, Kische S, Schmermund A et al (2006 Feb) Endovascular stent-graft placement in aortic dissection: a meta-analysis. Eur Heart J 27(4):489–498
3. Bockler D, Schumacher H, Ganten M, von Tengg-Kobligk H, Schwarzbach M, Fink C et al (2006 Aug 1) Complications after endovascular repair of acute symptomatic and chronic expanding Stanford type B aortic dissections. J Thorac Cardiovasc Surg 132 (2):361–368
4. Leurs LJ, Bell R, Degrieck Y, Thomas S, Hobo R, Lundbom J (2004 Oct) Endovascular treatment of thoracic aortic diseases: combined experience from the EUROSTAR and United Kingdom Thoracic Endograft registries. J Vasc Surg 40(4):670–679
5. Fattori R, Nienaber CA, Rousseau H, Beregi JP, Heijmen R, Grabenwoger M et al (2006 Aug) Results of endovascular repair of the thoracic aorta with the Talent Thoracic stent graft: the Talent Thoracic Retrospective Registry. J Thorac Cardiovasc Surg 132(2): 332–339

Aortic Injury

▶ Mediastinal Hematoma

Aortic Regurgitation

CHARLES S. BRUDNEY[1], SRINI PYATI[2]
[1]Department of Anesthesiology, Duke University Medical Center, Durham, NC, USA
[2]Division of Veterans Affairs, Duke University Medical Center, Durham, NC, USA

Definition

Aortic regurgitation is reflux of blood from the aorta through the aortic valve into the left ventricle during diastole. The overall prevalence of aortic regurgitation was about 5.0% in Framingham heart study [1] and 10% in the Strong heart study [2]. The prevalence increases with age because of degenerative changes in the aortic valve and the root. The most common causes can be subdivided into acute and chronic regurgitation with some significant overlap (Table 1).

The majority of the causes of aortic regurgitation (AR) present either acutely or sub acutely. Prior to aggressive antibiotic treatment of rheumatic fever and syphilis, AR was a common sequelae of these conditions. The most frequent cause of aortic regurgitation is endocarditis complicating a previously damaged valve. This can be a congenitally damaged valve or diseased valve secondary to rheumatic fever. The disease ranges from mild to severe regurgitation. However, the natural history of severe AR is poorly defined with wide disparity in the reporting of long-term survival that ranges from 50% to 96% at 10 years [3, 4].

The majority of patients with AR are men (75%). Symptoms and signs occur late and do not develop until left ventricular failure develops. Varying grades of dyspnea

Aortic Regurgitation. Table 1 Causes of aortic regurgitation

Congenital	Acquired
Marfan syndrome	Syphilis
Myxomatous degeneration	Rheumatic fever
Osteogenesis imperfects	Endocarditis
Turner syndrome	Failure of prosthetic valve
Bicuspid aortic valve	Aortic dissection
	Trauma
	Reiter syndrome
	Ankylosing spondylitis
	Rheumatoid arthritis
	Systemic Lupus Erythematosis
	Severe hypertension

Aortic Regurgitation. Table 2 Causes of acute AR

Rheumatic heart disease
Infective endocarditis
Ruptured sinus of valsalva
Trauma
Prosthetic valve malfunction

occur depending on the extent of the left ventricular dilatation and dysfunction. Angina pectoris is also a frequent complaint. Symptom presentation is quite different between acute and chronic regurgitation.

Characteristics

Acute Versus Chronic AR

Patients with chronic AR may have long intervals of asymptomatic period of nearly 20 years before the disease manifests with worsening symptoms. However, once symptoms develop, the progression to poor prognosis can occur with an expected survival rate of 5–10 years. The usual presenting symptoms are varying degrees of dyspnea, palpitations, abdominal discomfort, and syncopal attacks. Chronic regurgitation affords time for the ventricle to dilate and hence accommodate the regurgitant volume. The onset of AR leads to LV systolic and diastolic volume overload. Initially, this leads to adaptation that maintains forward stroke volume and cardiac output despite the addition of the regurgitant volume. The increased volume overload leads to eccentric hypertrophy of LV and gradual increase in LVEDP. Forward flow is aided by large stroke volume and compensatory peripheral vasodilatation. Symptoms are mild with regurgitant fraction less than 40% of stroke volume. When the regurgitant fraction exceeds 50% of stroke volume, increasing LV dilatation and hypertrophy occurs resulting in irreversible myocardial damage, the early sign of which is LVEDP more than 20 mmHg. As regurgitant fraction

increases, patients present with decreased aortic diastolic pressure, leading to inadequate coronary perfusion pressure and angina symptoms [5].

In acute AR the lack of time for adaptation for the regurgitant volume leads to the spiral of events seen in acute AR (Table 2). Patients usually present with severe dyspnea, hypotension, angina, and fatigue. The rapid and sudden increase in ventricular volume leads to limited compensatory mechanism to take effect. Once the left ventricle is unable to cope with the regurgitant volume and there is an excessive backward blood flow, with subsequent decrease in stroke volume. This initially leads to a compensatory tachycardia, which may preserve cardiac output, but eventually, there is development of hypotension, organ failure, and cardiogenic shock. Pulmonary artery occlusion pressure will also increase abruptly leading to pulmonary edema. The rapid deterioration in cardiac output can occur, necessitating emergent surgical intervention [6].

Signs of AR

The diastolic regurgitation and the increased systolic stroke volume result in the increased systolic pressure, widened pulse pressure, and bounding pulses, which are highly suggestive of aortic regurgitation. The rapid upstroke in arterial pressure tracing is due to increased LV preload and steep down stroke is a consequence of peripheral vasodilatation.

Signs of AR are many and are due to hyperdynamic circulation. These include the following:

- De Musset's sign – the head nods with each heart beat.
- Quincke's sign – capillary pulsation can be palpated in the nail beds.
- Durozier's sign – systolic bruit can be heard after light auscultation over the femoral arteries.
- Traube's sign (Pistol shot femoral arterial pulsations) – sharp and loud sounds can be heard on auscultation of femoral arteries.

- The apex beat is displaced downwards and laterally and is heaving in nature.
- On auscultation of the heart there is a high pitched diastolic murmur running from the aortic component of the second heart sound. A systolic murmur may also be heard because of increased stroke volume. The length of the diastolic murmur should be noted, as this reflects the severity of the leak until the late stages of the disease. Decrescendo diastolic murmur is best heard with patient leaning forward and on deep expiration.
- An Austin-Flint apical diastolic murmur may also be heard and represents significant AR. This is a mid-diastolic murmur, best heard at the apex and reflects ante grade flow across an incompletely opened mitral valve caused by the AR jet's effect on the anterior mitral leaflet.

Diagnosis

The majority of cases can be diagnosed clinically by the above-mentioned signs.

- ECG appearances are those of left ventricular hypertrophy (LVH) due to "volume overload" of LVH. There are tall R waves and deeply inverted T waves in the left sided chest leads and deep S waves in the right sided leads. Normally, sinus rhythm is present, but arrhythmias such as atrial fibrillation can be observed in chronic AR.
- Chest X-ray features are those of LV enlargement and possible dilatation of the ascending aorta. The LV enlargement is marked in chronic AR.
- Echocardiography will define the functional anatomy of the valve and aortic root, while Doppler imaging will demonstrate the severity of the leak. Echo will also demonstrate LV thickness, dilatation, and function.
- Ejection fraction is an unreliable index in patients with chronic regurgitation due to increases in LV compliance over time that allows maintenance of stroke volume.

Treatment

The underlying cause of the AR (e.g., syphilis or infective endocarditis) may require specific treatment. The treatment of chronic AR usually requires carefully timed surgical intervention (Table 3). Because symptoms do not start to develop until the myocardium fails, and the myocardial damage is irreversible it is imperative to start therapy as early as possible. The goals of hemodynamic management are to maintain forward flow by beta agonists to improve contractility and at simultaneously maintaining peripheral vasodilatation by decreasing

Aortic Regurgitation. Table 3 Indications for surgical intervention

Dyspnea class III and IV
Syncopal symptoms
Ejection fraction of <0.4
Cardiothoracic ratio of >0.64
End diastolic diameter of 55 mm or more
Cardiac index <2.2 L/min/m^2
Severe symptoms in young patients with rheumatic AR
Frank LV enlargement or moderate LV dysfunction

afterload [7]. Forward flow can also be augmented by slight increase in heart rate (around 90/min) without compromising coronary perfusion. Many patients are started on calcium channel blockers in an attempt to reduce the regurgitant fraction. In addition although beta blockers may prolong diastole many clinicians use modest doses. In contrast to chronic AR, acute AR necessitates immediate surgical intervention due to life threatening hypotension and pulmonary edema.

Most patients with chronic aortic regurgitation have a protracted clinical course, despite evidence of severe regurgitation. Nevertheless, long-term care of the asymptomatic individual with aortic regurgitation consists of carefully monitoring for the onset of symptoms or, more often, of left ventricular dysfunction or dilation. Asymptomatic patients with chronic severe aortic regurgitation and normal left ventricular systolic function should be assessed clinically and echocardiographically approximately every 6 to 12 months. There are no randomized controlled trials to guide surgical decision making [8].

Current guidelines suggest aortic valve surgery for chronic severe aortic regurgitation for patients with symptom onset (Class I indication), asymptomatic patients with left ventricular ejection fraction lower than 0.50 (Class I indication), patients undergoing coronary artery bypass grafting or surgery on the aorta or other heart valves (Class I indication), and patients with preserved ventricular function but left ventricular end-systolic dimension more than 55 mm or end-diastolic dimension more than 75 mm (Class IIa indication). Aortic valve surgery [9] may be considered in asymptomatic patients with preserved ventricular function but left ventricular end-systolic dimension more than 50 mm or end-diastolic dimension more than 70 mm, patients with declining exercise tolerance, and patients with moderate aortic regurgitation undergoing coronary artery bypass grafting or surgery on the aorta or other heart valves (Class IIb indications). The operative mortality of isolated aortic valve replacement is about 4% [10–12].

Much depends on the patients exercise tolerance as well as their ability to progress, or not deteriorate on medical management. Patients must be counseled that antibiotic prophylaxis is required once the valve has been fixed.

References

1. Singh JP, Evans JC, Levy D, Larson MG, Freed LA, Fuller DL Lehman B, Benjamin EJ (1999) Prevalence and clinical determinants of mitral, tricuspid, and aortic regurgitation (the Framingham Heart Study) [published correction appears in Am J Cardiol. 1999; 84:1143]. Am J Cardiol 83:897–902
2. Lebowitz NE, Bella JN, Roman MJ, Liu JE, Fishman DP, Paranicas M, Lee ET, Fabsitz RR, Welty TK, Howard BV, Devereux RB (2000) Prevalence and correlates of aortic regurgitation in American Indians: the Strong Heart Study. J Am Coll Cardiol 36:461–467
3. Padial LR, Oliver A, Sagie A, Weyman AE, King ME, Levine RA (1997) Two-dimensional echocardiographic assessment of the progression of aortic root size in 127 patients with chronic aortic regurgitation: role of the supraaortic ridge an relation to the progression of the lesion. Am Heart J 134:814–821
4. Bonow RO, Lakatos E, Maron BJ, Epstein SE (1991) Serial long-term assessment of the natural history of asymptomatic patients with chronic aortic regurgitation and normal left ventricular systolic function. Circulation 84:1625–1635
5. Bekeredjian R, Grayburn PA (2005) Valvular heart disease: aortic regurgitation. Circulation 112(1):125–134
6. Goldbarg SH, Halperin JL (2008) Aortic regurgitation: disease progression and management. Nat Clin Pract Cardiovasc Med 5 (5):269–279
7. Kleaveland JP, Reichek N, McCarthy DM, Chandler T, Priest C, Muhammed A, Makler PT Jr, Hirshfeld J (1986) Effects of six-month afterload reduction therapy with hydralazine in chronic aortic regurgitation. Am J Cardiol 57:1109–1116
8. Borer JS, Hochreiter C, Herrold EM, Supino P, Aschermann M, Wencker D, Devereux RB, Roman MJ, Szulc M, Kligfield P, Isom OW (1998) Prediction Of indications for valve replacement among asymptomatic or minimally symptomatic patients with chronic aortic regurgitation and normal left Ventricular performance. Circulation 97:525–534
9. Chaliki HP, Mohty D, Avierinos J-F, Scott CG, Schaff HV, Tajik AJ, Enriquez-Sarano M (2002) Outcomes after aortic valve replacement in patients with severe aortic regurgitation and markedly reduced left ventricular function. Circulation 106:2687–2693
10. Edwards FH, Peterson ED, Coombs LP, DeLong ER, Jamieson WR, Shroyer ALW, Grover FL (2001) Prediction of operative mortality after valve replacement surgery. J Am Coll Cardiol 37:885–892
11. Florath I, Rosendahl UP, Mortasawi A, Bauer SF, Dalladaku F, Ennker IC, Ennker JC (2003) Current determinants of operative mortality in 1400 patients requiring aortic valve replacement. Ann Thorac Surg 76:75–83
12. Henry WI, Bonow RO, Borer JS, Ware JH, Kent KM, Redwood DR, McIntosh CL, Morrow AG, Epstein SE (1980) Observations on the optimum time for operative intervention for aortic regurgitation, I: evaluation of the results of aortic valve replacement in symptomatic patients. Circulation 61:471–483

Aortic Stenosis

CHARLES S. BRUDNEY
Department of Anesthesiology, Duke University Medical Center, Durham, NC, USA

Definition

Aortic valve stenosis can be defined by restricted systolic opening of the valve leaflets, with a mean transvalvular pressure of at least 10 mmHg.

Characteristics

Prevalence and Causes

The majority of cases of aortic stenosis (AS) are due to calcific aortic stenosis and congenital bicuspid aortic valve stenosis. Aortic sclerosis occurs in up to 25% of people older than 75 years and involves mild thickening as well as some calcification of the tricuspid aortic valve without restricted leaflet motion. Calcified aortic stenosis, however, occurs in 2–3% of patients older than 75 years. Congenital aortic valve stenosis develops progressively because of turbulent blood flow through a congenitally abnormal (usually bicuspid) aortic valve. Rheumatic fever results in progressive fusion, thickening, and calcification of the aortic valve [3].

Valvular aortic stenosis should be differentiated from other causes of obstruction to left ventricular (LV) emptying such as

- Supravalvular obstruction
- Hypertrophic cardiomyopathy
- Subvalvular aortic stenosis

Pathophysiology

Obstructed left ventricular emptying leads to increased left ventricular pressure and a corresponding hypertrophy of the left ventricle. In turn, this action results in relative ischemia of the left ventricular myocardium, and subsequent angina, arrhythmias and left ventricular failure (LVF). The natural history of AS reflects the functional integrity of the mitral valve. As long as the mitral valve function is maintained, the pulmonary bed is protected from the systolic pressure overload imposed by the AS.

Eventually, however, left ventricular hypertrophy (LVH) causes either diastolic dysfunction with the onset of congestive symptoms or myocardial stress with subsequent angina. Some patients experience exertional syncope where the increased cardiac output of exercise is not able to be processed through the dysfunctional aortic valve. This leads to a relative decrease in cardiac output, decreased blood pressure, worsening coronary ischemia, and a failed myocardium.

Symptoms and Signs

There are usually no symptoms until aortic stenosis is moderately severe, when the aortic orifice is reduced by up to one third of its normal size. Most patients are picked up at routine screening prior to changes in their functional status. Once symptoms of exercise-induced, syncope, dyspnea, or angina occur, the disease is relatively advanced.

On physical examination AS is characterized by abnormalities of the pulse, precordial pulsation, and auscultation. The pulse is of small volume and rising or plateau in nature. Precordial palpation reveals an apex beat that may feel *heaving* and is sustained and clearly palpated. It is not usually displaced, as there is usually no associated ventricular dilatation. Auscultation reveals a mid-systolic ejection murmur. This is often loudest at the base of the heart and radiates to the carotids and is crescendo/decrescendo in nature.

Other findings may include a systolic ejection click, unless the valve is immobile or calcified. When the valve becomes immobile, there may be a soft or inaudible second heart sound. There may also be reversed splitting of the second heart sound, due to the fixed delay in left heart emptying. There may also be a fourth heart sound due to increased ventricular stiffness.

Evaluation/Assessment

Investigation

Chest x-ray usually reveals a small heart with a prominent, and dilated ascending aorta. The aortic valve may be calcified, and when the heart has failed, there may be an increased cardiothoracic ratio.

Electrocardiogram (ECG) shows LVH and left atrial delay, usually sinus rhythm is present but ventricular arrhythmias may be seen.

Echo demonstrates thickened, calcified or immobile valve cusps. LVH is also visualized. Echo will also highlight the valve gradient and subsequent treatment options.

Treatment

Patients with AS fall in to one of four categories of severity defined in Table 1 by echocardiography [1].

Asymptomatic patients are recommended to be screened every 2–3 years for mild AS and every year to 2 years for moderate and every 6–12 months for severe

Aortic Stenosis. Table 1

Severity	Valve area (cm²)	Maximum aortic velocity (m/s)	Mean pressure gradient (mmHg)
Mild	1.5–2.0	2.5–3.0	<25
Moderate	1.0–1.5	3.0–4.0	25–40
Severe	0.6–1.0	>4.0	>40
Critical	<0.6	–	–

stenosis. Patients with moderate to severe asymptomatic AS should be advised to refrain from exertion.

Symptomatic patients with severe AS should undergo valve replacement (class 1 indication) [2].

Other class 1 indications are where the patient is scheduled for coronary artery bypass grafting (CABG) and has severe AS. Also patients with severe AS and an ejection fraction below 50%.

Class 11a indications are where a patient is scheduled for valve replacement surgery or CABG and has moderate AS.

Class 11b is where surgery is considered in moderate AS patients who are intolerant of exertion.

Patients should be advised that valve replacement is palliative not curative. Patients should be made aware of the follow-up required post cardiac surgery, anticoagulation risks, endocarditic risks, as well as risks of malfunction of the new valve.

References

1. Nishimura RA et al (2006) Acc/Aha guidelines for the management of patients with valvular heart disease. J Am Coll Cardiol 48:e1–e148
2. Otto CM (2006) Valvular aortic stenosis. Disease, severity and timing of intervention. J Am Coll Cardiol 47:2141–2151
3. Stewart BF, Siscovick D, Lind BK, Gardin JM, Gottdiener JS, Smith VE (1997) Clinical factors associated with calcific aortic valve disease. J Am Coll Cardiol 29:630–634

Aortic Syndrome

▶ Aortic Dissection

Aortic Transection

▶ Torn Thoracic Aorta

Aortic Ulcer

▶ Aortic Dissection

APAP

▶ Acetaminophen Overdose

Apheresis

▶ Plasmapheresis

Arbovirus

Is an acronym (**AR**thropod-**BO**rne) used to refer to a group of viruses that are transmitted by the bite of arthopod vectors.

ARDS

The adult respiratory distress syndrome which is characterized by loss of lung volumes, increased pulmonary microvascular permeability and increased extravascular lung water.

Arenaviruses

▶ Biological Terrorism, Hemorrhagic Fever

Argentine Hemorrhagic Fever

▶ Biological Terrorism, Hemorrhagic Fever

Arginine

Juan B. Ochoa[1], Mary K. Miranowski[2]
[1]Trauma and Surgical Critical Care, University of Pittsburgh Medical Center, Pittsburgh, PA, USA
[2]Nestlé Health Care Nutrition

Introduction

Arginine plays pivotal roles in both innate and adaptive immunity being a substrate for the production of nitric oxide and an essential amino acid for the normal function of T-lymphocytes. In addition, arginine plays multiple metabolic roles including the detoxification of ammonia (being part of the urea cycle), as a precursor for the formation of ornithine, polyamines, and proline, and the production of creatine among many others. Arginine deficiency develops selectively in some illnesses making this a conditionally essential amino acid that mandates nutritional supplementation under some circumstances [1].

Arginine availability is uniquely determined by myeloid cells during immune activation through the induction and/or release of the enzyme arginase 1 (ARG1). Regulation of T-lymphocyte function through arginine depletion has been discovered as a novel function of myeloid cells expressing ARG1, thus giving them the name myeloid-derived suppressor cells (MDSC). Arginine deficiency by MDSC may also compromise nitric oxide production. Systemic activation of MDSC may lead to generalized arginine deficiency potentially compromising arginine-dependent metabolic processes outside the immune system [2].

The Identification of MDSC, and the arginine deficiency they cause, has led to dramatic growth in understanding the immune suppression observed in a diverse number of illnesses: renal cell carcinoma, H. pylori, Salmonella, Tuberculosis, and parasitic diseases such as Leishmaniasis. In the intensive care unit (ICU), arginine deficiency characteristically develops after physical injury (be it surgery or trauma) where MDSC upregulation has been described extensively. The presence of myeloid-derived suppressor cells expressing ARG1, and the pathologic role these play has not been observed in all illnesses. For example, in sepsis, a classic inflammatory response results in the production of large amounts of nitric oxide and appears to predominate over MDSC expressing ARG1. Consistent with this, and in contrast to trauma and surgery, a wide range of arginine plasma levels are observed in sepsis [3].

The identification of the causative factors of arginine deficiency and its biological consequences opens the possibility to understand the use of nutritional therapies aimed at arginine replacement, better known as immunonutrition. Arginine replacement therapy (ART) in the form of immunonutrition is of clear benefit in patients undergoing elective surgery with an approximate 40% decrease in postoperative infection rates, a decrease in length of stay and decreased cost. In these patients, ART is considered to be the standard of care and should be used routinely in patients undergoing high-risk surgical interventions, particularly those patients with cancer of the gastrointestinal tract. Similar trends are observed after trauma, but are dependent on how early the formula is initiated and on the volume of immunonutrition delivered [4, 5]. Immunonutrition with arginine is controversial in septic and other nonoperative medical critically ill patient populations where a significant amount of research is still necessary to determine if and when arginine deficiency is present.

Cellular Transport of Arginine

The capacity of cells to utilize arginine for metabolic activity depends on active transport across the cell membrane. A family of transporters termed Cationic Amino acid Transporters (CATs) actively moves arginine across the cell membrane. Three genes (CAT1, 2, and 3) encode four CAT proteins (the fourth one created through splicing of CAT2). The CAT expressed depends on the cell type and developmental stage, and CATs can be constitutively present or induced.

Cationic amino acid transporters are expressed in immune cells. Under resting conditions, CAT1, a low-efficiency transporter, is ubiquitously expressed across many cell types including cells of the immune system. Under immune activation, CAT2B, a high efficiency transporter is induced in lymphoid and myeloid cells providing arginine as a substrate for both inducible nitric oxide synthase (iNOS), arginase1 (ARG1), and other metabolic functions. The amount of arginine entering into the cell can increase dramatically upon induction of CAT2B.

Because of their function as gatekeepers, CATs may play important regulatory functions for biological processes such as the production of Nitric Oxide (·NO). Thus, when studying the functional aspects of arginine metabolism, cationic amino acid transport expression and activity need to be taken into account. Knowledge of CATs provides a unique opportunity for the regulation of biological functions. For example, agents that block arginine transport (such as Ng-monomethyl-L-arginine) are useful in regulating arginine-dependent metabolic functions such as nitric oxide production. Cationic amino acid transporters also have affinity for other amino acids (lysine and ornithine) which can compete with arginine [6].

Arginine Metabolism in Myeloid Cells

Arginine metabolism is an essential part of myeloid cells. There are several myeloid cell types including macrophages, neutrophils, and immature myeloid suppressor cells. Expression of arginine-metabolizing enzymes varies significantly between these cells. The predominance of one or another cell type is dictated by local and systemic inflammatory conditions.

Arginine metabolism by myeloid cells is an essential aspect of their function. Two divergent pathways for arginine metabolism are expressed. In the late 1980s and early 1990s an inducible isoenzyme of the nitric oxide synthase family (iNOS) was described in macrophages. Human neutrophils on the other hand express arginase 1 (ARG1), probably located in the azurophil granules and released as an active enzyme upon activation. Arginase 1 and iNOS can both be induced in immature myeloid cells.

Nitric oxide is a potent effector molecule with multiple biological functions. Produced in large quantities through iNOS, ·NO contributes significantly to inappropriate vasodilation and the hemodynamic instability of sepsis. Nitric oxide is important in the killing of parasites and bacteria but can also cause host-injury. Nitric oxide produced by myeloid cells may regulate T-lymphocyte function. Several inflammatory signals that upregulate iNOS expression, include IL-1, IL-2 (T-helper 1), TNF, IFNγ, and endotoxin.

Arginase 1 metabolizes arginine into ornithine and urea and as such, may provide substrate for several metabolic pathways including the production of polyamines and proline. It is however, in its capacity to deplete arginine, that ARG1 has gained significant notoriety in recent years. Released locally or systemically from neutrophils, ARG1 rapidly depletes arginine. The degree of arginine depletion appears proportional to the degree of neutrophil activation. Through arginine depletion, myeloid cells serve as regulatory cells, controlling nitric oxide production and cellular metabolic processes such as those observed in T-lymphocytes (see below). Like iNOS, ARG1 is also an inducible enzyme characteristically observed in immature myeloid cells expressing GR1+ markers (in mice) and CD33+ markers in humans. In contrast to iNOS, classic anti-inflammatory signals induce

ARG1 including IL-4/IL-13 (T-helper 2), IL-10, TGF-B, and GM-CSF among others.

In 2001 Gabrilovich isolated myeloid cells capable of suppressing T-lymphocytes; however the mechanisms of T-cell suppression remained unclear [7]. That same year, Bernard reported increased ARG1 expression in the spleens of mice subjected to surgical trauma. Soon thereafter, increased ARG1 expression was observed in circulating peripheral blood mononuclear cells after trauma, the amount proportional to the severity of injury [8]. Furthermore, in 2001, initial reports demonstrated the membrane expression of several T-cell receptor complexes including CD3, CD4, and CD8 were dependent on the amount of extracellular arginine available [9]. By 2006, the capacity of immature myeloid cells expressing ARG1 to deplete arginine became well established. Because of their capacity to regulate T-cell function through arginine depletion, these cells were officially called myeloid-derived suppressor cells (MDSC) [10].

In the last few years, there is a growing awareness of the immunosuppressive roles of MDSC, the arginine depletion they cause and their importance in playing pathologic roles in multiple illnesses. In cancer, MDSC infiltration of solid tumors is associated with a worse overall prognosis. In animal models, blocking arginase produced by MDSC inhibits tumor growth. In surgery and trauma, high arginase activity is associated with worse acute physiology scores. Thus, it is logical to believe strategies aimed at overcoming the suppressive role of MDSC should lead to improved arginine availability and better outcomes.

There is growing evidence that ARG1 can also regulate ·NO production through arginine depletion. Arginine is not only a substrate for all nitric oxide synthases including iNOS; it has also become progressively evident that arginine deficiency can block iNOS translation and assembly of enzyme monomers. Increased evidence has accumulated to demonstrate regulation of ·NO production by ARG1 is of significant importance in vivo. Decreased accumulation of nitric oxide metabolites in urine is observed in severely traumatized patients even if they become septic. Similarly, mice subjected to surgical trauma exhibit a significantly blunted accumulation of circulating nitric oxide metabolites in response to injection of endotoxin. Not surprisingly, ·NO production was restored in STAT6 knockout mice incapable of inducing ARG1 in response to trauma. Clinically, patients undergoing elective surgery operations that received supraphysiologic quantities of arginine exhibit improved microcirculation, tissue oxygenation, and an increase in circulating nitric oxide metabolites, which may translate into improved outcomes.

The converse may also be true. Hydroxy-L-arginine, an intermediate product in the generation of ·NO is a potent arginase inhibitor. The clinical significance of this finding remains to be defined. Co-induction of ARG1 and iNOS is possible and results in the accumulation of reactive nitrogen species (peroxynitrite among others), protein nitrosylation (nitrotyrosine), and cellular damage. Reactive nitrogen species can also result in T-cell dysfunction.

Arginine in T-Lymphocytes

Similar to myeloid cells, T-lymphocytes exhibit little uptake and utilization of arginine during resting conditions. However, arginine becomes an essential amino acid for normal T-lymphocyte proliferation, the production of interferon gamma and possibly the development of memory. Perhaps the most striking change observed in T-lymphocytes is the loss of the ζ chain, a mostly intracellular peptide of the T-cell receptor complex. The ζ chain plays essential roles in the signal transduction pathways for T-cell activation and in the export of the T-cell receptor complex to the cell membrane, after its intracellular assembly. Thus, T-cell receptor expression is proportional to the extracellular concentration of arginine. In the absence of arginine, T-lymphocytes will exhibit a characteristic loss in the ζ chain, a decrease in the number of T-cell receptors expressed on the cell surface and a lack of response to proliferative stimuli.

Loss of the ζ chain has become a hallmark of T-lymphocyte dysfunction in a growing number of illnesses. It was first described in animals and humans with cancer. Soon however, loss of ζ chain was also described in chronic infections such as tuberculosis, and in patients undergoing surgical interventions. Increased arginase activity has been described in all of these situations. Not surprisingly, other changes in T-cell function that are characteristic of arginine deficiency are also observed [11].

Not all protein and/or other metabolic activities are inhibited when arginine becomes deficient. Facing arginine deficiency, the T-lymphocyte upregulates the necessary mechanisms to synthesize arginine from citrulline and through this mechanism, maintains normal function. Citrulline uptake is increased by up to sixfold and argininosuccinate synthase (AS), the first of two enzymes in the pathway to convert citrulline to arginine, is upregulated significantly. Interestingly, argininosuccinate lyase (AL), the second enzyme in this pathway is constitutively present. As a result, in the absence of arginine, T-lymphocytes are able to perform normal biological functions if adequate citrulline concentrations are present.

The characteristic changes in T-cells observed with arginine deficiency and the preliminary identification of these changes in a number of illnesses suggests the possibility some of these could be utilized in the identification of arginine deficiency. The successful identification of adequate biomarkers could potentially lead to timely identification of arginine deficiency and allow for monitoring therapies aimed at restoring arginine availability.

A significant amount of confusion exists as to the question of whether T-lymphocyte function is *enhanced* by arginine supplementation, and if this could lead to an inappropriately activated T-lymphocyte and systemic inflammatory response. There is no clinical or laboratory evidence that supports this view. In vitro, T-lymphocyte function is normalized with arginine concentrations of 100 μM, a level within the range of circulating arginine concentrations in normal individuals. Increasing arginine concentrations up to tenfold fails to increase T-lymphocyte function any further. In addition, there is no clinical or animal evidence that arginine supplementation in vivo significantly enhances metabolic activity in normal individuals or animals. Thus, the concern about creating severe inflammatory response with arginine supplementation has no basis and is not a reason for withholding arginine replacement when indicated.

Arginine in Illness

A clear understanding that the physiology of arginine depends on the state of immune activation is extremely helpful in understanding the ultimate metabolic fates of this amino acid during illness. This is especially true if the patient is to receive nutritional therapy aimed at arginine supplementation. In the intensive care unit, trauma and sepsis are two diseases that illustrate the importance of understanding this concept.

Primary sepsis such as that observed in patients with colon perforation and peritonitis is associated with a characteristic inflammatory response that includes the release of tumor necrosis factor (TNF), interleukin (IL) 1, IL-2, IL-6, IL-12, and interferon gamma among others in response to increased circulating endotoxin (LPS). This inflammatory response reflects the activation of T-helper 1 (TH1) lymphocytes. Myeloid cells (and other nonimmune cells), in response to some of these signals, upregulate the expression of iNOS and generate massive amounts of ·NO. Excessive ·NO production is responsible, in part, for the excessive vasodilation and hemodynamic instability of septic shock. The response by macrophages to TH1 cytokines and sepsis (with induction of iNOS) has been termed "classic," M1, or "inflammatory" response.

Physical injury (be it trauma or surgery) is also associated with immune activation. There is a characteristic release of IL-4/IL-13, IL-6, IL-10, and TGF-beta, some of which are described as T-helper 2 (TH2) cytokines. In this case, upregulation of ARG1 is observed. In humans there is a characteristic increase in arginase activity in peripheral blood mononuclear cells while in mice, MDSC in the marginal (T-cell) zones of the spleen rapidly accumulate. As a result, ARG1 expression predominates over iNOS. Thus a myeloid response with regulation of ARG1 conforms to an "alternate," M2, or anti-inflammatory response.

It follows that understanding the predominance of the immune response through either a classic M1 or an alternate M2 response dictates the ultimate metabolic fate and biological effect of arginine. This is particularly important when considering enteral delivery of supplemental arginine. In addition, following the ultimate metabolic fate of arginine during illness potentially allows clinicians to determine whether they are facing a classic inflammatory response with predominance of ·NO or alternatively, the predominance of an alternative anti-inflammatory response with the predominance of arginine deficiency. There is an obvious significant overlap between these two extreme responses in many patients. In addition, a significant number of trauma patients become septic and many septic patients undergo surgery. Thus it is possible some septic patients are arginine deficient by virtue of having had previous surgical trauma, while upregulation of iNOS over ARG1 could be observed in patients with primary sepsis having to undergo surgery. Finally, immune responses change over time. It is thus, at this point, difficult to ascertain the predominance of one or other pathways for arginine metabolism in the immune system for a significant number of critically ill patients.

Nutritional Arginine Supplementation in Critical Illness

Identifying a state of arginine deficiency, the mechanisms that cause it, and the negative biological consequences that may ensue, dictate the physiological basis of arginine replacement therapy (ART). Understanding ART is based on logical biological principles of restoring arginine availability and is important for several reasons as it:

- Provides the basis for hypothesis-driven clinical research
- Helps to better interpret the multiple studies on ART that have already been performed, understanding their weaknesses and strengths
- Allows clinicians and investigators to identify patient populations that are not candidates to receive ART
- Acts instrumentally for the identification of clinically useful biomarkers that assist diagnosis of arginine deficiency and monitoring ART

It is reasonable to hypothesize therapies aimed at overcoming arginine deficiency caused by upregulation of MDSC should restore arginine-dependent biological processes leading ultimately to better clinical outcomes. Nutritional interventions tend to be significantly less expensive to develop than pharmacological treatments, and thus should also contribute to decreased health care costs.

Arginine has been incorporated into so called "immune-modulating diets (IMDs)," enteral formulas containing a blend of different nutrients shown to have some effect on immune function. Several commercial IMDs contain arginine at supraphysiologic concentrations. Of the commercial diets, one in particular has been tested in multiple clinical trials. In fact, IMDs containing arginine constitute the most extensively studied category of acute care formulas to date. These diets commonly contain 15 or more grams of total arginine per liter, significantly higher than the normal daily nutritional intake of 3–5 g. Use of IMDs with ~6 g arginine/L (~2% of energy) are associated with negative results in general, whereas those with >12 g/L (>4% of energy) often yielded positive results. Despite its efficient destruction in the gut, diets containing supraphysiologic quantities of arginine are associated with increased arginine plasma levels (Table 1).

Omega-3 fatty acids (ω-3) are frequently incorporated with arginine into IMDs at concentrations that vary between 1.5 and 3 g/1,000 cal. Omega-3 fatty acids come from different sources but are highly concentrated in fish oils. The major components of fish oils constitute eicosapentanoic acid (C20:5n3, EPA) and docosahexanoic acid (C22:6n3, DHA). Both EPA and DHA can be synthesized from alpha-linolenic acid (C18:3n3, ALA) contained in green leafy vegetables, flaxseed, and walnuts among other sources. Typical western diets are low in ω-3 fatty acids with the ratio of n6:n3 being approximately 10:1. In contrast, an n6:n3 ratio of 2:1 is documented for use in the critically ill patient.

Omega-3 fatty acids exhibit significant anti-inflammatory properties through multiple mechanisms including the production of resolvins and oxylipins. Modulating the fatty acid composition of immune cells affects phagocytosis, T-cell signaling, and antigen presentation capability. As a substrate for cyclooxygenases, ω-3 competes with other fatty acids to generate prostaglandin E3 (PGE3) over the more inflammatory prostaglandin (PGE2) and other prostaglandins such as (PGE1). Studies performed in our laboratory demonstrated that, when compared to PGE1 or PGE2, PGE3 blunted the induction of ARG1 by IL-13 in RAW264.7, a rodent myeloid cell line. In sum, prostaglandins from ω-6 increase ARG1 expression, whereas prostaglandins from ω-3 may increase arginine availability by decreasing ARG1 expression. Further, it appears that PGE2 production by certain tumors provide a key signaling molecule for the accumulation of MDSC. Thus, it is possible that ω-3 and arginine given together in IMDs synergize to overcome MDSC activity and restore arginine availability.

Arginine. Table 1 Comparison of enteral formulas containing supplemental arginine[a]

	Crucial®	Impact®	Impact advanced recovery®	Optimental®	Perative®	Pivot® 1.5 cal
Total L-arginine (g/1,000 kcal)	10	14	14.1	3.6	6.1	8.7
% of energy from L-arginine	4	5.6	5.6	1.4	2.4	3.5
EPA/DHA (g/1,000 kcal)	2.9	1.7	3.2	3.3	–	2.6
n6:n3	1.5:1	1.4:1	1.2:1	1:1	4.8:1	1.7:1
Supplemental nucleotides (mg/1,000 kcal)	–	1,200	1,265	–	–	–
Calories per liter	1,500	1,000	1,400	1,000	1,300	1,500
Protein (g/1,000 kcal)	62.7	56	53.2	51.3	51.3	62.5
Soluble fiber (g/1,000 kcal)	–	–	9.7	5.0	5.0	5.0
Tube feeding	Yes	Yes	No	Yes	Yes	Yes
Oral supplement	No	No	Yes	Yes	No	No

[a]Nutrition information is subject to change. Contact the manufacturer for the most current information
Optimental®, Perative®, and Pivot® are registered trademarks of Abbott Laboratories. Crucial®, Impact®, and Impact Advanced Recovery® are registered trademarks of Société des Produits Nestlé S.A.

Nucleotides, antioxidants, and retinoic acid are other nutrients that exhibit effects on immune function. For example, vitamin A forces MDSC to lose the expression of ARG1 in the process of maturation. It is, however, unknown as to whether these nutrients interact with arginine to restore arginine availability.

There have been dozens of trials using immunonutrition. These trials include different medical and surgical populations, different immunonutrients, and are of varying quality. Many suffer from basic problems with patient selection, inadequate numbers, and inappropriate controls. It is thus not surprising that confusing results coupled with the theoretical (though unfound) harm of IMDs have prevented clinicians from adopting adequate use of immunonutrition. Despite these problems, a clear picture has now emerged allowing to the benefit of multiple patients and the health care system in general.

Arginine replacement therapy in Elective Surgery. More than 30 trials using IMDs have been performed in patients undergoing elective surgery. Multiple patient populations (3,000+ patients) have been studied including patients undergoing head and neck surgical procedures, cardiothoracic surgery, and both upper and lower gastrointestinal surgery. Timing of delivery of the IMDs varies between trials with some investigators ordering IMDs as a nutritional supplement starting preoperatively (generally 5 days), while others ordered the diets both pre- and postoperatively or exclusively postoperatively.

Regardless of the site of surgery, the use of IMDs is associated with a clear and highly significant decrease in postoperative infections by 38–61% ($p<0.0001$). In addition, other complications such as anastomotic breakdown (colon) and formation of oro-cutaneous fistulae (H&N) are also significantly decreased ($p<0.0001$). Not surprisingly, patients receiving IMDs exhibit decreased hospital length of stay (LOS) of 2–3 days ($p<0.0001$). Best results are obtained when the IMDs are started preoperatively.

The effect of IMDs containing arginine on cost has been studied in patients undergoing colon surgery for cancer. Through a decrease in the number of infections, complications, and length of stay, IMDs are highly cost-effective, decreasing cost by thousands of dollars per patient. For example, when cost data from GI cancer surgery patient stays is analyzed in terms of a 2-day decrease in LOS, a potential cost savings of over $4,000 per patient can be calculated. (HCUP data URL accessed August 2009: http://hcup.ahrq.gov).

Based on both the basic science and clinical findings from multiple trials, utilization of IMDs is therefore now considered standard of care with a Grade A recommendation by different published guidelines. There is currently no controversy in these findings. A policy of systematic utilization of IMDs could potentially result in a significant decrease in health care costs. The use of IMDs in patients undergoing major elective surgery, ideally started preoperatively, is *standard of care* and should be advocated as an important initiative for reduction of infection.

Arginine replacement therapy in Trauma. Compared to elective surgery, only a few trauma patients have been enrolled into trials that test IMDs. Kudsk and colleagues in 1996 reported a trial in severely traumatized patients (ISS$\geq$21) randomizing them to three groups receiving either a diet high in arginine and omega-3 fatty acids versus an isonitrogenous enteral diet or a conventional control group. Despite the low numbers of patients in each group (17, 18, 19 patients), trauma patients receiving an IMD exhibited a significant decrease in intra-abdominal abscesses (6%) when compared to the group receiving an isonitrogenous diet (41%, $p<0.02$) and to the control group (58%, $p<0.002$). To date, this study remains a model of well-executed clinical research on nutritional therapy in the critically ill. Thus, the critical care guidelines published by both the Society of Critical Care Medicine (SCCM) and the American Society of Parenteral and Enteral Nutrition (ASPEN) also give a Grade A recommendation in trauma surgery for the use of IMDs containing supplemental arginine, among other immunonutrients: omega-3 fatty acids, nucleic acid, glutamine, and antioxidants.

Two other important observations in trauma patients deserve mention. The first is that the benefit of an IMD in trauma appears to be related to the volume of diet received and the severity of injury. Unfortunately, it is difficult to separate these variables to determine their independent importance as sicker patients tend to be more difficult to feed enterally. Interestingly, arginine, when given in the absence of omega-3 fatty acids and other immune nutrients appears to exert no benefit. This lack of benefit is also observed in elective surgery.

Arginine replacement therapy in sepsis. The use of arginine in sepsis, particularly in the nonoperative medical critically ill remains controversial. Observations under basic experimental settings (in vitro and in animal models) suggest that upregulation of classic inflammatory response leads to the predominance in the production of ·NO with associated hemodynamic instability. In addition, arginine varies widely in sepsis with reports of decreased, normal, or even significantly elevated levels in plasma, and thus it is impossible to predict whether a given septic patient would benefit from supplemental arginine. Furthermore, clinical outcomes data fail to show a consistent evidence of benefit. Not surprisingly, guidelines vary significantly in their

Arginine. Table 2 Differences in ICU nutritional guidelines [1]

	SCCM 2009	ASPEN 2009	ADA 2008	Canadian 2007	ESPEN 2006
Immune-modulating formulas for all critical care patients	Yes	Yes	No	No	Yes
Immune-modulating formulas for surgery/trauma	Yes	Yes	N/A	Yes	Yes

Martindale R. *Highlights from the 2009 Critical Care Nutrition Guidelines*. NNI Breakfast Symposium. Clinical Nutrition Week 2009

recommendations for arginine containing IMDs. SCCM and ASPEN guidelines caution the use of these formulas in patients with severe sepsis, but give a grade A in critically ill surgical patients and a grade B recommendation in nonoperative medical critically ill patients with mild to moderate sepsis. The Canadian Critical Care Nutrition Task force advises the avoidance of supplemental arginine in sepsis [12] (Table 2).

Conclusions: Arginine Deficiency Syndrome

Arginine deficiency as an important state of nutritional deficiency that develops during illness has been recognized for many years. It is only during the last few years, however, that the mechanisms of how arginine deficiency develops have been recognized. Arginine deficiency conforms to all requirements to be identified as a nutrition deficiency syndrome. Arginine deficiency syndrome (ADS) occurs when immune activation through alternative pathways is induced with the appearance of MDSC expressing high levels of ARG1. Arginine deficiency in turn affects several biological processes, namely T-cell dysfunction, possibly increasing susceptibility to infection. Not surprisingly, therapies aimed at overcoming arginine deficiency are associated with a significant decrease in infection rates.

Arginine replacement therapy (ART) in the form of an IMD should be standard of care in all major elective surgical patients, particularly if started before surgery, regardless of whether intensive care management is needed in the postoperative period. IMDs should also be given in trauma patients. The use of IMDs in sepsis is still controversial and further studies are necessary.

References

1. Morris SM Jr (2006) Arginine: beyond protein. Am J Clin Nutr 83:508S–512S
2. Popovic PJ, Zeh HJ III, Ochoa JB (2007) Arginine and immunity. J Nutr 137:1681S–1686S
3. Zhu X, Herrera G, Ochoa JB (2010) Immunosupression and infection after major surgery: a nutritional deficiency. Crit Care Clin 26:491–500, ix
4. Waitzberg DL, Saito H, Plank LD et al (2006) Postsurgical infections are reduced with specialized nutrition support. World J Surg 30:1592–1604
5. Marik PE, Zaloga GP (2010) Immunonutrition in high-risk surgical patients: a systematic review and analysis of the literature. JPEN J Parenter Enteral Nutr 34:378–386
6. Closs EI, Basha FZ, Habermeier A et al (1997) Interference of L-arginine analogues with L-arginine transport mediated by the y+ carrier hCAT-2B. Nitric Oxide 1:65–73
7. Gabrilovich DI, Velders MP, Sotomayor EM et al (2001) Mechanism of immune dysfunction in cancer mediated by immature Gr-1+ myeloid cells. J Immunol 166:5398–5406
8. Ochoa JB, Strange J, Kearney P et al (2001) Effects of L-arginine on the proliferation of T lymphocyte subpopulations. JPEN J Parenter Enteral Nutr 25:23–29
9. Ochoa JB, Bernard AC, O'Brien WE et al (2001) Arginase I expression and activity in human mononuclear cells after injury. Ann Surg 233:393–399
10. Gabrilovich DI, Bronte V, Chen SH et al (2007) The terminology issue for myeloid-derived suppressor cells. Cancer Res 67:425
11. Rodriguez PC, Ochoa AC (2008) Arginine regulation by myeloid derived suppressor cells and tolerance in cancer: mechanisms and therapeutic perspectives. Immunol Rev 222:180–191
12. McClave SA, Martindale RG, Vanek VW et al (2009) Guidelines for the provision and assessment of nutrition support therapy in the adult critically Ill patient: Society of Critical Care Medicine (SCCM) and American Society for Parenteral and Enteral Nutrition (A.S.P.E.N.). JPEN J Parenter Enteral Nutr 33:277–316

Arginine Metabolism

REBECCA M. DODSON[1], SANDRA L. KAVALUKAS[1], ADRIAN BARBUL[1,2]
[1]Department of Surgery, Sinai Hospital of Baltimore and the Johns Hopkins Medical Institutions, Baltimore, MD, USA
[2]Department of Surgery, Hackensack University Medical Center, Hackensack, NJ, USA

Arginine is a dibasic, semi-essential amino acid that has many physiologic functions. In humans, arginine is a nonessential amino acid with endogenous biosynthesis providing sufficient amounts for normal function such as growth, reproduction, and longevity. Supplemental arginine, above and beyond nutritional requirements, has been shown to be beneficial to wound healing, immune function, and maintenance of nitrogen balance. Conversely, trauma and sepsis are associated with decreased circulating and tissue arginine levels which may negatively affect many of the same functions; in these situations supplemental arginine has been shown to have many positive benefits which impact clinical outcomes such as increased wound collagen synthesis, enhanced T and B cell proliferation and function, and support of nitric oxide biosynthesis.

Endogenous arginine biosynthesis produces 15–20 g of arginine each day and is highly dependent on the intestinal-renal axis. The intestinal absorption of arginine occurs via a transport system shared with lysine, ornithine, and cysteine. These ingested amino acids are converted to citrulline for absorption, with the small intestine being the predominant source of circulating citrulline for endogenous arginine synthesis. The majority of endogenous arginine synthesis in adults involves the intestinal-renal axis. This also is known as the interorgan pathway. In this process, renal tubular cells extract circulating citrulline released into the blood from enterocytes. Argininosuccinate synthase and argininosuccinate lyase in the cytosol of the renal tubular cells sequentially metabolize citrulline to L-arginine. This endogenous synthesis of arginine from citrulline is not affected by dietary intake of arginine. Consequently, impairment of small bowel or renal function can reduce endogenous arginine synthesis, thereby increasing the dietary requirement [1]. Synthesis of arginine from citrulline also occurs at a low level in many other cells and cellular capacity for arginine synthesis can be markedly increased under circumstances that induce enzymes that synthesize nitric oxide (NO).

In mammals, catabolism of arginine primarily occurs through two enzymatic pathways: arginase, generating urea and ornithine, or nitric oxide synthase producing NO and citrulline. There are two types of arginases. Type I, cytosolic in location, is most prominent in the liver as part of the full urea cycle but is also present in macrophages, lymphocytes, and fibroblasts. The urea cycle is essential for ammonia and nitrogenous waste detoxification. Ornithine, the other end product of arginase degradation, can be used upon further decarboxylation for polyamine synthesis (critical for cell division and replication) or can function as a precursor for proline biosynthesis, which can be crucial for wound healing responses. Type II arginase is a mitochondrial enzyme in the kidney, small intestine, brain, lung, prostate, and lactating mammary gland.

Through the action of nitric oxide synthase (NOS) arginine is the unique substrate for the production of NO. This important pathway is present in many tissues and cells including endothelium, brain, inflammatory cells (lymphocytes, macrophages, neutrophils, mast cells), platelets, and hepatocytes. In addition to its role in vasodilatation, NO is a neurotransmitter and cytotoxic effector molecule. NO is formed by oxidation of one of the two identical terminal guanidino groups of L-arginine by the NOS, a dioxygenase, of which there are at least two identified isoforms. Both isoforms of NOS have been identified as flavoproteins, each containing flavine adenine dinucleotide and flavine adenine mononucleotide and both are inhibited by diphenyleneiodonium, a flavoprotein inhibitor. Neuronal NOS and endothelial NOS collectively referred to as cytosolic NOS (cNOS), are expressed constitutively and are activated by Ca^{2+}/calmodulin. Inducible NOS is calcium independent and is expressed in response to inflammatory cytokines and endotoxins including interleukin-1, tumor necrosis factor-α, γ-interferon, and lipopolysaccharide.

There are strong regulatory mechanisms between the different metabolic pathways of arginine. L-Hydroxyarginine and nitrite, intermediate end products of the NO pathway, are both strong arginase inhibitors. Furthermore, urea, an end product of arginase activity, inhibits NO formation. Each pathway is stimulated by a well-defined set of cytokines which then downregulates the alternate pathway, for example TGF-β stimulates arginase but inhibits iNOS [2, 3].

Arginine Supplementation and Critically Ill

It has been established that plasma arginine levels rapidly decline in critical illness, trauma, and sepsis and are correlated with a worse prognosis [4]. Several factors are responsible for this decrease including decreased dietary intake, decreased gastrointestinal absorption, increased tissue uptake, and increased metabolism of arginine by arginase and iNOS [4]. Several studies have shown that enteral supplement of 15–30 g of arginine is safe. L-arginine is important for cell-mediated immune function, protein synthesis, wound healing, and microcirculation maintenance. The potential benefits of arginine supplementation in the critically ill include (1) improved would healing, (2) stimulation of immune function via its effects on lymphocytes, macrophages, and dendritic cells, (3) increased organ perfusion, and (4) increased nitrogen balance. Arginine supplementation is hypothesized to aid in various disease conditions: increased collagen deposition in the surgical patient, normalization of vasomotor tone in the cardiac

Arginine Metabolism. Table 1 Effects of arginine and No [5]

Beneficial effects	Cytotoxic effects
Hepatic damage following septic insult	Metabolic pathway inactivation
GI injury and splanchnic permeability	Alterations in gene expression
Downregulator of intercellular adhesion molecules	Oxidation of sulfhydryl groups
Myocardial ischemia	Nitration of tyrosine
Secondary sinus infections	Lipid peroxidation
Inhibits apoptosis	DNA mutation
Anti-inflammatory mediator	DNA strand breaks
Lung neutrophil infiltration	Activates ADP polymerases
iNOS inhibitor in sepsis is harmful adhesion	Possible detrimental hypotension in sepsis
Inhibits NFKB	Damage to cell structure
Prevents endothelial damage	
Leukocyte adherence	
Free radical scavenger	
Enhances anastomotic healing	
Decrease in neutrophil	
Decrease in infection rate	
Decrease in hospital, ICU, and ventilator days	

Arginine Metabolism. Table 2 Nutritional formulas

Formula	(g/L)
Immun-Aid	15.4
Impact	12.5
Crucial	10
Perative	6.5
Alitraq	4.5
Traumacal	3.3
Osmolite	1.45
Oxepa	0

patient, improved nitrogen balance and decreased protein catabolism in the critically ill patient. However, there is a potential danger of arginine supplementation in the hemodyamically unstable patient secondary to increased NO production causing vasodilation and hypotension (Table 1).

Several meta-analyses of arginine supplementation in the critically ill have demonstrated decreased infectious morbidity, decreased ventilator requirement, and decreased length of stay, but no survival benefits (Tables 2–4) [5]. Thus far the consensus of the US summit on immune enhancing enteral therapy has established benefit of arginine supplementation in elective GI surgery, abdominal and torso trauma versus probable benefit in major surgery, severe head injury, burns >30% BSA, and non-septic ventilator dependent ICU patients.

Arginine in Sepsis

In addition to factors stated above, arginine levels in sepsis are decreased due to impairment of intestinal transporters for absorption of amino acid and impairment of intestinal cellular function in the conversion of amino acids to citrulline. A third factor for patients that have sepsis with renal impairment is reduced renal production of endogenous arginine from citrulline. De novo arginine production as well as the precursor nonprotein amino acid of arginine, citrulline, are also decreased in septic patients. Although much research has been devoted to determining the effects of arginine supplementation in varying critically ill populations including sepsis, trauma, burns, and surgical patients, the data from these studies have been conflicting. The major studies using an immune-modulating formula containing arginine have reported benefit, no benefit, and/or potential harm. One reason for the controversial data is that the immuno-nutritional formulas often consists of high amounts of arginine in addition to other active components including glutamine, fish oil, purines, and vitamins. Other flaws in these studies have included heterogeneous populations, supratherapeutic or subtherapeutic levels of arginine, and enteral versus parenteral supplementation [6].

In a canine model of sepsis with *E. coli* peritonitis, administration of intravenous L-arginine in the first 6 h resulted in significantly worsened hemodynamic parameters and increase in mortality. Although raising significant concerns, this model used IV arginine during the induction phases of shock and sepsis, was a short-term survival study and used infusion rates of less than half of that administered in standard formulations of total parenteral nutrition. Data on the clinical outcome on using arginine alone in sepsis are lacking.

Asymmetric Dimethylarginine (ADMA)

It has become apparent that NO biosynthesis is not only influenced by substrate availability but also can be affected by endogenous inhibitors of NOS, including ADMA (asymmetric dimethylarginine). Synthesis of nitric oxide by NOS is competitively inhibited by analogs of arginine

Arginine Metabolism. Table 3 Immunonutrition in critical illness [5]

Study		Population	Supplement	N	Results
Atkinson	1998	ICU	IMP/IC-IN	398	Mortality, ICU mortality, LOS, ICU days, vent days, SIRS days, renal support
Bower	1995	ICU	IMP	296	LOS, infection rate
Braga	1996	ICU	IMP	40	Mortality, LOS, infections
Braga	1998	Three GI surgical groups	IMP/IC-IN/TPN	166	Surgical infection/complications
Braga	1999	Surgical-GI	IMP/IN	206	Mortality, LOS, infections
Brown	1994	Trauma, NSICU	arg, linoleic acid, betacarotene	37	Wound infection, PNA, UTI
Cerra	1991	ICU	IMP/Osmolite	22	Bacteremia, mortality, infection
Daly	1992	Surgical	IMP/osmolite	85	Mortality, infection, complications
Daly	1998	Surgical	Arginine	30	Surgical complications
Daly	1995	Surgical	IMP/tramacal	60	LOS, infections
Di Carlo	1999	Surgical	IMP, IC-IN/TPN	100	Mortality, LOS, infections
Engel	1997	Trauma	IMP/std/TPN	30	ICU days, vent days, infections
Gadek	1999	ICU	oxepa/IC-IN	98	Mortality, LOS, ICU days, Vent days, MOF
Galban	2000	ICU	IMP/IN	176	Mortality, ICU days, vent days, infections
Gianotti	1997	Three surgical groups	IMP/IC/TPN	174	Mortality, LOS, infections, sepsis score
Gottschlich	1990	Three groups	Modular/IN-IC/traumacal	50	Mortality, LOS, ICU days, vent days, infections, antibiotic days
Joudijk	1999	Two trauma groups	alitraq/IC-IN	72	Mortality, ICU mortality, infections
Kudsk	1996	Trauma	IA/promote	33	Mortality, LOS, ICU days, vent days, infections, cost
Mendez	1997	ICU-trauma	Arginine-trace elements-canola oil; IC-IN	43	Mortality, cost
Moore	1994	ICU-trauma	IA/vivonex	105	Mortality, LOS, ICU days, vent days, infections, MOF
Rodrigo	1997	ICU	IMP/IC-IN	30	Mortality, LOS, ICU days, vent days, infections
Schilling	1996	ICU-surgery/general-surgical	IMP/STD/TPN	42	LOS, ICU days, infection
Senkal	1997	ICU-surgery	IMP/IC-IN	164	LOS, ICU days, infections
Senkal	1999	Surgical	IMP/IC-IN	154	Mortality, LOS, infections
Snyderman	1999	Surgical-Head and Neck	IMP/STD		Mortality, LOS, infections
Weimann	1998	ICU-trauma	IMP/IC-IN	32	Mortality, LOS, ICU days, vent days, infections, SIRS, MOF

IMP impact, *IM* immun-aid, *IC* isocaloric, *IN* isonitrogenous, *LOS* length of stay, *PNA* pneumonia, *MOF* multiple organ failure

Arginine Metabolism. Table 4 IV arginine use in disease states [5]

Author	Disease condition	IV Dose	Outcome
Barbul (1985)	Surgical wound	28 g/day	Increased collagen deposition
Mehta (1995)	Pulmonary HTN	0.5 g/kg	Decreased pulmonary HTN
Facchinetti (1996)	Preterm labor	30 g/30 min	Decreased uterine contractions
Campisi (1999)	Cardiac	30 g/45 min	Normalized smokers vascular tone
Berard (2000)	Surgical ICU	TPN + arginine	Increased nitrogen balance, decreased myofibrillar catabolism
Komorrowska (2004)	Free-flap blood flow	30 g/day	Increased blood flow, decreased flap loss
Luiking (2006)	Sepsis	1.2 μmol/min × 72 h	No adverse hemodynamics

that have guanidino substitution. These endogenous NOS inhibitors include ADMA and N-monomethylarginine (MMA). Recent research has focused on ADMA, since it is the predominant circulating NOS inhibitor with plasma levels tenfold greater than those of MMA. ADMA and L-NMMA are derived from the proteolysis of methylated arginine residues on various proteins. The methylation is carried out by a group of enzymes referred to as protein-arginine methyltransferases. Protein-arginine methylation has been identified as an important posttranslational modification involved in the regulation of DNA transcription, protein function, and cell signaling.

Early studies demonstrated that ADMA concentrations were increased in patients with renal failure. Subsequently, increased plasma ADMA concentrations have been noted in situations of endothelial dysfunction including hypertension, dyslipidemia, diabetes mellitus, atherosclerosis, hyperhomocysteinemia, aging, and coronary heart disease. Elevated levels of AMDA have been associated with peripheral artery disease, atherosclerosis, stroke, congestive heart failure, increased cardiovascular morbidity and mortality, and increased morbidity and mortality in critically ill ICU patients. Elevation of ADMA levels in animal models or human subjects correlate with endothelial dysfunction, decreased renal blood flow, increased renovascular resistance, renal sodium retention, and elevated systemic blood pressure. In part ADMA may partly counteract the NO-dependent hypotension, while simultaneously impairing NO-dependent host defense.

The CARDIAC (coronary artery risk determination investigating the influence of ADMA concentration) study determined that ADMA concentration is an independent risk factor for coronary artery disease. When administered to healthy volunteers, ADMA produces the expected effects corresponding to NO synthase inhibition

such as elevation of blood pressure, vasoconstriction, increased renovascular resistance, reduced forearm blood flow, reduced heart rate, and reduced cardiac output. Once a novel marker of cardiovascular risk, elevated ADMA levels may be key in the pathogenesis of endothelial dysfunction and not only an innocent biochemical marker.

ADMA Metabolism

There are two known metabolic pathways for the elimination of ADMA in mammals: (1) the major pathway is via the hydrolysis of ADMA to citrulline and dimethylamine in the cytoplasm by the dimethylarginine dimethylaminohydrolases (DDAH-1 and DDAH-2), and (2) the minor path way is via the transamination of ADMA to α-keto-δ-(N,N dimethylguanidino) valeric acid (DMGV) in the mitochondria by alanine-glyoxylate aminotransferase 2 (AGXT2). It has been shown that overexpression of AGXT2 increased basal NO generation and protected from ADMA-mediated impairment of NO production in endothelial cells. DDAH1 and DDAH2 may be downregulated in several pathological conditions, such as hyperhomocysteinemia, chronic kidney disease, pulmonary hypertension, and diabetes. The two isoforms of DDAH have unique tissue specificity. DDAH-1 is associated with tissues that express high levels of neuronal NOS, whereas DDAH-2 is associated with tissues that express eNOS.

Heterozygous deficiency of DDAH-1 in gene-targeted mice leads to accumulation of ADMA, impairment in nitric oxide (NO)-dependent endothelial function, and elevated systemic and pulmonary blood pressure. Studies of transgenic DDAH-1 mice have demonstrated that these mice are protected against cardiac transplant vasculopathy. Other laboratories have demonstrated that DDAH overexpression inhibits ADMA-mediated endothelial function in cerebral arteries and can enhance insulin sensitivity through modulation of nitric oxide. In distinction, overexpression of DDAH-1 in transgenic mice results in decreased levels of ADMA in plasma and protection from endothelial dysfunction and myocardial reperfusion injury. Dysregulation of ADMA metabolism may occur in hyperhomocysteinemia through an inhibitory effect of homocysteine on the expression and activity of DDAH. It has also been shown that overexpression of DDAH1 protects from hyperhomocysteinemia-induced alterations in cerebral arteriolar structure and vascular muscle function.

Arginine Supplementation

The inhibitory effect of ADMA on NOS activity can be overcome by this enzyme's natural substrate, L-arginine. The rationale to use a NOS inhibitor in critically ill patients was to attenuate a presumed excessive NO synthesis contributing to circulatory failure, since earlier studies demonstrated elevated concentrations of NO metabolites in patients with septic shock. These findings led to the generally accepted hypothesis that increased NO synthesis was responsible for the hypotension associated with sepsis. However, the NOS inhibitor NG-methyl-L-arginine was found to increase overall mortality in a large clinical trial, even though blood pressure and vascular resistance were improved. Contrary to previous hypotheses, these results suggest that NO may be beneficial in sepsis. These results add further support that ADMA may be more than a marker of disease and may play a role in its pathogenesis.

References

1. Wu G, Morris SM (1998) Arginine metabolism: nitric oxide and beyond. Biochem J 336(Pt 1):1–17
2. Arginine BA (1986) Biochemistry, physiology, and therapeutic implications. J Parenter Enteral Nutr 10:227–238
3. Witte MB, Barbul A (2002) Role of nitric oxide in wound repair. Am J Surg 183:406–410
4. Witte MB, Barbul A (2003) Arginine physiology and its implication for wound healing. Wound Repair Regen 11(6):419–423
5. Zhou M, Martindale RG (2007) Arginine in the critical care setting. J Nutr 137(6 Suppl 2):1687S–1692S
6. Cooke JP (2004) Asymmetrical dimethylarginine – the über marker? Circulation 109:1813–1818

Arginine Vasopressin (AVP)

▶ Vasopressin

Argipressin

▶ Vasopressin

Arrhythmic Disease in Children

JONATHAN R. EGAN, MARINO S. FESTA
The Children's Hospital at Westmead, Westmead, Australia

Definition

Important arrhythmias in pediatric patients include supraventricular tachycardia and postoperative nodal tachycardia. Typically, two thirds of arrests in pediatrics culminate in asystole–bradycardia.

Characteristics

Supraventricular tachycardiac (SVT) is usually well tolerated despite rates >220 bpm. Wolf–Parkinson–White syndrome is present in a proportion of patients.

Junctional ectopic tachycardiac (JET) is a potentially troublesome arrhythmia seen postoperatively in children following cardiac surgery, e.g., transposition of the great arteries, tetralogy of Fallot, or complete artrioventricular septal defect (AVSD). It typically presents abruptly with rates of >200 bpm, it usually has important hemodynamic implications and requires prompt attention.

Asystole typically results after worsening respiratory failure or in the setting of septic shock, culminating in cardiac decompensation and a cardiac arrest.

Management

Supraventricular tachycardiac (SVT) is treated with supportive measures, adenosine, sotalol, amiodarone, or synchronized defibrillation (0.5–2 J/kg). In the setting of hemodynamic compromise, synchronized defibrillation is necessary with temporizing external cardiac compressions or extracorporeal membrane support as required.

Junctional ectopic tachycardiac (JET) is definitively managed by slowing the ventricular output with amiodarone (5 mg/kg IV over 2 h) and then atrial pacing via epicardial leads at ~150–160 bpm for 24–48 h or until the underlying JET has resolved. Additional measures such as normalizing electrolytes, maintaining a temperature <36°C, reducing chronotropic agents, and ensuring adequate sedation and analgesia are all worth-while measures.

Asystole is treated with prompt and effective external cardiac compressions at 100 bpm and 15:2 ventilations together with 3 min adrenaline 0.1 ml/kg 1:10,000 that should lead to a return of spontaneous circulation. Hypovolaemia, hypothermia, and tension pneumothoraces can impede recovery of circulation and should be treated. Calcium should only be administered in documented low calcium states. VF that develops during an arrest has a poor prognosis and is managed with defibrillation 2–4 J/kg and amiodarone as well as effective cardiopulmonary resuscitation (CPR). ECMO is a potential option if feasible and is implemented in some centers if a third dose of adrenaline is required.

Arterial Blood Gas Analysis

► Arterial Blood Gases Interpretation

Arterial Blood Gases Interpretation

SAMIR H. HADDAD[1], YASEEN M. ARABI[2]
[1]Intensive Care Department, King Abdulaziz Medical City, Riyadh, Kingdom of Saudi Arabia
[2]Intensive Care Department, King Saud Bin Abdulaziz University for Health Sciences, King Abdulaziz Medical City, Riyadh, Kingdom of Saudi Arabia

Synonyms

ABG; Arterial blood gas analysis; Blood gases

Definition

Arterial blood gas (ABG) is a test that measures or estimates pH, partial pressure of oxygen, partial pressure of carbon dioxide, and bicarbonate in the arterial blood.

Application

ABG analysis is an essential diagnostic test to assess acid–base balance, ventilation, and oxygenation. It is especially important in the management of critically ill patients, and its usefulness depends on the correct interpretation of the results.

Stepwise Approach to Diagnosing Ventilation and Acid–Base Balance Disorders

Assessment of acid–base balance and ventilation are made together by evaluating pH, P_aCO_2, and HCO_3. pH and P_aCO_2 are directly measured by the ABG machine, while HCO_3 is a calculated value. Table 1 shows the normal ranges of pH and P_aCO_2 [1].

Several methods exist to guide the interpretation of acid–base balance and ventilation. The following is a six-step practical approach for the analysis of acid–base disorders utilizing the ABG and serum electrolyte data. It was originally proposed by Narins and Emmett [2].

Step 1: To determine whether there is acidemia or alkalemia
Assessment of acid–base balance starts with evaluating pH which identifies acidemia or alkalemia. The normal pH is 7.38–7.42; acidemia is defined as blood pH of <7.38 and alkalemia as blood pH of >7.42.

Step 2: To determine the type of primary disorder as respiratory or metabolic
Respiratory disorders alter the P_aCO_2 (normal: 38–42 mmHg; 40 ± 2). A P_aCO_2 of >42 mmHg is consistent with respiratory acidosis and a P_aCO_2 of <38 mmHg is consistent with respiratory alkalosis.

Metabolic disorders alter the serum HCO_3^- (normal: 22–26 mEq/L; 24 ± 2). A serum HCO_3^- of <22 mEq/L is consistent with metabolic acidosis while a serum HCO_3^- of >26 mEq/L is consistent with metabolic alkalosis.

Respiratory compensation for a metabolic disorder is verified using Step 6 (Table 3).

Step 3: To determine whether the respiratory disorder is acute or chronic
Once respiratory acidosis or alkalosis is diagnosed, the next step is to determine whether the disorder is acute or chronic by examining the renal compensation. Acute respiratory acidosis or alkalosis results initially in marked changes in pH with limited alteration in HCO_3^-. The process of renal compensation of increasing reabsorption of HCO_3^- (in acidosis) or increased elimination of HCO_3^- (in alkalosis) develops over several hours, reaching a maximum after 4 days. This process helps in bringing the pH back toward

Arterial Blood Gases Interpretation. Table 1 Normal ranges of pH and P_aCO_2

	Mean	1 Standard deviation	2 Standard deviations
P_aCO_2 (mmHg)	40	38–42	35–45
pH	7.40	7.38–7.42	7.35–7.45

Arterial Blood Gases Interpretation. Table 2 Summary of pH, P_aCO_2, and HCO_3^- changes in different acid–base disorders

Disorder	pH	P_aCO_2	HCO_3^-
Respiratory acidosis	Decreased	Increased	Normal or increased
Respiratory alkalosis	Increased	Decreased	Normal or decreased
Metabolic acidosis	Decreased	Decreased	Decreased
Metabolic alkalosis	Increased	Increased	Increased

Arterial Blood Gases Interpretation. Table 3 pH changes in acute and chronic respiratory disorders

Acute respiratory acidosis	pH decreases by 0.08	For each 10 mmHg increase in P_aCO_2
Chronic respiratory acidosis	pH decreases by 0.03	For each 10 mmHg increase in P_aCO_2
Acute respiratory alkalosis	pH increases by 0.08	For each 10 mmHg decrease in P_aCO_2
Chronic respiratory alkalosis	pH increases by 0.02	For each 10 mmHg decrease in P_aCO_2

normal, however, not completely. These relationships are expressed within the equations shown in Table 3.

Step 4: To determine whether the metabolic acidosis is with or without an anion gap

The anion gap (AG) is the calculated difference between the routinely measured major cation (sodium) and the routinely measured major anions (chloride and bicarbonate) (Table 4).

$$AG = Na^+ - (Cl^- + HCO_3^-)$$

Because blood is electroneutral, cations (including major and minor) are balanced by anions (including major and minor). Therefore, the AG (normal: 8–12 mEq/L) represents the unmeasured anions required to counterbalance sodium's positive charge.

An increase in the AG indicates the accumulation of acid in body fluids. Strong acid, HX, reacts with serum $NaHCO_3$ to form NaX and H_2CO_3; the latter converts to H_2O and CO_2, which is excreted by the lungs. The net result is to replace the HCO_3^- anion with the anion X^- of

Arterial Blood Gases Interpretation. Table 4 Anion gap reflects the minor anions and cations

Major cations	Major anions
Sodium	Chloride
	Bicarbonate
Minor cations	**Minor anions**
Calcium	Proteins, mostly albumin
Potassium	Organic acids
Magnesium	Phosphates
	Sulfates

the acid. If hydrochloric acid (HCl) is added, 1 mEq of Cl^- replaces 1 mEq of HCO_3^- resulting in *normal AG* (also called *hyperchloremic or non-AG*) *metabolic acidosis*. Addition of any other acid will lower the HCO_3^- level without affecting Na^+ or Cl^- levels, resulting in elevation of the AG, or *AG metabolic acidosis*.

As such, the calculation of the AG helps in the diagnosis of the cause for metabolic acidosis by determining whether the acidosis is associated with normal or elevated AG.

The calculation of the AG provides reliable data with a few exceptions. First, hypoalbuminemia, a finding observed in as frequent as 75% of critically ill patients [3], is associated with the reduction of normal AG. This is because the negatively charged albumin accounts for a significant proportion of the unmeasured anions. Therefore, in patients with severe hypoalbuminemia, AG metabolic acidosis may exist with the measured AG being normal. As such, it is recommended to correct for the albumin level as per the following formula:

$$AG_{corrected}(mmol/L)$$
$$= AG_{observed} + 0.25 \times (normal\ albumin$$
$$- observed\ albumin)(g/L)$$

This approach has been demonstrated to improve the diagnostic performance of the acid–base balance assessment [3, 4].

Second, alkalemic patients with pH >7.5 may have an elevated AG due to metabolic alkalosis and not because of an additional metabolic acidosis. This is probably due to the fact that the albumin surface becomes more negative in alkalemic conditions, thus increasing the unmeasured anions and in turn the AG.

Step 5: To determine whether other metabolic disorders coexist with an anion gap acidosis

In patients with pure AG metabolic acidosis, the amount of accumulated acid correlates with the amount of bicarbonate consumed to buffer the acid, and, therefore, each 1 mEq/L increase in the AG should be associated with 1 mEq/L decrease in HCO_3^-. This is reflected in the following formula:

$$\Delta AG = \Delta HCO_3^-$$

However, in the presence of other concomitant metabolic disorders that affect the bicarbonate level, this reciprocal relationship is disturbed. For example, in the presence of concomitant metabolic acidosis, the drop in bicarbonate is more profound than the change in the AG:

$$\Delta AG < \Delta HCO_3^-$$

On the other hand, concomitant metabolic alkalosis leads to a less profound change of bicarbonate compared to the AG:

$$\Delta AG > HCO_3^-$$

Step 6: To assess the respiratory compensation for a metabolic disorder
Metabolic acidosis results in a rapid and predictable respiratory response by hyperventilation. As the change in P_aCO_2 exhibits a linear correlation with the change in HCO_3^-, the expected P_aCO_2 for any given HCO_3^- can be calculated using an equation called Winter's formula:

$$\text{Expected } P_aCO_2 = (1.5 \times HCO_3^-) + (8 \pm 2)$$

As a result, if a patient with metabolic acidosis has a P_aCO_2 level that corresponds to HCO_3^- as calculated by Winter's formula, then he has a pure metabolic acidosis. However, if P_aCO_2 levels are higher or lower than that expected for the HCO_3^- level, then a concurrent respiratory disorder exists. In this case, respiratory disorders would be defined by the direction of the P_aCO_2 variation outside the range predicted by Winter's formula, and not by the P_aCO_2 variation from the normal value of 40 mmHg. Subsequently, if the measured P_aCO_2 is less than the low expected range, then concurrent respiratory alkalosis exists; and if the measured P_aCO_2 is more than the high expected range, then concurrent respiratory acidosis exists.

The respiratory response to a metabolic alkalosis is predicted by the following formula:

$$\text{Expected } P_aCO_2 = 0.7(HCO_2) + 20$$

As a rule, the increase in P_aCO_2 to compensate for metabolic alkalosis would not exceed 50–55 mmHg. The diagnosis of concurrent respiratory acidosis or alkalosis follows the general rules described above.

Other Approaches for the Acid–Base Balance Interpretation

The interpretation of acid–base balance can be further completed by assessing the base excess (BE). The BE is defined as the amount of acid (H^+) that would be required to return the pH to 7.4 at a P_aCO_2 of 40 mmHg (and thus eliminating respiratory disorders). As such, the BE provides an estimate of the metabolic component of the acid–base balance. A BE of >+3 indicates metabolic alkalosis and <−3 indicates metabolic acidosis. The BE is a calculated (not a measured) value, which may affect its accuracy. Additionally, there is a debate about the added value of BE. In a study by Fencl, the BE missed serious acid–base abnormalities in about one sixth of the patients, especially in the presence of hypoalbuminemia [4].

An alternative approach for the assessment of acid–base balance is the Stewart approach, which states that pH is primarily determined by PCO_2; strong ion difference (SID), which is the difference between the sums of all the strong cations (Na, K, Ca_2, Mg_2) and all the strong anions (Cl plus other strong anions); and nonvolatile weak acids. Dubin et al. studied a large cohort of critically ill patients and demonstrated that the diagnostic performance of the Stewart approach exceeded that of traditional approaches based on HCO_3^- and the BE [3]. However, when $AG_{corrected}$ was included in the analysis, the Stewart approach did not offer any diagnostic or prognostic advantages [3].

Specific Acid–Base Disorders and Diagnoses

Respiratory Acidosis
Respiratory acidosis results from the accumulation of CO_2 in the blood with a drop in blood pH. Specific causes include

- Hypoventilation
  - Depression of the respiratory center
    - Sedatives and narcotics
    - Structural lesions such as trauma or stroke
  - Disorders of the spinal cord and the motor nerves
    - Spinal cord trauma, ischemia, or tumors
    - Guillain–Barré syndrome
    - Polio
  - Disorders of the neuromuscular junction and respiratory muscles
    - Myasthenia gravis
    - Neuropathies
    - Severe hypokalemia
  - Disorders of the chest wall
    - Kyphoscoliosis
    - Scleroderma

- Restrictive hypoventilation: pain, chest injury, abdominal distension
- Respiratory muscle fatigue
- Upper airway obstruction
- Sleep-disordered breathing: obesity hypoventilation syndrome, obstructive sleep apnea
- Dead space ventilation
  - Pulmonary disease: chronic obstructive lung disease (COPD), asthma, atelectasis, severe pneumonia, pneumothorax, severe pulmonary edema

Respiratory Alkalosis

Respiratory alkalosis results from hyperventilation that is manifested by excess elimination of CO_2 from the blood and a rise in the blood pH. Specific causes include

- Psychological responses: anxiety, fear
- CNS lesions: stroke, infection
- Drugs: salicylates, progesterone, respiratory stimulants
- Fever, sepsis, pain
- Thyrotoxicosis
- Liver cirrhosis
- Pregnancy
- Hypoxemia: early interstitial lung disease, pulmonary embolism
- Profound anemia

Metabolic Acidosis

A. Anion gap metabolic acidosis: AG metabolic acidosis results from accumulation of acid in body fluids leading to drop in pH and HCO_3^- and increased AG. Specific causes include
   - Advanced renal failure
   - Ketoacidosis
     - Diabetic
     - Alcoholic
     - Starvation
   - Lactic acidosis
   - Drug intoxication
     - Salicylates
     - Methanol
     - Ethylene glycol
B. Non-anion gap metabolic acidosis: Non-AG metabolic acidosis results from bicarbonate loss from body fluids leading to drop in pH and HCO_3^- with a normal AG. Specific causes include
   - Early renal failure
   - Renal tubular acidosis
   - Diarrhea
   - Carbonic anhydrase inhibitors (acetazolamide)

- Ureteral diversion
- Post-hypocapnic acidosis

Metabolic Alkalosis

Metabolic alkalosis results from an excess of serum bicarbonate or a loss of acid within the body. Specific causes include

- Excess base results from antacid ingestion, alkali ingestion, or use of lactate in dialysis
- Loss of acids can occur secondary to protracted vomiting, gastric suction, or hypochloremia
- Volume contraction (overdiuresis)
- Severe hypokalemia
- Excess gluco- or mineralocorticoids, or aldosterone
- Bartter's syndrome

Oxygenation

Information about oxygenation is derived from P_aO_2 and SaO_2. P_aO_2 refers to the partial pressure of oxygen that is dissolved in the arterial blood, and SaO_2 refers to the arterial oxygen saturation. P_aO_2 is measured directly by the ABG machine while SaO_2 is a derived value. Some ABG machines have a built-in co-oximeter that measures SaO_2 directly.

Assessment of oxygenation is performed by evaluating P_aO_2 and examining whether it is adequate for the amount of inspired oxygen. The normal P_aO_2 on room air ($FiO_2 = 0.21$) is 90–100 mmHg. P_aO_2 decreases slightly with age and the following formula can be used as a reference:

$$P_aO_2 = 104.2 - (0.27 \times age)$$

Hypoxemia refers to reduced P_aO_2 below the normal values. It is also essential to check the correspondence of the calculated SaO_2 on the ABGs with the saturation estimated by pulse oximeter. Discrepancy may reflect incorrect probe measurement, related, for example, to low perfusion, venous sampling, or carbon monoxide poisoning.

Alveolar–Arterial Oxygen Gradient (A–a Gradient)

If P_aO_2 is lower than expected for the FiO_2, calculation of the alveolar–arterial oxygen gradient (A–a gradient) can help in differentiating the mechanism.

A normal gradient of 10 mmHg exists between the alveolar oxygen pressure (P_AO_2) and the arterial oxygen pressure (P_aO_2). The A–a gradient increases little with age (up to 21 in older individuals). Generally, there is no gradient between the alveolar carbon dioxide pressure (P_ACO_2) and the arterial carbon dioxide pressure (P_aCO_2). The A–a gradient is calculated using the following equation:

$$P_AO_2 = FiO_{2x}(\text{barometric pressure} - PH_2O) - (P_ACO_2/0.8)$$

In patients breathing room air at sea level, the formula becomes:

$$P_AO_2 = 150 - (P_ACO_2/0.8)$$

Hypoxemia occurs *without* structural lung disease via one of two mechanisms: reduced inspired oxygen (such as at high altitude) or hypoventilation that leads to increased CO_2 and reduced O_2 in the alveoli. In both mechanisms, the oxygen alveolar exchange is normal and, therefore, the A–a gradient remains normal.

On the other hand, hypoxemia occurs *with* structural lung disease through one of three mechanisms: impaired diffusion, ventilation/perfusion mismatch (V/Q mismatch), and shunt. In these mechanisms, oxygen alveolar exchange is impaired and, therefore, the A–a gradient increases.

Oxyhemoglobin Dissociation Curve

The oxyhemoglobin dissociation curve (Fig. 1) demonstrates the relationship between SaO_2 and P_aO_2.

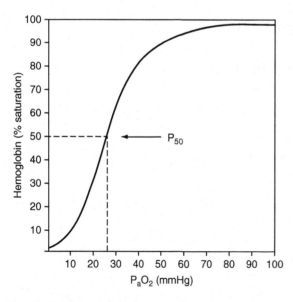

Arterial Blood Gases Interpretation. Figure 1
Oxyhemoglobin dissociation curve

The sigmoidal-shaped curve represents graphically the oxygen–hemoglobin affinity. At higher levels of P_aO_2, the curve is flat, and the arterial blood becomes fully saturated with P_aO_2 of 99.76 mmHg. A small drop of P_aO_2 has little effect on saturation. Once SaO_2 drops below 88%, which corresponds to a P_aO_2 of 50 mmHg, the oxygen dissociation curve enters its steep part where a small fall in P_aO_2 leads to a large drop in SaO_2. This is why a SaO_2 of 88% is used as a therapeutic target. As a usual reference point, a 50% SaO_2 corresponds to a P_aO_2 of 26.25 mmHg.

Several conditions influence the affinity of the oxygen molecule to hemoglobin. Factors that improve release of the oxygen molecule include acidosis, fever, hypercarbia, and increased 2,3-diphosphoglycerate (2,3-DPG). This change in affinity is called a shift to the right. Factors that hold the oxygen molecule tightly attached to hemoglobin include hypothermia, alkalosis, hypocarbia, and decrease in 2,3-DPG. This change is called a shift to the left and has more negative implications for the patient than a shift to the right.

References

1. Williams AJ (1998) ABC of oxygen: assessing and interpreting arterial blood gases and acid-base balance. BMJ 317(7167): 1213–1216
2. Narins RG, Emmett M (1980) Simple and mixed acid-base disorders: a practical approach. Medicine (Baltimore) 59(3): 161–187
3. Dubin A, Menises MM, Masevicius FD, Moseinco MC, Kutscherauer DO, Ventrice E, Laffaire E, Estenssoro E (2007) Comparison of three different methods of evaluation of metabolic acid-base disorders. Crit Care Med 35(5):1264–1270
4. Fencl V, Jabor A, Kazda A, Figge J (2000) Diagnosis of metabolic acid-base disturbances in critically ill patients. Am J Respir Crit Care Med 162(6):2246–2251

Arterial Desaturation

▶ Arterial Hypoxemia

Arterial Hemoglobin Oxygen Saturation

▶ Pulse Oxymetry and CO_2 Monitoring

Arterial Hypoxemia

DAVID W. COLLINS[1], YAHYA SHEHABI[2]
[1]The Prince of Wales Hospital, Randwick, NSW, Australia
[2]Clinical School, University New South Wales, The Prince of Wales Hospital, Randwick, NSW, Australia

Synonyms

Anoxic hypoxia; Arterial desaturation; Hypoxic hypoxia

Definition

Arterial hypoxemia is the state of low oxygen concentration in arterial blood. The concentration of oxygen in the blood is proportional to the partial pressure of oxygen (PO_2), and although the PO_2 of arterial blood (PaO_2) falls slowly with age, the lower limit of normal for an adult is usually accepted to be a PaO_2 of 60 mmHg (8.0 kPa). Normal PaO_2 in young healthy people is about 95 mmHg.

Arterial hypoxemia is important because it can cause tissue hypoxia (anoxic hypoxia) (Table 1). Almost all tissues of the body depend on arterial oxygen for survival, growth, and function, as it has a vital role in oxidative phosphorylation, which produces the basic energy substrate adenosine triphosphate (ATP). In the absence of oxygen, glycolysis may proceed to a limited extent in some tissues, but will result in lactic acid production and produce much less ATP than oxidative phosphorylation. Oxygen is also used in the functions of the cytochrome P-450 system and other oxidases. Tissue hypoxia may result in cellular death, stasis, and dysfunction.

The amount of oxygen delivered to the body each minute (oxygen flux) depends on cardiac output, hemoglobin concentration, and the extent of hemoglobin saturation with oxygen [1] (SaO_2) (Fig. 1). In arterial hypoxemia *less* hemoglobin is oxygen-saturated, and thus oxygen flux is reduced and tissue hypoxia may occur. It is unclear what degree of arterial hypoxemia is

Arterial Hypoxemia. Table 1 Causes of tissue hypoxia

Anoxic hypoxia	Inability to oxygenate hemoglobin
Anaemic hypoxia	Low hemoglobin concentration
Stagnant hypoxia	Inadequate tissue blood flow
Histotoxic hypoxia	Tissue poisoning preventing O_2 utilization

safe, but if it is combined with other causes of tissue hypoxia in Table 1 (e.g., anemia and/or low cardiac output) then even mild hypoxemia is dangerous.

Oxygen is very poorly soluble in plasma (0.03 mL O_2 per litre of plasma per mmHg O_2 tension). The vast majority of oxygen carried by blood (about 99%) is bound to hemoglobin. The relationship between SaO_2 and PaO_2 is seen in the oxyhemoglobin dissociation curve (Fig. 2). Hemoglobin is a complex molecule that changes its affinity for oxygen as it binds one, two, three, or four oxygen molecules. This change in affinity is responsible for the shape of the curve, and this is in turn important in the pathophysiology of arterial hypoxemia. It can be seen that when PaO_2 rises above 60 mmHg or so, the curve starts to flatten out, so increasing the PaO_2 of blood at this end of the curve does not markedly increase the *amount* of oxygen carried. Increases in temperature, 2,3-diphosphoglycerate (2,3-DPG) concentration, H^+ concentration, and partial pressure of carbon dioxide (PCO_2) will shift the oxyhemoglobin dissociation curve such that, at the same PaO_2, hemoglobin affinity for oxygen is lessened and oxygen offloading to the tissues is increased.

One can trace the path of oxygen delivery from atmosphere to alveolus to arterial blood to tissue mitochondria as the *oxygen cascade* (Fig. 3). One of the most important determinants of arterial oxygenation is the oxygen concentration in the alveolus (PAO_2). Room air usually contains 20.93% oxygen, resulting in an atmospheric PO_2 at sea level of 160 mmHg. In the alveolus, water vapor and carbon dioxide are also present so the PO_2 falls. Inhaled gases become saturated with water vapor, with a partial pressure of 47 mmHg, so PiO_2 is 21% $\times$ (760 − 47) = 150 mmHg. Carbon dioxide is evolved into the alveolus from the body at a slightly lower rate than O_2 is taken up (200 mL/min CO_2 produced vs 250 mL/min of O_2 used, giving a respiratory ratio (R) of 0.8), and a normal $PaCO_2$ is 40 mmHg. The alveolar PO_2 (PAO_2) is calculated from the simplified alveolar gas equation $PAO_2 = PiO_2 - PaCO_2/R$. Substituting normal values gives 150 − 40 / 0.8 = 100 mmHg. There is normally a small drop in PO_2 from alveolus to systemic artery (the "A-a gradient"); this worsens with age, posture, and pathology. The "normal" A-a gradient for age is quite variable, but can be estimated from $PAO_2 - PaO_2 = 2.5 + age \times 0.21$ [1].

Characteristics

Causes of Arterial Hypoxemia

The pathophysiological causes of arterial hypoxemia are low inspired partial pressure of oxygen (FiO_2), alveolar

O_2 Flux = Cardiac Output x Blood oxygen content
= Cardiac Output x ([Hb] x 1.34 x SaO_2 + 0.03 x PaO_2)

O_2 Flux: Amount of O_2 delivered to the body each minute (l/minute)
Cardiac output = Net forward flow from left ventricle each minute (l/minute)
[Hb] = Plasma concentration of haemoglobin (gm/l)
1.34 = Amount of oxygen carried by fully saturated haemoglobin (ml O_2/gm Hb)
0.03 = oxygen solubility in plasma (ml O_2/l plasma/mmHg partial pressure O_2)
PaO_2 = Partial pressure of oxygen in arterial blood (mmHg)
Approximate normal values: O_2 flux = 5 x (150 x 1.34 x 0.99 + 3) = 1000 mls O_2
delivered per minute

Arterial Hypoxemia. Figure 1 The oxygen flux equation

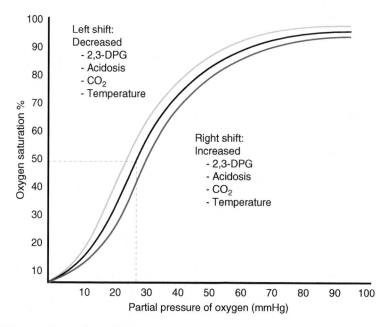

Arterial Hypoxemia. Figure 2 The oxyhemoglobin dissociation curve

hypoventilation, ventilation–perfusion (V/Q) mismatch, and veno-arterial ("right-to-left") shunting of blood.

Low inspired partial pressure of oxygen is an unusual cause of arterial hypoxemia in intensive care. It can occur if ventilatory equipment malfunctions, but is routinely seen at high altitudes. At an altitude of 4,600 m, as in the Andes, the barometric pressure is 430 mmHg, while FiO_2 is still 21% resulting in a moist PiO_2 of 80 mmHg. From the alveolar gas equation above, PaO_2 would be just 30 mmHg in the absence of compensatory hyperventilation. Adaptation to altitude is by hyperventilation to increase PAO_2, and by the development of polycythemia, shift in the oxygen-hemoglobin curve position, increased capillary density, and altered mitochondrial efficiency.

Causes of hypoventilation reside in the brain, brainstem, spinal cord, nerves, neuromuscular junction,

muscle, chest wall, or upper airway. The PAO_2 depends on the balance of oxygen delivery by ventilation and its removal by perfusion. Hypoventilation lessens delivery and thus lowers PAO_2 and causes arterial hypoxemia. Hypoventilation results in an accumulation of CO_2. The alveolar PO_2 can be quantified by use of the alveolar gas equation, which to a first approximation is given above. It can be seen that if, for example, hypoventilation results in a PCO_2 of 64 mmHg, then the alveolar PO_2 will be decreased from its usual value of 100 to 70, and arterial hypoxemia will often result. Equally it is clear that elevation in FiO_2 by nasal prongs or face mask will easily overcome arterial hypoxemia caused by hypoventilation.

In relation to pulmonary gas exchange, diffusion is the process whereby the energy of molecular motion of gases enables them to cross permeable cell membranes and

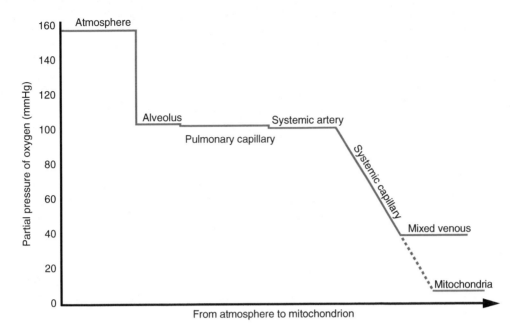

Arterial Hypoxemia. Figure 3 The oxygen cascade

tissue fluids. Oxygen becomes dissolved in body fluids en route to the red blood cell, wherein it binds to hemoglobin. The rate of diffusion is described by Fick's law. Oxygen diffuses across the alveolar cells very rapidly compared to the rate of hemoglobin transit through the alveolar capillary, and the hemoglobin reaches its maximal saturation after traversing only 30% of the capillary length. Diffusion has not been shown to be a common barrier to oxygenation in clinical practice, however in the context of high cardiac output and markedly desaturated mixed venous blood, especially if PAO_2 is limited then diffusion limitation may begin to occur.

In young, healthy people ventilation and perfusion are well-matched in the lung. However, if parts of the lung are relatively underventilated (have a low V/Q ratio), blood from those areas will have low PO_2, approaching the PO_2 of mixed venous blood (40 mmHg) in very low V/Q units. Because of the shape of the top of the oxyhemoglobin curve (Fig. 1) and the low solubility of O_2 in plasma, mixing well-saturated blood from higher V/Q lung units with desaturated blood from low V/Q lung units will only marginally improve desaturation of the resultant blood. Arterial saturation is defended by the process of hypoxic pulmonary vasoconstriction (HPV), diverting blood flow away from hypoxic alveoli to better ventilated alveoli. However, when vasodilatory inflammatory mediators are present in areas of low V/Q ratio (e.g., in pneumonia), blood will flow through those areas, remain poorly saturated and cause arterial hypoxemia.

Shunt is the extreme of low V/Q ratio, such that some blood enters the systemic arteries without any exposure to oxygenated alveoli. There is normally a very small amount of shunt due to Thebesian and bronchial venous drainage, contributing to the A-a gradient. Pathological shunt may be through anatomical abnormalities (e.g., congenital or acquired cardiac disease or pulmonary arteriovenous fistulae) or via fully consolidated alveoli as may exist in severe pneumonia. Hypoxemia due to moderate shunt will persist despite increased FiO_2 as the shunted blood is never exposed to the higher FiO_2, and blood from the normal lung cannot make up for that (see above). The larger the shunt fraction, the less effect any increase in FiO_2 will have.

Arterial hypoxemia may be complex, for example, in a patient with atelectasis who develops pneumonia. The atelectatic lung has low V/Q and this contribution to arterial hypoxemia will respond to increased FiO_2. The pneumonic areas act as shunt and so this contribution to arterial hypoxemia will be unresponsive to oxygen. The impact of arterial hypoxemia in this situation is worsened by the markedly increased work of breathing and any reduction in cardiac output.

Effects of Acute Arterial Hypoxemia
Symptoms and signs will depend on the severity and rate of onset of arterial hypoxemia, as well as on other factors that affect oxygen flux. Severe arterial hypoxemia (PaO_2 <50 mmHg) stimulates the arterial chemoreceptors

in the carotid bodies and the aortic arch causing an increase in ventilatory drive and dyspnoea may be acute. Arterial hypoxemia actually depresses the central chemoreceptors in the brain, but if lactic acidosis occurs in the brain this will stimulate the respiratory centre. Arterial hypoxemia will cause autoregulatory vasodilation in most tissues, but the lungs will have widespread hypoxic pulmonary vasoconstriction and the pulmonary vascular resistance will rise. Cerebral hypoxia will cause headache, confusion and agitation, and sympathetic activation with hypertension and an initial tachycardia. Direct effects on the cardiovascular system become prevalent as hypoxemia worsens and bradycardia and hypotension will indicate imminent cardiac arrest. Brain is critically dependent on oxygen for energy, and coma, seizures, then neuronal death will begin within minutes of acute profound hypoxia ($PaO_2 < 30$ mmHg) [1].

Central cyanosis has a poor negative predictive value for hypoxemia and so oxygenation must be measured. If there is doubt about oxygenation, treating as if hypoxemia is present is the safest approach.

Diagnosis and Assessment of Arterial Hypoxemia

Severe arterial hypoxemia should be treated on suspicion without awaiting test results. Management of the hypoxemia and diagnosis of the cause should proceed simultaneously.

The quickest and most readily available tool for diagnosis of arterial hypoxemia is pulse oximetry. All patients at risk of arterial hypoxemia should have continuous pulse oximetry monitoring. A tissue is transilluminated with radiation of different wavelengths. The pulsatile component of the transmitted radiation is taken to represent the arterial blood signal, and the absorption ratios of red and infrared radiation wavelengths are used to derive an arterial hemoglobin saturation (called SpO_2 when derived from pulse oximetry) from a look-up table of ratio values. Pulse oximetry gives a rapid and accurate estimate of true saturation (± 1–2%) down to about 80%, but poor peripheral perfusion, probe malposition, motion, and ambient light artifact can affect the SpO_2 reading. The presence and concentration of dyshemoglobins is important as they interfere with oxygen carriage and with SpO_2. Carboxyhemoglobin tends to make the SpO_2 read 100%, while methemoglobin tends to push the value towards 85%. New generation oximeters can measure (dys) hemoglobin concentrations.

PaO_2 is measured in the blood gas machine by amperometric techniques. An oxygen-selective membrane allows O_2 from the specimen into an electrode, where the current that flows in the circuit is proportional to the partial pressure of O_2 in the sample (less the zero current).

In the blood gas machine, spectroscopy based on the Beer-Lambert law (relating absorption to the extinction coefficient for a species, species concentration, and the path length) estimates the concentration of O_2Hb, reduced Hb, and dyshemoglobins. Measurement of light absorption over a wide spectrum is used to construct the absorption spectrum of the sample and the concentration of each species is calculated, and hence the fractional and functional hemoglobin saturations. Transcutaneous PO_2 monitoring is available and relies on "arterialization" of cutaneous blood by local heating. It is more effective in neonates and infants than in adults due to the latter's thicker epidermis. It has been shown to have good correlation with PaO_2 but requires skill and care in application to prevent cutaneous burns, probe dislodgement, and artifact generation.

PaO_2 or SpO_2 assess the end result of attempts to increase arterial oxygenation, but do not give an idea of how hard it is to achieve that level of arterial oxygenation. To assess the severity of the oxygenation deficit, other indices weighup the factors in effect to increase oxygen carriage against the oxygenation they are achieving (Fig. 4). One assessment tool is the ratio of PaO_2 to FiO_2 (P/F ratio). It is over 500 mmHg in normal people. P/F ratio is used in the definition of acute lung injury (ALI), but does not give an accurate assessment of the severity of lung pathology, as its value may change when FiO_2, oxygen extraction, or airway pressures change even if the lung pathology remains the same. Nonetheless it is a useful index often quoted in expressing a patient's oxygenation deficit. Another score is the

$$\text{P/F Ratio} = \frac{PaO_2}{FiO_2}$$

$$\text{Oxygenation Index} = \frac{PaO_2}{FiO_2 * MAP}$$

$$\text{A-a gradient} = PAO_2 - PaO_2$$
$$= (PiO_2 - 47 - PaCO_2/R) - PaO_2$$

$$\text{Shunt fraction } \frac{Qs}{Qt} = \frac{CCO_2 - CaO_2}{CCO_2 - CvO_2}$$

Abbreviations: MAP = mean airway pressure; R = respiratory ratio; C_CO_2 is pulmonary capillary, C_aO_2 is arterial, and C_v is mixed venous O_2 content.

Arterial Hypoxemia. Figure 4 Indices of oxygenation

oxygenation index (OI), which does include the mean airway pressure (P/F ratio/MAP).

If the alveolar gas equation is used to estimate the alveolar pO_2 the alveolar to arterial (A-a) gradient can be calculated and will give further assessment of the severity of oxygenation impairment in the lung and of any contribution of hypercarbia to arterial hypoxemia.

Shunt fraction is an expression of the oxygenation deficit in terms of what amount of pure shunt would be required to produce a given degree of arterial hypoxemia, even if that hypoxemia is due to a number of different causes. It is most accurate when the FiO_2 is 1, but this FiO_2 will itself increase shunt fraction through absorption atelectasis. Shunt fraction will give a reasonable estimate of true anatomical shunt but is inaccurate if the arterial hypoxemia is due to variable degrees of V/Q mismatch.

Investigations in Arterial Hypoxemia

Imaging has a vital role in assessing the cause of hypoxemia, the progress of the pathology, and some aspects of treatment. The chest X-ray is an indispensable part of the initial management of arterial hypoxemia. It may reveal pulmonary parenchymal disease (e.g., collapse, edema, or consolidation), intrapleural pathology (e.g., fluid or air), or endotracheal tube malposition. It is also important in detecting complications of the disease process (e.g., lung abscess) or of treatment (e.g., barotrauma). Transthoracic or transesophageal echocardiogram are often performed in hypoxemic patients, especially if hemodynamic instability is present. It can reveal causes of arterial hypoxemia (e.g., left ventricular failure, valve disease, intracardiac shunt, pulmonary embolus) and reveal cardiac effects of hypoxemia such as right ventricular failure. Other chest ultrasound modalities may reveal evidence of raised lung water, or pleural pathology (pneumothorax or pleural effusion). Bronchoscopy of the airway can be extremely beneficial when sputum plugging causes arterial hypoxemia, and can also assist in obtaining specimens for culture and histology. Computerized tomogram (CT) scanning of the chest is a part of the management of complex disease processes causing arterial hypoxemia, and can be of assistance in diagnosis of lung or pleural disease. CT-guided aspiration of abscess or loculated pneumothorax may be indicated in the medium-term management of arterial hypoxemia. Patients who are very unstable often do not tolerate transport to the CT scanner, and the risks should be weighed against any perceived benefit. Lung biopsy can be of assistance in the diagnosis of intrinsic lung disease when etiology is in doubt. As lung biopsy has the significant potential to worsen respiratory function it must be performed only if diagnostic information has a high likelihood of altering the patient's clinical course.

Treatment of Arterial Hypoxemia

If pathology causes arterial hypoxemia by hypoventilation, diffusion impairment, V/Q mismatch, and/or shunt, then the treatment of arterial hypoxemia is to reverse the pathology and attend to these mechanisms. The arterial hypoxemia of hypoventilation is easily abolished with oxygen, but reversal of the pathology causing the hypoventilation itself may be more difficult. Diffusion impairment, if present, will be overcome to some extent by increased FiO_2 and also by increasing mixed venous oxygenation (e.g., by abolishing spontaneous ventilation if work of breathing is profound). V/Q mismatch lends itself somewhat to oxygen therapy alone, but also requires improvement in the ventilation of low V/Q units, which requires that alveolar collapse be reversed and alveolar volume maintained throughout the respiratory cycle. V/Q matching is sometimes improved by increasing the perfusion of open lung. Shunt requires reopening of airways or direct attention to the anatomical lesion. Thus, oxygenation support is mostly about reversing the pathology, giving extra oxygen and matching ventilation with perfusion.

Acute lung injury (ALI) can be defined as acute hypoxemic respiratory failure (P/F ratio less than 300 mmHg) with bilateral pulmonary infiltrates on X-ray and not caused by left atrial hypertension. Acute respiratory distress syndrome (ARDS) is a subset of ALI with a P/F ratio less than 200 mmHg. ALI/ARDS is not an independent disease entity, but because it is a common endpoint of many disease processes and has a high mortality it has been the focus of many investigations into the treatment of arterial hypoxemia [3], and many of the treatments outlined below have been best investigated in the context of ALI/ARDS.

Oxygen Therapy

Delivery Systems

Any system that allows entrainment of room air with the delivered gases will give a variable and unpredictable FiO_2 due to the highly variable peak inspiratory flow rate of patients (compare a frail, narcotized old lady with chronic airways disease to a tall, strong young man with a pulmonary embolus). Table 2 shows a list of common delivery techniques and the FiO_2 they may deliver in normal tidal breathing. Medical gases are essentially dry so it should be remembered that if the upper airway is bypassed or if little room air is entrained then inspired

Arterial Hypoxemia. Table 2 Inspired oxygen fraction according to delivery system

Oxygen appliance	FiO$_2$ (normal tidal breathing)
Nasal prongs 2 L/min	0.33*
Nasal prongs 4 L/min	0.40*
Hudson mask 3 L/min	0.29*
Hudson mask 7.5 L/min	0.41*
Hudson mask 15 L/min	0.59*
Venturi mask set to 0.28	0.29*
Venturi mask set to 0.40	0.40*
Non-rebreathing face mask	0.80
Anesthesia, ventilator or CPAP circuit set to 1.0	1.00

Numbers marked* are tabulated from [2]

gases should be humidified to prevent upper airway desiccation with mucus inspissation and loss of ciliary function.

Adverse Effects of Oxygen

Lung Toxicity
In animals, prolonged exposure to high inspired oxygen levels causes lung toxicity. In humans it seems that lung disease itself provides some protection against high FiO$_2$, and whether high FiO$_2$ is clinically important, and what level and duration of exposure is safe in any individual is unknown. It is thought that the generation of reactive oxygen species in lung exposed to high oxygen concentrations causes cell injury and death through direct toxic effects and by alterations in intra- and extracellular signalling [5]. Many clinicians aim to keep FiO$_2$ below 60%, and if higher levels are needed then often they will first introduce positive pressure to reduce the need for supplemental oxygen. There is animal evidence of an interaction between mechanical ventilation and raised FiO$_2$ such that ventilator-induced lung injury (VILI) is much worse in animals receiving higher FiO$_2$ than in those exposed to less oxygen. Parallels between hyperoxia and VILI include the cellular targets (the type I pneumocyte and pulmonary vascular endothelium) and promotion of polymorphonuclear leukocyte aggregation. In patients previously exposed to bleomycin or paraquat, increased PiO$_2$ can result in significant lung injury.

Oxygen therapy has unique problems in pediatrics. In neonatal practice the development of hyperoxia should be avoided due to its ability to stimulate retrolental fibroplasia, and it is recommended to keep PaO$_2$ below 80 mmHg in premature infants. Bronchopulmonary dysplasia, a disease in low birth weight premature infants, has complex etiology but minimizing FiO$_2$, aiming for SpO$_2$ only in the low 90s and minimizing intubation duration and pressures seem prudent.

Absorption atelectasis
In arterial hypoxemia mixed venous blood is always desaturated (very low PO$_2$) so there will be a rapid uptake of oxygen from the alveolus. If there is no nitrogen in the alveolus to maintain its volume, i.e., if PAO$_2$ is very high, there will be loss of alveolar volume and absorption atelectasis may ensue with subsequent increase in shunt fraction. In acute severe hypoxemia none of these considerations should prevent administration of 100% oxygen until safe (SpO$_2$ >88%) levels of oxygenation are reached.

Chronic Airflow Limitation
In patients with chronic airflow limitation the respiratory center can become acclimatized to high PaCO$_2$, and ventilatory drive becomes dependent on hypoxia. The abolition of the hypoxic drive to breathe can thus result in further hypoventilation and CO$_2$ narcosis. In these patients, initial therapy should include adequate oxygen to prevent dangerous desaturation (i.e., aim for SpO$_2$ over 88%) while assessment of CO$_2$ levels proceeds. If PaCO$_2$ rises more than 10 mmHg (some rise is common, perhaps due to increased dead space), oxygen therapy should not be withheld but instead delivered by a system that helps to maintain minute alveolar ventilation (e.g., face mask BIPAP).

Maintaining an Open Lung

Aspects of Positive Pressure Ventilation
At the end of a normal exhalation the volume of gas left in the lung is called the functional residual capacity (FRC). When flow ceases at end-expiration, the airway pressure is close to atmospheric pressure, i.e. zero. Positive end-expiratory pressure (PEEP) is the raising of this airway pressure to a positive value. Continuous positive airway pressure (CPAP) is the maintaining of a fixed airway pressure above atmospheric pressure throughout the respiratory cycle. Both PEEP and CPAP will result in an increase in FRC. This improves V/Q matching and oxygenation because it increases the amount of gas in open alveoli (i.e., increases oxygen reservoir) and reduces the tendency of alveoli to collapse at the end of expiration (i.e., decreases shunt). It may also aid in opening up

(recruiting) collapsed alveoli but it takes greater transmural force to reopen an alveolus than to keep it open.

Holding the alveoli open throughout the respiratory cycle is a lung-protective effect of PEEP (see below).

The increase in lung volume may mean that tidal breathing is on a steeper part of the pressure–volume curve such that the lung is more compliant. Spontaneously breathing patients may benefit from the decreased work of breathing that this affords, but adding too much PEEP or CPAP will push the lung onto the less-compliant upper end of the curve. Patients with significant intrinsic PEEP may benefit from the decrease in early-inspiratory work that CPAP or PEEP gives, provided the lung is not overdistended.

Raising the mean airway pressure by increasing inspiratory volume, time or pressure will increase alveolar volume and improve oxygenation, so in ventilated patients techniques such as long inspiratory times or inverse-ratio ventilation are sometimes added to PEEP to further raise mean airway pressure. The adverse effects are similar to those of PEEP/CPAP.

Raised mean airway pressure will raise intrathoracic pressure and decrease venous return, This can be advantageous in the context of congestive cardiac failure and CPAP can be a very helpful adjunctive therapy in cardiogenic pulmonary edema. PEEP will redistribute lung water out of alveoli into the interstitium.

Adverse Effects of Positive Pressure

In treating arterial hypoxemia, positive airway pressure is often life-saving but can have deleterious effects. In some patients the decrease in venous return and therefore cardiac output can result in decreased organ perfusion and oxygen flux even if arterial saturation is improved.

Whilst PEEP may maintain recruitment of alveoli, positive pressure can overdistend other alveoli, especially if large tidal volumes are added to PEEP. Overstretching alveoli can cause volutrauma, and excessive pressure, barotrauma which may be manifest macroscopically (as pneumothorax or pneumomediastinum) or microscopically (as alveolar damage and inflammation). If alveoli repetitively collapse and reopen with each breath, as the alveolar walls come in contact with each other they "stick" through surface tension forces, and as the alveoli open again they are torn, becoming inflamed and damaged. This has been called atelectotrauma. The inflammatory mediators thus liberated in so-called VILI (ventilator-induced lung injury) have been implicated in multiple organ dysfunction syndrome. Avoiding VILI is important – studies [3] have shown decreased mortality

and increased ventilator-free days with a ventilation strategy that aimed to limit tidal volume (to 6 mL/kg) and plateau pressure (under 30 cmH$_2$O), compared with tidal volumes of 12 mL/kg and plateau pressures of up to 50 cmH$_2$O. Tidal volume was not increased to control PaCO$_2$ unless pH was under 7.15. Although this was performed in patients with ALI/ARDS, similar lung-protective principles may be applicable to any patient with arterial hypoxemia.

The "best" PEEP in any given patient is still an unknown quantity. The balance must be struck between a PEEP level that improves oxygenation, prevents tidal alveolar collapse, and decreases work of breathing versus a PEEP level that is associated with alveolar overdistension and/or decreased cardiac output. Whilst the FiO$_2$/PEEP tables used by the ARDS Network for their low tidal volumes study are often used as a starting point, some clinicians consider using higher PEEP levels for a given FiO$_2$.

An Approach to Arterial Hypoxemia

A suggested empirical approach to arterial hypoxemia is seen in (Fig. 5). The first priority is a clear airway, to allow alveolar ventilation with a high FiO$_2$. In the intubated patient, endotracheal tube obstruction or malposition must be excluded immediately: passage of a suction catheter will exclude obstruction, while continuity of the tube with the airway is confirmed visually and by the presence of an end-tidal CO$_2$ trace on the monitor. A trial of manual ventilation will eliminate mechanical ventilator dysfunction. Rapid, focused clinical examination to rule out acute conditions is indicated, for example, pneumothorax or endobronchial intubation. Oxygen is given, at high flow rates initially while response is assessed.

The benefit of facemask CPAP in acute, non-cardiogenic hypoxemic respiratory failure is contentious, and a few caveats should be observed. The patient must be alert, the CPAP device should provide whatever inspiratory flow the patient requires, the unit staff should be familiar with the technique, the presence of shock makes failure likely, and if hypoxemia persists despite 10 cmH$_2$O pressure in 60% oxygen, then intubation should occur electively, as if these patients worsen then sedation and intubation are more often associated with acute cardiorespiratory collapse.

When mild arterial hypoxemia occurs despite high PEEP/mean airway pressure and high FiO$_2$ it can be hard to decide whether to further stress the lung with PEEP or FiO$_2$, or to accept borderline SaO$_2$. In managing this situation, cardiac output and hemoglobin concentration must be optimized to prevent dangerous falls in oxygen

A

Arterial Hypoxaemia
Increase FiO$_2$
Improve V/Q Matching
Treat The Cause

Add Oxygen - increase
FiO$_2$ prn to 0.5

Increase FiO$_2$

Hypoxaemia Persists
OR work of breathing high

Add non-invasive
CPAP at 10 cmH$_2$O

Improve V/Q Matching

Hypoxaemia Persists

Increase FiO$_2$ prn to 0.6

Increase FiO$_2$

Hypoxaemia Persists

Intubate patient and use lung-protective ventilation
Increase PEEP prn to 18cmHO$_2$

Decrease oxygen demand and risk of loss of consciousness
Improve V/Q Matching

Hypoxaemia Persists

Check oxygen flux and evidence
of tissue hypoxia; consider
decrease SpO$_2$ target

Consider adding recruitment manoeuvres
to other ventilation strategies

Improve V/Q Matching

Hypoxaemia Persists

Change to HFOV

Improve V/Q Matching

Hypoxaemia Persists

Consider prone ventilation

Improve V/Q Matching

Hypoxaemia Persists

Add inhaled vasodilators

Improve V/Q Matching

Hypoxaemia Persists

Change to ECMO
Continue lung-protective ventilation

Examine Patient
Monitoring
Early Investigations
    Chest X-Ray
    Arterial Blood Gas
    Echocardiogram
    Others as indicated eg CTPA
Treat The Cause eg:
    Check equipment
    Drain pleural collections
    Change to BIPAP for ventilatory failure
    Afterload reduction and diuretics for LV failure
    Bronchodilators and steroids for asthma
    Antibiotics and drainage for pneumonia
    Thrombolysis in Pulmonary Embolus
    Treat cause of ARDS

Arterial Hypoxemia. Figure 5 An empirical algorithm for the management of arterial hypoxemia

flux. A high or rising serum lactate implies inadequate tissue oxygenation, and suggests that the current degree of arterial hypoxemia is unacceptable, but as it may also come from fatiguing muscle, from drugs, or from sepsis it should be interpreted with an understanding of the patient's physiology in mind. Symptoms and signs of organ dysfunction (the brain is the most sensitive and important) are a clear signal to augment oxygen delivery. There is an emerging role for tissue oxygenation monitoring, and this may in the future be used as a marker for the adequacy or otherwise of oxygen flux. Because of uncertainty about oxygen toxicity it is unclear at what stage of the schema (Fig. 5) inspired oxygen fraction should be increased to 100%.

Recruitment Maneuvers

A recruitment maneuver is the application of very high airway pressures to the lung for long inspiratory times, with the aim of recruiting lung that is not recruitable by normal airway pressures. Various combinations of inspiratory time, PEEP, and peak inspiratory pressure have been studied, often with peak pressures of 40–60 cmH$_2$O, with PEEP of 20–30 cmH$_2$O performed for 30–60 s or more. They are usually performed via a mechanical ventilator with the patient deeply sedated and paralyzed to prevent coughing. Recruitment maneuvers have been shown to improve oxygenation and respiratory mechanics, as well as reducing atelectasis, but also to overdistend inflated lung. Recruitment maneuvers can result in dramatic falls in cardiac output and blood pressure. When first using recruitment maneuvers in each patient they must be done under close supervision by the bedside clinician who must decrease the airway pressure quickly if marked hypotension occurs. The cardiovascular changes are complex but may differ in the presence of different pulmonary compliances. While the place of recruitment maneuvers is not yet clear with data from human clinical trials, using it to recruit all available alveoli and then maintaining that recruitment with PEEP (and decreasing the FiO$_2$ as tolerated to prevent absorption atelectasis) appears to be a reasonable approach. This would include use of recruitment maneuvers to reverse lung collapse after each episode of endotracheal suction. The effectiveness of recruitment maneuvers in recruiting lung varies between patients, and may vary depending on the etiology of arterial hypoxemia.

High Frequency Oscillatory Ventilation

High frequency oscillatory ventilation [4] (HFOV) is the use of very high frequency but very low tidal volume breaths. Oscillation is generated in the ventilator by pistonic movement of a diaphragm similar to a loudspeaker. HFOV has been thought to provide good lung protection, as the small tidal volumes makes tidal alveolar collapse unlikely, whilst oxygenation (via FiO2 and mean airway pressure) can be treated separately from CO$_2$ clearance (via frequency and amplitude). The rate of ventilation in adults is usually 4–7 Hertz. Oxygenation is improved because of the high mean airway pressure, while CO$_2$ is thought to be cleared by a number of mechanisms including bulk flow and chaotic gas movement within and between lung units. CO$_2$ clearance increases with increased amplitude but, in contrast to standard ventilation, *decreases* with increasing frequency of oscillation. The optimal settings for all these parameters at this stage are empirical. Initial settings might be frequency of 7 Hz, amplitude of 45 cmH$_2$O and mean airway pressure of 5–6 cmH$_2$O higher than the patient's conventional ventilator mean airway pressure. Frequency is often then decreased to cause greater "thigh wiggle," however it may be that lung protection is maximized if less wiggle than this is produced, so frequency and amplitude are manipulated such that PaCO$_2$ rises to the tolerable limit. One disadvantage of HFOV is the absence of an endtidal CO$_2$ signal, so blood gas analysis is used for PaCO$_2$ estimation. HFOV has not been shown to improve mortality but often improves oxygenation.

Patient Positioning

As gravity will increase perfusion of the dependent lung there is oxygenation benefit in nursing a patient with unilateral disease "good lung down." This is a useful temporizing measure but the need for pressure-area care, postural drainage, and wishing to protect the good lung from dependent atelectasis and soiling mean that it is not a long-term treatment. Appropriate positioning will ameliorate the effect of chest wall factors whose decrease may collapse alveoli, such as in abdominal compartment syndrome or obesity. Prone ventilation has been shown to improve oxygenation and lung compliance in the majority of ARDS patients. The full mechanism of this is unclear. The prone position not only redistributes blood flow during proning but the effects of prone ventilation have been shown to persist for some time. The logistics of turning a patient whilst preventing dislodgement of the endotracheal tube, intercostal catheters, and other invasive devices requires thought, planning, and practice. Consideration must be given to prevent pressure areas especially ocular injury. Although studies to prove mortality reduction from prone ventilation are lacking as yet, it is a useful, if cumbersome, technique to improve oxygenation while other measures take effect.

Inhaled Vasodilators

When vasodilators are delivered in inhaled gas, they dilate blood vessels in areas that are ventilated, thus increasing blood flow through these areas with a subsequent improvement in V/Q matching and a rise in PaO_2. One available option is nitric oxide (NO). When administered in doses from 1 to 20 parts per million NO causes direct vasodilation of pulmonary vessels and has been shown to improve oxygenation. It requires specialized devices for administration and monitoring of room gas for toxic oxidation products of NO. It is very expensive. Prostacyclin (prostaglandin I_2) and its analogue iloprost are available for nebulization and can improve V/Q matching with subsequent rise in PaO_2. Prostacyclin is delivered at 20–60 ng/kg/min to an ultrasonic nebulizer in the breathing circuit. It does not require environmental monitoring. No studies as yet show improved mortality with inhaled vasodilators in adults but they may have a role in maintaining safe oxygenation while other therapies become effective.

Extra-corporeal Membrane Oxygenation

Extra-corporeal membrane oxygenation (ECMO) of the blood is a technique in which blood is pumped from the body via venous catheters at high flow rates, and returned to the body after passing through a gas-permeable, high-surface area interface with oxygen gas. The blood can return by an artery or vein. When gas-exchange is the main aim, venovenous ECMO is becoming more common, with drainage from the IVC and return to the IVC-RA junction. Because ECMO takes the place of the gas-exchanging function, it allows ventilatory pressures, rates, and oxygen fractions to be titrated to lung protection, not to other organ function. Improved technology for the tubing, oxygenator, and pump systems has improved performance and safety of ECMO since its inception in the 1970s. ECMO is currently indicated for short-term support of patients with a life-threatening reversible lung injury (P/F ratio $<$ 50 mmHg), and is usually instituted as a last resort when other measures fail. However, with recent increased experience due to the recognition of the factors above and increased demand due to viral pneumonitis ECMO may be poised to be instituted earlier in critically ill patients of the future.

References

1. Nunn's Applied Respiratory Physiology Nunn JF Butterworth-Heinemann, Oxford 1993
2. Waldau T, Larsen VH, Bonde J (1998) Evaluation of five oxygen delivery devices in spontaneously breathing subjects by oxygraphy. Anaesthesia 53(3):256–263
3. The ARDS Network (2000) Ventilation with lower tidal volumes as compared with traditional tidal volumes for acute lung injury and the acute respiratory distress syndrome. NEJM 342(18):1301–1308
4. Chan KPW, Stewart TE, Mehta S (2007) High frequency oscillatory ventilation for adult patients with ARDS chest 131(6):1907–1916
5. Altemeier WA, Sinclair SE (2007) Hyperoxia in the intensive care unit: why more is not always better. Curr Opin Crit Care 13:73–78

Arterial Pulse Cardiac Output (APCO)

▶ Cardiac Output, Measurements

Arterial Pulse Power Analysis

▶ LiDCO

Arteriobiliary Fistula

▶ Hematobilia

Arteriography with Therapeutic Embolization

▶ Musculoskeletal Trauma, Pelvic Angioembolization

Arterioles

▶ Microcirculation

Arteriovenous Fistula (AVF)

▶ Vascular Access for RRT

Arteriovenous Graft (AVG)

▶ Vascular Access for RRT

Arthritis, Septic

Steven E. Carsons
Division of Rheumatology, Allergy and Immunology,
Winthrop–University Hospital, Mineola, NY, USA
Stony Brook University School of Medicine, Stony Brook,
NY, USA

Definition

Joint infection is an important and sometimes overlooked source of a septic process. The incidence of septic arthritis ranges between 2 and 5 per 100,000 in the general population and approximately 6 and 12 per 100,000 in children. Rates for patients with rheumatoid arthritis (RA) and prosthetic joints are approximately 10- and 20-fold higher, respectively. A patient may require admission to the critical care unit for bacteremia and sepsis secondary to a community-acquired infected joint, or else a critical care unit patient may develop a septic joint as a complication of critical care unit admission. Chronic illness, indwelling catheters, immunosuppression, cutaneous breakdown, and end-stage renal disease, conditions common to critical care unit patients, all may predispose to septic arthritis and subsequent bacteremia and sepsis.

Characteristics

Types of Septic Arthritis

Two-thirds of septic joints caused by Gram-positive organisms are secondary to *S. aureus*. The knee is a common site, although involvement of nearly all peripheral joints and the spine has been described. If not promptly detected and treated, *S. aureus* septic arthritis may lead to severe functional disability, continued bacteremia, and increased mortality. Irreversible articular damage may occur within a time frame as short as 2 weeks. A recent history of joint replacement surgery should raise suspicion for a septic joint in a febrile or bacteremic patient. *S. epidermidis*, usually a nonpathogenic contaminant, frequently becomes pathogenic in the setting of a prosthesis where the foreign material is hypothesized to be conducive to biofilm formation. Another common Gram-positive organism responsible for joint infection is *S. pnumoniae*. Fifty percent of pneumococcal joint infections occur concomitantly with lung and/or meningeal infection. Overall, 10% of pneumococcal septic arthritis episodes are polyarticular, although this percentage rises to 50% in RA patients.

Beta hemolytic streptococci also may be associated with septic arthritis. *S. pyogenes* has been reported to be associated with septic arthritis, occurring in the context of toxic shock syndrome as well as with fasciitis. Group B streptococcus (*S. agalactiae*, GBS) infections are more commonly seen in pregnant and immunocompromised adults. Two-thirds of GBS joint infections are monoarticular, most often involving the knee, followed by the shoulder. Prosthetic joints may also become infected with GBS. Two-thirds of nonpregnant adult patients with GBS septic arthritis have a predisposing underlying illness most often diabetes mellitus, chronic liver disease, and cancer. Septic arthritis secondary to Enterococcus (Group D streptococcus) is less common but is increasingly seen following endoscopic procedures and in patients with underlying malignancy.

Approximately 10% of septic joints are caused by Gram-negative bacillary organisms. Aerobic Gram-negative bacillary arthritis may be seen in the context of neonates, immunosuppression, older individuals with gastrointestinal infections, or following GU procedures. In contrast, it has been estimated that up to 70% of episodes of septic arthritis in individuals under 40 years of age are due to infections caused by Gram-negative intracellular diplococci, i.e., gonococcal arthritis.

While it is rare to encounter GC arthritis in a critical care unit, it may be seen in the setting of disseminated gonococcal infection (DGI) associated with gonococcal endocarditis. A mono- or oligoarthritis characterized by tenosynovitis and accompanied by pustular skin lesions on the palms and trunk should raise suspicion for DGI. Pregnancy, menstruation, and late classical complement component deficiencies predispose to GC arthritis.

Patients with Lyme disease who are sufficiently ill to require critical care usually suffer from neuroborreliosis. As this is most often a manifestation of late Lyme disease, it can be accompanied by chronic Lyme arthritis. This form of Lyme arthritis is usually a monoarthritis and often involves the knee. In contrast, musculoskeletal manifestations of early Lyme infection include myalgia and migratory polyarthralgia. Patients with early Lyme disease may require monitoring in a critical care setting for heart block and myocarditis.

Critical care unit patients are often immunosuppressed. These patients may be at risk for opportunistic joint infections. Such infections may include mycobacterial species including *M. tuberculosis* and fungal organisms. Any suspected septic joint that is repeatedly negative upon routine bacterial culture should be re-aspirated and examined for the presence of acid-fast bacilli and fungal species. Synovial biopsy may be required for diagnosis in the rare setting where all smears and cultures are negative. Pathology revealing granulomatous synovitis is a clue to the presence of mycobacterial, nocardial, or brucella infection.

Predisposing Factors

In addition to immunosuppression from cancer chemotherapy and high-dose corticosteroid administration, other factors may predispose patients to septic arthritis. Any joint which has incurred prior damage is at risk for hematogenous seeding during episodes of bacteremia. This is particularly true for patients with rheumatoid arthritis. In an RA patient, any joint that is disproportionately inflamed and swollen should be suspected of concomitant infection and undergo aspiration for bacteriologic diagnosis. The advent of effective anti-cytokine therapy for RA has also resulted in an increased risk of infection including septic arthritis. In addition to routine bacterial infections, RA patients undergoing therapy with inhibitors of TNF-α are at increased risk for infections caused by mycobacterial and fungal organisms. TNF-α is required for intracellular killing of these organisms even in the presence of effective opsonization and phagocytosis. It appears that TNF-α monoclonal antibodies confer a higher risk for Mycobacterial infections as compared to TNF-α receptor antagonists. Thus, RA patients on TNF-α inhibitors have an increased risk of septic arthritis and a greater risk of infection with opportunistic organisms, particularly *M. tuberculosis*. Joint aspiration and/or intra-articular injection of corticosteroid are frequently used as ancillary therapies for RA patients as well as for patients with other forms of arthritis. Elderly patients with osteoarthritis of the knees frequently receive intra-articular injections of hyaluronic acid. Introduction of a needle into the joint space carries a risk for inoculation with bacteria, most frequently *S. aureus*. Although not necessarily undergoing treatment with immunosuppressive drugs, patients with chronic disease, especially diabetes mellitus and cancer, are at increased risk for the development of a septic joint.

Septic Arthritis in Children

Septic joints in infants up to 3 months are often caused by *S. aureus* but may also be secondary to Group B streptococcus and Gram-negative bacteria. Newborns may have had exposure to *N. gonorrhea* during delivery. In addition to septic arthritis secondary to *S. aureus*, children greater than 3 months of age may be admitted to the hospital with joints infected by Group A streptococcus, *S. pneumoniae*, *K. kingae*, and *H. influenza b*.

Differential Diagnosis

Since most cases of septic arthritis present as a monoarthritis, by far, the most common differential diagnostic scenario in adults is crystalline arthritis. The critical care setting, in fact, is fraught with clinical conditions that predispose to flares of crystalline arthritis including rapid shifts in fluid balance (particularly postoperatively), diuretic use, tissue catabolism, renal insufficiency, hypercalcemia, and administration of medications that induce hyperuricemia. Acute crystalline arthritis is often accompanied by fever, occasionally reaching 102–103°F. Therefore, in most instances, differentiation between crystalline and septic arthritis is not possible without examination and culture of synovial fluid. Gout is by far the most common form of crystalline arthritis; however, the incidence of acute arthritis secondary to calcium pyrophosphate deposition disease (CPPD) appears to be increasing in some centers, perhaps due to aging of the population and an increased prevalence of chronic renal insufficiency. Patients in the PACU or SICU following thyroid or parathyroid surgery are at particular risk for acute CPPD arthritis triggered by perturbations in calcium homeostasis.

Reactive arthritis syndromes, particularly those presenting as monoarthritis or oligoarthritis may be confused with septic arthritis. These include acute rheumatic fever and reactive arthritis itself (formerly Reiter's syndrome, ReA). The latter may be particularly difficult to distinguish from septic arthritis when presenting as a monoarthritis since ReA patients have often had recent gastrointestinal or genitourinary infections which have served as triggers for the ReA episodes. Septic arthritis may also be confused with monoarthritis secondary to occult trauma. Hospitalized patients on anticoagulant therapy may develop a hemarthrosis spontaneously or with minimal trauma such as striking a knee on a bed rail. Such joints are painful, warm, and may be erythematous or in an early stage of ecchymosis formation.

Septic arthritis should be suspected in children with acute arthritis who are sufficiently ill to require admission to the hospital. Nonetheless, other pediatric diagnoses may masquerade as septic arthritis. Acute leukemia may present with a painful swollen joint. This often involves a knee joint and frequently occurs in the setting of pallor, fever, and easy bruisability. Juvenile idiopathic arthritis (formerly JRA) may occur as several subtypes. Children who present with the systemic onset (Still's disease) subcategory may have high spiking fevers, monoarthritis, and a leukemoid reaction. These children may require admission to a critical care unit for management of pericarditis or myocarditis.

Diagnostic Studies

The most crucial diagnostic study in the workup of an infected joint is arthrocentesis. There is no blood test or imaging study that is diagnostic of septic arthritis. Most peripheral joints are readily accessible by needle aspiration at the bedside. Centrally located joints such as the hips, sacroiliac joints, and spine can be aspirated under imaging guidance. The availability of portable ultrasound provides assistance with arthrocentesis in more technically difficult cases, i.e., small or loculated effusions. Once obtained, synovial fluid (SF) should be examined by Gram stain, culture, and sensitivity. In appropriate cases, it is prudent to culture SF on special media for gonococcal organisms, although the yield of gonococcal cultures from SF is relatively low, frequently in the order of 50%. Urethral, rectal, and pharyngeal cultures for gonococcus should also be obtained since they have a higher probability of growth. When suspected, culture for fungal and mycobacterial organisms should be obtained. Blood cultures should be obtained in most if not all cases of suspected septic arthritis to rule out concurrent bacteremia. The likelihood of septic arthritis increases with the degree of SF leukocytosis; however, the predictive value of the SF WBC count is poor. Not all patients with extremely elevated SF WBC ($>50,000/mm^3$) have septic arthritis. Conversely, some patients with relatively low SF WBC ($10–25,000/mm^3$) have infected joints. Baseline SF WBC counts are also useful to gauge improvement and efficacy of therapy since they can be compared to values obtained from SF samples obtained during subsequent drainage procedures. SF should also be examined for crystals under polarized light microscopy. It is important to remember, however, that joints affected by crystalline arthropathy are also more susceptible to infection which may occur during episodes of trauma or bacteremia. Thus, it is not unusual to find bacteria and crystals in the same synovial fluid specimen. Therefore, the identification of crystals in SF does not automatically preclude a diagnosis of septic arthritis. SF glucose may be depressed and SF LDH may be elevated in septic arthritis; however, neither is sufficiently specific to warrant routine testing. If arthrocentesis yields only a few drops of SF, the most important tests to obtain are Gram stain, culture, and crystal analysis.

While imaging studies are not definitively diagnostic for septic arthritis, they are invaluable for localizing areas of inflammation and/or collection, defining the anatomy of involved structures and providing guidance for needle aspiration and biopsy. Imaging studies also can identify complications of septic arthritis such as dissected popliteal cysts and osteomyelitis. Magnetic resonance imaging, CT scanning, and ultrasound are all capable of identifying joint effusions, bursal effusions, and/or other periarticular fluid collections. MR is superior for imaging cartilage, menisci, and tendons, but certain patients have contraindications to MR scanning such as implanted permanent pacemakers and intracardiac defibrillators. Ultrasonography has the advantage of portability and has become the standard imaging modality for guiding arthrocentesis of peripheral joints. Identification of osteomyelitis adjacent to a septic joint is critical for optimal management, including determination of the duration of antibiotic therapy and the necessity for debridement procedures. Technicium 99 bone scanning is sensitive for areas of bone involvement but is relatively nonspecific. Labeled leukocyte scanning, usually with indium 111 oxime, is more specific, but its usefulness has been questioned in chronic infection. Identification of marrow changes on MR imaging is extremely useful for the detection of early osteomyelitis. MR imaging is indispensable for the identification of septic joints and areas of osteomyelitis in inaccessible areas such as the spine and sacroiliac joints.

Treatment

The two major principles of septic arthritis treatment are: (1) prompt administration of antibiotics and (2) drainage of septic effusions. The choice of antibiotic will be determined in part by the clinical circumstances surrounding acquisition of the infection, the initial Gram-stain findings, and local microbial antibiotic sensitivities. Critical care unit patients require careful evaluation for special risk factors such as exposure to resistant organisms and immunosuppression. Broad spectrum antibiotics are preferred for initial therapy until specific sensitivities are known. Currently, third-generation cephalosporins or vancomycin are recommended for Gram-positive infections of which approximately three-fourths will be S. aureus. The choice is in part dependent upon the prevalence of methicillin resistant S. aureus in the community. Third-generation cephalosporins are also good first choices for suspected Gram-negative bacillary infections. Gonococcal infections should be managed with intravenous ceftriaxone. Since nearly all parenteral and some oral antibiotic regimens achieve excellent synovial fluid antibiotic levels, there is no role for the administration of intra-articular antibiotic. Antimicrobial treatment of M. tuberculosis septic arthritis usually requires a four drug regimen due to the occurrence of isoniazid resistance.

Joint drainage is an integral part of the management of septic arthritis as infected joints are analogous to closed space abscesses. Drainage of peripheral joints is most easily accomplished by bedside arthrocentesis. This is particularly suited to critical care management where transport of a patient to an imaging unit may be difficult. Daily aspiration may be required to ensure the removal of recurrent septic effusion. Synovial fluid should be re-cultured to assess the efficacy of antibiotic therapy. Serial WBC counts may be useful in documenting improvement in inflammation. Alternates to needle arthrocentesis include open arthrotomy or arthroscopic drainage. While data supporting the efficacy of needle arthrocentesis for drainage is well established in the literature, small studies suggest that arthroscopic drainage is also effective. Aspiration of a para-spinal abscess requires axial imaging and thus access to CT or MRI.

References

1. Goldenberg DL, Reed JI (1985) Bacterial arthritis. N Engl J Med 312:764–771
2. De La Torre IG, Nava-Zavala A (2009) Gonococcal and nongono-coccal arthritis. Rheum Dis Clin N Am 35:63–73
3. Weston CC, Jones AC, Bradbury N et al (1999) Clinical features and outcome of septic arthritis in a single UK Health District 1982–1991. Ann Rheum Dis 58:214–219
4. Atkins BL, Bowler IC (1998) The diagnosis of large joint sepsis. J Hosp Infect 40:263–274
5. Barton LL, Dunkle MM, Habib FH (1987) Septic arthritis in child-hood; a 13-year review. Am J Dis Child 141:898–900

Artificial Kidney

▶ Renal Replacement

Artificial Nutrition

▶ Enteral Nutrition

Ascending Mediastinitis

▶ Mediastinal Infections

Ascending Part of the DO$_2$/VO$_2$ Relationship

▶ Oxygen Supply Dependency

Aseptic Meningitis

▶ Meningitis

Aspergillosis (Invasive)

WOUTER MEERSSEMAN
Department of General Internal Medicine, University Hospital, Leuven, Belgium

Introduction

Apart from pneumonia caused by endemic mycoses, *Pneumocystis jiroveci* and *Cryptococcus* species, fungal pneumonia is almost always caused by filamentous fungi. Over the past two decades, the range of people at risk of pulmonary mold infections has been expanding with the wider use of immunosuppressive agents in the treatment of cancer and autoimmune disorders, the grow-ing number of patients undergoing transplantation, and the aging of the population. Many of these at-risk patients are hospitalized in hematology wards and transplantation units. Invasive aspergillosis (IA), by far the most common mold infection involving the respiratory tract, may affect up to 10% of patients with acute leukemia, up to 30% of solid organ transplant recipients, and up to 15% of allogeneic hematopoietic stem cell transplant patients. Fortunately, in these specific patient groups, a significant decrease of the fungal infection-related mortality has been observed over the last decade.

However, parallel with improvements in medical care, the spectrum of patients at risk for respiratory fungal infections is also expanding. Recent studies have focused on these nonclassic risk groups; these include "apparently immunocompetent" hosts whose mild-to-moderate immune deficits may be transiently worsening to a net state of immunosuppression severe enough to cause life-threatening fungal infections. Nowadays, many of these latter patients reside in intensive care facilities and units of respiratory medicine, including patients with chronic obstructive lung disease, recipients of low doses of corti-costeroids, and patients with cirrhosis, iron overload, and diabetes. Besides classic risk factors as neutropenia and (prolonged) use of immunosuppressive drugs, the impor-tance of additional transient attacks to the immune system such as poorly controlled glycemia, sepsis-associated immunoparalysis, malnutrition, and moderate to severe renal or hepatic impairment is now well recognized.

Epidemiology of Invasive Aspergillosis in the ICU

In a medical ICU, a high incidence of IA was observed in two separate, retrospective, autopsy-controlled studies. In the larger study, 127 (6.9%) of 1,850 hospitalized patients had microbiologic or histopathologic evidence of aspergillosis during their ICU stay, including 89 cases (70%) in which there was not an underlying hematological malignancy. The observed mortality rate of 80% was much higher than the mortality rate predicted on the basis of the Simplified Acute Physiology Score II (48%) [1]. An earlier study sought unsuspected causes of death in the same medical ICU and revealed that, among 100 autopsies, there were 15 cases of IA, of which 5 were missed before death [2]. These data are in line with previous autopsy findings, suggesting that invasive fungal infections are among the most commonly missed diagnoses in ICU patients. During a 6-year period, Cornillet et al. [3] found that a mean number of 15 patients per year received a diagnosis of IA; approximately one-half of these patients were in the ICU. Intercenter differences can be explained by differences in underlying patient characteristics, case mixes, and autopsy policies.

Pathogenesis of Invasive Aspergillosis

Over the past two decades, IA has emerged as a life-threatening fungal infection in patients with hematological diseases. Although many infected patients will eventually be admitted to the ICU for advanced supportive care, it seems that IA has also gained a foothold in less severely immunocompromised ICU patients. So, can a threshold of immunosuppression needed for the development of IA be defined?

Various factors, including the prolonged use of antibiotics and the use of central venous catheters and/or mechanical ventilation, adversely affect the defense systems of previously healthy individuals. Although these factors are present in most ICU patients, many of these patients do not develop IA. One of the intriguing hypotheses for immunosuppression in the apparently immunocompetent patient with multiple-organ dysfunction relates to the biphasic response to sepsis. The initial hyperinflammatory phase is followed by relative immunoparalysis. This latter process is characterized by neutrophil deactivation, and it may put the patient at risk of developing opportunistic infections, such as IA. Additional epidemiological studies are warranted to better delineate this phase of immunoparalysis.

Patients in the ICU (medical and surgical) are often treated with steroids. However, in vitro pharmacological concentrations of hydrocortisone accelerate the growth of *Aspergillus* species. Clearly, high steroid intake diminishes both lines of cellular defense against IA (i.e., macrophages and neutrophils). This has been demonstrated in hematopoietic stem cell transplant recipients who received prolonged courses of steroids for the treatment of graft-versus-host disease. Palmer et al. [4] reported that the threshold steroid concentration varies according to the type of patient, and they emphasized that underlying lung disease is a risk factor for IA even when low doses of steroids are administered. Cases of IA have even been reported in association with inhaled steroids. Additional studies are needed to investigate whether administration of the 7-day course of hydrocortisone (200 mg/day) to patients with septic shock puts them at risk of developing IA, knowing that recognition of fungal infection may be delayed, because the anti-inflammatory properties of steroids blunt the signs of infection.

Two at-risk groups not included in the EORTC/MSG definitions stand out with regard to IA: patients with chronic obstructive pulmonary disease (COPD) and patients with cirrhosis. Patients with COPD have an increasingly recognized risk of developing IA, and in some institutions, cases of IA among patients with COPD treated with steroids outnumber those cases in "classic" patients.

Hepatic failure is generally not recognized as a risk factor for IA. A literature review revealed that 5 of 14 previously reported cases of IA in seemingly immunocompetent hosts were associated with liver disease. Patients with cirrhosis experience depressed phagocytosis, which may increase their risk for severe infections.

It is expected that new risk categories of IA will arise as new immunosuppressive agents, such as alemtuzumab and etanercept (a TNF-α blocker), are used widely.

There are numerous sources of *Aspergillus* species for patients in the ICU. Some studies suggest that fungal colonization of the lungs is present before entry into the hospital. It is believed that the primary ecological niche is decomposing material. However, aerosolized spores may become a potential source of infection through improperly cleaned ventilation systems, water systems, or even computer consoles. The use of high-efficiency particulate air filtration reduces the risk of IA but does not reduce it to zero, probably in part because patients may be colonized before admission to the ICU, and partly because of breaks in airflow. In addition to the airborne route, contaminated water has been implicated as a source of infection. Of note, the development of IA depends on an interplay between the inoculating dose, the ability of the host to resist infection, and the virulence of the organism.

Disease Manifestations in the ICU

There are several manifestations of IA disease in the ICU. There are three types of pulmonary pathogen–host interactions. The most frequent interaction is colonization of the airways; this can be present in patients with defective mucociliary clearance and structural changes in the bronchial wall. These changes are present in almost every patient who is undergoing mechanical ventilation, making them particularly susceptible to colonization. IA will not develop in these patients unless a critical level of immunodeficiency has been reached. The second type of interaction is "allergic" in nature and is beyond the scope of this review. The most relevant form of interaction for ICU physicians is the invasive disease that develops in persons with impaired immunity. The lungs and sinuses are implicated in >90% of these cases. The aggressive angioinvasive form of IA is frequently encountered in neutropenic patients, whereas cavitating infiltrates are observed most frequently in patients who are receiving steroids, patients with COPD, patients with cirrhosis, solid-organ transplant recipients, etc. In lung transplant recipients, anastomotic infections are the most frequently occurring presentations. Other, rarer presentations include endocarditis, wound infection, mediastinitis (after cardiac surgery), infection of vascular grafts, and osteomyelitis; these are occasionally a problem in immunocompromised patients or during epidemic outbreaks. Infection of the CNS is frequently an ominous sign and may arise from hematogenous seeding (for which the lung is the most common primary site), from spread of the pathogen from the sinuses, or after neurosurgery.

The pathogenesis of IA in patients with steroid-associated immunosuppression differs greatly from that in neutropenic patients. Data demonstrate that pathologic lesions are often widespread, and that death is related to a high fungal burden in neutropenic animals, whereas the pathogenesis in nonneutropenic, steroid-treated animals is driven by an adverse inflammatory host response that is frequently confined to the lungs, with a low fungal burden in the lung parenchyma and other organs.

Clinical signs are usually nonspecific and do not necessarily differ from those for other causes of nosocomial pneumonia. Fever, increasing sputum production, and evolving pulmonary infiltrates despite antibiotics are frequently present but nonspecific. In addition, critically ill patients with prolonged stays in the ICU often develop pulmonary infiltrates, atelectasis, and/or acute respiratory distress syndrome (ARDS), whereas patients with prior lung disease (e.g., COPD) may present with preexisting cavities noted by conventional chest radiography. These features may obscure the classical halo sign or air crescent sign that is present in hematological patients suffering from invasive aspergillosis.

Diagnosis of IA in the ICU

Making a timely diagnosis of IA in the ICU population is probably even more challenging than establishing an early diagnosis in patients with hematologic disease. Basically, this is because the index of suspicion is lower in the ICU population because most patients do not belong to one of the well-established risk groups. Moreover, the diagnostic tools were developed in hematology patients. In general, a diagnosis is made on the basis of a combination of compatible clinical findings, abnormal radiologic findings, and microbiologic confirmation or on the basis of histologic proof of tissue invasion by the fungus.

Over the past few years, lung CT has become one of the most important diagnostic tools. Diagnostic signs of angioinvasive pulmonary mycosis – not only those due to Aspergillus species, but occasionally those due to Mucorales species – include single or multiple small nodules with the halo sign. It should be recognized that the utility of this sign has been evaluated almost exclusively in neutropenic patients. In other groups, including ICU patients, similar CT findings are frequently absent, and if the signs are present, they are far less specific. Many ICU patients have nonspecific interfering radiologic abnormalities associated with atelectasis or ARDS.

A positive result of a culture of a respiratory specimen or positive findings of a direct microscopic examination is present in only one-half of patients with IA. The predictive value of a positive culture result depends largely on whether the patient is immunocompromised and ranges from 20% to 80%. Given the ubiquitous nature of Aspergillus spores, differentiation of colonization from infection remains problematic. Two studies have examined the significance of isolation of Aspergillus species in ICU patients and have confirmed the poor positive predictive values. However, although culture and microscopic examination of respiratory tract samples are performed on a regular basis in most ICUs (once or twice weekly, as a means of surveillance), it is not an appropriate guide for clinical practice.

Serologic testing techniques based on the detection of circulating fungal cell wall components, such as galactomannan (GM) or β-D-glucan, and detection of circulating fungal DNA by PCR techniques hold promise for patients with hematologic malignancy, but they have not been systematically studied for the diagnosis of IA in the ICU. GM and β-D-glucan are polysaccharide fungal cell wall components that are released during tissue invasion and that can be detected in specimens of body fluids (e.g., serum and bronchoalveolar lavage fluid) obtained from patients with IA. Studies of neutropenic patients have revealed high rates of sensitivity (67–100%) and specificity (86–99%). However, in a retrospective observational study of a medical ICU population, serum GM was elevated in only 53% of patients with IA. Detection of serum GM is probably not a sensitive marker for IA (especially in nonneutropenic patients), as demonstrated in lung and liver transplant recipients. Viable fungi can endure in the lung tissue (with encapsulation by an inflammatory process), whereas circulating markers can remain undetectable because of clearance by circulating neutrophils. Bronchoalveolar lavage fluid could be a better specimen for GM detection as has been demonstrated in a medical ICU setting [5]. The use of β-D-glucan detection in the ICU is hampered by false-positive results (associated with the use of albumin, wound gauze, hemodialysis, and bacterial infections). GM detection yields fewer false-positive results, although the use of β-lactam antibiotics, such as piperacillin-tazobactam, may also pose a problem. Thus far, no prospective data on PCR detection are available for ICU patients.

Critical-care physicians need a helpful instrument to guide clinical practice. A combination of host status (number of organ failures, length of stay, intake of immunosuppressive drugs, etc.) and diagnostic markers (e.g., galactomannan level in bronchoalveolar lavage fluid, clinical signs, and chest X-ray) should be used for decision making regarding start of antifungal drugs.

Treatment of IA in the ICU

Amphotericin B has been the mainstay of the treatment of IA for a long time. However, this formulation is renowned for being associated with serious adverse effects (e.g., nephrotoxicity, hypokalemia, and fever). These events often result in the use of suboptimal dosing regimens. Fortunately, over the past few years, lipid-based formulations of amphotericin B and new antifungal drugs with more favorable tolerability and safety profiles (including voriconazole, posaconazole, and the echinocandins) have become available as alternatives.

Recently, voriconazole, a derivative of fluconazole, has become the new standard of care for treating IA. A significantly better outcome (response rate, 52.8% vs. 30.6%) was demonstrated in a randomized study that compared initial treatment with voriconazole versus conventional amphotericin B [6]. Posaconazole is a new, oral, broad-spectrum triazole that is effective against several fungi that are resistant to most other antifungals; it is well tolerated and holds promise as a prophylactic agent in neutropenic patients. It can be used as an alternative agent in salvage therapy. Caspofungin, micafungin, and anidulafungin belong to a new class of antifungal drugs, the echinocandins, which act by inhibiting the synthesis of β-(1,3)-D-glucan in the fungal cell wall. Echinocandins display activities against Aspergillus species, as demonstrated in several studies of salvage therapy, but convincing data on its use as first-line treatment are still lacking. (The latter criticism also applies to first-line treatment with lipid-based formulations of amphotericin B.)

However, most patients who were recruited in these first- and second-line treatment studies were experiencing an underlying hematological disorder or were transplant recipients. These studies usually exclude patients with baseline characteristics that are commonly seen in ICU patients, including patients with liver function abnormalities, coagulation disorders, or renal dysfunction, and patients in need of advanced cardiovascular or pulmonary support, including mechanical ventilation. Nonneutropenic ICU patients and patients who are not transplant recipients largely tend to be underrepresented in all major trials; and given the impact of these comorbidities, lower response rates can be anticipated.

In addition, many aspects of antifungal therapy that are relevant to the ICU population have not been sufficiently addressed in clinical studies, including the pharmacokinetic profile of antifungals in patients with underlying renal, hepatic, and/or cardiac dysfunction; the dose–response relationship; the best route of administration (oral, enteral, or parenteral); the monitoring of drug-related toxicities (e.g., how to monitor voriconazole-induced visual disturbances in sedated patients); and, especially, drug interactions with frequently used "ICU drugs." The echinocandins have not been studied as first-line therapy but offer the advantage of being free of nephrotoxicity; dose adjustments are not required in the event of renal failure or in patients who are undergoing continuous hemofiltration. In addition, few clinically significant drug–drug interactions have been reported.

Prognosis

In an era of increased availability of new immunosuppressive drugs and better intensive care, with prolonged patient survival, we can expect a continuing increase in the incidence of IA. The occurrence of IA in the ICU usually entails a poor prognosis despite major recent improvements in the diagnosis and treatment of IA in patients with hematologic diseases. Mortality rate is above 80% for mechanically ventilated patients with proven aspergillosis. Multicenter studies are warranted, to explore the exact incidence of IA in the ICU, and to better delineate the difference between hospital-acquired, ICU-acquired, and community-acquired aspergillosis.

Evaluating the value of galactomannan, β-D-glucan, and PCR in nonneutropenic, critically ill patients with different sample types (and, especially, with respiratory samples) are needed, as is a better delineation of the patient population at risk for IA in the broad group of critically ill patients. Finally, antifungal pharmacokinetics, pharmacodynamics, and interactions with other drugs need to be explored more thoroughly. These elements can eventually result in a better prognosis.

References

1. Meersseman W, Vandecasteele SJ, Wilmer A, Verbeken E, Peetermans WE, Van Wijngaerden E (2004) Invasive aspergillosis in critically ill patients without malignancy. Am J Respir Crit Care Med 170:621–625
2. Roosen J, Frans E, Wilmer A, Knockaert D, Bobbaers H (2000) Comparison of premortem clinical diagnoses in critically ill patients and subsequent autopsy findings. Mayo Clin Proc 75:562–567
3. Cornillet A, Camus C, Nimubona S et al (2006) Comparison of epidemiological, clinical and biological features of invasive aspergillosis in neutropenic and nonneutropenic patients: a 6-year survey. Clin Infect Dis 43:577–584
4. Palmer LB, Greenberg HE, Schiff MJ (1991) Corticosteroid treatment as a risk factor for invasive aspergillosis in patients with lung disease. Thorax 46:15–20
5. Meersseman W, Lagrou K, Maertens J et al (2008) Galactomannan in broncho-alveolar lavage fluid: a tool for diagnosing invasive aspergillosis in intensive care unit patients. Am J Respir Crit Care Med 177:27–34
6. Herbrecht R, Denning DW, Patterson TF et al (2002) Voriconazole versus amphotericin B for primary therapy of invasive aspergillosis. N Engl J Med 347:408–415

Aspiration Pneumonia

Is defined as the misdirection of oropharyngeal or gastric contents into the larynx and lower respiratory tract.

▶ Burns, Pneumonia

Aspirin Overdose

▶ Salicylate Overdose

Asplenia Infection

▶ Overwhelming Postsplenectomy Sepsis

Assessment of Preload Responsiveness or Fluid Responsiveness

▶ Functional Hemodynamics

Asthma Attack

▶ Acute Asthma

Asthma Exacerbation

▶ Acute Asthma

ATA

The combination (or the sum) of the atmospheric pressure and the hydrostatic pressure is called atmospheres absolute (ATA). In other words, the ATA or atmospheres absolute is the total weight of the water and air above us.

Atherosclerotic Aneurysm

▶ Vascular, True Aneurysms

Atlantoaxial Dislocation

DANIEL K. RESNICK, BASHEAL M. AGRAWAL
Department of Neurological Surgery, University of Wisconsin, Madison, WI, USA

Synonyms
Atlantoaxial subluxation

Definition
Atlantoaxial dislocation (AAD) is characterized by a loss of bony or ligamentous stability between the first cervical

vertebra (C1), the atlas, and the second cervical vertebra (C2), the axis. Varying degrees of myelopathy can occur given the severity of vertebral translation; however, death is rare with appropriate treatment.

Anatomy

Stability of the atlantoaxial joint is greatly dependent on the ligamentous integrity at this level. The odontoid process is approximated to the anterior arch of C1 by the transverse ligament. The transverse ligament is the primary restraint against anteroposterior translation of the dens relative to the arch of C1. Additional ligamentous support is provided by the alar ligaments, which course from the posterolateral surface of the dens to the occipital condyles, the apical ligament extending from the tip of the dens to the foramen magnum, and the tectorial membrane (an extension of the posterior longitudinal ligament) [1].

Mechanism

Atlantoaxial dislocation is caused by excessive motion around the C1-2 articulation. Symptomatic AAD occurs when the spinal cord is compressed either ventrally by the odontoid process or posteriorly by the arch of C1.

Imaging

AAD can be diagnosed using plain radiographs of the cervical spine. Three view x-rays (anteroposterior, lateral, and open-mouth odontoid) are utilized. Special attention is given to the atlanto-dens interval (ADI). An ADI of greater than 3 mm in adults or greater than 5 mm in children is indicative of AAD. The integrity of the transverse ligament is evaluated by calculating the spread of the lateral masses of C1 on C2. The cumulative distance should be less than 7 mm with an intact transverse ligament. Additional indications of instability include displacement of greater than 3.5 mm in flexion–extension films and prevertebral soft tissue swelling. Computed tomography can provide additional definition of bony abnormalities, and magnetic resonance imaging can further demonstrate ligamentous injury.

Treatment

Atlantoaxial dislocation requires evaluation and treatment by a spine specialist. Consultation with a neurosurgeon or orthopedic spine surgeon is advised. Treatment may consist of immobilization, traction, surgical fixation, or some combination thereof [2].

Differential Diagnosis

Trauma
Rheumatoid arthritis
Connective tissue disorders
Ankylosing spondylitis
Neurofibromatosis
Os odontoideum
Osteogenesis imperfecta
Mucopolysaccharidosis

Cross-reference to Disease

Trauma

Cervical trauma can result in disruption of either the bony or ligamentous structures of the C1-2 joint. In adults, approximately 10% of cervical fractures involve the atlantoaxial joint with 15% of these resulting in neurologic manifestation. This low number is attributable to the wide canal diameter at this level. In children younger than 8 years, the incidence of AAD is higher because of increased ligamentous laxity, the horizontal orientation of facets, less mature bone, and forces associated with larger head/body ratio [3].

Classic injuries resulting in traumatic AAD occur in motor vehicle accidents when a patient's head strikes a windshield or steering wheel. Biomechanically, three general patterns of AAD include flexion-extension, distraction, and rotation.

Atlantoaxial rotation is produced by hyperrotation or lateral bending and can vary from subluxation to dislocation. It often manifests with unilateral locked facets. A four-part classification scheme (Fielding and Hawkins Classification) has been devised to evaluate rotatory displacement [4]. Injuries involving greater than 5 mm of anterior displacement or posterior displacement of C1 on C2 are considered highly unstable injuries.

Rheumatoid Arthritis

Greater than two million individuals in the USA suffer from rheumatoid arthritis (RA). Twelve to fifteen percent of patients will have atlantoaxial instability. AAD occurs because of loss of tensile strength of the transverse ligament. Increased ligamentous laxity coupled with erosive bony changes common to RA lead to translation. Moreover, rheumatoid pannus formation further destabilizes the joint. In addition to myelopathy, basilar invagination may lead to brainstem findings [5].

Grisel's Syndrome

Grisel's syndrome is a spontaneous atlantoaxial subluxation following a pharyngeal infection. While the vast majority of patients are children, similar mechanisms exist in adults. The presumed pathophysiology involves a local inflammatory reaction in the cervical spine derived from shared pharyngeal and prevertebral venous plexuses.

Grisel's syndrome is treated with appropriate antibiotics and external immobilization versus traction and immobilization [3].

Down Syndrome

Down syndrome is characterized with systemic ligamentous laxity. Between 15% and 25% of patients with Down syndrome have some evidence of atlantoaxial instability. Treatment is usually reserved for patients with symptomatic subluxation. Consultation with a spine specialist is commonly performed when such instability is discovered as part of a screening for athletic competition. Operative intervention is uncommonly required in asymptomatic children.

Mucopolysaccharidoses

Mucopolysaccharidoses cause metabolic abnormalities in complex carbohydrate metabolism. Generalized ligamentous laxity contributes to the atlantoaxial subluxation described in a variety of mucopolysaccharidoses.

References

1. Van Gilder J, Menezes A (2006) Craniovertebral abnormalities and their neurosurgical management. In: Schmidek HH, Sweet WH (eds) Operative neurosurgical techniques: indications, methods, and results, 5th edn. Elsevier, Philadelphia, PA
2. Claybrooks R, Kayanja M, Milks R, Benzel E (2007) Atlantoaxial fusion: a biomechanical analysis of two C1–C2 fusion techniques. Spine J 7(6):682–688
3. Rahimi S, Stevens A, Yeh D, Flannery A, Choudhri H, Lee M (2003) Treatment of altlantoaxial instability in pediatric patients. Neurosurg Focus 15(6):1–4
4. Fielding JW, Hawkins RJ (1977) Atlanto-axial rotatory fixation. (Fixed rotatory subluxation of the atlanto-axial joint). J Bone Joint Surg Am 59(1):37–44
5. Boden SD, Dodge LD, Bohlman HH, Rechtine GR (1993) Rheumatoid arthritis of the cervical spine. A long-term analysis with predictors of paralysis and recovery. J Bone Joint Surg Am 75(9):1282–1297

Atlantoaxial Subluxation

▶ Atlantoaxial Dislocation

Atlantooccipital Dislocation

▶ Occipitocervical Dissociation

Atlantooccipital Dissociation

▶ Occipitocervical Dissociation

Atrial Fibrillation

Griet van Thielen, Susanna Price
Department of Intensive Care, Royal Brompton Hospital, London, UK

Synonyms

Auricular fibrillation

Definition

Atrial fibrillation (AF) is a supraventricular tachyarrhythmia characterized by chaotic atrial activity, and is the commonest documented arrhythmia on the intensive care unit (ICU). AF can be paroxysmal (self-terminating), recurrent (≥ 2 episodes), or persistent (potentially requiring cardioversion to terminate) [7]. Postoperative AF is a secondary arrhythmia where treatment of the underlying precipitant in parallel with the episode of AF is usually sufficient to terminate the arrhythmia without recurrence.

Epidemiology

AF occurs in up to 15% of patients in the general ICU population, however, the literature regarding AF-related mortality in this patient population is controversial [7]. In the postoperative ICU setting, the incidence of AF is 6.7%. AF is the most common arrhythmia complicating cardiothoracic surgery, with prevalence between 20% and 40% following cardiac surgery [5, 6]. In surgical patients, most arrhythmias occur within 5 days, with a peak incidence on the second postoperative day [5, 6]. AF increases the risk of stroke, hemodynamic instability, and mortality. In addition, it can precipitate ICU admission, prolong ICU and hospital length of stay (LOS) significantly, and thus increase hospital costs [5].

Characteristics

The onset of any tachyarrhythmia requires both an initiating trigger and an underlying substrate. Automatic focal triggers (atrial tachycardia or atrial premature beats) and propagation of multiple reentry wavelets throughout the atria are both mechanisms contributing to AF. In the critically ill, altered automaticity and conductivity are frequently encountered. Factors that contribute to this altered state include high catecholaminergic state, atrial stretch, transcellular fluid and electrolyte shifts, metabolic changes, acute atrial enlargement, ischemia, infarction, and hypertension. In postcardiac surgical patients additional factors include trauma from cannulation, pulmonary vein venting, pericarditis, hypothermia, cardioplegia, and an increased inflammatory response due to cardiopulmonary bypass and cross-clamping [5]. In contrast to AF occurring outside the postoperative period, the initiating triggers are often reversible in this patient population, with sinus rhythm restored in 90% of patients within 6–8 weeks postoperatively [5–8].

Risk Factors for AF in the ICU

Several clinical risk factors for the development of AF have been identified. These include age, history of AF, chronic obstructive pulmonary disease, atrial enlargement, hypovolemia, left ventricular dysfunction, congestive heart disease, valvular heart disease, withdrawal of either beta-blocker or angiotensin-converting enzyme (ACE) inhibitor, obesity, and P-wave duration. In patients undergoing noncardiac surgery, an elevated right atrial pressure (RAP), and presence of a pro-inflammatory state has been shown to correlate with the onset of AF. Among these risk factors, age is probably the most important; age-related atrial fibrosis and increasing age-related atrial refractoriness support the onset of AF. With an increasingly aging population, this constitutes a current and increasing clinical burden in the future [5, 6].

Evaluation and Assessment

The onset of AF is marked by an abrupt change in ventricular rhythm with loss of the normal P-wave morphology, and often an abrupt change in ventricular rate. The atrial rate is usually above 350 beats per minute with irregular fibrillatory waves on the surface electrocardiogram (ECG). By contrast, in atrial flutter the atrial rate is between 240 and 320 beats per minute with a sawtooth pattern (). The diagnosis of an atrial arrhythmia is confirmed by telemetry, 12-lead ECG, or definitively with an atrial electrocardiogram (AEG). Here, the atrial pacing wires, placed during surgery (or a standard endocardial pacing wire positioned in the esophagus), can be connected to a 12-lead ECG and hence amplify the atrial activity seen on the surface ECG. Alternatively, where a permanent pacemaker with an atrial lead is implanted, interrogation may reveal the underlying arrhythmia. Special attention is needed to diagnose AF during ventricular

pacing because the pacing spikes may mask AF with slow ventricular rate or an accelerated junctional rhythm.

In addition to the diagnosis of arrhythmia, an assessment of potential associated risk factors should be performed to determine potentially reversible precipitants. This is particularly important in the postoperative patient. (see Fig. 1)

Prevention Strategies

The evidence for pharmacological prophylaxis to prevent AF varies according to the patient population. In the medical ICU, there is no evidence that any agent is effective in preventing AF. The situation in postoperative patients is different. Multiple studies have shown a consistent benefit in the prophylactic administration of beta-blockers, including metoprolol, atenolol, carvedilol, timolol, and propanolol. Nevertheless they are rarely used, particularly in patients with impaired ventricular systolic function, due to their side effect profile, although this is changing with more recent treatment algorithms in heart failure [5, 4]. Sotalol, a Class III antiarrhythmic agent with beta-blocker activity, may be more effective, but requires monitoring of the QTc [1]. Amiodarone has been shown to reduce the incidence of postoperative AF, and different dosing regimens have been proposed [5]. The prophylactic use of amiodarone has been shown to reduce stroke, LOS, and the cost of admission, especially in the high-risk patients [8, 1]. Other antiarrhythmics proposed include propafenone 675 mg daily, however, it is not widely used. The preoperative use of digoxin or verapamil does not reliably decrease the incidence of postoperative AF. Finally, despite initial enthusiasm, there is only limited evidence that atrial and particularly biatrial overdrive pacing prevents postoperative AF [5, 8, 1]. Thus, in patients undergoing non-cardiothoracic surgery, current guidelines recommend the prophylactic use of beta-blockers and amiodarone to prevent postoperative AF, although this is rarely undertaken. Current recommendations for the prevention of AF in postcardiac surgical patients are the use of beta-blockers (Class I indication, level of evidence A). Additionally, these guidelines suggest that preoperative administration of amiodarone should be considered for high-risk (Class IIa indication, level of evidence A). There is discrepancy in the guidelines regarding the prophylactic use of Sotalol (level of evidence A NICE guidelines, ACC/AHA/ESC gave only a Class IIb indication) [5, 8] (Table 1).

Patients undergoing cardiac surgery develop a high inflammatory response and antioxidant stress perioperatively. Recent studies have highlighted the use

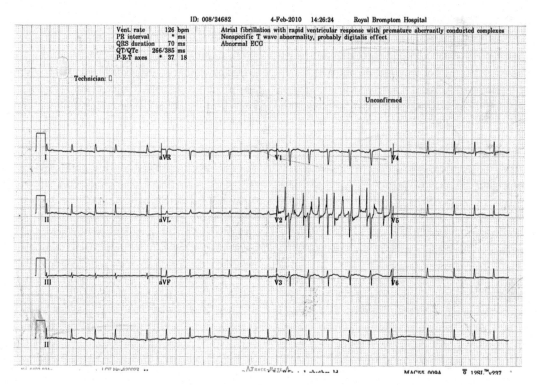

Atrial Fibrillation. Figure 1 Twelve-lead surface electrocardiogram in a patient with atrial fibrillation (AF) postcardiac surgery. Lead V2 is connected to the atrial epicardial pacing wires and the fibrillatory waves are clearly seen

of HMG CoA-reductase inhibitors (statins) and omega-3 fatty acids in primary prevention of AF, possibly due to their pleiotropic (anti-inflammatory) effects. Further studies are needed to further elucidate their role [5, 6].

Treatment

If symptoms of ischemia, hemodynamic instability, or heart failure occur in the context of new AF, an immediate attempt should be made to restore sinus rhythm with direct current cardioversion (DCCV). In the absence of the requirement for urgent cardioversion, rate control can be considered; however, rhythm control is almost always the preferred option [8]. In conjunction with the treatment of the AF, other potential exacerbating causes should generally be corrected. Patients with complex congenital heart disease may initially tolerate AF well, however, the potential for sudden and catastrophic hemodynamic deterioration exists (for more detail, see chapter on ▶ Anti-Arrhythmic Therapy). Here, expert advice should be sought early. This is particularly relevant to those with pulmonary hypertension, a univentricular heart or a systemic right ventricle.

Pharmacological Management

The heightened adrenergic state and other confounding factors, such as electrolyte, fluid and metabolic disturbances, pain, hypoxia, anemia, make it sometimes difficult to cardiovert and/or maintain sinus rhythm, and therefore rate control may have to be accepted. The following AV nodal blocking agents have proven efficacy: beta-blockers, non-dihydropyridine calcium channel antagonists, and amiodarone when hemodynamic stability is particularly of concern. Digoxin can be used, although its effect not reliable in states of high sympathetic drive. The target ventricular rate is generally between 70 and 100 beats per minute with normal cardiac function; however, rates above this may be required where specific cardiac physiology demands [5, 8]. Where pharmacological cardioversion is attempted, procainamide, amiodarone (together with magnesium), and ibutilide have all been used with similar conversion rates. In postcardiac surgery patient, AF is often self-limiting and self-terminates within 24 h. If AF persists for >24 h despite attempts to pharmacologically cardiovert and/or with inadequate rate control, a reconversion strategy should be considered. A number

Atrial Fibrillation. Table 1 Pharmacologic antiarrhythmic drugs

Drug	Class	Dose	Side effects
Amiodarone	III	300 mg loading +	Bradycardia
		900–1,200 mg/24 h iv	Mild negative inotrope
			Nausea
Sotalol	III+Beta-blocker activity	80 mg bid orally	QTc prolongation
		120 mg bid (>70 kg)	Renally excreted
			Hypotension/bradycardia
			Negative inotrope
Ibutilide	III	1 mg/10′ iv (repeat 1 mg)	QTc prolongation
		(0.01 mg/kg if <60 kg)	Hypotension
Procainamide	I A	10 mg/kg/1 h loading +	Negative inotrope
		1–2 mg/min/24 h iv	Renally excreted
			Proarrhythmogenic
			Nausea

of pharmacological agents, with or without repeated attempts to electrically cardiovert (see below), including amiodarone, although the efficacy in acute cardioversion is often modest, ibutilide, procainamide, and sotalol have been shown to be effective [5, 3, 8].

In postoperative AF, recurrence of the arrhythmia is not uncommon due to the ongoing secondary triggers. The decision for starting antiarrhythmic maintenance therapy depends on the tolerance, the risk factors and the number of episodes of AF of each individual patient. Because of its efficacy and safety profile, amiodarone is most commonly used.

Direct Current Management

The most effective way to achieve sinus rhythm is DCCV. Anteroposterior defibrillation pad position provides a better vector for cardioversion of AF. If DC cardioversion does not result in a single beat of sinus rhythm, a second attempt with higher delivered energy should be considered. If, however, sinus rhythm after DC shock is accomplished (even one beat), but early reinitiation of AF occurs, antiarrhythmic drugs should be considered. After loading the antiarrhythmic agent, a further attempt of DC cardioversion can be performed. In patients following cardiac surgery, relatively high-rate atrial pacing (for example rates of 85–100 bpm) anecdotally may reduce the recurrence rate of AF.

Anticoagulation Management

AF increases the risk of stroke/thromboembolic events, hence the need for anticoagulation for patients with AF

lasting longer than 48 h or with recurring episodes. Where sinus rhythm is restored within 48 h, anticoagulation should be considered for patients with underlying structural heart disease (left ventricular dysfunction and valve disease) and with risk factors indicating an increased risk for stroke (previous history of ischemic stroke/TIA, age >75 years with hypertension or diabetes or vascular disease) [8].

When cardioversion is attempted after 48 h of AF, or when the onset is not known, transesophageal echocardiography (TOE) should be performed to exclude an intracardiac thrombus. Studies show that when AF persists for 48 h even with a negative TOE pre-cardioversion to sinus rhythm, stunning of left atrium or left atrial appendix can persist up to 10 days and more with risk of thrombus formation. Therefore, anticoagulation should be continued for a minimum of 3–4 weeks [5]. In all cases, the decision to start oral anticoagulation needs to be balanced with the bleeding risk of each individual patient.

The management of atrial flutter is similar to AF, except that performing atrial overdrive pacing should be the first strategy in attempt to cardiovert the patient.

References

1. Artucio H, Pereira M (1990) Cardiac arrhythmias in critically ill patients: epidemiologic study. Crit Care Med 18:1383–1388
2. Burgess DC, Kilborn MJ, Keech AC (2006) Interventions for prevention of post-operative atrial fibrillation and its complications after cardiac surgery: a meta-analysis. Eur Heart J 27:2846–2857
3. Chung MK (2000) Cardiac surgery: postoperative arrhythmias. Crit Care Med 28:136–144

4. DicksteinK, Cohen-Solal A, Filippatos G et al (2008) ESC 2008 guidelines for the diagnosis and treatment of acute and chronic heart failure. Eur Heart J 29:2388 – 2442
5. Fuster V, Rydén LE, Cannom DS et al (2006) ACC/AHA/ESC 2006 guidelines for the management of patients with atrial fibrillation. Europace 8:651–745
8. NICE guidelines atrial fibrillation http://www.nice.org.uk/nicemedia/pdf/cg036fullguideline.pdf
6. Rho RW (2009) Treatment of atrial fibrillation after cardiac surgery. Heart 95:422–429
7. Sleeswijk M, Van Noord T, Tulleken J et al (2007) Clinical review: treatment of new-onset atrial fibrillation in medical intensive care patients: a clinical framework. Crit Care 11:233. doi:10.1186/cc6136

Atrial Natriuretic Factor (ANF)

▶ ANP

Atrial Natriuretic Hormone (ANH)

▶ ANP

Atrial Natriuretic Peptide (ANP)

▶ ANP
▶ Renal Blood Flow Regulation

Atriopeptin

▶ ANP

ATS

American Thoracic Society.

Atypical HUS

▶ Hemolytic Uremic Syndrome and Thrombotic Thrombocytopenic Purpura

Atypical Pneumonia Syndrome

▶ Severe Acute Respiratory Syndrome, Viral (SARS)

Auriculin

▶ ANP

Auricular Fibrillation

▶ Atrial Fibrillation

Autochthonous

Refers medically to something that originates or forms in the place where it is found.

Autoimmune Disorder of the Neuromuscular Junction

▶ Myasthenia Gravis

B

B2M

▶ Serum and Urinary Low Molecular Weight Proteins

Bacillus anthracis

▶ Biological Terrorism, Anthrax

Bacillus anthracis Infection

▶ Anthrax

Bacteremia, Primary of Unknown Origin

Vikas P. Chaubey, Kevin B. Laupland
Department of Critical Care Medicine, University
of Calgary and Calgary Health Region, Calgary,
AB, Canada

Definition

While many definitions for bacteremia exist, it may be defined by the growth of a microbe from an aseptically obtained blood culture specimen associated with symptomatic infection. Determining if an infection is symptomatic is based on multiple factors, including history of the patient, physical examination, body temperature, peripheral leukocyte count and differential, clinical course, results of cultures from other sites, and percentage of blood cultures positive [1]. The term bacteremia may be considered synonymous with bloodstream infection. An important aspect in defining bacteremia is that contamination of blood culture specimens must be ruled out. Common skin contaminants including diphtheroids, *Bacillus* spp., *Propionibacterium* sp., coagulase-negative staphylococci, and micrococci generally require isolation from two different blood cultures drawn from separate sites to be considered as significant. A positive blood culture is requisite for bacteremia; if the test is not performed the diagnosis cannot be made. In addition, prior administration of systemic antimicrobials may sterilize blood culture specimens and result in the under recognition of bacteremia.

Bacteremia may be classified as being either primary or secondary. In the former, the origin of the bacteremia is either associated with an intravascular catheter or is of unknown origin. In the latter, the bacteremia is associated with infection concurrently diagnosed at another body site, such as with pneumonia, meningitis, or bone and joint infection. Catheter-related bacteremia is a special case of primary bacteremia that occurs in a patient with an intravascular catheter. Such bacteremia is still considered primary even if localized signs of infection are present at the access site. A primary bacteremia that is not catheter-related is also referred to as a bacteremia of unknown origin.

Traditionally, bacteremias that were present or incubating at the time of hospital admission were classified as community-acquired and those that developed as a complication of hospitalization as nosocomial (usually first identified more than 48 h after admission). However, over the recent years, there has been a shift in delivery of healthcare with an increasing number of sicker patients with multiple comorbidities managed in the community setting. When community onset bacteremia occurs in patients that have had extensive healthcare exposure, it tends to be associated with higher rates of antimicrobial resistance and mortality [2]. Bacteremias that occur in either community-based outpatients or that are first identified within 48 h of admission are now generally classified as healthcare-associated if there is a significant history of healthcare exposure as evidenced by recent admissions to hospital, residence in a nursing homes or long-term care facility, hemodialysis, recent intravenous therapy, or specialized medical care in the home. Community-acquired bacteremias are diagnosed when these factors are not present [2].

Jean-Louis Vincent & Jesse B. Hall (eds.), *Encyclopedia of Intensive Care Medicine*, DOI 10.1007/978-3-642-00418-6,
© Springer-Verlag Berlin Heidelberg 2012

Epidemiology

While a number of large observational and surveillance studies have reported on the epidemiology of bacteremia among critically ill patients, most have focused on nosocomial infections and have not separated ICU patients from the general inpatient population. Furthermore, it must be emphasized that considerable differences exist at the national, regional, and local levels with respect to the epidemiology of bacteremia. In most cases, ICU-acquired primary bacteremias are similar to nosocomial primary bacteremias in the hospital population at large, with the exception of an increased risk for antimicrobial resistance. Gram-positive organisms including coagulase-negative staphylococci and *Staphylococcus aureus* are the most common etiologies of ICU-acquired bacteremia. Community onset primary bacteremic disease (including healthcare-associated and community-acquired disease) is less well defined among patients admitted to ICU, but *Escherichia coli, S. aureus,* and *Streptococcus pneumoniae* are predominant pathogens in most studies. While coagulase-negative staphylococci are regularly listed as a major etiology of bacteremia in critically ill patients, these bacteremias are almost exclusively healthcare or nosocomially associated and are invariably related to intravascular catheters or other implanted prosthetic materials.

The diagnosis of bacteremia of unknown origin is made by exclusion of a secondary infected source. Therefore, its identification will depend in part on the degree of effort made to localize a source by clinical, laboratory, and radiological means. As a result, there is considerable variability in reported rates of bacteremia of unknown origin among critically ill patients and ranges from 10% to 50% of all bacteremias.

Risk factors specifically for primary bacteremia in critically ill patients have not been studied extensively. However, even if not recognized as a focal source, intravascular catheters likely represent the main risk factor for development of healthcare-associated, nosocomial, and ICU-acquired bacteremias. Factors associated with development of catheter-related bacteremia include inexperience of the operator, high patient-to-nurse ratios, catheter insertion with less than maximal sterile barriers, placement in the internal jugular or femoral vein rather than subclavian vein, placement in an old site by guidewire exchange, heavy colonization of the insertion site or contamination of a catheter hub, and prolonged duration of use.

It is well documented that ICU-acquired bacteremia increases cost, length of ICU and hospital stay, and mortality. However, few studies have looked specifically at the effect of primary bacteremia on outcomes. Generally speaking, primary bacteremia is associated with a significantly lower mortality rate than with secondary bacteremia. This may in part be due to a lower mortality attributable to catheter-related bacteremias where the infectious source is easily removed. In one case-control study of 111 episodes of bacteremia in 15 French ICUs, the authors found that the excess mortality was 20% in patients with primary bacteremia and was 55% for secondary bacteremia. The excess mortality for those with catheter-related bacteremia was considerably lower at 12% [3].

Diagnosis

At least two cultures of blood should be taken from separate blood draws at different sites in patients suspected of having bacteremia. Increasing the number of culture sets will improve the detection rate for pathogens. While the sensitivity of two sets of blood cultures has been reported to be 80–90%, three and four sets may be required to detect >95% and >99% of bacteremias, respectively. At least one culture should be drawn by peripheral venipuncture. Cultures may be obtained through intravascular devices but should not be taken through multiple ports of the same intravascular catheter. Another advantage of multiple blood culture draws is that it can aid in the assessment of the potential significance of common contaminants. Isolating common contaminants from multiple samples increased the probability that true bacteremia is present [4]. Markers such as procalcitonin may also help distinguish blood culture contaminants from true positive blood cultures. However, the current clinical standard involves integration of all available clinical and microbiological data.

In patients where bacteremia is documented, a thorough evaluation must be undertaken to determine the source of infection as this can considerably influence management. Common secondary sources for bacteremia in critically ill patients include pneumonia, vascular catheters, intra-abdominal and surgical site infections, and to a much lesser degree sinusitis and urinary tract infections. Catheter-associated bacteriuria is not commonly symptomatic and rarely causes bacteremia. A detailed clinical examination should be performed, and basic investigations should include a chest roentgenogram and cultures of suspected body sites (i.e., urine, wounds, cerebrospinal fluid, synovial fluid) as appropriate. Depending on the suspected clinical source and the pathogen, further specific radiologic investigations may be indicated [4].

Endocarditis is an important diagnosis to consider in any patient with bacteremia. While classical clinical signs such as Janeway lesions, Osler nodes, and splinter hemorrhages are important when present, they are insensitive and their absence does not rule out this diagnosis with any certainty. Other clues that may suggest a diagnosis of endocarditis include persistently positive blood cultures (particularly while on adequate therapy), persistent fever after 72 h of appropriate therapy, and long-term intravascular and hemodialysis catheter use. The specific etiology of bacteremia is also important. This is especially so with *Staphylococcus aureus* as approximately 10–20% patients with bacteremia due to this organism may have occult endocarditis, with the rate highest in those with community acquired disease. All patients with *Staphylococcus aureus* bacteremia and those with other organisms and clinical concern should undergo echocardiography. Increased sensitivity of transesophageal echocardiography makes it the diagnostic modality of choice to reliably rule out endocardial complications of *S. aureus* bacteremia [5].

Upon suspicion of catheter-related bacteremia, the catheter should be promptly removed under usual circumstances. A confirmation of line-sepsis can be done by one of several methods including sonication, vortexing, and the semiquantitative "Maki" roll-plate method. Although there is concern about the sensitivity of the Maki-method in detecting endoluminal infection, this method performs well. Each of these methods has a sensitivity of ~90%. The specificity of both sonication and the Maki-method are similar at approximately 80%, while vortexing has a higher specificity of ~90%. However, the simplicity of the Maki-method frequently makes it the procedure of choice in many laboratories. Briefly, the Maki-method involves rolling the catheter tip across a blood agar plate and uses a cut-off of 15 colony forming units (CFUs) to diagnose true infection versus colonization [5].

Controversy exists as to whether all central line tips that are removed should be cultured or only those that are removed after identifying bacteremia. On one hand, culturing all removed lines may lead to over treatment of many patients with uncomplicated line colonization. On the other hand, such an approach may lead to preemptive treatment of bacteremia with a reduction in associated complications. It is prudent to at least culture those central line tips that are suspected of being infected or removed following an associated positive blood culture.

In most critically ill adults, removal of a catheter suspected of being the source of infection is a low-morbidity procedure. However, an approach where a catheter could be classified as infected or not while in situ with removal of only those infected catheters would be preferred. Several methods have been developed in an attempt to define whether a line may be infected prior to

removal and include differential quantitative blood cultures and the differential time to positivity. Differential quantitative blood cultures with a ratio ≥5:1 (comparing colony counts from peripheral blood samples with colony counts of blood samples from catheter hubs) has a sensitivity of 70% and specificity of 95% relative to the Maki-method. Differential time to positivity (comparing time to positivity between cultures of blood samples obtained from peripheral veins and from catheter hubs) has a sensitivity of 95% and a specificity of 90% relative to the Maki-method. It must be recognized that these approaches require maintaining potentially infected catheters in situ while cultures are incubated. While this may be done safely in selected stable patients, suspected infected catheters should be promptly removed in hemodynamically unstable patients or in those where complications are suspected prior to the availability of blood culture results.

Diagnostic imaging procedures frequently play an important role in evaluating potential sources for bacteremia. Roentgenograms of the chest may identify pneumonia. Free air due to a perforated viscus is readily identified by typical views of the abdomen. Plain radiographs may also be useful to identify bone and joint sources. While often a reasonable first investigation, plain radiographs suffer from limited sensitivity, and other modalities may be indicated. Computed tomography has generally good sensitivity and specificity to detect infective foci at most body sites. Ultrasound is readily available at the bedside and is particularly valuable for assessing the liver and biliary tree, and can potentially identify infected large vessel thrombi using Doppler mode. Magnetic resonance imaging has markedly improved resolution as compared to computed tomography and is particularly valuable in defining infections of the head, neck, and spine. A main limitation of these mentioned modalities is that they require the clinician to select the body site to be imaged. In many cases, clinical clues may suggest a potential focus of infection, but in many cases, the site of infection is clinically unapparent.

Nuclear medicine scans have been employed in evaluation of bacteremia of unknown origin, and it may allow a full body assessment. Traditionally, [67]Gallium, [111]Indium, and [99m]Technetium radiotracers have been employed but are limited in their specificity for localizing bacterial infection. Scans using autologous leukocytes labeled with either [111]Indium or [99m]Technitium, while specific for leukocyte infiltration, do not detect infection per se. Several newer nuclear technologies are now being evaluated in the diagnosis of bacterial infections.

18-Fluorodeoxyglucose positron emission tomography (18-FDG PET) scans have been investigated with considerable success in identifying metastatic foci of infection. However, 18-FDG is poorly taken up into the brain, heart, kidneys, and bladder and therefore is complementary to other imaging modalities. In addition, 18-FDG PET may have similar specificity issues as the radiotracers mentioned above. Another new imaging technology using ^{99m}Technitium-ciprofloxacin has also been developed. This tracer has the advantage of being specific to bacterial enzymes. Performance in defining sources of bacteremia as compared to other techniques is limited.

Treatment

The treatment of primary bacteremia depends on a number of factors not limited to patient factors including severity of disease and comorbid illness, microbiological factors including infecting species and in vitro antimicrobial susceptibilities, evidence of metastatic foci of infection, and whether the primary bacteremia is catheter-related or is of unknown origin.

In patients suspected of having primary bacteremia, or among those where preliminary blood culture results indicate a presumptive infection, empiric therapy should be initiated pending confirmation of true bacteremia. Numerous observational studies have emphasized the importance of early administration of effective antimicrobial therapies on the mortality outcome of serious infections including bacteremia. The selection of empiric therapy involves an evaluation of the most likely agent(s) causing disease and expected antimicrobial susceptibilities. While generally one or more agents may be required to cover a broad spectrum of potential bacterial pathogens, it should be recognized that evidence is emerging that *Candida* species are frequent causes of primary bloodstream infection in critically ill patients and that delays in providing adequate antifungal therapy are associated with adverse outcome. Once the etiology of bacteremia has been established, antimicrobial therapy should be revised to provide optimum coverage. Generally speaking, high doses of bactericidal/fungicidal agents are preferred and, with few exceptions, should be administered at least initially through the intravenous route.

Catheter-related bacteremias may be classified as uncomplicated or as complicated being associated with one or more metastatic foci of infection. Complicated catheter-related infections are secondary bacteremias that require treatment directed at both the catheter source and the complicated focus, and are discussed elsewhere in the *Encyclopedia*. Of note, a negative transesophageal echocardiogram is required to define an uncomplicated episode of *S. aureus* bacteremia. The approach to management of primary (uncomplicated) catheter-related bacteremia involves prompt removal of the infected catheter source in addition to providing optimal antimicrobial therapy [5].

The duration of antimicrobial therapy for primary bacteremia has not been well defined in clinical trials and is largely based on anecdotal experience. In uncomplicated primary catheter-related bacteremia, the duration of therapy will depend on clinical response and the infecting organism. A typical therapy duration for a primary "uncomplicated" catheter-related bacteremia is 2 weeks following catheter removal as long as there is good clinical response. However, it is common practice to prescribe either no antimicrobials or only a brief course of therapy in primary catheter-related bacteremias specifically due to coagulase-negative staphylococci after catheter removal in patients who do not have implanted prosthetic material. On the other hand, 4 or more weeks of treatment is considered standard in primary catheter-related bacteremia due to most multidrug resistant organisms, including methicillin-resistant *Staphylococcus aureus* [5]. The treatment duration for primary bacteremia of unknown origin is less well defined, but because a possible deep body site focus has potentially not been recognized, treatment durations are frequently prolonged as a precaution, particularly with Gram-positive and antimicrobial resistant pathogens. Primary bacteremia of unknown origin caused by susceptible Gram-negative organisms can generally be treated for shorter courses (10–14 days).

References

1. Weinstein MP, Reller LB, Murphy JR, Lichtenstein KA (1983) The clinical significance of positive blood cultures: a comprehensive analysis of 500 episodes of bacteremia and fungemia in adults. I. Laboratory and epidemiologic observations. Rev Infect Dis 5:35–53
2. Friedman ND, Kaye KS, Stout JE, McGarry SA, Trivette SL, Briggs JP et al (2002) Health care–associated bloodstream infections in adults: a reason to change the accepted definition of community-acquired infections. Ann Intern Med 137:791–797
3. Renaud B, Brun-Buisson C (2001) Outcomes of primary and catheter-related bacteremia cohort case control study critically ill patients. Am J Respir Crit Care Med 163:1584–1590
4. O'Grady NP, Barie PS, Bartlett JG, Bleck T, Carroll K, Kalil AC et al (2008) Guidelines for evaluation of new fever in critically ill adult patients: 2008 update from the American college of critical care medicine and the infectious diseases society of America. Crit Care Med 36:1330–1349
5. Mermel LA, Allon M, Bouza E, Craven DE, Flynn P, O'Grady NP et al (2009) Clinical practice guidelines for the diagnosis and management of intravascular catheter-related infection: 2009 update by the infectious diseases society of America. Clin Infect Dis 49:1–45

Bacterial Endocarditis

▶ Cardiac and Endovascular Infections

Bacterial Meningitis

▶ Meningitis

Bacterial Pneumonia

▶ Burns, Pneumonia

Bacteriuria

▶ Urinary Tract Infections

Bag-Valve-Mask Ventilation

▶ Airway Management

Bailout Surgery

▶ Damage Control Surgery

BAL

Bronchoalveolar Lavage (BAL).

Bang's Disease

▶ Brucellosis

Barlow's Disease

▶ Mitral Valvular Disease

Barotrauma

▶ Diving Sickness
▶ Pleural Disease and Pneumothorax

Basic Life Support

Christopher B. Colwell, Gina Soriya
Department of Emergency Medicine, Denver Health
Medical Center, Denver, CO, USA

Synonyms
EMT-basic; Field medicine; First responder; Out-of-hospital care

Definition
Basic life support (BLS) is defined as a variety of noninvasive emergency procedures performed to assist in the immediate survival of a patient, including cardiopulmonary resuscitation, hemorrhage control, stabilization of fractures, spinal immobilization, and basic first aid. Some of these procedures can be lifesaving and are often important to implement early. Specifically in the case of cardiopulmonary resuscitation (CPR) and defibrillation with automatic external defibrillators (AEDs), BLS procedures can have a significant impact on survival, and are typically delivered by initial responders (sometimes referred to as first-responders) until more advanced and definitive medical care can be implemented. BLS is typically provided by either ▶ first responders or emergency medical technician (EMT)-basics.

Characteristics
BLS can be provided by first responders or EMTs. EMTs are classified as ▶ EMT-basic (EMT-b), EMT-advanced, or EMT-paramedic (please see ▶ Prehospital Care for a more detailed description of each level of provider).

Cardiopulmonary resuscitation (CPR) integrates ventilations and chest compressions in the setting of a patient who is pulseless and/or apneic. The purpose of performing these maneuvers in sequence is to provide oxygenation and circulation in an attempt to prevent brain injury in patients whose heart has stopped. Recent research has suggested the early access to quality CPR and defibrillation may be the most significant determinants of whether or not someone survives and recovers from cardiac arrest [1].

An automatic external defibrillator (AED) is a portable computerized device that can diagnose a life-threatening arrhythmia, direct the provider if an electric shock is indicated, and deliver that electric shock. It can detect pulseless ventricular tachycardia (VT) and ventricular fibrillation (VF), which then stimulates the machine to indicate to the provider that a shock is advised. The AED is also able to recognize a non-shockable rhythm, such as asystole and pulseless electrical activity (PEA), and will not designate a shock advisory. The AED is designed for use by first responders or laypeople that have ideally been trained in the use of the machine although the use of AEDs by members of the public that have not been previously trained in its use has been increasing. Lack of training on AEDs should never discourage a member of the public from using these machines. Early use of AEDs in the appropriate setting by trained or untrained responders can have a significant impact on mortality [2].

Pre-existing Condition

1. Unconsciousness/apnea/pulselessness
2. Foreign body obstruction/choking
3. Drowning
4. Hypothermia
5. Stabilization of basic injuries

Application

1. Adult BLS/CPR sequence for the unconscious/apneic/pulseless patient:
   - Establish scene safety.
   - Assess victim's level of consciousness: (1) ask "are you okay?" (2) stimulate the patient physically to check responsiveness.
   - Activate local emergency system: instruct a bystander to call 911.
   - Apply an AED if available, and shock if advised.
   - If no suspected spinal injury, open the airway via head-tilt/chin-lift (image). If spinal injury is suspected, open the airway via jaw-thrust (image).
   - Look, listen, and feel for 10 s: (1) Look for foreign body; if any are visible, remove with finger-sweep technique. Blind finger sweep is not

recommended. Look for chest rise. (2) Listen for breath sounds. (3) Feel for breath; feel for chest rise.
   - If the patient is breathing normally, place patient in the lateral recumbent (recovery) position and await transport. Continue to check for breathing.
   - If the patient is not breathing, administer two artificial ventilations using mouth-to-mouth technique, mouth-to-mask technique, or bag-valve-mask. If using mouth-to-mouth technique, close the patient's nostrils between the thumb and forefinger on one hand, covering the mouth with that of the rescuer's, forming a seal. Ensure chest rise with ventilations.
   - If no chest rise occurs, reposition the airway utilizing the appropriate technique and attempt artificial ventilations again. If ventilations continue to be unsuccessful, and the patient is unresponsive, consider an airway foreign body. Begin chest compressions. Check airway after each set of 30 compressions, removing any foreign body found, and reattempting ventilations.
   - If ventilations are successful, check for a carotid pulse. If a pulse is found, continue with appropriate ventilations and await immediate transport. If there is no pulse, begin CPR with 30 compressions followed by two ventilations at 100 compressions per minute for five cycles.
   - After five cycles of CPR have been completed, the cycle should be repeated, starting with reassessing the patient's airway, breathing, and circulation.
   - The BLS sequence should be continued until one of the following conditions has been met: (1) the patient regains a pulse, (2) the initial provider is relieved by another rescuer of equal or higher medical training, (3) the rescuer is physically unable to continue with CPR, or (4) the patient is pronounced dead by a physician.

2. Foreign body obstruction/choking:
   Airway obstruction from a foreign body may present in a variety of ways, ranging from minimal symptoms to respiratory compromise and death. The death rate nears 2,000 annually in the USA, with children aged 1–3 as the primary victims. Mortality rates are up to 3.3% [3].
   - Assess severity of obstruction. If the patient is able to cough effectively, the patient should be encouraged to cough and monitored for deterioration.
   - If the patient is unable to speak or breathe, is cyanotic, or has a silent cough, abdominal thrusts should be administered in rapid progression until the obstruction is relieved. If the patient is

pregnant or obese, chest thrusts should be delivered as an alternative to abdominal thrusts. In infants under 1 year of age, the rescuer should alternate between back blows and chest thrusts.

- If the patient subsequently becomes unresponsive, the patient should be lowered to the ground, EMS activated, and CPR initiated. The airway should be assessed for foreign body and removed if visualized.

3. Drowning:

Death from drowning reaches over 8,000 annually in the USA, almost 25% of those being children.

- Remove the patient from the body of water, maintaining cervical spine immobilization if trauma is suspected.
- Assess airway, breathing, and circulation as outlined under Sect. I. Proceed with CPR. Compression-to-ventilation ratio is 30:2.
- There is no need to clear aspirated water from the airway, as the amount is minimal and does not obstruct the trachea.
- There is no need to perform the Heimlich maneuver or abdominal thrusts in an attempt to clear water from the lungs, as these moves are ineffective and can be dangerous for the patient.
- Patient emesis is not uncommon during resuscitation of the drowning victim. If this occurs, vomitus from the airway should be removed via finger sweep with the patient's head turned laterally. If the patient has a suspected cervical spine injury, the patient should be logrolled to the side, and vomitus swept from the airway.

4. Hypothermia:

For hypothermic patients with a perfusing rhythm:

- Assess airway, breathing, and circulation. The pulse and respiratory rate may be difficult to detect, therefore it may take longer to adequately assess, such as 45–60 s.
- Remove wet garments and prevent any further exposure to the cold environment.
- Apply warm dry blankets, hot packs, or other modality to warm the patient. If available, administer warm, humidified oxygen.

For hypothermia patients with no perfusing rhythm:

- Assess the ABCs, keeping in mind it may take longer to detect a pulse or respiratory rate.
- If no respirations are detected, begin rescue breathing. If there is no detectable pulse, or if there is any doubt that a pulse may be present, begin compressions. Compression-to-ventilation ratio is 30:2.

- If an AED is available, it should be applied. If the machine advises a defibrillation, the shock should be delivered one time, then CPR immediately resumed. The number of defibrillation attempts in the hypothermic cardiac arrest is controversial; however, further defibrillation attempts should be postponed until the patient's core body temperature warms, in order to improve the chance of conversion to a normal rhythm.

5. Stabilization of basic injuries

(a) Bleeding control

- Check airway, breathing, and circulation. Resuscitate as indicated.
- Expose area by removing or cutting clothing.
- Apply direct pressure to the bleeding wound.
- Check for circulation distal to the wound by assessing pulse or capillary refill.
- Elevate the wound if possible.
- Apply a clean dressing and bandage firmly in place.
- Do not remove debris from the wound. If there is a protruding foreign object, such as a knife, leave in place and bandage securely so the object is immobilized.
- For chest wounds, seal open sucking wounds with hand or an air-tight dressing.
- For abdominal wounds, cover with clean bandage. Do not replace protruding intestines into the wound.

(b) Fracture splinting

- Immobilize the joints above and below the fracture site with a splint.
- Check distal circulation, motion, and sensation (CMS) before and after immobilization.
- If the fracture is angulated and there is no noted distal circulation, attempt to straighten the fracture into anatomical alignment and recheck circulation. If there continues to be lack of circulation, splint in alignment and seek immediate help.
- If there is an open wound at the site of the fracture, cover the wound and apply direct pressure for bleeding control. Splint as above and elevate.
- If there is a suspected spinal injury, do not move the patient unless assisted by trained medical personnel.

(c) Burn care

- Extinguish the burn with a large amount of water.

- Check airway, breathing, circulation, and resuscitate as indicated.
- Remove smoldering clothing, as well as jewelry, belts, and shoes.
- Cover with sterile burn dressing if available; otherwise use any clean dry dressing.
- Do not open or drain blisters.

References

1. Eisenberg MS, Psaty BM (2009) Defining and improving survival rates from cardiac arrest in US communities. JAMA 301:860–862
2. Bobrow BT et al (2008) Minimally interrupted cardiac resuscitation by emergency Medical services for out-of-hospital cardiac arrest. JAMA 299:1158–1165
3. Soroudi A et al (2007) Adult foreign airway obstruction in the prehospital setting. Prehosp Emerg Care 11(1):25–29

Basic Life Support (BLS)

▶ Cardiopulmonary Resuscitation

Bed Sore

▶ Pressure Ulcer Evaluation, Prevention and Treatment

Bedside Hemodynamic Monitoring

SHELDEN MAGDER
Critical Care Division, McGill University Health Centre, Royal Victoria Hospital, Montreal, QC, Canada

Synonyms

Hemodynamic monitoring; Pressure monitoring; Vital signs

Definition

Bedside monitoring refers to the systematic recording of physiological data over time. This extends from the technologically very simple and noninvasive collection of vital signs such as heart rate, blood pressure, respiratory rate, temperature, and urine output, to the more technologically demanding noninvasive techniques such pulse oximetry, end-tidal CO_2, and techniques for the assessment of cardiac output, and to invasive intravascular measurements of pressures such as the central venous pressure (CVP), arterial pressure, pulmonary artery pressure, measurements of cardiac output, airway pressures and flows, and cerebrospinal pressure. Measurement of variables over times allows trend analysis so that changes in the patient's underlying condition or changes in response to therapy can be assessed. In this entry, I will concentrate on the hemodynamic components of bedside monitoring. *(I assume that respiratory and neuro monitoring are covered elsewhere).* For the purpose of this discussion, a central assumption is that for an individual patient there is a range of parameters such as heart rate, blood pressure, cardiac output, and markers of metabolic stability (e.g., arterial oxygen, lactate, base excess, central venous oxygen content) that have been identified by the treating team and there is a desire to maintain the patient's values in a given range. When a patient's values are in the desired range, the patient is defined as "hemodynamic stabile."

Pre-existing Condition

Indications

Hemodynamic monitoring has the following roles. (1) It alerts the medical team to deterioration in a patient's hemodynamic status and the requirement for urgent interventions. This includes the development of an inadequate heart rate response or rhythm disturbance, excessively high or low blood pressure or inadequate cardiac output for tissue needs. (2) It can be used to predict potential responses to therapeutic interventions. (3) It allows assessment of the response to therapeutic interventions. (4) The pattern of hemodynamic wave patterns themselves can have diagnostic information for the underlying condition.

In choosing a monitoring tool one must consider potential benefits, costs, and risks. Costs and risks generally are more readily available but the benefits are much harder to define. Although there is no rigorous evidence that supports the utility of any hemodynamic tools including vital signs, it is important to appreciate that a monitoring tool is only as good as the algorithm that makes use of the information. This is well illustrated by studies in which investigators have tried to assess the roles of the pulmonary artery catheters for the management of critically ill patients [1, 2]. No benefit has been observed in these studies, but in reality they have only tested the presence of a catheter and not an algorithm and there is no reason to expect that the catheter itself should have a benefit. Even a stethoscope has no value if the clinician does not know how to interpret the sounds that are heard and to put them into the context of the patient's overall condition.

Perhaps the most significant use of hemodynamic monitoring is that it allows physicians to continuously assess responses to therapeutic interventions and to correlate these responses with the patient's overall condition. The important phrase here is "overall condition." When the predefined targets have been met as assessed by the monitoring tool, the physician can limit further interventions and potentially prevent harm from excess use of the interventions. Physicians deal with individual patients, not populations and hemodynamic monitoring allows the physician to determine the response to a therapy in an individual patient. If the expected response does not occur, it does not make sense to continue the therapy in that patient even if it is recommended as a standard treatment from large population studies.

Conditions in which there is a greater potential for hemodynamic instability to occur and close monitoring is warranted include: (1) patients with known cardiovascular disease who have either developed new cardiac dysfunction or who are under increased risk of hemodynamic or rhythmic instability because of surgery or a new medical condition; (2) patients undergoing high-risk surgical procedures and who are expected to have major fluid losses as well as large fluctuations in blood pressure and cardiac output and in whom the subsequent use of careful volume resuscitation and vasoactive drugs are likely to be required to maintain hemodynamic stability; (3) Patients with recent large blood losses from trauma, gastrointestinal sources, or large surgical losses; (4) patients with severe sepsis or septic shock, (5) patients with major burns and who will have challenging volume management; (6) patients requiring ongoing analysis of their respiratory status. In all these conditions the changing pattern of the measurements are more important than the actual values.

Applications

Techniques

Measurements can be categorized as those related to (1) rhythm and rate, (2) pressure, (3) flow measurements, and (4) metabolic consequences of flow and oxygen delivery.

Rhythm and Rate

Heart rate and rhythm are easily assessed with surface electrodes and the amplified signal of the electrocardiogram. The identification of rapid or bradycardic rhythms is a subject by itself and will not be dealt with here. However, a cautionary note is worthwhile related to the significance of rapid sinus rhythm. A rapid heart rate is always abnormal and should alert the physician to look for causes. However, it does not necessarily indicate that the rate should be slowed pharmacologically and I would suggest that unless the patient manifests evidence of myocardial ischemia or is known to be at high risk of myocardial ischemia, there currently is no evidence that slowing the rate pharmacologically is beneficial. Tachycardia also is not a reliable indicator of a patient's intravascular volume status. Patients with inflammation in the area of the celiac axis (e.g., pancreatitis, post-surgery, or who has abdominal abscesses), can often be tachycardic but volume replete. This likely occurs from activation of sympathetic afferents from local sympathetic ganglia, which increase central sympathetic output. On the other side, a normal heart rate does not rule out hypovolemia.

Pressures

General Principles

Pressures that we measure are primarily due to the elastic force that stretches the walls of vessels and the heart [3]. A key principle is that measured pressures are relative to a reference value. Since we are normally surrounded by atmospheric pressure, we are interested in deviations from atmospheric pressure and atmospheric pressure actually is the reasonable starting value or "zero" for our measurements. A pressure of zero is actually not zero but around 760 mmHg and an arterial systolic pressure of 120 mmHg is really about 880 mmHg. The commonly used units of pressure as millimeters of mercury (mmHg) or centimeters of water (cmH$_2$O) are based on the force produced by the height of a column of fluid and the density of that fluid. The density of mercury is 13.6 times greater than that of water and this value can be used to interconvert the values in cmH$_2$0 and mmHg.

The use of fluid-filled tubes to connect the patient to a transducer introduces an additional gravitational component to the pressure measurement. The difference in height of the column of fluid between the reference level on the patient and the transducer produces an addition pressure of around 8 mmHg for every 10 cm height. Standard and consistent leveling of the transducer to the patient is thus essential for the comparison of values in a particular patient to other patients and for trending measurement over time in the same patient. The generally accepted (although arbitrary) "physiological" reference level is the midpoint of the right atrium for that is where the blood comes back to the heart before it is pumped out again. That level is approximately 5 cm vertical distance below the sternal angle which is where the second rib meets the sternum and is valid when the patient is flat or sitting at up to 60°. Accurate measurement of this level requires a carpenter's leveling device and a marker of 5 cm below the device so that it is more popular to reference transducers to the midpoint of the thorax at the fourth rib. This position, though, should only be used in the supine position for it will vary relative to the midpoint of the right atrium when the upper body is elevated. Referencing at this level gives values of vascular pressures that are approximately 3 mmHg higher than the value obtained by using 5 cm below the sternal angle. The appropriate level on the transducer is the level of the stopcock that is used to open the system to atmospheric pressure for zeroing.

It is the pressure across the wall of elastic structures that determines the stretch of the wall; this is called transmural pressure. The pressure outside the heart is pleural pressure and not atmospheric pressure and pleural pressure changes relative to atmospheric pressure during the ventilator cycle. However, transducers that are used to measure intrathoracic pressure are outside the chest and referenced to atmospheric pressure and it is not possible to easily obtain the pleural pressure to calculate the transmural pressure. To minimize the error produced by of changes in pleural pressure during the ventilatory cycle, pressures are measured at the end of expiration (which is also the point just before inspiration) whether ventilation occurs with negative or positive pressure ventilation. However, this does not account for positive end-expiratory pressure and there is no simple solution for this error. Although expiration is normally passive, critically ill patients often have active expiratory efforts and if these increase during the expiratory phase, they increase the end-expiratory pressure that is measured relative to atmosphere. In these situations, the valid pressure is likely at the beginning of the expiratory phase, before the patient begins to recruit expiratory muscles.

Arterial Pressure

Arterial pressure is the most commonly measured vascular pressure and can be measured invasively with intravascular catheters or noninvasively by the classic auscultation method or by devices that use oscillometry. These latter devices are frequently used for repeated automatic measurements, but it is important to appreciate that the values obtained with these devices need to be validated with occasional auscultatory measured pressures for they can sometimes produce artifactual values of pressure.

In patients in the ICU following surgical procedures upper limits for pressure are often set to reduce the risk of bleeding. Identification of high pressure is also important in patients with hypertensive crisis, aortic dissection, or an unstable aneurysm, but not as important in the short run in most other patients. In the majority of cases, decreased arterial pressure is the primary concern. Despite the frequency of the hypotension and its aggressive treatment, it is amazing how little empiric knowledge there is for acceptable limits of low pressures and whether the important pressure is the systolic, mean, or diastolic pressure. It is important to remember that flow to the tissues, or even more precisely delivery of oxygen and nutrients and clearance of waste is what counts and not pressure. The pressure is used as a surrogate for potential flow. The patient's clinical status provides an important guide. A low pressure in patient who is awake with normal sensorium, who has stable renal function, and no acidosis, is likely of no consequence. However, in many patients some or all of these are abnormal. The pressure may or may not be a contributor and empiric values must be chosen to guide therapy.

There are advantages and disadvantages for the choices of any one of systolic, diastolic, or mean pressure. When the pressure is measured by auscultation, it is generally a low systolic pressure that triggers clinical responses and provides a convenient signal. When arterial catheters and transducers are used to measure pressure, the characteristics of the measuring device can affect the observed systolic pressure and one must be careful to make sure that the waveform of the signal is appropriate and not over- or under-damped. The mean pressure should be related to overall flow to organs with higher flows, but does not give a good guide to regions that receive more of their flow in systole. There are some patients who also have a low diastolic pressure but high systolic pressure and targeting the mean can result in high doses of vasopressor. Finally, diastolic pressure is important for coronary flow, but excess use of vasopressors to raise the diastolic pressure could end up increasing myocardial oxygen demand by increasing systolic pressures and cardiac ionotropy and also decrease coronary flow by constricting the coronary arteries.

Ideal pressures really need to be established empirically, but there are few rigorous studies to provide guidance. Optimal arterial pressures have been studied best for the kidney and it is suggested that a minimal mean pressure of 80 mmHg is required for normal renal function. However, this value is primarily derived from animal studies over short periods of time and without underlying vascular or intrinsic renal disease. Septic patients are an interesting example where monitoring pressure and urine output can allow individualization of pressure targets. Elevation of arterial pressure with vasopressors can restore renal blood flow and function and this individualized pressure thus provides a useful pressure target for the use of vasopressors in these patients.

One must be careful of some potential measurement problems that can occur. Patients with a stenosis proximal to the measuring device will appear to have low arterial pressures, when in fact central pressure is normal. In patients who have a distal arterial catheter and who are receiving high doses of vasopressors, constriction of the vessel can lead to underestimates of the central pressure.

Central Venous Pressure

Central venous pressure (CVP) is a commonly used measure and can even be estimated without a catheter by examining the level of jugular venous distension [4]. A fuller discussion of the use of CVP with changes in cardiac output will be given below for the CVP is only useful in conjunction with an estimate of cardiac output. It is also the change in CVP in relation to other hemodynamic events that is helpful. Importantly, CVP by itself is not an indicator of blood volume.

Pulmonary Arterial and Pulmonary Arterial Occlusion Pressure

Pulmonary artery pressure is an important indicator of the load on the right ventricle. It is also an indicator of pathology in the pulmonary vasculature. The pulmonary artery pressure can be elevated passively because of high left heart pressures, high pulmonary flow and reactive pulmonary vascular changes, obstructive processes, or obliterative processes.

Inflation of a balloon at the end of a pulmonary catheter or advancing a pulmonary catheter until the end-hole occludes the vessel gives the pressure distal to the end-hole which after equilibration is equal to the left atrial pressure. This "wedged" pressure provides diagnostic information about the behavior of the left side of the heart. It also gives an indication of the minimal pressures in the pulmonary capillaries and thus the hydrostatic force that drives pulmonary capillary filtration. On the other hand it does not give an indication of the preload status of the heart as a whole for that is related to the CVP for the left heart can only put out what the right heart gives it. An important use of these catheters is that they provide a simple tool for measuring cardiac output which is discussed below.

Cardiac Output

The cardiac output, liter per minute, is a major component of the ultimate clinical end-point which is the delivery of nutrients to the tissues and removal of waist and thus a very desirable value to measure [5, 6]. Unfortunately, flow is not as easy to measure as pressure. One of the most reliable methods but a cumbersome one is based on the dilution of an indicator that is injected at a proximal site such as a major vessel and detected by a sensor at a downstream site. Indocyannine green was one of earliest indicators, but the development of thermal sensing catheters allowed the use of temperature which is a much simpler indicator to use although it has more potential errors. Small doses of lithium can also be used as an indicator. Placement of the thermistor in the pulmonary artery allows injection of a solution that is cooler than blood into the right atrium and sensing the change in temperature in the pulmonary artery but this requires passing a catheter through the right heart and the risks of arrhythmias and perforation. The alternative is to place the sensor in an artery which generally needs to be bigger than a radial artery so that it also has an invasive component and is not without risks. Two key requirements for the use of an indicator dilution technique are that there must be immediate complete mixing and no loss of "indicator." This can be a problem when the injection is made in the right atrium and the patient has tricuspid insufficiency for some of the indicator (temperature) is potentially lost when the blood goes back and forth and mixing may not be complete because of the regurgitant flow. Pulmonary catheters can also be equipped with a sensor for oxygen saturation and these catheters allow the measurement of cardiac output continuously.

Flow can also be measured with Doppler techniques which detect the velocity of blood by the phase shift of the Doppler wave when it hits the flow pulse and gives a measure of the stroke volume which is then converted to cardiac output by multiplying by the heart rate. The calculation of flow from velocity requires a measure of the cross-sectional area of the vessel for flow is equal to the product of velocity and the cross-sectional area of the vessel. The latter is not always easy to obtain and is often assumed, which is reasonable under basal conditions but not when a patient is in shock. Continuous assessment of flow by Doppler probes can be made with a probe placed in the esophagus but this is really only tolerable in a heavily sedated or unconscious patient. Appropriate positioning of the catheter must also be made.

Devices have also been developed to measure the electrical impedance related to blood volume and the changes during the cardiac cycle give a measure of stroke volume.

This too is multiplied by heart rate to give cardiac output. These devises give reasonable estimates in normal subjects but there are potential problems in critically ill patients who have increased chest wall edema, pleural or pericardial effusions, or hyperinflated chests

A number of techniques have been developed to try to estimate stroke volume from the pulse pressure. This requires knowledge of the elastic properties of the patient's vessels which is hard to predict in individual patients. It will also vary with disease and likely be very sensitive to the volume in the vessel for elastance is curvilinear against the radius of vessels. These techniques can give trends in patients who do not have major pathology but likely will not be useful in patients who are hemodyanmically unstable which is when you really need them.

All techniques that attempt to measure stroke volume and calculate cardiac output by multiplying stroke volume by heart rate will always show at least a moderate relationship to direct measurements of cardiac output for populations but one must be cautious about extrapolating this to individual patients. This is because the heart rate, which provides a very reliable measure, is a large percentage of the product and therefore drives a large part of the correlation. However, it is often the smaller changes in stroke volume that are important for that it identifies changes in cardiac muscle function.

Therapeutic Application

As discussed above, the values of pressures and flow that are adequate for a patient's metabolic need are not well empirically established and need to be customized to the individual patient. However, hemodynamic monitoring that includes a measure of cardiac output can be useful for detecting a decrease from the values that the patient had when deemed stable or becomes "stable" and also to identify the dominant hemodynamic process. Clinical responses are most often triggered by decreases in arterial blood pressure. Arterial pressure is approximately equal to the product of cardiac output and systemic vascular resistance (SVR) (Fig. 1). The two measured values are arterial pressure and cardiac output (or a surrogate) so that SVR is a derived variable. This means that it is changes in cardiac output that are key. If the blood pressure is low and cardiac output is normal or elevated, the primary problem is a decrease in SVR and the differential diagnosis for the problem is specific. If the cardiac output is depressed, then the next question is why is it decreased? The steady-state cardiac output is determined by the interaction of cardiac function (based on the Frank–Starling relationship) and the function that determines venous return. These two

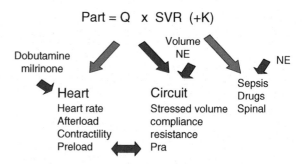

Bedside Hemodynamic Monitoring. Figure 1 Predictions of changes of cardiac output and changes in CVP

functions intersect at the working cardiac output and the working right atrial pressure which is approximately the same as the CVP. A low cardiac output with a high CVP indicates that the cardiac function is the primary limiting factor, whereas a low cardiac output with a low CVP indicates that the return function is the primary limiting factor and the most common cause is inadequate vascular volume. The specific values are not as useful as the change in values. A fall in cardiac output with a rise in CVP indicates a decrease in cardiac function and a fall in cardiac output with a fall in CVP indicates a return problem, which is most commonly insufficient vascular volume (Fig. 2).

If inadequate volume is thought to be the primary problem then the best test is to do a volume challenge [4]. In this procedure, a small bolus is given quickly with the aim of raising CVP. The faster the fluid is given the less fluid that is needed. The hemodynamic variable that one is trying to correct needs to be reassessed as soon as the CVP is increased. A reasonable value for the increase in CVP is 2 mmHg because that is a value that can be detected with certainty on a monitor. It also should produce an obvious increase in cardiac output if the heart is functioning on the ascending part of its function curve. If the cardiac output increases, more volume can be given to try to maintain the desired values, but importantly a positive response only means that the patient is volume responsive but it does not indicate that the patient actually needs volume. That is a clinical decision. If the cardiac output does not increase with a bolus that increased the CVP by 2 mmHg or more, the patient should be considered volume unresponsive and further volume loading will not help and may be harmful no matter what the starting CVP value. This situation indicates limitation of right ventricular output and even if the left heart is deemed to be underfilled based on the pulmonary artery occlusion pressure or by

Implications of changes in cardiac output and CVP

Cardiac Output	CVP	Indicates
Decreased	Decreased	Decreased return (most often volume $\downarrow$)
Decreased	Increased	Decreased Pump function
Increased	Increased	Increased return (likely volume $\uparrow$)
Increased	Decreased	Increased pump function

Bedside Hemodynamic Monitoring. Figure 2 Approach to assessment of cause of hypotension and simplified approach to management. *Part* arterial pressure, *Q* cardiac output, *SVR* systemic vascular resistance, *K* a constant representing the "downstream" value of pressure because the true equation is "upstream minus downstream" *pressure Q x SVR, Pra*right atrial pressure (= CVP), *NE* norepinephrine. Cardiac output is determined by the interaction of the cardiac function and return function; the preload of the cardiac function is the Pra which is also the outflow pressure for the venous return ("circuit")

echocardiography, volume will not solve the problem for the left heart can put out what the right heart gives it. This raises an important limitation of the use of echocardiography for "hemodynamic monitoring" as is sometimes advocated [7]. Besides not being able to provide easy and rapid assessment of serial values, it mainly assesses left heart function, but the output of the left heart is totally dependent upon right heart function which often does not functioning well in critically ill even though left ventricular function is intact. In that situation, the volume status of the left ventricle is no help for fluid management.

There have been many attempts to use the respiratory variations in arterial pressure or pulse with positive pressure ventilation to predict volume responsiveness [8]. These techniques can be effective but are only valid if there are no spontaneous inspiratory or expiratory ventilatory efforts by the patients. The various values given for these variations also are only valid when the patient is ventilated with the same ventilator parameters as in the original study and when the rhythm is regular. Their use is thus limited.

An inspiratory fall in CVP with a spontaneous (negative pressure swing) breath, whether the patient is on a ventilator or not, has also been shown to predict volume responsiveness [4]. The test works best in the negative. Absence of an inspiratory fall in CVP in a patient with an adequate effort indicates that the patient will not have an increase in cardiac output in response to an infusion of volume. When using this technique, one must be careful to make sure that the inspiratory fall in CVP is not in fact the release of a forced expiration that looks like an inspiratory fall and produces an apparent false positive.

Information can also be gathered by examining waveforms. As some examples, a wide arterial pulse pressure is suggestive of a low SVR. Prominent "y" descents in the CVP tracing suggest that the right heart is volume limited

and will not respond to further volume loading. A large C-V wave in the CVP tracing is indicative of tricuspid regurgitation. A prominent "v" in the pulmonary artery occlusion pressure is indicative of mitral regurgitation but is seen when there is excessive filling of the left heart. A loss of a "y" descent in the CVP can be a sign of the development of cardiac tamponade.

Conclusion

The important part of bedside monitoring is not the actual values but the changes in the values as they related to changes in the patient's condition. In a sense, the meaning of a patient's values should be "calibrated" to the clinician's impression of the patient's overall status. This is especially important when trying to gauge the impact of therapeutic interventions. The value of the information obtained by bedside monitoring can only be as good as the skill of the clinicians and nurses receiving them.

References

1. Vincent JL, Pinsky MR, Sprung CL, Levy M, Marini JJ, Payen D, Rhodes A, Takala J (2008) The pulmonary artery catheter: in medio virtus. Crit Care Med 36:3093–3096
2. Hadian M, Pinsky MR (2006) Evidence-based review of the use of the pulmonary artery catheter: impact data and complications. Crit Care 10(Suppl 3):S8
3. Magder S (2007) Invasive intravascular hemodynamic monitoring: technical issues. Crit Care Clin 23:401–414
4. Magder S (2006) Central venous pressure: a useful but not so simple measurement. Crit Care Med 34:2224–2227
5. Magder S (1997) Cardiac output measurement. In: Tobin MJ (ed) Principles and practice of intensive care monitoring. McGraw-Hill, Chicago, pp 797–810
6. de Waal EE, Wappler F, Buhre WF (2009) Cardiac output monitoring. Curr Opin Anaesthiol 22:71–77
7. Vignon P (2005) Hemodynamic assessment of critically ill patients using echocardiography doppler. Curr Opin Crit Care 11:227–234
8. Magder S (2004) Clinical usefulness of respiratory variations in arterial pressure. Am J Resp Crit Care Med 169:151–155

Bedside Ultrasonography

► Ultrasound: Uses in ICU

Bedside Ultrasound

► Shock, Ultrasound Assessment

Being the Active Part of "Fish Oil"

► Omega-3 Fatty Acids

Beta-2-Microglobulin

► Serum and Urinary Low Molecular Weight Proteins

Beta-Blockers

JONATHAN BALL
General Intensive Care Unit, St. George's Hospital &
Medical School, University of London, London, UK

Introduction

Beta-adrenoceptor blocking drugs (β-blockers) have been a mainstay of therapy for hypertension, myocardial ischemia, and, more recently, cardiac failure. The current British National Formulary [1] lists 15 β-blockers while the medical literature contains at least as many agents again, either in development or consigned to history. Unlike most other classes of drugs, the heterogeneity between β-blockers involves marked differences in their pharmacodynamics as well as differences in their pharmacokinetics. Our understanding of adrenergic receptors and the myriad roles the sympathetic nervous system plays, in both health and disease, continues to increase. Coupled with the extensive body of trial data examining, the role of β-blockers in a diverse group of settings has resulted in much ongoing controversy. In critical care, not only do we need a clear understanding of the risks and benefits of acute therapy with β-blockers, but we must also be aware of the consequences of chronic therapy in our patients.

Basic Science

The sympathetic nervous system has two principal transmitters, noradrenaline (norepinephrine) and adrenaline (epinephrine). The receptors for these endogenous agonists have been classified into alpha and beta with more recent identification of a number of subtypes. Beta-adrenoceptors are found in nearly every human organ and tissue. There are three subtypes: β_1, β_2, and β_3. A β_4 subtype was believed to exist but has been proven to be the β_1-receptor in a different conformational state with distinct agonist/antagonist binding [2]. Their tissue location and agonist binding responses are detailed in Table 1. Pathophysiologically and therapeutically cardiac beta-adrenoceptors have been studied in the greatest detail [3, 4]. A review of beta-adrenoceptor physiology, pathophysiology, and polymorphisms can be found here [12]. Despite this body of research many questions remain unanswered.

An important property of beta-adrenoceptors is the autoregulatory process of receptor desensitization. This process operates to prevent overstimulation of receptors in the face of excessive beta-agonist exposure. Desensitization occurs in response to the association of receptor with the agonist molecule, and is prevented by the interaction of the receptor with an antagonist. The mechanisms by which desensitization can occur consist of three main processes: (1) uncoupling of the receptors from adenylate cyclase, (2) internalization of uncoupled receptors, and (3) phosphorylation of internalized receptors. The extent of desensitization depends on the degree and duration of the receptor agonist or antagonist response [13]. From the perspective of β-blockade, the physiological process of desensitization results in an increase in sensitivity in subjects exposed to chronic blockade.

Indications

β-blockers have been used for multiple indications for many decades. Perhaps surprisingly therefore, many gaps remain in our knowledge with regard to the optimal use of currently available agents. Commonly used β-blockers exhibit variable degrees of relative affinity to β_1-, β_2-, and β_3-receptors [14]. The effect of drug receptor binding also produces variable effects with some agents producing universal antagonism, while others produce partial

Beta-Blockers. Table 1 Subtypes of beta-adrenoceptors. Adapted from [3–7]

Receptor	Tissue	Response to agonist
β_1	Heart (β_1:β_2 70:30 atria, 80:20 ventricles)	Increases heart rate (sinoatrial firing), impulse conduction through the atrioventricular node, cardiac contractility ($>\beta_2$), and rate of relaxation Ubiquitous coupling to stimulatory G-proteins Pro-apoptotic
		Chronic stimulation results in endocytosis and reduction in functional density
	Lung (~20%) [8]	Bronchodilatation [9]?
	Juxtaglomerular cells	Increases rennin secretion
	Innate and adaptive immune cells	Pro-inflammatory
	Coagulation system	May increase platelet aggregability; may decrease fibrinolytic activity
	Brain	Poorly characterised [10]
β_2	Heart (β_1:β_2 70:30 atria, 80:20 ventricles)	Increases heart rate (sinoatrial firing), impulse conduction through the atrioventricular node, cardiac contractility ($<\beta_1$), and rate of relaxation Coupled to both stimulatory and inhibitory G-proteins Anti-apoptotic
		Chronic stimulation results in uncoupling from adenylyl cyclase (stimulatory) pathway
	Lung (~180%) [8]	Bronchodilatation and alveolar sodium and water clearance
	Smooth muscle	Relaxation of smooth muscle in vasculature, gastrointestinal tract, and genitourinary tract
	Skeletal muscle	Glycogenolysis; uptake of potassium
	Liver	Glycogenolysis; gluconeogenesis
	Pancreas	Insulin and glucagon secretion
	Thyroid	T_4 to T_3 conversion
	Innate and adaptive immune cells	Downregulate the synthesis of pro-inflammatory cytokines and upregulate synthesis of anti-inflammatory cytokines
	Coagulation system	Reduces platelet aggregability; increases factor VIII and von Willebrand factor concentration; increases fibrinolytic activity
	Brain	Poorly characterized [10]
β_3	Heart	Inactive during normal physiologic conditions but upregulated in cardiac failure Stimulation seems to produce a negative inotropic effect opposite to that induced by β_1- and β_2-receptors [11]
	Smooth muscle	Relaxation of smooth muscle in vasculature, bronchi, gastrointestinal tract, and genitourinary tract
	Brain	Present in discrete regions including hippocampus, hypothalamus, amygdala, and cerebral cortex areas known to be involved in thought processes and possibly responsible for the negative thoughts associated with depressive episodes of bipolar disorder
	Adipose tissue	Lipolysis; thermogenesis

agonism or inverse agonism [15, 16]. Table 2 summarizes the pharmacology of the most commonly used β-blockers. It should be stressed that β-blockers are a very heterogeneous group of drugs. Indeed, much of the controversy surrounding their optimal use results from the wide-ranging pharmacodynamic and pharmacokinetic properties of available agents and the lack of comparative studies in patients. Thus, for each indication, the choice of β-blocker significantly influences the balance of risks and benefits.

Beta-Blockers. Table 2 Commonly used β-blockers and their pharmacology [17, 18]

Drug	Relative receptor affinity			Lipo*	PB (%)	Enteral	IV	$T_{1/2}$	Metabolism and elimination	Notes
	$\beta_1{:}\beta_2$	$\beta_2{:}\beta_3$	$\beta_1{:}\beta_3$							
Atenolol	4.7:1	76:1	355:1	+	10	50% absorption	✓	6–8 h	100% GF	Removed by hemodialysis
Bisoprolol	13.5:1	10.7:1	145:1	++	30	100% absorption 10% FPM		9–12 h	50% GF. Remainder CYP450 to inactive metabolites	
Carvedilol	1:4.5	12.6:1	2.8:1	+++	98	100% absorption 75% FPM		6–10 h	98% CYP450 to active metabolites, mostly excreted in bile	Racemic mixture, only S(–) enantiomer has β-blocking activity. Both enantiomers are selective α_1-adrenergic antagonists. Ca^{2+} entry blockade. Antioxidant. Antiproliferative. Vasodilating. Weak membrane stabilizer
Esmolol	32:1			+	55		✓	9 min	Rapidly and extensively metabolized via RBC esterases. Inactive metobilte 100% GF	Moderately β_1 selective
Labetalol	1:2.5	71:1	28:1	+	50	100% absorption 75% FPM	✓	4–8 h	95% converted to inactive glucuronide of which 60% GF and remainder in bile	Racemic mixture with two optical centers. Selective α_1-adrenergic antagonist. β_2 partial agonist. Vasodilating
Metoprolol	2.3:1	54:1	126:1	++	12	100% absorption 50% FPM	✓	3–4 h	5–10% GF. Remainder CYP450 to inactive metabolites	Crosses normal BBB (CSF levels 78% of serum). Despite minimal protein binding not significantly removed by haemodialysis

Drug										
Nevibolol	47:1			+++	98	100% absorption Extensive FPM	8–27 h		CYP450 to 3 metabolites, one of which is active. Subject to polymorphisms hence wide spectrum of $T_{1/2}$. Active metabolite is dependant upon GF for elimination	Racemic mixture. Highly β_1 selective antagonist and β_3 agonist. Vasodilating properties by direct action on endothelium, possibly by NO production / release
Propranolol	1:8.3	141:1	17:1	+++	90	100% absorption Extensive FPM	3–4 h	✓	Eight metabolites, at least 1 active. Elimination independent of GF	Racemic mixture, only l-isomer active. Moderate membrane stabilizing effect. Decreases Hb O_2 affinity. Decreases platelet aggregability. Crosses normal BBB
Sotalol	1:12	63:1	5.2:1	+	10	100% absorption	10–20 h	✓	100% GF	Racemic mixture. Class II and III anti-arrhythmic activity. Potentially pro-arhythmic in the presence of hypokalaemia. Partially removed by haemodialysis
Timolol	1:26	758:1	2.1:1	++	10–30	90% absorption 50% FPM	4–5 h		80% CYP450 to inactive metabolites. 20% + metabolites via GF	Commonly used in ophthalmic preparations but associated with significant systemic effects

Notes: Relative receptor affinity data taken from [14]. Lipo* = lipophilicity. Lipophilicity is associated with CNS penetration and better CVS outcomes [19]. PB(%) = percentage protein bound. IV = intravenous preparation available in the UK. $T_{1/2}$ = elimination half life. GF = glomerular filtration/renal clearance

Hypertension

The optimal role of β-blockers as a class, and specific agents in particular, in the management of chronic hypertension, remains controversial [20]. However, in patients with hypertensive crises (malignant hypertension and pre-eclampsia) or those in whom rapid reduction/control is indicated (aortic dissection and spontaneous Intracerebral hemorrhage) β-blockers have an established role. In these setting, intravenous (IV) labetolol, usually as an infusion (15–160 mg/h titrated to response), is commonly employed as a first-line agent. Of the commonly available β-blockers, labetolol has several pharmacodynamic and pharmacokinetic properties that make it the optimal choice. In addition to its β_1 antagonism, it is also a β_2 partial agonist and α_1-adrenergic antagonist thus produces a significant vasodilating effect. It is available as an intravenous preparation and has a relatively short elimination half-life.

Ischemic Heart Disease (IHD)

β-blockers have an established role in the management of acute and chronic angina, acute coronary syndromes, myocardial infarction [20], and during percutaneous coronary intervention (PCI) [21]. Most of these effects are mediated through β_1 antagonism, which results in [20]:

1. A reduction of myocardial oxygen requirements by a decrease in heart rate, systolic pressure, and ventricular contractility
2. Bradycardia, which prolongs the coronary diastolic filling period
3. A reduction in arrhythmogenic free fatty acids
4. A redistribution of coronary flow to vulnerable subendocardial regions
5. A reduction of platelet stickiness
6. An increase in the threshold to ventricular fibrillation
7. A reduction in infarct size
8. A reduction in risk of cardiac rupture
9. A reduction in the rate of reinfarction

However, the evidence of efficacy of the use of β-blockers, especially in the acute setting, has been questioned by some authors [22, 23]. Atenolol, metoprolol, and bisoprolol are the most widely investigated and utilized β-blockers in the management of IHD. Each agent has its strengths and weaknesses and no comparative trials exist. Optimal dosing remains controversial; however, up-titration to maximal tolerated doses is widely advocated. Adequate dosing can be judged by both resting heart rate (target <70 beats per min, sinus rhythm) and lack of both angina and fatigue symptoms on exertion. The latter may

of course be influenced by multiple factors other than an excessive dose of β-blockade. In the acute setting, many advocate rapid IV loading with immediate enteral therapy. Indeed, many authorities consider this intervention to be underutilized. The strongest evidence for such therapy does predate the modern rapid thrombolytic/primary PCI era. However, biological plausibility would suggest that this approach is still valid as long as cardiogenic shock is not present.

The use of perioperative β-blockers to prevent cardiovascular morbidity and mortality (in both cardiac and noncardiac surgery) has been another area of marked controversy. The most recent consensus guidelines [24] conclude that such a strategy may have a role but only in high-risk patients and if started long enough before surgery to achieve optimal dosing/heart rate control.

Cardiac Tachyarrhythmias [25]

β-blockers are the prototypical class II antiarrhythmics. They are considered first-line therapy in acute onset atrial and ventricular tachycardias in hemodynamically stable patients. This advice is based largely on expert opinion [26, 27]. Their mechanism of action goes beyond simple beta-adrenoceptor antagonism [28]. There is limited data directly comparing available β-blockers. Due to their availability in intravenous formulations and comparatively short duration of action, metoprolol and esmolol are widely used to initiate therapy and achieve rapid rate/rhythm control. Landiolol, a comparatively novel, ultra-short acting β-blocker, with a very high β_1 selectivity, has shown potential as the preferred agent for this indication but this hypothesis remains untested and the drug widely unavailable [29].

Chronic rate control, in atrial fibrillation, many be best achieved with combination therapy of β-blockers and digoxin [30] or amiodarone [25] although recent evidence questions the previously accepted therapeutic target rate [31]. Perhaps surprisingly, non-cardioselective β-blockers, in particular, carvedilol may be the optimal choice [25, 32].

Sotalol is unique among β-blockers in exhibiting class II and III antiarrhythmic properties. There is some, albeit limited evidence, to suggest this action has significant clinical benefits in some settings [33–35].

Chronic Cardiac Failure

It is now clearly established that combination therapy of angiotensin converting enzyme inhibitors and β-blockers (that lack intrinsic sympathomimetic activity) have markedly beneficial effects on patients with cardiac failure

(New York Heart Association class II, III and IV), regardless of etiology [36, 37]. β-blockers improve myocardial performance (increase in ejection fraction of 5–10%) and prevent complications of cardiac failure by the following means [20]:

1. Bradycardia, leading to increased diastolic coronary filling time (particularly relevant to ischemic heart failure)
2. Reduction in myocardial oxygen requirements
3. Antiarrhythmic activity
4. Upregulation of β_1 receptors
5. Inhibition of the rennin/angiotensin system
6. Increasing atrial and brain naturetic peptide secretion
7. Inhibition of catecholamine-induced necrosis. This is an effect of both β_1 antagonism and β_2 agonism

There have been positive outcome trials for carvedilol, metoprolol, bisoprolol, and nevibolol and even a trial comparing carvedilol and metoprolol. Whether β_1 selectivity is an advantage or disadvantage remains controversial, however, carvedilol may be the optimal agent [32]. Of note, nevibolol, in addition to its marked β_1 selectivity, is a β_3 agonist. Whether β_3 agonism is a good or bad thing in chronic cardiac failure remains unclear [11].

β-blocker therapy should not be initiated in patients with acute decompensation of cardiac failure, until their condition has been stabilized, however, long-term therapy should not be stopped unless shock is evident. Therapy should be started/restarted at the earliest opportunity. Therapy should commence at a low dose and be up-titrated to the maximal tolerated dose. Again, controversy exists as to the best determinant of effective dose in an individual.

Portal Hypertension and Variceal Hemorrhage

Nonselective β-blockers have an established role both in the primary and secondary prevention of variceal hemorrhage [38]. Propranolol is the most widely used agent. The recommended starting dose is 40 mg twice daily, increased as tolerated up to 160 mg twice daily. Carvedilol [39] and nadolol [40] have also been investigated but their place in therapy remains undefined.

To prevent bleeding/re-bleeding, nonselective β-blockers must reduce the hepatic venous pressure gradient (HVPG) to <12 mmHg or by ≥10% from baseline [40]. However, only ~30–70% of patients achieve this [40, 41] and even among responders, undesirable/intolerable side effects, in particular hypotension and fatigue, are common and may result in cessation of therapy.

Nonselective β-blockers may have other/additional beneficial effects in patients with portal hypertension. By a separate effect on intestinal beta-receptors, they decrease intestinal permeability thereby reducing bacterial translocation [42]. This not only reduces the incidence of spontaneous bacterial peritonitis in patients the ascites it may contribute to the prevention of variceal hemorrhage which is linked to local infection.

In cirrhosis, β_3-receptors are upregulated both in hepatic stellate cells and mesenteric blood vessels. Whether β_3 agonists have a therapeutic role in the prevention or treatment of cirrhosis warrants investigation [43].

Traumatic Brain Injury (TBI) [44]

Non-neurological organ dysfunction is a common sequelae of TBI and may be provoked or exacerbated by a hyperadrenergic state. Though difficult to quantify, this non-neurological organ dysfunction probably makes a significant contribution to short- and medium-term morbidity, mortality, and functional neurological outcome. Advocates of the eponymous Lund strategy, which includes the early use of metoprolol (and clonidine), together with a series of retrospective cohort analyses strongly suggests that exposure to β-blockers is associated with a decreased mortality and improved functional outcome. Prospective studies are warranted to establish guidance on indications for, and timing of, therapy, choice of agent, and dose titration before a meaningful and pragmatic randomized trial can be designed.

Hypercatabolism Post Burns/Major Injury [45]

Major burns and other causes of major tissue injury can result in a prolonged (up to 1 year) hypercatabolic state, which is associated with a significant morbidity and mortality. Catecholamines, though by no means the only players, appear to have a central role in its evolution and perpetuation. From both basic science and clinical reports, there is significant evidence that β-blockers ameliorate this condition and appear to confer both morbidity and mortality benefits in such patients. As with other critical care interventions, we appear to lack both prospective randomized control trials and the equipoise to perform them to clearly establish the role of β-blockers in the post-injury hypercatabolic syndrome.

Sepsis and Immunomodulation [6]

Sepsis, like the systemic inflammatory response syndrome secondary to traumatic injury and burns, is associated with a hyperadrenergic state that may result in more harm than good. The effects of selective or nonselective β-blockade on the innate and adaptive immuno-inflammatory systems, remains speculative, but β$_1$-blockade coupled with β$_2$ stimulation is a potentially attractive therapeutic target.

Thyroid Storm [46]

β-blockers relieve the symptoms of thyrotoxicosis but do not modify the underlying disease. Their use is advocated in the acute management of a thyrotoxic crisis (storm) as part of package of endocrine care. Nonselective β-blockers are usually recommended though this is predominantly based on historical president.

Useful Neuropsychiatric effects?

Agitation and aggressive behavior, following acquired brain injury is a common and complex problem for which numerous pharmacological and therapeutic strategies have been trialled. There is some evidence from small-scale trials to suggest propranolol and possibly pindolol may form part of a useful strategy in reducing agitation and aggression following moderate to severe brain injury [47]. Early studies also suggest a potential role for propranolol in both the prevention and treatment of post-traumatic stress disorder [48].

β-blockers appear to cause measurable neuropyschiatric effects including sleep disturbance, vivid dreams, anxiolysis, and subtle effects on memory. When administered during general anesthesia, they appear to exhit antinociceptive and anesthetic-sparing effects [49, 50]. Whether this is a synergistic effect or merely a result of β-blockers altering the pharmacokinetics of opiates and anesthetic agents remains unclear.

Contraindications [1]

- Second- and third-degree heart block
- Cardiogenic shock
- Peripheral arterial insufficiency (relative contraindication as vasodilating agents may be well tolerated)
- Asthma (relative contraindication as highly β$_1$ selective agents may be tolerated)
- Recurrent hypoglycemia

Adverse Reactions [1]

β-blocker therapy may be associated with the following adverse reactions:

- Generalized fatigue.
- Cardiovascular – hypotension, bradycardia, asystole, cardiogenic shock. A deterioration in symptoms of peripheral arterial insufficiency.

- Respiratory – bronchospasm, due to β$_2$-blockade, which may be averted by using highly β$_1$ selective agents. β-blockers are generally well tolerated in chronic obstructive pulmonary disease. The respiratory effects of β-blockers in chronic cardiac failure are complex and reviewed here [51]. In short, the overall effect is beneficial but some drug-specific effects may have detrimental effects in some individuals. Monitoring of pulmonary function is advised.
- Brain – sleep disturbances with nightmares, believed to be less common with the less lipophilic agents.
- Metabolic – a small deterioration of glucose tolerance and interference with the metabolic and autonomic responses to hypoglycemia. They may also cause an increase in serum triglycerides, low density and very low density lipoprotein cholesterol, and a decrease in high density lipoprotein cholesterol.

β-Blocker Toxicity and Overdose [52]

In addition to supportive care beta-adrenoceptor agonists, phosphodiesterase inhibitors (e.g., milrinone), glucagon, and hyperinsulinemic euglycemia have been investigated as antidotes. Individually, none are reliably effective and only anecdotal reports support combination therapy. Atenolol and sotalol may be significantly cleared by hemodialysis.

Drug Interactions – Class Effects [1]

Synergistic effects with other antihypertensives can lead to symptomatic hypotension. Synergistic effects with other negative chronotropes can lead to symptomatic bradycardia and even asystole. Synergistic effects with other negative inotropes can lead to cardiogenic shock. Use with α$_1$ agonists can result in severe hypertension.

Drug Interactions – Specific Agents [1]

Propranolol decreases the threshold for lidocaine and bupivacaine toxicity. Sotalol increases the risk of ventricular arrhythmias when coadministered with any drug that causes QT prolongation.

References

1. British National Formulary [online]. BMJ and Pharmaceutical Press. http://bnf.org. Accessed 9 May 2010
2. Granneman JG (2001) The putative beta 4-adrenergic receptor is a novel state of the beta 1-adrenergic receptor. Am J Physiol Endocrinol Metab 280:E199–E202, http://ajpendo.physiology.org/cgi/content/abstract/280/2/E199
3. Saucerman JJ, McCulloch AD (2006) Cardiac beta-adrenergic signaling: from subcellular microdomains to heart failure. Ann NY Acad Sci 1080:348–361, http://dx.doi.org/10.1196/annals.1380.026

4. Triposkiadis F, Karayannis G, Giamouzis G, Skoularigis J, Louridas G, Butler J (2009) The Sympathetic nervous system in heart failure: physiology, pathophysiology, and clinical implications. J Am Coll Cardiol 54:1747–1762, http://www.sciencedirect.com/science/article/B6T18-4XJF21G-2/2/1ee152e807507d734280554ab1e53046

5. Mason RPP, Giles TDMD, Sowers JRMD (2009) Evolving mechanisms of action of beta blockers: focus on nebivolol. J Cardiovasc Pharmacol 54:123–128, http://www.ncbi.nlm.nih.gov/pubmed/19528811

6. de Montmollin E, Aboab J, Mansart A, Annane D (2009) Bench-to-bedside review: beta-adrenergic modulation in sepsis. Crit Care 13:230, http://ccforum.com/content/13/5/230

7. Ursino MG, Vasina V, Raschi E, Crema F, De Ponti F (2009) The beta 3 adrenoceptor as a therapeutic target: current perspectives. Pharmacol Res 59:221–234, http://www.sciencedirect.com/science/article/B6WP9-4VFK7X6-4/2/d31298d83445a213648a1b324d3e7548

8. Abraham G, Kottke C, Dhein S, Ungemach FR (2003) Pharmacological and biochemical characterization of the beta-adrenergic signal transduction pathway in different segments of the respiratory tract. Biochem Pharmacol 66:1067–1081, http://www.sciencedirect.com/science/article/B6T4P-499FDD0-3/2/a01f998a74ff63fe89a3b91f2a8c75c6

9. Reinhardt D (1989) Adrenoceptors and the lung: their role in health and disease. Eur J Pediatr 148:286–293, http://dx.doi.org/10.1007/BF00444116

10. van Waarde A, Vaalburg W, Doze P, Bosker FJ, Elsinga PH (2004) PET imaging of beta-adrenoceptors in human brain: a realistic goal or a mirage? Curr Pharm Des 10:1519–1536, http://www.ncbi.nlm.nih.gov/entrez/query.fcgi?cmd=Retrieve&db=PubMed&dopt=Citation&list_uids=15134573

11. Balligand J-L (2009) Beta 3 adrenoceptor stimulation on top of beta 1 adrenoceptor blockade: "Stop or Encore? J Am Coll Cardiol 53:1539–1542, http://www.sciencedirect.com/science/article/B6T18-4W46RCC-B/2/4a5009f41ddfb1f516864abdc3c72350

12. Brodde O-E, Bruck H, Leineweber K (2006) Cardiac adrenoceptors: physiological and pathophysiological relevance. J Pharmacol Sci 100:323–337, http://www.jstage.jst.go.jp/article/jphs/100/5/323/_pdf

13. Johnson M (1998) The beta -adrenoceptor. Am J Respir Crit Care Med 158:S146–S153, http://ajrccm.atsjournals.org/cgi/content/abstract/158/5/S2/S146

14. Baker JG (2005) The selectivity of beta-adrenoceptor antagonists at the human beta1, beta2 and beta3 adrenoceptors. Br J Pharmacol 144:317–322, http://dx.doi.org/10.1038/sj.bjp.0706048

15. Hoffmann C, Leitz MR, Oberdorf-Maass S, Lohse MJ, Klotz KN (2004) Comparative pharmacology of human β-adrenergic receptor subtypes—characterization of stably transfected receptors in CHO cells. Naunyn-Schmiedebergs Arch Pharmacol 369:151–159, http://dx.doi.org/10.1007/s00210-003-0860-y

16. Hanania NAA, Dickey BFB, Bond RAC (2010) Clinical implications of the intrinsic efficacy of beta-adrenoceptor drugs in asthma: full, partial and inverse agonism. Curr Opin Pulm Med 16:1–5, http://www.ncbi.nlm.nih.gov/pubmed/19887938

17. AHFS Drug Information [online]. American Society of Health-System Pharmacists, Inc. http://www.medicinescomplete.com/mc/ahfs/current/. Accessed 5 May 2010

18. Sweetman SC: Martindale: The Complete Drug Reference [online]. The Pharmaceutical Press. http://www.medicinescomplete.com/mc/martindale/current/. Accessed 5 May 2010

19. Hjalmarson A (2000) Cardioprotection with beta-adrenoceptor blockers. Does lipophilicity matter? Basic Res Cardiol 95(1):41–45, http://www.ncbi.nlm.nih.gov/entrez/query.fcgi?cmd=Retrieve&db=PubMed&dopt=Citation&list_uids=11192352

20. Cruickshank JM (2007) Are we misunderstanding beta-blockers. Int J Cardiol 120:10–27, http://www.sciencedirect.com/science/article/B6T16-4NGB9WF-5/2/860cff792d0b3e10401a7ab816aa539c

21. Uretsky BF, Birnbaum Y, Osman A, Gupta R, Paniagua O, Chamoun A, Pohwani A, Lui C, Lev E, McGehee T et al (2008) Distal myocardial protection with intracoronary beta blocker when added to a Gp IIb/IIIa platelet receptor blocker during percutaneous coronary intervention improves clinical outcome. Catheter Cardiovasc Interv 72:488–497, http://www.ncbi.nlm.nih.gov/entrez/query.fcgi?cmd=Retrieve&db=PubMed&dopt=Citation&list_uids=18814223

22. Messerli FH, Bangalore S, Yao SS, Steinberg JS (2009) Cardioprotection with beta-blockers: myths, facts and Pascal's wager. J Intern Med 266:232–241, http://dx.doi.org/10.1111/j.1365-2796.2009.02140.x

23. Brandler E, Paladino L, Sinert R (2010) Does the early administration of beta-blockers Improve the in-hospital mortality rate of patients admitted with acute coronary syndrome? Acad Emerg Med 17:1–10, http://dx.doi.org/10.1111/j.1553-2712.2009.00625.x

24. Fleisher LA, Beckman JA, Brown KA, Calkins H, Chaikof EL, Fleischmann KE, Freeman WK, Froehlich JB, Kasper EK, Kersten JR et al (2009) ACCF/AHA focused update on perioperative beta blockade incorporated into the ACC/AHA 2007 Guidelines on perioperative cardiovascular evaluation and care for noncardiac surgery. J Am Coll Cardiol 54:e13–e118, http://www.sciencedirect.com/science/article/B6T18-4XPWPGW-R/2/5661775886126303431ea020-89af4675

25. Singh BN (2005) Beta-adrenergic blockers as antiarrhythmic and antifibrillatory compounds: an overview. J Cardiovasc Pharmacol Ther 10:S3–S14, http://cpt.sagepub.com/cgi/content/abstract/10/4_suppl/S3

26. Kanji S, Stewart R, Fergusson DA, McIntyre L, Turgeon AF, Hebert PC (2008) Treatment of new-onset atrial fibrillation in noncardiac intensive care unit patients: a systematic review of randomized controlled trials. Crit Care Med 36:1620–1624

27. Khoo CW, Lip GY (2009) Acute management of atrial fibrillation. Chest 135:849–859, http://www.chestjournal.org/content/135/3/849.long

28. Dorian P (2005) Antiarrhythmic action of{beta}-blockers: potential mechanisms. J Cardiovasc Pharmacol Ther 10:S15–S22, http://cpt.sagepub.com/cgi/content/abstract/10/4_suppl/S15

29. Atarashi H, Kuruma A, Yashima M, Saitoh H, Ino T, Endoh Y, Hayakawa H (2000) Pharmacokinetics of landiolol hydrochloride, a new ultra-short-acting beta-blocker, in patients with cardiac arrhythmias. Clin Pharmacol Ther 68:143–150

30. Nikolaidou T, Channer KS (2009) Chronic atrial fibrillation: a systematic review of medical heart rate control management. Postgrad Med J 85:303–312, http://pmj.bmj.com/content/85/1004/303.abstract

31. Dorian P (2010) Rate control in atrial fibrillation. N Engl J Med 362:1439–1441, http://content.nejm.org

32. Reiffel JA (2005) Drug and drug-device therapy in heart failure patients in the post-comet and SCD-HeFT Era. J Cardiovasc Pharmacol Ther 10:S45–S58, http://cpt.sagepub.com/cgi/content/abstract/10/4_suppl/S45

33. Patel A, Dunning J (2005) Is Sotalol more effective than standard beta-blockers for the prophylaxis of atrial fibrillation during cardiac surgery. Interact Cardiovasc Thorac Surg 4:147–150, http://www.ncbi.nlm.nih.

gov/entrez/query.fcgi?cmd=Retrieve&db=PubMed&dopt=Citation&list_uids=17670378

34. Furushima H, Chinushi M, Okamura K, Komura S, Tanabe Y, Sato A, Izumi D, Aizawa Y (2007) Effect of dl-sotalol on mortality and recurrence of ventricular tachyarrhythmias: ischemic compared to nonischemic cardiomyopathy. Pacing Clin Electrophysiol 30:1136–1141, http://www.ncbi.nlm.nih.gov/entrez/query.fcgi?cmd=Retrieve&db=PubMed&dopt=Citation&list_uids=17725758

35. Chaki AL, Caines AE, Miller AB (2009) Sotalol as adjunctive therapy to implantable cardioverter-defibrillators in heart failure patients. Congest Heart Fail 15:144–147, http://www.ncbi.nlm.nih.gov/entrez/query.fcgi?cmd=Retrieve&db=PubMed&dopt=Citation&list_uids=19522964

36. Klapholz M (2009) Beta-blocker use for the stages of heart failure. Mayo Clin Proc 84:718–729, http://www.mayoclinicproceedings.com/content/84/8/718.full.pdf

37. McMurray JJV (2010) Systolic heart failure. N Engl J Med 362:228–238, http://content.nejm.org/cgi/reprint/362/3/228.pdf

38. de Franchis R (2005) Evolving Consensus in portal hypertension report of the Baveno IV consensus workshop on methodology of diagnosis and therapy in portal hypertension. J Hepatol 43:167–176, http://www.sciencedirect.com/science/article/B6W7C-4G7DXYB-2/2/beeec811dc19e07c248956564d486ef8

39. Hemstreet BA (2004) Evaluation of carvedilol for the treatment of portal hypertension. Pharmacotherapy 24:94–104, http://www.ncbi.nlm.nih.gov/entrez/query.fcgi?cmd=Retrieve&db=PubMed&dopt=Citation&list_uids=14740791

40. Villanueva C, Aracil C, Colomo A, Hernández-Gea V, López-Balaguer JM, Alvarez-Urturi C, Torras X, Balanzó J, Guarner C (2009) Acute hemodynamic response to beta-blockers and prediction of long-term outcome in primary prophylaxis of variceal bleeding. Gastroenterology 137:119–128, http://www.sciencedirect.com/science/article/B6WFX-4VYXMJ2-2/2/8a94fd55572b0befbfecae298-998a8cf

41. De-Madaria E, Palazon JM, Hernandez FT, Sanchez-Paya J, Zapater P, Irurzun J, Espana FD, Pascual S, Such J, Sempere L et al (2010) Acute and chronic hemodynamic changes after propranolol in patients with cirrhosis under primary and secondary prophylaxis of variceal bleeding: a pilot study. Eur J Gastroenterol Hepatol 22(5):507–12, http://www.ncbi.nlm.nih.gov/pubmed/20150817

42. Senzolo M, Cholongitas E, Burra P, Leandro G, Thalheimer U, Patch D, Burroughs AK (2009) beta-Blockers protect against spontaneous bacterial peritonitis in cirrhotic patients: a meta-analysis. Liver Int 29:1189–1193, http://www.ncbi.nlm.nih.gov/pubmed/19508620

43. Trebicka J, Hennenberg M, Schulze Probsting A, Laleman W, Klein S, Granzow M, Nevens F, Zaagsma J, Heller J, Sauerbruch T (2009) Role of beta3-adrenoceptors for intrahepatic resistance and portal hypertension in liver cirrhosis. Hepatology 50:1924–1935

44. Tran TY, Dunne IE (2008) German JW: Beta blockers exposure and traumatic brain injury: a literature review. Neurosurg Focus 25:E8, http://thejns.org/doi/abs/10.3171/FOC.2008.25.10.E8

45. Atiyeh B, Gunn S, Dibo S (2008) Metabolic implications of severe burn injuries and their management: a systematic review of the literature. World J Surg 32:1857–1869, http://dx.doi.org/10.1007/s00268-008-9587-8

46. Kearney T, Dang C (2007) Diabetic and endocrine emergencies. Postgrad Med J 83:79–86, http://pmj.bmj.com/content/83/976/79.abstract

47. Fleminger S, Greenwood RJ, Oliver DL (2006) Pharmacological management for agitation and aggression in people with acquired brain injury. Cochrane Database Syst Rev. doi:CD003299, http://www.ncbi.nlm.nih.gov/entrez/query.fcgi?cmd=Retrieve&db=PubMed&dopt=Citation&list_uids=17054165

48. Cukor J, Spitalnick J, Difede J, Rizzo A, Rothbaum BO (2009) Emerging treatments for PTSD. Clin Psychol Rev 29:715–726, http://www.sciencedirect.com/science/article/B6VB8-4X6FNP8-2/2/685352841-60f7a36815568708e6c94b3

49. Kadoi Y, Saito S (2009) Beta-Blockers in the perioperative period: are there indications other than prevention of cardiac ischemia? Curr Drug Targets 10:842–849, http://www.ncbi.nlm.nih.gov/entrez/query.fcgi?cmd=Retrieve&db=PubMed&dopt=Citation&list_uids=19799538

50. Tanabe T, Fukusaki M, Fujinaga A, Ando Y, Yamashita K, Terao Y, Sumikawa K (2009) Landiolol, a new ultra-short-acting beta1-blocker, reduces anaesthetic requirement during sevoflurane/N(2)O/fentanyl anaesthesia in surgical patients. Eur J Anaesthesiol 26:39–42, http://www.ncbi.nlm.nih.gov/pubmed/19122550

51. Agostoni P, Palermo P, Contini M (2009) Respiratory effects of β-blocker therapy in heart failure. Cardiovasc Drugs Ther 23:377–384, http://dx.doi.org/10.1007/s10557-009-6195-2

52. Kerns Ii W (2007) Management of beta-adrenergic blocker and calcium channel antagonist toxicity. Emerg Med Clin North Am 25:309–331, http://www.sciencedirect.com/science/article/B75J3-4NN0V9V-5/2/00bb40a9a00beaa94934dfdc64bc574f

Beta-Trace-Protein

▶ Serum and Urinary Low Molecular Weight Proteins

BG

(1,3)-b-D-Glucan.

Bilemia

▶ Biliovenous Fistula

Bilevel Positive Airway Pressure (BiPAP)

▶ Noninvasive Ventilation

Bilhemia

Is the flow of bile into the bloodstream. It is usually due to a fistulous connection between a bile duct and hepatic or portal vein. Bilhemia is much less common than hemobilia.

▶ Biliovenous Fistula

Biliary-Venous Fistula

▶ Biliovenous Fistula

Biliovenous Fistula

Jennifer M. DiCocco[1], Timothy C. Fabian[2]
[1]General Surgery Resident, University of Tennessee Health Science Center, Memphis, TN, USA
[2]Surgery – General, University of Tennessee Health Science Center, Memphis, TN, USA

Synonyms

Bilemia; Bilhemia; Biliary-venous fistula

Definition

Biliovenous fistula (BVF) is a fistulous connection between a bile duct and hepatic or portal vein. This connection can result in bile entering the bloodstream, a phenomenon known as ▶ bilhemia (or bilemia). A better-known entity is ▶ hemobilia, hemorrhage into the biliary tract. Hemobilia is usually the result of a bile duct to hepatic artery fistula. Hemobilia and bilhemia are distinct entities with different treatments and outcomes. This entry will focus on the pathophysiology and management of bilhemia resulting from biliovenous fistulas.

Literature regarding biliovenous fistulas is a collection of case reports only, due to the rarity of this disease. The first report of biliovenous fistula was from 1559, describing gallstones found in the portal vein of a patient on autopsy. Since then, less than 100 cases have been reported.

Pathophysiology

Normal common bile duct pressure is about 10–15 mmHg and can be greater than 20 mmHg during sphincter of Oddi contraction. Hepatic vein pressure is 0–6 mmHg. The vena cava, during diastole, can have pressures of −5 mmHg. When a biliovenous fistula occurs, the differences in these pressures allows for bile to flow from the bile duct system to the venous system, leading to bilhemia. Bilhemia cannot exist in an arterial-biliary fistula due to the high pressures in the arterial system. Pressure gradients cause blood to flow from arterial to biliary system, causing hemobilia.

Several case reports note that patients have an abrupt rise in bilirubin after mechanical ventilation is discontinued. Mechanical ventilation increases venous pressures secondary to positive end-expiratory pressures. Once a patient is extubated, central venous pressures return to normal, below pressures in the biliary system. This allows the bile to be shunted into the venous system when a fistula is present. Several authors have reported a delay in presentation of bilhemia, and contribute this to changes in pressure gradients associated with mechanical ventilation.

The most common cause for biliovenous fistula is blunt liver trauma. Mechanisms with rapid deceleration are typical, such as motor vehicle collisions. Central rupture of liver venules and bile ducts can lead to hematomas and necrotic liver parenchyma. Within these necrotic cavities, intrahepatic biliovenous fistulas may form.

There are reports of biliovenous fistulas occurring during interventional procedures on the liver such as tranjugular intrahepatic portosystemic shunt (▶ TIPS) or liver biopsy. TIPS is used to decompress the portal venous system for treatment of uncontrolled varices, recurrent bleeding, refractory ascites, and hepatic hydrothorax. The development of biliovenous fistula is even more rare in these patients because many have elevated portal pressures, above 20 mmHg, even after TIPS procedures. The pressure difference favors hemobilia, not bilhemia. Thrombosed shunts lead to lower pressures and allow the shunt to reverse causing bilhemia. There ehave also been a few reported cases of gallstone erosion into hepatic veins resulting in fistula formation. Common bile duct obstruction with gallstones elevates the biliary pressures to increase the likelihood of bilhemia.

Evaluation/Assessment

Successful treatment of biliovenous fistula depends on accurate and prompt diagnosis; however, many cases are identified on autopsy. Patients typically present with acute asymptomatic jaundice. Laboratory findings include severe hyperbilirubinemia, greater than 50 mg/dL in many cases. This rise in bilirubin is rapid, usually taking place in just days. Direct bilirubin predominates due to bile dissolving into the bloodstream. Liver enzymes will remain normal because there is no functional impairment of the liver. Trauma patients will have elevated liver enzymes relating to the degree of parenchymal injury. Patients often have normal hemoglobin levels, as opposed to hemobilia, where the patient is bleeding into their biliary system, and may present with anemia.

In a review of more than 50 cases, the most common source of biliovenous fistula was blunt trauma (23 cases). Less common reasons include iatrogenic injuries, liver biopsy, stab wounds to the abdomen, manipulation during surgery, and gallstone erosion into hepatic veins. The diagnosis of biliovenous fistula should be suspected in patients with a rapid rise in direct bilirubin after liver trauma or manipulation, such as biopsy or TIPS procedures, especially in the face of normal enzyme levels.

In order to confirm the diagnosis of biliovenous fistula, endoscopic retrograde cholangiopancreatography (▶ ERCP) is generally performed. This allows for direct visualization of the fistula and the direction of flow. Additionally, definitive treatment may be attempted at during the same procedure. Intraoperative cholangiogram (IOC) is an option when ERCP is unavailable.

Treatment

Since biliovenous fistula is a very rare disease, it is difficult to recommend specific treatments. Various authors have made recommendations based on review of case reports. There are three general techniques used to treat biliovenous fistulas: liver resection, fistula occlusion, and relief of bile duct obstruction.

Liver Resection

Though highly morbid, some patients can only be treated by liver resection. Large hepatic hematomas can lead to areas of necrosis and abscess formation. These complications may be difficult to treat with stents or prosthetic devices due to recurrent infection. Operative management allows for examination of the fistula, which can be sutured closed. The patient must have adequate liver function after the resection to prevent liver failure. Liver transplant was used for at least one case, in which the diagnosis of biliovenous fistula was made on examination of the explanted liver. More conservative treatments are usually attempted first and liver resection is reserved for cases in which the diagnosis is unclear or other treatments have failed.

Fistula Occlusion

Direct occlusion of biliovenous fistulas is possible during hepatic venography. Endoscopic placement and occlusion of biliovenous fistula is accomplished by positioning a balloon catheter in the affected hepatic vein. This will allow for clot formation and closure of the fistula. Endoscopic retrograde cholangiopancreatography (ERCP) with stent placement in the bile duct across the area of fistula can also be used to occlude biliovenous fistulas.

Relief of Ductal Obstruction

The theory behind this treatment is if the pressure in the biliary system is decreased to below the venous system, then bile will not be able to flow into the bloodstream and the fistula can heal. Some authors fear this will lead to shunt reversal and result in massive hemobilia. However, there have been case reports that were successfully treated in this manner without complications.

Several methods for relieving biliary obstruction exist. While performing an ERCP to confirm the diagnosis of biliovenous fistula, sphincterotomy or stent placement in the common bile duct can be done. Stents can be removed after documenting the fistula has healed. Other options include nasobiliary drainage and external drainage creating a percutaneous bile fistula. T-tube drain is difficult in children due to the small size of their common bile ducts. Closed suction drainage of the necrotic cavity or bile cyst has been used to shunt bile before reaching the venous system in children and adults.

After-care

The care required for patients with biliovenous fistula is dependent on the treatment used. Bilirubin levels should be obtained to ensure an appropriate decrease following intervention. Most patients return to normal levels within days of adequate therapy. If bilirubin remains elevated, alternate therapy should be considered.

Prognosis

Biliovenous fistula is highly lethal with early reports having a near 100% mortality. More recent literature, especially in pediatric populations, have shown improved survival. However, there is still an approximately 50% mortality associated with biliovenous fistulas. Most deaths are rapid, with only a few reports resulting in death months after the diagnosis. Late deaths are generally due to complications of the treatment used, not the fistula itself. Sudden, early deaths resemble right-sided heart failure. Bile emboli to the lungs are blamed for the death in these cases. Autopsy reveals bile staining in lungs and kidneys. In survivors, morbidity is generally related to the underlying cause of bilhemia, such as trauma or liver disease, not the disease itself. When treatment of biliovenous fistula is successful, patients have excellent outcomes and follow-up studies reveal normal liver anatomy and function.

References

1. Antebi E, Adar R, Zweig A, Barzilay J, Mozes M (1973) Bilemia: an unusual complication of bile ducts stones. Ann Surg 177(3):274–275
2. Gable DR, Allen JW, Harrell DJ, Carrillo EH (1997) Endoscopic treatment of posttraumatic "bilhemia": case report. J Trauma 43(3):534–536
3. Glaser K, Wetscher G, Pointner R et al (1994) Traumatic bilhemia. Surgery 116(1):24–27
4. Haberlik A, Cendron M, Sauer H (1992) Biliovenous fistula in children after blunt liver trauma: proposal for a simple surgical treatment. J Pediatr Surg 27(9):1203–1206
5. Sandblom P, Jakobsson B, Lindgren H, Lunderquist A (2000) Fatal bilhemia. Surgery 127(3):354–357

Bioincompatible Membrane

The interaction of blood with dialysis membranes made of cellulose or cellulose polymers results in complement activation. These membranes are thus deemed "bioincompatible." Newer, synthetic dialysis membranes cause less complement activation and so are more "biocompatible."

Biological Terrorism

The deliberate or threatened release of viruses, bacteria, or toxins derived from living organisms in an attempt to cause fear, illness, or death in a population.

Biological Terrorism, Anthrax

Gregory J. Moran, Raul Easton-Carr
Department of Emergency Medicine, Olive View-UCLA Medical Center, Sylmar, CA, USA

Synonyms

Bacillus anthracis; Bioterrorism

Definition

Anthrax is caused by *Bacillus anthracis*, a gram-positive organism that is well suited for use as a biological weapon because it can form spores that are stable over long periods and can withstand exposure to air, sunlight, and even some disinfectants. Anthrax also occurs naturally as a zoonotic disease of persons who handle contaminated animal products, such as hair or hides. Anthrax has been used as a bioterrorism agent, most notably in 2001 when 18 people were infected via intentional exposure through the United States mail.

Clinical Presentation

Anthrax can present as three distinct clinical syndromes in humans: cutaneous, inhalation, and gastrointestinal. The key to diagnosis in all three syndromes consists of a high clinical suspicion and a history of exposure or proximity to an area with a known outbreak.

Cutaneous anthrax, the most common naturally occurring form, is usually spread through contact with infected animals, particularly cows, sheep, and horses, or their products. Greater than 95% of all anthrax cases are cutaneous [1, 2], most commonly on the head, neck, and extremities. There have also been case reports of transmission by insect bites [3]. After inoculation, there is an incubation period of 1–5 days, after which erythematous papular lesions form, progressing to vesicles and then large black eschars. The lesion is usually painless and may be surrounded by varying degrees of edema, which can sometimes be quite severe [1, 3]. Patients may also experience lymphadenopathy, fever, malaise, and nausea.

Gastrointestinal anthrax is rare in humans [2]. It is acquired by ingesting inadequately cooked meat from infected animals. The ingested spores germinate with an incubation period of 2–5 days. The infected person may then develop ulcers in the mouth or esophagus, or may develop lesions lower in the intestinal tract causing them to present with abdominal pain, fever, and bloody diarrhea that progresses to a sepsis syndrome with high mortality [1, 3]. Although the initial presentation may be that of an acute abdominal syndrome, there may also be substantial dysphagia and respiratory distress associated with GI exposure to anthrax [1].

A far greater threat is posed by the inhalational form of anthrax. This type of anthrax, also known as woolsorter's disease when it occurs naturally, is only rarely seen among wool or tannery workers, but is the form of anthrax most likely to be spread through a terrorist attack [2]. Inhalational anthrax can be rapidly fatal once symptoms begin. After a 1–6 day incubation period, symptoms typically begin as a nonspecific prodrome resembling influenza, with malaise, dry cough, and fever. This progresses to chills, diaphoresis, vomiting, chest pain, and respiratory distress. Patients will often have some abnormality on chest radiograph or CT scans, including infiltrates, pleural effusion, or mediastinal widening [1–4]. This widening may be due to necrosis and hemorrhage of the mediastinal lymph nodes and surrounding tissues [1]. Some patients develop meningitis, which is a poor prognostic indicator [3]. Inhalation anthrax can also sometimes present as a sepsis syndrome without the usual symptoms of chest pain and shortness of breath. The illness often progresses to septic shock and death approximately 24–36 h after the appearance of respiratory distress [1].

Treatment and Prophylaxis

The mainstay of treatment is antibiotic therapy, but the regimen should be started as early as possible to be effective. Although penicillin is usually regarded as the preferred treatment for naturally occurring cutaneous anthrax [3], penicillin-resistant strains are known to occur, and the belief is that terrorists would be likely to use a resistant strain (although this was not the case in the 2001 attack). Penicillin is not recommended as empiric treatment until susceptibility of the organism is known. Naturally occuring B. anthracis is also susceptible to tetracyclines, erythromycin, chloramphenicol, gentamicin, and fluoroquinolones. Initial empiric treatment with ciprofloxacin (400 mg IV every 12 h) or another fluoroquinolone is recommended until susceptibility is known [2, 5]. Some authors have recommend that inhalation, oropharangeal, or gastrointestinal anthrax should be initially treated with two IV antibiotics, one of them being a flouroquinolone or doxycycline (100 mg IV every 12 h), and for the second agent clindamycin, rifampin, penicillin, ampicillin, vancomycin, imipenem, linezolid, clarithromycin, chloramphenicol, or an aminoglycoside [1, 5]. This would be a reasonable approach, since the particular susceptibilities and virulence of a bioterrorism agent may not be known at the beginning of an outbreak. Supportive therapy to maintain the airway, replenish fluids, and alleviate shock is also crucial. Because spores can be dormant for a long time, a 60-day course of antibiotics is recommended for treating anthrax [1, 2, 5]. Although, in theory, cutaneous anthrax without systemic symptoms can be successfully treated with a 7–10 day course of oral penicillin, cutaneous anthrax in the setting of a bioterrorism attack would also likely be associated with inhalation exposure. Therefore it is prudent to treat any potential systemic exposure initially with the IV regimen recommended above.

Prophylaxis

In patients who were exposed to anthrax but are not yet sick, illness and death can be prevented with prophylactic antibiotics. The CDC recommends ciprofloxacin (500 mg orally twice daily) or doxycycline (100 mg orally twice daily) as first-line prophylaxis after inhalational exposure to anthrax and for presumptive treatment of mild symptoms after anthrax exposure [2].

A vaccine for anthrax, derived from an attenuated anthrax strain, has been licensed by the US Food and Drug Administration since 1970. This vaccine has been used mostly for military personnel, and might not be generally available to the public in adequate amounts in the event of a large biological attack. The vaccine is given repeatedly in a series of six subcutaneous injections over 18 months and can cause several adverse effects. It is not licensed for use against inhalational anthrax exposure, but some limited animal data suggest protection.

Evaluation and Assessment

Generally, diagnosis must be suspected on clinical grounds for treatment to be initiated in time to be beneficial. By the time the disease is confirmed through laboratory tests, many patients will be beyond help [2]. B. anthracis is detectable through Gram stain of the blood and blood culture on routine media, but often not until the patient is seriously ill. An enzyme-linked immunosorbent assay (ELISA) for the anthrax toxin exists, but most hospital laboratories do not have it readily available. The organism may also be identified in CSF, as many patients exposed to inhalational or gastrointestinal anthrax will develop hemorrhagic meningitis [1–4].

After-care

Anthrax does not spread person-to-person, and standard precautions are recommended. However, persons who present shortly after exposure may still be contaminated with spores. Any persons coming into direct contact with a substance alleged to be anthrax spores should simply bathe with soap and water and store contaminated clothing in a plastic bag, but decontamination procedures for other persons in the area should not be necessary. Disinfectants such as bleach solutions can be used to decontaminate inanimate objects, but are not recommended for skin.

Prognosis

Cutaneous Anthrax

Local cutaneous anthrax has a mortality rate of less than 1% if treated, but can occasionally become systemic, with mortality rates approaching 20% [1], although this is the exception rather than the rule. Eighty to ninety percent of cutaneous infections can be expected to recover without complications or scarring.

Gastrointestinal and Oropharyngeal Anthrax

After development of severe abdominal symptoms, mortality may be as high as 50%. Severe infections are associated with significant blood loss, electrolyte abnormalities, hypotension, and shock. Death can result from bowel perforation and toxemia. If the patient is able to survive this stage, recovery usually takes 10–14 days [3].

Inhalation Anthrax

Treatment is usually successful early in the course of the disease, but mortality is much higher once respiratory symptoms have developed, with 90% succumbing to death within 24–72 h in most case series [4]. Anthrax meningitis is a bad prognostic sign as it is almost universally fatal, with death occurring 1–6 days after the onset of illness, despite intensive antibiotic therapy [3]. In the absence of appropriate treatment, mortality from inhalational anthrax is essentially 100% [1, 2]. However, the case fatality rate was 45% among the 11 confirmed inhalational cases resulting from bioterrorism in the fall of 2001, largely attributed to earlier and more aggressive supportive care and antibiotic therapy [2].

References

1. Purcell BK, Worsham PL, Friedlander AM (2007) Anthrax. In: Dembek ZF (ed) Medical aspects of biological warfare. Office of the Surgeon General, Washington, DC, pp 69–90, http://www.bordeninstitute.army.mil/published_volumes/biological_warfare/biological.html. Accessed 25 Jul 2009
2. Moran G, Talan D, Abrahamian F (2008) Biological terrorism. Infect Dis Clin North Am 22(1):145–187, vii
3. Dixon T, Meselson M, Guillemin J, Hanna P (1999) Anthrax. N Engl J Med 341(11):815–826
4. Bossi P, Garin D, Guihot A, Gay F, Crance J, Debord T et al (2006) Bioterrorism: management of major biological agents. Cell Mol Life Sci 63(19–20):2196–2212
5. Inglesby T, O'Toole T, Henderson D, Bartlett J, Ascher M, Eitzen E et al (2002) Anthrax as a biological weapon, 2002: updated recommendations for management. JAMA 287(17):2236–2252

Biological Terrorism, Botulinum Toxin

GREGORY J. MORAN, RAUL EASTON-CARR
Department of Emergency Medicine, Olive View-UCLA Medical Center, Sylmar, CA, USA

Synonyms

Bioterrorism; Botulism; Clostridium botulinum

Definition

Botulism is a syndrome caused by exposure to one or more of the seven neurotoxins produced by the bacillus *Clostridium botulinum*, a spore-forming, obligate anaerobic, gram-positive bacillus. The botulinum toxins are among the most potent toxins in existence. Theoretically, enough toxin is present in a single gram of crystallized botulinum toxin to kill more than one million people [1].

C. botulinum spores are found ubiquitously in soil and marine sediments and can often be found in the intestinal tracts of domestic grazing animals [2]. Terrorists could conceivably contaminate food supplies with the botulinum toxins or initiate a large-scale attack by dispersing the toxins through aerosol over a vast area [3].

Clinical Presentation

Botulism is a neuroparalytic disease, resulting from the inhibition of presynaptic acetylcholine release at the neuromuscular junction, which results in neuromuscular paralysis. The time until symptom development as well as the severity and duration of symptoms are dependent upon the serotype and amount of toxin to which the person has been exposed [2].

Unlike most other bioterrorism-related illness, botulism has a fairly characteristic presentation and therefore can usually be diagnosed from the clinical signs and symptoms alone. The clinical syndrome is similar regardless of whether the botulinum toxins are ingested or inhaled.

After an initial food-borne exposure to botulism, there is a variable incubation period of 2 h–8 days [1, 2], after which the patient may initially present with nonspecific gastrointestinal symptoms such as nausea, vomiting, abdominal cramps, and diarrhea. The prompt diagnosis of botulism will depend on the recognition of the cardinal signs of the disease: *a acute symmetric descending flaccid paralysis with prominent bulbar palsies in an afebrile patient with normal sensorium.* The bulbar palsies classically associated with botulism are diplopia, dysarthria, dysphonia, and dysphagia. These are often followed by muscle weakness in the following order: muscles involving head control, muscles of the upper extremities, respiratory muscles and, lastly, muscles of the lower extremities. Weakness generally occurs in a proximal-to-distal pattern and is usually symmetric [2].

On physical examination, infected patients are generally afebrile, alert, and oriented. They may have postural hypotension, and some complain of dry mouth, sore throat, or dizziness. Although some paresthesias have been reported, botulism is not thought to cause objective sensory deficits.

Treatment and Prophylaxis

The mainstay of treatment is hemodynamic and ventilatory support, including intensive care monitoring and mechanical ventilation, often for several weeks. Unfortunately, this strategy would present insurmountable logistical problems in the event of a large-scale terrorist attack affecting thousands of people. Mechanical ventilators would be in short supply, and bag-ventilation would be impractical for weeks to months. The sudden demand for limited resources could make proper care for the many victims nearly impossible. Suspected exposures who are breathing spontaneously should be carefully monitored for impending respiratory failure, including frequent assessment of vital capacity and negative inspiratory force. Because a biological weapon would likely use the toxin rather than the organism itself, antibiotics have no utility. For wound botulism, in which *C. botulinum* is reproducing in damaged tissue and producing toxin, surgical debridement and antibiotics such as metronidazole are used.

A trivalent equine botulinum antitoxin is available from limited sources such as the U.S. Centers for Disease Control and Prevention, as well as some state health departments [4]. Unfortunately, it is effective only in preventing further deterioration; it will not reverse muscle weakness that has already developed. It would not be available in adequate amounts to treat the number of people resulting from a large-scale exposure. Because the antitoxin is a horse serum product, skin testing for horse serum sensitivity is recommended before the drug is administered.

A newer human botulism immunoglobulin, BabyBIG, has been shown to be effective for infant botulism [5] and may be effective for preventing progression of botulism related to bioterrorism events. Since it is derived from humans, it does not have the high risk of anaphylaxis observed with equine products or the risk of lifelong hypersensitivity to equine antigens [2].

Evaluation and Assessment

Laboratory testing is generally not helpful. The diagnosis usually must be made on clinical and epidemiological grounds. Botulinum toxins are generally difficult to detect, and most patients do not have a measurable antibody response because the amount of toxin required to produce clinical symptoms is so small. Some bioassay tests are available, such as a mouse bioassay, in which the specimen is injected into mice that are then observed for changes. These assays are labor intensive and take several days, and are only available in a few laboratories.

After-care

Standard universal procedures should be taken whenever a patient presents with botulism. Patients who may have the toxin on their skin as a result of aerosol exposure should bathe thoroughly with soap and water and discard their clothes.

Prognosis

Most patients who have botulism will survive if they are given proper ventilatory assistance. Those who die from the disease usually succumb to respiratory failure or secondary infections from prolonged mechanical ventilation. Of those who survive, full recovery generally takes several weeks or months, during which the patient is required to remain on a ventilator, because new synapses must grow to replace the ones damaged by the botulinum toxin. Cranial nerve dysfunction and some autonomic dysfunction may persist a year or longer [2]. In the 1950s, mortality from botulism was approximately 60%, but with adequate ventilatory support and improvements in ICU care, case fatality rates are now as low as 5–10%.

References

1. Moran G, Talan D, Abrahamian F (2008) Biological terrorism. Infect Dis Clin North Am 22(1):145–187, vii
2. Dembek ZF, Smith LA, Rusnak JM (2007) Botulinum toxin. In: Medical aspects of biological warfare. Office of the Surgeon General, Washington, DC, pp 337–353, http://www.bordeninstitute.army.mil/published_volumes/biological_warfare/biological.html. Accessed 25 Jul, 2009
3. Arnon SS, Schechter R, Inglesby TV, Henderson DA, Bartlett JG, Ascher MS et al (2001 Feb 28) Botulinum toxin as a biological weapon: medical and public health management. JAMA 285(8):1059–1070
4. Shapiro RL, Hatheway C, Becher J, Swerdlow DL (1997 Aug 6) Botulism surveillance and emergency response: a public health strategy for a global challenge. JAMA 278(5):433–435
5. Arnon SS, Schechter R, Maslanka SE, Jewell NP, Hatheway CL (2006 Feb 2) Human botulism immune globulin for the treatment of infant botulism. N Engl J Med 354(5):462–471

Biological Terrorism, Hemorrhagic Fever

GREGORY J. MORAN, RAUL EASTON-CARR
Department of Emergency Medicine, Olive View-UCLA
Medical Center, Sylmar, CA, USA

Synonyms

Arenaviruses; Argentine hemorrhagic fever; Bioterrorism; Brazilian hemorrhagic fever; Bunyaviruses; Ebola; Filoviruses; Flaviviruses; Hantavirus; Lassa fever; Marburg; Venezuelan hemorrhagic fever; Yellow fever

Definition

Viral hemorrhagic fever is an acute febrile syndrome caused by several viruses and characterized by systemic involvement which, in severe cases, includes generalized bleeding and can result in death [1]. The exact nature of the disease depends on the virulence, strain characteristics, route of exposure, dose, and host factors [2]. Many of these viruses cause rapidly progressive illnesses that carry extremely high mortality rates. Laboratory cultures can yield sufficient concentrations of organisms to provide a credible terrorist weapon if disseminated as an aerosol [3].

Clinical Presentation

The main target of viral hemorrhagic fevers is the vascular bed, therefore, while the clinical presentations of different viral hemorrhagic fevers vary, all can involve diffuse hemorrhage and bleeding diatheses as a consequence of the microvascular damage and changes in vascular permeability [2]. The incubation periods of the hemorrhagic fevers range from 2 to 35 days [1, 2, 4]. The more severe diseases such as Ebola or Marburg generally have shorter incubation periods. Patients typically present with a nonspecific prodrome that includes malaise, headache, myalgias, arthralgias, abdominal pain, nausea, vomiting, diarrhea, and a high fever. This prodrome typically lasts less than a week. On physical examination, the only findings may be conjunctival injection, mild hypotension, flushing, and scattered petechiae.

Laboratory testing may show thrombocytopenia or other signs of disseminated intravascular coagulation or elevated levels of liver enzymes or creatinine.

Within hours or days after the initial presentation, patients with the more severe hemorrhagic fevers will experience a rapid deterioration of their status, followed by mucous membrane hemorrhage and shock, often with signs of neurologic, pulmonary, renal and hepatic involvement [2, 4].

Treatment

Good supportive care is the mainstay of therapy for patients who have any viral hemorrhagic fever. Special care must be taken during fluid resuscitation because fluid transudation into the lungs will occur in some patients. In addition, because the risk for hemorrhage is high among these patients with fragile vascular endothelium, caution is necessary when performing invasive procedures such as intravenous lines, as well as when transporting patients. It has also been recommended to avoid air transport, due to the effects of drastic pressure changes on lung water balance [2]. Secondary infections are thought to be quite common, and should be assessed and treated aggressively. Patients with profuse bleeding should similarly be assessed and treated for disseminated intravascular coagulation. Shock should be treated with crystalloid fluid resuscitation and vasoactive agents; however, due to a combination of myocardial impairment and increased pulmonary vascular permeability, these patients may more easily develop pulmonary edema [2].

For patients who have Lassa fever, Bolivian hemorrhagic fever, Congo–Crimean hemorrhagic fever, or Rift Valley fever, the antiviral agent ribavirin may offer some benefit [4]. The suggested dose for adults and children is 30 mg/kg IV (max. 2 g) once, followed by 16 mg/kg IV (max. 1 g) every 6 h for 4 days, then 8 mg/kg IV (max. 500 mg) every 8 h for 6 days. An alternative dosing strategy for mass casualty settings is 2 g PO once, followed by 1,200 mg/day PO in 2 divided doses for 10 days (for patients weighing >75 kg) [4]. This may be given empirically to patients with suspected viral hemorrhagic fever until the causative agent can be identified.

Evaluation and Assessment

The most valuable tool for the prompt diagnosis of a hemorrhagic fever virus is to have a high index of suspicion, especially in the early phases of a bioterror attack. Viral hemorrhagic fevers should be suspected in any patient presenting with a severe febrile illness and evidence of diffuse vascular dysfunction (hypotension, petechiae, nondependent edema, and hemorrhage) who has traveled to an endemic area, or one where known or suspected biological attacks may have taken place. Specific tests for some hemorrhagic fevers exist, but are not available at most hospital laboratories. Specific identification requires

ELISA detection of antiviral IgM antibodies or direct culture of the viral agent from blood or tissue samples. These tests can only be performed at specialized laboratories, such as those available at the US Centers for Disease Control and Prevention or military labs. If the agent remains unknown, it may be visualized through electron microscopy followed by immunohistochemical techniques. The laboratory should be notified if severe hemorrhagic fever viruses such as Ebola or Marburg are suspected because specimens should be handled under biosafety level 4 precautions.

After-care

Contact precautions are necessary for all persons with hemorrhagic fever. All body fluids should be considered infectious. In several outbreaks in Africa, hospital personnel were able to prevent transmission to themselves and other patients simply through wearing gowns, gloves, and masks. Respiratory isolation, however, may be necessary for patients who experience massive hemorrhage into the lungs. Aerosol transmission of hemorrhagic fever has been shown in animal studies, but does not appear to be a significant mode of transmission among humans. Under ideal conditions, each patient should be cared for in a private room. The room should be entered through an adjoining anteroom that is used for decontamination and hand washing.

Prognosis

The overall mortality rate from the hemorrhagic fever viruses varies from 5 to 20%, although certain outbreaks, such as the Ebola and Marburg outbreaks in sub-Saharan Africa, had case-fatality rates approaching 90% [2]. Poor prognostic indicators include elevated liver enzymes, bleeding, and neurologic involvement.

References

1. Moran G, Talan D, Abrahamian F (2008) Biological terrorism. Infect Dis Clin North Am 22(1):145–187
2. Jahrling PB, Marty AM, Geisbert TW (2007) Viral hemorrhagic fevers. In: Dembek ZF (ed) Medical aspects of biological warfare. Office of the Surgeon General, Washington, DC, pp 271–310, http://www.bordeninstitute.army.mil/published_volumes/biological_warfare/biological.html. Accessed 25 Jul 2009
3. Darling R, Catlett C, Huebner K, Jarrett D (2002) Threats in bioterrorism. I: CDC category A agents. Emerg Med Clin North Am 20 (2):273–309
4. Borio L, Inglesby T, Peters CJ, Schmaljohn AL, Hughes JM, Jahrling PB et al (2002) Hemorrhagic fever viruses as biological weapons: medical and public health management. JAMA 287(18):2391–2405

Biological Terrorism, Plague

GREGORY J. MORAN, RAUL EASTON-CARR
Department of Emergency Medicine, Olive View-UCLA Medical Center, Sylmar, CA, USA

Synonyms
Bioterrorism; Bubonic plague; Yersinia pestis

Definition
Plague is an infectious disease caused by the pleomorphic gram-negative bacillus *Yersinia pestis*. Bubonic plague is the most common naturally occurring form. It is a zoonotic infection spread from the rodent reservoir to humans through the bites of infected fleas. Plague, like anthrax, also has a pneumonic form that can be transmitted through inhalation of droplets spread by cough. *Y. pestis* has potential to be used as an agent of bioterrorism, most likely, via inhalation. As with anthrax, the pneumonic form of the disease is far more dangerous. Plague is more difficult to use as a biological weapon compared with anthrax because *Y. pestis* is susceptible to drying, heat, and ultraviolet light. However, unlike anthrax, secondary cases may result from person-to-person transmission with as little as 1–10 *Y. pestis* organisms being sufficient to cause infection by respiratory or parenteral routes.

Clinical Presentation
Bubonic plague begins as painful adenopathy, usually 2–8 days after the infecting flea bite. Between 4% and 10% of patients will have a pustule or ulcer at the site of inoculation. Common initial symptoms in decreasing order of incidence include malaise, headache, vomiting, chills, altered mental status, cough, abdominal pain, and chest pain [1]. Other findings include bladder distention, apathy, confusion, anxiety, oliguria, anuria, tachycardia, hypotension, leukocytosis, and fever. By the day following the onset of symptoms, patients begin to develop visible swollen, painful, tender lymph nodes, usually in the groin, axilla, or cervical region. These nodes are commonly called buboes. They are extremely tender, warm, nonfluctuant nodes associated with overlying skin erythema and often surrounding edema [2].

Septicemic plague may be the primary manifestation of plague, or it may arise secondarily to hematogenous dissemination. Sepsis caused by plague presents similarly to that caused by other gram-negative organisms.

Symptoms include fever, chills, sweats, nausea, vomiting, diarrhea, and it eventually may progress to acral cyanosis and disseminated intravascular coagulation [1]. Patients in the terminal stages of septicemic or pneumonic plague can develop large ecchymoses on the back, possibly leading to this disease being referred to as "the Black Death." Due to the nonspecific presentation of primary septicemic plague, diagnosis may be delayed compared to bubonic plague, thus contributing to a higher mortality. Approximately 5–15% of patients will develop a secondary pneumonia that can spread plague through droplets from coughing.

Pneumonic plague, like septicemic plague, may occur primarily by exposure to aerosols or by hematogenous dissemination. Pneumonic plague would be the most likely presentation after a bioterrorism attack, as the agent would be most effectively spread to large numbers of individuals via aerosol [3–5]. After an incubation period of 1–6 days, patients who have pneumonic plague typically develop fulminant pneumonia characterized by dyspnea, chest pain, malaise, high fever, cough, hemoptysis, and septicemia with ecchymoses and extremity necrosis. Findings on chest radiographs are generally typical of patients who have pneumonia, although bilateral alveolar infiltrates may be the most common finding [1]. The disease progresses rapidly, leading to dyspnea, stridor, cyanosis, and septic shock. Death results from respiratory failure and circulatory collapse.

Plague meningitis is most commonly seen in children, usually 9–14 days after ineffective treatment [1]. The presentation is similar to meningitis caused by other bacterial etiologies.

Treatment and Prophylaxis

Early treatment with antibiotics, within 24 h of the appearance of symptoms, is crucial to the survival of patients who have pneumonic plague. Streptomycin (15 mg/kg IM twice daily) is the traditional preferred agent but may not be readily available in some facilities. Gentamicin (5 mg/kg IV/IM once daily) may be similarly efficacious and more readily available [1, 2]. Doxycycline (100 mg IV twice daily or 200 mg IV once daily), ciprofloxacin (400 mg IV twice daily), and chloramphenicol (25 mg/kg IV four times daily) should also be effective [1, 5]. Chloramphenicol has been suggested as the preferred treatment for plague meningitis due to its theoretical ability to better penetrate the blood–brain barrier; however, this has not been confirmed by clinical trials [2]. Treatment should be continued for a minimum

of 10 days, or for 4 days after clinical recovery, whichever is longer. Pregnant patients should be treated with gentamicin or doxycycline if gentamicin is not available. Although both gentamicin and doxycycline are potentially teratogenic, aminoglycosides are the most effective treatment for plague and a large case-control study of doxycycline in pregnancy showed no teratogenic risk to the fetus [2]. Given the high potential mortality rate of bubonic plague, its use in this setting likely justifies the risk. Patients who have mild illness can be treated with oral doxycycline or fluoroquinolones [5].

Prophylaxis

Persons exposed to plague should receive postexposure prophylaxis with oral doxycycline (100 mg twice daily) or ciprofloxacin (500 mg twice daily) for 7 days [1, 2, 5]. Doxycycline is recommended as prophylaxis for children and pregnant women [2]. Medical personnel who practice good infection control precautions should not require prophylaxis. A recombinant vaccine is under development and seems to protect against pneumonic plague.

Several mammals are known to harbor plague, including bears, cats, pigs, mice, rats, prairie dogs, and squirrels, with cats being particularly efficient at transmitting the disease to humans [1]. While no specific recommendations are made regarding these animal vectors, this knowledge may target antibiotic prophylaxis.

Evaluation and Assessment

As with other bioterrorism agents, generally, the diagnosis must be suspected on clinical grounds for treatment to be initiated in time to be beneficial. Once suspected, a presumptive diagnosis can often be made by identifying *Y. pestis* in Gram's, Wayson's, or Wright–Giemsa stain of blood, sputum, or lymph node aspirate samples. The organism has a characteristic bipolar "safety pin" appearance (Fig. 1). A definitive diagnosis is generally made with culture studies. An ELISA test for plague exists, but it is not widely available. Direct fluorescent antibody staining of the capsular antigen is also available.

Buboes may be aspirated with a small-gauge needle for diagnostic purposes, but incision and drainage should not be performed because of the risk for aerosolization of the organism [5]. Sputum samples in pneumonic plague may contain gram-negative rods, but the yield is variable [1].

Hematologic studies show leukocytosis with left shift. Bilirubin levels and serum aminotransferases are often elevated. Antibody studies are not useful for diagnosing disease during the acute phase. Blood, sputum, bubo

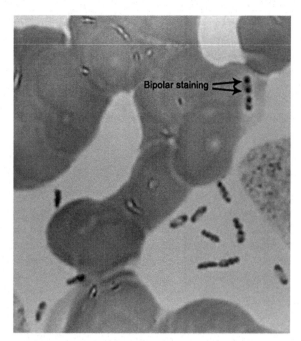

Biological Terrorism, Plague. Figure 1 *Yersinia pestis.* Giemsa stain of blood smear (Source: American Society for Microbiology. Available at: http://archive.microbelibrary.org/ASMOnly/Details.asp?ID=1423)

Septicemic plague can result in disseminated intravascular coagulation, small vessel necrosis, purpura, and gangrene of the nose and digits [2]. In a group of patients in New Mexico with plague, mortality was 33.3% for septicemic plague compared to 11.5% for bubonic plague [1]. Without treatment, the mortality rate approaches 100% [4].

Pneumonic plague is rapidly fatal unless antibiotics are administered during the first day of illness [1].

References

1. Worsham PL, McGovern TW, Vietri NJ, Friedlander AM (2007) Plague. In: Dembek ZF (ed) Medical aspects of biological warfare. Office of the Surgeon General, Washington, DC, 2007:91–119, http://www.bordeninstitute.army.mil/published_volumes/biological_warfare/biological.html. Accessed 25 Jul 2009
2. Inglesby T, Dennis D, Henderson D, Bartlett J, Ascher M, Eitzen E et al (2000) Plague as a biological weapon: medical and public health management. JAMA 283(17):2281–2290
3. Darling R, Catlett C, Huebner K, Jarrett D (2002) Threats in bioterrorism. Emerg Med Clin N Am 20(2):273–309
4. Bossi P, Garin D, Guihot A, Gay F, Crance J, Debord T et al (2006) Bioterrorism: management of major biological agents. Cell Mol Life Sci 63(19–20):2196–2212
5. Moran G, Talan D, Abrahamian F (2008) Biological terrorism. Infect Dis Clin North Am 22(1):145–187, vii

aspirate, and CSF cultures on normal blood agar media are often negative at 24 h but positive by 48 h. The colonies of *Y. pestis* are usually 1–3 mm in diameter and have been described as having a "beaten copper" or "hammered metal" appearance.

After-care

Unlike pulmonary anthrax, pneumonic plague is very contagious. Strict respiratory isolation is necessary until infected patients have undergone treatment for at least 3 days [3, 5]. Unfortunately, because the initial presentation resembles that of severe pneumonia caused by other agents, the actual diagnosis may not be known for several days. Therefore, patients who present with fulminant pneumonia after a suspected biological attack should be held in respiratory isolation until the cause has been determined. Bubonic plague in humans, without secondary pneumonia, is not considered to be contagious [4].

Prognosis

Without treatment, the mortality rate for bubonic plague is 60% [1, 4], while some studies suggest that with appropriate treatment, mortality may be as low as 5–14% [2, 4]. With appropriate treatment, buboes typically resolve in 10–14 days [3].

Biological Terrorism, Smallpox

GREGORY J. MORAN, RAUL EASTON-CARR
Department of Emergency Medicine, Olive View-UCLA Medical Center, Sylmar, CA, USA

Synonyms

Bioterrorism; Poxvirus; Variola virus

Definition

Smallpox (variola) is a DNA orthopoxvirus that was a common cause of serious illness throughout recorded human history. No nonhuman reservoirs or human carriers exist for smallpox; the disease was spread only through continual person-to-person transmission. The disease was declared eradicated by the World Health Organization (WHO) in 1980 and routine vaccination was stopped soon after.

Because of its suitability for airborne dispersal, propensity for secondary human-to-human transmission, relative stability, and retention of infectivity outside the host, smallpox is one of the most feared agents that could be unleashed in a biological attack [1]. Because routine vaccination is no longer given, most persons today are susceptible to infection. Even those who were vaccinated as children are likely to be susceptible because immunity wanes over time.

Clinical Presentation

The incubation period associated with smallpox is approximately 12 days (range 9–14 days). Smallpox begins with a febrile prodrome, followed by viremia and a rash that may also be accompanied by malaise, chills, head and body aches, nausea, vomiting, and abdominal pain [2]. Fifteen percent of patients develop delirium [3]. The characteristic rash develops on the extremities and spreads centrally. Skin lesions evolve slowly from macules to papules to vesicles to pustules, with each stage lasting 1–2 days. Unlike chickenpox, all smallpox lesions are at the same stage of development.

The first lesions are often on the oral mucosa or palate, face, or forearms. The vesicles or pustules tend to be distributed with the greatest concentration on the face and distal extremities, including the palms and soles. Vesicles and pustules are deep-seated, firm, or hard, round, well-circumscribed lesions; they are sharply raised and feel like small round objects embedded under the skin. As they evolve, the lesions may become umbilicated or confluent and will scab over in 1–2 weeks, leaving hypopigmented scars.

If a biological attack is not known to have occurred, some early smallpox cases are likely to be mistaken for chickenpox or other diseases. Chickenpox differs from smallpox in that the prodrome is milder, the vesicles are superficial (i.e., easily collapse on puncture) and more heavily distributed on the trunk as opposed to the distal extremities, and active and healing lesions occur simultaneously.

Treatment and Prophylaxis

No known effective treatment exists against smallpox. The drug cidofovir, used to treat cytomegalovirus infections, may be active against variola virus, but no data currently show the drug's efficacy in humans [4]. Gleevec (imatinib), a drug traditionally used to treat certain leukemias, has been suggested as a possible treatment due to its observed ability to slow viral progression in mice; however, no human studies have been done [3]. Management of smallpox is largely supportive care.

A vaccine based on the live vaccinia virus is effective for immunizing against smallpox and has been the mainstay of smallpox control. Unlike many other vaccines,

smallpox vaccine can be effective in preventing disease even up to several days after exposure.

Smallpox vaccination is not without risk. Risks are higher for those who have never been previously vaccinated. Complications from the use of the current smallpox (vaccinia) vaccine range from the relatively benign autoinoculation and generalized vaccinia through the more severe progressive vaccinia. The most serious complications include postvaccinial encephalopathy and encephalitis, but fortunately, these are rare [4]. Because vaccinia is a live virus, potential exists for secondary transmission after vaccination. In the era of routine smallpox vaccination, contraindications to vaccination included pregnancy, certain immunocompromised conditions, and eczema. In the setting of a bioterrorism-related smallpox outbreak, those believed to have been exposed to the virus would have no absolute contraindications to vaccination since the benefit would likely outweigh the risk.

Health-care workers would be prioritized for smallpox vaccination in the event of a bioterrorism-related outbreak. Optimal infection-control practices and appropriate site care should prevent transmission of vaccinia virus from vaccinated individuals to others. Health-care personnel providing direct patient care should keep their vaccination sites covered with gauze in combination with a semipermeable membrane dressing to absorb exudates and provide a barrier for containment of vaccinia virus to minimize the risk of transmission. The dressing should also be covered by a layer of clothing.

Patients should be isolated with both airborne and contact precautions, and considered infectious until all scabs separate [3].

Evaluation and Assessment

The United States Centers for Disease Control and Prevention (CDC) have an excellent website (http://www.bt.cdc.gov/agent/smallpox/diagnosis/riskalgorithm/) to assist clinicians in the early diagnosis of a rash suspicious for smallpox. The algorithm can be used to quickly identify patients at risk of smallpox when an outbreak is not known.

The diagnosis of smallpox can be confirmed with electron microscopy or gel diffusion on vesicular scrapings, but these modalities are not available in most hospital laboratories. If smallpox is suspected, the laboratory must be notified to take proper precautions. Smallpox specimens should be handled under biosafety level four conditions. Because testing for varicella virus is usually available, a vesicular eruption in which varicella cannot be identified should alert clinicians to possible smallpox. Specimens could then be forwarded for testing at a specialized laboratory, such as at the CDC or U.S. Army Medical Research Institute of Infectious Diseases (USAMRIID).

Electron microscopy cannot reliably differentiate between variola, vaccinia (cowpox), and monkeypox. New polymerase chain reaction (PCR) techniques that can rapidly diagnose smallpox may soon be available.

After-care

Identification of even a single case of smallpox would signal an infectious disease emergency of worldwide significance. Clinicians who suspect smallpox should immediately contact their local health department and their hospital infection-control officer. If an initial outbreak cannot be contained within a single community, an arduous worldwide eradication effort may need to be begun anew.

Smallpox is readily transmitted person-to-person through respiratory droplets. Because delays in the initial diagnosis are likely, some secondary exposures may already have occurred by the time smallpox virus is identified as the cause of illness. Although people are generally not considered infectious until the rash begins, they can shed virus in early stages of the rash before it can be readily identified as smallpox.

Aggressive quarantine measures will be necessary to prevent further spread. Anyone who has had direct contact with an infected person should undergo strict quarantine with respiratory isolation for 17 days. In large-scale outbreaks, infected individuals may need to be kept at home.

Virions can also remain viable on fomites for up to 1 week. All laundry, including bedding of infected individuals, should be autoclaved or washed in hot water with bleach. Standard hospital antiviral surface cleaners are adequate for disinfecting surfaces (e.g., counters, floors). Viable virus has been found in scabs that have been stored for up to 13 years, so meticulous decontamination is crucial. If possible, all bodies should be cremated to prevent subsequent exposure of individuals who have had contact with the deceased, such as funeral home workers.

Prognosis

Mortality for variola major, the more severe form of the disease, is reported as approximately 30% overall among unvaccinated persons and 3% among those vaccinated, but this reflects historical data in populations without modern medical care. Mortality is higher in infants and elderly individuals, and would likely be much lower among healthy adults and older children. Death occurs late in the first week or during the second week of the illness and is caused by the toxemia induced by the overwhelming viremia.

There is a rare hemorrhagic form seen in less than 3% of all smallpox patients which is associated with extensive petechie, toxemia, and massive bleeding into the skin and gastrointestinal tract followed almost universally by death within a few days. This form occurs more commonly in pregnant patients and small children [3, 4]. Other described complications include bacterial superinfection (more common in the preantibiotic era), arthritis, osteomyelitis, pulmonary edema (more common in the hemorrhagic form), orchitis, encephalitis, and keratitis [3].

Variola minor, the less severe form of the disease, carries a 1% mortality in the vaccinated and unvaccinated alike [5].

References

1. Henderson D, Inglesby T, Bartlett J, Ascher M, Eitzen E, Jahrling P et al (1999) Smallpox as a biological weapon: medical and public health management. Working Group on Civilian Biodefense. JAMA 281(22):2127–2137
2. Henderson D (1999) Smallpox: clinical and epidemiologic features. Emerg Infect Dis 5(4):537–539
3. Jahrling PB, Huggins JW, Ibrahim MS, Lawler JV, Martin JW (2007) Smallpox and related orthopoxviruses. In: Dembek ZF (ed) Medical aspects of biological warfare. Office of the Surgeon General, Washington, DC, pp 215–240, http://www.bordeninstitute.army.mil/published_volumes/biological_warfare/biological.html. Accessed 25 Jul 2009
4. Moran G, Talan D, Abrahamian F (2008) Biological terrorism. Infect Dis Clin North Am 22(1):145–187, vii
5. Darling R, Catlett C, Huebner K, Jarrett D (2002) Threats in bioterrorism. I: CDC category A agents. Emerg Med Clin North Am 20(2):273–309

Biological Terrorism, Tularemia

GREGORY J. MORAN, RAUL EASTON-CARR
Department of Emergency Medicine, Olive View-UCLA Medical Center, Sylmar, CA, USA

Synonyms

Bioterrorism; Deer fly fever; Francisella tularensis; Rabbit fever

Definition

Tularemia is a disease caused by *Francisella tularensis*, an aerobic intracellular gram-negative coccobacillus. *F. tularensis* remains viable for weeks in water, soil, carcasses, and hides, and for years in frozen meat. It is easily killed by heat and disinfectants, but can survive for months in temperatures of freezing and below.

F tularensis has been weaponized by both the United States and the former Soviet Union [1], and other countries are also suspected to have weaponized the organism [2]. F tularensis could potentially be stabilized for weaponization and produced in either a wet or dried form for delivery in a terrorist attack [3]. As few as 10–50 organisms may cause disease if inhaled or injected into skin; however, approximately 10^8 organisms are required to cause infection after oral ingestion.

Tularemia is considered to have the potential to be an especially effective bioterror weapon due to its nonspecific disease presentation, high morbidity, significant mortality if untreated, limited ability to obtain a rapid diagnosis, and the potential to develop antibiotic-resistant strains which may make standard treatments ineffective [1].

Clinical Presentation

Tularemia can manifest in several ways, depending on the route of infection and organ systems involved. These presentations are typically divided into ulceroglandular, oculoglandular, glandular, oropharyngeal, typohoidal, and pneumonic tularemia. Any of these types may progress into septic shock known as septic tularemia, which will not be considered here as a separate entity.

Ulceroglandular Tularemia

Ulceroglandular tularemia resulting from contact with infected animals is the most common form, accounting for up to 85% of cases. After an incubation period of 3–6 days, patients typically present with fever, chills, headache, cough, and myalgias (in decreasing order of incidence). There is usually associated malaise, an ulcerated skin lesion, and painful regional lymphadenopathy. Skin ulcers typically begin in the area of exposure to the organism, most commonly on the hands. The ulcers range in size from 0.4 to 3.0 cm and occasionally have raised borders. Pulse-temperature dissociation has also been reported, although this sign is neither sensitive nor specific for tularemia. Other nonspecific complaints include chest pain, vomiting, arthralgias, sore throat, abdominal pain, diarrhea, dysuria, back pain, and nuchal rigidity [1].

Oculoglandular Tularemia

Oculoglandular tularemia is distinguished from the ulceroglandular form by ocular erythema and exudative conjunctivitis. Otherwise, it is quite similar to ulceroglandular tularemia. It is typically acquired through contact with infected animals, although it has also been reported with exposure to contaminated food or water.

Glandular Tularemia

Although ulceroglandular and oculoglandular tularemia typically present with ulcerative skin lesions, there is also a form referred to as glandular tularemia which is similar to the two presentations described above, with the exception of skin lesions. This syndrome typically includes lymphadenopathy greater than 1 cm [1].

Oropharyngeal Tularemia

While pharyngitis has been observed in approximately one quarter of patients with tularemia, oropharyngeal tularemia as a separate entity is recognized by the predominance of a severe exudative pharyngitis as opposed to the nonspecific and mild symptoms of pharyngitis seen with the other forms. This form typically results from the ingestion of contaminated food or water.

Pneumonic Tularemia

Lower respiratory tract symptoms are present in 47–95% of patients with tularemia of any type. There is also a distinct pneumonic form which can result a few days to several months after the appearance of non-pulmonary symptoms in ulceroglandular or glandular tularemia [1]. This form is characterized by an abrupt onset of fever, headache, sore throat, malaise, myalgia, coryza, and cough. Chest radiograph findings are nonspecific, and may be confused with other bacterial pneumonias, tuberculosis, lymphoma, or lung carcinomas. Pulmonary disease from a naturally occurring tularemia outbreak is uncommon, and if a significant number of cases are reported, it would be highly suspicious for a bioterrorism attack [1].

Typhoidal Tularemia

Typhoidal tularemia, which is caused by infectious aerosols, is the form most likely to appear after a terrorist attack. After an incubation period of 2–10 days, most victims present with fever, headache, chills, myalgia, nausea, vomiting, and diarrhea. Lymphadenopathy is not necessarily present. Patients may also have cough and other respiratory symptoms.

Treatment

The Working Group on Civilian Biodefense [3] describes various treatments for tularemia in both contained and mass casualty settings for adults, children, and pregnant women. Their recommendations are summarized below Table 1.

Treatment with streptomycin, gentamicin, or ciprofloxacin should continue for 10 days. Treatment with doxycycline or chloramphenicol should continue for 14–21 days. A 2-week course should be effective as postexposure prophylaxis when given within 24 h of aerosol exposure. A live attenuated vaccine against tularemia is in development [4].

Evaluation and Assessment

Initial laboratory evaluations are generally nonspecific. These nonspecific signs and symptoms would make a specific diagnosis of tularemia difficult in the event of a terrorist attack, possibly leading to increased mortality. A definitive diagnosis can be made by culturing the organism from blood, ulcers, conjunctival exudates, sputum, gastric washings, and pharyngeal exudates, although culture is difficult and the yield is low. The organism grows poorly on standard media, but can be grown on media containing cysteine or other sulfhydryl compounds (e.g., glucose cysteine blood agar, thioglycollate broth). The laboratory should be notified if tularemia is suspected because the organism requires specialized culture techniques and represents a hazard to laboratory personnel. Culture should only be attempted using biosafety level 3 precautions. Tularemia is usually diagnosed serologically using bacterial agglutination or ELISA. Antibodies to *F. tularensis* appear within the first week of infection, but levels adequate to allow confidence in the specificity of the serologic diagnosis (titer > 1:160) do not appear until more than 2 weeks after infection. Cross-reactions can occur with other organisms, such as Brucella, Proteus, and Yersinia. Because antibodies may persist for years after infection, serologic diagnosis depends on a fourfold or greater increase in the tularemia tube agglutination or microagglutination titer during the course of the illness. Titers are usually negative during the first week of infection, become positive during the second week in 50–70% of cases, and achieve a maximum level in 4–8 weeks.

Although person-to-person transmission of tularemia is rare, health-care personnel should follow standard universal precautions whenever managing patients who have the disease.

Prognosis

Tularemia can be quite lethal, with case fatality rates of untreated naturally acquired typhoidal tularemia being about 35% [2]. However, with prompt and appropriate

Biological Terrorism, Tularemia. Table 1 Recommendations for the treatment and prevention of Tularemia

| | Contained casualty setting | | Mass casualty setting or PEP* |
	Preferred agents	Alternative agents	Preferred agents
Adults	Streptomycin 1 g IM once daily, or	Doxycycline 100 mg IV once daily, or	Doxycycline 100 mg PO twice daily, or
	Gentamicin 5 mg/kg IV/IM once daily	Chloramphenicol 15 mg/kg IV 4 times daily, or	Ciprofloxacin 500 mg PO twice daily
		Ciprofloxacin 400 mg IV twice daily	
Children	Streptomycin 15 mg/kg IM twice daily (<2 g/day), or	Doxycycline: <45 kg, 2.2 mg/kg IV twice daily. >45 kg 100 mg IV twice daily, or	Doxycycline: <45 kg, 2.2 mg/kg PO twice daily. >45 kg 100 mg PO twice daily, or
	Gentamicin 2.5 mg/kg IV/IM three times daily	Chloramphenicol 15 mg/kg IV 4 times daily, or	Ciprofloxacin 15 mg/kg PO twice daily
		Ciprofloxacin 15 mg/kg IV twice daily	
Pregnant women	Gentamicin 5 mg/kg IV/IM once daily, or	Doxycycline 100 mg IV twice daily, or	Ciprofloxacin 500 mg PO twice daily, or
	Streptomycin 1 g IM once daily	Ciprofloxacin 400 mg IV twice daily, or	Doxycycline 100 mg PO twice daily

Adapted from [3]

*PE postexposure prophylaxis

antibiotic treatment mortality rates of 1–2.5% have been reported. This rate varies depending on the type of infection, premorbid conditions, and the time interval between infection and the initiation of appropriate antimicrobial therapy [1].

References

1. Hepburn MJ, Friedlander AM, Dembek ZF (2007) Tularemia. In: Dembek ZF (ed) Textbooks of military medicine: medical aspects of biological warfare. Borden Institute, Washington, DC, pp 167–184, Available at: http://www.bordeninstitute.army.mil/published_volumes/biological_warfare/biological.html. Accessed 25 Jul 2009
2. Moran G, Talan D, Abrahamian F (2008) Biological terrorism. Infect Dis Clin North Am 22(1):145–187, vii
3. Dennis DT, Inglesby TV, Henderson DA, Bartlett JG, Ascher MS, Eitzen E et al (2001) Tularemia as a biological weapon: medical and public health management. JAMA 285(21):2763–2773
4. Mann BJ, Ark NM (2009) Rationally designed Tularemia vaccines. Expert Rev Vaccines 8(7):877–885

Biomarkers

The characteristic biological properties that can be detected and measured in parts of the body like the blood or tissue. They may indicate either normal or diseased processes in the body.

Biopsy by Thoracotomy

▶ Bronchial Fibroscopy and Lung Biopsy

Bioreactance®

Pierre Squara[1], Daniel Burkhoff[2]
[1]CERIC – ICU, Clinique Ambroise Paré,
Neuilly-sur-Seine, France
[2]Department of Medicine, Columbia University,
New York, NY, USA

Definition

Bioreactance® refers to the electrical resistive, capacitive, and inductive properties of blood and biological tissue that induce phase shifts between an applied electrical current and the resulting voltage signal [1]. This is distinguished from *bioimpedance*, which refers to the electrical properties of blood and tissue that determine the amplitude of the voltage field resulting from an applied electrical current. Bioreactance has proved to be useful clinically because changes in thoracic blood volume occurring during the heartbeat induce instantaneous changes in the phase shift between an applied current and the measured voltage signal that can be quantitatively related to stroke volume and thus can be used to measure cardiac output.

Signal Analysis

In practice, four double-electrode stickers are placed on the chest wall (Fig. 1).

The exact location of the electrodes is not critical, but the goal is to place the stickers so as to encase the heart and thoracic aorta. Typically, the electrodes are placed in the mid clavicular line, two at the level of the clavicles and two just below the lower margin of the rib cage. For certain applications, electrodes can be placed on the side (e.g., during surgery to be outside of the surgical field) or on the back (e.g., during exercise testing so that arm movement is not impeded). The electrodes are connected by wires to the signal processor that delivers an electrical current ($I(t)$) of known amperage and frequency between the outer set of electrodes, measures the voltage ($V(t)$) between the inner two sets of electrodes and analyzes the phase shift between the current and voltage signals. The phase shift varies instantaneously in relation to the amount of blood ejected by the heart in the aorta, which varies during the cardiac cycle.

An example of the Bioreactance signal in relation to the electrocardiogram and a directly measured aortic flow signal is shown in Fig. 2. As seen, the phase signal (Φ) increases once flow starts in the aorta (refer to the AoF signal), reaching a peak at approximately the end of ejection. Since Φ varies in relation to the volume of blood in the aorta, it follows that the derivative of the phase signal ($d\Phi/dt$) resembles the aortic flow signal, which indeed is the case. It is seen that the positive portion of the $d\Phi/dt$ signal (the portion above the zero line shown in red) is in phase with the aortic flow signal and these two signals start and end at approximately the same time. Once ejection is complete, the $d\Phi/dt$ signal becomes negative, reflecting the discharge of blood stored in the aorta during diastole.

One of the advantages of the Bioreactance approach is that analysis of phase shifts can be done with very high precision while allowing a high degree of filtering of electrical noise, be it from ambient signals from other

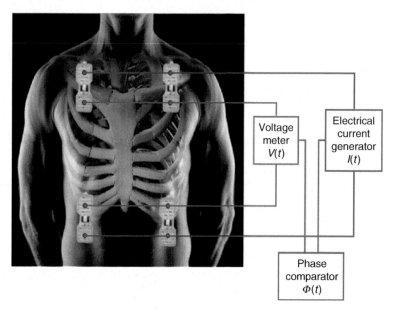

Bioreactance®. Figure 1 Typical electrode position and schematic representation of Bioreactance technology

electronic devices or due to patient movement. As a result, the signal-to-noise ratio is very high with Bioreactance compared to other electrical approaches that are based on analysis of voltage amplitudes.

From Transthoracic Bioreactance to Cardiac Output

The basic assumption underlying transformation from the measurement of Bioreactance signals to estimation of cardiac output is that the area under the positive portion of the $d\Phi/dt$ signal is proportional to stroke volume (SV) (Fig. 3).

Since the $d\Phi/dt$ is roughly triangular, the area under the curve is estimated from the peak value of $d\Phi/dt$ ($d\Phi/dt_{max}$) and the duration of ejection (or ventricular ejection time, VET, which can be measured directly from the $d\Phi/dt$ signal) so that: SV = $CF\frac{1}{2}\cdot d\Phi/dt_{max}\cdot$VET, where CF is a correlation factor that is mainly based on body size, gender, and age. Once SV is obtained, cardiac output (CO) is determined by the heart rate (HR): CO = SV·HR. The value of the correlation factor (CF) and its variation with body size, gender, and age was initially determined in a cohort of post-cardiac surgery patients who had a pulmonary artery catheter for routine continuous cardiac output (CCO) monitoring by thermodilution. The age-, height-, weight-, and gender-dependent CF derived from these patients was then tested

prospectively in another cohort of 119 patients [2] that compared the Bioreactance system (NICOM™, Cheetah medical, Portland, OR, USA) to continuous cardiac output by pulmonary artery catheter-based thermodilution (PAC–CCO, Edwards Life Sciences, Irvine CA, USA). In these 119 post-cardiac surgery patients [2], the bias was optimally analyzed during 40 periods of stable PAC–CCO to minimize the effects of both natural changes in CO and time responsiveness differences of the two devices. This included more than 9,000 minute-by-minute CO values. The average bias was negligible (0.16 L/min) and the limits of agreement were ±0.88 L/min (Fig. 4) indicating a high degree of accuracy of Bioreactance for measuring CO compared to PAC–CCO.

Also, precision (random fluctuation) assessed by the variability of measurements around the trend line slope (2SD/mean) was always better for the NICOM than for PAC–CCO. When the 40 periods of stable CO were considered, the variability of the averaged PAC–CCO measurements (2SD) was 0.66 ± 0.20 L/min and the precision (2SD/mean) was 14% ± 4%, versus 0.62 ± 0.29 L/min and 12% ± 7% for the NICOM respectively, $p = 0.08$. When CO was consistently changing (PAC–CCO slope > ±10%), the precision was better for NICOM than PAC–CCO: 16% ± 10 versus 23% ± 9, ($p < 0.0001$) for increasing CO and 16% ± 10 versus 20% ± 7, ($p = 0.002$) for decreasing CO. Bioreactance has also been validated as a reliable method for cardiac output monitoring by

B

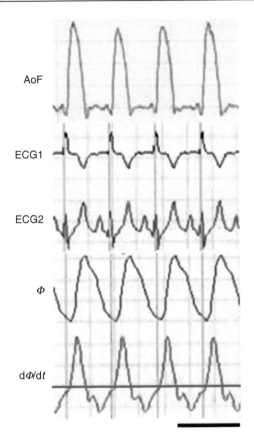

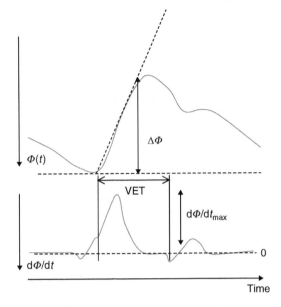

Bioreactance®. Figure 3 The upper part shows an idealized Bioreactance phase shift signa $\Phi(t)$ and its first derivative $d\Phi/dt$ with maximal value $d\Phi/dt_{max}$ and ventricular ejection time (VET)

Bioreactance®. Figure 2 Experimental recordings from an animal instrumented with an aortic flow probe and a Bioreactance system. The relation between aortic flow (AoF), the Bioreactance phase shift (Φ) and its first derivative ($d\Phi/dt$) are shown. The positive deflection of the $d\Phi/dt$ signal mimics the AoF tracing

comparison with other available technologies in different clinical situations [3, 4].

Pre-existing Condition

The only requirement for use of the Bioreactance technique is that the electrodes (stickers) be appropriately applied to the body so that there is good and stable electrical contact. Also, the wires that connect from the stickers to the electronic signal conditioner box should also be fixed (e.g., taped near the connection) to ensure stable connection.

There are certain clinical scenarios in which the technique has not been fully tested for accuracy of absolute values. This is especially the case when the relationship between change in aortic volume and stroke volume are different than encountered in a majority of patients. Such

settings include severe aortic regurgitation, thoracic aortic prosthesis, large thoracic aortic aneurysm, and intra-aortic balloon pumping. In most of these settings, it is still expected that the Bioreactance technology will appropriately track trends in cardiac output. Another potential limitation includes patients with continuous flow left ventricular assist devices where there are no aortic pulsations.

Applications

The ability to measure CO, along with other hemodynamic parameters, can play an important role in diagnosis, establishment of the optimal treatment plan, monitoring treatment effectiveness, and guiding refinement of treatment in real time to achieve therapeutic goals. Therefore, there are many situations in which information about CO is desired but use of invasive techniques are not fully justified or feasible and availability of an accurate noninvasive approach can provide significant value. These include circulatory shock (of any cause), trauma, pre-, intra- and postoperative monitoring and hemodynamic optimization for high-risk surgical procedures, in patients with heart failure (acute and chronic), during hemodialysis in patients at high risk for hemodynamic compromise and high-risk obstetric patients. Application to pediatric populations is also feasible, a setting in which CO monitoring is typically

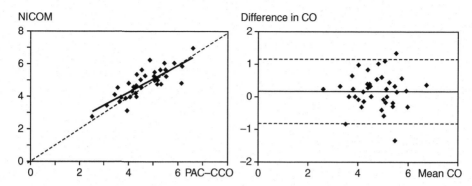

Bioreactance®. Figure 4 Accuracy of the Bioreactance (NICOM)-based cardiac output (CO) as compared to continuous thermodilution (PAC–CCO). *Left* panel correlation (*r* = 0.87) not significantly different from the identity line, *Right* panel, Bland and Altman schema showing mean bias = 0.2L and limits of agreements (2SD) = 1L (Reprinted from [2])

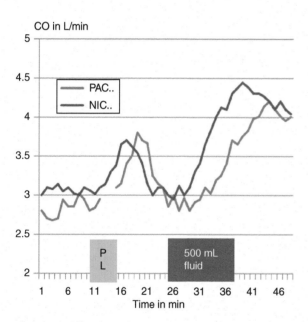

Bioreactance®. Figure 5 Continuous cardiac output: in *blue* continuous thermodilution and in *red* Bioreactance. Passive leg raise test is indicated by the *green bar* and rapid fluid infusion (500 ml) by the *blue bar*

not available especially in neonates and very small children. Other, less often considered applications include cardiac output monitoring during stress testing (especially in patients with chronic heart failure) and optimization of cardiac resynchronization therapy (CRT) devices. Settings in which these applications arise span the entire spectrum of clinical practice: outpatient clinics, emergency rooms, routine hospital wards, intensive care units, operating rooms,

and cardiac catheterization laboratories. Also, availability of noninvasive cardiac output monitoring opens many avenues for clinical research that are not otherwise feasible. An appreciation for how this approach can be helpful is illustrated by the examples shown in Fig. 5 obtained from a patient following cardiac surgery that demonstrate the responsiveness of Bioreactance-based cardiac output monitoring to standard acute hemodynamic interventions.

First, consider the response to a passive leg raise (PLR) followed by a 500 ml infusion of colloid as indicated in Fig. 5. The PLR maneuver is used by some investigators as a means of assessing fluid responsiveness. After steady state was established, the legs were raised to 45° for ~5 min. A gradual rise in CO is detected. When the legs are lowered, CO returns to baseline. The PLR maneuver has been suggested as a simple, reversible means of assessing whether or not a patient would respond to fluid administration. As seen, the COs provided by the two modalities start at nearly the same values. With the introduction of PLR and the ensuing fluid infusion, CO detected by NICOM increases almost immediately, followed by a comparable increase detected by PAC–CCO; the ~5 min delay in the PAC–CCO measurement is likely due to filters incorporated in the PAC–CCO technology. Despite this time delay, the two technologies both indicate comparable increase in CO once steady conditions are established several minutes later. Similarly the Bioreactance-based tracking of CO has been shown to be comparable to other technologies for CO monitoring during lung recruitment maneuvers using high external positive end expiratory pressure (PEEP) and for inotrope drug titration in patient with heart failure [3, 4]. Assessment of change in cardiac output in response to drugs and fluids and ability to assess fluid responsiveness provide the opportunity for

B

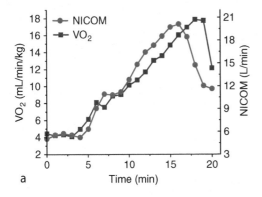
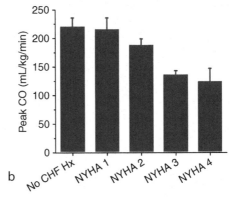

a   b

Bioreactance®. Figure 6 (**a**) Bioreactance-based measurement of CO during treadmill exercise in a heart failure patient showing parallel changes in CO and oxygen consumption (VO_2). (**b**) Peak CO during exercise declines as the clinical severity of heart failure (indexed by New York Heart Association Class) increases (Reprinted from [5])

development of goal-directed therapy (GDT) algorithms based fully on noninvasive measurements.

In addition to these examples demonstrating appropriate hemodynamic responses to standard hemodynamic interventions, data obtained during treadmill exercise testing further serve to illustrate the versatility and robustness of Bioreactance for CO measurement in challenging, complex settings (Fig. 6). During exercise, there is an almost immediate gradual rise of CO; as shown in Fig. 6a, the rise in CO very closely parallels the rise of total oxygen consumption (VO_2). Upon cessation of exercise, both CO and VO_2 decrease abruptly. When performed in a cohort of normal volunteers and patients with chronic heart failure spanning the spectrum of disease severity (from New York Heart Association Class I through IV), it is appreciated that the value of CO achieved at the peak of exercise declines with clinical severity of disease. Other indexes of cardiovascular performance (such as cardiac power and stroke work, values dependent upon measurement of stroke volume during exercise) have been shown to provide even greater ability to discriminate disease severity than peak CO or even peak VO_2, Fig. 6b. Therefore, noninvasive Bioreactance may provide a new tool for assessing disease severity, for following response to treatment and for prognostication in chronic heart failure and other cardiovascular diseases.

CO monitoring is a key component in intensive care, anesthesia, and many other clinical settings. CO and related parameters are used to guide diagnosis and decisions on fluid administration and drug titration. The NICOM Bioreactance-based technology has been proven accurate and reliable in monitoring CO in clinical studies when compared to the gold standard of continuous

cardiac output (CCO) and bolus thermodilution. The noninvasiveness and high degree of accuracy of the NICOM device may lead to early recognition of clinical situations that call for aggressive fluid resuscitation.

References

1. Keren H, Burkhoff D, Squara P (2007) Evaluation of a noninvasive continuous cardiac output monitoring system based on thoracic bioreactance. Am J Physiol Heart Circ Physiol 293:H583–589
2. Squara P, Denjean D, Estagnasie P, Brusset A, Dib JC, Dubois C (2007) Noninvasive cardiac output monitoring (NICOM): a clinical validation. Intensive Care Med 33:1191–1194
3. Marqué S, Cariou A, Chiche J, Squara P (2009) Non invasive cardiac output monitoring (NICOM) compared to minimally invasive monitoring (VIGILEO). Crit Care 13(3):R73
4. Squara P, Rotcajg D, Denjean D, Estagnasie P, Brusset A (2009) Comparison of monitoring performance of Bioreactance vs. pulse contour during lung recruitment maneuvers. Crit Care 13:R125
5. Maurer M, Burkhoff D, Maybaum S, Franco V, Vittorio T, Williams P, White L, Kamalakkannan G, Myers J, Mancini D (2009) A multicenter study of noninvasive cardiac output by bioreactance during symptom-limited exercise. J Card Fail 15:689–699. Epub 2009 Jun 2018

Bioterrorism

- ▶ Biological Terrorism, Anthrax
- ▶ Biological Terrorism, Botulinum Toxin
- ▶ Biological Terrorism, Hemorrhagic Fever
- ▶ Biological Terrorism, Plague
- ▶ Biological Terrorism, Smallpox
- ▶ Biological Terrorism, Tularemia

Bioterrorism Agent

An organism characterized by easy dissemination, high mortality rate, potential to cause public panic and social disruption, and the necessity of special action for public health preparedness.

BIS Monitoring System

Rolf Dembinski
Klinik für Operative Intensivmedizin,
Universitätsklinikum Aachen, Aachen, Germany

Synonyms
Bispectral Index (BIS) Monitoring

Definition
BIS monitoring is one method to control anesthetic depth by continuous automated analysis of the Electroencephalogram (EEG). In 1996, the US American Food and Drug Administration approved BIS monitoring as an accepted adjunct measure of the hypnotic effect of anesthetics and sedative drugs. Today, BIS monitoring is the most frequently used system of EEG monitoring during general anesthesia and is presently applied in intensive care units and some emergency departments as well. However, there is no official recommendation to use BIS monitoring routinely in clinical practice.

Conventional Clinical Assessment of Anesthetic Depth
Since the introduction of general anesthesia into clinical practice in 1846, the assessment of anesthetic drug effects is challenging due to the complexity of brain function, drug effects, individual response variability, and clinical requirements during surgical procedures.

It has to be taken into account in this context that adequate anesthetic depth is not only characterized by ▶ sedation but also by ▶ analgesia and for numerous interventions by muscle relaxation as well. Therefore, it is difficult to define but even more demanding to assess and control the optimal anesthetic depth.

In the early years, anesthesia was induced and maintained with only one inhalational anesthetic such as nitrous oxide, ether, or chloroform. However, due to pharmacodynamic properties high doses of a single anesthetic drug had to be administered to achieve adequate sedative, analgesic, and relaxant effects. Therefore, anesthesia at that time was associated with a high risk of overdosage and concomitant toxic side effects of anesthetic drugs.

With the aim to establish a clinical guide for the assessment of anesthetic depth, Arthur E. Guedel was the first to present a detailed description of different anesthetic stages (Fig. 1). Originally, his classification was solely derived from observations during ether anesthesia but in the following Guedel's classification has also been applied to anesthesia induced by other inhalational anesthetic agents.

Today, general anesthesia is usually induced and maintained by several different and more specific drugs to influence sedation, analgesia, and muscle relaxation separately according to particular requirements. This technique of balanced general anesthesia is based on the concept that administration of a mixture of small amounts of anesthetics summates the advantages but not the disadvantages of the individual components of the mixture. As a consequence, dosage and concomitant *side effects* of each drug could be clearly reduced due to the introduction of this technique. However, in the course of balanced anesthesia some of the specific characteristics of ether anesthesia such as the stage of excitement (Fig. 1) cannot be observed anymore. Nowadays, assessment of anesthetic depth by Guedel's classification is therefore no longer suitable in modern anesthesia.

Nevertheless, assessment of anesthetic depth is of course still necessary to minimize drug administration thereby further decreasing side effects, recovery time, and costs.

On the other hand, anesthetic depth should be sufficient to prevent intraoperative awareness. Until today, unintended intraoperative awareness occurs rarely but frequently during general anesthesia. Overall, intraoperative awareness occurs in 0.1–0.4% of all patients but in cardiac surgery intraoperative awareness may be observed in up to 4% and in trauma patients even in up to 11% of all cases. It is characterized by different degrees of consciousness with or without postoperative recall. In the most severe cases, patients suffer full consciousness during surgery with pain and explicit recall of intraoperative events. Frequently, these patients develop post-traumatic stress disorders lasting for years. From the patient's perspective, prevention of intraoperative awareness is therefore certainly the most important reason for precise control of anesthetic depth.

At present, most anesthesiologists rely on somatic signs (motor response, changes in respiratory pattern)

Stage I (Stage of Analgesia or the stage of disorientation)
from beginning of induction of anesthesia to loss of consciousness.

Stage II (Stage of Excitement of the stage of Delirium)
from loss of consciousness to onset of automatic breathing.
➤ Eyelash reflex disappear but other reflexes remain intact and coughing, vomiting and struggling may occur; respiration can be irregular with breath-holding.

Stage III (Stage of Surgical anesthesia)
from onset of automatic respiration to respiratory paralysis.
• *Plane I* : from onset of automatic respiration to cessation of eyeball movements. Eyelid reflex is lost, swallowing reflex disappears, marked eyeball movement may occur but conjunctival reflex is lost at the bottom of the plane
• *Plane II* : from cessation of eyeball movements to beginning of paralysis of intercostal muscles. Laryngeal reflex is lost although inflammation of the upper respiratory tract increases reflex irritability, corneal reflex disappears, secretion of tears increases (a useful sign of light anesthesia), respiration is automatic and regular, movement and deep breathing as a response to skin stimulation disappears.
• *Plane III* : from beginning to completion of intercostal muscle paralysis. Diaphragmatic respiration persists but there is progressive intercostal paralysis, pupils dilated and light reflex is abolished. The laryngeal reflex lost in plane II can still be initiated by painful stimuli arising from the dilatation of anus or cervix. This was the desired plane for surgery when muscle relaxants were not used.
• *Plane IV* : from complete intercostal paralysis to diaphragmatic paralysis (apnoea).

Stage IV
from stoppage of respiration till death.
➤ Anesthetic overdose cause medullary paralysis with respiratory arrest and vasomotor collapse. Pupils are widely dilated and muscles are relaxed.

BIS Monitoring System. Figure 1 Guedel's classification

and autonomic signs (tachycardia, hypertension, lacrimation, and sweating) to guide the dosage of anesthetic agents. These signs have also been used to develop a clinical scoring system, presented by Evans and coworkers in 1983 (Fig. 2): According to this score, a sum of 2 and more score points denotes that anesthesia is too light and should be deepened. Furthermore, somatic signs are still used to describe the potency of inhaled anesthetics until today: Thus, one of the most important pharmacologic variables of inhaled anesthetics is the minimum alveolar concentration (MAC), which is defined as the alveolar gas concentration that is needed to prevent motor response in 50% of subjects in response to a surgical stimulus.

However, clinical somatic and autonomic signs provide only a poor correlation to the conscious state of anesthetized patients or to the likelihood of awareness because somatic signs may be depressed or even completely interrupted by muscle relaxation and autonomic signs may be considerably influenced by widely used cardiovascular drugs such as ▶ beta-blockers. Therefore, the use of these clinical signs in judging dosage of anesthetic agents can also lead to either overdosage or underdosage, which can result in adverse effects due to too deep or too light anesthesia.

Index	Condition	Score
Systolic blood pressure	<control + 10%	0
	<control + 20%	1
	>control + 20%	2
Heart rate	<control + 10%	0
	<control + 20%	1
	>control + 20%	2
Sweating	Nil	0
	Skin moist to touch	1
	Visible beads of sweat	2
Tears	No excess tears in open eye	0
	Excess tears in open eye	1
	Tears overflow closed eye	2

BIS Monitoring System. Figure 2 Evans' classification

Goals of Alternative Methods for the Assessment of Anesthetic Depth

According to the problems described above, alternative methods for the assessment of anesthetic depth should meet several requirements:

• A clear relationship between anesthetic dosage and subsequent response by the assessment system
• Independency of the anesthetic drug

- Reliable results during induction, maintenance, and recovery of anesthesia
- Detection of intraoperative awareness
- Prevention of over- and underdosage
- Detection of malfunction
- Little costs for acquisition and support

EEG-Derived Assessment of Anesthetic Depth

Electroencephalography, EEG

Electroencephalography (EEG) is the recording of cerebral electrical activity from multiple electrodes placed on the scalp, displayed in waves typically changing in amplitude and frequency in correlation to the state of consciousness (Fig. 3). Accordingly, typical EEG changes have been described during general anesthesia: Waves slow down, shift to lower frequencies, and become closely synchronized with one another. In a relaxed state before induction of anesthesia there is an alpha wave predominance. Light anesthesia is accompanied by a decrease in alpha and increase in beta waves. With deepening of anesthesia, slow delta- and theta-wave activity predominates whereas

alpha and beta activities simultaneously decrease as a sign of cortical activity depression. All these changes are usually reversed in the same order with the return of consciousness.

Processed EEG Parameters

Developed at the beginning of the twentieth century several attempts were made in the 1980s and 1990s to use EEG for the assessment of anesthetic depth. However, due to its complexity usual EEG recordings appeared not suitable to control consciousness during general anesthesia. However, various mathematical algorithms were developed to analyze specific EEG wave patterns automatically thereby simplifying the use of this technique [1].

Initially, power spectrum analyses were performed by using fast Fourier transformation to transform EEG signals in sinus waves. This transformation allows to calculate the spectral edge frequency (SEF), defined as the frequency above 95% (SEF 95) of the total power spectrum and the median frequency (MF), based on the median frequency of the EEG signal at any given moment. However, due to a lack of a clear correlation to the degree of consciousness, similar SF 95 and MF values could be obtained in awake and

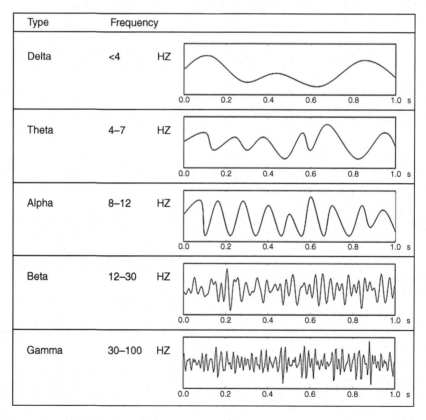

BIS Monitoring System. Figure 3 EEG wave patterns

sedated patients, these systems could finally not be implemented in clinical anesthesiology.

Later on the computer-aided topographical electroencephalometry (CATEEM) was developed providing a high-resolution topographical illustration of cerebral activity. From this technique, the spectral frequency index (SFx) was derived, a single value between 0% and 100% with normal values of more than 80% for awake subjects and a threshold value of 45% for the lose of consciousnesses. CATEEM has been used to determine the effect of neurology, anesthesia, and sleep medicine.

Entropy monitoring is another newer method based on EEG irregularity. The underlying observation of this technique is that the irregularity within an EEG signal decreases with increasing anesthetic drug effects. The calculation of two variables, a state entropy (SE) and a response entropy (RE), is suggested to provide additional information about muscle activity and upcoming arousal and awareness. Entropy monitoring is actually used in clinical anesthesiology.

Development and Features of BIS Monitoring

In view of experimental and clinical research data and contemporary use in clinical practice, BIS monitoring is the best evaluated and most popular method for EEG-derived assessment of anesthetic depth so far.

BIS monitoring is derived by the mathematical method of bispectral analysis, which provides a more complex analysis of the relationship between EEG signals when compared to power spectrum analyses with Fourier transformation alone. For clinical use, the BIS algorithm was developed in the early 1990s by multivariate analysis of numerous processed EEG signals compared to the ▶ Glasgow Coma Scale and similar scoring systems in a large number of patients and volunteers. In a first step, those variables with the best predictive value in view to a movement on surgical stimulation were included. Further analysis used additional end points such as losing consciousness and intraoperative awareness. As a result, BIS monitoring now includes analyses of the degree of high-frequency activation, the amount of low-frequency synchronization, the presence of nearly suppressed periods within the EEG, and the presence of fully suppressed, isoelectric periods. However, it should be noted that the algorithm is proprietary information, which means that details are kept secret by the company that developed it.

The analysis of processed EEG signals is transformed into one sole parameter, the BIS index, which is a 100 point index score where values close to 100 indicate the awake state, and values close to 0 indicate very deep general anesthesia (Fig. 4). Thus, the BIS index should decrease linearly with increasing doses of anesthesia. The recommended range on this scale for general anesthesia is between 40 and 60 [2].

Worth notable, the bispectral index is a work in progress. With new anesthetic agents being developed and used, the BIS algorithm is continually retested and refined. As a result, BIS monitoring has undergone several software developments since its initial release. Therefore, the reported performance of a certain BIS model might not necessarily apply to other models.

Application

Before induction of anesthesia the special BIS sensor is applied to the patient's forehead after an alcohol wipe to provide good electrical contact. The BIS sensor consists of four connected sensors, which must be applied carefully according to anatomic landmarks. No additional gels or electrodes are required. Usually, the BIS system itself is integrated into patient monitoring devices produced by a number of different manufacturers. The BIS system displays both raw data from the EEG and the BIS Index between 0 and 100.

Clinical Evidence

BIS monitoring has becoming widely used in anesthesia practice and has been evaluated in several clinical studies [3]. Taken their results together, BIS-guided anesthesia may reduce anesthetic drug requirement and recovery times for eye opening, response to verbal command, time to extubation, and orientation in the range of 2–3 min compared to controls. Moreover, BIS may shorten the length of stay in the recovery room by an average of about 7 min but could not be demonstrated to reduce

BIS Monitoring System. Figure 4 BIS Index

time to home readiness. Finally, BIS monitoring has been shown to significantly reduce the incidence of intraoperative recall awareness in surgical patients with high risk of awareness. Only two studies reported a significantly increased use of opioids or muscle relaxants due to BIS monitoring. Data on cost effectiveness are limited. However, at least total anesthetic drug costs have been shown to be lower during BIS monitoring.

Limitations

BIS monitoring does not account for all anesthetic drugs, including ketamine, nitrous oxide, and halothane [4]. Moreover, high electromyographic activity and electric device interference may create signal artifacts not necessarily being displayed as artifacts. Furthermore, data processing time produces a lag in the computation of the BIS index. Moreover, the EEG effects of anesthetic drugs are not good predictors of movement in response to a surgical stimulus because the main site of action for anesthetic drugs to prevent movement is the spinal cord. Finally, the use of BIS monitoring is not sufficiently evaluated in children.

References

1. Palanca BJA, Mashour GA, Avidan MS (2009) Processed electroencephalogram in depth of anesthesia monitoring. Curr Opin Anesthesiol 22:553–559
2. Rampil IJ (1998) A primer for EEG signal processing in anesthesia. Anesthesiology 89:980–1002
3. Punjasawadwong Y, Phongchiewboon A, Bunchungmongkol N (2009) Bispectral index for improving anaesthetic delivery and postoperative recovery. Cochrane Database Syst Rev 4:1–53
4. Dahaba AA (2005) Different Conditions That Could Result in the Bispectral Index Indicating an Incorrect Hypnotic State. Anesth Analg 101:765–773

Bispectral Index (BIS) Monitoring

▶ BIS Monitoring System

Bite Injuries

Esther H. Chen
Department of Emergency Medicine, San Francisco General Hospital, San Francisco, CA, USA

Synonyms

Animal bite wounds; Clenched-fist injury

Definition

A bite injury is defined as a skin wound that is produced by an animal's teeth (i.e., dog or cat bite) or mouthparts (i.e., insect bite) and may manifest as puncture wounds, lacerations, or crush wounds. A specific type of bite wound is the clenched-fist injury, in which the skin, and sometimes tendons, of a person's closed fist is punctured by the teeth of the person being punched.

The injury pattern of bite wounds differs between adults and children and by the type of animal. Injuries to the head, face, neck, and trunk are more commonly seen in children whereas upper-extremity injuries are more common in adults. Almost all bat bites and 84% of rodent bites involve the hand or arm. In pediatric patients, two thirds of wounds are superficial compared with 50% of adult wounds. In addition, dogs are more likely to cause lacerations because they have large teeth that can crush and tear tissue whereas the small sharp teeth of cats are more likely to cause puncture wounds. Because most injuries are caused by dog, cat, and human bites, this article will focus primarily on the treatment of these wounds.

Treatment

The goals of treatment are to promote healing, prevent infection, restore function, and maintain esthetics. Local wound care begins with a thorough evaluation of the injury and documentation of the location, number, type, and depth of the wounds, as well as any signs of wound infection. Bite wounds are notoriously deceptive and wounds that appear minor may actually be more extensive and involve deeper structures. Wounds should be explored for foreign bodies and concurrent injury to tendons, joint spaces, and bone. Special attention should be paid to clenched-fist injuries. Because they are injured when the hand is clenched, the site of skin penetration will move proximal to the metacarpal head when the hand is extended during evaluation and the underlying joint capsule and tendon sheath may appear normal. To avoid missing a deeper tissue injury involving the joint space, the wound must be explored throughout the entire range of motion. In addition, if bony penetration or embedded foreign bodies (e.g., embedded teeth in cat bites) are suspected, a radiograph of the site of injury should be performed.

After examination, all wounds should be thoroughly cleaned and irrigated with normal saline. Some wounds require generous debridement, with a scalpel, of devitalized tissues – tissue embedded with organisms, soil, and clots that may be difficult to remove by mechanical irrigation. After débridement, the wound should be irrigated again to remove any remaining contamination.

Superficial abrasions and puncture wounds should be covered with a topical antimicrobial agent. Alternatively, abrasions may be covered with an absorbent, occlusive dressing, which creates a moist environment to promote healing. Patients should change the dressing daily and be followed closely for wound infection.

Most lacerations, even on the extremities, may undergo primary closure after good local wound care. Infection rates after wound closure have been reported in the literature to be from 5.5% to 7.7% [1, 2]. These rates are acceptable in wounds where cosmesis is important, such as facial wounds or large extremity wounds. In a study of dog bites to the head and neck, the infection rate of wounds that were primarily repaired and not treated with antibiotics was 1.4% [3]. Very small lacerations (<1.5 cm) may behave as puncture wounds and should be allowed to heal by secondary intent. Large wounds requiring reconstructive surgery should be referred to the appropriate specialist. Delayed primary closure may be used to treat lacerations that are heavily contaminated or that involve the hand, where bacteria are inoculated into the wound and trapped within the small compartments and numerous fascial planes. Injured extremities should be immobilized and elevated.

Antibiotics

Infected wounds should be treated with antibiotics (Table 1). Patients with local cellulitis, no deep structure involvement, or who lack systemic symptoms may be treated as outpatients. Amoxicillin–clavulanate is a good initial oral antibiotic of choice that provides broad coverage for all bite wounds. Patients with a penicillin and cephalosporin allergy may be given a fluoroquinolone, doxycycline, or macrolide antibiotic. Alternative regimens include clindamycin and either a fluoroquinolone (adults) or trimethoprim–sulfamethoxazole (children). Outpatient oral treatment should continue for 7–10 days. Patients should be reevaluated every few days.

Patients with systemic symptoms and signs, complicated infections (e.g., tenosynovitis, osteomyelitis, lymphangitis), or failed outpatient therapy should be admitted for parenteral antibiotics and surgical consultation. Ampicillin–sulbactam, nafcillin, or imipenem–cilastatin with gentamicin (if one suspects a gram-negative organism) are good antibiotic regimens.

Uninfected, superficial bite wounds in adults and children do not benefit from antibiotic prophylaxis. Uninfected, high-risk wounds (Table 2) should be considered for antibiotic prophylaxis, even though prophylactic antibiotics have not been shown to significantly reduce infection rates of most bite wounds [4]. There was no difference in infection rates when analyzed by animal type (dog versus human versus cat bites), injury type (puncture versus lacerations), or wound location (forearm versus head and neck). The only subgroups for which antibiotic prophylaxis decreased the infection rate included patients with hand bites (2% [antibiotic] versus 28% [control]) and human bites (0% [antibiotic] versus 47% [control]). Hand bites and human bites, especially clenched-fist injuries, have such a high risk of infection

Bite Injuries. Table 1 Antibiotic recommendations for outpatient therapy and prophylaxis

Bite	Predominant pathogens	Oral outpatient antibiotic regimen	
		Primary	**Alternate**
Dog	*Pasteurella multocida* *Streptococcus* species *Staphylococcus aureus* *Capnocytophaga canimorsus* Anaerobes	Amoxicillin–clavulanate 875/125 mg, BID (adults) or 10–15 mg/kg TID (children)	Clindamycin 300 mg QID + ciprofloxacin 500 mg BID (adults) or clindamycin 10–25 mg/kg/day divided QID + TMP/SMX 30–60 mg/kg/day SMX divided BID (children)
Cat	*P. multocida* *S. aureus*	Amoxicillin–clavulanate 875/125 mg BID (adults) or 10–15 mg/kg TID (children)	Cefuroxime axetil 500 mg BID or doxycycline 100 mg BID (adult) or cefuroxime axetil 15–30 mg/kg/day divided BID (children)
Human	*S. aureus* *Eikenella corrodens* Anaerobes	Amoxicillin–clavulanate 875/125 mg BID (adults) or 10–15 mg/kg TID (children)	Clindamycin 300 mg QID + ciprofloxacin 500 mg BID (adults) or Clindamycin 10–25 mg/kg/day divided QID + TMP/SMX 30–60 mg/kg/day SMX divided BID (children)

TMP/SMX = trimethoprim–sulfamethoxazole

Bite Injuries. Table 2 Recommendations for antibiotic prophylaxis

Wound location
Hand or wrist; penetration into joint space
Wound type
Deep puncture wounds; extensive crush injury; involvement of underlying tendon, muscle, or bone; retained foreign body
Patient characteristics
Orthopedic prosthesis; immunocompromised state; prosthetic or diseased cardiac valve
Animal type
Large wild cats, pigs

that those patients should be given prophylaxis. Dog and cat bite wounds that are full-thickness and deep, contain devitalized tissue, or are heavily contaminated should also be given prophylactic antibiotics. Cat bites often penetrate deeper than they appear and these puncture wounds have a high infection rate; these types of bites should be treated with antibiotics.

Once the decision is made to give antibiotics, some clinicians recommend that the first dose of antibiotics be administered parenterally to ensure rapid tissue penetration, despite the lack of supporting data. This approach is reasonable but should not be considered the standard of care. The same antibiotics used to treat infections are also given for prophylaxis. Patients should be prescribed a 3–5-day course.

Wild Animals

Wild animals can cause tearing, penetrating, and crushing injuries, combined with falls and other blunt trauma. All patients should have a thorough trauma evaluation for injuries that are less obvious than the bite wound. The management of wild animal bites is either extrapolated from studies of dog and cat bites or anecdotal. Because many exposures occur in remote or wilderness settings, the delay in seeking medical care increases the risk of infection. Moreover, certain animals (e.g., wild cats, pigs, large carnivores) inflict wounds that are prone to infection. Similar to other animal bites, puncture wounds and wounds that are heavily contaminated or involve the hand should be treated with delayed primary closure or left to heal by secondary intent. All other lacerations may be repaired primarily. Prophylactic antibiotics are reasonable for extremity injuries, immunocompromised patients, large cat and pig exposures, puncture wounds, and severe crushing injuries.

Tetanus and Rabies Immunoprophylaxis

Bite wounds should be considered tetanus-prone injuries. In addition, patients should be assessed for the need for postexposure rabies immunoprophylaxis. The rabies virus is transmitted through a bite from a clinically ill animal, enters the central nervous system, and causes an acute, progressive encephalomyelitis. In the USA, most cases of human rabies occur from exposure to wild animals, primarily raccoons, skunks, foxes, and bats. Rodents and lagomorphs (i.e., rabbits and hares) rarely harbor rabies. Over the past few years, the majority of cases have been from bat exposures. The Advisory Committee on Immunization Practices' recommendations for rabies prophylaxis should be followed (Table 3). Local and state public health officials may be consulted for individual cases.

Postexposure prophylaxis consists of human rabies immunoglobulin and the 4–5-dose series of rabies vaccine. In 2009, the Advisory Committee on Immunization Practices removed the fifth dose of vaccine for all immunocompetent persons; the fifth dose is still recommended for immunocompromised persons [5]. Immunization with rabies immunoglobulin provides passive immunity for a few weeks (half-life of 21 days) until the active antibody response to the vaccine develops (within 7–10 days). As much of the immunoglobulin (20 IU/kg) should be administered into the wound as possible and the remainder intramuscularly in the gluteal region. In adults, the vaccine should be administered in the deltoid region whereas in younger children, the outer aspect of the thigh should be used to ensure intramuscular administration. Patients should return for the remainder of the series on days 3, 7, and 14, and, if immunocompromised, on day 28.

Reactions to the rabies vaccine are predominantly local and mild, including pain at the injection site, redness, swelling, and induration. Systemic symptoms include headache, dizziness, myalgias, nausea, and weakness. Serious systemic reactions such as anaphylaxis and neuroparalytic reactions are rare.

Mandatory Reporting

Finally, remember that many local governments mandate reporting of all domestic and wild animal bites to the health department. Public health departments can assist in coordinating follow-up with the animal, its owner, and the patient that was bitten.

Epidemiology

The true incidence of bite wounds from domestic and wild animals is difficult to estimate because many who sustain minor injuries do not seek medical evaluation unless an

Bite Injuries. Table 3 Postexposure rabies immunoprophylaxis guide: advisory committee on immunization practices recommendations, 2009

Animal type	Animal characteristics	Recommendations
Domestic dogs, cats, and ferrets	Rabid	Immediate prophylaxis
	Healthy and can be confined and observed for 10 days	No prophylaxis unless the animal develops signs of rabies
	Unknown	Consult local health officials because rabies risk has regional variation
Raccoons, skunks, foxes, and most carnivores	All are considered to be rabid unless the animal is available for testing	Immediate prophylaxis unless the animal tested negative for rabies
Bats	Regarded as rabid unless the animal has tested negative; includes any bite or non-bite exposure (e.g., sleeping with a bat in the room)	Immediate prophylaxis
Small rodents (squirrels, mice, hamsters, gerbils), large rodents (chipmunks), and lagomorphs (rabbits, hares)	Rarely infected with rabies; risk only in areas where raccoon rabies is enzootic	Consult public health officials; rarely requires prophylaxis

infection or other complication occurs. In the USA, an estimated 1–2 million animal bites are treated each year, most often for dog bites, followed by cat bites.

Compared with adults, children have a higher risk of being bitten by dogs and less likely by cats. Children often are bitten because they are small and ignorant about what is considered provocative behavior to a dog. Simple play or teasing may provoke a dog bite. Children are also three times more likely to be injured by other pets such as hamsters, gerbils, and rabbits.

By contrast, 80% of non-dog and non-cat bites (e.g., raccoon, rats, mice) occur in adults. In particular, people in certain occupations (e.g., veterinarians, animal control workers, laboratory workers, zookeepers) and those that keep wild animals as pets have the highest risk of wild animal bites. Because most pediatric injuries occur in the home, more often than not the involved animal may be observed or its immunization history may be obtainable. In adult patients, however, one third of animal exposures occur in the park or public streets, where information about the animal would be difficult to obtain.

Bacteriology

Infected dog and cat bite wounds typically have mixed aerobic and anaerobic bacteria, with a few pathogens that are unique to the biter's oral flora. The most common pathogen is *Pasteurella* species, isolated from 50% of dog and 75% of cat bites. In infected dog bites, the most common strain is *Pasteurella canis* (26%) whereas *P. multocida* (75%) is most commonly implicated in cat bites. Oral flora (e.g., *Streptococcus* species) dominate

human skin flora (i.e., *Staphylococcus aureus*) in bite infection isolates, particularly for puncture wounds. Infections from dog and cat bites that develop within 24 h are likely caused by *P. multocida* whereas symptoms that develop after 24 h are more likely caused by *Staphylococcus* or *Streptococcus* species.

An important pathogen associated with dog bites is *Capnocytophaga canimorsus*, a gram-negative bacillus found in the normal oral flora. It is a fastidious organism that can cause severe sepsis with disseminated intravascular coagulopathy, cutaneous gangrene, and multiorgan failure, especially in asplenic, immunocompromised, and chronic alcoholic patients, but also in healthy patients.

P. multocida, the major pathogen in cat bite infections, is a gram-negative coccobacillus that can incite an intense inflammatory response, typically within 24 h of injury. It can cause serious infections such as necrotizing fasciitis, septic arthritis, and osteomyelitis. Less commonly, it has been implicated in a variety of systemic illnesses including pneumonia in patients with underlying pulmonary disease, meningitis and brain abscesses in infants and elderly patients, spontaneous bacterial peritonitis in AIDS patients, and bacteremia in patients with liver dysfunction.

Similar to animal bite infections, human bite infections are typically caused by mixed anaerobic and aerobic bacteria, most commonly *Streptococcus* species (84%). *Eikenella corrodens*, a gram-negative rod, is the infecting organism in 7–29% of human bites and is very common in clenched-fist injuries. *Eikenella* is an important cause of chronic infection, osteomyelitis, and loss of joint function in the hand, but has also been associated with abdominal abscesses, meningitis, endocarditis, and fatal gram-negative sepsis.

Evaluation/Assessment

As mentioned previously, bite wounds that appear minor may actually be more extensive and involve injury to deeper structures. All wounds require a thorough exploration for foreign bodies and concurrent injury to tendons, joint spaces, and bone. Extremities, in particular, have deep complex fascial planes that may hide foreign bodies, such as cat teeth, so extremity wounds have a very high risk of infection. The clenched-fist injury is a good example of these notoriously deceptive, high-risk wounds. To avoid missing a deeper tissue injury, the wound must be explored throughout the entire range of motion. In addition, if bony penetration or embedded foreign bodies (e.g., embedded teeth in cat bites) are suspected, a radiograph of the site of injury should be performed.

Prognosis

The most frequent complication of bites is wound infection, although the majority of bite injuries heal well. Severe systemic diseases such as sepsis, osteomyelitis, meningitis, endocarditis, and peritonitis are uncommon. Moreover, animal bites can potentially transmit other diseases including cat-scratch fever (*Bartonella henselae*), tularemia (*Franciscella tularensis*), leptospirosis, brucellosis, and rat-bite fever (*Spirillum minus*) and human bites can transmit hepatitis B, hepatitis C, syphilis, herpes simplex, tuberculosis, actinomycosis, and HIV.

References

1. Chen E, Hornig S, Shepherd SM, Hollander JE (2000) Primary closure of mammalian bites. Acad Emerg Med 7(2):157–161
2. Maimaris C, Quinton DN (1988) Dog-bite lacerations: a controlled trial of primary wound closure. Arch Emerg Med 5(3):156–161
3. Oehler RL, Velez AP, Mizrachi M, Lamarche J, Gompf S (2009) Bite-related and septic syndromes caused by cats and dogs. Lancet Infect Dis 9(7):439–447
4. Medeiros I, Saconato H (2001) Antibiotic prophylaxis for mammalian bites. Cochrane Database Syst Rev 2:CD001738
5. Rupprecht CE, Briggs D, Brown CM et al (2010) Use of a reduced (4-dose) vaccine schedule for postexposure prophylaxis to prevent human rabies: recommendations of the advisory committee on immunization practices. MMWR Recomm Rep 59(RR-2):1–9

Biventricular Assist Device (BVAD)

▶ Circulatory Assist Devices

Blackout

▶ Coma

Black-out

▶ Syncope

Blakemore Tube

ANDREW D. YEOMAN, JULIA A. WENDON
Liver Intensive Therapy Unit, Institute of Liver Studies, Kings College Hospital, London, UK

Synonyms

Bleeding; Hemorrhage

Definition

Variceal hemorrhage remains one of the most feared and dramatic complications of cirrhosis and ▶ portal hypertension. Esophageal ▶ varices occur in 40% of patients with cirrhosis and up to 50% of these will subsequently bleed, with the risk being greatest in the first 2 years after diagnosis [1]. Predictors of variceal hemorrhage in cirrhotic patients include: the presence of ▶ Child-Pugh grade C cirrhosis and high-risk endoscopic features such as large varices or red wale signs. In the context of cirrhosis, varices tend to bleed only when the pressure gradient between the portal venous and systemic venous circulation exceeds 12 mmHg with variceal pressure broadly equating to portal pressure [1]. Although this threshold value has limited sensitivity, it has a high specificity for the development of variceal hemorrhage and its clinically relevance is predominantly a target to aim for in portal pressure lowering attempts via pharmacologic therapy, TIPPS, or surgical shunts. It is important to emphasize that the onset of variceal hemorrhage in a cirrhotic patient is a highly significant event, which frequently heralds a poor prognosis. Indeed, mortality following the first variceal bleed approaches 50% [1, 2].

Pre-existing Condition

While major technological advances (such as video endoscopy, band ligation, and ▶ TIPSS) have been made over the past 2 decades, adequate volume resuscitation, including correction of any coagulopathy, remains the mainstay of the early management of the patient bleeding from varices. In addition, consideration should be given to elective endotracheal intubation for airway control in all patients with torrential variceal hemorrhage. Only once hemodynamic stability has been achieved and the airway is secure, should the focus shift toward attempts at bleeding cessation. Therapies that have been proven beneficial in reducing bleeding and mortality in variceal hemorrhage include:

(a) Pharmacotherapy with octreotide or terlipressin
(b) Endoscopic therapy with band ligation, sclerosant, or histoacryl glue injection
(c) Balloon ▶ tamponade with ▶ Sengstaken–Blakemore tube (SBT)
(d) Transjugular intrahepatic portosystemic shunts (TIPSS)
(e) Surgery (surgical shunts, esophageal transaction, underrunning of varices)

Therapeutic options used to achieve hemostasis in variceal hemorrhage can also be divided into attempts at lowering portal pressure (pharmacotherapy, TIPSS, surgical shunts), disconnecting the site of hemorrhage from the portal circulation, either through thrombosis of the varix (sclerosant, band ligation, or glue) or mechanical dissociation (transection) and, finally, by balloon tamponade of relatively low-pressure varices. This review will now focus on the indications, technique, efficacy, and complications of the use of SBT and other balloon tamponade devices in the management of variceal hemorrhage.

The choice of therapeutic option will, however, depend on both the severity of bleeding and the local expertise. For example, while pharmacotherapy is almost universally available, expert therapeutic endoscopy may not always be readily available. In contrast, endoscopic therapy may have been attempted but failed. Failure of endoscopic therapy has been precisely defined and is subdivided into failure before and after 6 h following treatment [1]. Failure within 6 h is a transfusion requirement of 4 units or more and failure to achieve a 20 mmHg increase in systolic blood pressure/systolic <70 mmHg, or failure to reduce heart rate to <100 or a 20 beat/min overall reduction [1]. In contrast, failure of hemostasis after 6 h is defined by any of the following: hematemesis after 6 h, a fall in BP by >20 mmHg, or a 20 beat/min increase in heart rate on two consecutive readings 1 h apart, the need for a further 2 units of blood to increase the hemoglobin content above 9 g/L [1].

Application

Broadly speaking, two situations exist where emergency therapy is required to stop major hemorrhage and in which balloon tamponade with an SBT may be successfully utilized. The first of these situations relates to failure to control variceal hemorrhage following initial endoscopic therapy as previously defined or the inability to identify a precise bleeding point amenable to targeted endoscopic therapy. Secondly, if ongoing major bleeding occurs and advanced therapeutic endoscopy is unavailable, then the use of a balloon tamponade device, such as a Sengstaken–Blakemore tube, may be considered as an interim measure to achieve hemostasis. Contraindications to SBT insertion include esophageal stricture or recent esophageal surgery, although these are relative rather than absolute.

The use of a modified naso/orogastric tube to balloon tamponade bleeding varices in the distal esophagus/proximal stomach was first described in the 1930s. However, the type of device in clinical use today was first introduced by Sengstaken and Blakemore in 1950. Consequently, the majority of balloon tamponade devices are now referred to as SBT even if they have undergone modification and are officially known by another name. A modified SBT (Minnesota tube) is displayed in Fig. 1.

The basic features of the SBT are a multilumen latex tube that has a circumferential esophageal balloon and a distal gastric balloon, each with an inflation port. The original SBT only carried one aspiration port (gastric) and therefore a theoretical risk existed of blood pooling in the esophagus and subsequent aspiration pneumonia. Therefore, a modified four-lumen tube was developed in the 1950s with an esophageal aspiration port, known as a Minnesota tube. Another modification of the SBT is that of a single, large capacity (700 mL), gastric balloon known as the Linton–Nachlas tube, which has been

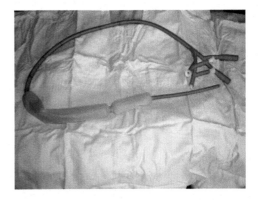

Blakemore Tube. Figure 1 A four-lumen modified Sengstaken–Blakemore tube (Minnesota tube)

suggested to be more effective for the tamponade of gastric fundal varices. For patients with a latex allergy, both silicone SBT and Linton–Nachlas tubes have been used, which, in addition, have one-way valves that prevent leakage and enable pressure monitoring of the esophageal and gastric balloons to be undertaken. Other features relevant to balloon tamponade devices are that they are radio-opaque, typically 85–115 cm in length and include insertion depth markings in centimeters. They are also available in sizes 16, 18, and 20 French gauges (5.3, 6.0, and 6.7 mm circumference), although a pediatric 12F (4 mm) tube is produced by some manufacturers. As all balloon tamponade devices have identical modes of action and require the same technique for insertion and monitoring, henceforth, for consistency of presentation, the term SBT will refer to all devices, unless explicitly stated.

Efficacy and Safety of SBT

SBT insertion results in cessation of hemorrhage in the vast majority of patients with hemostasis lasting 24 reported in 80–90% [2, 3]. However, it should be made clear that all published studies have evaluated the efficacy of SBT as primary rather than rescue therapy for variceal hemorrhage. As a consequence, its efficacy among patients who have failed initial pharmacologic or endoscopic therapy may be lower as these individuals represent a higher-risk group. Furthermore, the use of SBT is merely a temporizing measure prior to the application of definitive procedures to achieve hemostasis either via endoscopic therapy or by measures that lower portal pressure (TIPSS, surgical shunts). Highlighting this issue is the reported risk of rebleeding, which occurs in 50% within 24 h of deflating the gastric balloon [1, 3, 4].

While effective as a bridge to definitive therapy, clinicians must remain cognizant. of the risks attendant upon the use of SBT. The most common complication related to SBT use is the development of aspiration pneumonia, which occurs in around 10% [3]. The risk of aspiration pneumonia is further exacerbated by the presence of hepatic encephalopathy, which is common in these patients. However, most of the published data related to this complication refers to patients who were not intubated [2, 3] for the procedure and the risk of aspiration will probably be ameliorated, though not abolished, by endotracheal intubation. Indeed, there is a good argument to be made for all major variceal bleeds to be intubated prior to endoscopy to secure the airway. Less common, but far more serious, is esophageal perforation/rupture, which usually occurs as a result of misplacement of the tube tip, inflation of the gastric balloon within the esophagus with subsequent esophageal rupture, which is usually fatal. If ongoing bleeding occurs in a patient who has suffered an esophageal perforation consideration must be given to the risks and benefits of repeat endoscopic treatment. While perforation represents only a relative contraindication to another endoscopic attempt at achieving hemostasis, repeat intubation may further contaminate the mediastinum.

Figure 2a presents a plain chest radiograph from a patient with an esophageal perforation following insertion of an SBT, which led to subcutaneous emphysema, bilateral pneumothoraces, and pneumomediastinum.

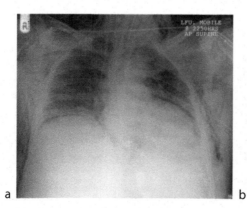
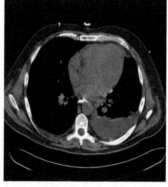

a   b

Blakemore Tube. Figure 2 (**a**) Plain chest radiograph of a patient with esophageal perforation following SBT insertion. Note the presence of bilateral intercostal chest drains used to treat pneumonthoraces and the presence of subcutaneous emphysema and pneumomediastinum. (**b**) Computerized tomography of the thorax in another patient with esophageal perforation following SBT placement. Extravasation of oral contrast medium into the mediastinum is clearly visualized

Figure 2b demonstrates the computerized tomography appearance of extravasated oral contrast in the mediastinum.

Other reported complications include rupture of the trachea, jejunal perforation, and SBT impaction. Although the precise incidence and mortality associated with these complications remains unknown, they appear to be uncommon. Thus, in spite of the potentially serious risks, in uncontrollable variceal hemorrhage, placement of an SBT probably represents the safest and most efficacious therapy, unless access to rescue TIPSS is immediately available. Although surgical interventions such as esophageal transection may prevent exsanguination, these procedures require significant experience in themselves and the short-term rebleeding rate and mortality remain extremely high, as is usually the case for any patient with advanced liver disease undergoing surgical intervention.

Technical Aspects of SBT Insertion

Once it has been determined that an SBT is indicated, and the risks and benefits considered, attention must turn toward its safe insertion. Despite almost 60 years experience of the use of SBT in the management of variceal hemorrhage, there is remarkably scant evidence to guide clinicians in regards their safe and effective insertion. Consequently, the optimal techniques for initial placement, implementation, and removal of SBT have not been fully determined.

For example, historical reports have suggested a significant increased risk of aspiration pneumonia following placement of an SBT in patients with more advanced grades of hepatic encephalopathy. However, there are a number of concerns regarding the placement of SBT in a conscious patient. Firstly, SBT placement is an extremely unpleasant procedure in a conscious patient. Also, patients actively bleeding have a high intrinsic adrenergic drive, which leads to distress and agitation. This, unsurprisingly, renders them poorly compliant of attempts to place a large bore (16–20 French gauge) tube nasally or orally. Furthermore, stimulation of the gag reflex by insertion of an SBT only tends to provoke further episodes of emesis, exacerbating patient distress and possibly increasing the risk of aspiration. In addition, these wide bore tubes may splint the crico-pharyngeus and therefore leave the airway unprotected, irrespective of the presence of hepatic encephalopathy, which may further compromise the airway. Consequently, the risk of aspiration is probably highest at the time of SBT insertion and therefore it is felt mandatory, in terms of patient safety, that all patients are sedated, intubated, and ventilated prior to the placement of an SBT. The major technical issue this presents is the resistance to the passage of the tube due to the presence of an inflated endotracheal tube cuff.

As already stated, an SBT is placed either nasally or as an orogastric tube, although if endotracheal intubation is undertaken, the orogastric route is preferable as the wide bore of these tube may not permit entry into the nares and, in addition, the potential for nasopharyngeal trauma is significant, especially so in patients who frequently are coagulopathic.

Prior to insertion both esophageal and gastric balloons should be inflated (to ensure that there is no leak) and fully deflated. The tube should then be suitably lubricated and advanced orally beyond the crico-pharyngeus. While many practitioners keep the tubes in refrigerators to improve stiffness, there is no objective evidence that this actually improves stiffness and, indeed, the tubes rapidly rewarm when removed from refrigeration. It should be noted that SBT made from silicone is stiffer than those made manufactured from latex.

Typically, these tubes are inserted "blind" as per regular naso/orogastric tube placement. A concern exists that particularly among inexperienced operators, a blind technique could lead to the SBT coiling in the esophagus or upper airways. Subsequent gastric balloon inflation could then lead to rupture of the trachea or esophagus with disastrous consequences. Again, we assert that the prior undertaking of appropriate patient sedation and endotracheal intubation facilitates not only patient compliance, but also the operators' ability to gently guide rather than "blindly" pass the tube. This is particularly useful if pharyngeal resistance is encountered as, in this instance, the use of a laryngoscope and Magill's forceps allows visualization of the endotracheal tube and feeding of the SBT posteriorly into the upper esophagus and beyond.

Methods reported in the literature to try and improve the likelihood of correct tube placement include the use of guidewires, ultrasonography, direct visualization at endoscopy, or plain chest radiography. Most of these techniques are designed to confirm balloon position prior to maximal inflation with the aim of preventing major complications. Importantly, no head-to-head comparisons exist, however, as to whether any of these technical modifications improve either ease of insertion or the incidence of serious complications when compared to "blind" insertion. However, if an SBT is inserted due to failure of endoscopic therapy, then it seems reasonable to confirm its position under direct endoscopic visualization prior to gastric balloon inflation. It must be acknowledged, though, that it remains virtually impossible for individual centers to perform such studies due to the relative infrequency of SBT usage and, to date, collaborative studies have not been performed.

Once inserted the tube is advanced to at least 50–60 cm from the teeth (as the gastro-oesophageal junction (GOJ) usually exists at 35–40 cm) [4], and, once satisfied that no pharyngeal coiling has occurred, the gastric balloon should be inflated. To inflate the gastric balloon, a 60 mL) catheter tip syringe and an artery clamp are needed. The latter is required, as the inflation ports in many devices lack nonreturn valves. Consequently, after inflation, the clamp should be used prior to disconnecting the syringe to prevent leakage of the injectate. Although either air or water may be insufflated into the gastric balloon, it is our policy to inflate the gastric balloon with 200 mL of water [5] as leakage from the gastric balloon may then be easier to detect. In addition, it is also our policy to mix contrast agents with the water [5] to allow clear identification of the gastric balloon on plain chest radiography. If excessive resistance to gastric balloon inflation is encountered, any fluid injected should be withdrawn, the presence of any coiling in the oropharynx checked for, and, if any uncertainty persists about correct positioning, the device should be removed and a further attempt at placement be made. Assessing what constitutes excessive resistance to gastric insufflation relies partly on operator experience of placing such devices, and also strongly reinforces the concept and practice of a test inflation of the gastric balloon prior to insertion of the SBT into the patient. This allows the clinician to gauge the inflation forces required when no external resistance is present. Finally, once inflation is complete, the injected volume should be recorded and a spigot be placed firmly in the gastric inflation port.

Once the SBT is satisfactorily placed, the tube should be slowly withdrawn until resistance is encountered at the gastro-oesophageal junction (GOJ) and the distance from the teeth is measured, recorded, and monitored to detect tube displacement. Tube displacement may occur as a consequence of normal gut peristalsis or following patient turning as part of their nursing care. The SBT should then be secured to the side of the face, preferably by tape [4, 5] or onto a helmet. Heavy traction (such as attaching a hung weight to the device) should not be routinely applied as this could lead to significant pressure necrosis of the GOJ and may produce only variable traction. The tape fixation should then be removed approximately every 4 h and the SBT taped to the opposite side of the face to prevent pressure necrosis.

Once again, the optimal duration of continuous tamponade applied at the GOJ is not known. However, it is generally accepted that continuous tamponade is applied for less than 12 h and certainly not more than 24 h [4, 5]. Deflation of the gastric balloon should virtually always be attempted only when definitive treatment options are in place. These options usually consist of repeat attempts at endoscopic therapy or consideration of TIPSS or, less commonly, surgical shunts. The period during which balloon tamponade is being applied may also be used to buy time for definitive therapy to be organized, which in many instances, necessitates the transfer of the patient to a specialist liver unit.

The vast majority of severe variceal bleeds will be stemmed by gastric tamponade and if this fails to achieve hemostasis, the position of the SBT must be checked, the integrity of the gastric balloon evaluated, and the amount of traction applied reviewed. If following these checks hemostasis is not achieved, then consideration should be given to inflation of the esophageal balloon. Although generally speaking, the esophageal balloon should almost never be inflated, due to the risk of pressure necrosis in extreme circumstances, and under expert guidance, this may be considered with the tacit acknowledgment of the increased risk. Such circumstances would include the nonavailability of definitive treatment measures and/or the inability to stop torrential variceal hemorrhage in an unstable patient or the presence of high esophageal perforator vessels, which effectively bypass tamponade at the GOJ.

If this maneuver is to be undertaken, then the esophageal balloon should only be inflated to a maximum pressure of 40 mmHg [4, 5]. The pressure should then be frequently monitored with a sphygmomanometer (attached to the esophageal aspiration port by a Y connector) and the esophageal balloon should be deflated regularly to prevent pressure necrosis, which could lead to bleeding or perforation. The optimal time intervals for pressure monitoring, deflation of the balloon, and duration of deflation remain unknown, but it has been suggested that esophageal balloon pressure measurements be taken hourly [4]. Continued failure to obtain hemostasis should lead to a search for bleeding from another source such as an ectopic varix (usually duodenal), Dieulafoy lesion, or a peptic ulcer.

Once the SBT is secured in place, a plain chest radiograph should be obtained to check its position. An example of this is demonstrated in Fig. 3. Finally, low-pressure suction (~5 cm H_2O) should be applied to the esophageal aspiration port to prevent existing blood in the esophagus being aspirated. The gastric aspiration port should be manually aspirated fully, and then left on free drainage. Evacuating the stomach of blood is important, as although aspiration of its contents is unlikely if the SBT is correctly

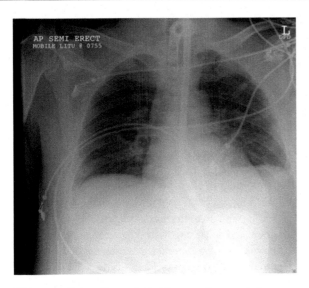

Blakemore Tube. Figure 3 Satisfactory placement of a Sengstaken–Blakemore tube in a tracheostomized patient with contrast material clearly demonstrated within the gastric balloon

sited, it can prove useful in detecting fresh hemorrhage indicative of therapeutic failure.

Summary and Conclusion

Despite advances in endoscopic technology and the emergence of TIPSS, the SBT continues to play an essential role in the management of the patients with acute variceal hemorrhage. These devices predominantly serve as an emergency, temporizing, measure to achieve hemostasis while definitive interventions are arranged. Although highly effective, their use is not without significant risk. However, the commonest complication, that of aspiration pneumonia, can be minimized by the routine use of endotracheal intubation prior to SBT insertion. This will also render subsequent attempts at endoscopic treatment easier for the endoscopist and, ultimately, safer for the patient. Endotracheal intubation will not prevent other serious complications such as esophageal perforation due to tube misplacement and the specter of such complications reinforces both the need for a thorough understanding of the harms that SBT can cause and the application of sound insertion technique, for which there is no substitute for experience. Finally, the increasing burden of liver disease, particularly among Western populations, will undoubtedly lead to greater numbers of patients presenting with variceal hemorrhage in the coming years. Therefore, the future use of an SBT is likely to become more, rather than less, common. Future work should focus on the efficacy of SBT, specifically among patients who have failed other therapies, and how we can improve their safe use. This will require collaborative studies reporting complication rates and type, the optimal duration of tamponade application and subsequent clinical outcomes including mortality rates.

References

1. Jalan R, Hayes PC. UK guidelines on the management of variceal haemorrhage in cirrhotic patients. Available at http://gut.bmj.com/cgi/content/extract/46/suppl_3/iii1
2. Panes J, Teres J, Bosch J, Rodes J (1988) Efficacy of balloon tamponade in treatment of bleeding gastric and esophageal varices. Dig Dis Sci 33:454–459
3. Haddock G, Garden OJ, McKee RF, Anderson JR, Carter DC (1989) Esophageal tamponade in the management of acute variceal haemorrhage. Dig Dis Sci 34:913–918
4. McCormick PA, Burroughs AK, McIntyre N (1990) How to insert a Sengstaken–Blakemore tube. Br J Hosp Med 43:274–277
5. Vlavianos P, Gimson AE, Westaby D, Williams R (1989) Balloon tamponade in variceal bleeding: use and misuse. BMJ 298:1158

Blast Injuries

▶ Bomb Injuries

Blast Injury

ERIC R. FRYKBERG
Department of Surgery, University of Florida Health Science Center, Jacksonville, FL, USA

Synonyms

Blast lung; Blast lung injury; Blast trauma; Explosion-induced trauma; Explosion-induced tympanic membrane rupture; Explosive barotrauma; Explosive injury; Pulmonary barotrauma; Tympanic membrane barotrauma

Definition

Blast injury refers to the anatomic and physiologic damage caused to organic tissues and the human body by the physical properties of an explosion, or *blast*. Since the invention of gunpowder in the last millennium, the magnitude and destructive potential of explosions have increased exponentially. They have increasingly been used to deliberately inflict death and disability on large populations in the settings of war and terrorism. The growing availability of explosives has led to an increasing confrontation of medical providers with the injuries they impart. This has led to abundant research and knowledge of the pathophysiology and unique clinical manifestations of blast injury that differ in many ways from other more common forms of trauma.

Blast Physics

An explosion is the sudden release of energy from the rapid conversion of solids or liquids into gas. Low energy explosives, such as gunpowder, release this energy relatively slowly in the process termed *deflagration*, and do not cause major bodily injury. They are generally used as propellants. High energy explosives (e.g., TNT, dynamite, C-4, Semtex) cause a virtually instantaneous transformation of solids and liquids into the gaseous state in the process of *detonation*, or what is commonly called an explosion. This creates a sudden intense compression of the surrounding medium that propagates radially from the source as a shock wave at speeds that may reach 3,000–8,000 m/s. This is the *blast wave*. The instantaneous pressure rise, lasting only 2–10 ms, is the *peak overpressure*, the magnitude of which depends on the strength of the explosion. The leading edge of the blast wave, or *blast front*, imparts a shattering force known as *brissance*, as a result of the high magnitudes of energy involved. The destructive capacity of the blast wave is measured by the mathematically calculated force called *blast loading*, which is the major determinant of destruction and bodily injury imparted to objects and organisms in its path [1–3].

High-energy explosions are also characterized by an intense fireball that is localized to only a small area around the blast source, which further magnifies the severe destruction in the immediate locale of a blast. This represents the highest levels of the intense energy release of detonation. The rapid dissipation of this thermal energy in a very short distance results in the remaining energy continuing radially outward beyond the fireball as the blast wave. As this energy continues to dissipate, the blast wave degrades into the lower pressure and velocity range of sound waves, giving rise to the sound of the explosion [2].

The blast wave dissipates rapidly in open-air explosions, according to the cube of the distance from the blast, so that moving three times further away reduces its magnitude 27-fold. The instantaneous peak overpressure is followed by a more gradual decline, lasting ten times longer, to the point of actually falling below ambient pressure in a negative pressure, or *under pressure* phase, before then returning to ambient pressure. This under-

pressure phase explains the implosive effects commonly seen in major explosions (Fig. 1). Blast wind refers to the resulting rapid back and forth movements of air after the blast wave passes, which can reach hurricane strength within a fraction of a second, and which creates ongoing destruction beyond that of the blast wave itself [1, 2].

Blasts that occur in confined spaces are more destructive than in open air as the blast wave is magnified, rather than dissipated, due to its reflection off floors, walls and ceilings. The magnitude of confined space explosions is directly related to the magnitude of the blast force, and indirectly related to the volume of the space and the degree of venting and decompression allowed by open doors, windows, and collapsing walls. The orientation of objects to the blast wave is another determinant of destructive potential. A large enough blast inside a building may collapse the entire structure to further magnify the level of destruction of objects, and injury and death among people in it, beyond the effects of the confined-space blast alone [1–4]. These principles have been demonstrated in a number of major terrorist bombings of the past 30 years, and explain why bombs are deliberately detonated in confined spaces and crowded buildings (Table 1). Busses have been a common location of suicide bombings in Israel, in which setting mortality approaches 50%, compared to only 8% following open-air bombings. The open-air terrorist bombings at the Centennial Olympics in Atlanta and the Khobar Towers in Saudi Arabia in 1996, and at a Helsinki shopping mall in 2002, resulted in death rates of 3% or less.

Blast Pathophysiology and Epidemiology

The highly injurious effects of blasts on the human body are understandable from the above physical

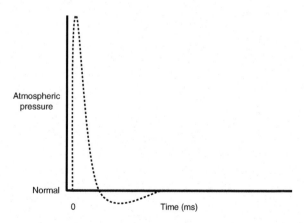

Blast Injury. Figure 1 Friedlander curve showing pattern of pressure changes with time following high energy explosions

Blast Injury. Table 1 Terrorist bombing events and outcomes

Event	Year	No. Total Casualties (Deaths)
Train terminal Bologna[b]	1980	291 (85)
U.S. Marine barracks Beirut[a,b]	1983	346 (241)
World Trade Center, New York City[b]	1993	1,042 (6)
AIMA Buenos Aires[a,b]	1994	286 (85)
Murrah Building Oklahoma City[a]	1995	759 (168)
Centennial Olympics, Atlanta	1996	111 (2)
Khobar Towers Saudi Arabia	1996	574 (20)
U.S. Embassies Tanzania and Kenya[a]	1998	4,100 (223)
USS Cole Yemen	2000	52 (17)
World Trade Center, New York City[a]	2001	2,839 (2,819)
Shopping mall Helsinki[b]	2002	166 (7)
U.N. Headquarters Baghdad[a,b]	2003	100 (17)
Train terminals Madrid[b]	2004	2,092 (191)
Subways and bus London[b]	2005	>700 (55)

[a]Involved some element of building collapse
[b]Confined space explosions

characteristics, and tend to result in more severe and lethal trauma than the standard forms of blunt and penetrating trauma seen routinely in hospitals. Studies from Israel have documented among victims of blast injury significantly younger ages, more females, more children, higher Injury Severity Scores, more complex injuries involving more than three body regions, more major operations, more ICU and hospital days, and higher mortality than among those with non-blast trauma. There are four recognized categories of blast injury, each with distinct etiologies, clinical manifestations, and treatment implications.

Primary Blast Injury (PBI)

The destruction of tissues caused by the blast wave itself traversing the body results in this category. A distinctive feature PBI is the absence of any external evidence of trauma despite significant internal damage. Air-containing tissues and organs are most susceptible to the destructive effects of the hypersonic blast wave, especially at air–liquid interfaces where disruptive shearing forces, known as *spalling*, occur due to differences in compressibility of these two media. Solid organs tend to be spared from PBI due to their homogeneous densities. This explains the high incidence of injury to the ear structures, lung, and hollow viscera of the abdomen following exposure to major blasts [1].

Tympanic Membrane Rupture (TMR)

This is probably the single most common injury found among casualties of major blasts, as the ear is the most sensitive organ to PBI. It results from the substantial pressure gradients that develop between the inner and external ear compartments, and generally requires 20–50 pounds per square inch (PSI) of pressure to occur. It is often absent in victims of PBI. Its occurrence relates to a number of variables, including proximity to the blast, ear protection, and orientation of the ears to the blast wave. Following the Madrid terrorist bombings in 2004, less than 50% of hospitalized survivors had TMR, and the majority of those were not seriously injured [5]. TMR may be associated with middle and inner ear damage, with disruption of the bony ossicles, auditory and vestibular damage, and conductive and sensorineural hearing loss, cranial nerve palsy, and the long-term sequelae of cholesteatoma, brain abscess, or meningitis. Clinical manifestations include tinnitus, hearing loss, earache, and vertigo, although these symptoms are most often temporary. Hearing loss commonly complicates the initial care of blast victims.

Blast Lung Injury (BLI)

This is among the most common organ injuries found among blast victims, especially in open-air blasts.

However, the great majority of casualties with BLI die immediately due to the close proximity they must be to the blast to be subjected to the effects of the blast wave, and therefore it is quite uncommon among survivors. In a collective review of injury patterns resulting from terrorist bombings published in 1988 (Table 2), only 0.6% of all survivors had BLI. Following the 2004 Madrid terrorist bombings, only 0.84% of survivors had BLI. However, the 11–12% mortality among BLI victims in both reports is far out of proportion to its incidence, indicating how severe is the tissue damage, and how important is the rapid identification and intense treatment of these victims [4, 5]. The cause of immediate deaths is multifactorial, as the proximity of the victim to the blast causes severe multisystem injuries. The pulmonary injury is characterized by disruption of the alveolar: vascular interface, resulting in fatal air embolism. The most common cause of late death among afflicted survivors is intractable respiratory failure [3]. Open-air blasts typically cause unilateral BLI on the side of the blast origin, while confined space blasts result in bilateral BLI [6].

The clinical and radiological manifestations of BLI are similar to those of pulmonary contusions. Victims develop progressive respiratory insufficiency characterized by

Blast Injury. Table 2 Patterns of injury and mortality in 3,357 victims of terrorist bombings

Specific injury	Incidence in immediate deaths (%)	Incidence in survivors (%)	Specific mortality(%)[a]	% Survivor deaths with specific injury[b]
Head	71	31	1.5	52
Chest	25	2	15	21
Blast lung	47	0.6	11	4
Abdomen	30	1.4	19	21
Traumatic Amputation	–	1.2	11	10
Skeletal	–	11	0	0
Soft tissue	–	55	0	0

[a]Percentage of all survivors with specific injury who died of that injury
[b]Percentage of all late deaths among survivors who had specific injury
Source: Adapted from [4]. With permission from Lippincott, Williams and Wilkins

increased work of breathing and hypoxia. Alveolar disruption commonly results in pneumothorax, pneumomediastinum, bronchopleural fistula and hemoptysis. Chest x-rays show a spectrum of heterogenous alveolar-interstitial infiltrates and consolidation, which may progress to a classic "butterfly" pattern. Sustained hypotension may be due to a vagal response to the force of the blast wave. This clinical picture evolves over a period of 48 h or more, emphasizing the importance of close observation and serial physical and radiologic examinations of casualties who have been exposed to the primary blast wave, regardless of how stable, comfortable and uninjured they may appear initially [3, 6].

Other PBI Organ Injuries
The air-containing hollow viscera of the abdomen are susceptible to PBI, more so in underwater blasts than open-air blasts. The colon is the most frequently injured organ. In a collective review of terrorist bombings (see Table 2), abdominal injuries were identified in as many as 34% of immediate fatalities and only 1.4% of survivors, but these survivors had a 19% incidence of late mortality [4]. All victims of the 2005 bus and train bombings in London with abdominal injuries were immediately killed and only 5% of surviving casualties of the 2004 Madrid bombings had abdominal injuries [5]. Confined space bombings have resulted in abdominal injuries in as many as 14% of victims. The two major etiologies of PBI of abdominal viscera include direct bowel wall microcirculatory disruption leading to perforation, and mesenteric lacerations leading to infarction. In both settings, symptoms and signs may not manifest until hours or days after the blast, as with BLI, increasing the risks of mortality and morbidity if these victims are not monitored carefully [2].

Traumatic amputation of limbs is a devastating injury caused by the direct coupling of the primary blast wave into extremity tissues, weakening the long bones from powerful axial stresses. The subsequent blast wind then causes a flailing of the limb with fracture and soft tissue shearing to complete the amputation. These fractures are typically midshaft and not joint dislocations. As with other forms of PBI, most casualties with this injury are immediately killed. The disproportionately high mortality (11%) among the small minority of afflicted survivors (1.2%) makes this injury another marker of severity that should be recognized early as requiring urgent treatment (see Table 2) [4]. Traumatic amputation of the ears and nose are similarly devastating injuries with the same management implications.

PBI of the central nervous system (CNS) affects the brain, spinal cord, and vertebral skeleton. The concussive effects of the blast wave on the brain may cause altered mental status, abnormal EEG activity with characteristic theta-waves, and a spectrum of sensorimotor deficits. Air emboli to the CNS from BLI may indirectly contribute to these problems. The classic manifestations of "shell shock" and post-traumatic stress disorder (PTSD) among blast victims may have an organic basis from PBI. *Spinal shock* from PBI is best distinguished from that caused by air embolism or direct trauma to the spinal cord by a rapid and complete resolution without anatomic or radiological signs of injury. This form of spinal shock is uncommon, documented in only 1.6% of hospitalized survivors of the 2004 Madrid bombings. Spinal vertebral fractures from PBI are characterized by involvement of multiple levels of the spinal column and an association with severe torso injuries. Among the 5% of afflicted survivors of the 2004 Madrid bombings, 65% involved the upper thoracic spine [5].

Secondary and Tertiary Blast Injury

These are the most common forms of blast injuries found among survivors of explosive events [4]. *Secondary blast injury* is caused by the impact on the body of objects and projectiles that are propelled by the blast wave and blast wind, or that result from *secondary fragmentation* of other objects struck by this debris. *Tertiary blast injury* results from the body itself being propelled into objects and structures by the blast wind, and tends to occur more in children than adults due to their lighter weight. Both result in typical though severe blunt and penetrating trauma and impalement. Skeletal and soft tissue injuries with little risk of mortality predominate (see Table 2).

Glass shards from shattered windows are among the most common projectiles causing secondary blast injury. In recent years, destructive metal fragments have increasingly been placed in bombs by terrorists to magnify the wounding capacity (Fig. 2). One bizarre injury pattern recently reported involves biologic projectiles of tissue and bone from the exploded bodies of suicide bombers which penetrate victims. In some cases these human remains projectiles have been found to be infected with hepatitis B, further magnifying the level of injury and terror.

Quaternary Blast Injuries

Also known as *miscellaneous* blast injuries, this category includes injuries only indirectly related to the blast, such as thermal burns from the fireball immediately surrounding an explosion, crush injuries from structural collapse, and inhalation injuries from dust and toxic chemicals [2]. The explosive disaster with the highest incidence of inhalation injuries among casualties (93%) was the 1993 terrorist bombing of the World Trade Center in New York City. A substantial number of rescue personnel developed long-term pulmonary problems years after the September 11, 2001, World Trade Center collapse, due to inadequate use of personal protection.

The dissemination of biologic, chemical, or radiologic agents through dirty bombs falls under this category, although these agents are very difficult to effectively weaponize. The bomb used in the 1993 World Trade Center explosion contained enough cyanide to contaminate the whole building, but was destroyed by the blast. There was also a failed release of cyanide in the 1995 Sarin gas attack in Tokyo.

Psychological sequelae of explosive disasters are also included in this category. This may affect casualties, responders and medical providers and can result in long-term debilitating problems. Untreated *acute stress reactions* could progress to posttraumatic stress disorder (PTSD).

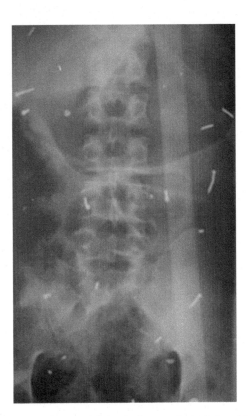

Blast Injury. Figure 2 Abdominal x-ray of suicide bombing victim showing multiple destructive metal objects in abdomen that were packed in the bomb

Treatment

The two major therapeutic challenges for blast victims are the multiplicity and complexity of the injuries, and the probability that they will present in a mass casualty setting. Optimizing the outcome of each casualty may be impeded by competing, or contradictory treatment modalities for different injuries, with the treatment of one injury making another worse. Further adding to this challenge is the fact that major explosions typically result in a large number of casualties, unlike conventional forms of trauma which afflict only one patient at a time. The complex decision-making required for each blast victim is therefore magnified exponentially and may be substantially altered by the resource limitations of a mass casualty event. *Triage* assumes major importance in this setting in allocating and rationing scarce resources where they are judged to maximize overall casualty outcome to achieve the greatest good for the greatest number [4]. Initial management should follow the basic trauma principles of assuring airway, breathing, and circulation before addressing specific organ system injuries.

Tympanic Membrane Rupture/Ear Injuries

There is no specific intervention required for most cases of external, middle, or inner ear blast trauma. TMR usually heals spontaneously without significant long-term consequences. Tympanoplasty may be beneficial in some cases to prevent infectious complications and hearing problems. Cholesteatomas may develop over time, and do require surgical intervention to prevent the danger of erosion through the skull with the possibility of direct invasion and infection of CNS structures. Regular follow-up examinations of the ear are recommended to prevent these long-term problems [5].

Blast Lung Injury

The goal of BLI therapy is to maximize oxygenation while minimizing air embolism. The challenge lies in the complexity of this injury, which may include elements of barotrauma from PBI, bronchopleural and alveolar-venous fistulae, pneumothorax, hemothorax, blunt and penetrating injuries to the chest wall and lungs, inhalation injury, and shock. The standard treatment of these problems tend to be contradictory, such as the need for high ventilatory pressures to expand functional residual capacity to improve oxygenation, while the risk of air embolism and pneumothorax require lower pressures. The volume expansion required for shock tends to worsen pulmonary congestion and hypoxia. Ventilatory and shock management must therefore be judicious to achieve a fine balance between these different therapeutic requirements. Effective ventilation strategies include maintenance of low tidal volumes (5–7 cc/kg) that restrict peak inspiratory pressure and plateau pressure to <20 cmH$_2$O and <40 cmH$_2$O, respectively. Pressure control ventilation is recommended for difficult cases, with PEEP at 10–20 cmH$_2$O, and keeping FiO$_2$ as low as possible to maintain arterial oxygen saturation above 90%. Permissive hypercapnia may be necessary in refractory cases, in which setting pH should be kept >7.25. Prone positioning and nitric oxide may be used to enhance oxygenation. Extracorporeal membrane oxygenation (ECMO) is one intervention to consider in cases refractory to these methods [6].

Adding to these difficulties is the relatively slow evolution of some cases of BLI over hours to days, requiring a high index of suspicion, and close observation of those blast victims with evidence of PBI or thoracic wounds. Early administration of high flow oxygen is recommended in these cases, with intubation for the standard indications to support oxygenation or ventilation.

Research has shown that BLI is associated with an intense inflammatory response, and that antioxidant and vasodilating agents such as heme-oxygenase-1 (HO-1), hemin, and manganese superoxide dismutase (MnSOD) enhance resolution of the lung damage and inflammation, improving recovery from BLI. Effective prevention of BLI has been developed in the form of ballistic vests that disrupt and dissipate the stress, shock, and shear components of the blast wave before it exerts destructive effects on the thoracic viscera [3].

Abdominal Blast Injury

All blast victims should be examined for external markers and physical signs of intra-abdominal injury. Serious injuries may be delayed in their presentation, emphasizing the importance of close observation and radiologic imaging for any development of abdominal pain, peritoneal signs, hypotension and free intraperitoneal air. In mass casualty settings imaging must be minimized, although abdominal ultrasound has proven useful in this setting for its sensitivity, safety, and rapidity. Any penetrating wounds to the torso, no matter how small, should prompt a low threshold for exploratory laparotomy, due to their association with foreign body damage to the viscera (see Fig. 2) [1–3].

Soft Tissue and Extremity Blast Injury

These injuries are generally noncritical and nonfatal but may lead to long-term morbidity. Standard shock management and hemorrhage control should be applied to these victims initially. Open and closed fractures should be cleansed, covered, and splinted until definitive treatment can be initiated. Soft tissue wounds should be vigorously managed with debridement and thorough exploration for foreign body removal, followed by closure or skin grafting. Crush injuries and associated renal failure, hyperkalemia and rhabdomyolysis should be managed with aggressive volume repletion and debridement of nonviable tissue. Extremity vascular injuries should be addressed once life-threatening problems have been stabilized, with shunting to restore perfusion and maintain limb viability until definitive repair can be undertaken. Long-term rehabilitation should be planned [2].

Severe thermal burns are found in victims close to the blast source from the intense fireball. This is the one form of soft tissue blast injury that has a high mortality. Standard burn management should be applied to afflicted survivors, including volume repletion, topical antibiotics, and burn wound excision and debridement. There is a high risk of compartment syndrome in circumferentially burned extremities due to the destructive effect of PBI on the underlying muscle tissue. Therefore, unlike standard burns not related to blasts, blast-induced circumferential extremity burns require routine fasciotomy rather than simple escharotomy [3].

Blast CNS Injury
Open skull fractures and penetrating wounds to the head and spine in blast victims should be managed as aggressively as resources permit. The entire spine should be immobilized due to the known pattern of multiple spine fractures associated with blast, until a full radiologic and clinical assessment excludes these injuries. This is one of the few indications for early CT scan evaluation, as rapid identification of major intracranial hemorrhage or foreign body implantation should prompt immediate surgery to maximize survival. Facial fractures and eye injuries may be delayed in their diagnosis and definitive management.

Obstetric Blast Injuries
Pregnant women have a unique susceptibility to blast injury. Although the fetus and gravid uterus do not contain air, the strong amplification of the blast wave through the amniotic fluid poses risks of fetal injuries from PBI. Sonographic assessment should focus on detection of uterine rupture or placental abruption, and can also monitor fetal heart tones and fetal movement. Secondary and tertiary blast phases threaten the uterus with direct trauma. Rh-negative pregnant women should be given anti-D-immunoglobulin to protect against isoimmunization in this setting.

Psychological Trauma
Assessment of casualties, prehospital responders, and medical providers for mental health issues should be an integral part of any response to an explosive event. In the acute phase of casualty management, medical personnel should be evaluated regularly for critical signs of stress which could impair their own mental health as well as their care of casualties. Any person who is judged to be impaired should then be pulled out of the care system for a brief rest. Long-term follow-up of victims and providers is also important in order to identify signs of acute stress reaction, including irritability, withdrawal, insomnia, and personality changes. Early treatment interventions for this could reduce the chance of progression to the more long-term PTSD. Psychological follow-up could also identify those problems that may have an organic basis from PBI effects on the brain.

Prognosis
There are several external markers of exposure to the blast wave that should be recognized on physical examination of blast victims. Ear examination should be performed on all blast victims for TMR. Although TMR is a sensitive marker of exposure to the primary blast wave, and therefore indicates the need to observe afflicted survivors closely, it does not significantly correlate with severity of injury or prognosis. Markers that have been associated with significant mortality risk in victims of blast injury include chest and abdominal trauma, blast lung injury, severe head injury, and traumatic amputation of limbs

Blast Injury. Table 3 Prognostic factors in major explosions

Blast-related factors
Magnitude of explosive energy
Proximity to blast
Extent of secondary fragmentation
Biologic, chemical or radiologic dissemination
Occurrence of building collapse
Environmental factors
Surrounding medium – underwater versus air
Confined space versus open-air explosion
Rural or isolated locale
Toxic fumes, dust and debris
Anatomic and physiologic factors
Number of body systems injured
Injury Severity Score >15
Age and comorbidities
Treatment delay
Primary Blast Injury
Tympanic membrane rupture
Blast lung injury with respiratory failure
Bowel injury
Brain injury
Spine and spinal cord injury
Traumatic amputation
Secondary and Tertiary Blast Injury
Blunt and penetrating torso injuries
Impalement
Skull fractures
Glasgow Coma Score <10
Foreign body implantation (metallic, glass, human remains)
Quarternary Blast Injury
Extensive and deep burns
Crush injuries
Toxic inhalation injuries
Biologic, chemical, radiologic exposure/contamination/ingestion

and other body parts. Soft tissue and skeletal injuries do not generally pose a risk of mortality (see Table 2), although major burns are a marker of mortality risk in survivors, as this indicates close proximity to the blast [4]. In victims who were in close proximity to a blast, studies have shown that the presence of sustained hypotension and two or more of the elements of multiple (>2) long bone fractures, penetrating head injury, and associated fatalities correlate with significant risk of mortality. All victims of confined space explosions, especially involving building collapse, have higher risks of mortality than those from open-air blasts [1–3]. Several other nonanatomic and non-physiologic prognostic factors also correlate with the outcome of blast victims (Table 3).

The prognosis of BLI is related to the severity of tissue damage and the rapidity of provision of oxygenation and ventilatory support. The Pizov scale is an objective measure of BLI prognosis that correlates with outcome, using the following three elements of mortality risk: worsening PaO_2:FiO_2 ratio, extent and duration of pulmonary air leaks and bronchopleural fistulae, and the extent of radiographic infiltrates on chest x-ray [6]. This could be useful in making clinical decisions regarding aggressive interventions to support lung function, such as altering I/E ratios, prone positioning, use of nitric oxide, and ECMO.

References

1. Wightman JM, Gladish SL (2001) Explosions and blast injuries. Ann Emerg Med 37:664–678
2. Born CT (2005) Blast trauma: the fourth weapon of mass destruction. Scand J Surg 94:279–285
3. Champion HR, Holcomb JB, Young LA (2009) Injuries from explosions: physics, biophysics, pathology, and required research focus. J Trauma 66:1468–1477
4. Frykberg ER, Tepas JJ (1988) Terrorist bombings: lessons learned from Belfast to Beirut. Ann Surg 208:569–576
5. Turegano-Fuentes F, Caba-Doussoux P, Jovier-Navalon JM et al (2008) Injury patterns from major urban terrorist bombings in trains: the Madrid experience. World J Surg 32:1168–1175
6. Pizov R, Oppenheim-Eden A, Matot I et al (1999) Blast lung injury from an explosion on a civilian bus. Chest 115:165–172

Blast Lung

▶ Blast Injury

Blast Lung Injury

▶ Blast Injury

Blast Trauma

▶ Blast Injury

Blastomycosis

JULIE P. CHOU[1], TOM LIM[1], ANDREW G. LEE[2]
CHRISTOPHER H. MODY[3]
[1]Department of Internal Medicine, University of Calgary, Calgary, AB, Canada
[2]Department of Radiology, University of Calgary, Calgary, AB, Canada
[3]Departments of Internal Medicine and Microbiology, Immunology and Infectious Disease, University of Calgary, Calgary, AB, Canada

Synonyms

Chicago disease; Gilchrist's disease; North American blastomycosis

Definition

Blastomycosis is a multisystem disease caused by *Blastomyces dermatitidis*, a dimorphic fungus. Blastomycosis is endemic in southeastern and southcentral states bordering the Mississippi and Ohio River basins, the Midwestern states in the USA, and Canadian provinces bordering the Great Lakes. Cases have also been encountered in Africa, Mexico, and Central and South America.

The clinical presentation ranges from asymptomatic infection to acute, subacute, or chronic pneumonia and extrapulmonary disease. Although *B. dermatitidis* has been reported to involve any organ, the lung is the most commonly affected, followed by skin, bones, and genitourinary system.

The lungs are the portals of entry for blastomycosis. Diverse pulmonary presentations including lobar pneumonia (Fig. 1), mass lesions, single or multiple nodules, and chronic fibronodular or fibrocavitary infiltrates have been described. Rarely, patients might present with an infectious acute respiratory distress syndrome (ARDS) [1].

Dissemination from the lung resulting in multiorgan involvement occurs in approximately 20% of cases. Extrapulmonary disease is either concurrent with active pulmonary disease or occurs after resolution of a clinical or subclinical primary infection, often within 1 or 2 years [2].

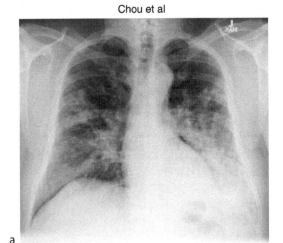

Chou et al

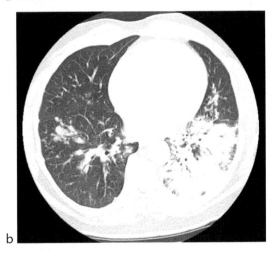

Blastomycosis. Figure 1 Blastomycosis in two different patients. (**a**) A chest radiograph of acute blastomycosis resembling bacterial pneumonia. (**b**) Computed tomography showing lobar infiltrate in acute blastomycosis

Skin is the second most common site of infection after the lung. The lesions can be verrucous or ulcerative in appearance. Subcutaneous nodules are also possible. Osteomyelitis can occur in up to a quarter of patients with disseminated blastomycosis. Vertebrae, pelvis, and sacrum are the most common sites. Genitourinary disease manifests in the form of prostatitis or epididymo-orchitis in men. Rare cases of tuboovarian abscess or endometritis have been reported in women. In immunocompetent individuals, less than 5% of patients with disseminated disease present with central nervous system (CNS) involvement. In contrast, the CNS is commonly affected in immunocompromised patients, especially those with AIDS [3].

Treatment

Immunocompetent Host

Patients with mild to moderate disease involving the lung, skin, and/or bone, which can be treated with itraconazole, are unlikely to present to the intensive care unit. By contrast, life-threatening pulmonary infections, such as those that require intensive care therapy can be treated with intravenous amphotericin B deoxycholate (0.7–1.0 mg/kg/day) to a total cumulative dose of 1.5–2.5 g. Treatment can be delivered daily until there is clinical improvement and then three times weekly. Since renal function is often impaired in critically ill patients, liposomal amphotericin B (5 mg/kg/day) often becomes the preferred agent. Once clinical stability has been achieved with intravenous therapy, a sequential course of therapy with itraconazole 200 mg orally twice daily is administered for at least 6 months [4].

Meningeal infections require therapy with amphotericin B deoxycholate at a dose of 0.7 mg/kg/day, to a total dose of at least 2.0 g, or, when indicated, liposomal amphotericin B as described above. High-dose fluconazole (400–800 mg daily intravenously or orally) can be used in combination with amphotericin B from the onset or used in sequence after initial improvement. The duration of therapy is for a minimum of 6 months. Fluconazole is used in lieu of itraconazole because of its superior CNS penetration.

Immunosuppressed Host

Patients with immunosuppression are known to have higher mortality and therefore require more aggressive treatment strategies. For treating pulmonary and nonmeningeal blastomycosis, amphotericin B (or liposomal amphotericin B) is used as the first line agent, followed by oral itraconazole 200 mg twice daily for a minimum of 12 months. Recommended treatment for mild to moderate clinical infections is oral itraconazole from onset. In patients with AIDS, lifetime maintenance is required.

CNS involvement is treated with amphotericin B deoxycholate (or liposomal amphotericin B) in combination with high-dose fluconazole (400–800 mg/daily) from onset. The sequential therapy with fluconazole is continued for an additional 12 months.

Special Circumstances

In patients presenting with fulminant pneumonia and/or ARDS, the initial therapy consists of amphotericin B deoxycholate (or liposomal amphotericin B) often in combination with itraconazole 200 mg intravenously twice daily until clinical improvement, followed by oral itraconazole for 6 months (immunocompetent), 12 months (immunocompromised), or indefinitely (AIDS).

CNS blastomycosis that progresses on amphotericin B deoxycholate or develops while the patient is on itraconazle will require a change in treatment strategy. The recommended regime includes liposomal amphotericin B plus fluconazole 800 mg/day to clinical improvement followed by fluconazole for 6 months, 12 months, or indefinitely in immunocompetent, immunocompromised, and AIDS patients, respectively.

For a more complete discussion of therapy with references, the reader is referred to the ATS Statement on the management of fungal infections [5].

Evaluation/Assessment

Once suspected, the diagnosis of blastomycosis can be supported by the appearance of broad-based budding yeasts in sputum, bronchoalveolar lavage, or tissue biopsy. A commercially available urine antigen testing kit is quite sensitive for diagnosis; however it demonstrates cross-reactivity with *Histoplasma* antigen. A culture of *B. dermatitidis* remains the definitive diagnostic standard.

After-care

In patients with AIDS, maintenance therapy with itraconazole is required indefinitely.

Prognosis

The mortality rate in appropriately treated blastomycosis is ≤15%, but exceeds 50% in patients presenting as ARDS.

References

1. Lemos L, Baliga M, Guo M (2001) Acute respiratory distress syndrome and blastomycosis: presentation of nine cases and review of the literature. Ann Diagnostic Pathol 5:1–9
2. Sarosi GA, Davies SF (1979) Blastomycosis. Am Rev Respir Dis 120:911–938
3. Pappas PG, Pottage JC, Powderly WG, Fraser VJ, Stratton CW, McKenzie S, Tapper ML, Chmel H, Bonebrake FC, Blum R et al (1992) Bastomycosis in patients with the acquired immunodeficiency syndrome. Ann Intern Med 116:847–853
4. Chapman SW, Bradsher RW, Jr., Campbell GD, Jr., Pappas PG, Kauffman CA (2000) Practice guidelines for the management of patients with blastomycosis. Infectious Diseases Society of America. Clin Infect Dis 30:679–683
5. Limper AH, Knox KS, Sarosi GA, Ampel NM, Bennett JE, Catanzaro A, Davies SF, Dismukes WE, Hage C, Marr K, Mody CH, Perfect JR, Stevens DA (2011) An official American Thoracic Society statement on the treatment of fungal infections in adult pulmonary and critical care patients. Am J Respir Crit Care Med 183:96–128

Bleeding

▶ Blakemore Tube
▶ Hematologic Complications of Children on the ICU

Bleeding and Hemostasis in Acute Renal Failure

GEORGES OUELLET, MARTINE LEBLANC
Service de néphrologie, Hôpital Maisonneuve-Rosemont
Centre hospitalier affilié à l'Univ. de Montréal, Montréal, QC, Canada

Synonyms

Alterations in coagulation in acute renal failure; Impact of renal replacement therapy on coagulation; Thrombotic diathesis in acute renal failure; Uremic bleeding; Uremic coagulopathy

Trade Names

Desmopressin
DDAVP®, Stimate®, Minirin®

Conjugated Estrogens
Premarin®

Erythropoietin
Eprex®, Epogen®, Procrit®

Tranexamic Acid
Cyklokapron®

Class and Category

Desmopressin
Vasopressin analog

Conjugated Estrogens
Hormone replacement therapy

Erythropoietin
Erythropoiesis-stimulating agent (ESA)

Tranexamic Acid
Antifibrinolytic agent

Indications

Bleeding

Alterations in hemostasis in acute renal failure (ARF) are numerous and may expose the patient to serious risks. The clinical spectrum of bleeding complications in acute and chronic renal failure (CRF) ranges from petechia, ecchymoses, and oozing at puncture sites, to life-threatening gastrointestinal, cerebral, or retroperitoneal hemorrhage. The intensity and aggressiveness of the interventions taken to control the bleeding will be dictated by its severity and acute character. In acute or life-threatening hemorrhage, the hemostasis should be quickly corrected. Treatments with short onset of action (desmopressin, cryoprecipitate) should thus be selected, pending more definitive measures to control the bleeding diathesis. Subacute or chronic low-grade bleeding in uremia should be addressed with longer-lasting interventions, such as conjugated estrogens, initiation or optimization of dialysis, and correction of anemia.

Invasive Procedure

Patients with ARF are also at particular risk of bleeding complications while submitted to an invasive procedure, such as central venous catheterization, surgery, or renal biopsy. Agents with a short onset of action (desmopressin, cryoprecipitate) may be particularly useful in this context. Screening for abnormal hemostasis may be considered before performance of any invasive procedure. However, coagulation tests such as activated partial thromboplastin time, prothrombin time, and thrombin time are frequently normal in uremia. Prolongation of the cutaneous ▶ bleeding time is regarded as the best indicator of uremic coagulopathy by many nephrologists, despite controversies regarding lack of reproducibility and of clear correlations of abnormal results with post-procedure bleeding. The in vitro ▶ closure time (PFA), or platelet function analyzer, is a more recent test presenting less technical variability and patient discomfort. In a small case-control study comparing this assay with a historic cohort of patients screened with cutaneous bleeding time, a better positive predictive value and a comparable negative predictive value were shown for hemorrhagic complications following kidney biopsy [1]. The same study also showed that bleeding complications were not significantly more frequent in patients with prolonged bleeding time than in patients with a normal test. Systematic administration of desmopressin or cryoprecipitate prior to invasive procedure is probably not cost-effective in most institutions [2]. It should be emphasized that the utilization of both the cutaneous bleeding time and the platelet function analyzer has been described in patients requiring dialysis, but not specifically in the critically ill patient with ARF.

Abnormal Coagulation Test

An abnormal coagulation test, in the absence of bleeding or anticipated invasive procedure, is not an indication for a corrective intervention per se.

Dosage

Desmopressin is usually administered intravenously at a dose of 0.3 µg/kg. The same dosage is recommended for subcutaneous administration. The intranasal route is also effective at a dose of 3 µg/kg. Desmopressin effect on bleeding time appears within 1 h, lasts for 4–8 h, and disappears within 24 h. The efficacy of desmopressin decreases over the course of repeated administration.

When cryoprecipitate is selected for correction of uremic bleeding, 10 units are usually infused, and can be repeated every 12–24 h. Cryoprecipitate corrects bleeding time in approximately 50% of patients, within 1 h of administration. Its effect lasts for 4–24 h.

Different dosages have been described for conjugated estrogens in uremic bleeding, all of them in patients on chronic hemodialysis [3]. One single 25 mg oral dose of conjugated estrogens can normalize bleeding time for 3–10 days. Intravenous administration might be more practical and result in better absorption in the critically ill patient with ARF. The recommended dose is 0.6 mg/kg for five consecutive days; the effect on bleeding time lasts for 14 days. The maximal effect of a single dose is reached within 24 h. Transdermal estradiol patches application twice weekly at a dose of 50–100 µg/kg is also effective.

Correction of anemia improves platelets rheology by promoting their laminar flow along the endothelial surface, increasing platelets-vessel wall interactions. Depending on the clinical context, use of ESA or packed red blood cells to raise the hemoglobin above 100 g/l (hematocrit > 30%) has been advocated in patients on chronic hemodialysis. It should however be emphasized that there is no evidence of clear benefits for ESA administration in ARF.

Uremic toxins play a key role in platelets functional abnormalities. Therefore, uremic bleeding is an indication for initiation or optimization of dialysis in CRF. While the beneficial effect of uremic toxins clearance on hemostasis is logical, no optimal dialysis dose has been described for that matter in chronic hemodialysis patients. As well, bleeding complications were either not addressed or not significantly different between groups in the large randomized studies that investigated the outcome of different dialysis doses in ARF.

Although tranexamic acid can shorten bleeding time [4], its role in the treatment of uremic bleeding is not well characterized. Successful treatment of intracranial or upper gastrointestinal hemorrhage was described in chronic hemodialysis patients, but there is no evidence for its utilization in ARF. Various dosages have been reported. Tranexamic acid accumulates in renal insufficiency. Therefore, this medication should be used in the presence of acute bleeding when other measures have failed.

Preparation/Composition

Desmopressin (1-deamino-8-D-arginine vasopressin) is a synthetic derivative of arginine vasopressin, the antidiuretic hormone. Oral tablet and liquid forms are available. The liquid form can be administered by the intranasal route with a metered spray pump. When administered intravenously, it should be diluted in 50 ml of normal saline and given over 30 min.

Cryoprecipitate is obtained from centrifugation of a thawed fresh frozen plasma unit. Virtually all of factor VIII, von Willebrand factor (vWF), factor XIII, fibrinogen, and fibronectin of the fresh frozen plasma are found in a cryoprecipitate unit, in a volume of 10–15 ml instead of 250 ml.

Conjugated estrogens contain a mixture of different estrogens. The formulations available on the market are derived from plants or pregnant mares' urine. The conjugation of estrogens allows for better digestive absorption.

Tranexamic acid is a synthetic analog of the amino acid lysine. It is available in tablet and injectable forms. The intravenous formulation may be injected directly, without previous dilution.

Recombinant human erythropoietin (rHuEPO) is produced by transfer of the human erythropoietin gene in a mammalian cell line culture. Darbepoietin alfa (Aranesp®), an analog of erythropoietin, has two extra N-linked glycosylation chains that confer longer half-life and is manufactured in the same manner as rHuEPO. ESA are available in pre-filled, fixed-dose preservative-free syringes, and in multi-dose vials, which contain a preservative.

Contraindications

Although not a formal contraindication, a prolonged bleeding time or closure time, in the absence of active bleeding or anticipated invasive procedure, should not be regarded as an indication for treatment of uremic coagulopathy.

Estrogens should be avoided in patients with a history of or an active venous thromboembolic event, with an active or recent arterial thromboembolic event, or with an estrogen-dependant tumor.

Tranexamic acid is contraindicated in patients with active thrombosis or subarachnoid hemorrhage, due to risk of secondary hydrocephalus.

Hypersensitivity to human albumin, a history of acquired ESA-related ▶ pure red cell aplasia, and uncontrolled hypertension are contraindications for administration of erythropoietin analogs.

Adverse Reactions

Although not frequent, a vasopressor effect of desmopressin is possible when administered intravenously. Facial flushing and local discomfort at site of injection may occur. Mild to moderate thrombocytopenia may develop. Thrombotic events, especially in patients with pre-existent vascular disease, have been rarely reported following the administration of desmopressin. When desmopressin is used to treat central diabetes insipidus, hyponatremia and water intoxication may become a concern. However, the risk for these complications is virtually inexistent when the medication is employed to control uremic bleeding in an oligo-anuric ARF patient.

Cryoprecipitate is a blood product and is thus associated with the risk of viral transmission. Since each cryoprecipitate is obtained from a different plasma specimen, the transmission risk increases with the number of cryoprecipitate units administered.

No significant adverse reactions were observed in the studies describing the use of conjugated estrogens to control uremic bleeding, since the hormone is administered for a relatively short time. Long-term administration of conjugated estrogens has nevertheless been associated with deep vein thrombosis, myocardial infarction, stroke, and aggravation of hypertension. Caution is thus advised when prescribing this medication to a patient with a positive history for these conditions.

Tranexamic acid can cause hypotension when rapidly infused. Arterial and venous thromboses have been reported.

Besides usual transfusion risks, packed red blood cells can cause volume overload in ARF patients not receiving renal replacement therapy, or on intermittent hemodialysis.

Intravenous administration of ESA is associated with aggravation of hypertension. In chronic hemodialysis patients, normalization of the hematocrit with ESA has been associated with increased mortality and increased incidence of stroke, cardiovascular events, and arteriovenous access thrombosis. These potential complications are less concerning in the critically ill patient with ARF, since ESA was not shown to have a significant impact on the anemia of acute kidney injury.

Drug Interactions

Beta-lactam antibiotics and third-generation cephalosporins are commonly prescribed in the intensive care unit. Their accumulation in uremia may alter platelet membrane function and adenosine diphosphate (ADP) receptors, thereby further disturbing hemostasis. Since their effect lasts up to 10 days after the last dose, any antiplatelet drug taken by the patient prior to its intensive care unit admission may also have an adverse impact on its coagulation. Nonsteroidal anti-inflammatory drugs, on top of their deleterious renal effects, may have an antiplatelet effect.

Dialysis has a beneficial effect on hemostasis in the uremic patient. However, in order to avoid coagulation of the extracorporeal circuit, heparin is part of a standard dialysis prescription and therefore exposes the patient to an increased risk of bleeding. Heparin can also cause mild, transient thrombocytopenia or florid heparin-induced thrombocytopenia with positive anti-heparin antibodies. Heparin utilization should thus be minimized, and ideally avoided in the ARF patient with bleeding. In this regard, different strategies, such as ▶ saline flushes, hemofiltration in ▶ predilution mode, or citrate ▶ regional anticoagulation, can be employed. The interaction between blood and the dialysis membrane may result in chronic platelet activation, ultimately resulting in their exhaustion. This phenomenon is probably more important with the use, nowadays infrequent in most units, of ▶ bioincompatible membranes, which resulted in increased complement activation and cytokine release.

Desmopressin, when used to control uremic bleeding, is not subject to significant drug interactions since repeated administration is unusual. Enhancement of the thrombogenic effect of fibrinogen and activated prothrombin complex concentrates with tranexamic acid is possible and their combination should consequently be avoided. Conjugated estrogens induce the metabolism of CYP 1A2 and CYP 3A4 substrates, leading to many potentially significant interactions. ESA are associated with no known significant interactions.

Mechanisms of Action

Normal Hemostasis

The three phases of normal hemostasis are primary hemostasis, coagulation, and fibrinolysis.

In primary hemostasis, the interaction of platelet receptors glycoprotein Ib and glycoprotein IIb-IIIa with vWF and fibrinogen results in adherence to the breached endothelium. Adhesion of the platelets to the vessel wall is followed by a conformational change. ADP, thromboxane, vWF, fibrinogen, thrombin, serotonin, and epinephrine are released from platelets granules. These substances generate further platelet activation and aggregation, and cause vasoconstriction. Uremic bleeding, mainly a problem of primary hemostasis, is associated with defects in most steps of the hemostatic plug formation, probably due to interactions of uremic toxins with platelet receptors and granules [3].

The coagulation cascade consists of two pathways. The intrinsic pathway is activated by contact with negatively charged surfaces, and the extrinsic pathway is activated by tissue factor. Tissue factor is a cell membrane protein exposed after endothelial injury. The complexation of tissue factor and factor VIIa is the trigger that activates the cascade that leads to formation of fibrin polymers. Antithrombin, protein C, the tissue factor pathway inhibitor, and glycosaminoglycans regulate the coagulation cascade. Despite a net bleeding tendency, procoagulant abnormalities in the coagulation cascade are observed in uremia [3].

Fibrinolysis, the final step of normal hemostasis, leads to fibrin dissolution through the proteolytic action of plasmin. The action of tissue plasminogen activator or urokinase initiates fibrinolysis by activating plasminogen to plasmin. Abnormalities in the fibrinolytic system in uremia are complex, but activation is likely, as suggested by reports of positive results with tranexamic acid in the treatment of uremic bleeding [4].

Therapeutic Interventions

Desmopressin exerts its effect on hemostasis by inducing the release of factor VIII:vWF multimers from the endothelial cells stores. The decrease in desmopressin efficacy over repeated administration appears to result from depletion of these stores.

The effect of cryoprecipitate on bleeding time is mediated by the presence of vWF multimers.

The mechanism of action of conjugated estrogens in the treatment of uremic bleeding is not well described. Inhibition of nitric oxide (NO) synthesis, an inhibitor of platelet function, seems to be important. Indeed, the effect of conjugated estrogens on bleeding time is abolished by the administration of L-arginine, a precursor of NO.

Tranexamic acid may reduce uremic bleeding by inhibiting fibrinolysis. Binding of plasminogen to fibrin and activation of plasminogen to plasmin are inhibited, resulting in stabilization of the hemostatic clot.

ESA and packed red blood cells, by increasing the hematocrit, have a favorable effect on the platelets rheology. Erythrocytes displace platelets toward the vessel wall, thereby facilitating platelet–vessel wall interactions.

References

1. van den Hoogen M, Verbruggen B, Polenewen R, Hilbrands L, Nováková I (2009) Use of the platelet function analyzer to minimize bleeding complications after renal biopsy. Thromb Res 123:515–522
2. Mattix H, Singh A (1999) Is the bleeding time predictive of bleeding prior to a percutaneous renal biopsy? Curr Opin Nephrol Hypertens 8:715–718
3. Galbusera M, Remuzzi G, Boccardo P (2009) Treatment of bleeding in dialysis patients. Semin Dial 22:279–286
4. Mezzano D, Panes O, Muñoz B, Pais E, Tagle R et al (1999) Tranexamic acid inhibits fibrinolysis, shortens the bleeding time and improves platelet function in patients with chronic renal failure. Thromb Haemost 82:1250–1254

Bleeding Patient

MARCEL M. LEVI

Department of Medicine, Academic Medical Center, University of Amsterdam, Amsterdam, The Netherlands

Synonyms
(Excessive) blood loss; Hemorrhage

Definition
Blood loss, either spontaneously or upon an invasive procedure. Bleeding may be minor, major, or excessive; for this classification various criteria are used. Commonly, excessive blood loss is (arbitrarily) defined as bleeding at a rate of >200 mL/h, and or bleeding leading to hemodynamic instability, and/or bleeding leading to transfusion of >5 U red cell concentrate within 3 h. For major bleeding, a more consensual definition is used, that is, any bleeding leading to a clinically significant intervention (such as transfusion, hospital admission, a procedure (e.g., endoscopy)) and any intracranial, intra-abdominal, retroperitoneal, or intrathoracic bleeding. Minor bleeding is all other bleeding that does not meet the criteria for major bleeding.

Characteristics
The leading causes of major blood loss (20% of total blood volume or more) are surgical operations, among which the most frequently implicated are cardiovascular operations, liver transplantation and resection, major orthopedic procedures, including hip and knee replacement, and spine surgery [1]. Nonsurgical causes of excessive blood loss may also occur. For instance, bleeding is the second most important cause of death in patients with trauma, contributing to approximately 30% of trauma-related mortality. There are also situations in which bleeding poses a major clinical challenge due to its critical localization, as illustrated by intracerebral hemorrhage.

Severe bleeding often results in the need of allogeneic blood transfusion. Even if benefits of transfusion outweigh the still existing risks (allergic reactions, transmission of infections, acute lung injury, and immunosuppression), the implementation of strategies meant to minimize the use of a limited community resource is mandatory (see further entry on ▶ Blood Transfusion). The most obvious and probably most effective strategy is the improvement of surgical and anesthesiological techniques. A successful example is liver transplantation, which required huge amount of blood products in the past, but is now performed with minimal transfusion requirements.

In the bleeding patient, it is first important to rule out abnormalities of hemostasis that can usually be corrected by replacement of the defective components. However, there are cases for which no surgical or hemostatic cause can be identified and yet excessive blood loss warrants the adoption of pharmacological strategies, broadly divided in perioperative prophylaxis during at-risk operations or intervention should bleeding occur.

Most experience with pro-hemostatic therapy has been accumulated in the prevention and treatment of bleeding in patients with congenital and acquired coagulation defects. Indeed, specific correction of a hemostatic defect is highly effective in this situation, as, for example, has been shown in the management of hemophilia with coagulation factor concentrates. There is, however, increasing evidence that also in patients with less specific abnormalities or even a normal coagulation status and who encounter severe bleeding or are at high risk for bleeding, promoting hemostatic function may be of benefit. Interestingly, there seems in general not to be a strong need to specifically target a factor or pathway in the coagulation or fibrinolytic system that is causally related to the hemostatic defect, since interference in one part of the system may be able to compensate for a defect in another part.

The safety of pro-hemostatic therapy also deserves some consideration. Interfering in the balance between coagulant and anticoagulant mechanisms can indeed result in undesirable adverse effects. The best illustration may be the higher risk of bleeding in patients receiving anticoagulant therapy. Conversely, pro-hemostatic agents may, at least theoretically, predispose for thrombotic complications. The occurrence of such complications, which are fortunately relatively rare, seems to be very much dependent on considerate clinical use of this therapy. Obviously, the expected benefit of the application of pro-hemostatic agents in distinct clinical situations should be balanced with the risk of thrombosis in that particular patient population. Ideally, the benefit/risk ratio should be evaluated in properly controlled clinical trials.

Desmopressin (DDAVP)

De-amino D-arginine vasopressin (DDAVP, desmopressin) is a vasopressin analog that despite minor molecular differences has retained its antidiuretic properties but has much less vasoactive effects. DDAVP induces release of the contents of the endothelial cell associated Weibel Palade bodies, including von Willebrand factor. Hence, the administration of DDAVP results in a marked increase in the plasma concentration of von Willebrand factor (and associated coagulation factor VIII) and (also by yet unexplained additional mechanisms) a remarkable augmentation of primary hemostasis as a consequence. A rare but important adverse effect of DDAVP is the occurrence of acute coronary syndromes, such as myocardial infarction and unstable angina, particularly in patients with preexisting unstable coronary artery disease, probably due to the remaining vasoactive effect of the drug. Hence, in these patients the use of DDAVP is contraindicated. The antidiuretic effect of a single or once repeated dose of DDAVP is clinically not very significant and may be dealt with by fluid restriction for some time. Exceptions to this rule are children, who may experience a severe dilution hyponatremia after the administration of DDAVP, which should be monitored clinically for 24 h after its administration.

Recombinant Activated Factor VII

Based on the current insight that activation of coagulation in vivo predominantly proceeds by the tissue factor/factor VIIa pathway, recombinant factor VIIa (NovoSeven®) has been developed as a pro-hemostatic agent and is now available for clinical use. Indeed, recombinant factor VIIa appears to exert potent pro-hemostatic effects. Most experience with recombinant factor VIIa has been accumulated in patients with severe coagulation defects that are difficult to treat, such as patients with antibodies to coagulation factors (e.g., so-called inhibitors to factors VIII or IX) and excessive bleeding. In addition, in patients with severe thrombocytopenia or disorders of primary hemostasis that fail to respond to conventional treatment, recombinant factor VIIa has been applied. In most of these

situations, administration of recombinant factor VIIa was shown to be effective in controlling bleeding, although most of the reports are uncontrolled series. Recombinant fVIIa has been licensed for the prevention and treatment of bleeding in patients with antibodies to coagulation factors and complex platelet disorders. Nevertheless, there is an abundant number of case reports and case series on the hemostatic efficacy of rFVIIa in patients undergoing surgery. However, virtually all these reports did not include adequate controls, which makes it very hard to draw any clinical conclusion from them. Notwithstanding this lack of sound evidence, there is widespread off label use of rFVIIa in patients with excessive blood loss that is hard to treat by conventional measures. The first controlled trial of recombinant fVIIa was done in patients undergoing prostatectomy. This study demonstrated that the administration of recombinant factor VIIa was associated with a 50% reduction in perioperative blood loss, thereby completely eliminating the need for blood transfusion. Preliminary trials in patients with liver cirrhosis undergoing laparoscopic liver biopsies or liver transplantation indicated that the use of recombinant factor VIIa may limit blood loss and prevent transfusion, and subsequently large trials in major liver surgery were performed. In parallel, based on successful case reports and encouraging preclinical studies, administration of recombinant factor VIIa to trauma patients with excessive blood loss has also been evaluated in large controlled multicenter clinical trials. Generally, all trials show that administration of relatively high doses of recombinant factor VIIa is effective in reducing blood loss and reducing (excessive) transfusion, however, the intervention is not significantly effective at clinically directly more relevant outcomes, including mortality. A recent phase II dose-escalation and placebo-controlled study in 172 patients with major blood loss after cardiac surgery showed that the administration of rFVIIa resulted in less blood loss, a significant reduction in the need for reoperation (25% in the placebo group, 14% in the group receiving rFVIIa 40 μg/kg, and 12% in the group receiving rFVIIa 80 μg/kg), and a significant larger proportion of patients not needing any transfusion after the administration of rFVIIa (10% in the placebo group, 28% in the group receiving rFVIIa 40 μg/kg, and 32% in the group receiving rFVIIa 80 μg/kg). However, there were more serious adverse events in the patients treated with rFVIIa (13% versus 7% in the placebo group, not significant). Indeed, in view of its pro-hemostatic potency, the safety of rFVIIa, in particular as related to the potential occurrence of thrombosis, has been the subject of attention and surveillance. In controlled clinical trials, administration of this agent resulted in a relatively low incidence of thrombotic complications, comparable to placebo-treated patients [2, 3]. However, most of these studies were carried in patients with impaired coagulation or at low risk for thrombosis. In the trial carried out in patients with a much higher risk, such as those with intracerebral hemorrhage, serious thromboembolic events, mainly myocardial or cerebral infarction, occurred in 7% of patients treated with rFVIIa, as compared with 2% of placebo-treated patients. Hence, there is some indication that rFVIIa may heighten the risk of thrombotic complications and this needs to be offset to its potential benefit in patients with severe blood loss. More randomized controlled trials are needed to establish efficacy and safety in patients undergoing cardiac surgery.

Antifibrinolytic Treatment

Agents that exert anti-fibrinolytic activity are aprotinin and the group of lysine analogues. The pro-hemostatic effect of these agents proceeds not only by the inhibition of fibrinolysis (thereby shifting the procoagulant/anticoagulant balance towards a more procoagulant state), but also due to a protective effect on platelets, as has been demonstrated at least for aprotinin [1]. Aprotinin is a 58 amino acid polypeptide, mainly derived from bovine lung, parotid gland or, pancreas. Aprotinin directly inhibits the activity of various serine proteases, including plasmin, coagulation factors or inhibitors, and constituents of the kallikrein-kinin and angiotensin system. This rather nonspecific mode of action of aprotinin is frequently considered as a disadvantage for its use, however, the interactions of aprotinin with proteases other than plasmin have never been demonstrated to cause clinically important adverse effects. The clinically most important side effect of aprotinin is a rarely occurring but sometimes serious allergic or anaphylactic reaction. The use of aprotinin is contraindicated in case of ongoing systemic intravascular activation of coagulation, as in disseminated intravascular coagulation (DIC), and in patients with renal failure. Although many meta-analyses of controlled clinical trials with aprotinin have confirmed the potency of this agent to reduce (perioperative) blood loss and transfusion requirements [4], the safety of aprotinin was questioned by a study in 4,374 patients who underwent elective coronary-artery bypass surgery. The study was observational and non-randomized but used a propensity score method to balance the covariates. Compared with untreated controls, aprotinin (but neither aminocaproic acid nor tranexamic acid) doubled the occurrence of severe renal failure, increased the incidence of myocardial infarction or heart failure by 55%, and was associated with a nearly twofold increase in stroke or other cerebrovascular events. Subsequently, similar results were found in two other studies and in an observational survey conducted by the manufacturer of aprotinin in 67,000 patients undergoing cardiac surgery. A prospective randomized trial comparing aprotinin and lysine analogues in 2,331 high risk cardiac surgery patients confirmed a higher 30 day mortality in the aprotinin group (6.0%) in comparison with 3.9% in the tranexamic acid group and 4.0% in the aminocaproic acid group. Based on all these findings, the FDA has suspended the license of aprotinin in the USA and the manufacturer has stopped the distribution of the agent in the rest of the world.

Lysine analogues, that is, ε-aminocaproic acid and tranexamic acid are potent inhibitors of fibrinolysis. The antifibrinolytic action of lysine analogues is based on the competitive binding of these agents to the lysine-binding sites of a fibrin clot, thereby competing with the binding of plasminogen. Impaired plasminogen binding to fibrin delays the conversion of plasminogen to plasmin and subsequent plasmin-mediated fibrinolysis, which then proceeds at an inefficient and slow rate. Subtle molecular variations between different lysine analogues may have important consequences for their fibrinolysis-inhibiting capacity. Indeed, tranexamic acid (Cyklokapron®) is at least ten times more potent than ε-aminocaproic acid (Amicar®). The use of lysine analogues is contra-indicated in situations with ongoing systemic activation of coagulation (such as in DIC) and, furthermore, in case of macroscopic hematuria, since the inhibition of urinary fibrinolysis due to the high concentrations of the antifibrinolytic agent in the urine may result in deposition of urinary tract-obstructing clots. In view of the studies showing an efficacy in reducing blood loss of tranexamic acid that is similar to that of aprotinin, tranexamic acid (most frequently used total dose 3–10 g, usually divided in a loading dose of 2–7 g, and a maintenance dose of 20–250 mg/h, or given as bolus doses of 1 g, four times daily) is the most appropriate antifibrinolytic agent for use in patients with major blood loss or patients undergoing surgery, that is, high risk for bleeding.

References

1. Mannucci PM, Levi M (2007) Prevention and treatment of major blood loss. N Engl J Med 356:2301–2311
2. Levi M, Peters M, Buller HR (2005) Efficacy and safety of recombinant factor VIIa for the treatment of severe bleeding: a systematic review. Crit Care Med 33:883–890

3. Levi M (2009) Use of recombinant factor VIIa in the perioperative
    period. Hamostaseologie 29:68–70
4. Levi M, Cromheecke ME, de Jonge E, Prins MH, de Mol BA, Briet E,
    Buller HR (1999) Pharmacological strategies to decrease excessive
    blood loss in cardiac surgery: a meta-analysis of clinically relevant
    endpoints. Lancet 354:1940–1947

Bleeding Time

The cutaneous bleeding time is used to evaluate primary hemostasis, mainly in uremic patients. The test is performed by making an incision of a standardized depth and length on the skin of the forearm. A fixed pressure (usually 40 mm Hg) is applied with a blood pressure cuff above the level of the incision and the blood is regularly absorbed with a piece of filter paper. The time necessary for bleeding to completely stop is recorded and is the bleeding time. The normal bleeding time is 2–9 min.

ß-Blocker Toxicity

▶ ß-Adrenergic Antagonist Toxicity

Blood and Body Fluid Exposures

▶ Blood and Body Fluid Exposures and Postexposure Prophylaxis

Blood and Body Fluid Exposures and Postexposure Prophylaxis

James C. O'Neill
Department of Emergency Medicine, Wake Forest University Baptist Medical Center, Winston-Salem, NC, USA

Synonyms

Blood and body fluid exposures; Healthcare personnel exposures; Needle stick exposure; Occupational exposures

Characteristics

▶ Healthcare personnel (HCP) are constantly at risk of exposure to patient blood and body fluids. Preventing contact with these fluids by means of barrier protection most successfully minimizes this risk. Even with barrier protection, it is not usual for HCP to experience contact with patient bodily fluid through a splash or a needle stick injury at some point in their career. This entry will discuss the risks of various types of contact with bodily fluid and the post exposure prophylaxis (PEP) for Human Immunodeficiency Virus (HIV) that is currently recommended by the Centers for Disease Control (CDC). It is essential to follow local hospital recommendations when dealing with ▶ body fluid exposures. All PEP should be started with either local experts or with help from University of California PEPline hotline at 888 448 4911. All PEP should be started within hours rather than days to be effective [1].

Healthcare personnel are paid or unpaid hospital workers that are at risk of exposure to body fluids, tissue, or equipment and surfaces contaminated with such fluids. HCP are at risk for exposure to Hepatitis B, Hepatitis C, and HIV viruses. Most hospital workers are immunized against Hepatitis B. If an exposed employee is not immunized against Hepatitis B, they are given Hepatitis B vaccine and Hepatitis B immune globulin if a source patient is found to be positive for Hepatitis B surface antigen. There is no current PEP, vaccine, or immunoglobulin for Hepatitis C. If a source patient is found positive for Hepatitis C infection the HCP is tested monthly for a period of 6 months to determine if they are infected. PEP is given for HIV if the source patient is found to be HIV positive. The type of medications given for HIV PEP is determined by assessing whether the exposure is of high or low risk [2].

The average risk of HIV transmission is 0.3% due to percutaneous exposure of a needle infection with HIV infected blood. Several factors have been shown to increase the risk of developing HIV infection after percutaneous needle injury. These factors include: (1) a deep injury, (2) injury with a device that was visibly contaminated with the source patient's blood, (3) a procedure with a needle being placed in the source patient's artery or vein, (4) a high HIV viral load in the source blood, and (5) failure to undergo PEP after an exposure [3].

The risk of HIV transmission due to mucous membrane exposure is 0.09%. There is currently no good estimation of the risk of ▶ non-intact skin coming in contact with HIV infected body fluid, but the risk is thought to be less than that of mucous membrane exposure. In addition, the risk of contracting HIV from a "found" needle without a known source patient is extremely low. There have been no cases of transmission reported from a found needle outside a medical setting. In the medical setting, a "found" needle with no source patient has only been reported to cause three cases of HIV in 2 decades. Of note, saliva, urine, feces, respiratory secretions, and gastric fluid that are not visibly bloody cannot transmit HIV [4]. Risk of different exposures is found in Table 1.

Occupational Safety and Health Administration (▶ OSHA) requirements have been set to ensure that hospitals and clinics have an exposure control plan that minimizes employee exposures. OSHA requires that employers maintain a log of occupational blood exposures as well as provide expert advice to healthcare personnel who have come into contact with patient body fluids. OSHA dictates that the employer is responsible for providing and paying for postexposure evaluation and follow-up [5].

Steps to Take when Exposed to Blood or Body Fluid

1. Remove yourself from the area in which you are exposed. If you have a needle injury, ensure that the needle device has been removed from the area so that there is no danger to others. If you are exposed to a piece of equipment, reporting the danger to others is essential. Ensure patient and worker safety at the site of the incident.
2. Wash the area carefully with soap and water. There has been no evidence that washing with antiseptics such as alcohol reduces the risk, but it is not contraindicated. Caustic substances such as bleach solution are contraindicated. Mucous membranes should be flushed with water. If you have experienced an eye splash, use eye wash station that has been provided by your facility.

Blood and Body Fluid Exposures and Postexposure Prophylaxis. Table 1 Risk of different exposures

Type of exposure	Risk of contracting HIV from HIV positive source
Percutaneous	1/300
Mucous membrane	1/1,000
Skin with compromised integrity	<1/1,000

3. After washing the area carefully, contact the employee health center or officer at your workplace. Your workplace is required by law to have staff to advise you in this situation.
4. If the needle injury or blood splash is from an identifiable patient, blood is often drawn from the patient per hospital policy. This blood is tested for HIV and Hepatitis C antibody to obtain a baseline on the HCP.
5. If the HIV test is a rapid test that will be complete in an hour, it is reasonable to wait for this test to decide whether or not PEP for HIV is necessary. If there is no rapid test (<1–2 h) PEP should be started immediately. If there is no physician available to help with the ordering of this medicine, call the PEP hotline at 888 448 4911 for assistance. Rapid PEP has been shown in studies to reduce the transmission of HIV and should not be delayed.
6. If Hepatitis C test is positive the healthcare worker will often have serial blood tests over the upcoming months to determine if they have contracted Hepatitis C. Since there is no PEP for Hepatitis C the test results often take longer than the HIV results.
7. Blood is drawn from the exposed healthcare personnel to obtain baseline HIV and Hepatitis testing. This helps determine the need for PEP.
8. Extensive history will be taken as to when and why the accident occurred. This information can help determine the type of PEP needed. Employee health centers take this information very seriously and use it to prevent similar exposure incidents from occurring.
9. Healthcare workers that are exposed are told to practice safe sexual practices (condom use) with their partners until the final tests are determined.

HIV Postexposure Prophylaxis

Guidance for PEP should be obtained from local employee health clinic, infectious disease specialist, or PEP hotline. These types of drug recommendations are subject to change and local variation. The type of PEP regimen used for this type of exposure depends on whether or not the exposure is determined to be a high-risk or a low-risk event. As noted above, the needle stick injury is thought to be of higher risk when it is from a larger bore needle (such as one used in obtaining a central line), if the needle stick injury was a deep puncture wound, if the needle had been in a vein or an artery, or if the patient is known to have HIV and a high viral load. The basic PEP for low-risk exposures includes a two-drug therapy with either the combination tablet of emtricitabine 200 mg and tenofovir 300 mg (Truvada) or a combination tablet of lamivudine 150 mg and zidovudine 300 mg (Combivir). The patient is given one tablet each day for 28 days.

The expanded PEP for high-risk exposures includes one additional combination pill to the above regiment. This pill is a combination of lopinavir/ritonavir (200mg/50mg) formulation (Kaletra). This additional pill is given twice a day with the low risk once a day drug. Of course, recommendations change rapidly and the start of PEP should be done in consultation with an expert. The above dosing instructions are given as examples. If there is confusion or disagreement about whether or not the exposure is of low or high risk, it is recommended to start the expanded dosing for high-risk exposures.

There has been concern about the possibility that the source patient may have HIV infection but could still be in the window in which they do not test positive. There has never been a reported infection from a source still in the window before seroconversion. In addition, pregnancy is not a contraindication to start PEP in an exposed HCP. But, there are risks to these medication and the risks should be discussed with a knowledgeable expert on these matters before PEP is begun.

One limitation to the success of PEP is the occurrence of side effects such as nausea, vomiting, drug interactions, diabetic exacerbation, and nephrolithiasis. Side effects causing non-adherence may lead to drug resistant strains if the healthcare worker becomes infected. It is essential that once the PEP is started for HIV, the HCP tries to finish the medications as directed.

Body fluid contact and needle stick injuries are a source of anxiety for all HCP who experience them. It is essential that workers act quickly to protect themselves and their family members when they are exposed to patient blood and body fluids. As required by law, all hospitals and health care centers are required to provide equipment to protect their personnel. They are also required to test and evaluate both the source patient and the HCP in event of an exposure. The HCP should find appropriate help and education in this situation from their employee health center or from online and phone resources.

References

1. Panlilio AL et al (2005) Updated U.S. public health service guidelines for the management of occupational exposures to HIV and recommendations for postexposure prophylaxis. MMWR Recomm Rep 54(RR-9):1–17

2. Updated U.S. Public Health Service (2001) Guidelines for the management of occupational exposures to HBV, HCV, and HIV and recommendations for postexposure prophylaxis. MMWR Recomm Rep 50(RR-11):1–52

3. Cardo DM et al (1997) A case-control study of HIV seroconversion in health care workers after percutaneous exposure centers for disease control and prevention Needlestick Surveillance group. N Engl J Med 337(21):1485–1490

4. National HIV/AIDS Clinicians' Consultation Center. 2010 [cited 2010 August 12]; Available from: http://www.nccc.ucsf.edu/home/

5. Occupational Safety and Health Standards: Bloodborne pathogens 1910.1030 [cited 2010 August 10]; Available from: http://www.osha.gov/pls/oshaweb/owadisp.show_document?p_table=standards&p_id=10051

Blood Gas Analysis

▶ Acid–Base Evaluation

Blood Gases

▶ Arterial Blood Gases Interpretation

Blood in Urine

▶ Hematuria

Blood Pressure Support

▶ Inotropic Therapy

Blood Purification

▶ Renal Replacement

Blood Transfusion

ANNE-CORNÉLIE J. M. DE PONT
Academisch Medisch Centrum, Academisch Ziekenhuis
bij de Universiteit van Amsterdam, Amsterdam,
The Netherlands

Synonyms

Transferring one or more blood components from a donor
into the circulation of a patient

Definition

Blood component transfusion aims at correcting blood
loss or shortage of one or more blood components.

Pre-existing Condition

In critically ill patients, massive bleeding is a common
indication for the transfusion of all blood components:
red cells, plasma, and platelets. Even fresh whole blood
may be transfused. In other conditions, blood components are usually transfused for specific indications. Historically, red cells were transfused to correct anemia,
platelets in case of low platelet count or planned invasive
procedures, and fresh frozen plasma in case of hemostatic
disorders or invasive procedures. However, transfusion of
allogenic blood is associated with the risk of allergic reactions, infection transmission, immunosuppression,
increased intensive care unit and hospital lengths of stay,
and increased mortality [1]. Moreover, a hemoglobin level
(Hb) as low as 7 g/dL (4.3 mmol/L) is well tolerated by
critically ill patients and the use of a liberal transfusion
strategy targeting a Hb > 10 mg/dL (6.2 mmol/L) may in
fact lead to a worse clinical outcome. Recently, international guidelines for the transfusion of red cells in adult
trauma and critical care have been developed [1] and
a recent review article summarized five international
guidelines for the transfusion of fresh frozen plasma [2].
Several national guidelines for the transfusion of platelets
have been published, among which two recent guidelines
are in English [3, 4].

Common Indications

The clinical practice guideline for red blood cell transfusion in adult trauma and critical care gives level 1 recommendations for the transfusion of red cells in general
critically ill patients [1]. In addition, risks and alternatives
of transfusion are formulated, as well as strategies to
reduce transfusion.

Red Blood Cell Transfusion

In general critically ill patients, red blood cell transfusion
is indicated for patients with evidence of hemorrhagic
shock and may be indicated for patients with evidence of
acute hemorrhage and hemodynamic instability or inadequate oxygen delivery. In critically ill patients with hemodynamically stable anemia and without acute coronary
syndromes, such as acute myocardial infarction or unstable angina, a target Hb of 7 g/dL (4.3 mmol/L) is as
effective as a target Hb of 10 mg/dL (6.2 mmol/L). In
patients with acute coronary syndromes and a Hb < 8.0
mg/dL (5.0 mmol/L) on hospital admission, red blood cell
transfusion may be beneficial. Level 1 recommendations
for red blood cell transfusion are listed in Table 1.

Plasma Transfusion

Plasma transfusion is generally indicated to correct deficiencies of clotting factors for which a specific concentrate is
not available, in patients with active bleeding or in preparation for surgery or other invasive procedures [2, 3].
An additional indication is apheretic treatment for
microangiopathies, such as thrombotic thrombocytopenic purpura. The indications for plasma transfusion in the
critically ill are summarized in Table 2.

Platelet Transfusion

The transfusion of platelets is indicated for the prevention
and treatment of hemorrhage in patients with thrombocytopenia or platelet function defects [3, 4]. The indications for the transfusion of platelets are summarized in
Tables 3 and 4.

Risks of Transfusion

Blood component transfusion carries several risks with an
impact on morbidity and mortality, such as risk of infection, inflammatory response, and organ failure [1].

Blood Transfusion. Table 1 Level 1 recommendations for the
transfusion of red blood cells in the critically ill

Recommendation
Red blood cell transfusion is indicated for patients with evidence of hemorrhagic shock
Red blood cell transfusion may be indicated for patients with evidence of acute hemorrhage and hemodynamic instability or inadequate oxygen delivery
A target Hb of 7 g/dL (4.3 mmol/L) is as effective as a target Hb of 10 g/dL (6.2 mmol/L) in critically ill patients with hemodynamically stable anemia, except possibly in patients with acute myocardial ischemia

Blood Transfusion. Table 2 Indications for the transfusion of plasma in the critically ill

Clinical condition
Inherited or acquired deficiencies of clotting factors in case of active bleeding or in preparation for surgery or other invasive procedures, when specific factors are not available
Disseminated intravascular coagulation (DIC), in case of active bleeding
Thrombotic thrombocytopenic purpura, during plasma exchange
Anticoagulation with vitamin K antagonists, in case of severe bleeding
Massive transfusion

Blood Transfusion. Table 3 Indications for the therapeutic transfusion of platelets in the critically ill

Clinical condition	Transfusion threshold platelets
Surgical patient with active bleeding	$50–100 \times 10^9$/L
Massive transfusion	75×10^9/L
Acute disseminated intravascular coagulation with major bleeding and thrombocytopenia	50×10^9/L
Extracorporeal circulation with bleeding in the absence of a surgical cause or other coagulopathy	Not set
Platelet function defects with perioperative bleeding	Not set
Auto-immune thrombocytopenia with major or dangerous bleeding	Not set
Post transfusion purpura with severe hemorrhage	Not set
Peripheral blood stem cell autologous transplantation with grade II or higher bleeding according to the WHO bleeding scale	Not set

Blood Transfusion. Table 4 Indications for the prophylactic transfusion of platelets in the critically ill

Clinical condition	Transfusion threshold platelets
Unstable patients with acute leukemia, except acute promyelocytic leukemia	20×10^9/L
Unstable patients with bone marrow aplasia or myelodysplasia	10×10^9/L
Patients after allogeneic bone marrow transplantation	10×10^9/L
Patients after autologous peripheral blood stem cell transplantation	10×10^9/L
Patients with active treatment for bladder cancer or necrotic tumors	20×10^9/L
Patients with active treatment for solid tumors	10×10^9/L
Patients scheduled for ocular surgery or neurosurgery	100×10^9/L
Patients scheduled for major surgery	50×10^9/L
Patients scheduled for lumbar puncture, epidural anesthesia, endoscopy with biopsy, liver biopsy, or placement of a central venous catheter	50×10^9/L
Patients scheduled for bone marrow biopsy or marrow aspiration	Not set

(range 5.03–5.43). Blood transfusions change the immune response of the acceptor, enhancing the production of prostaglandin E2, interleukin (IL)-4 and IL-10, while decreasing the production of IL-2, IL-12, and interferon γ. The transfusion effect is superimposed on the T helper 2 skewing associated with trauma and surgery. This results in impaired monocyte and natural killer cell functions with reduced phagocytosis and killing of micro-organisms, as well as a lack of pro-inflammatory response to bacterial endotoxin. Some studies have demonstrated an association between prestorage leukocyte reduction and a lower incidence of infectious complications, but because of conflicting results, the evidence is not definitive.

Risk of Infection

A recent meta-analysis including 20 articles demonstrated the relationship between allogenic red blood cell transfusion and postoperative infections, such as sepsis, pneumonia, and wound infection. The odds ratio (OR) for postoperative bacterial infection was 3.45 in the transfused group (range 1.43–15.15) and was even higher in trauma patients who received red blood cell transfusion: 5.26

Risk of SIRS and MODS

Several studies in trauma patients have demonstrated an association between red blood cell transfusion and the occurrence of the systemic inflammatory response syndrome (SIRS) and the multiple organ dysfunction syndrome (MODS) [1]. In a prospective observational study, logistic regression identified transfusion of >4 units of blood as a significant risk factor for SIRS. In another large observational study, a dose–response relationship between early blood transfusion and the later development of MODS was demonstrated. Subsequent studies confirmed this finding and documented that the age of the transfused blood was an independent risk factor for post-injury MODS [1].

Risk of Acute Lung Injury (ALI) and Adult Respiratory Distress Syndrome (ARDS)

Transfusion related acute lung injury (TRALI) is an immune mediated transfusion reaction leading to acute respiratory distress, non-cardiogenic pulmonary edema, and hypoxemia [5]. It is the most common cause of transfusion-related death worldwide, with a mortality rate ranging from 5% to 35%. TRALI occurs within 6 h of transfusion with the majority of cases presenting during the transfusion or within the first 2 h. The onset is insidious and presents with tachypnea, cyanosis and dyspnea with acute hypoxemia, and decreased pulmonary compliance despite normal cardiac function. The chest X-ray shows diffuse, fluffy infiltrates consistent with pulmonary edema. Although all blood components have been implicated in TRALI, fresh frozen plasma and whole blood derived platelet concentrates have caused the largest number of cases. Neutrophil-priming agents released in stored cellular blood components, leukocyte antibodies present in fresh frozen plasma, and platelet concentrates of multiparous donors have all been considered to be causative. Autopsy specimens have demonstrated widespread neutrophil infiltration with interstitial and intra-alveolar pulmonary edema, hyaline membrane formation, and destruction of the normal lung parenchyma consistent with adult respiratory distress syndrome. The treatment of TRALI is supportive with supplemental oxygen and mechanical ventilation. Most cases recover within 72 h.

Risk of Alloimmunization

After ABO and Rhesus-D, antibodies against human leukocyte antigen (HLA) are most frequently found after blood transfusion. Platelet transfusions are most immunogenic. Platelets and lymphocytes carry a similar density of HLA class I antigens on their surface, representing 70% of the HLA class I in the peripheral blood. By strict leukocyte removal from all transfusions, HLA antibody production can be reduced by two thirds. However, approximately 15–20% of the recipients of leukocyte depleted red cell and platelet transfusions still produce HLA antibodies. This most often occurs in females after prior sensitization by pregnancies. HLA alloimmunization is the most frequent cause of a poor response to platelet transfusion.

Contraindications

Relative contraindications to the transfusion of blood components are heart failure and pulmonary edema [1, 3]. Absolute contraindications to the transfusion of fresh frozen plasma are documented intolerance to plasma or its components and congenital deficiency of immunoglobulin A (IgA) in the presence of IgA antibodies [3]. Transfusion of platelets is contraindicated in thrombotic thrombocytopenic purpura and in heparin-induced thrombocytopenia [3, 4].

Strategies to Reduce Blood Component Transfusion

Strategies to reduce red blood cell transfusion include:

- Use of intraoperative and postoperative blood salvaging methods
- Intraoperative use of antifibrinolytic agents such as aprotinin and tranexamic acid
- Use of recombinant factor VIIa for the management of intractable nonsurgical bleeding unresponsive to routine hemostatic therapy
- Use of reduced volume blood sampling tubes and the elimination of automatic daily laboratory orders
- Administration of recombinant human erythropoietin

These strategies are listed as level 2 recommendations in the clinical practice guideline for red blood cell transfusion in adult trauma and critical care [1] and as level I and II recommendations in the perioperative blood transfusion and blood conservation in cardiac surgery: the society of thoracic surgeons and the society of cardiovascular anesthesiologists clinical practice guideline [6].

Strategies to reduce the use of platelet transfusions include:

- Lowering of the platelet transfusion threshold to $10 \times 10^9/L$
- Use of local audits of the use of platelet transfusions
- Use of tranexamic acid during consolidation treatment for acute leukemia
- Use of cytokine growth factors in thrombocytopenia after chemotherapy or stem cell transplant
- Correction of concurrent coagulopathy in bleeding thrombocytopenic patients
- Preoperative cessation of anti-platelet therapy whenever possible

- Avoidance of prophylactic use of platelet transfusions in patients undergoing cardiopulmonary bypass
- Intraoperative monitoring of platelet count and thrombelastography with appropriate correction of abnormalities according to an agreed algorithm
- Intraoperative use of aprotinin and tranexamic acid
- Early return to theatre for surgical bleeding

These strategies are recommended in the guidelines for the use of platelet transfusions [4].

Applications

Red Blood Cell Transfusion

In the absence of acute hemorrhage, red blood cell transfusion should be given as single units [1]. Since transfusion-associated graft versus host disease (TA-GvHD) is the most frequent cause of transfusion-associated death, patients at risk of TA-GvHD should be given gamma-irradiated red blood cell transfusions [4].

Plasma Transfusion

Fresh frozen plasma must be ABO-compatible, whereas Rhesus compatibility is not necessary [3]. The plasma must be thawed between 30°C and 37°C in a water bath under continuous agitation or with another system to ensure a controlled temperature. Fresh frozen plasma must be transfused as soon as possible after thawing, but in any case within 24 h, if stored at $4°C \pm 2°C$. The plasma must not be refrozen after thawing. The recommended dose of fresh frozen plasma is 10–15 mL/kg body weight. However, the dose depends on clinical situation and laboratory parameters, which may justify the administration of higher doses.

Platelet Transfusion

The platelet concentrate must be ABO identical or at least ABO compatible to give a good yield [3]. The average dose of platelet concentrate for each transfusion consists of 300×10^9 platelets (one apheretic platelet concentrate or one platelet concentrate from a pool of five to eight platelet concentrates from whole blood or from a buffy coat pool). This should increase the platelet count by at least 20×10^9/L [3, 4]. The platelet concentrate should be administered over a 30 min period through a standard blood or platelet administration set that has not been used for blood [4]. It is essential to monitor the efficacy of platelet transfusions in order to guide the use of subsequent transfusions. The corrected platelet count increment (CCI) can be calculated from the platelet counts before and after transfusion, corrected for body surface area. The CCI should be $>7.5 \times 10^9$/L at 1 h and 4.5×10^9/L at 20–24 h. A low CCI ($<7.5 \times 10^9$/L) already in the first hour, is often associated with alloimmunization to leukocyte and platelet antigens. A normal CCI at 12 h and a low one ($<4.5 \times 10^9$/L) at 20–24 h is usually associated with non-immunological platelet consumption such as splenomegaly, sepsis, diffuse intravascular coagulation, or treatment with amphotericin B. Patients with a low CCI on two or more occasions should be screened for immunological causes of their platelet transfusion refractoriness. The use of ABO compatible fresh platelet concentrates (produced within 48 h before transfusion) is important to determine whether platelet refractoriness is antibody-mediated. Platelets collected more than 48 h before transfusion have a shortened survival in patients with non-immunological platelet refractoriness. Since transfusion-associated graft versus host disease (TA-GvHD) is the most frequent cause of transfusion-associated death, patients at risk of TA-GvHD should be given gamma-irradiated platelet concentrates [4].

Management of Adverse Effects

Hospitals should have policies for the management and reporting of adverse events following transfusion, including reporting to Serious Hazards of Transfusion (SHOT). If a transfusion reaction is suspected, the transfusion should be stopped immediately, and the patient's temperature, pulse, and blood pressure recorded. Further management depends on the type and severity of the reaction [4].

References

1. Napolitano LM, Kurek S, Luchette FA et al (2009) Clinical practice guideline: red blood cell transfusion in adult trauma and critical care. Crit Care Med 37:3124–3157
2. Iorio A, Basileo M, Marchesini E et al (2008) The good use of plasma. A critical analysis of five international guidelines. Blood Transfus 6:18–24
3. Liumbruno G, Bennardello F, Lattanzio A et al (2009) Recommendations for the transfusion of plasma and platelets. Blood Transfus 7:132–150
4. British Committee for Standards in Haematology, Blood Transfusion Task Force (Chairman P. Kelsey) (2003) Guidelines for the use of platelet transfusions. Br J Haematol 122:10–23
5. Silliman CC, Lin Fung Y, Ball JB et al (2009) Transfusion-related acute lung injury: current concepts and misconceptions. Blood Rev 23:245–255
6. Spiess BD, Shore-Lesserson L, Stafford-Smitm M et al (2007) Perioperative blood transfusion and blood conservation in cardiac surgery: the society of thoracic surgeons and the society of cardiovascular anesthesiologists clinical practice guideline. Ann thorac Surg 83:S27–S86

Blunt Abdominal Trauma

▶ Abdominal Trauma

Blunt Avulsion of the Scapula

▶ Scapulothoracic Dissociation

Blunt Cardiac Injury

▶ Myocardial Contusion

Blunt Carotid Injury (BCI)

▶ Blunt Cerebrovascular Injury

Blunt Cerebrovascular Injury

Walter L. Biffl
Department of Surgery, Denver Health Medical Center,
Denver, CO, USA

Synonyms
Blunt carotid injury (BCI); Blunt vertebral artery injury (BVI)

Definition
Blunt cerebrovascular injury (BCVI) is an injury to the carotid or vertebral artery due to a blunt force such as direct pressure, crushing, or stretching.

Mechanism/Pathophysiology
There are four fundamental mechanisms of BCI [1]. The first, originally thought to be most common, is a direct blow to the neck, including clothesline-type,

strangulation, and near-hanging injuries. The most common mechanism appears to be due to hyperextension and contralateral rotation of the head and neck. This may be explained by anatomical relationships: the lateral articular processes and pedicles of the upper three cervical vertebrae project more anteriorly than do those of the lower four cervical vertebrae. The overlying distal cervical internal carotid artery is prone to stretch injury during cervical hyperextension. Rotation at the atlantoaxial joint may result in anterior movement of the contralateral C1 lateral mass, further exacerbating a stretch injury. The third type of mechanism results from intraoral trauma, and may be seen in children who have fallen with a hard object (such as a toothbrush) in their mouth. The fourth mechanism is injury from bony fragments in the setting of a basilar skull fracture involving the carotid canal. The primary mechanism of vertebral artery injury is stretch or laceration during cervical spine fracture or distraction injury [1].

Regardless of the underlying mechanism of injury, the final common pathway of BCVI in most cases is intimal disruption. This exposes the thrombogenic subendothelial collagen, promoting platelet aggregation with subsequent thrombosis or embolization. In addition, the intimal tear offers a portal of egress for a dissecting column of blood. Dissection may result in progressive luminal narrowing and subsequent vessel occlusion. Whether it is due to thromboembolism or vessel occlusion, the end result, particularly in the setting of multisystem trauma with hypotension, is cerebral ischemia. Less commonly, partial or complete transection of the artery occurs, resulting in pseudoaneurysm formation or free rupture. The former may increase in size to compress and occlude the vessel lumen; it may be the source of platelet thromboembolism; or it may rupture. Rupture may result in intra- or extra-cranial hemorrhage, or arteriovenous fistula formation. The clinical manifestations of BCVI depend upon the type of injury, but ultimately the involved artery and the collateral circulation determine the manner in which the injury presents.

Incidence
Early multicenter reviews suggested an incidence of BCI of 0.08–0.17% among patients admitted to trauma centers following blunt trauma, but more recent series reported incidences of 0.24–0.33%. The argument that the incidence actually is increasing is supported by the fact that nearly all the patients in the series published through 1997 were symptomatic at the time of diagnosis. By screening asymptomatic individuals, many centers have reported BCVI in 1.0–1.6% [2].

Treatment

Acute

The primary management strategies for BCVI include observation, surgical repair, antithrombotic drugs, and endovascular therapy. In determining the treatment for an individual, the location and grade of the injury (Table 1), as well as symptomatology, must all be considered [1]. Given the high morbidity and mortality rates associated with BCVI, observation should not be chosen unless there are contraindications to alternative strategies. Extrapolating from penetrating trauma literature, wherein neurologic morbidity and mortality were better in those undergoing operation, early reports recommended surgery in the absence of completed hemiplegic deficits. However, the vast majority of BCVI are not surgically accessible, involving the carotid artery at the base of the skull. Thus, inaccessibility precludes direct surgical repair in most patients. Extracranial-intracranial bypass has been successfully employed in select patients, but this remains a controversial concept. Consequently, nonsurgical management is the first-line treatment of BCVI. There have been no published prospective randomized studies comparing treatment strategies; management recommendations have been made based on retrospective analyses of patients managed per institutional protocols. Early reports recommended systemic anticoagulation with heparin, demonstrating improved neurologic outcomes among symptomatic patients, as well as stroke prevention among asymptomatic patients. A few retrospective, uncontrolled case series, as well as more recent large reports, suggest that systemic heparinization and antiplatelet therapy are equally efficacious in stroke prevention [3, 4]. In the absence of controlled data, systemic heparin may be preferred among patients with neurologic symptoms and in those who have no contraindications [2]. Many case reports tout endovascular interventions for various types of BCVI, but there have been no controlled trials. Case series offer discrepant results [2, 3]. It is clear that controlled trials are needed, that caution should be used during stent deployment to avoid dislodging unstable thrombus, and that post-stent antithrombotic therapy is critical.

Treatment recommendations are based on injury location and grade [5]. Grade I injuries have a low stroke risk and high rate of resolution with antithrombotic therapy [2]. Their lack of flow-limiting potential makes surgery or endovascular treatment unnecessary; thus, antithrombotic therapy is recommended. Higher-grade (II-V), surgically accessible lesions should be approached surgically. Nonsurgical management recommendations are as follows. Grade V injuries are associated with high mortality and mandate immediate attempts at control. Given their relative inaccessability, this typically involves endovascular techniques. Grade IV injuries – occlusions – may have a lower stroke rate when treated with antithrombotic therapy [2]. Although it seems to be performed occasionally, there is no good literature support for embolization to "reduce the pressure head" proximal to an occlusion. Grade II and III injuries are typically treated with antithrombotic therapy. In the setting of progressive vessel narrowing or pseudoaneurysm enlargement, stents have been deployed in an effort to maintain vascular patency [2, 3]. As stated, the literature base for this is not robust. A follow-up imaging study is recommended 7–10 days after injury, or for any change in neurologic status. Therapy may be changed in 65% of Grade I and 51% of Grade II injuries, and the imaging may help plan therapy for Grade III injuries [2].

Long Term

There are no good long-term outcome data. It has been recommended that patients receive long-term antithrombotic therapy [5], but the optimal drug and duration have not been studied. In the absence of documented healing of the vessel, it is reasonable to provide some treatment, as stroke has been reported as long as 14 years after injury. Coumadin was recommended in early series [2, 3], but with the apparent efficacy of antiplatelet therapy in the early period, it seems that long-term antiplatelet therapy is preferable to warfarin for its safety and cost profile. Aspirin and clopidogrel have different mechanisms of action; in addition, some individuals are resistant to the effects of one or both drugs. Several studies have evaluated the safety and efficacy of dual antiplatelet therapy (aspirin combined with clopidogrel) in various clinical situations, primarily related to cardiovascular disease. However, based on the

Blunt Cerebrovascular Injury. Table 1 Blunt carotid and vertebral arterial injury grading scale [1]

Injury grade	Description
I	Luminal irregularity or dissection with <25% luminal narrowing
II	Dissection or intramural hematoma with ≥25% luminal narrowing, intraluminal thrombus, or raised intimal flap
III	Pseudoaneurysm
IV	Occlusion
V	Transection with free extravasation

increased bleeding risk, and the lack of benefit or increase in mortality in various clinical situations, dual therapy is not recommended for BCVI until more data become available.

Evaluation/Assessment

Clinical Presentation

Premonitory signs and symptoms associated with the vessel injury itself may suggest the presence of BCVI prior to manifestations of cerebral ischemia [1]. Pain (neck, ear, face, or periorbital) can be a common symptom, present in up to 60% of patients, and is believed to reflect either mural hemorrhage or dissection of the vessel wall. Complaints of such pain are often difficult to elicit in the multiply injured patient and may be attributed to other injuries; however, BCVI must be considered in the differential diagnosis of post-traumatic neck pain and headache. Horner's syndrome or oculosympathetic paresis (partial Horner's syndrome) may result from disruption of the periarterial sympathetic plexus. Pupillary asymmetry can have several etiologies in the injured patient. However, if the larger of the pupils is reactive and the smaller pupil is not, BCVI should be suspected on the side of the smaller pupil.

Systematic neurologic examination will help to localize the distribution of cerebral ischemia. No single neurologic finding allows a precise diagnosis, but the constellation of findings may identify the involved artery. A detailed review of the manifestations of cerebral ischemia has been presented elsewhere [1]. Cerebral ischemic signs or symptoms may be absent in many patients with acute BCVI. A latent period between the time of injury and the appearance of clinical manifestations is characteristic of BCVI, and relates to its pathophysiology. Unless the vessel is immediately occluded, time is required for a platelet plug to form and either limit flow or embolize. In various series, 23–50% of patients first developed signs or symptoms of BCI more than 12 h after the traumatic event. Delayed recognition may occur in the face of multisystem trauma, with critical injuries demanding immediate attention, or head injury, which may preclude a meaningful neurologic examination. In order to make the early diagnosis of BCVI it is imperative that the surgeon recognize the signs and symptoms in a trauma patient. These include: arterial hemorrhage from neck, mouth, nose, ears; large or expanding cervical hematoma; cervical bruit in a patient <50 years old; focal or lateralizing neurologic deficit, including hemiparesis, transient ischemic attack, Horner's syndrome, oculosympathetic paresis, or vertebrobasilar insufficiency; evidence of cerebral infarction on computed tomography (CT) or magnetic resonance imaging (MRI) scan; or neurologic deficit that is incongruous with CT or MRI findings.

Screening

Stroke rates are significantly lower in treated patients when compared to untreated patients, and screening appears to be cost-effective [2, 3]. Identification of a high-risk group for screening has been debated in the literature. Analyses of screening have identified the following list of high-risk factors for BCVI: (a) an injury mechanism compatible with severe cervical hyperextension/rotation or hyperflexion; (b) Lefort II or III midface fractures; (c) basilar skull fracture involving the carotid canal; (d) closed head injury consistent with diffuse axonal injury with Glasgow Coma Score <6; (e) cervical vertebral body or transverse foramen fracture, subluxation, or ligamentous injury at any level, or any fracture at the level of C1-C3; (f) near-hanging resulting in cerebral anoxia; or (g) seat belt or other clothesline-type injury with significant cervical pain or swelling or altered mental status. In such high-risk groups, 15–30% of screened patients will be found to have BCVI. With the improved accuracy of noninvasive screening modalities, there is a tendency to liberalize screening in an attempt to capture all injuries, rather than restricting screening to the highest-risk groups. Broadened screening guidelines may include combined thoracic and cervical or cranial injuries, but there have not been any large-scale analyses to determine the yield of such protocols.

Imaging

Four-vessel biplanar cerebral arteriography (ART) has been considered the gold standard for diagnosis of BCVI. Unfortunately, it is invasive and resource-intensive, and its risks include complications related to catheter insertion (1–2% hematoma; arterial pseudoaneurysm), contrast administration (1–2% renal dysfunction; allergic reaction), and stroke (less than 1%) [2]. Duplex ultrasonography (US) is widely considered the modality of choice for imaging the extracranial carotid arteries; however, experience in diagnosing BCVI is limited. In a multicenter review, US had 86% sensitivity for identifying ICA injuries. In that series it was noted that the lesions missed by US were located at the base of the skull. Since the large majority of BCI involve the artery at or near the base of the skull, this is a major limitation of US. It is also unreliable in imaging the vertebral artery. Furthermore, while duplex can provide indirect evidence of injuries by detecting turbulence and other flow disturbances, these findings are not reliable in the presence of stenoses <60%. More recently, in a series of 1,451 blunt trauma patients, US missed eight injuries that resulted in stroke, and its overall sensitivity was just 39%. Consequently, there is virtually no role for US for BCVI screening. At one time, magnetic resonance angiography (MRA) held great promise to supplant ART. Potential advantages of MRA include the capability to simultaneously image the entire head and neck and to detect cerebral infarction earlier than CT scanning, and avoid contrast. The successful demonstration of BCVI by MRA has been reported by a number of investigators. However, prospective trials documented poor sensitivity and specificity of MRA when compared directly to ART. Given issues such as timeliness of availability and incompatibility of equipment, MRA is not considered a standard screening test for BCVI.

Recently, computed tomographic arteriography (CTA) has gained popularity in the evaluation of the cervical vessels. There are many features of CTA that make it an attractive screening tool for BCVI. First and foremost, patients who are identified for screening typically have indications for CT scanning of other regions. Thus, additional "road trips" are unnecessary. The BCVI can be visualized along with associated brain injuries, facial or basilar skull fractures, or cervical spine injuries. In addition, the study is noninvasive, examination times are relatively short, and the image can be manipulated in three dimensions. Finally, the required dye load is less than that used for cerebral arteriography. The first two prospective studies performed in trauma patients to assess the accuracy of CTA versus ART were unfavorable, with poor sensitivity of CTA for BCVI. However, these studies evaluated early-generation (1- and 2-slice) scanners. More recently, investigators have reviewed cohorts of patients undergoing multidetector-row (4- and 8-slice) CTA as well as ART. Sensitivity for BCI was better, ranging from 83% to 92%, and sensitivity for BVI ranged from 40% to 60%. Sixteen-slice CTA has been adopted by a number of centers and appears to reliably identify clinically significant BCVI. Three published studies have evaluated the accuracy of 16-slice CTA compared with ART. The first reported 100% sensitivity of 16-slice CTA for carotid, and 96% sensitivity for vertebral artery injuries. In another study, ART was performed on a subset (30%) of patients with normal CTA, and it was found that CTA missed seven BCVI among 82 patients, for a negative predictive value of 92%. However, on retrospective review of the CTA images, the investigators found that the injuries were evident in six

of the seven patients, and that the seventh patient's abnormality was most likely not traumatic in origin. Still more recently, a group has offered a note of caution, reporting 43% false (+) and 9% false (−) rates for CTA. However, the inaccuracy of CTA once again appeared to be related in large part to the radiologists' experience, as all of the missed BCVI occurred in the first half of the study period. Thus, it appears that 16-slice CTA is reliable for screening for clinically-significant BCVI, but that the accuracy diminishes with fewer detector-rows. Although a relatively high false (+) rate suggests CTA may be oversensitive, ART may be warranted in the setting of high clinical suspicion but a normal CTA, to definitively exclude an injury [4]. A relatively high false (+) rate suggests CTA may be oversensitive. However, ART may be warranted in the setting of high clinical suspicion and a normal CTA, to definitively exclude an injury.

After-care

As noted above, long-term antiplatelet therapy is recommended. Patients may be referred for follow-up imaging 3 months after discharge. If the lesion is healed, treatment may be discontinued. If the injury is still evident, antiplatelet therapy is continued. It might be argued that simply continuing lifelong antiplatelet therapy with aspirin is a low-risk, cost-effective alternative to follow-up imaging. This should be individualized [5].

Prognosis

In early reports, BCVI-related stroke was associated with 28% mortality, and permanent neurologic deficits persisted in 58% of survivors. In recent series, stroke-related mortality has not improved. Asymptomatic patients do well, with a late stroke rate approaching 0%. The incidence of bleeding complications related to treatment is less than 10%.

References

1. Biffl WL, Moore EE, Elliott JP et al (1999) Blunt cerebrovascular injuries. Curr Probl Surg 36:507–599
2. Biffl WL, Ray CE, Moore EE et al (2002) Treatment-related outcomes from blunt cerebrovascular injuries: importance of routine follow-up arteriography. Ann Surg 235:699–707
3. Edwards NM, Fabian TC, Claridge JA et al (2007) Antithrombotic therapy and endovascular stents are effective treatment for blunt carotid injuries: results from longterm followup. J Am Coll Surg 204:1007–1015
4. Cothren CC, Biffl WL, Moore EE et al (2009) Treatment for blunt cerebrovascular injuries: equivalence of anticoagulation and antiplatelet agents. Arch Surg 144:685–690
5. Biffl WL, Cothren CC, Moore EE et al (2009) WTA critical decisions in trauma: screening for and treatment of blunt cerebrovascular injuries. J Trauma 67:1150–1153

Blunt Chest Trauma

▶ Flail Chest

Blunt Injury

▶ Patterns of Injury

Blunt Injury Thoracic Aorta

▶ Torn Thoracic Aorta

Blunt Vertebral Artery Injury (BVI)

▶ Blunt Cerebrovascular Injury

BMT

Bone marrow transplantation. A procedure in which bone marrow that is diseased (or damaged) is replaced by healthy bone marrow. The bone marrow to be replaced may be deliberately destroyed by high doses of chemotherapy and/or radiation therapy. The replacement marrow may come from another person, or it may be the patient's own marrow (which was removed and stored before treatment). When marrow from an unrelated donor is used, the procedure is an allogeneic bone marrow transplantation. If the marrow is from an identical twin, it is termed "syngeneic." Autologous bone marrow transplantation uses the patient's own marrow.

BMT Infections

▶ Bone Marrow Transplant: Infectious Complications

BNP

▶ B-Type Natriuretic Peptide

Body Fluid Exposure

A percutaneous injury (needle stick exposure or skin laceration with needle), mucous membrane or non-intact skin exposure to blood, tissue, or other bodily fluids that could place a health-care worker at risk for HIV.

Body Fluids Noninfectious for HIV

Feces, nasal secretions, saliva, sputum, sweat, tears, urine, and vomitus (unless visibly bloody).

Body Fluids Possibly Infected with HIV

Blood, semen, vaginal secretions, cerebrospinal fluid, pleural fluid, peritoneal fluid, pericardial fluid, and amniotic fluid.

Boerhaave's Syndrome

Emesis-induced rupture of the esophagus leading to mediastinitis.

▶ Mediastinal Infections

Bomb Explosions

▶ Multidimensional Injury

Bomb Injuries

C. Crawford Mechem
Department of Emergency Medicine, Hospital of the University of Pennsylvania, Philadelphia, PA, USA
Philadelphia Fire Department, Philadelphia, PA, USA

Synonyms

Blast injuries; Explosive injuries

Definition

A bomb is a device containing a solid or liquid material that can undergo rapid conversion to a gas with the generation of tremendous amounts of heat and pressure. Necessary components include an oxidizing agent, such as ammonium nitrate; a fuel, such as fuel oil; and an initiating stimulus. Potential stimuli include friction, direct impact, shock, heat, or an electrostatic discharge. Radio waves, such as from a handheld radio or cell phone, can also function as remote stimuli.

Bomb injuries result from exposure to explosions in a variety of settings including the workplace (forestry, mining, oil exploration, and ordinance disposal personnel), warfare, and terrorist attacks. The latter category is perhaps of greatest concern for civilian medical providers. While much attention has been placed on the medical consequences of chemical, biological, or radiological weapons of mass destruction, terrorist attacks involving explosives continue to generate far more casualties. The increasing death toll among American and other coalition soldiers in the Middle East as a result of improvised explosive devices (IEDs) illustrates the popularity of explosives as a terrorist weapon. Their appeal is based on their low cost, relatively low risk, ease of manufacture, predictable results, ready availability of component parts, and the variety of delivery options.

Explosives are classified as "high-order" and "low-order." High-order explosives "detonate," meaning they are almost instantaneously converted to gases at very high pressures. The gases expand at greater than 1,000 m/s, producing a supersonic, overpressurization blast wave and very high winds. The overpressurization wave leaves behind a relative vacuum at the site of detonation. This in turn causes an underpressurization wave that tends to pull objects back inward. Examples of high-order explosives are C-4, Semtex, TNT (trinitrotoluene), and dynamite.

Unlike high-order explosives, low-order explosives undergo "deflagration," meaning they burn rather than detonate. Energy is released more slowly, so an overpressurization wave is not generated. While still potentially deadly, low-order explosives do not cause the characteristic injuries associated with the rapid pressure changes and shearing forces seen with high-order explosives. Examples of low-order explosives are black powder and fireworks.

Injuries from explosives are categorized as "primary," "secondary," "tertiary," "quaternary," and "quinary" [1].

Primary Blast Injuries

Primary blast injuries result from the direct effect of overpressurization and underpressurization waves. They most commonly involve air-filled structures, specifically the ears, lungs, and bowels. The tympanic membrane (TM) is the most susceptible, with damage occurring from as little as 5 lb per square inch above atmospheric pressure. Patients may present with decreased hearing. On physical exam, hemotympanum or TM rupture may be noted. At higher pressures, injury to the middle and inner ear may occur. Consequences include tinnitus, vertigo, ossicle dislocation, and perforation of the oval or round window. In severe cases, hearing loss may be permanent.

The lungs are the structures next most frequently injured by a bomb blast wave. Pulmonary injuries are also the most common critical primary blast injury. They include hemo- or pneumothorax, pneumomediastinum, air emboli, and pulmonary contusions. Patients may present with dyspnea, chest pain, cough, or hemoptysis. Findings on physical exam include hemodynamic instability, tachypnea, hypoxia, cyanosis, wheezing, decreased breath sounds, subcutaneous emphysema, and respiratory arrest. A characteristic butterfly pattern is frequently seen on chest radiograph.

Acute air embolism is another manifestation of pulmonary blast injury. Emboli most frequently occlude blood vessels in the brain or spinal cord and may produce acute neurologic symptoms. Emboli to the coronary vessels can produce ST-segment elevation and hypotension.

Primary blast injuries of the bowel most commonly result from underwater explosions and often involve the colon, producing perforation or mesenteric ischemia. Symptoms may be delayed and include nausea, abdominal pain, and hematemesis.

While primary blast injuries most commonly affect hollow viscera, solid organs can be injured as well. Examples are cardiac contusion or myocardial infarction, renal contusion or laceration, concussion or air emboli to the brain, globe rupture or hyphema, and testicle rupture.

Secondary Blast Injuries

Secondary blast injuries are the leading cause of death and injury in military and civilian terrorist bombings. They result from projectiles from the explosion, such as flying debris from IEDs, shrapnel from military explosives, and glass from shattered windows.

Tertiary Blast Injuries

Tertiary blast injuries result from individuals being thrown by the blast wind and can affect any part of the body. Common injuries include fractures, traumatic amputations, blunt trauma to the chest and abdomen, and open and closed head injuries.

Quaternary Blast Injuries

Quaternary blast injuries are most others and include toxic inhalation, radiation exposure, asphyxiation (including carbon monoxide and cyanide), dust inhalation, and chemical and thermal burns. While the heat generated by an explosion generally dissipates rapidly, thermal burns may still be extensive and are often associated with significant inhalational injury. In the context of an explosion causing structural collapse, crush syndrome, characterized by rhabdomyolysis, hyperkalemia, and oliguric renal failure, is frequently encountered. Compartment syndrome is also a serious concern.

Quinary Injury

The fifth category, the quinary injury pattern, was recently introduced based on a case series of casualties who were in close proximity to the detonation of a terrorist bomb in Israel. This injury results from an immediate hyperinflammatory state characterized by hyperpyrexia, sweating, low central venous pressure, and a positive fluid balance.

Treatment

Victims of bombings can suffer a wide variety of injuries. For example, the most frequently encountered injuries among survivors of the 2004 Madrid train bombings were ruptured TMs; chest trauma including rib fractures, pneumothorax, and hemothorax; shrapnel wounds; fractures; burns; eye injuries; head trauma; abdominal trauma; amputations; and stress reactions [2]. Management of the more commonly encountered conditions will be discussed.

Ruptured Tympanic Membrane

Initial management of ruptured TMs consists of removal of debris from the auditory canal and referral to an otolaryngologist for further evaluation and definitive care. The patient should be instructed to keep the ears dry. The role of prophylactic antibiotic drops is subject to debate. However, if used, ototoxic medications such as gentamicin, neomycin, or tobramycin, should be avoided.

In the majority of cases, TM perforations will heal spontaneously. In the remaining cases, paper patch myringoplasty or tympanoplasty may be required.

Pulmonary Blast Injury

Management consists of respiratory support and avoidance of further barotrauma. Because physical activity can worsen symptoms, the patient should be encouraged to rest. Most hemo- and pneumothoraces require immediate decompression. High-peak inspiratory pressures should be avoided in patients requiring respiratory support due to the risk of exacerbating underlying injuries such as air embolism. Likewise, overly aggressive fluid resuscitation must be avoided because of the risk of precipitating pulmonary edema.

Acute Air Embolism

High-flow oxygen is administered with a tight-fitting mask. As is the case with other pulmonary blast injuries, positive pressure ventilation should be avoided or minimized. Placing the patient on his or her left side may prevent further embolization of bubbles. The value of placing the patient in the Trendelenberg position is now in question. Aspirin administration may hasten recovery by blunting the associated inflammatory response [3]. Finally, hyperbaric oxygen therapy should be considered as definitive treatment.

Shrapnel Wounds

The treatment is similar to that of low-velocity gunshot wounds, including local wound care and appropriate tetanus prophylaxis. Because IEDs and other devices containing nails, bolts, or other small, sharp objects can leave deceptively benign-appearing wounds, radiographs should be used liberally to identify foreign bodies and associated injuries.

Rhabdomyolysis and Crush Syndrome

Crush forces can cause localized muscle injury along with systemic abnormalities such as electrolyte disturbances, hypovolemia from third-spacing, and renal failure. Treatment consists of aggressive intravenous fluid administration, initially using isotonic saline to maintain a urine output off at least 200–300 mL/h. Success of therapy may be monitored with serial creatine kinase (CK) determinations. To enhance diuresis, intravenous mannitol can be added after volume deficits are corrected. Alkalinization of the urine is recommended to minimize the deposition of myoglobin casts in the kidneys with resultant nephrotoxicity. This can be accomplished by adding three ampules (44 mEq each) of sodium bicarbonate to a liter of 5% dextrose in water. This is infused at 100 mL/h, titrating to maintain a urine pH of 6.5.

Because of the risk of life-threatening hyperkalemia, serum electrolytes should be closely monitored. Depending on the severity, hyperkalemia is treated with calcium chloride, sodium bicarbonate, glucose, insulin, sodium polystyrene, and an inhaled β_2 agonist. In refractory cases, hemodialysis may be required. Calcium and phosphate abnormalities may also be noted but generally only require treatment if the patient becomes symptomatic [4].

Compartment Syndrome

Compartment syndrome is a limb-threatening and potentially life-threatening emergency that results when tissue pressure within a fascia-enclosed compartment exceeds perfusion pressure. It often occurs in the setting of long-bone fractures or crush injury. Symptoms and physical findings are frequently unreliable. Therefore, when suspected, intracompartment pressures should be measured in coordination with the appropriate consultant. If elevated, emergent fasciotomy should be performed to restore tissue perfusion.

Burns

The management of blast injury victims with burns consists of airway support, fluid resuscitation, tetanus prophylaxis, adequate analgesia, wound care, and prevention of complications. When inhalation injury is suspected, early endotracheal intubation is prudent. Inhalation injury should be suspected in patients who were in an enclosed-space explosion or those with facial burns, carbonaceous sputum, voice change, or respiratory distress. Fluid resuscitation should be initiated early to avoid burn shock. This is a combination of hypovolemic and distributive shock characterized by hypovolemia, increased systemic vascular resistance, and decreased cardiac output. Delays in fluid resuscitation of just 2 h can increase mortality. Appropriate fluid administration requires an accurate determination of the total body surface area (TBSA) affected by the burn. Therefore, a Lund–Browder chart should be completed early in the patient's care. Lactated Ringer's solution is then administered in accordance with the Parkland formula, 4 mL/kg/TBSA burned. Half of this volume is infused over the first 8 h, with the rest given over the next 16 h. Target physiological parameters are a urine output of 0.5 mL/kg/h and a pulse less than 110. While under-resuscitation can increase morbidity and mortality, overly aggressive fluid administration can also be harmful, with consequences including pulmonary edema and abdominal compartment syndrome.

Once the patient has been stabilized, local burn care should be initiated. This involves daily hydrotherapy with debridement of devitalized tissue. A topical antibiotic, such as silver sulfadiazine, is then applied to reduce the risk of infection. Escharotomy and skin grafting may be required. The patient's nutritional needs should be addressed early. Finally, the patient should be observed for complications such as hypothermia, compartment syndrome, stress ulcers, and deep venous thrombosis [5].

Eye Injuries

Serious eye injuries are seen in up to 28% of survivors of explosions. They include lacerations, orbit fractures, hyphema, optic nerve injury, thermal or chemical burns, and globe rupture. Visual acuity should be assessed. Chemical burns are initially managed with irrigation with sterile saline for up to 60 min. If injury due to an acid or base is suspected, pH of the eye should be monitored until it reaches 7–7.4. In the case of penetrating trauma to the globe, a protective convex shield should be applied pending definitive care. A CT of the brain and orbits can help to localize foreign bodies and identify associated injuries. Tetanus prophylaxis, intravenous antibiotics, and antiemetics may be warranted. Early ophthalmologic consultation is recommended for all but the most minor eye injuries.

Evaluation/Assessment

The vast majority of fatalities from a bombing incident are instantaneous. These deaths are usually due to shrapnel injuries; brain trauma; multiorgan system trauma, particularly involving the brain and thorax; and long-bone fractures. An estimated 9–22% of survivors have critical injuries. Thus, most survivors have injuries that are not life-threatening and can be managed as outpatients. These are generally minor secondary and tertiary blast injuries, such as soft tissue trauma and minor fractures. Contamination of these wounds with debris or, in some cases, body fluids from other victims, is a strong possibility.

Multiple factors affect the severity of bomb injuries. These include the amount of explosive used, the intensity and duration of the overpressurization and underpressurization waves, the distance of the victim from the explosion, and whether the bomb contained shrapnel. Injuries will generally be less severe if the victim is shielded by a substantial structure or object. Similarly, the use of body armor will be protective against shrapnel. However, it may also paradoxically increase the risk of pulmonary blast injuries. Explosions that cause structural collapse may lead to crush injuries or compressive asphyxia. Explosions occurring in water can result in greater severity of injury and have a lethal radius three times that of explosions in air. Likewise, explosions within confined spaces can be more devastating, as the blast wave tends to reverberate off of walls and around corners, increasing in intensity two- to ninefold. To illustrate this, a study from Israel showed a mortality of 7.8% among victims of open-air bombings compared with 49% among victims of bombings on buses. Finally, injuries can be made more complicated if toxic or radioactive materials have been combined with the explosive.

Prehospital Assessment

Prehospital assessment of victims should only be initiated once the safety of providers is ensured. Secondary devices and booby-trapped victims may be a very real concern. Local policies should guide the use of handheld radios and cell phones, which can remotely detonate another explosive device. With the help of law enforcement, a perimeter around the area should be established to limit access by Good Samaritans and the media. Patient care consists of triage followed by standard trauma interventions. Personal protective equipment should be worn because of potential exposure to body fluids and tissues. Triage can be complicated by the fact that patients may be unable to hear due to ruptured TMs. Unless providers have experience with victims of bombings, there is a tendency to overestimate the severity of injuries, which can tax limited trauma center resources. This can be minimized by ongoing training, drills, and close onsite supervision. Depending on the context, decontamination of victims may be necessary either before or at the same time as patient care. Finally, while not a primary concern, emergency responders should be cognizant of the fact that they are working in a crime scene and so should try to avoid moving or destroying what could be important evidence for the associated law enforcement investigation.

Emergency Department Assessment

As a rule, half of all victims of bombings will arrive at the emergency department (ED) in the first hour following the incident. The least injured generally arrive first, often bypassing Emergency Medical Services (EMS), coming in on foot or by private vehicle. Hospitals closest to the incident will be most heavily impacted, receiving 50–80% of all casualties. This is regardless of whether they are trauma centers.

Assessment and management are guided by standard trauma principles. The patient's airway, breathing, and circulation should be addressed and resuscitation initiated as indicated. The fully exposed patient should then be examined from head to toe and definitive care administered. The lungs, abdomen, and TMs of all victims should be carefully examined. If the TMs are intact and the patient is asymptomatic, primary blast injury is unlikely. If the TMs are ruptured, but the patient is otherwise asymptomatic, a chest radiograph should be obtained and the patient observed for approximately 6 h. Pulmonary injuries may evolve over time, so despite a normal initial chest radiograph, repeat imaging is recommended if the patient develops respiratory symptoms.

In addition to chest radiographs, frequently ordered diagnostic tests include spine and extremity films, and computerized tomograms (CTs) of the head, chest, abdomen and pelvis. Laboratory studies will be guided by the severity of injuries and any preexisting medical conditions. A baseline complete blood count may be considered, along with electrolytes, type and cross, coagulation studies, urinalysis, and, if rhabdomyolysis is a consideration, a total CK.

After-care

Patients exposed to an open-air explosion who remain asymptomatic after a 6–8 h period of observation can be discharged from the ED. Those exposed to a closed-space explosion, an in-water explosion, and those with ruptured TMs should be watched longer, with a low threshold for admission. The disposition of other patients will be guided by symptoms and associated injuries. Aftercare of patients discharged either from the ED or inpatient service will likewise be determined by their specific injuries. All patients should be educated on the symptoms of post-traumatic stress disorder and other stress reactions and appropriate referrals given when indicated.

Prognosis

The prognosis of victims of bomb injuries is greatly dependent on the injuries sustained. In the combat arena, increased use of body armor has resulted in the survival of victims who would previously have died of their wounds. Many of their injuries, such as traumatic brain injuries and mangled extremities, may be devastating and require complicated and long-term care. However, increasing familiarity with these injuries combined with advances in medicine is helping to decrease mortality and long-term morbidity.

References

1. DePalma RG, Burris DG, Champion HR, Hodgson MJ (2005) Blast injuries. N Engl J Med 352:1335–1342
2. Ceballos J, Turégano-Fuentes F, Perez-Diaz D, Sanz-Sanchez M, Martin-Llorente C, Guerrero-Sanz JE (2005) Casualties treated at the closest hospital in the Madrid, March 11, terrorist bombings. Crit Care Med 33(1):S107–S112
3. http://emergency.cdc.gov/masscasualties/afterbombing-ecp.asp. Accessed 21 Jun 2010
4. Khan FY (2009) Rhabdomyolysis: a review of the literature. Neth J Med 67:272–283
5. Latenser BA (2009) Critical care of the burn patient: the first 48 hours. Crit Care Med 37:2819–2826

Bone Infections

▶ Osteomyelitis

Bone Marrow Transplant: Infectious Complications

ANA VELEZ[1], MARCIE TOMBLYN[2]
[1]Division of Infectious Diseases and International Medicine, Department of Medicine, Tampa, FL, USA
[2]H. Lee Moffitt Cancer Center & Research Institute, Department of Blood and Marrow Transplantation, Associate Professor of Oncologic Sciences, USF, Tampa, FL, USA

Synonyms

BMT infections; Immune compromised hosts

Definition

Bone marrow transplant, now more commonly referred to as hematopoietic cell transplant (HCT), describes the procedure in which damaged marrow is replaced with healthy hematopoietic stem cells obtained from marrow, peripheral blood, or umbilical cord blood units. This damage can be iatrogenic, as in the setting of high dose chemotherapy followed by autologous hematopoietic cell infusion, or due to inherent damage from malignancy requiring a donor hematopoietic cell graft. Over time, the traditional conditioning regimens have expanded dramatically to include reduced intensity or non-myeloablative conditioning, reduced toxicity conditioning, as well as the conventional ablative regimens. Variations in stem cell source and conditioning intensity have resulted in disparities in the duration of neutropenia (i.e., longer with umbilical cord blood) and immune recovery (i.e., longer with T-cell depleting agents or T-cell depleted grafts). Other factors that contribute to infectious complications include increasing age of recipients and complications such as graft versus host disease (GVHD).

Treatment

Tremendous advances have occurred in the prevention and treatment of infectious complications after HCT. In part, the success is due to screening and preemptive strategies used to prevent late infections. Despite these efforts, bacterial, viral, and fungal infections remain an important cause of morbidity and mortality. A recent publication extensively details guidelines for prevention of infection in HCT patients [1].

Viral Infections

Screening and Prevention

The Herpes viruses account for a significant component of viral infections after HCT. These infections often occur after reactivation of latent virus. Pertinent Herpes viruses with known sequelae in HCT patients include Herpes Simplex Viruses (HSV), Varicella zoster virus (VZV), Cytomegalovirus (CMV), Epstein–Barr virus (EBV), and Human Herpes Virus 6 (HHV6). Serologic testing for evidence of prior exposure to HSV, VZV, CMV, and EBV is strongly recommended prior to transplant. Respiratory viruses such as influenza, parainfluenza, respiratory syncytial virus (RSV), and metapneumovirus also cause significant morbidity and mortality. Other viruses such as BK virus and adenovirus can cause severe hemorrhagic cystitis. Additionally, adenovirus can also cause conjunctivitis, pneumonitis, and hepatitis [1].

In general CMV diseases have severe impact in HCT recipients. To reduce the risk of CMV transmission, blood products from CMV seronegative donors or leukocyte-depleted blood products should be used in CMV seronegative HCT recipients. It is recommended that CMV seropositive HCT recipients or CMV seronegative recipients with a seropositive donor follow either preemptive or prophylactic therapy [2]. Preemptive therapy, designed to treat early viremia prior to development of CMV disease, includes close monitoring for the presence of CMV viremia by using CMV pp65 antigen in leukocytes or by CMV DNA polymerase chain reaction (PCR) viral load. Patients should be screened at least weekly from 10 days until 100 days after HCT. Prophylactic therapy includes ganciclovir, high doses of acyclovir, or valacyclovir from engraftment until 100 days after HCT. If acyclovir or valacyclovir is used, it is recommended that patients have frequent viral load monitoring as with preemptive therapy.

The most feared complication related to EBV is post-transplant lymphoproliferative disease (PTLD). EBV disease typically results from reactivation of latent virus or primary transmission from the graft. EBV viremia is usually asymptomatic but may lead to organ disease including encephalitis, pneumonitis, hepatitis, and PTLD. This malignancy results from proliferation of clonal B cells due to profound T cell immunodeficiency.

The incidence of PTLD ranges from 0.45% to as high as 29% depending on the type of transplant. High risk patients include recipients of T-cell depleted grafts or those receiving anti-T-cell antibodies such as antithymocyte globulin (ATG). Monitoring EBV viremia by quantitative PCR once per week for at least 3 months is recommended in high risk patients [1].

HSV reactivation post transplant can result in significant morbidity and, occasionally, mortality due to dissemination. Patients who are seronegative should be aware of behaviors that decrease HSV exposure [2]. Prior to the use of prophylactic acyclovir, the rate of HSV reactivation among HCT patients was reported to be 80%. Acyclovir prophylaxis should be offered to all HSV-seropositive HCT patients to prevent reactivation during the early post-transplant period. Patients should continue on acyclovir until a minimum of 30 days after transplant but continued use of acyclovir appears to prevent later HSV reactivation. Routine use of acyclovir is not indicated for HSV-seronegative HCT recipients. Valacyclovir is not approved for the use of preventing HSV disease among HCT recipients but studies have shown effective suppression following autologous HCT.

Long term acyclovir prophylaxis is recommended during the first year after HCT for all VZV seropositive patients to prevent reactivation. The use of acyclovir for longer than a year may be indicated if there is evidence of GVHD. HCT recipients should avoid exposure to persons with active VZV infections. However, in the event of exposure, patients with active GVHD and/or those within 24 months following HCT should receive Varicella zoster immunoglobulin (VZIG) within 96 h of contact with a person with chicken pox or shingles. Post exposure prophylaxis with acyclovir or valacyclovir is acceptable if VZIG is not available.

The prevention of respiratory viruses such us influenza, parainfluenza, RSV, and metapneumovirus includes screening with throat viral cultures as soon as symptoms occur. These patients should be placed under contact and droplets precautions [2]. Adenovirus screening by weekly PCR during the first 6 months after HCT has also been suggested for patients with T-cell lymphopenia, refractory GVHD, and/or who have received anti-T-cell antibodies.

Pharmacologic Therapy

Intravenous acyclovir is the treatment of choice for severe forms of mucocutaneous or visceral HSV disease. Oral acyclovir, valacyclovir, or famciclovir are available for less severe forms of disease. Resistant strains have been documented in patients with severe forms of mucocutaneous, esophageal, life threatening meningoencephalitis, and pneumonia. Such strains of HSV are usually susceptible to foscarnet.

VZV infection can be lethal in HCT recipients, particularly primary infection. These patients are at risk for visceral dissemination. Intravenous acyclovir is the drug of choice for disseminated VZV. Oral acyclovir, valacyclovir, or famciclovir can be an option if there is no evidence of visceral dissemination such us encephalitis, pneumonia, or hepatitis.

Prior to the availability of antiviral drugs, the mortality related to CMV infection in HCT was 90–100%. CMV can present as viremia or disease. CMV disease includes bone marrow suppression, pneumonitis, gastroenteritis, hepatitis, nephritis, cystitis, and encephalitis. CMV encephalitis can be suspected if the MRI reveals a periventricular hyperintense signal. The diagnosis is made after PCR for CMV is detected in the cerebrospinal fluid (CSF). The definitive diagnosis of CMV pneumonitis and/or gastroenteritis requires tissue biopsy demonstrating the viral inclusion "owl's eye cells." Evidence of CMV by PCR from a bronchoalveolar lavage may also be considered evidence of CMV pneumonitis. Currently most transplant centers use ganciclovir 5 mg/kg intravenous every 12 h for 2–3 weeks followed by an additional 2 weeks of maintenance therapy with ganciclovir at lower doses. Combined therapy with intravenous immunoglobulin (IVIG) is recommended for patients with CMV pneumonitis. Foscarnet and cidofivir have been used as alternatives for ganciclovir resistant CMV disease or in patients unable to tolerate the marrow suppression associated with ganciclovir.

Reactivation of HHV6 has been associated with disease. Clinical syndromes associated with HHV6 include fever, rash, hepatitis, pneumonitis, encephalitis with temporal lobe enhancing lesions, and bone marrow suppression with delayed platelet engraftment. Indications for treatment of HHV6 reactivation remain unclear and further study is warranted. However, treatment with either ganciclovir or foscarnet can be used.

Reactivation of EBV virus can lead to encephalitis, pneumonitis, hepatitis, and PTLD. The recommended first line therapy for EBV reactivation includes anti-CD20 immunotherapy (rituximab), and reduction of immunosuppressive therapy.

Adenovirus infection can present as conjunctivitis, pneumonitis, gastrointestinal disease, nephritis, cystitis, and meningoencephalitis. The therapy of choice is cidofivir.

BK virus can cause severe cystitis and nephritis in HCT patients. The treatment of choice is intravenous cidofivir.

Other options include cidofivir bladder installation, leflunomide, and the fluoroquinolones.

The respiratory viruses including influenza A and B, parainfluenza, and Respiratory Syncytial Virus (RSV) are commonly encountered in the general population. HCT patients can easily acquire them with lethal outcomes. Influenza and RSV occur mainly in winter months and parainfluenza in summer. Clinical syndromes include upper or lower respiratory infections. Antiviral therapy for influenza A and B includes neuraminidase inhibitors such us oseltamivir and zanamivir. Amantadine and rimantadine are only active against influenza A. Treatment for RSV infections include ribavirin and the monoclonal antibody palivizumab [2].

Bacterial Infections

Screening and Prevention
Bacterial infections occur throughout all periods of hematologic and immune recovery after HCT. The spectra of bacterial infections seen during the pre-engraftment period are primarily related to neutropenia. In the peri-transplant period, risk factors for infections include primarily mucositis and indwelling catheters. The most common gram positive cocci are coagulase negative staphylococcus. *Streptococcus viridans* is seen in the setting of severe mucositis. Dental procedures should be done prior to HCT to minimize *Streptococcus viridans* infections

Screening for Methicillin Resistant *Staphylococcus aureus* (MRSA) and vancomycin resistant enterococcus (VRE) should be considered for infection control purposes and to appropriately tailor therapy if neutropenic fever or specific disease develops. Antibacterial prophylaxis with a fluoroquinolone to prevent bacterial infections should be strongly considered for patients undergoing HCT with an anticipated period of neutropenia lasting longer than 7 days and the fluoroquinolone therapy continued until the neutropenia resolves. The emergence of fluoroquinolone resistant pathogens including *Klebsiella* species, *Escherichia coli*, *Pseudomonas* species, *Staphylococcus aureus*, and *Streptococcus viridans* remains a concern. The role of antibacterial prophylaxis to prevent gram positive cocci infections is unclear. The extensive use of vancomycin in this population has led to an increase of VRE [1]. Metronidazole for prophylaxis and to reduce the anaerobic bacterial growth is not recommended.

Pharmacologic Therapy
Broad spectrum antimicrobial therapy for the management of febrile neutropenia is well established. Options include single agent therapy with a third or fourth generation cephalosporin or a carbapenem with antipseudomonas activity. Some physicians add vancomycin, particularly if there is a concern for line infection, or if mucositis is present.

The antibiotic of choice can be modified depending on clinical symptoms; history of recent cultures from blood, respiratory tract, gastrointestinal tract, or genitourinary tract; and local resistance patterns. If there is evidence of VRE colonization, daptomycin or linezolid may be used in place of vancomycin. Anaerobic coverage with metronidazole is frequently added for patients with fever and enterocolitis. Aminoglycosides are reserved for treatment of documented resistant organisms or septic shock. The frequent use of fluoroquinolone prophylaxis in HCT patients has limited their utility for empiric therapy in neutropenic fever for this group of patients due to potential fluoroquinolone resistant organisms.

The risk of bacterial infections continues after engraftment. Bacterial infections including pneumonia, blood stream, genitourinary tract, or gastrointestinal tract can emerge, especially in the setting of severe immune suppression from GVHD. Such cases should be managed in an individual basis using clinical symptoms, physical examination, past cultured organisms, and local resistance patterns as guidance [1]. Long term antimicrobial prophylaxis against *Streptococcus pneumoniae* is indicated for patients with chronic GVHD and ongoing immune suppression [1].

Fungal Infections

Screening and Prevention
Over the past 2 decades the epidemiology of fungal infections has changed. Organisms previously thought to be nonpathogenic or rare are now increasing. In the past *Candida* species, specifically *Candida albicans*, were the most common cause of fungal blood stream infections and *Aspergillus* species were the most common cause of invasive fungal pneumonia. Recently other emerging mold infections such as fusarium, zygomycetes, and scedosporium continue to increase. Several factors are contributing to this change in epidemiology: changes in medical treatments and prophylaxis, aggressive new therapies for HCT and malignancies, and extended survival of critically ill patients [3].

The risk of *Candida* species infections is significantly higher early during the post-transplant period because of ongoing neutropenia, mucositis, and the presence of central venous catheters. The presence of severe GVHD of the gastrointestinal tract results in additional continued risk of infection with *Candida* species. Classically, fluconazole has been the drug of choice to prevent *Candida* infection in HCT patients but there are emerging species that are less susceptible or resistant such as *Candida glabrata* and *Candida kruseii*.

Opportunistic invasive fungal infections (IFIs) such as aspergillus, fusarium, scedosporium, and zygomycetes are a major cause of morbidity and mortality in immune compromised patients. Potential risk factors for the development of IFI include a history of mold infections prior to HCT, prolonged periods of neutropenia either before HCT or due to delayed engraftment, and GVHD. In patients at high risk for mold infections, posaconazole or voriconazole can be used for prophylaxis.

Pneumocystis jiroveci previously known as *Pneumocystis carini* pneumonia (PCP) is a preventable complication of HCT. Prophylaxis should be continued for longer than 6 months in patients who continue to receive immune suppressive therapy. The preferred regimen for PCP prophylaxis is trimethoprim–sulfamethoxazole (TMP-SMX). Other medications that can be used to prevent PCP include aerosolized pentamidine, oral dapsone, or oral atovaquone [2].

Pharmacologic therapy

The diagnosis of IFIs remains a challenge. Diagnostic criteria are based on tissue culture or histopathology. If tissue culture and/or histopathology are not available or are difficult to obtain, host risk factors plus radiologically demonstrable lesions (halo sign, reverse halo sign) can be used as a probable diagnosis [4].

Treatment of mold infections such as *Aspergillus* spp., *Fusarium* spp., and *Scedosporium* spp. includes voriconazole or posaconazole. Some species of fusarium may be resistant to the new generation of azoles such as voriconazole and posaconazole but remain susceptible to amphotericin B. The treatment of choice for zygomycetes is amphotericin B. Posaconazole can also be used for patients unable to tolerate amphotericin B [3].

Combination therapy for severe mold infections has being described. For refractory cases of fusarium, the combination of voriconazole or posaconazole plus amphotericin B has been reported to be successful. Additionally the combination of terbinafine plus an azole, or amphotericin B plus pentamidine, or amphotericin B plus voriconazole has been studied for the therapy of scedosporium. Innovative treatment options have also been reported for the treatment of zygomycetes including deferasirox, granulocyte growth factors (GCSF, GM-CSF), and the combination of amphotericin B with an echinocandin [3].

The length of therapy for mold infections is generally prolonged. Antifungals should be continued until clinical response is evident and improvement of the immunosuppressed status is appreciated. Close follow-up is indicated to prevent relapses.

References

1. Tomblyn M et al (2009) Guidelines for preventing infectious complications among hematopoietic cell transplant recipients: a global perspective. Recommendations of the Center for International Blood and Marrow Transplant Research (CIBMTR®), the National Marrow Donor Program (NMDP), the European Blood and Marrow Transplant Group (EBMT), the American Society of Blood and Marrow Transplantation (ASBMT), the Canadian Blood and Marrow Transplant Group (CBMTG), the Infectious Disease Society of America (IDSA), the Society for Healthcare Epidemiology of America (SHEA), the Association of Medical Microbiology and Infectious Diseases Canada (AMMI), the Centers for Disease Control and Prevention (CDC), and the Health Resources and Services Administration (HRSA). Jointly published in Biol Blood Marrow Transplant 15(10), 1143–1238; Bone Marrow Transplant 44(8), part 2
2. Hiemenz JW (2009) Management of infections complicating allogeneic hematopoietic stem cell transplantation. Semin Hematol 46(3):289–312
3. Naggie S, Perfect JR (2009) Molds: hyalohyphomycosis, phaeohyphomycosis, and zygomycosis. Clin Chest Med 30(2):337–353, vii–viii
4. Ascioglu S et al (2002) Defining opportunistic invasive fungal infections in immunocompromised patients with cancer and hematopoietic stem cell transplants: an international consensus. Clin Infect Dis 34(1):7–14

Borderline Patient

The term "borderline patient" describes a specific subgroup of trauma patients who, although hemodynamically stable, are at particular risk when subject to the additional physiologic insult sustained from prolonged surgical procedures.

Botulism

▶ Biological Terrorism, Botulinum Toxin

Bovine Heparin

▶ Heparin

Box Jellyfish

▶ Jellyfish Envenomation

Brain Abscess

HITOSHI HONDA[1], DAVID K. WARREN[2]
[1]Department of General Internal Medicine and Infectious Diseases, Teine Keijinkai Medical Center, Teine, Sapporo, Japan
[2]Division of Infectious Diseases, Department of Medicine, Washington University School of Medicine, Saint Louis, MO, USA

Synonyms

Infectious mass lesion in the central nervous system

Definition

Brain abscess is defined by the presence of focal infection in the brain parenchyma commonly caused by bacterial, fungal, and parasitic pathogens [1]. The entity of brain abscess may include other central nervous system (CNS) infections, such as subdural empyema, since they may coexist with brain abscess. Subdural empyema is defined as a purulent infection of the space between the cranial dura and arachnoid membrane. Clinical symptoms in patients with brain abscess range from constitutional symptoms to significant neurological deficits. Given the lack of hallmark clinical findings for brain abscesses, the combination of radiographic and microbiological evaluation are important in the definitive diagnosis of brain abscess.

Treatment

Brain abscess is a life-threatening infectious disease requiring urgent medical attention. A multidisciplinary approach, including surgical and medical management, is required for definitive therapy. Antimicrobial therapy is the mainstay of medical management. Empiric antimicrobials should cover likely pathogens in the context of the individual clinical settings. Choice of empiric antimicrobials should be determined by several factors. These include the known or presumed original source of infection (i.e., contiguous spread from adjacent structures vs hematogenous origin). Patient factors (e.g., age and immune function) and pharmacological factors (i.e., the degree of penetration of particular

antimicrobial agents into the cerebrospinal fluid) also influence the choice of antimicrobials. For brain abscess arising from a contiguous source, such as sinuses or the oral cavity, empiric antimicrobial therapy should be broad-spectrum and have activity against Gram-positive (i.e., *Streptococci* and *Staphylococci*), Gram-negative (i.e., *Enterobacteriaceae* with or without *Pseudomonas* spp.), and anaerobic (e.g., *Bacteroides*) bacteria. The combination of a third- or fourth-generation cephalosporin and metronidazole, with or without vancomycin, is a reasonable choice. Using empiric antipseudomonal agents should be strongly considered for brain abscess associated with penetrating trauma, intravenous illicit drug use, and severe immunocompromised status, including poorly controlled diabetics with malignant otitis externa. A carbapenem can be used instead of the combination of cephalosporin and metronidazole since this drug class covers the wide range of causative pathogens, including Gram-positive (except methicillin-resistant Staphylococci), Gram-negative, and anaerobic bacteria. However, carbapenems should be used cautiously since they can be associated with a lowered seizure threshold. Vancomycin is recommended to treat methicillin-resistant Gram-positive bacteria (e.g., methicillin-resistant *Staphylococcus aureus*). Newer agents with activity against resistant Gram-positive bacteria, such as linezolid, daptomycin, or telavancin are also available, but limited clinical data currently exist regarding their use in the treatment of brain abscesses.

In addition to empiric antimicrobial coverage for common bacterial pathogens, antimicrobial therapy may need to be expanded to treat relatively uncommon pathogens, depending on the clinical scenario. Several opportunistic pathogens can cause brain abscesses in immunocompromised patients. Nocardial brain abscess should be considered in immunocompromised patients who presented with focal neurological signs and symptoms, or infection due to *Nocardia* spp. at another body site. Brain abscess due to *Listeria monocytogenes* can be seen in immunocompromised or elderly individuals. Fungal brain abscesses caused by yeast, dimorphic fungi, and molds are associated with severely immunocompromised individuals, such as solid organ or stem cell transplant patients, and in the case of brain abscess, due to *Rhizopus* spp., in poorly controlled diabetes. Patients with acquired immunodeficiency syndrome (AIDS) have a risk for developing brain abscesses due to *Toxoplasma gondii*. Other, less common causes of brain abscess, (e.g., *Mycobacterium tuberculosis*, *Taenia solium*, and *Trypanosoma cruzii*) should be considered in individuals from endemic regions or with the appropriate exposure history.

A neurosurgical evaluation is warranted on patients with a brain abscess. Although the surgical treatment for brain abscesses has significantly evolved over recent decades, the indications for surgical therapy remain controversial. Surgical therapy included open craniotomy, stereotactic abscess drainage and ventriculostomy for elevated intracranial pressure. Surgical therapy for brain abscesses is recommended if the size of the abscess is greater than 2.5 cm, given the poor response to antimicrobial therapy alone [2]. Also, surgical drainage of periventricular abscesses or abscesses in the posterior fossa is usually indicated due to the risk of intraventicular rupture or cranial herniation. Foreign bodies or bone fragments associated with a traumatic brain abscess should be surgically removed. Difference in clinical outcome between stereotactic drainage versus open craniotomy remains unclear; however, minimally invasive surgical techniques are generally preferred. A coexisting subdural empyema with a brain abscess is an absolute indication for emergent surgical evacuation due to the risk of rapid expansion and herniation [1].

Dexamethasone is generally given to patients with brain abscesses to reduce intracranial pressure, especially in patients with impending brain herniation. Dexamethasone reduces vasogenic edema around a brain abscess and may also reduce inflammatory response associated with the infection. However, the overall benefit (i.e., improvement of morbidity and mortality) of dexamethasone therapy remains unclear. Non-randomized studies for assessing the efficacy of dexamethasone in patients with brain abscess may be confounded by selection bias since patients who received dexamethasone are more likely to have impending herniation, which is independently associated with morbidity and mortality.

Seizures can occur in patients with brain abscesses. Seizures may lead to altered mental status and complications such as aspiration pneumonia. Incidence of seizure may be influenced by the size and location of an abscess. Institution of prophylactic anticonvulsants (e.g., fosphenytoin, phenytoin, valproate, and levetiracetam) should be considered, especially in the early course of therapy. Anticonvulsant therapy should always be given to patients with a brain abscess who present with a seizure.

Evaluation and Assessment

The diagnosis of brain abscess requires the high index of suspicion. The classic clinical trial of brain abscess (headache, mental status changes, and focal neurological deficits) is insensitive and nonspecific.

Definitive diagnosis of brain abscesses consist of radiographic and microbiological evaluation. Computed tomography (CT) or magnetic resonance imaging (MRI) is commonly used for the diagnosis of brain abscess.

Rim-enhancing mass lesions are the common finding in cranial imaging with intravenous contrast. There are both advantages and disadvantages to these two imaging modalities: CT is widely available and useful for assessing brain abscess associated with penetrating trauma, and orbital or sinus fractures, but MRI is generally preferable for detecting smaller lesions or lesions in the posterior fossa.

A microbiological diagnosis is important for determining appropriate antimicrobial therapy. Advanced techniques in neurosurgery, such as stereotactic aspiration, enable clinicians to obtain microbiological specimens in a relatively noninvasive manner. While empiric antimicrobial therapy should not be delayed in patients presenting with sepsis or impending herniation, antimicrobial therapy can be held in neurologically stable patients until a microbiological and histological diagnosis is made. This is because the use of preoperative antimicrobials may reduce the diagnostic yield of cultures. Microbiological specimens should be sent for aerobic, anaerobic, fungal, and mycobacterial cultures. Histopathological evaluation for biopsy specimen should be performed as well. Since empiric antimicrobials are may be started before obtaining a microbiological culture, a causative pathogen may not be recovered. Newer molecular methods (e.g., 16 S ribosomal DNA sequencing) may help identify pathogens and tailor antimicrobial therapy in cases of culture-negative abscesses [3]. Serological testing, for parasitic or fungal brain abscess, should be ordered when clinical history warrants.

Evaluation of a patient with brain abscess should be done in an expedited manner and involve regular neurological exams. A grave complication of brain abscess is cerebral herniation due to increased intracranial pressure. Deteriorating neurological exams, vital sign changes (e.g., Cushing phenomenon), or papilledema on fundoscopic exam should prompt immediate cranial imaging with CT and neurosurgical evaluation. An emergent ventriculostomy may need to be performed, or surgical decompression, especially in case of cerebellar or brain stem abscesses, given the small volume of the posterior fossa. Intensive care is required for patients who need frequent neurological exams, are intubated for airway protection due to altered mental status, have intraventricular catheters, or are septic. Periodic, thorough neurological exams and close monitoring are essential in the early course of therapy. Besides infection, various factors can alter a patient's mental status, including seizures, hyponatermia due to salt wasting or syndrome of inappropriate antidiuretic hormone (SIADH), antimicrobial toxicity, and fever. Patients with a brain abscess associated with a mycotic aneurysm or endoarteritis may be a risk of intracranial bleeding. Serial imaging studies might be necessary in case of prolonged altered mental status to evaluate for new complications, such as bleeding.

After-care

After patients received adequate surgical evaluation or treatment, continuing antimicrobial therapy is a mainstay of long-term management. The optimal duration of antimicrobial therapy is unclear and differs individually. Traditionally, antimicrobial therapy for pyogenic brain abscess has been for at least 6–8 weeks, depending on the patient's clinical response, radiographic improvement, and the causative pathogens. For brain abscess caused by common bacterial pathogens, such as *Streptococcus* spp., antimicrobial therapy can be continued until the abscess has resolved radiographically and clinical improvement is achieved. For more atypical pathogens, such as *Nocardia* spp., or *Actinomyces* spp., prolonged courses of antimicrobial therapy (e.g., 12 months) are required to minimize the risk of recurrence, regardless of radiographic resolution.

Once the causative pathogens are identified, empiric therapy should be modified to pathogen-targeted therapy. Definitive therapy should be based upon the in vitro susceptibility of the pathogen and the penetration of antimicrobial agents into central nervous system. Many physicians prefer simplified antimicrobials, which allow for once- or twice-a-day dosing. Periodic blood test (i.e., complete blood count and comprehensive metabolic profile) are necessary to detect side effects due to long-term antimicrobial therapy. Antimicrobial therapy for pyogenic abscesses requires parenteral agents. Switching to oral antimicrobials with excellent bioavailability may be possible, in the chronic phase of treatment; however, it should be done in consultation with an infectious diseases specialist.

Although many physicians utilize periodic imaging studies to determine the duration of antimicrobial therapy, there is no guidance how often and how frequent radiographic imaging should be performed. The resolution of radiographic findings after treatment varies and is hard to predict. Moreover, it may be difficult to distinguish scar tissue from residual infection, especially after surgical resection. A repeat imaging bimonthly or monthly during long-term therapy is reasonable [1].

Prognosis

Because of advancements in critical medicine and surgical management, the mortality associated with brain abscess has substantially decreased over the last 30 years [4]. However, it continues to result in substantial morbidity and mortality. In a large case series of patients with brain abscess over an 18-year time period, the unfavorable outcomes (death, persistent vegetative status, and severe disability) occurred in 26% of patients [5]. Factors associated with morbidity and mortality in brain abscesses include the anatomical location and size of the abscess, altered mental status on presentation, patient underlying comorbidities, intraventricular rupture of the abscess, delayed diagnosis, and suboptimal accessibility of advanced care (i.e., timely neurosurgical management).

Summary

Prompt diagnosis and timely medical and surgical therapy are key to the successful management of brain abscesses. An intensive monitoring of patients with brain abscess early in treatment is important. Comprehensive care involving critical care physicians, neurosurgeons, and infectious diseases specialists optimizes clinical outcome.

References

1. Mathisen GE, Johnson JP (1997) Brain abscess. Clin Infect Dis 25(4): 763–779
2. Mamelak AN, Mampalam TJ, Obana WG, Rosenblum ML (1995) Improved management of multiple brain abscesses: a combined surgical and medical approach. Neurosurgery 36(1):76–85, discussion 85–76
3. Al Masalma M, Armougom F, Scheld WM et al (2009) The expansion of the microbiological spectrum of brain abscesses with use of multiple 16S ribosomal DNA sequencing. Clin Infect Dis 48(9): 1169–1178
4. Tattevin P, Bruneel F, Clair B et al (2003) Bacterial brain abscesses: a retrospective study of 94 patients admitted to an intensive care unit (1980 to 1999). Am J Med 115(2):143–146
5. Tseng JH, Tseng MY (2006) Brain abscess in 142 patients: factors influencing outcome and mortality. Surg Neurol 65(6):557–562

Brain Death

Lars Widdel[1], Kathryn M. Beauchamp[2]
[1]Department of Neurosurgery, University of Colorado Denve Health Medical Center, Denver, CO, USA
[2]Department of Neurosurgery, Denver Health Medical Center, University of Colorado School of Medicine, Denver, CO, USA

Synonyms

Brainstem death; Coma depasse; Neurologic death

Definition

The definition of brain death is "the irreversible loss of function of the brain, including the brainstem" or in a much more refined manner "the irreversible loss of the capacity for consciousness combined with the irreversible loss of all brainstem functions including the capacity to breathe."

The concept of brain death is a relatively young one. First described in 1959, Mollaret and Goulon presented a series of patients who had lost consciousness, brainstem reflexes, as well as the ability to breathe and had a flat electroencephalogram. They described this condition as irreversible coma – coma depasse. Subsequent separate reviews on the issue by an ad hoc committee of the Harvard Medical School, the Conference of Medical Royal Colleges, and their Faculties in the United Kingdom and by Mohandas and Chou further clarified the diagnosis and the concept of irreversible coma placing emphasis on the complete and irreversible injury to the brain stem as a main factor in the diagnosis of this condition and calling it "brain death." They made the statement that "without brain stem there is no life." As a result, some define brain death as irreversible brainstem injury while others require global brain injury to be present before the diagnosis may be established. Some countries have embraced the concept of only requiring demonstration of irreversible complete brainstem injury and not global brain injury as in other countries.

In the 1980s and 1990s, the President's Commission and the American Academy of Neurology published guidelines regarding the diagnosis of brain death. Similar guidelines have been published since that date by different medical societies throughout the world. However, there is currently no global consensus on the diagnosis criteria and medicolegal implications of brain death.

Clinical Determination of Brain Death

The clinical determination of brain death requires an exhaustive and precise evaluation and understanding of the process that led to complete and irreversible damage of the brain stem, a thorough neurologic examination of the patient, and the exclusion of any conditions that may mimic brain death.

This process can vary from country to country, from state to state, or even from hospital to hospital within the same city. Additionally, practices may vary based on patient age. Adults are often viewed differently in terms of brain death than children or neonates. In some locations, these guidelines have been made into laws and any variation from them can be considered criminal. These differences are most commonly related to the number of observers required to determine brain death, the specialty

of the assessing physician, the duration of observation, and the use of confirmatory tests. Therefore, it is strongly advised that, prior to initiating a brain death determination evaluation on a patient, one get accustomed to the local brain death diagnosis guidelines.

To begin with, the determination of brain death should be done by somebody with the knowledge and understanding of neurologic disease. In many places, it is required that the person conducting the evaluation should be a board certified neurologist or neurosurgeon. The most common causes of brain injuries leading to brain death include traumatic brain injury (TBI), hypoxic or anoxic brain injury, spontaneous intracerebral hemorrhages due to either arterial hypertension, amyloid angiopathy, cerebral aneurysms, arterious venous malformations, hydrocephalus, and brain tumors or other space occupying lesions. The diagnosis of the conditions leading up to brain death require a full understanding of the events, signs and symptoms, a thorough physical examination of the patient, and an evaluation of any associated studies. Cerebral imaging either by computed tomography (CT) or magnetic resonance imaging (MRI) is important. These will often indicate the cause of the brain injury. Often a cause for the brain damage cannot be identified initially and requires observation over time, repetition of studies, and/or evaluation by more specialized practitioners. It is important to know and understand the cause of the brain injury in each individual patient prior to proceeding with brain death diagnosis, and be able to rule out conditions that may mimic brain death. Severe systemic disease leading to acid–base or electrolyte alterations can lead to coma suggestive of brainstem injury. Severe hypothermia below 32°C, hypotension, drug intoxication, poisoning, and anesthetic and neuromuscular blockade can all induce a profound coma. These reversible causes of coma must be ruled out prior to the examination of brain death.

Coma is a state of absolute willful or centrally regulated unresponsiveness to external stimuli. In a coma, a patient may not open or close the eyes spontaneously or have any purposeful movement. It is evaluated by evaluating the absence or presence of the movement to painful stimuli such as pressing on the supraorbital rim, the temporomandibular joint, sternal rub, or by applying pressure to the nail bed. At times, it might be difficult to differentiate between a withdrawal reaction that is centrally mediated and would exclude brain death and an entirely spinally mediated reflex such as the triple flexion response in the lower extremities that is not centrally mediated and does not exclude the diagnosis of brain death. The lack of spontaneous respiratory efforts should also be documented.

Once coma has been established, one should proceed with the evaluation of the brainstem reflexes:

1. Pupillary reflex: This reflex is mediated by an afferent CNII and efferent CNIII reaction. In brain death, the pupils can be midpoint or fully dilated without constrictive response to light. This reflex is usually still present even with deep sedation, but conditions such as prosthetic globe, pseudophakia, intentional or incidental topical application of midriatic agents, Adie's pupils, bilateral isolated CN III palsies, among others may mimic the condition.

2. Corneal reflex: This reflex is mediated through an afferent CN V and efferent CN III and VII reaction. It is evaluated by applying soft cotton on the cornea and evaluating if the patient's eye lid contracts. It is important to apply the corneal stimulus lateral to the pupil and to avoid applying too much pressure on the eyelid while trying to open the patient's eye as it may obscure the response.

3. Occulo-cephalic reflex: This evaluates the vestibular system in the brain stem. When turning the head on a comatose patient in whom this reflex is not impaired the eyes will turn the opposite way, while in a brain-dead patient they will remain fixed in a mid position – doll's eyes. This test cannot be performed on patients with suspected cervical spinal injuries or in awake patients.

4. Occulo-vestibular reflex or caloric testing: In a patient with this reflex intact the irrigation of the external auditory canal with ice water will cause the eyes to turn toward that ear. This test cannot be done if the ear canal is obstructed by wax or blood, or if the eardrum is perforated. This reflex is absent in brain-dead patients.

5. Gag reflex: Also called pharyngeal reflex is a reflex contraction of the back of the throat, evoked by touching the soft palate. The afferent limb is supplied by CN IX and the efferent limb by CN X. It is elicited by applying pressure onto the soft palate.

6. Cough reflex: This reflex is mediated by the CN X for both the afferent and efferent pathways. In intubated patients, it can be elucidated by inserting a suction tubing through the endotracheal tubing to irritate the bronchial airways.

All reflexes should be evaluated as they evaluate different aspects of the brain stem: The pupillary reflex evaluates the midbrain, the corneal reflex the pons, the occulo-cephalic and occulo-vestibular reflex both the pons and midbrain, and the gag and cough reflex evaluate the medulla. They all need to be absent in the case of brain death.

Apnea Test

The final step in the clinical evaluation and determination of a patient with suspected brain death is the apnea test. This test is done with the rationale that a functional medulla will induce a respiratory effort if the patient's pCO_2 rises above 60 or 20 mmHg above the patient's baseline.

In order to perform this test, initially the physician needs to establish the patient's hemodynamic status that is stable enough to tolerate an apnea test. It needs to be ensured that the patient's core temperature is within normal range, the patient has no significant metabolic or electrolyte disturbance that might interfere with the test, there are no sedatives or toxins that could interfere or masquerade the results of the test, the patient's pCO_2 is near a normal level and that the patient has no high cervical spine injury, maxillofacial or thoracic injury that may interfere with the physiological response of a ventilatory effort.

The patient should be pretreated with 100% oxygen for about 10 min and a baseline arterial blood gas level should be obtained. Thereafter, the patient should be disconnected from ventilator support, either by placing him on a CPAP setting or disconnecting him completely from the ventilator and placing a large bore catheter with oxygen into the endotracheal tube. The patient's chest and abdomen should be uncovered and carefully watched for any respiratory efforts for a period of 10 min. It is noted that one must differentiate respiratory effort movements from cardiac pulsations or ventilatory support caused by a CPAP ventilator with very sensitive trigger settings. If after 10 min no respiratory efforts have been noted, a new arterial blood gas should be obtained and the patient should be reconnected to ventilatory support. If the patient's pCO_2 has risen above 60 mmHg or greater than 20 mmHg above the baseline level without any obvious respiratory effort, the test is considered positive and consistent with brain death. Any respiratory effort should render the test as negative and rule out the diagnosis of brain death.

Confirmatory Tests

The diagnosis of brain death is considered a sole clinical diagnosis. In most countries, the use of confirmatory test for the diagnosis of brain death is considered optional, although in other places it is mandatory. There currently exist a wide variety of confirmatory tests, some of which are better established in the literature than others. Most guidelines recommend performing confirmatory tests in the following conditions:

- Inability to establish a diagnosis of coma due to sedation, use of paralytics, systemic neuropathies
- Inability to perform a thorough brainstem reflexes exam due to extensive maxillofacial trauma, suspicion of cranial neuropathies, drug-induced paralysis
- Inability to perform an apnea test due to patient's hemodynamic and/or respiratory instability, high cervical spine injury, or in patients who are high carbon dioxide retainers
- In children, especially those under 1 year of age

The ideal confirmatory test is a test that would have no false positives to minimize the risk of overdiagnosing brain death and very few false negatives. In addition, it should be readily accessible and require minimal intervention on a patient who is most likely hemodynamically unstable. At present, the ideal confirmatory test does not exist.

There are two types of confirmatory tests. The electro-encephalogram (EEG) that evaluates the presence or absence of cerebral electrical activity and those studies that evaluate intracranial blood flow.

The use of EEG bases itself on the theory that in case of brain death, there will be no recordable electrical activity. It is one of the most studied and most validated confirmatory tests of brain death. Its advantages include the fact that it is usually readily available, it can be applied on the patient at bedside, and it is not invasive. Recordings are obtained for at least 30 min with a 16- or 18-channel instrument. In a brain-dead patient, electrical activity is absent at levels higher than 2 μV with the instrument set at a sensitivity of 2 μV per millimeter. The drawbacks of this test are that it requires that the patient should not be under any sedative medication, as well as not be in supratherapeutic levels of any antiepileptic medication. The presence of multiple monitoring devices, as usually found in most ICU settings, can also introduce artifacts into the EEG that can interfere with the interpretation.

The other line of confirmatory tests constitutes those that evaluate cerebral blood flow and perfusion. The basis of these is that a condition that leads to brain death will most commonly cause severely elevated intracranial pressure, either due to the presence of a volume occupying lesion such as a hematoma, a tumor, or a cerebrospinal fluid in case of hydrocephalus or due to diffuse cerebral edema in case of diffuse trauma or anoxic brain injury. In order to ensure that there is no intracranial blood flow, the intracranial pressure must surpass the arterial pressure. The most common and most studied blood flow studies are cerebral angiography, transcranial doppler, and cerebral scintigraphy. In the case of cerebral angiography, pressure injections should be done at both the anterior and posterior circulations and no flow should be detected past the entry point into the intracranial vault of the carotid or vertebral arteries. External carotid flow and delayed longitudinal sinus flow can however be visible. In the case of transcranial doppler, it needs to be established if the patient has insonation windows, because if these are absent a different study needs to be selected. Once established, the presence of small systolic peaks with absent diastolic flow or reverberating flow is consistent with brain death. For the cerebral scintigraphy with technetium-99m hexamethyl-propylene-amineoxime, no intracranial uptake of isotope should be noted.

More recently, other blood flow studies such as computed tomography angiography and magnetic resonance angiography have been coming in vogue, mainly because of their availability and ease of interpretation. However, there are not enough studies yet to fully justify their use.

Differential Diagnosis

Although the diagnosis of brain death seems straightforward, there are several conditions that may mimic it. Examples of this include the use of sedatives, anesthetics, antidepressant (especially large quantities of tricyclics), and paralytics. Though these medications will rarely cause suppression of brainstem reflexes, care needs to be taken when determining brain death on a patient for the clinical evaluation may be influenced by these medications. Often, one must wait until these medication levels are below their respective therapeutic levels or their effects are reversed to proceed with brain death evaluation.

Patients who are in status epilepticus or who are postictal may also be in profound coma and evaluations such as an EEG should be undertaken if this condition is suspected.

Other neurologic states such as coma, vegetative state, and locked-in syndrome demonstrate profound states of unresponsiveness, but these patients do not have absent brainstem reflexes, unless they have individual cranial nerve palsies. The presence of any brainstem reflex during evaluation should rather suggest one of these conditions.

In patients with brain death, there are certain physiological responses that are often disconcerting but still compatible with brain death. They may exhibit spontaneous movement of limbs or body other than pathologic extension or flexion movements that are mediated by the spine. These have been referred also as "Lazarus signs" and are especially evident after discontinuation of ventilatory support. Brain-dead patients may also present sweating, blushing, tachycardia, deep tendon reflexes, triple flexions responses, superficial abdominal reflexes, back arching, shoulder elevation and adduction and Babinski responses. In addition, the persistence of pituitary function does not exclude the diagnosis of brain death as the blood supply of the pituitary gland is often supplied by extracranial vessels.

Overall, the medicolegal implications of brain death are far reaching. Once a patient is pronounced dead, legal issues such as probate proceedings, organ donations, insurance claims, or actions for wrongful death and criminal prosecution may be initiated. In addition, many laypeople remain suspicious of the concept of brain death, fearing that premature determination of death may be prompted by the need for donor organs. Therefore, the diagnosis of this condition should be done with absolute attention to detail and documented extremely well. The misdiagnosis or misnomer of this condition can have serious implications in the future.

Cross Reference
▶ Death by Neurologic Criteria

References
1. The Quality Standards Subcommittee of the American Academy of Neurology (1995) Practice parameters for determining brain death in adults (summary statement). Neurology 45:1012–1014
2. Wijdicks EF (2001) The diagnosis of brain death. N Engl J Med 344(16):1215–1221
3. Morenski JD, Oro JJ, Tobias JD, Singh A (2003) Determination of death by neurological criteria. J Intensive Care Med 18:211

Brain Injury Prognosis
▶ Glasgow Coma Scale

Brain Natriuretic Peptide
▶ B-Type Natriuretic Peptide
▶ Renal Blood Flow Regulation

Brain Trauma
▶ Traumatic Brain Injury, Initial Management

Brainstem Death
▶ Brain Death

Brazilian Hemorrhagic Fever
▶ Biological Terrorism, Hemorrhagic Fever

Breakbone Fever
▶ Dengue

Bright's Disease
▶ Glomerulonephritis

Bronchial Endoscopy
▶ Bronchial Fibroscopy and Lung Biopsy

Bronchial Fibroscopy
▶ Bronchial Fibroscopy and Lung Biopsy

Bronchial Fibroscopy and Lung Biopsy

Stéphane Y. Donati[1], Laurent Papazian[2]
[1]Service de Réanimation Polyvalente, Hôpital Font-Pré, Toulon, France
[2]Service de Réanimation médicale, Assistance Publique Hôpitaux de Marseille, URMITE CNRS-UMR 6236, Université de la Méditerranée Aix-Marseille II, Marseille, France

Synonyms

Biopsy by thoracotomy; Bronchial endoscopy; Bronchial fibroscopy; Bronchoscopy; Fibrobronchoscopy; Open lung biopsy; Surgical lung biopsy

Definition

Fibrobronchoscopy is performed with a flexible cylindrical tube (whose external diameter is 3 to 6 mm) that is mounted on a handle, connected to a light source with optic fibers that transmit this light and produce an image in an eyepiece. A swing bar on the handle enables the operator to orient the last 5 cm, which is more flexible and thinner. The fibroscope is also equipped with a suction intake and an operator conduit for diagnostic or therapeutic procedures. A watertight sheath contains and isolates the optic fibers and the operator conduit. Bronchoscopy in the ICU is performed in spontaneously breathing or mechanically ventilated patients and is used for various diagnostic (bronchoalveolar lavage, protected specimen brushing, transbronchial, or bronchial biopsies) and therapeutic procedures (tracheal intubation, atelectasis, hemoptysis). In this chapter, only its diagnostic use within the framework of bronchoalveolar lavage (BAL) and protected specimen brush (PSB) will be described.

Lung biopsy by thoracotomy is one of the techniques to obtain a lung tissue sample for diagnostic purposes (postaggressive fibrosis from acute respiratory distress syndrome, diffuse infectious or noninfectious pathologic process) in ICU patients under sedation and invasive mechanical ventilation and in whom less invasive methods such as fibroscopic BAL are not contributive. It is an invasive surgical procedure that consists of a thoracotomy and the harvesting of a sample of pulmonary parenchyma for multimodal analysis.

Pre-existing Condition

Fibroscopy in the ICU

Fibroscopy with a flexible endoscope is used since 1967 and intensivists rapidly adopted it for therapeutic acts (which will not be described in this chapter) such as difficult intubation, verification for hemoptysis, or atelectasis. Fibroscopy is also an indispensable diagnostic tool that enables bronchial or alveolar sampling: transbronchial and bronchial biopsies, simple suction, and especially protected specimen brushing (PSB) and bronchoalveolar lavage (BAL), which are by far the two most frequently used fiberoptic procedures in the ICU.

Bronchoalveolar lavage: the principal studies that have shown the interest of fibroscopic BAL in the diagnosis of nosocomial pneumonia have been performed in spontaneously breathing and often immunodepressed patients. Within the framework of ventilator-associated pneumonia (VAP), a comparison of BAL with histological examination revealed the sensitivity of BAL at a threshold of 10^4 CFU/mL ranged from 47% to 58%. In patients who do not receive antibiotics before their death, this sensitivity can reach 91%. Specificity, however, has been diversely determined. If one refers to studies with a histological standard, it ranges from 45% to 100%. In a meta-analysis of 23 studies, there was a sensitivity of 73% $\pm$ 18% and a specificity of 82% $\pm$ 19% for the diagnosis of VAP [1]. Moreover, the dilution of secretions carries the risk of false-negative results. Thus, in a study of 47 patients presenting a suspicion of VAP, the rate of potential false-negative results linked to dilution was evaluated at 17%. The reproducibility of BAL is also in question. In 44 patients with suspected VAP, two BALs were consecutively performed in the same pulmonary region by the same operator. The patients were matched for the presence or absence of pneumonia at the usual threshold of 10^4 CFU/mL in only 75% of the cases. However, the interest of BAL is based on the possibility of detecting other pathogens such as intracellular germs. Molecular biology makes it possible to examine the nucleic acid of these intracellular bacteria, thanks to specific PCR amplification, and appears to be of greater interest than cultures that are difficult to perform. Viral diagnosis, in particular *Herpes simplex virus* and *Cytomegalovirus* can also benefit from PCR amplification parallel to usual cultures and cytologic analysis. Fungal culture (Aspergillus, yeasts, Cryptococcus) and detection of parasitosis (pneumocystosis, toxoplasmosis, strongyloidosis) are even possible with BAL. BAL cytology (see Tables 1 and 2) is also a valuable tool in pneumonia. BAL also enables the diagnosis of

Bronchial Fibroscopy and Lung Biopsy. Table 1 Alveolar cell numeration and formula in normal nonsmoking subjects

	n/mL	%
Epithelial cells	Rare	
Cellular viability		86 ± 1
Cellularity	$129 \pm 20/10^3$	
Macrophages	$99 \pm 8/10^3$	85 ± 2
Lymphocytes	$15 \pm 2/10^3$	12 ± 1
Neutrophiles	$1 \pm 0.001/10^3$	2 ± 0.07
Eosinophiles	$0.2 \pm 0.012/10^3$	0.2 ± 0.06

Bronchial Fibroscopy and Lung Biopsy. Table 2 BAL results for noninfectious pneumopathies

Diffuse neoplastic infiltration	Presence of neoplastic cells
Intraalveolar hemorrhage	Presence of siderophages
Hypersensitivity pneumonia	Presence of lymphocytosis (>50%), and presence of mastocytes and eosinophiles
Alveolar proteinosis	Milky aspect, PAS-positive proteinated material
Histiocytosis X	Numerous Langerhans cells (Birbeck bodies)
Eosinophilic pneumonia	Presence of over 40% eosinophiles
Pneumoconioses: Asbestosis/berylliosis/silicosis	Analyses for crystals (mineralogy)
Sarcoidosis	Predominance of T lymphocytes with elevated CD4/CD8 ratio

noninfectious pulmonary pathologies that are sometimes found in ICU patients. Specific analyses for crystals, alveolar cytokines or procollagen (the precursor of collagen involved in pulmonary fibrosis) dosage, neoplastic cells, or cells that are specific to systemic diseases can be performed according to the clinical picture.

Protected specimen brushing (PSB): as opposed to BAL, this technique, developed *in vitro* by Wimberley, is only useful for pneumonia. Human histologic studies [2] have shown a sensitivity of PSB ranging between 33% and 57%. The usual threshold of 10^3 CFU/mL, the low volume of secretions collected (approximately 1 μL), and the difficulty to perform a direct examination

associated with culture on the same brush could explain the number of false-negative results. A repetition of the PSB in case of a negative first result if associated with a clinical suspicion of VAP has been proposed. Repetition of PSB after a borderline result ($\geq 10^2$ and $< 10^3$ CFU/mL) made it possible to make a diagnosis of VAP following the second PSB at a threshold of 10^3 CFU/mL in 35% of the cases. This concept of a threshold at 10^3 CFU/mL is all the more open to criticism since numerous differences, above and below this threshold, are noted when two PSB are performed during the same fiberoptic procedure and in the same territory. The specificity of PSB is the object of almost as much controversy as its sensitivity [2]. When the reproducibility of PSB was studied (two PSB performed successively), differences in 14% of the cases at a threshold of 10^3 CFU/mL were reported. The concentration of each germ varied by a factor of at least 10 in 59% to 67% of the sample pairs. This would appear to be due to the heterogeneity of the pneumonia lesions and to the low volume of collected secretions. Finally, from the twelfth hour after administration of adapted antibiotherapy, PSB was negativated in almost one third of the cases, thereby justifying sampling before the administration of any new antibiotherapy.

All in all, within the framework of pulmonary infectious pathology, no guidelines have been established for the choice of a fiberoptic diagnostic technique. Nevertheless, it appears that BAL in the ICU can be considered as superior given the possibilities it offers in terms of a direct examination that can facilitate the choice of empiric antibiotherapy and the diversity of examinations that can be performed on the sample in order to approach an infectious or noninfectious pathology (inflammatory, neoplastic, etc.).

Open-Lung Biopsy

In order to best treat unresolving acute respiratory distress syndrome (ARDS) after making sure that prior treatment has been optimal vis-à-vis plateau pressure and volemia, three questions must be asked: Was the initial cause insufficiently treated? Is there an additional cause (nosocomial pneumonia)? Is post-aggressive fibrosis developing? There are two essential reasons for the clinician to harvest a sample of the lung parenchyma: to diagnose an etiology that is potentially curable when less invasive examinations such as BAL were not contributive and/or reveal post-aggressive fibrosis in order to administer corticoids which could improve survival or at least improve lung physiologic parameters. In current practice, such corticotherapy is readily "blindly" administered in cases of unresolved ARDS on approximately the seventh day of evolution. This therapy is potentially immunosuppressive. In case of pulmonary infection, the classic sampling techniques for microbiological examinations lack sensitivity and specificity to contraindicate or delay corticosteroids after the beginning of an adequate anti-infectious treatment. In particular, the viral risk is far from being negligible as reported by the authors of a study in which *Cytomegalovirus* was identified in 50% of the 36 patients presenting ARDS and undergoing surgical lung biopsy [3]. In addition, the dosing of alveolar markers for post-aggressive fibrosis is not yet in current practice and lacks specificity. Procollagen III has yet to be correlated with histologically proven post-aggressive fibrosis. The clinical consequences of the results of a lung biopsy performed within the framework of ARDS can therefore be major. On the one hand, therapeutic modifications can be dictated by the anatomopathological and/ or microbiological results: administration of corticosteroids in case of post-aggressive fibrosis, administration or modification of anti-infectious treatment, and in particular, administration of antiviral treatment for a *Cytomegalovirus* infection or another *Herpes virus* [3]. On the other hand, the prognosis can be totally modified if a potentially curable etiology is detected (infectious, in particular) or on the contrary, owing to a tumoral cause (e.g., carcinomatous lymphangitis). Detection of post-aggressive fibrosis can worsen the vital prognosis although the patient can benefit from an anti-inflammatory treatment. The time it takes to implement a specific treatment can be shortened by carrying out a rapid analysis of a fresh biopsy fragment that has been immediately transported to the anatomopathologic laboratory before fixation and more exhaustive analysis. In the same manner, this immediate analysis makes it possible to avoid potentially deleterious empiric corticotherapy if signs of active infection, in particular viral, have been detected. In a recent study, 100 surgical lung biopsies for unresolving ARDS with noncontributive BAL made it possible to detect the presence of fibrosis in only 53% of the cases [1]. Moreover, of the patients with fibrosis, more than half had a concomitant infection requiring anti-infectious treatment before the administration of corticotherapy. This biopsy was contributive in the sense that it made it possible to make a specific therapeutic modification in 78% of the cases. The main result of this study was that the outcome in terms of survival is significantly better with a contributive biopsy (67% survival versus 14% with noncontributory biopsies $p < 0.001$) [3]. One can therefore consider that without this histological proof, almost half of the patients with unresolving ARDS would have received unjustified corticotherapy. The recent randomized prospective study performed by the ARDS network, which studied the benefit of corticotherapy for unresolving ARDS, did not report a decrease in mortality in the treated group. In this study, no proof of the presence of fibrosis was provided by lung biopsy. Nevertheless, in the treated subgroup with low alveolar procollagen III, a comparatively high death rate was noted which suggests that the patients without fibrosis did not undergo corticotherapy (although the correlation between this marker and fibrosis has not been absolutely established). Moreover, when corticosteroid treatment is delayed (beyond the 13th day), one can also observe an increased mortality which argues for early lung biopsy in order to avoid administering corticotherapy for an irreversible lung fibrosis. Lachapelle and Morin have already reported a better outcome in patients for whom a therapeutic modification was based on early biopsy with a more specific diagnosis. Given our experience and recent recommendations, we propose a practical attitude in cases of unresolving ARDS. A lung biopsy can be proposed on approximately the seventh day of evolution if, despite treatment adapted for an initial cause, ARDS persists and post-aggressive fibrosis is suspected. If no etiology is found initially despite BAL, it is consequently desirable to perform an earlier biopsy. Specific treatment (antibiotic, antiviral, chemotherapy, etc.) is then administered as soon as the results are known. In cases of post-aggressive fibrosis, corticotherapy is administered but possibly delayed after adapted treatment in case of concomitant infection. Lung biopsy remains, pending less invasive but equally specific examinations, the best diagnostic tool for unresolving ARDS.

Application

Flexible Fibroscopy

We only consider flexible fibroscopy for its diagnostic use with BAL and PSB. Therefore, we will not discuss the possible therapeutic acts in the ICU (difficult tracheal intubation, hemoptysis, or atelectasis), see Fig. 1.

Flexible fibroscopy requires preparation of both the patient and the equipment. It is a clean but not sterile procedure. Nevertheless, it is indispensable that the operator be equipped with a cap, a mask, sterile gloves, and a disposable paper gown. The operator positions himself or herself next to the patient who can remain positioned between 30° and 45° on the bed. An assistant, positioned on the other side of the bed, is useful for this procedure to help maintain the intubation tube in position, handle the equipment required for collection of samples, monitor vital signs, modify ventilator adjustments, and optimize

B

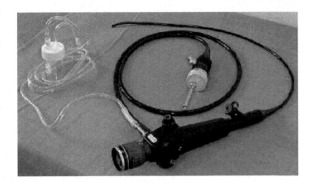

Bronchial Fibroscopy and Lung Biopsy. Figure 1 Flexible fibroscopy

sedation. A cold light source is necessary (plugged into the mains or on battery and positioned directly on the fiberscope).

Fibroscopy can be performed in conscious patients on spontaneous ventilation with a mask with a high concentration of oxygen or under continuous positive airway pressure (CPAP). Given the considerable progress and the now very broad use of noninvasive ventilation (NIV), this technique should be considered for fibroscopy. Under these conditions, the patient has been fasting for at least 4 h and the use of a local anesthetic such as lidocaine at 5% in the nasal fossa and the pharynx is necessary before the insertion of the fiberscope. This anesthesia is completed by the instillation of lidocaine at 1% through the operator channel of the fiberscope, in the larynx and then the trachea. The patient then continues fasting for 2 h after administration of the local anesthetic. However, fibroscopy in the ICU concerns patients under sedation and invasive mechanical ventilation in the majority of the cases.

In case of mechanical ventilation, fibroscopy increased the frequency of asynchronies between the patient and the ventilator, thereby decreasing the efficacy of mechanical ventilation. During aspirations by the fibroscope and given the reduction in tidal volume, PaO_2 can decrease by 40% and $PaCO_2$ increase by 30%. Whatever the breathing mode, it is necessary to increase the FiO_2 in order to obtain an SpO_2 that is superior to 90% during the fibroscopy. If this objective is not reached before the beginning of the procedure, the benefits of the fibroscopy should be weighed with the elevated risks of the procedure. Moreover, the placing of a fiberscope in an intubation tube triggers excess pressure that can reach 80 cmH_2O. This high pressure is recorded at the level of the intubation tube but does not represent the real alveolar pressure. It is due to the reduction in the diameter of the intubation

tube caused by the fiberscope that increases the resistive component of airway pressure. On the other hand, this excess pressure persists at the level of the trachea on expiration, thereby creating an auto positive end expiratory pressure (PEEP). This was also noted in 18 mechanically ventilated ICU patients after BAL was performed. A fiberscope with a 5.7 mm external diameter occupies 51% of the surface of a tube with an internal diameter of 8 mm and 66% of a 7-mm tube. It was therefore recommended to take off the external PEEP applied by the ventilator in order to limit this effect. However, this attitude is controversial, particularly in cases of ARDS, because repeated aspirations during fibroscopy provoke drops in pressure in the distal airways and therefore a risk of alveolar derecruitment and hypoxemia. The compromise setting is probably represented by maintaining external PEEP level and a maximum inspiratory pressure level set to the superior level, in order to limit alarms, and in modern ventilators, to not be responsible for a limitation of current volume delivered once the recommended intratracheal pressure has been reached. Moreover, the use of a fiberscope with an external diameter that is at least 2 mm inferior to the internal diameter of the intubation tube and in particular, the shortest endoscopy time possible with limited aspirations must be respected.

ARDS represents a risk factor for increasing hypoxemia during this procedure. However, if hypoxemia occurs, it is transitory and rarely serious. In a series of 110 patients with ARDS (defined by a PaO_2/FiO_2 ratio inferior to 200) who underwent fiberoptic bronchoscopy with BAL, only one patient had a major reduction in SpO_2 (<80%) during the procedure and only one pneumothorax occurred. In this series, there were no cases of alteration in respiratory mechanics or hemodynamic status. Fiberoptic bronchoscopy can generate an increase in intrathoracic pressures which could potentially be deleterious in patients with intracranial hypertension (by increasing intracranial pressure). During 26 fiberoptic bronchoscopies performed in patients with an intracranial hypertension, there was an elevation in intracranial pressure in 21 of the patients, 38 mmHg on average, there was a concomitant elevation in mean arterial pressure such that there was no variation in cerebral perfusion pressure. These changes were also transitory and no neurologic deterioration was reported during fibroscopy in this series. Here again, while caution is the rule, fiberoptic bronchoscopy is not contraindicated but must be performed with maximum safety under sedation and paralysis. Finally, the risk of fiberoptic bronchoscopy in patients with cardiopathy has not been specifically evaluated but in the American College of Chest Physicians (ACCP) registry of 48,000 procedures in all kinds of patients, six deaths out of the ten reported occurred in patients with ischemic cardiopathy. Moreover, out of the 29 patients over 50 years of age (including 45% smokers, 34% hypertensive, 17% ischemic heart disease, and 14% with histories of myocardial infarction), 5 (17%) presented a modification in ST segment on EKG during fiberoptic bronchoscopy and only 1 of these 5 patients had a history of coronaropathy. The benefit/risk ratio must therefore be carefully evaluated in mechanically ventilated patients with severe ischemic cardiopathy. In patients under invasive mechanical ventilation, reinforcement of sedation or even the addition of paralysis is necessary to ensure the safety and effectiveness of the procedure, particularly in ARDS patients suffering from intracranial hypertension or ischemic cardiopathy.

After optimizing the ventilator settings, it is indispensable to insert a mouthpiece in patients with an orotracheal tube in order to avoid biting the fiberscope through the tube which could damage the watertight sheath and in particular the optic fibers. In addition, the fiberscope sheath must be coated with silicon spray to facilitate passage in the tracheal interface.

The fiberoptic bronchoscopy is inserted through an orifice made in the oxygen mask or through the annular orifice of the CPAP or NIV mask or through the endotracheal interface that has first been decontaminated with an iodized solution, for example. The eyepiece must then be adjusted to the operator's view. Right-left identification in the bronchial tree is easily obtained by anterior visualization of the tracheal rings and the anatomic appearance.

Bronchoalveolar lavage (BAL) consists in instilling sterile saline solution at an ambient temperature through the internal channel of the fiberscope, which is positioned in the third- or fourth-generation bronchus ventilating the pulmonary territory that the operator wishes to analyze. It is then no longer moved during the entire procedure in order to avoid contamination by bronchial secretions and thereby preserve the alveolar specificity of the examination. In this manner, only the distal bronchioles and the alveoli are sampled. A total volume of 100 to 400 mL is administered, ideally by 50-mL adapted syringes. In fact, there is no established consensus on the quantity to administer by aliquot, the number of aliquots, or whether to keep or eliminate the first aliquot that is supposed to represent the bronchial fraction of BAL. Nevertheless, BAL is considered as effective and representative in a patient on mechanical ventilation if at least 40% to 50% of the instilled liquid is collected. Aspiration must be smooth to avoid damaging the bronchial mucosa and the risk of hemorrhagic contamination. The administration of a local anesthetic in the bronchi being sampled can

diminish coughing in the patient with little or no sedation but must be avoided given the bacteriostatic character of this type of product. After collecting the instilled fluid in a single-use receptacle, whose volume is adapted to the procedure and observing the macroscopic aspect, the sample is divided up and sent to the various laboratories concerned (microbiology, virology, biochemistry, pathology, immunology, etc.). The sampled alveolar liquid must be cultured within less than an hour to avoid the risk of a false-negative result. Refrigeration at 4°C can buy time when the sample cannot rapidly be processed. BAL tolerance in ventilated patients can limit its use and fever can follow its use and be associated with arterial hypotension. However, a study of 12 ventilated patients (mean PaO_2 at 100 mmHg with PEEP $\geq$ 10 cmH_2O and $FiO_2 \geq 0.5$) did not reveal an alteration in hemodynamic status after BAL. On the other hand, a prolonged reduction in PaO_2 was noted after the return of FiO_2 to its level prior to the fibroscopy. During performance of the procedure, as for any fiberoptic bronchoscopy, it would therefore appear to be necessary to increase the FiO_2 to 1 and then only reduce progressively over a period of several hours after the end of the examination. In patients on invasive mechanical ventilation, the level of sedation must in all cases be optimized to avoid the hemodynamic and in particular, the respiratory consequences of this act.

Protected specimen brush (PSB) is a double catheter sealed with a polyethylene-glycol plug. After inserting the catheter through the operator conduit until the area to be analyzed, the internal catheter is released from its covering, thereby ejecting the polyethylene-glycol plug (which will gradually be destroyed in the bronchial tree), then enabling a brushing of the distal bronchial mucosa. Before withdrawing the device, the internal catheter containing the sample is again retracted into the external catheter in order to avoid contamination. The volume of collected secretions is low (approximately 1 µL). This technique could theoretically be performed blindly by inserting the catheter directly into the tracheal interface but its precision and the occasional necessity to harvest the sample in the left bronchial tree (inaccessible by blind technique) requires the use of an endoscope. In addition to the risks linked to the fibroscopy, the use of this catheter only rarely causes complications such as bronchial hemorrhage or pneumothorax.

Open-Lung Biopsy

Lung biopsies can be performed by percutaneous, transbronchial (under endoscopy), or pleural (medical or surgical thoracoscopy) approach, but for reasons of safety and/or effectiveness, these techniques are poorly adapted to the context of ARDS. Only surgical pulmonary biopsy by thoracotomy fulfills the conditions required in this framework, see Fig. 2.

The majority of open-lung biopsies are performed at bedside in the ICU, which is of great interest since such patients are often difficult to transport [4]. The most pathologic lung area is usually chosen for the biopsy. The only ventilator adjustment required is to increase FiO$_2$ to 1 with deep sedation and the administration of neuromuscular blocking agents is often necessary. The patient therefore is positioned in supine position with a pad placed under the scapula homolateral to the biopsy in order to tilt the patient approximately 15° [4]. The homolateral upper limb is held in abduction with the forearm folded up over the head. An anterolateral thoracotomy of approximately 10 cm is performed in the fifth intercostal space with access facilitated by means of a small retractor [4]. Exploration of the pulmonary parenchyma and pleural cavity is first performed. Pleural liquid is sampled (for cytologic and microbiologic analysis), drained, and quantified. Extreme care must be taken in handling the lung tissue to avoid alveolar rupture, with

particular attention (monopolar electrocoagulator) given to preventing bleeding. A single but broad biopsy is performed in an area that appears to be macroscopically pathologic (usually at the level of the dependent zones) with mechanical forceps with linear stapling [4]. The ventilator must be temporarily disconnected in order to limit tissue thickness to ensure better aerostasis. The parenchymatous sample is then cut into five parts and each fragment is packaged in a specific manner for histologic, bacteriologic, virologic, parasitologic-mycologic, and immunologic analyses [4]. Two chest drains, anterior and posterior, are inserted and then placed on aspiration. Verification by chest X-ray is performed at the end of the procedure. The mean duration of the procedure is 30 min [4]. Pulmonary parenchymatous leaks are evaluated, blood loss through the drains is evaluated daily, and the surgical wound is examined regularly for any local complications. Thoracic X-ray is performed daily until the drains are taken out which is usually after weaning from the mechanical ventilator. It is very rare that the biopsy cannot be performed because of poor respiratory or hemodynamic tolerance. There have been no cases of preoperative death

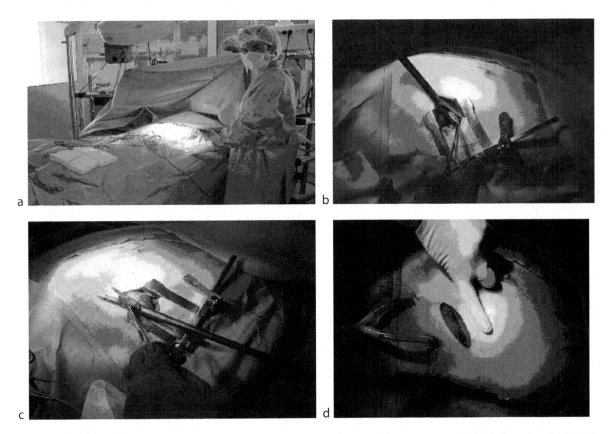

Bronchial Fibroscopy and Lung Biopsy. Figure 2 Pulmonary biopsy by lateral thoracotomy at the bed of a patient in the ICU

directly attributable to the biopsy reported in the litera-ture. The postoperative complication generally reported is prolonged bubbling at the level of thoracic drain (15–20% of the cases) which is rarely associated with pneumotho-rax. The evolution of these complications which is usually spontaneously favorable can require a mobilization of the thoracic drains, a new chest drain, and in rare cases, surgery. Other complications such as hemorrhages, pleu-ral, or parenchymatous infections are rarely observed. This surgical lung biopsy technique by thoracotomy was recently recommended by the French Society of Intensive Care in order to sample lung tissue [5].

References

1. Torres A, El-Ebiary M (2000) Bronchoscopic BAL in the diagnosis of ventilator-associated pneumonia. Chest 117:198S–202S
2. Timsit JF, Misset B, Francoual S, Goldstein F, Vaury P, Carlet J (1993) Is protected specimen brush a reproducible method to diagnose ICU-acquired pneumonia? Chest 104:104–108
3. Papazian L, Doddoli C, Chetaille B et al (2007) A contributive result of open-lung biopsy improves survival in acute respiratory distress syndrome patients. Crit Care Med 35:755–762
4. Donati SY, Doddoli C, Chetaille B, Papazian L (2004) La biopsie pulmonaire au cours du syndrome de détresse respiratoire aiguë. Réanimation 13:71–78
5. Richard JC, Girault C, Leteurtre S et al (2005) Prise en charge ventilatoire du syndrome de détresse respiratoire aiguë de l'adulte et de l'enfant (nouveau-né exclus) - Recommandations d'Experts de la Société de Réanimation de Langue Française. Réanimation 14:2–12

Bronchitis and Bronchiectasis

JAMES D. CHALMERS[1], ADAM T. HILL[2]
[1]Centre for Inflammation Research, Queens Medical Research Centre, Edinburgh, Scotland, UK
[2]Department of Respiratory Medicine, Royal Infirmary and University of Edinburgh, Edinburgh, Scotland, UK

Synonyms

Chronic bronchial sepsis; Non-cystic fibrosis bronchiectasis

Definition

Chronic Bronchitis

The term chronic bronchitis refers to a symptom, rather than a disease, and is defined as daily cough with produc-tion of sputum for 3 months of the year, for more than 2 consecutive years. The principal cause of chronic bronchitis is cigarette smoking, and the majority are cured with smoking cessation. Chronic bronchitis with associated predominantly fixed airflow obstruction forms part of the clinical syndrome of Chronic Obstruc-tive Pulmonary Disease (COPD).

Bronchiectasis

The term bronchiectasis may be used to describe a clinical syndrome, a radiological appearance, or a pathological finding. The clinical syndrome of bronchiectasis is char-acterized by symptoms of chronic cough, chronic sputum production, and recurrent respiratory infections. It is a disease of children and adults. The disorder is associated with impaired mucociliary clearance and frequent chronic colonization of the normally sterile airway with bacteria. Approximately two-thirds of patients with bronchiectasis are chronically colonized with microorganisms, most fre-quently *Haemophilus influenzae* and *Pseudomonas aeruginosa*, but also *Streptococcus pneumoniae*, *Staphylo-coccus aureus*, *Moraxella catarrhalis*, and gram-negative *Enterobacteriacae*. Patients are also susceptible to coloni-zation with environmental mycobacteria. Recurrent exac-erbations lead to increased utilization of health-care resources and hospitalization in severe cases.

Pathologically, bronchiectasis is characterized by per-manently damaged and dilated airways. Lung damage is typically the result of a vicious cycle of inflammation, infection, and tissue destruction caused by one of a large number of inherited and acquired disorders (discussed later). The disease may be localized to a single anatomical lobe or be more generalized.

Radiologically, bronchiectasis is now defined by a characteristic appearance of bronchial dilatation on high-resolution chest computed tomography. In health, the overall diameter of a bronchus is approximately equal at any given level to its adjacent pulmonary artery and a ratio of bronchus diameter: vascular diameter >1 denotes abnormal dilatation. Cylindrical/tubular bronchi-ectasis is the mildest form of bronchiectasis, where the diameter of the bronchus exceeds that of the adjacent blood vessel. In varicose and cystic bronchiectasis, there is further bronchial dilatation, and this is seen in patients with more advanced disease. There may be associated mucus plugging, atelectasis, subsegmental, segmental or lobar collapse, and emphysema.

An exacerbation of bronchiectasis that would benefit from antibiotic therapy is defined as deterioration in a patient with known bronchiectasis from their stable condition, associated with increased cough, increased sputum production, increased sputum purulence, and/or increased dyspnea/wheeze. In addition to these subjective symptoms, patients may have objective evidence of reduction in forced expired volume in 1 s (FEV_1) or a reduction in exercise capacity.

Treatment

Treatment in Stable Patients
In stable patients, the priority of management is as follows

- Promote airway clearance
- Maximize exercise capacity and lung function
- Prevent exacerbations
- Treat exacerbations promptly
- Manage complications

Identifying and treating the underlying cause is also important [1]. More specific management may be required in special circumstances, such as immunoglobulin replacement therapy in patients with common variable immunodeficiency, but this is not the case in the majority of patients with bronchiectasis.

Patient Education
Patient should be given information about the disease and educated in how to recognize an exacerbation. The need to promptly treat exacerbations with antibiotic therapy is emphasized. Patients should be encouraged not to smoke and to adhere to their prescribed treatment regime. Pneumococcal vaccination and annual influenza vaccination are encouraged.

Airway Clearance
Effective airway clearance can reduce distressing symptoms of retained secretions. Airway clearance is achieved through a combination of physical therapy and pharmacotherapy.

Physiotherapy
Commonly used physiotherapy techniques to promote airway clearance include the active cycle of breathing technique and postural drainage. Positive pressure assist devices, such as Acapella and Flutter are also used, and may be more convenient than traditional methods. Aerobic exercise is also recognized as an effective means of mobilizing secretions. In patients with more advanced disease, twice daily physiotherapy is recommended, while in milder disease, physiotherapy may only be required during exacerbations.

Pharmacological Management
Bronchodilators prior to physiotherapy may aid sputum clearance and avoid bronchospasm post physiotherapy.

Some physiotherapists advocate the use of nebulized 0.9% saline to promote chest clearance in patients admitted with an exacerbation. Further studies are needed before we could advocate the use of hypertonic saline (3% or higher) as routine therapy to aid chest clearance. Recominant human DNase has been used as an aid to airway clearance in cystic fibrosis with good clinical efficacy. It is not, however, recommended in adults with non-CF bronchiectasis as a well-designed randomized controlled trial found no evidence of benefit, and a worsening of lung function in patients randomized to DNase [2].

There is an absence of trial evidence to support the use of mucolytics or osmotic agents such as mannitol currently.

Exercise Capacity and Lung Function

Exercise
Aerobic exercise maintains cardiovascular fitness, promotes well-being and, in the context of bronchiectasis, may aid airway clearance.

Pulmonary rehabilitation is effective in Chronic Obstructive Pulmonary Disease, and there is some evidence of benefit following pulmonary rehabilitation in patients with bronchiectasis. Patients with bronchiectasis should be encouraged to remain active, and patients with limiting breathlessness should be offered pulmonary rehabilitation if facilities are available.

Bronchodilators
Bronchiectasis may coexist with Chronic Obstructive Pulmonary Disease or asthma where the benefit of short-acting and long-acting bronchodilator medications are established. Patients with bronchiectasis may have impaired lung function, particularly in advanced disease. In patients with impaired lung function, reversibility testing with inhaled or nebulized bronchodilators may provide evidence of airway reversibility and can guide which bronchodilator to use ($beta_2$-agonists and/or anticholinergics). Even in those without significant airways reversibility, patients with impaired lung function and reduced exercise capacity are often offered a trial of inhaled bronchodilators, either $beta_2$-agonists and/or anticholinergics, with these medications continued if there is evidence of clinical benefit.

Inhaled Corticosteroids (ICS)
Similarly, inhaled corticosteroids have an established role in asthma and COPD. Patients with these conditions in addition to bronchiectasis will frequently be prescribed these medications. In patients without asthma or COPD,

small studies have suggested ICS may reduce sputum volume but without significant effects on lung function or exacerbation frequency. Patients may be offered a 6-month trial of inhaled corticosteroids, with the medication continued if there is evidence of clinical response.

Preventing Exacerbations

Maximizing patients physical fitness, maintaining good airway clearance, and maintaining good lung function are likely to minimize exacerbations. The role of long-term antibiotics and surgery is discussed next.

Long-Term Oral Antibiotic Therapy

In cystic fibrosis, the efficacy of long-term antibiotic therapy is well established. The evidence in adult non-CF bronchiectasis is less clear, and the benefit of preventing exacerbations must be balanced against the risks of antibiotic side effects and encouraging antibiotic resistance. In a 12-month Medical Research Council sponsored trial (conducted in 1957) of tetracycline, long-term therapy was associated with reduced sputum volume, sputum purulence, and fewer days absent from work due to ill health. Similarly, in 1990, an 8-month trial of high dose oral amoxicillin observed a reduction in 24 h sputum volume, sputum purulence, and a reduction in days absent from work. Other studies using an open label design have shown a reduction in exacerbation frequency.

The British Thoracic Society Guidelines recommend consideration of long-term antibiotics to patients experiencing 3 or more exacerbations per year [3].

In general, long-term antibiotic therapy should be tailored to individual patient need, with the class of antibiotic chosen based on the patient's usual microbiology.

Nebulized Antibiotic Therapy

Nebulized antibiotic therapy has the potential to deliver bacteriocidal doses of antibiotic to the lungs while minimizing systemic absorption. Treatment with nebulized therapy is more expensive than oral treatment and carries a risk of bronchospasm, even when administered with inhaled bronchodilators.

Nebulized tobramycin has been shown to reduced bacterial density and reduce hospitalization in patients chronically colonized with *Pseudomonas aeruginosa*. Nebulized gentamicin over 1 year in patients chronically colonized with two or more exacerbations per year reduced the microbial burden, exacerbation frequency, improved time to next exacerbation and improved health related quality of life [4]. Further studies are needed.

The British Thoracic Society Guidelines recommend consideration of long term antibiotics to patients experiencing 3 or more exacerbations per year [3]. Further studies are needed. Options currently for patients with *Pseudomonas aeruginosa* are nebulized gentamicin, tobramycin, or colomycin, the choice being decided by sensitivity results and local availability.

Surgery

Localized bronchiectasis that has a significant effect on health-related quality of life, not responding to medical management, may be considered for surgical resection. In practice, bronchiectasis is now an unusual referral for surgical management except in the context of life-threatening haemoptysis.

Treatment – Exacerbations

Prompt antibiotic therapy for exacerbations prevents further airway damage and speeds clinical recovery. Antibiotic therapy should be tailored to individual patients taking into account their previous sputum bacteriology and severity of disease. It is essential to send a sputum sample at the beginning of exacerbations so that treatment can be altered if necessary and to monitor changes in bacterial pathogens and antibiotic resistance (see Table 1).

Assessment of Severity

The majority of exacerbations are mild and can be managed with oral antibiotics in the community. Medical indications for hospitalization include: hypotension, confusion, hypoxaemia, respiratory distress, systemic sepsis, large volume haemoptysis, culture of a pathogen only sensitive to intravenous antimicrobials, failed response to oral antibiotics.

Antimicrobial Treatment

Table 1 suggests first- and second-line antimicrobial treatments for patients with bronchiectasis based on current UK recommendations. Resistance patterns for organisms such as *Streptococcus pneumoniae*, *Haemophilus influenzae*, and *Pseudomonas aeruginosa* vary substantially in different countries. Antibiotic choice should be personalized based on knowledge of the patient's usual pathogens, and knowledge of local organism susceptibilities and local practice.

As shown in Table 1, oral monotherapy is recommended for the majority of patients, but dual therapy is recommended for patients with MRSA and in hospitalized patients with *Pseudomonas aeruginosa*. Dual therapy is recommended to reduce the chance of development of antimicrobial resistance. Severe exacerbations are treated with intravenous antibiotic therapy (see above).

Bronchitis and Bronchiectasis. Table 1 Antimicrobial recommendations

Usual colonizing organism	First-line treatment	Second-line treatment	Severe exacerbation
Haemophilus influenzae-Beta lactamase negative	Amoxicillin or Doxycycline	Clarithromycin	Intravenous amoxicillin or Intravenous third-generation cephalosporin
Haemophilus influenzae-Beta lactamase positive	Amoxicillin with clavulanic acid or Doxycycline	Clarithromycin	Intravenous third-generation cephalosporin or Amoxicillin with clavulanic acid
Streptococcus pneumoniae	Amoxicillin or Doxycycline	Clarithromycin	Intravenous third-generation cephalosporin or Amoxicillin with clavulanic acid
Moraxella catarrhalis	Amoxicillin with clavulanic acid or Doxyxycline	Ciprofloxacin or Clarithromycin	Intravenous Amoxicillin with clavulanic acid
Staphylococcus aureus	Flucloxacillin	Clarithromycin	Intravenous flucloxacillin
Methicillin resistant Staphylococcus aureus	Rifampicin + Doxycycline	Rifampicin + Trimethoprim	Intravenous Vancomycin or Teicoplanin or Linezolid
Coliforms (e.g., klebsiella, enterobacter)	Amoxicillin with clavulanic acid	Ciprofloxacin	Intravenous Amoxicillin with clavulanic acid or third-generation cephalosporin
Pseudomonas aeruginosa	Ciprofloxacin	Intravenous Ceftazidime or Piperacillin with tazobactam or Meropenem, +/− Aminoglycoside	Intravenous Ceftazidime or Piperacillin with Tazobactam or Meropenem, +/− Aminoglycoside

The optimum duration of therapy is unknown, but the majority of studies have used 10–14 days. Longer antibiotic courses are recommended because of the higher airway bacterial load in patients with bronchiectasis compared to patients with other infections.

Adjunctive Treatment in Exacerbations

Patients should perform at least twice daily chest physiotherapy duration exacerbations to aid expectoration of increased sputum volumes. Bronchodilators are recommended for patients with airway obstruction, and systemic corticosteroids may be prescribed for patients with coexistent asthma or Chronic Obstructive Pulmonary Disease or if lung function is reduced.

Evaluation/Assessment

History

Bronchiectasis should be considered as a diagnosis in any patient presenting with persistent cough and sputum production, or recurrent respiratory infections. Symptoms of airways obstruction such as wheeze and breathlessness may also be present. There may or may not be a history of an associated disorder (see below).

Imaging

The gold standard investigation for diagnosis of bronchiectasis is high-resolution chest computed tomography. Bronchiectasis is defined as bronchial dilatation and is recognized radiologically as the internal diameter of the bronchial lumen exceeding that of the adjacent artery. Dilatation can be classified as tubular, varicose, or cystic. Varicose and cystic dilatation is often associated with a greater disease severity. Examples of tubular, varicose, and cystic dilatation are shown below (Figs. 1–3).

Sputum Bacteriology

Sputum should be sent for culture in all patients with bronchiectasis complaining of productive cough. Two-third of patients will be chronically colonized with organisms even when well, and the presence of these organisms helps to guide antibiotic therapy during exacerbations (Table 1).

Lung Function

Spirometry can be normal even in advanced bronchiectasis but both obstructive and restrictive patterns can also be seen.

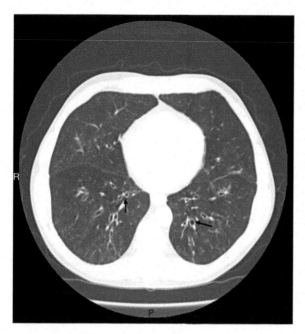

Bronchitis and Bronchiectasis. Figure 1 Mild tubular bronchiectasis in both lower lobes (*arrows* show two examples where the diameter of the bronchus is larger than the adjacent vessel)

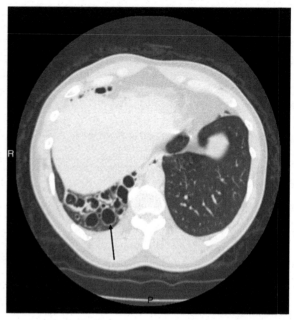

Bronchitis and Bronchiectasis. Figure 3 Cystic bronchiectasis- marked cystic dilatation in the right lower lobe – one cyst highlighted – see *arrow*

Underlying Cause

A specific underlying cause is only identified in a minority of patients with bronchiectasis. Performing investigations to find associated disorders is important, however, as some have specific treatments. Many patients are classified as having "post-infective" bronchiectasis based on a previous history of respiratory infection such as pneumonia or whooping cough. It is important to investigate these patients for other underlying causes as these histories are not specific. Specific therapies are available for some underlying disorders, for example, immunoglobulin replacement for common variable immunodeficiency, and corticosteroids +/− antifungal therapy for active allergic bronchopulmonary aspergillosis (Table 2).

After-care

Patients with frequent exacerbations, patients treated with long-term oral or nebulized antibiotic therapy, patients colonized with *Pseudomonas aeruginosa*, and patients requiring specialist management for an underlying disorder (e.g. immune deficiencies) should have follow-up in secondary care. This is best achieved in a respiratory unit with access to a multidisciplinary team

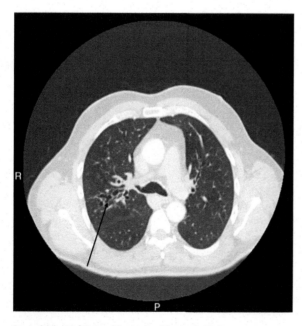

Bronchitis and Bronchiectasis. Figure 2 Varicose bronchiectasis in the right upper lobe – see *arrow* – the bronchus is enlarged and saccular

Bronchitis and Bronchiectasis. Table 2 Underlying causes identified in adults with bronchiectasis

Underlying disorder	Frequency	Confirmatory test or physical findings
Idiopathic and post-infective	60%	Diagnosis of exclusion
Post-tuberculous	25%	Radiological evidence (CXR or CT) of previous pulmonary tuberculosis
Rheumatoid arthritis and other connective tissue diseases(systemic sclerosis, systemic lupus erythematosus, ankylosing spondylitis)	3–6%	Positive autoantibodies. Some other clinical evidence of connective tissue disease is usually required for diagnosis
Allergic bronchopulmonary aspergillosis (ABPA)	1–7%	History of asthma + aspergillus hypersensitivity + radiological change (fleeting infiltrates and/or central bronchiectasis)
Immunodeficiency	1–8%	Typical disorders associated with bronchiectasis are IgG subclass deficiencies (particularly subclass 2), common variable immunodeficiency, X-linked agammaglobulinamia, IgA deficiency. Early onset bronchiectasis, or bronchiectasis in the context of recurrent non-pulmonary infections should lead to consideration of inherited or acquired immunodeficiency
Cystic fibrosis	2–4%	Suspect in patients aged <40 years with associated malabsorption, male infertility, upper lobe bronchiectasis, colonization with *Staphylococcus aureus*, and/or *Pseudomonas aeruginosa*. Confirm by CFTR genotyping and/or sweat test
Recurrent aspiration or inhaled foreign body	2–10%	Bronchiectasis may occur in the context of any cause of aspiration
		Foreign body may be located at bronchoscopy
Primary ciliary dyskinesia	2–4%	Suspect in patients with a history of upper respiratory tract infections, otitis media, or male infertility. Confirm by ciliary function testing or saccharin test
Inflammatory bowel disease	1–2%	Patients will usually have an established diagnosis of inflammatory bowel disease
Congenital airway structural abnormality	<1%	Usually identified on chest radiograph or HRCT

of respiratory physicians, physiotherapists, microbiologists, and nursing staff.

Patients with mild bronchiectasis, or patients in whom the disease has been stable for many years may be managed in primary care, provided that the basic principles of bronchiectasis managed are followed, such as airway clearance and regular monitoring of sputum bacteriology. Bronchiectasis may remain stable for many years, but patients should have access to specialist secondary care if they experience increasing symptoms, frequent exacerbations, or an important change in their disease such as acquisition of *Pseudomonas aeruginosa*.

Prognosis

Historically, patients with bronchiectasis had markedly reduced life-expectancy with the majority of patients with bronchiectasis dying before the age of 40 in the pre-antibiotic era. More recently, the long-term outcome for

patients with bronchiectasis appears to be good, and some studies suggest that life-expectancy is not reduced in patients receiving modern management. This will largely depend on the severity of patient's disease and their adherence to follow-up and treatment. In a recent investigation of 120 patients with bronchiectasis followed-up for 13 years, risk factors for death were age, male gender, colonization with *Pseudomonas aeruginosa*, reduced lung function, and poorer activities on the St. George's Respiratory health-related quality of life Questionnaire [5].

References

1. Pasteur MC, Helliwell SM, Houghton SJ et al (2000) An investigation into causative factors in patients with bronchiectasis. Am J Respir Crit Care Med 162(4):1277–1284
2. O'Donnell AE, Barker AF, Ilowite JS, Fick RB (1998) Treatment of idiopathic bronchiectasis with aerosolized recombinant human DNase I. Chest 113(5):1329–1334

3. Pasteur MC, Bilton D, Hill AT (2010) British thoracic society bronchiectasis non-CF guideline group. British Thoracic Society guideline for non-CF bronchiectasis. Thorax 65(Suppl 1):i1–58
4. Murray MP, Govan JR, Doherty CJ, Simpson AJ, Wilkinson TS, Chalmers JD, Greening AP, Haslett C, Hill AT (2010) A randomised controlled trial of nebulised gentamicin in non-cystic fibrosis bronchiectasis. Am J Respir Crit Care Med. http://www.ncbi.nlm.nih.gov/pubmed/20870753. Accessed 24 Sep 2010
5. Loebinger MR, Wells AU, Hansell DM et al (2009) Mortality in bronchiectasis: a long term study assessing the factors influencing survival. Eur Respir J 34:843–849

Bronchopleural Fistula

LAURA J. MOORE
Department of Surgery, The Methodist Hospital Research Institute, Houston, TX, USA

Definition

Bronchopleural fistula (BPF) is defined as an abnormal connection between the bronchial tree and the pleural cavity. This is a rare but highly morbid condition that can be extremely difficult to manage. BPF is most commonly seen in patients that have undergone pulmonary resection, with a reported incidence of 1.5–28% [1]. Other causes of BPF include lung necrosis after pulmonary infection, tuberculosis, chemotherapy or radiation therapy for pulmonary malignancy, iatrogenic or traumatic injury, and persistent spontaneous pneumothorax. The development of BPF is associated with an increased risk of death, with an associated mortality rate of 18–67% [2].

The clinical presentation of BPF is variable in both time of presentation and clinical findings. BPF can be divided into the categories of acute (postoperative days 1–7), sub acute (postoperative days 8–30), and delayed/chronic (postoperative day >30) depending upon the time of presentation [3]. Acute BPF typically presents with the classic findings of a tension pneumothorax (PTX) with acute onset of dyspnea, chest pain, hypotension, subcutaneous emphysema, jugular venous distention, mediastinal shift, and pulsus paradoxus. The clinical presentation of sub acute and delayed BPF is not typically as impressive in presentation, with the most common findings being cough and a change in appearance of the chest x-ray. In the postsurgical setting, most BPFs will present between postoperative days 7 and 15.

Differential Diagnosis

The diagnosis of BPF should be suspected in any patient with a persistent postoperative air leak. Other causes of postoperative air leak may include technical problems with the pleural drainage system, misplacement of tube thoracostomy, and benign air leak from the cut surface of the lung parenchyma. The diagnosis of BPF can be made based upon clinical and radiographic findings. The presence of a persistent air leak after excluding other possible etiologies is suggestive of the diagnosis. Radiographic findings include steady increase in the volume of intrapleural air, the appearance of a new air-fluid level in the chest or changes to a pre-existing air-fluid level, and the development of a tension PTX. Multidimensional computed tomography may be helpful and allows for visualization of the fistula tract. Bronchoscopy may also be diagnostic and can be employed to visualize the site of the fistula in the bronchial tree. Methylene blue may also be selectively instilled under bronchoscopic guidance into the bronchial tree, with subsequent drainage of the Methylene blue from the pleural space being diagnostic for BPF.

Cross-Reference to Disease

Lung Cancer Patients

Patients with lung cancer represent the vast majority of BPF patients. This is because BPF most commonly occurs after surgical resection. The development of BPF can also occur as a result of tumor necrosis following chemotherapy or radiation therapy. In the surgical patient, development of a BPF results from failure of the bronchial stump to properly heal after resection. This can be seen following any type of lung resection but is more commonly seen in pneumonectomy patients, occurring in up to 20% of patients [4]. It can also be seen following lobectomy, but the incidence is much lower at 0.5% [4]. Failure of the bronchial stump to heal can be due to technical complications at the initial surgery, inadequate blood supply to the bronchial stump, of persistence of tumor at the bronchial stump. Risk factors for the development of BPF include diabetes mellitus, malnutrition, steroid use, performance of a mediastinal lymph node dissection, high dose preoperative radiation therapy, residual tumor at the bronchial margin, performance of a right-sided resection, and need for prolonged positive pressure mechanical ventilation.

Treatment of BPF should initially focus on stabilizing the patient, particularly in patients presenting with a tension PTX. If the patient does present with a tension PTX, emergent decompression of the chest is critical. Pulmonary flooding may also occur as a result of entry of fluid from the pleural cavity into the bronchial tree. This can be addressed by placing the patient with the affected side down and establishing adequate drainage of the pleural space with a tube thoracostomy. In the acute, postoperative setting, surgical management of BPF is often utilized. Surgical repair of BPF should include coverage of the new bronchial suture line with some type of tissue flap. Available options include muscle flaps, pericardial fat flaps, and omental pedicle flaps.

Pulmonary Infections

Patients presenting with BPF in the setting of infection are initially managed medically. These patients are often chronically debilitated as a result of their underlying infectious state. Management of these cases of BPF includes adequate drainage of the associated empyema allowing for reduction of the pleural space, aggressive antimicrobial therapy, and optimization of the patient's nutritional status. Initially, these patients are managed medically. If the patient requires mechanical ventilation, maintaining airway pressures below the critical opening pressure of the BPF may improve closure of the BPF. In the event that the patient does not respond to a trial of medical therapy, surgical consultation may be necessary. The surgical management of BPF in the setting of infection abides by the same principles described above.

References

1. Lois M, Noppen M (2005) Bronchopleural fistulas: an overview of the problem with special focus on endoscopic management. Chest 128(6):3955–3965
2. Hollaus PH, Lax F, el-Nashef BB et al (1997) Natural history of bronchopleural fistula after pneumonectomy: a review of 96 cases. Ann Thorac Surg 63(5):1391–1396, discussion 1396–1397
3. Varoli F, Roviaro G, Grignani F et al (1998) Endoscopic treatment of bronchopleural fistulas. Ann Thorac Surg 65(3):807–809
4. Sarkar P, Chandak T, Shah R, Talwar A (2010) Diagnosis and management bronchopleural fistula. Indian J Chest Dis Allied Sci 52 (2):97–104

Bronchopneumonia

▶ Burns, Pneumonia
▶ Pneumonia, Aspiration
▶ Pneumonia, Empiric Management
▶ Pneumonia, Ventilator-Associated

Bronchoscopy

▶ Bronchial Fibroscopy and Lung Biopsy

Bronchoscopy, Role in Suspected Infection

John G. Muscedere
Department of Medicine, Kingston General Hospital, Kingston, ON, Canada

Introduction

The diagnosis of pulmonary infections in the intensive care unit (ICU) can be challenging for critical care practitioners since the clinical signs and symptoms for pulmonary infection are nonspecific. As in noncritically ill patients, the suspicion of a respiratory infection in ICU patients is based on the development of clinical signs such as increasing sputum production, fever, or hypothermia and findings on physical examination such as bronchial breath sounds, if any. These may be accompanied by laboratory abnormalities such as abnormalities in white blood cell count or gas exchange. However, in critically ill patients these clinical signs and symptoms may also arise from systemic inflammation secondary to their underlying disease and not from infection. As an example, an ICU patient with severe pancreatitis may have fever, leukocytosis, and respiratory failure secondary to acute respiratory distress syndrome without having a respiratory infection. Moreover, as in this example, abnormal chest X-rays in patients in the ICU are nonspecific and the majority of patients with abnormal chest X-rays in the ICU do not have pulmonary infection. Common noninfectious etiologies of an abnormal chest X-ray in the ICU which may be mistaken for pneumonia include pulmonary edema both cardiogenic and non-cardiogenic, atelectasis, pulmonary hemorrhage, and pulmonary infarction.

Given the nonspecific clinical and radiological findings of respiratory infection in the critically ill, the diagnosis of a respiratory infection has been traditionally based on microbiological confirmation. In mechanically ventilated patients access to respiratory tract secretions is straightforward and endotracheal aspirates (ETA) are commonly sent for culture. However, the difficulty with cultures of ETA aspirates is that the organisms isolated may be colonizers or pathogens. That is, they may be present on biofilms present on the endotracheal tube or on the trachea or larger airways without tissue invasion. Further, many cultures of ETA are negative and the possibility of inadequate sampling arises. To circumvent these difficulties, the focus has been on bronchoscopic methods of obtaining secretions from the lower respiratory tract with quantitation of microorganisms in order to improve the sensitivity and specificity of cultures obtained. In this entry we will discuss bronchoscopy and associated techniques as a means of diagnosing respiratory tract infections in the critically ill. We will then discuss their applicability to the diagnosis of ventilator-associated pneumonia (VAP), ventilator-associated tracheobronchitis (VAT), and the evaluation of pulmonary infection in critically ill immunocompromised patients.

Bronchoscopy and Associated Techniques

While rigid bronchoscopy was first described in the 1890s, it was not until the 1960s that technological advances allowed the advent of flexible fiber-optic bronchoscopy (FOB). While FOB did not come into common use until the 1970s, improvements in technology and affordability have led to its widespread use, particularly in the ICU and over time video bronchoscopes have gradually replaced standard bronchoscopes. In the ICU, bronchoscopy is utilized for both therapeutic and diagnostic purposes. We will only discuss the use of bronchoscopy for the diagnosis of pulmonary infectious diseases in this entry.

Bronchoscopy-Intubated Patient

The technique in an intubated mechanically ventilated patient is relatively straightforward. The presence of an endotracheal tube or tracheotomy tube allows the upper airway and associated reflexes to be bypassed thereby minimizing the amount of sedation/analgesia required. Further, the majority of these patients are already sedated for the facilitation of mechanical ventilation and may only require small amounts of additional sedation and analgesia. Similar to bronchoscopy in outpatients, cough reflexes can be blunted through the application of aqueous lidocaine 1% through the suction port of the bronchoscope. Care must be taken to avoid toxic levels of lidocaine in the bloodstream as it is well absorbed through the bronchial mucosa and for this reason the maximum dose of lidocaine in adults should be limited to 8.2 mg/kg in adults with

lower maximum doses in patients with impairments in hepatic function or at risk from cardiac suppression [1]. If additional sedation is required, short-acting agents such as midazolam or propofol along with short-acting narcotics such as fentanyl for analgesia are the agents of choice.

In a mechanically ventilated patient the bronchoscope is introduced through the endotracheal tube or tracheotomy tube using an adapter which allows for a tight seal around the bronchoscope and minimal air loss. The major consideration is the diameter of the artificial airway since the insertion of the bronchoscope through the airway can cause functional obstruction. For example, the insertion of a bronchoscope with an external diameter of 5.1 mm in a No. 7.5 endotracheal tube (ETT) will obstruct 46% of the cross-sectional area and in a No. 7 ETT, it will obstruct 53%. Narrowing of the effective size of the ETT may reduce the ability to ventilate the patient and cause acute increases in positive end expiratory pressure (PEEP). These, along with loss of lung volume from suctioning along with de-recruitment at the initiation of the study procedure if the patient is disconnected to place the adapter on the ETT, may cause significant hypoxemia during the procedure. These may be mitigated by having as large an ETT as possible, maintaining the same amount of minute volume during the procedure and increasing the amount of supplemental oxygen. Further, acute increases in PEEP along with coughing during the procedure may increase intrathoracic pressure thereby decreasing venous return and cause hypotension during the procedure. This may be minimized by fluid loading if no contraindications are present and avoiding acute increases in PEEP along with adequate sedation and topical anesthesia to avoid coughing.

Overall, bronchoscopy in the critically ill is very well tolerated with minimal complications but significant morbidity and mortality have been reported. Reported complications include hypoxemia, bronchospasm, arrhythmias, pneumothoraces, and hemorrhage. In addition, reduction in mesenteric blood flow during bronchoscopy may occur and put patients at risk for mesenteric ischemia and bacterial translocation. In outpatients in which there is more information but which may have fewer complications because of their greater cardiorespiratory reserve, rates of major complications have been reported as occurring in only 0.5% of all cases [2].

Bronchoscopy-Non-intubated Patient

In contrast to patients who are intubated and mechanically ventilated, bronchoscopy in the critically ill who are not intubated poses more challenges. For the diagnosis of infection, access to lower respiratory tract secretions may not be available as in patients who have an endotracheal tube or a tracheostomy in place and this may be the indication for bronchoscopy. These patients may require high levels of supplemental oxygen and hemodynamic support. Topical anesthesia of the upper airway is important such the sedative and analgesia use may be minimized and respiratory depression avoided. Since it may be difficult to spray the upper airway in a patient who is in respiratory distress or receiving high levels of supplemental oxygen, an alternative technique that can be used for topical anesthesia of the airway is the nebulization of 4cc of 4% lidocaine while delivering high flow oxygen prior to bronchoscopy. Recognizing that oxygen requirements will increase during the procedure, the provision of supplemental oxygen can be accomplished with high flow oxygen through a face mask in which a port is made to accommodate the bronchoscope or commercially available facemasks specifically designed for this purpose. For patients whose respiratory status is unstable bronchoscopy utilizing noninvasive ventilation during the procedure or through a laryngeal mask have been described [3]. To facilitate bronchoscopy with noninvasive ventilation, commercial facemasks with extra ports for the introduction of the bronchoscope are available. These techniques may be beneficial in patients in which there is a desire not to intubate such as in immunocompromised patients with pulmonary infiltrates.

Bronchoscopic Techniques

Bronchial Lavage

Bronchial lavage involves the injection of saline and aspiration of secretions from the larger airways. With bronchial lavage, no attempts are made to sample the alveoli. It is unclear if secretions obtained in this manner are superior to ETA. The major indication for bronchial lavage is for the detection of cancerous cells and in non-intubated patients' infectious agents. Unless there is another indication for bronchoscopy, in a critically ill patient, performing a bronchoscopy just for bronchial lavage does not justify the risks involved with the procedure.

Bronchoalveolar Lavage

Bronchoalveolar lavage (BAL) is a procedure designed to be able to obtain material from the smaller airways and alveoli. To perform a BAL, the bronchoscope is wedged into a distal bronchial segment and saline is instilled into that lung segment in 20–40 ml aliquots until 100–120 ml is reached. This amount of saline is sufficient to sample up to the alveolar level. Although 100 ml is a usual amount of

saline instilled for a BAL, larger amounts have been safely used and may sample larger amounts of lung. Smaller amounts may only sample the proximal airways; there should be at least 40–70% recovery of total instillate. In order to maximize returns, intermittent suction may be more effective than continuous suction or excessive suction will collapse the airway and thereby decrease BAL fluid return. If BAL is being performed for the evaluation of a pulmonary infection, the channel of the bronchoscope is first lavaged with 20 ml of saline to minimize the influence of upper airway secretions that may have been suctioned prior to wedging the bronchoscope. Complications of BAL include transient fever, bronchospasm, transient pulmonary infiltrates, worsening gas exchange, and increased hypoxemia or requirement for supplemental oxygen. In non-intubated critically ill patients the transient worsening of lung function may lead to intubation.

Protected Specimen Brush

Similarly to BAL, a protected specimen brush (PSB) is used to minimize the influence of upper airway secretions on culture results. This is done by having the sampling brush enclosed in a protective catheter closed off with a polyethylene glycol plug which quickly dissolves when extruded. To sample using a protected specimen brush, the catheter containing the brush is advanced through the suction channel of the bronchoscope until it protrudes from the end of the bronchoscope. When the desired area is reached, the brush is advanced and the plug is extruded. The area is then brushed and the brush is withdrawn into the catheter. The catheter is then removed and the brush is cultured. Problems with PSB include variability in the technique, small amount of secretions sampled with possibility of sampling error, patient selection, and comparisons with which the PSB is compared to [4]. For these reasons, it is felt to have high specificity but low sensitivity in the diagnosis of VAP. In spite of these difficulties, both PSB and BAL are used interchangeably in the diagnosis of respiratory tract infections in the critically ill.

Transbronchial Biopsies

There is limited information on the utility of transbronchial biopsies for the diagnosis of pulmonary infections in non-immunocompromised critically ill patients. Concerns about the risk of complications such as hemorrhage and pneumothoraces in patients who have respiratory compromise along with the requirement for specialized expertise have made this procedure fairly uncommon in the ICU. Not surprisingly, published series on the conduct of transbronchial biopsies in mechanically ventilated patients have reported pneumothorax, hemorrhage, and worsening hypoxemia as the most common complications. It is not clear if transbronchial biopsies add to the diagnostic efficacy of ETA or BAL for the diagnosis of infection in the non-immunocompromised critically ill although it may add to the diagnostic utility of BAL in immunocompromised patients. Further a high percentage of critically ill patients with a suspicion of pulmonary infection will have absolute or relative contraindications to transbronchial biopsy such as coagulopathy, high levels of PEEP, and severe gas-exchange abnormalities. Given the potential for significant complications, lack of evidence for utility and that the diagnosis may be available from less invasive procedures, transbronchial biopsy for the diagnosis of pulmonary infection in immunocompetent critically ill patients should be reserved only for experienced clinicians when BAL fails to arrive at a diagnosis.

Non-bronchoscopic Sampling

Since bronchoscopy and its associated procedures requires specialized equipment and expertise that may not be available at all centers, non-bronchoscopic methods for sampling the distal airways for infection have been developed. These are "blind" BAL and "blind" PSB and are conducted at the bedside without using a bronchoscope. For the sake of completeness they will be discussed here although an extensive discussion is beyond the scope of this review. For blind PSB, the brushing catheter is advanced blindly through the ETT until resistance is met and the airway is brushed similarly as when the procedure is conducted through the bronchoscope. Blind BAL is conducted by inserting either a single lumen or double lumen protected catheter through the ETT until resistance is met and at that point saline is instilled and then aspirated. The amount of saline instilled is usually 20 ml although volumes from 10 to 100 ml have been described. It has been reported as being highly reproducible although it is a blind technique.

The degree of correlation between bronchoscopic PSB and blind PSB has been reported to be approximately 80% in all pneumonias and to be higher when the suspected pneumonia was suspected on the right. Blind PSB has been reported as having the same sensitivity and specificity as bronchoscopic BAL. Variable efficacy in the diagnosis of VAP has been reported for blind BAL [5].

Overall these techniques are effective in obtaining microbiological sampling of the lower airways without bronchoscopic guidance. However, the difficulty in interpreting these studies is the lack of a reference standard for pulmonary infection and there is no evidence that they are superior to ETA in guiding therapy and improving patient outcomes.

Disease Considerations

Ventilator-Associated Pneumonia

The clinical suspicion of ventilator-associated pneumonia (VAP) is based on clinical and radiological criteria. As these criteria are nonspecific, microbiological confirmation is necessary. The method of obtaining samples for microbiological confirmation has been the focus of extensive study. Methods that have been studied have included noninvasive techniques such as ETA without quantitation and techniques with quantitative cultures including BAL and PSB, both blind and bronchoscopic. The threshold levels for quantification of BAL are greater than 10^5 colony forming units (cfu)/ml and greater than 10^3 cfu/ml for PSB. These techniques have reported variable sensitivity and specificity depending on the technique, patient population, and comparator to which the test was compared [6].

In discussions of diagnostic tests and methods of microbiological sampling for VAP, it is important to note that there is no accepted reference test for VAP. In the absence of a reference standard for VAP it is impossible to know which test or diagnostic strategy is superior and the question then becomes which test is associated with the best patient outcomes and management when VAP is suspected. In considering bronchoscopic tests with quantitation, these tests require specialized equipment and training, laboratory support, and may not be available at all institutions or if they are available may not be accessible at all times of the day.

Five randomized controlled trials have examined the question of the best diagnostic strategy for VAP [7–11]. Two randomized trials have compared the results of quantitative cultures from BAL to quantitative cultures from ETA [7, 8] and three randomized trials have compared results from quantitative cultures from BAL to nonquantitative ETA [9–11]. When these studies are combined in a meta-analysis (Fig. 1), a diagnostic approach for suspected VAP using bronchoscopy and quantitative cultures of BAL and/or PSB compared to nonquantitative cultures of endotracheal aspirates does not lead to differences in hospital mortality, length of stay, or duration of mechanical ventilation. Given the higher costs, higher risk of complications and lower availability for bronchoscopy and BAL, ETA are favored for microbiological sampling in

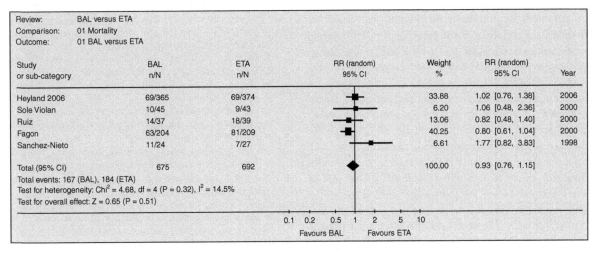

Bronchoscopy, Role in Suspected Infection. **Figure 1** Meta-analysis of randomized controlled trials comparing the effect of bronchoalveolar lavage (BAL) and endotracheal aspirates (ETA) on mortality

VAP. An important consideration is that all of the five trials evaluated immunocompetent patients and four of the five trials used empiric antibiotic therapy initiated at the time of suspected VAP.

Ventilator-Associated Tracheobronchitis

Ventilator-associated tracheobronchitis (VAT) is defined using the following criteria: the presence of fever (>38°C) with no other recognizable cause, purulent sputum production, and positive cultures of respiratory specimens without radiographic signs of new pneumonia. This entity is controversial but is felt to be a precursor of VAP before the radiographic signs of pneumonia develop. It is not known whether bronchoscopic techniques and quantitative cultures add to the specificity of diagnosing VAT and what threshold of bacterial growth should be used. At this time, there is not enough evidence to choose over the various techniques for microbiological sampling of the airways although it stands to reason that techniques that sample the alveoli such as BAL would have less of a role in the diagnosis of VAT. Quantitative ETA cultures have been suggested for the diagnosis of VAT but again it is not clear that they add to diagnostic specificity over standard cultures of ETA [12].

Immunocompromised Patient

The diagnosis of the cause of pulmonary infiltrates in the setting of critical illness and immunodeficiency is difficult. These patients have many potential causes of abnormal

chest radiography including infectious and noninfectious causes. Infectious causes may include usual pathogens, difficult to culture organisms or opportunistic pathogens. Noninfectious causes include alterations of pulmonary permeability such as acute respiratory distress syndrome, pulmonary hemorrhage, drug reactions, or neoplastic diseases. Because of the wide spectrum of diagnostic possibilities, alveolar sampling increases the diagnostic yield and bronchoscopy with BAL has become the procedure of choice. In cohorts of immunocompromised patients with pulmonary infiltrates, infection accounts for 50–70% of the final diagnosis and BAL can identify up to 80% of the infectious etiologies [13].

The yield of bronchoscopy in patients who are immunocompromised and have respiratory infiltrates depends on the etiology of the immunosuppression with the major distinction being immunosuppression secondary to human immunodeficiency virus (HIV) and all other causes. In patients with immunosuppression from HIV and diffuse pulmonary infiltrates, diagnostic yields of BAL for *Pneumocystis jiroveci* have been reported to be 90% and yields for other pathogens have been reported to be in the range of 60–85%. In contrast to the diagnosis of pulmonary infections in the critically ill, transbronchial biopsies along with BAL do increase the diagnostic yield. For *Pneumocystis* yields of close to 100% have been reported using a combination of BAL and a transbronchial biopsy with a negative predictive value over 90%. Fortunately, the frequency of patients with HIV being admitted to the ICU has dropped dramatically with the use of highly active antiretroviral therapy.

Although the frequency of patients with HIV has declined, the incidence of patients with non-HIV-related immunosuppression admitted to the ICU is increasing. With non-HIV-related disease immunosuppression, the diagnostic yield from BAL is lower. The requirement for bronchoscopy in immunocompromised patients is dependent on the pathogen suspected and in intubated immunocompromised patients the yield for ETA is high for bacterial disease. The yield for bronchoscopy with BAL has been reported to be as high as 80% in patients with infectious causes for pulmonary infiltrates. The yield in noninfectious causes of pulmonary infiltrates in the immunocompromised is lower and this patient population where both infectious and noninfectious etiologies are possible transbronchial biopsy may be additive to BAL. However, as discussed previously many of these patients will have significant contraindications to transbronchial biopsy. A relatively frequent relative concern for the conduct of bronchoscopy and BAL in patients who are immunosuppressed is the presence of thrombocytopenia. However, with the support of platelet transfusions, both of these procedures have been shown to be safe even in the presence of severe thrombocytopenia.

Conclusion

Bronchoscopy for the diagnosis of pulmonary infection is not indicated for all critically ill patients. As a routine, in non-immunocompromised patients the incremental benefit of bronchoscopic microbiological sampling over ETA is minimal and should only be done when there are other indications or unusual pathogens are suspected. For immunocompromised critically ill patients, bronchoscopy with BAL is the procedure of choice with or without transbronchial biopsies, dependent on the presence of contraindications.

References

1. Honeybourne D, for the British Thoracic Society Bronchoscopy Guidelines Committee (2001) British thoracic society guidelines on diagnostic flexible bronchoscopy. Thorax 56(suppl):i1–i21
2. Pue C, Pacht E (1995) Complications of fiberoptic bronchoscopy at a university hospital. Chest 107:430–432
3. Maitre B, Jaber S, Maggiore S, Bergot E, Richard J, Bakthiari H, Housset B, Boussignac G, Brochard L (2000) Continuous positive airway pressure during fiberoptic bronchoscopy in hypoxemic patients. A randomized double-blind study using a new device. Am J Respir Crit Care Med 162:1063–1067
4. Baughman RP (2000) Protected-specimen brush technique in the diagnosis of ventilator-associated pneumonia. Chest 117:203S–206S
5. Campbell G (2000) Blinded invasive diagnostic procedures in ventilator-associated pneumonia. Chest 117:207S–211S
6. Michaud S, Suzuki S, Harbarth S (2002) Effect of design-related bias in studies of diagnostic tests for ventilator-associated pneumonia. Am J Respir Crit Care Med 166:1320–1325
7. Sanchez-Nieto JM, Torres A, Garcia-Cordoba F et al (1998) Impact of invasive and noninvasive quantitative culture sampling on outcome of ventilator-associated pneumonia: a pilot study. Am J Resp Crit Care Med 157:371–376
8. Ruiz M (2000) Noninvasive versus invasive microbial investigation in ventilator-associated pneumonia: evaluation of outcome. Am J Resp Crit Care Med 162:119–125
9. Sole Violan J, Fernandez JA, Benitez AB, Cardenosa C, Rodriguez D (2000) Impact of quantitative invasive diagnostic techniques in the management and outcome of mechanically ventilated patients with suspected pneumonia. Crit Care Med 28:2737–2741
10. Fagon J, Chastre J, Wolff M et al (2000) Invasive and noninvasive strategies for management of suspected ventilator-associated pneumonia. A randomized trial. Ann Inter Med 132:621–630
11. Heyland D, Dodek P, Muscedere J, Day A, Cook D for the Canadian Critical Care Trials Group (2006) A multi-centre trial of invasive diagnostic techniques for ventilator associated pneumonia. New Engl J Med 355:2619–2630
12. Craven D, Chroneou A, Zias N, Hjalmarson K (2009) Ventilator-associated tracheobronchitis; the impact of targeted antibiotic therapy on patient outcomes. Chest 135:521–528
13. Shorr A, Susla G, O'Grady N (2004) Pulmonary infiltrates in the non-HIV infected immunocompromised patient. Chest 125:260–271

Bronchovenous Air Embolism

Christopher C. Baker
The Isidore Cohn, LSU Health Sciences Center – LSUHSC, New Orleans, LA, USA

Synonyms

Air embolus; Pulmonary venous air embolism; Systemic air embolism

Definition

This syndrome occurs when there are concomitant injuries to a pulmonary vein and a bronchus leading to the passage of air to the left side of the heart.

Historical Perspective

Air embolism has been known to occur during cardiopulmonary bypass, neurosurgical procedures in the sitting position, and diving accidents. Nonetheless, part of the first description of air embolism from penetrating chest trauma was reported in 1974 [1] by Art Thomas, a thoracic and trauma surgeon at San Francisco General, and Boyd Stephens, the Medical Examiner for the City and

County of San Francisco. They described four cases of bronchovenous air embolism following penetrating chest trauma involving a lung injury. In the first two cases, they did not see the air in coronary arteries, but air was aspirated from the left ventricle. In the other two cases, air was found in the coronary arteries and the left ventricle. Neither one of these cases survived. They previously reported four other cases at the American Association for Thoracic Surgery meeting in 1973. The mechanism of air embolism was found to be a concomitant injury to the bronchus and the pulmonary vein, which allows air to travel into the left side of the heart. Although a moderate amount of air can be tolerated on the right side of the heart, as little as one cc of air in the coronary artery can lead to ventricular fibrillation. Perhaps the most important clinical observation that the authors made was that all eight of their patients had positive pressure ventilation when the embolism was recognized, which caused the air to be pushed from bronchus into the pulmonary vein. Working in the autopsy lab, Dr. Stephens pointed out that the only way to detect an arterial air embolism was to perform an autopsy anaerobically or under water, which he did on several occasions.

Clinical Manifestations of Bronchovenous Air Embolism

A high index of suspicion should be maintained regarding bronchovenous air embolism when patients sustain penetrating chest trauma. The important tipoff is that the patient will deteriorate once positive pressure ventilation has begun. This can occur because pulmonary venous pressure may be low due to thoracic blood loss. This can promote passage of air from a bronchial injury into pulmonary circulation when positive pressure ventilation has begun. These findings may be seen in the pre-hospital setting, in the emergency department, or in the operating room, and air embolism should be suspected if the patient deteriorates after positive pressure ventilation. The majority of the patients with air embolus have penetrating trauma. In my experience, we treated one patient with air embolus from blunt trauma (a forklift injury), who required a pneumonectomy in order to be salvaged.

Treatment and Outcomes

Emergency Department (ED) thoracotomy may sometimes be required to salvage patients with air embolus. In our original series from San Francisco General [2] of 168 patients who underwent ED thoracotomy for trauma, only 11 patients had air embolism. Only one of these patients survived (9%) compared to the 14% survival for

patients with hypovolemic cardiac arrest, and a 38% survival for pericardial tamponade. In addition to cross clamping the pulmonary hilum, other resuscitative measures that have been advocated are placing the patient in Trendelenburg's position with the aspiration of air from the apex of the left ventricle, or aspiration of air from the root of the aorta.

Salvage of these patients requires prompt recognition of the clinical syndrome of bronchovenous air embolism. A rapid thoracotomy on the affected side, followed by clamping the pulmonary hilum is the key to success. In addition, it may be necessary to aspirate air from the left ventricle, which may be more easily accomplished with a left thoracotomy. The pulmonary injury and the bronchial injury can then be repaired. The patient will usually tolerate cross clamping as long as oxygenation can be maintained by ventilating the other lung. A review from San Francisco General, published in 1983 by Yee, Verrier, and Thomas, identified 61 patients (from 1970 to 1981) who had air embolism [2]. Interestingly, 15 of these patients had blunt trauma, but the majority of the patients had gunshot wounds or stab wounds to the chest. The air embolism was recognized by visualizing air in the coronary arteries (57%) or aspiration air from the heart (30%). Again, the key to diagnosis was early thoracotomy and cross clamping of the pulmonary hilum on the affected side. In a number of these cases, aortic cross clamping was also necessary. Interestingly, the overall survival rate was 44% in this group of critically injured patients.

A recent paper from Harbor–UCLA Medical Center described 24 patients who required thoracotomy for trauma, 3 (13%) of whom required pulmonary hilar cross clamping [3]. In this series, this maneuver was done for massive hemothorax. The major point of this article was that the authors described a "hand-over-hand" technique that allowed control of the pulmonary hilum with control of hemorrhage and prevention of air embolism prior to definitive cross clamping.

Another article from Parkland Hospital in Dallas described systemic arterial air embolism, which is a synonym for bronchovenous air embolism [4]. Over an 8-year period, they had nine patients with penetrating lung injuries with this syndrome. Eight of these patients had sustained gunshot wounds to the chest and then developed cardiac arrest after receiving positive pressure ventilation. Air was visualized in coronary arteries in all nine patients, and in three of these patients, air was aspirated from the apex of the left ventricle and the aortic root. In seven of the nine patients, the only injury was to the lung. Six of the patients in this series died (66%). It is clear that prompt recognition of air embolism in the setting of patients with penetrating chest trauma, since clinical deterioration often follows the institution of positive pressure ventilation.

Conclusion

Bronchovenous air embolism is particular clinical syndrome that occurs primarily in patients with penetrating lung injuries. The pathophysiology of this syndrome is related to entraining of air from an injured bronchus into the nearby pulmonary vein. The air is then embolized into the coronary arteries leading to cardiac decompensation. The tipoff in these patients is that they may be stable initially, but they then decompensate when they receive positive pressure ventilation (either by bag valve mask technique, or after endotracheal intubation). The key to salvaging these patients is rapid thoracotomy (either in the emergency department or in the operating room), with clamping of the pulmonary hilum. The mortality rates have varied widely between 91% [2], 66% [4], and 44% [5]. The last series is the largest, and the better survival rate probably reflects increased recognition of the syndrome. In summary, early diagnosis of the syndrome of bronchovenous air embolism requires a high index of suspicion followed by rapid thoracotomy and cross clamping of the pulmonary hilum in order to salvage these patients.

References

1. Thomas AN, Stephens RG (1974) Air embolism: a cause of morbidity and death after penetrating chest trauma. J Trauma 14(8):633–638
2. Baker CC, Thomas AN, Trunkey DD (1980) The role of emergency room thoracotomy in trauma. J Trauma 20(10):848–855
3. Van Natta TL, Smith BR, Bricker SD, Putnam BA (2009) Hilar control in penetrating chest trauma: a simplified approach to an underutilized maneuver. J Trauma 66:1564–1569
4. Estera AS, Pass LJ, Platt MR (1990) Systemic arterial air embolism in penetrating lung injury. Ann Thorac Surg 50(2):257–261
5. Yee ES, Verrier ED, Thomas AN (1983) Management of air embolism in blunt and penetrating thoracic trauma. J Thorac Cardiovasc Surg 85(5):661–668

Broselow Pediatric Emergency Tape

This is a tape that allows measurement of the height or length of the patient and from this, the tape indicates the sizes of tubes, doses of drugs, and rates of fluid administration.

Brown Sequard Syndrome

▶ Spinal Cord Injury Syndromes

Brucellosis

Jaffar A. Al-Tawfiq[1], Ziad A. Memish[2]
[1]Speciality Internal Medicine, Saudi Aramco Medical Services Organization, Kingdom of Saudi Arabia
[2]Ministry of Health, Riyadh, Kingdom of Saudi Arabia

Synonyms

Bang's disease; Gibraltar fever; Malta fever; Mediterranean fever; Undulant fever

Definition

Brucellosis is a zoonotic disease with a worldwide distribution. The disease is caused by infection with the bacterial genus Brucella. *Brucella* spp. are small aerobic intracellular coccobacilli. All *Brucella* spp. belongs to a monospecific genus termed *B. melitensis,* and all other species are subtypes as they pose a high interspecies homology of >87%. Based on antigenic variation and primary host, the genus *Brucella* is classified into seven species and include *Brucella melitensis* (sheep and goats), *B. suis* (hogs), *B. abortus* (cattle), *B. ovis* (sheep), *B. canis* (dogs), *B. neotomae* (wood rats), and *B. maris* (marine mammals). The species responsible for causing disease in humans are *B. abortus, B. suis, B. melitensis,* and *B. canis* [1].

Epidemiology

The most common species to cause human disease worldwide is *B. melitensis.* The route of acquisition of human brucellosis is variable and include direct inoculation through cuts and skin abrasions, ingestion of contaminated food such as raw milk, raw meat, or soft cheeses made from non-pasteurized milk, or by inhalation of infected aerosols. Consumption of unpasteurized dairy products is the most common mean of transmission. In addition, occupational acquisition of brucellosis is of particular importance in shepherds, abattoir workers, veterinarians, dairy-industry professionals, and personnel in microbiologic laboratories.

Brucellosis is a worldwide disease; however, hot zones for the disease with high rates of occurrence are observed in countries of the Mediterranean basin, Arabian Gulf, the Indian subcontinent, parts of Mexico, Central and South America [2]. In 2003, most cases were reported from Syria (23,297), Iran (17,765), Turkey (14,435), Mexico (3,008), and Algeria (2,766) [2].

Evaluation/Assessment

None of the symptoms of brucellosis is specific enough to make a definite diagnosis. Moreover, brucellosis may present with variable signs and symptoms. Although nonspecific, fever seems to be the most common sign and symptom of brucellosis. Constitutional symptoms including anorexia, asthenia, fatigue, weakness, and malaise are common manifestations of brucellosis. In one study, the most common symptoms were fever (78.3%), arthralgia (77.5%), and sweating (72.5%) [3]. A localized disease such as endocarditis and spine infection may also occur in brucellosis.

A positive culture from blood, bone marrow, liver biopsy specimens, or other sites would indicate a definite diagnosis. However, the sensitivity of blood cultures for brucellosis is about 80% [3]. Serology is the most common method for the diagnosis of brucellosis. Serological tests include the Rose Bengal agglutination, serum agglutination (standard tube agglutination) (SAT), complement fixation, anti-brucella Coombs, and enzyme-linked immunosorbent assay (ELISA). Titers of $\geq$ 1:160 in conjunction with compatible clinical presentation are highly suggestive of infection. However, titers of >1:320 are more specific in endemic areas.

Polymerase chain reaction (PCR): PCR testing for brucellae allows for rapid and accurate diagnosis of brucellosis. However, after completion of the standard treatment, Brucella DNA may persist in the serum weeks to months.

Treatment

The mortality rate of untreated brucellosis was reported historically to be 2% in *B. melitensis* infection [3]. In addition, monotherapy is associated with a high relapse rate. The use of combination therapy allows for a lower relapse rate and reduction in treatment failure. The World Health Organization (WHO) recommended the use of a combination therapy of doxycycline-streptomycin (DOX-STR) or doxycycline-rifampicin (DOX-RIF). WHO recommended the use of rifampicin and doxycycline daily for a minimum of 6 weeks and, alternatively, rifampicin could be replaced with streptomycin,

intramuscularly, for the initial 2 weeks [3]. In a meta-analysis, the efficacy of DOX-STR regimen was superior to DOX-RIF regimen. Superiority of DOX-STR regimen is also supported by pharmacokinetic data [1].

In some studies, the combination of quinolone plus doxycycline showed a similar relapse rate of 8.3% compared to rifampin and doxycycline [3]. However, those studies included heterogeneous study populations, different combinations of antibiotics used and their dosages, variable duration of treatment, and periods of follow-up [3]. Fluoroquinolones in combination with rifampin or doxycycline, however, could be used for the treatment of acute uncomplicated brucellosis [4]. Other studies recommend the use of these antibiotics only in the context of properly designed prospective clinical trials [1].

The treatment of brucellosis in children less than 8 years of age is usually with a combination of trimethoprim-sulfamethoxazole (TMP-SMX) and rifampin orally for 45 days or TMP-SMX plus rifampin and a short course of an aminoglycoside [3]. For children aged 8 years and older, a combination of doxycycline and rifampin with gentamicin or streptomycin is recommended.

The treatment of brucella spondylitis varies widely. However, aminoglycoside-containing regimens seem to be superior to rifampicin-containing ones and a longer duration of treatment of not less than 3 months [1]. Brucellar endocarditis is associated with a high mortality rate; however, there are no randomized studies on the optimal therapy. Surgical intervention seems to be necessary in the majority of reported cases [1]. Therapy of such conditions is based on case repots only and includes long-term combination antimicrobial therapy and surgical valve replacement when required [3]. There are no randomized trials for treatment of brucellosis in pregnancy; however, most series support the use of TMP-SMX alone or in combination with rifampicin [1].

After-care

The compliance of patients with the recommended therapy is an important aspect of the road to cure. After adequate therapy of brucellosis, recurrent symptoms should prompt a search for localized disease or relapse of the initial condition. Serologic testing using ELISA or other methods may be used to document response to therapy. Persistently high IgG agglutinating antibodies or ELISA may reflect inadequate treatment and persistent infection. However, persistently elevated IgG titers are not an uncommon finding in cured patients who had high titers or focal disease on presentation. Rising agglutinating titers or levels of IgG may suggest relapse [5].

Prognosis

The outcome of brucellosis is usually good; however, relapse may occur. The relapse is characterized by reappearance of symptoms or signs of the disease or new positive blood cultures in the following 12 months after therapy. Predictors of relapse include presence of positive blood cultures at baseline, presence of symptoms for <10 days before treatment, and fever of $\geq 38.3°C$ [6]. The mortality rate of human brucellosis is low (<5%) and is usually related to endocarditis.

Prevention

In almost all countries, effective prevention of brucellosis among humans and other animals is based on disease control programs in domestic animals, involving vaccination and slaughter of infected animals. Most of the successful disease control programs in animals have occurred in developed countries. Despite the existence of effective brucella vaccine for cattle and goats, control efforts in poor developing endemic countries have failed due to lack of funding and infrastructure. The best preventive strategies for human brucellosis are based on occupational food hygiene since no human vaccines are available to prevent disease transmission to humans. Heavy education campaigns about the avoidance of consumption of raw milk or products made from raw milk is highly valuable in interrupting the chain of disease transmission.

References

1. Ariza J, Bosilkovski M, Cascio A, Colmenero JD, Corbel MJ, Falagas ME, Memish ZA, Roushan MR, Rubinstein E, Sipsas NV, Solera J, Young EJ, Pappas G (2007) International Society of Chemotherapy; Institute of Continuing Medical Education of Ioannina. Perspectives for the treatment of brucellosis in the 21st century: the Ioannina recommendations. PLoS Med 4(12):e317
2. Pappas G, Papadimitriou P, Akritidis N, Christou L, Tsianos EV (2006) The new global map of human brucellosis. Lancet Infect Dis 6(2):91–99
3. Al-Tawfiq JA (2008) Therapeutic options for human brucellosis. Expert Rev Anti Infect Ther 6(1):109–120
4. Kalo T, Novi S, Nushi A, Dedja S (1996) Ciprofloxacin plus doxycycline versus rifampicin plus doxycycline in the treatment of acute brucellosis. Méd Mal Infect 26:587–589
5. Ariza J, Pellicer T, Pallares R, Foz A, Gudiol F (1992) Specific antibody profile in human brucellosis. Clin Infect Dis 14(1):131–140
6. Ariza J, Corredoira J, Pallares R et al (1995) Characteristics of and risk factors for relapse of brucellosis in humans. Clin Infect Dis 20(5):1241–1249

BTP

▶ Serum and Urinary Low Molecular Weight Proteins

B-Type Natriuretic Peptide

Andrew K. Roy, Patrick T. Murray
School of Medicine and Medical Science,
University College Dublin, Dublin, Ireland

Synonyms

Brain natriuretic peptide; BNP; Endogenous natriuretic hormones; Natriuretic peptides

Trade Names

Natrecor, Nesiritide, Noratek.

Class and Category

Recombinant human BNP intravenous vasodilator therapy.

Indications

For the treatment of acutely decompensated heart failure in patients presenting to hospital who have dyspnoea at rest or at minimal activity.

Dosage

The licensed dose for nesiritide is an IV *bolus* of 2 mcg/kg, followed by a continuous *infusion* of 0.01 mcg/kg/min (nesiritide product information).

Drug Interactions

Nesiritide is physically and/or chemically incompatible with injectable formulations of heparin, insulin, ethacrynate sodium, bumetanide, enalaprilat, hydralazine, and furosemide. These drugs should not be co-administered as infusions with nesiritide through the same IV catheter. The preservative sodium metabisulfite is incompatible with nesiritide. Injectable drugs that contain sodium metabisulfite should not be administered in the same infusion line as nesiritide. The catheter must be flushed between administration of nesiritide and incompatible drugs.

Contraindications

1. Hypersensitivity to any of its components.
2. Nesiritide should not be used as primary therapy for patients with cardiogenic shock, patients with systolic blood pressure <90 mmHg, or those with, or suspected of having, low filling pressures.

Definition

Natriuretic peptides are produced as a result of increased myocardial (atrial and ventricular) wall stretch, to act as counterregulatory hormones with antagonistic effects on the renin-angiotensin-aldosterone and sympathetic nervous systems. They have potent vasodilating properties, maintain salt and water homeostasis, and have been shown to influence cardiac remodeling, fibrosis, and myocyte hypertrophy. In humans, the family of natriuretic peptides consists of atrial natriuretic peptide (ANP – see previous chapter), B-type natriuretic peptide (BNP) (both of myocardial cell origin), C-type natriuretic peptide (CNP) derived from endothelium, and urodilatin (Uro) originating from the kidney. Human recombinant ANP (Carperitide) and BNP (Nesiritide) are available in certain countries for therapeutic use, and recombinant Uro (Ularitide) is currently in advanced phase III trials in Europe and the US. Measurements of circulating BNP and its N-terminal pro-BNP have also been shown to be useful biomarkers for the diagnosis and prognostic evaluation of heart failure, particularly in the emergency department. This chapter describes the cardiorenal physiological effects of BNP, in the context of the therapeutic actions of the recombinant BNP Nesiritide, and reviews some of the clinical trials and issues surrounding its US FDA approval for use in acute heart failure in 2001.

Synthesis, Structure, and Secretion

BNP was originally described by Sudoh et al. in 1990, in extracts of porcine brain tissue, hence the original name "brain natriuretic peptide." Thereafter it was discovered in much higher concentrations in cardiac tissues (Mukoyama, 1991). It shares the common feature of the natriuretic peptide family, a 17 amino acid disulfide ring structure, with different biological activity being conferred by its unique N and C terminal portions. Human BNP is encoded for by the NPPB gene (GeneID 4879), located on chromosome 1 at 1p36.2. Similar to ANP and CNP, BNP is secreted as a preprohormone. PreproBNP is 134 amino acids long, made up of a 26 amino acid signal sequence, followed by the proBNP consisting of 108 amino acids. Cleavage by several peptidases results in circulating mature, active 32 amino acid BNP, and other smaller BNP fragments which are presumed to possess some degree of biological activity as well. The majority of BNP is found in ventricular myocardial tissue, with very small amounts also stored with ANP in atrial granules. BNP release occurs constitutively, with continuous secretion under the control of transcription factor GATA4, as determined by left ventricular pressure and volume overload. It is also released in a pulsatile fashion through the coronary sinuses in response to left ventricular wall stretch, volume overload, and tissue hypoxia, along with multiple neurohormonal factors. Plasma levels of BNP under normal conditions are negligible.

Mechanism of Action

The natriuretic peptide receptors NPR-A, NPR-B, NPR-C are binding proteins with varying affinities for the different natriuretic peptides. ANP, BNP, and Uro bind to the natriuretic peptide-A receptor (NPR-A) binding protein. This in turn catalyzes synthesis of 3′,5′-cyclic guanosine monophosphate (cGMP) to mediate cell signal for natriuresis, vasodilatation, renin and aldosterone inhibition, anti-mitogenesis, and positive lusitropic effects. To a lesser degree, BNP also binds NPR-B and NPR-C. The importance of natriuretic peptides in cardiorenal homeostasis has been demonstrated using genetically altered knockout mice, with ANP modification or NPR-A/B antagonism having profound effects on hypertension, renal responsiveness to volume expansion, and ventricular hypertrophy. Mouse BNP gene knockout models demonstrate significant ventricular fibrosis. Targeted receptor antagonists resulting in activated renin-angiotensin-aldosterone system, increases in cardiac filling pressures, and excess sodium retention. In human studies nesiritide produces dose-dependent reductions in pulmonary capillary wedge pressure, and systemic arterial pressure in patients with heart failure. No improvements in cardiac contractility have been demonstrated in animal models, and tachyphylaxis does not occur during infusions of BNP for up to 48 h; however, this may occur during longer exposure. As NPR-A is a membrane-resident protein dependent on phosphorylation, Potter et al. have reported dephosphorylation as a possible mechanism of desensitization in response to prolonged natriuretic peptide exposure or protein kinase C activation. NPR-A is found in kidney, brain, heart, lung, adrenal, and vascular smooth muscle tissue.

Clearance

All four peptides are cleared by NPR-C, the clearance receptor, and eventually degraded by 24.11 neutral endopeptidase (NEP), both of which are widely expressed in heart, kidney, lung, and vascular wall. BNP first requires cleavage of its 6 amino-terminal amino acids by a metalloprotease in the kidney brush border before NEP degradation. The half-life of circulating human BNP is 20 min. The half-life of nesiritide is 18 min, with time to approach steady state level accordingly less than 90 min. Clearance for nesiritide is similar to endogenous BNP, with no dosage modification needed for impaired renal function.

Synthetic BNP Therapy for Congestive Heart Failure

Nesiritide is a human purified form of BNP manufactured from Escherichia Coli using recombinant DNA technology. It has been extensively studied as a therapeutic tool in a number of clinical trials for management of heart failure. Nesiritide has been shown to lower filling pressures, decrease pulmonary and systemic vascular resistance, and increase cardiac output in a dose- dependent manner. Two major clinical trials led to the approval of human recombinant BNP/nesiritide by the FDA in the US in 2001 – the multicenter Vasodilatation in the Management of Acute Congestive Heart Failure (VMAC) trial by Young et al. [1], and the Efficacy and Comparative trials published by Colucci et al. [2]. Patients hospitalized for heart failure requiring intravenous therapy were recruited into either the Efficacy (double-blind design) or Comparative (open-label) trials (Colucci et al.). In the Efficacy trial, 127 patients with a Swan-Ganz catheter and pulmonary wedge pressures of ≥ 18 mmHg and cardiac index ≤ 2.7 l/min/m^2 were randomized to placebo or nesiritide 0.3 μg/kg IV bolus followed by infusion of 0.015 μg/kg/min, or nesiritide 0.6 μg/kg/min bolus, followed by an infusion of 0.03 μg/kg/min for 6 h. A dose-dependant decrease in systemic vascular resistance was seen, as well as a decrease in PCWP of 6 mmHg and 9.6 mmHg, respectively, compared with placebo. A dose-dependant increase in cardiac index was seen, with no change in heart rate noted. Global clinical status improved by up to 40% compared with placebo, with reductions in dyspnoea and fatigue. The Comparative trial reported improved global status, dyspnoea, and fatigue for up to 7 days, similar to that observed for standard therapy. Nonetheless, symptomatic and asymptomatic hypotension were reported more frequently in the nesiritide group (Safety). Lower doses of nesiritide were used in the VMAC trial [1], a randomized, double-blind study to compare efficacy of intravenous nesiritide, nitroglycerin, and placebo in 489 patients with decompensated heart failure and dyspnoea at rest. Bolus dosing of 2 μg/kg followed by an infusion of 0.01 μg/kg/min was administered, with primary endpoints of change in dyspnoea and absolute change in PCWP at 3 h. Nesiritide improved PWCP and dyspnoea at 3 h compared with placebo, and the incidence of hypotension was similar between groups. Taken together, these data led to the approval of nesiritide for treatment of dyspnea in patients with acute decompensated heart failure.

Nesiritide Use for Preservation of Renal function

Several small nesiritide studies have demonstrated improvements in renal function indices, particularly with low-dose "nonhypotensive" nesiritide infusions in cardiac surgery patients. The reported beneficial effects of nesiritide on renal function include increases in renal blood flow (via vasodilatation of the afferent arteriole and vasoconstriction of the efferent arteriole of the glomerulus), improvements in GFR, enhanced natriuresis via decreased sodium reabsorption in the proximal tubule and collecting duct, and diuresis. Furthermore, in contrast to the effects of other diuretics, aldosterone inhibition occurs during BNP-induced natriuresis. The NAPA [3] study randomized patients undergoing cardiopulmonary bypass for cardiac surgery with preoperative impaired LV systolic function (EF <40%) to placebo or nesiritide 0.01 μg/kg/min without bolus. They found that the nesiritide group had better indices of renal function post-op. Specifically, in the immediate postoperative period there was less increase in serum creatinine (0.15 ± 0.29 mg/dl versus 0.34 ± 0.48 mg/dl; $p \leq .001$), a smaller fall in GFR, and greater urine output, without significant systemic or pulmonary hemodynamic changes. Some improvements in LOS and mortality were seen at 180 days. Interestingly, Mentzer Jr. et al. suggest that some beneficial results may be due to dosing with no bolus given, and also make the (debatable) point that these patients are stable in compared with the decompensated heart failure population. As was seen with ANP, the effects of blunting neurohormonal activation (sympathetic overactivity, increased circulating norepinephrine levels) in response to cardiopulmonary bypass initiation might account for some of the observed beneficial effects on renal function. Conversely acute decompensated heart failure patients may indeed rely on some of these physiological mechanisms for maintaining GFR. Similarly, in another pilot study, Chen and colleagues [4] studied low-dose nesiritide doses (0.005 μg/kg/min) in a small group of patients ($n = 40$) with preoperative renal insufficiency (CrCl < 60 ml/min), receiving nesiritide infusion for 24 h after anesthesia induction and during cardiopulmonary bypass cardiac surgery. Cystatin C was used as more sensitive endogenous GFR marker than creatinine. Proof of biological activity was demonstrated by increased plasma second messenger cGMP, plasma BNP, and reduced plasma aldosterone in the nesiritide group compared with placebo. The placebo group had a greater decline in renal function at 48 and 72 h as measured by increase in plasma cystatin ≥0.3 mg/l 26% placebo versus 12% nesiritide. Postoperative outcomes were improved, with 37% placebo versus 12% nesiritide requiring inotropic support >48 h. Although encouraging, these studies are limited by small sample size and a lack of clinical endpoints and long-term follow-up. Unfortunately, the NAPA II/CS trial that was planned to confirm and extend these findings was withdrawn prior to subject enrollment, and will apparently not be conducted [5].

Nesiritide Safety Issues

Renal Function

Post-hoc analyses of clinical trial data have raised concerns about potential adverse renal effects and increased in mortality in nesiritide-treated patients. Thirty day follow-up data in the 2000 Colucci trial [2] showed a deterioration in renal function in nesiritide-treated patients, with serum creatinine values more than three times higher than patients treated with placebo ($p = .04$). Wang et al. (2004) reported no effect (positive or negative) of nesiritide on GFR or urine output in a crossover study of 15 patients with heart failure and worsening renal function. However, Sacker-Bernstein and colleagues [6] performed a meta-analysis of FDA data from five trials, and suggested that nesiritide therapy might be associated with an increased risk of acute serum creatinine elevation >0.5 mg/dl in patients with heart failure. They point out that increases in SCr often occurred days after cessation of study infusions, and 11.1% (32 of 288) of nesiritide patients required a "medical intervention" for worsening renal failure in comparison with 4.2% (6 of 144) in the control group. There was no change in the need for dialysis between both groups (nesiritide 2.5% vs. control 2.2%). The manufacturer notes – "doses higher than 0.01 µg/kg/min increase the rate of elevated serum creatinine over baseline compared with standard therapies." In follow-up analysis of the VMAC trial at day 30, the incidence of elevation of SCr to >0.5 mg/dl over baseline was 27% vs. 21% ($p = .11$) with GTN.

Excess hypotension is a known adverse effect of nesiritide, with a VMAC trial incidence of 4% for a mean duration of 2.2 h – in some cases causing syncope, nausea, and dizziness requiring volume resuscitation. It is this significant reduction in systemic blood pressure which may, along with other factors, be a contributor to worsening renal function via reduced renal perfusion pressure and paradoxical hypotension-induced activation of the RAAS and SNS. This has led to promising data examining lower dose nesiritide, both in intravenous, and subcutaneous forms, with reno-protective properties reported in elective cardiac surgery patients on cardiopulmonary bypass with left ventricular dysfunction, the NAPA [3] trial (discussed above).

Mortality

Concerns regarding the potential adverse effects of nesiritide on mortality are significant, in addition to possibly worsening renal function. 30 day follow-up data in the 2000 Colucci trial [2] suggest nesiritide associated mortality was 7.1% as compared with 4.8% in the placebo group ($p = .62$). 30 day mortality rates in the VMAC trial were 8.6% in the nesiritide group versus 5.5% among controls (relative risk, 1.56; 95% confidence interval, 0.75–3.24; $p = .20$). A meta-analysis conducted by Sacker-Bernstein et al. [7] of short-term risk of death in three large, randomized controlled trials found treatment with nesiritide was associated with a 74% increased risk of death within 30 days (although the trend was marginal; $p = .059$). Notably this meta-analysis only included 3 of the 12 randomized controlled trials, as their intention was to focus only on FDA's approved indication for nesiritide.

Clinical Conclusion

The clinical roles of the natriuretic peptides and their synthetic analogs are evolving, and current ACC/AHA guidelines for acute decompensated heart failure recommend a role for nesiritide as vasodilator therapy, in conjuction with standard treatments. Future targets and candidates for therapy include chimeric natriuretic peptides, specific cyclic GMP activators, and low-dose nesiritide for aldosterone suppression in acute myocardial infarction. Given the significant safety concerns, and pharmacoeconomic implications, "off-label" use of nesiritide should be strongly discouraged. For the indication of treatment of those patients presenting to hospital with acute decompensated heart failure with dyspnoea at rest, physicians should carefully consider the potential risk and benefits and the availability of alternative therapies. Further clinical trials with prospective mortality evaluations, re-hospitalization rates, and pharmacoeconomic analyses, such as the European Evaluating Treatment with Nesiritide in Acute Decompensated Heart Failure (ETNA) [5], and the ASCEND-HF [5] trial, will provide important information to fully define safety parameters, dosages, and utility of these therapies.

References

1. Publication Committee for the VMAC Investigators (Vasodilatation in the Management of Acute CHF) (2002) Intravenous nesiritide vs nitroglycerin for treatment of decompensated congestive heart

failure: a randomized controlled trial. JAMA 287:1531–1540 [Erratum, JAMA (2002) 1288:1577]

2. Colucci WS, Elkayam U, Horton DP, Abraham WT, Bourge RC, Johnson AD, Wagoner LE, Givertz MM, Liang CS, Neibauer M, Haught WH, LeJemtel TH (2000) Intravenous nesiritide, a natriuretic peptide, in the treatment of decompensated congestive heart failure. Nesiritide study group. N Engl J Med 343:246–253
3. Mentzer RM Jr, Oz MC, Sladen RN, Graeve AH, Hebler RF Jr, Luber JM Jr, Smedira NG on behalf of the NAPA Investigators (2007) Effects of perioperative nesiritide in patients with left ventricular dysfunction undergoing cardiac surgery. J Am Coll Cardiol 49:716–726
4. Chen HH, Thoralf MS, Cook DJ, Heublein DM, Burnett JC Jr (2007) Low dose nesiritide and the preservation of renal function in patients with renal dysfunction undergoing cardiopulmonary-bypass surgery. Circulation 116(I):I–134–I–138
5. www.clinicaltrials.gov; NCT00530361
6. Sackner-Bernstein JD, Skopicki HA, Aaronson KD (2005) Risk of worsening renal function with nesiritide in patients with acutely decompensated heart failure. Circulation 111:1487–1491
7. Sackner-Bernstein JD, Kowalski M, Fox M, Aaronson K (2005) Short-term risk of death after treatment with nesiritide for decompensated heart failure: a pooled analysis of randomized controlled trials. JAMA 293:1900–1905
8. Wang W, Ou Y, Shi Y (2004) AlbuBNP, a recombinant B-type natriuretic peptide and human serum albumin fusion hormone, as a long-term therapy of congestive heart failure. Pharm Res 21:2105–2111
9. Mukoyama M, Nakao K, Hosoda K, Suga S, Saito Y, Ogawa Y et al (1991) Brain natriuretic peptide as a novel cardiac hormone in humans. Evidence for an exquisite dual natriuretic peptide system, atrial natriuretic peptide and brain natriuretic peptide. J Clin Invest 87: 1402–1412
10. Sudoh T, Minamino N, Kangawa K, Matsuo H (1990) C-type natriuretic peptide (CNP): a new member of natriuretic peptide family identified in porcine brain. Biochem Biophys Res Commun 168:863–870

Bubonic Plague

▶ Biological Terrorism, Plague

Bumetanide

▶ Diuretics for Treatment of Acute Kidney Injury

Bunyaviruses

▶ Biological Terrorism, Hemorrhagic Fever

Burn Fluid Resuscitation

DEVASHISH J. ANJARIA, EDWIN A. DEITCH
Department of Surgery, UMDNJ-New Jersey Medical School, Newark, NJ, USA

Synonyms
Correction of burn shock; Fluid resuscitation

Definition
Burn injury of any etiology including thermal, chemical, or electrical can have profound cardiovascular effects. Significant burns are associated with hemodynamic changes including depressed cardiac output, vasodilation, extravascular fluid shifts, and fluid loss. Collectively, these changes result in burn shock or hypoperfusion at the tissue level. The purpose of fluid resuscitation post-burn is to restore and/or maintain tissue perfusion in the patient with major burns.

Pre-existing Condition
Any patient with >10% total body surface area (TBSA) thermal or chemical burns or any high-voltage electrical burns is at risk for the development of requiring fluid resuscitation. For thermal or chemical burns, second or third degree, but not first degree, burns are considered in calculating burn size, since superficial first-degree burns do not contribute significantly to the metabolic/hemodynamic response.

After major burn injury, vasoactive mediators are released that cause decreased cardiac output while increasing vascular permeability, resulting in leakage of intravascular fluid into the interstitial space with formation of edema. The loss of intravascular fluid results in intravascular hypovolemia with a compensatory vasoconstrictive response. This leads to an interesting combination of distributive shock and hypovolemic shock. If untreated, the compensatory mechanisms will eventually fail, leading to hypotension, organ dysfunction, and ultimately death [1].

Because of this, after a major burn, it is imperative to initiate volume resuscitation therapy promptly. Delay in resuscitation for more than 2 h after a major burn has been shown to complicate resuscitation and increase mortality [2].

Application

Calculation of Resuscitation Requirement
The amount of fluid resuscitation required is dependent on the extent of the burn and the size of the patient.

The extent of second- and third-degree burn should be estimated by the rule of nines or any available burn diagram. With the rule of nines, each body part is divided into a multiple of 9% TBSA (Fig. 1a, b). Each upper extremity is 9% TBSA while a lower extremity is 18% TBSA. Of note, the rule of nines is accurate at estimating burn extent in adults; however, it can be inaccurate in children due to changing body proportions. Therefore, many burn centers use a Lund and Browder chart to determine burn percentage in children (Fig. 2). This chart can be used for increased accuracy of estimating burns in adults, but the rule of nines still provides a useful tool for rapid assessment of the extent of burn injury [3]. A patient's baseline weight should be determined as soon after injury as possible, preferably prior to dressing of the burns. Ideally, a pre-burn weight can be

Rule of nines

Head	9%
Anterior Trunk	18%
Posterior Trunk	18%
Right Upper Extremity	9%
Left Upper Extremity	9%
Right Lower Extremity	18%
Left Lower Extremity	18%
Perineum	1%

a

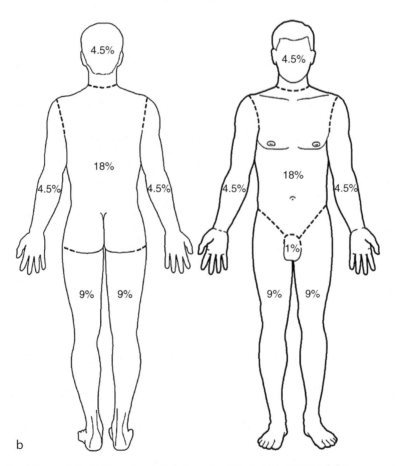

b

Burn Fluid Resuscitation. Figure 1 (**a, b**) The rule of nines for estimating burn extent in adults

Area Burned	Age in years					
	1	1 to 4	5 to 9	10 to 14	15	Adult
	Percentage of Total Body Surface					
Head	19	17	13	11	9	7
Neck	2	2	2	2	2	3
Anterior Trunk	13	13	13	13	13	13
Posterior Trunk	13	13	13	13	13	13
Left Buttock	2.5	2.5	2.5	2.5	2.5	2.5
Right Buttock	2.5	2.5	2.5	2.5	2.5	2.5
Genitals	1	1	1	1	1	1
Right Upper Arm	4	4	4	4	4	4
Left Upper Arm	4	4	4	4	4	4
Right Lower Arm	3	3	3	3	3	3
Left Lower Arm	3	3	3	3	3	3
Right Hand	2.5	2.5	2.5	2.5	2.5	2.5
Left Hand	2.5	2.5	2.5	2.5	2.5	2.5
Right Thigh	5.5	6.5	8	8.5	9	9.5
Left Thigh	5.5	6.5	8	8.5	9	9.5
Right Lower Leg	5	5	5.5	6	6.5	7
Left Lower Leg	5	5	5.5	6	6.5	7
Right Foot	3.5	3.5	3.5	3.5	3.5	3.5
Left Foot	3.5	3.5	3.5	3.5	3.5	3.5

Burn Fluid Resuscitation. Figure 2 Lund and Browder chart for estimating the extent of burns in children

obtained from the patient or family. Accurate determination of burn extent and weight will increase the accuracy of calculation of estimated resuscitation requirements.

The fluid requirement for a given patient is then calculated as follows [4].

- Adults: 2–4 ml Ringer's lactate × kg body weight × % TBSA burn
- Children: 3–4 Ringer's lactate × kg body weight × % TBSA burn – with small children or greater than 40% TBSA burns, this will underestimate needs and should be given in addition to maintenance requirements
- Infants < 12 months and small children: fluid with 5% dextrose at a maintenance rate in addition to the resuscitation fluid calculated above

For adults, the traditional formula used for calculation is the Parkland formula, which calls for 4 ml/kg/% TBSA burn. The fluid requirement calculated with the appropriate formula above provides an estimate of the fluid requirement in the first 24 h post-burn. Half of this total calculated resuscitation is given in the first 8 h post-burn injury, and the other half is administered over the subsequent 16 h. For example, for a 100 kg man with a 50% TBSA burn the total calculated resuscitation requirement would be 4 ml × 100 kg × 50% TBSA = 20,000 ml of Ringer's lactate. This would be

administered with 10,000 ml given in the first 8 h post-burn and the subsequent 10,000 ml given over the next 16 h. If the patient's presentation or resuscitation is delayed, the initial rate of resuscitation is increased to administer the prescribed fluid by the time goals. It is important to note that the above formulas provide estimates of fluid requirement for the burn patient and clinical therapy must be tailored to efficacy of restoring perfusion. As a rule of thumb, these formulas work in about 70–80% of patients, but may either over- or underestimate fluid needs in the other 20–30%.

Access for Resuscitation

Peripheral intravenous lines are the ideal access for fluid resuscitation. Ideally, peripheral IVs are placed in areas without burn involvement. If necessary, peripheral lines can be placed through burned skin into underlying veins. If peripheral access is unobtainable, central venous access can be used, preferably through non-burned skin given the increased risk of infection.

Monitoring Adequacy of Resuscitation

As the calculated resuscitation requirement is an estimate, monitoring for adequacy of resuscitation becomes extremely important. Urine output is the most important measure of resuscitation and volume status in the burn patient. Urine output should be monitored with an indwelling urinary catheter. Adequate urine output is:

- Adults: 0.5 ml/kg/h
- Children: 1 ml/kg/h

Using urine output, approximately 20% of patients are observed to have fluid administered in excess of what is required to restore intravascular euvolemia and tissue perfusion. These patients are usually young and healthy with second-degree burns. A high urine output (greater than 2 ml/kg/h) with hemodynamic stability can be the first sign of potential over-resuscitation. In these patients, hourly resuscitation should be decreased by 25% and if urine output is maintained above 0.5 ml/kg/h for adult patients, the reduced resuscitation rate is continued. If at any point, the hemodynamic status deteriorates or urine output drops, the volume of resuscitation is increased.

Conversely, in approximately 10% of the patients these formulas will underestimate resuscitation requirements. Specific conditions that may lead to an increased fluid volume requirement include older patients, associated non-burn injuries, deeper burn injuries, electrical injury, inhalational injury, preexisting dehydration, and/or delays in treatment or resuscitation. Need for increased fluid volume is often initially seen as a persistent low urine output less than 0.5 ml/kg/h for more than 2 h. In these patients, the calculated resuscitation rate should be increased by 25% with continued monitoring of urine output and volume status and additional titration of resuscitation as required. It should be noted that in the setting of an acute burn, the treatment of oliguria should be additional resuscitation and never diuretics.

Traditional hemodynamic parameters such as heart rate and blood pressure have their limitations as end points of resuscitation. Tachycardia of 100–120 is common in patients after burns in whom intravascular euvolemia has been reached with adequate resuscitation. However, a heart rate of greater than 120 may be indicative of inadequate resuscitation. Blood pressure tends to be lower in the burn patient due to a potentially decreased cardiac output and increased peripheral vasoconstriction and therefore a systolic blood pressure of greater than 100 mmHg is considered adequate. Of note, measurement of blood pressure can be limited in noninvasive routes secondary to edema and therefore if significant resuscitation is required, a peripheral arterial catheter is recommended for continual pressure monitoring.

Refractory Burn Shock

Although the majority of patients can be successfully resuscitated with the guidelines above, there is a small group of patients who may be refractory despite aggressive fluid resuscitation (greater than 6 ml/kg/%TBSA). This includes patients with limited cardiovascular reserve and/or preexisting cardiac disease and patients with massive burns (i.e., greater than 80% TBSA). In these patients, if perfusion is limited despite adequate volume resuscitation, then consideration should be given to the use of ionotropic agents, such as dopamine or dobutamine. Additionally, in these patients, early administration of colloid resuscitation, specifically albumin, may be successful in treating the refractory shock.

Special Considerations in Burn Resuscitation

Smoke Inhalation

Inhalational injury superimposed on a major burn causes a major increase in the physiologic effect of a burn regardless of extent. Patients with inhalational injuries can require up to 50% more fluid for adequate resuscitation in the initial 24 h post-burn period (therefore up to 6 ml/kg/% TBSA). Attempts at under-resuscitating these patients in order to decrease pulmonary edema are ineffective and can result in increased pulmonary sequestration of fluid in the lungs. Therefore, resuscitation of these patients should be titrated according to the guidelines described above.

Electrical Burns

There are two factors making resuscitation of major high-voltage electrical injuries challenging. First is the under appreciation of the extent of tissue injury. Electrical injuries often have minimal cutaneous signs with significant injury to the underlying muscle and tissues. It has been estimated that these patients can require two to three times (8–12 ml/kg/% TBSA) the amount of fluid resuscitation as calculated by the Parkland formula based on their cutaneous burns [3].

Second, injury to the muscle results in release of myoglobin and myoglobinuria. To lessen the nephrotoxic effects and decrease the incidence of acute renal failure, urine output must be maintained at 1–1.5 ml/kg/h (>100 ml/h in adults). This is continued until the myoglobinuria clears. If the patient fails to have adequate urine output despite aggressive fluid administration, the addition of 12.5 g of mannitol as an osmotic diuretic to each liter of resuscitation fluid can be considered to augment clearance of myoglobin and maintain urine output. If myoglobin persists or continues to increase despite all resuscitative measures, a search should be made for an unrecognized compartment syndrome.

Complications of Inadequate Resuscitation

Continued burn shock with tissue hypoperfusion leads to organ failure. The most commonly effected organ is the kidney. Untreated burn shock and organ failure will lead to increased mortality if shock is inadequately appreciated and treated.

Complications of over Resuscitation

Although the traditional emphasis on evaluating resuscitation has been on preventing under-resuscitation, increasing evidence is present that over-resuscitation is not without significant complication. The patients most sensitive to excessive fluid administration include children, the elderly, and patients with preexisting cardiac disease. The most common complication is excessive tissue edema. This edema decreases cellular oxygen availability in tissues and may worsen injury to already damaged tissues. This can result in the conversion of superficial burns into deep burns. In addition, there is recognition that excessive fluid resuscitation may increase the incidence of pulmonary edema and/or ARDS. More recently, excessive fluid resuscitation has been recognized as a cause of compartment syndromes including abdominal compartment syndrome, whose treatment may require surgical intervention.

This has brought to question whether the Parkland formula should be the gold standard for burn resuscitation in the average burn patient given the significant rate of overestimation of fluid resuscitation observed with its use. In a recent retrospective analysis of the use of the Parkland formula (4 ml/kg/% TBSA) versus a modified Brook formula (2 ml/kg/%TBSA) in the military showed significantly decreased fluid resuscitation in the group resuscitated with the Brook formula without any increase in organ failure or mortality [5]. It should be noted that the population included young healthy individuals and therefore self-selecting the population more likely to be overestimated by the Parkland formula.

Summary

The goal of fluid resuscitation after burn injury is to restore tissue perfusion and maintain organ function. It begins with determining the extent of burn and using a standard formula such as the Parkland formula in adults as a guide to initiate prompt therapy. However, appropriate resuscitation is tailored to the specific patient scenario keeping in mind complicating factors and adjusting resuscitation based on clinical response. With watchful and attentive resuscitation, burn shock can be successfully corrected without the morbidity of under- or over-resuscitation.

References

1. Deitch EA (1990) The management of burns. NEJM 323:1249–1253
2. Latenser BA (2009) Critical care of the burn patient: the first 48 hours. Crit Care Med 37:2819–2826
3. Sittig K, Deitch EA (1989) Principles and practices in the fluid resuscitation of thermally injured patients. Trauma Quarterly 5:7–18
4. American Burn Association. Advanced burn life support course provider manual. Copyright © 2007, American Burn Association
5. Chung KK, Wolf SE, Cancio LC et al (2009) Resuscitation of severely burned military casualties: fluid begets more fluid. J Trauma 67:231–237

Burn Injury

Body injury due to flames and or combustion products.

Burn Injury, Compartment Syndromes

DEVASHISH J. ANJARIA, EDWIN A. DEITCH
Department of Surgery, UMDNJ-New Jersey Medical School, Newark, NJ, USA

Synonyms

Abdominal compartment syndrome; Muscle compartment syndrome; Secondary compartment syndrome

Definition

A compartment syndrome is a disease process where the pressure within a compartment, such as the fascial compartment surrounding the muscle tissue, exceeds the vascular perfusion pressure of that compartment resulting in decreased blood flow of the muscle contents of the compartment and hence tissue ischemia. In the case of a burn injury, this can be caused by the accumulation of tissue fluid or by the extrinsic compression by the burned tissue acting as a tourniquet and resulting in high pressures in a closed fascial space. This results in impaired perfusion of the tissues within the compartment compromising their viability if left untreated.

Specifically, compartment syndromes are most commonly observed in patients with high-voltage electrical burns or patients with circumferential third-degree burns. In high-voltage electrical burns, the underlying muscle tissue through which the current passes is frequently injured and hence becomes swollen and edematous.

The rigid fascial compartments that surround this injured muscle cannot distend and hence the pressure within this fascial compartment increases. A second common clinical scenario resulting in a compartment syndrome is seen in patients with circumferential third-degree extremity burns where the rigid burn eschar does not expand as tissue fluid accumulates and thus causes extrinsic compression of the extremity and a compartment syndrome.

Major burn injury can also cause secondary compartment syndromes in body parts not directly affected by the burns. This is a side effect of the high-volume crystalloid resuscitation often required to correct burn shock. This secondary compartment syndrome can occur in the extremities but can also present as an abdominal compartment syndrome.

Most compartment syndromes associated with burn injury do not present in the immediate postburn period unless there is associated traumatic injury or the patient presents in a delayed fashion. As such, compartment syndromes after burns are not commonly observed in the emergency department. Instead, they develop during the first 6–12 h of the initial volume resuscitation period as the administered intravascular volume goes into the interstitial and intracellular spaces resulting in tissue edema in or under the burned tissue.

Treatment

High clinical suspicion leading to early diagnosis is the most important factor in the treatment of compartment syndromes. Once a compartment syndrome is diagnosed, prompt surgical treatment is required [1]. Treatment of extremity compartment syndrome whether primarily due to electrical injury or secondary to resuscitation is with a surgical fasciotomy of the affected portion of the extremity [2]. A surgical fasciotomy can be performed in the operating room or at the bedside, if necessary, but should be performed with the patient asleep on mechanical ventilation due to concerns about patient comfort and pain control. Minimal instruments are required although an electrocautery is recommended as bleeding can be encountered. Although fasciotomies can be technically easy procedures for the experienced surgeon, a thorough understanding of the anatomy and location of the fascial compartments is required to decompress all potentially affected compartments. If a documented compartment syndrome is being treated, it is recommended to perform full decompression of the compartment with skin as well as the fascia so as to obviate any potential of untreated compartment syndrome in that specific extremity. A "skin sparring" fasciotomy with a full fascial incision under a limited skin incision can be complicated by incomplete

decompression of the compartment and a recurrent compartment syndrome and therefore is not recommended. Once the fasciotomy is completed, the open wounds are covered and dressed with sterile dressing.

For circumferential third-degree burns causing extrinsic compression and decreased perfusion, the therapy is an escharotomy (Fig. 1). An escharotomy is a bedside procedure requiring only a scalpel. An incision is made dividing the eschar down to the subcutaneous tissue, NOT through the fascia. The incision is created only through eschar and does not continue onto non-third-degree burned skin. As such, it is a relatively painless and bloodless procedure that is well tolerated at the bedside. Once the escharotomy is completed, an assessment of distal perfusion is completed to assess the efficacy of the procedure and any need for additional surgical intervention. It should be noted that a circumferential third-degree burn is not mutually exclusive from a traditional compartment syndrome and it is possible to have both processes concurrently, especially with high-voltage electrical injuries. Therefore, even after an escharotomy is performed, if perfusion to the extremity is not restored or diminishes after initial restoration, an evaluation must be made for a "subfascial" muscle compartment syndrome and fasciotomy performed for decompression [3]. Once perfusion is restored, the escharotomy incision(s) are covered in antimicrobial cream such as silver sulfadiazine and sterile dressings applied.

For abdominal compartment syndrome secondary to burns, the primary question prior to deciding which therapeutic option should be employed is to determine whether or not there is a significant amount of abdominal free fluid [4] A CT scan or bedside ultrasound may assist in making the diagnosis. Multiple studies have shown that in cases where the interstitial leak after burn presented as significant abdominal free fluid, paracentesis is an effective method for alleviation of abdominal compartment syndrome. However, it is recommended to repeat a bladder pressure after paracentesis to assess the efficacy of treatment. If paracentesis is effective, but significant resuscitation is ongoing, it is possible to have a recurrence of the abdominal compartment syndrome and therefore due diligence must be observed in monitoring fluid reaccumulation. In cases of abdominal compartment syndrome that do not have significant free fluid, or if elevated intra-abdominal pressures persist despite paracentesis, a decompressive laparotomy is the therapy of choice. The laparotomy is combined with a temporary abdominal closure (whether utilizing a commercially designed product for that purpose or noncommercial approach such as a silo or Bogota bag). This combination of laparotomy with temporary wound closure ensures

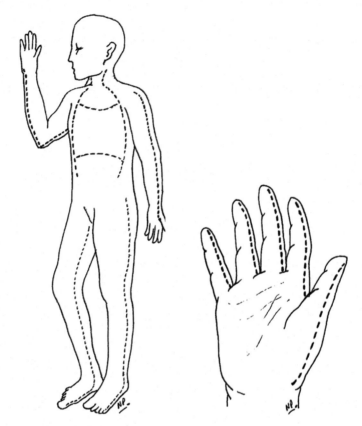

Burn Injury, Compartment Syndromes. Figure 1 Standard location for escharotomy for circumferential burns on the body and hands

adequate decompression of the intra-abdominal contents while providing protection to the viscera and allowing drainage and collection of abdominal fluid.

Evaluation/Assessment

Diagnosis of an extremity compartment syndrome requires a high degree of clinical suspicion. The clinical signs include pain, pallor, paresthesias, and coolness of the distal extremity with the loss of pulses being a late finding. Thus, the diagnosis should be made before loss of arterial flow has occurred. Physical examination, while potentially helpful, may be limited secondary to the significant edema that occurs with a major burn injury and is especially difficult in high-voltage electrical injuries where the injury causing the compartment syndrome occurs in the muscle compartment. Thus, individuals with high-voltage electrical injuries should be monitored with serial measurements of creatinine phosphokinase (CPK). A persistently rising CPK or a failure to clear myoglobinuria may indicate a developing compartment syndrome. In case of clinical suspicion, a definitive diagnosis can be made with by directly measuring the compartment pressures of the extremity in question. Pressure measurements of the fascial compartments can be performed with a commercial pressure monitoring device such as a Stryker Intra-Compartmental Pressure Monitor, more commonly known as a Stryker Needle. If this is not available, one can use a critical care monitor with a pressure transducer system as one would use for central venous pressure monitoring that is attached to an 18 gauge needle for pressure measurements. A thorough understanding of the anatomy of the region in question is necessary to ensure that the pressures in all at risk compartments are measured. Compartmental pressures of greater than 30 mmHg are worrisome and warrant either decompression or continued invasive monitoring depending on the clinical scenario.

In patients with circumferential third-degree burns of the extremities, pain and/or paresthesia distal to the burn may be the earliest symptoms of vascular compromise. In these patients, serial Doppler examinations of distal arterial flow are recommended [5]. Escharotomy is required for patients in whom distal arterial flow diminishes or becomes absent. After escharotomy is completed, restoration of arterial flow must be documented to ensure that the escharotomy is complete.

Intra-abdominal hypertension progressing to abdominal compartment syndrome can have many signs. The two most frequently seen signs are oliguria and elevation of peak inspiratory pressures. Oliguria is secondary to decreased cardiac output secondary to decreased venous return as well as direct compression of the kidneys and the venous outflow. In the setting of a major burn, oliguria is first assumed to be secondary to inadequate resuscitation and therefore the rate of fluid resuscitation is increased. If the problem is an abdominal compartment syndrome, increased fluid resuscitation will potentially improve the oliguria in the short term, however increased tissue edema due to capillary leak will potentially perpetuate and worsen the process. Respiratory insufficiency is a second common presenting sign in patients with an abdominal compartment syndrome and will present as respiratory distress in non-ventilated patients and as elevation of peak inspiratory pressures in patients on mechanical ventilation. This occurs secondary to elevation of the diaphragm from the increased intra-abdominal pressure with a resulting decrease of vital capacity and pulmonary compliance. Physical examination is limited in the diagnosis of abdominal compartment syndrome with a sensitivity of only 50%. The definitive diagnosis is made by the determination of the intra-abdominal pressure, most commonly via measurement of a bladder pressure. This is performed through an indwelling Foley catheter as follows: After complete drainage of the bladder, 50–100 ml of sterile saline is infused through the catheter and then clamped. The catheter is then attached via an 18 gauge needle or a needleless access system and transduced by a pressure transducer with the zero reference being the pubic symphysis. Pressures over 20 mmHg are worrisome for intra-abdominal hypertension and a pressure over 25 mmHg warrants intervention. For the burn patient, approximately 20% will be amenable to paracentesis, while the remainder will require a decompressive laparotomy. Therefore, if the diagnosis of abdominal compartment syndrome is made, an abdominal ultrasound should be obtained to determine if there is significant peritoneal fluid allowing for a "minimally invasive" therapeutic option.

After-care

After decompression of an extremity compartment syndrome, local wound care is provided to the open fasciotomy with clean dressings applied to the open wounds. The extremity is maintained elevated. As edema of the extremity resolves, delayed primary closure, often in staged procedures may be possible. When delayed primary closure is not feasible, closure of the fasciotomy wounds often require split thickness skin grafting for coverage.

For patients requiring escharotomy, initial care requires the application of antimicrobial cream such as silver sulfadiazine and sterile dressings. The third-degree burns will require operative excision and skin grafting for definitive therapy of the affected extremity.

In cases of abdominal compartment syndrome, if the intra-abdominal hypertension was relieved with paracentesis, continued serial monitoring of intra-abdominal pressure continues until such time that it is clear that repeated paracenteses will not be required. If decompressive laparotomy was required, the patient is maintained with a temporary abdominal closure with return to the operating room every 2 to 3 days for evaluation. Patients with a decompressive lararotomy should remain on mechanical ventilation and heavily sedated, since otherwise the risk of visceral evisceration is greatly increased. If the patient's visceral edema resolves, primary fascial closure is possible. However, if there is a concern that complete closure of the laparotomy incision will result in recurrence of the abdominal compartment syndrome, then staged procedures with sequential partial closure of the laparotomy should be attempted. If fascial closure is attempted, either partial or complete, the change in peak inspiratory pressures on the ventilator can be used as a real-time surrogate for intra-abdominal pressure to determine if further closure will risk recurrent abdominal compartment syndrome. If fascial closure is completed, skin closure is not recommended as the skin and subcutaneous tissues are colonized with skin flora and have a high rate of superficial wound infection. The open skin wound is treated with local wound care, allowing the skin incision to heal by secondary closure. If complete closure of the abdominal wall is not possible, the patient will require split thickness skin grafting of the viscera with delayed reconstruction of the abdominal wall at 9–12 months.

Prognosis

Although the extent of tissue injury directly caused by the burn injury is an important prognostic factor, in patients with extremity compartment syndromes, prognosis is improved by early diagnosis and prompt therapy. Delays in diagnosis and definitive treatment can be associated with significant preventable morbidity including long-term nerve injury and myonecrosis as well as acute renal failure secondary to prolonged or excessive myoglobinuria. Likewise, delayed recognition and treatment of an abdominal compartment syndrome increases the risk of the patient developing multiple organ failure with a significant increase in mortality.

References

1. Li X, Liang D, Liu X (2002) Compartment syndrome in burn patients: a report of five cases. Burns 28:787–789
2. Tremblay LN, Feliciano DV, Rozycki GS (2002) Secondary extremity compartment syndrome. J Trauma 53:833–837
3. Burd A, Noronha FV, Ahmed K et al (2006) Decompression not escharotomy in acute burns. Burns 32:284–292
4. Anjaria DJ, Hoyt DB (2007) Abdominal compartment syndrome. In: Wilson WC, Grande CM, Hoyt DB (eds) Trauma Critical Care Volume 2. Informa Heathcare, New York, p 619
5. American Burn Association (2007) Advanced Burn Life Support Course Provider Manual. Copyright © 2007, American Burn Association

Burn Injury, Inhalation Injury

GABRIEL A. MECOTT[1], MARC G. JESCHKE[2],
AHMED M. AL-MOUSAWI[3], DAVID N. HERNDON[3]
[1]Division of Plastic Surgery, Universidad Autonoma de Nuevo Leon, Monterrey, NL, Mexico
[2]Department of Surgery, Division of Plastic Surgery, University of Toronto, Sunnybrook Research Institute, Toronto, ON, Canada
[3]Department of Surgery, University of Texas Medical Branch and Shriners Hospital for Children, Galveston, TX, USA

Synonyms

Smoke inhalation injury

Definition

Inhalation injury (INH-INJ) is a complex entity that comprises local and systemic alterations (e.g., physical damage to the airway, release of oxygen radicals, and proinflammatory cytokines to the systemic circulation) caused by the inhalation of physical and chemical agents. It is considered one of the major predictors of mortality following severe burns [1, 2]. Isolated INH-INJ accounted for 0.3% of admissions to burn centers in the USA [1], and is observed concomitantly with burns in 7–30% of cases [1, 3], with the incidence of INH-INJ increasing with age [1].

Pathophysiology

The extent of injury is determined by the origin, temperature, water solubility, and size of inhaled substances and particles (fumes, gasses, and mists). The most common toxic compounds associated with inhalation injury include, but are not limited to, carbon monoxide (CO), cyanide, hydrogen chloride (HCl), phosgene (COCl$_2$), ammonia, sulfur dioxide (SO$_2$), acrolein, formaldehyde, isocyanates, and acrylonitriles [3]. These substances are typically produced by combustion of upholstery (CO, cyanide, HCl, phosgene, ammonia, acrolein, isocyanates, and acrylonitriles), wood (CO, acrolein), and clothing and fabrics (CO, cyanide, HCl, ammonia, and SO$_2$) [4].

Inhalation injury is classified according to the extent of injury as follows [3]:

(a) Upper airway injury
(b) Lower airway injury
(c) Pulmonary parenchymal injury
(d) Systemic toxicity

The upper airway is usually affected by heat and chemicals, and the subsequent edema formation follows the same behavior seen in thermal burns of other regions of the body [3]. Following resuscitation, rapid and massive edema can be life-threatening, obstructing the airway and making intubation of the patient very difficult, if not impossible, in this scenario.

Due to heat dissipation and the highly effective temperature regulation within the upper airway, direct thermal injury of the lower airway is unusual. Chemicals present in smoke are commonly responsible for injuries observed in this area. These lead to inflammation and subsequent hyperemia, shedding of the respiratory epithelia, and profuse transudate formation [3]. The accumulation of this exudate/transudate obstructs the airway and induces further inflammation, perpetuating the injury (Fig. 1).

In the pulmonary parenchyma, the inflammation produced leads to pulmonary edema and pulmonary dysfunction, with loss of hypoxic pulmonary vasoconstriction, and is reflected clinically as reduced arterial partial pressure of oxygen/fraction of inspired oxygen ratio (PaO$_2$/FIO$_2$) (Fig. 1).

For study purposes, INH-INJ can be viewed in three clinical stages [5]:

1. First phase (0–36 h): Manifested as upper airway obstruction, bronchospasm, and acute pulmonary insufficiency. Usually observed with CO poisoning, thermal injury, and hypoxia.
2. Second phase (24–72 h): Characterized by damage to the respiratory epithelium, sloughing of mucosa, and formation of plugs and casts. Clinically manifested with pulmonary edema, atelectasis, and tracheobronchitis.

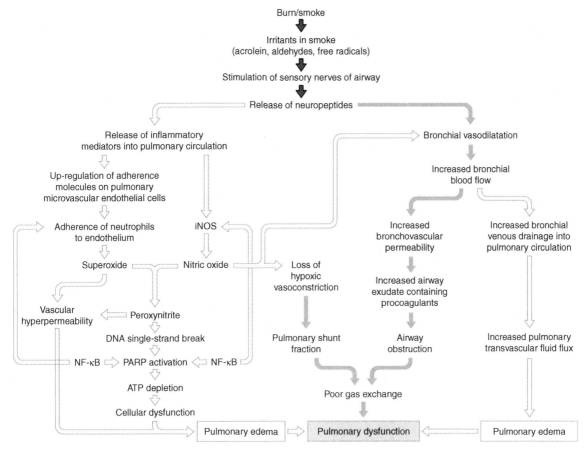

Burn Injury, Inhalation Injury. Figure 1 Pathophysiology of burn and smoke inhalation-induced acute injury. iNOS, inducible nitric oxide synthase; PARP, poly(ADP-ribose) polymerase. (Reprinted from Total Burn Care [3] Copyright 2007, with permission from Elsevier)

3. Third phase (3–10 days): Lung defenses are impaired, usually resulting in bronchopneumonia. The perpetuated injury can lead to acute respiratory distress syndrome (ARDS).

Evaluation/Assessment

The diagnosis of INH-INJ is based on the following aspects:

- Clinical
- Bronchoscopical
- Clinical imaging
- Toxicological

It is imperative to obtain a detailed history of the event, including the source of fire or incident, time of exposure, and history of loss of consciousness. A history of

entrapment in a closed space, facial burns, singed nasal hair, hoarseness, stridor, and carbonaceous sputum (sooty sputum) are early findings that should raise suspicion of the presence of INH-INJ. However, it is important to remember that INH-INJ can be present without cutaneous burns. In the case that both history and clinical findings are suggestive of INH-INJ, the patient should be considered to present with this until proven otherwise. On arrival, the patient can be disorientated or present with altered mental status as a result of CO, cyanide, drug and alcohol intoxication, or head injury [5].

Fiberoptic bronchoscopy is the most useful diagnostic tool for the assessment of the airway and should be performed in every patient with clinical suspicion of INH-INJ. Furthermore, it has an advantage of facilitating intubation if needed. Typical bronchoscopic findings include hyperemia, edema, and presence of carbonaceous material along the airway [3, 5]. Bronchoscopic findings can be classified into five grades of severity based on the Abbreviated Injury Score (AIS) criteria[6]:

- Grade 0 (no injury): absence of carbonaceous deposits, erythema, edema, bronchorrhea, or obstruction
- Grade 1 (mild injury): minor or patchy areas of erythema, carbonaceous deposits in proximal or distal bronchi (any or combination)
- Grade 2 (moderate injury): moderate degree of erythema, carbonaceous deposits, bronchorrhea, with or without compromise of the bronchi (any or combination)
- Grade 3 (severe injury): severe inflammation with friability, copious carbonaceous deposits, bronchorrhea, bronchial obstruction (any or combination)
- Grade 4 (massive injury): evidence of mucosal sloughing, necrosis, endoluminal obliteration (any or combination)

Other studies that are useful for diagnosis and follow-up, which should be obtained once the patient is admitted, include:

- Chest radiography
- Arterial blood gasses
- Carboxyhemoglobin
- Cyanide levels

Arterial gasses and chest radiographs are often normal at admission, so this situation does not exclude INH-INJ, but are valuable as a baseline and necessary to monitor the evolution of the patient. Carboxyhemoglobin levels are used to identify CO poisoning and cyanide levels to assess exposure to hydrogen cyanide.

Treatment

Patients from a burn scene should be managed similar to any other trauma patient, following the basic ABC approach. If the airway is patent and there is no need for intubation at the site of the accident, 100% oxygen should be administered until arrival to the hospital.

At arrival, once inhalation injury is diagnosed, the patient must be closely monitored. The airway must be secured before edema jeopardizes the intubation.

Specific treatment includes:

- High-flow humidified oxygen (100%), maintaining oxygen saturation (SaO$_2$) >90–95%
- Chest physical therapy
- Tracheal suction

- Aerosolized heparin
- *N*-acetylcysteine

Aerosolized heparin and *N*-acetylcysteine have improved mortality and reduced the incidence of atelectasis and reintubation [2]. Frequent position changes and early ambulation are warranted. Early extubation is encouraged, but without jeopardizing the patient.

CO poisoning requires 100% oxygen until carboxyhemoglobin levels are under 10% [5]. The half-life of CO is dependent on oxygen tension. The half-life is 320 min in room air, and approximately 75 min with 100% oxygen at atmospheric pressure. There are some reports that hyperbaric oxygen decreases the half-life of CO even further, but its utility in patients with INH-INJ has not been clearly demonstrated.

Cyanide treatment is controversial and requires close monitoring. Amyl nitrite or sodium nitrite is used as an antidote by inducing methemoglobin, which binds to the cyanide-forming cyanmethemoglobin. It further metabolizes to thiocyanate and is excreted in the urine.

Pharmacoeconomics

Inhalation injury increases hospital length of stay, need for intensive care, days on respiratory support, and the incidence of complications such as pneumonia. All these variables increase the in-hospital costs to a great extent.

Prognosis

Inhalation injury is one of the most important predictors of morbidity and mortality in burn patients. When present, INH-INJ increases mortality by up to ten times [1, 2]. Inhalation injury most likely requires endotracheal intubation, which in turn increases the incidence of pneumonia. Pneumonia is a common complication of INH-INJ, and increases mortality by up to 60% in these patients [2]. Patients usually recover full pulmonary function and late complications are not the rule. Complications can be secondary to the INH-INJ or to the endotracheal or tracheostomy tube. Hyperreactive airways and altered patterns of pulmonary function (obstructive and restrictive) have been described following INH-INJ [5]. Scarring of the airway can cause stenosis and changes in the voice, requiring voice therapy and occasionally surgery.

Future Directions

Advances in critical care, respiratory support, and the use of novel therapies have led to reduced morbidity and mortality in patients with INH-INJ. High-frequency

Burn Injury, Primary Wound Excision 415

B

percussive ventilation, airway pressure release ventilation, and extracorporeal membrane oxygenation are some of the newer strategies used to improve oxygenation while decreasing trauma to the airway. In CO poisoning, drugs including thiosulfate and hydroxycobalamin seem to be useful options with fewer side effects than nitrites. Inhaled nitric oxide (NO) dilates the capillaries of the ventilated areas, increasing the PaO_2/FiO_2 ratio. Tocopherol is a reactive oxygen scavenger and has been used successfully in ovine models, with promising results. Large clinical trials are needed to assess the clinical impact of these therapies.

References

1. 2009 National Burn Repository. In: American Burn Association; 2009
2. Shirani KZ, Pruitt BA Jr, Mason AD Jr (1987) The influence of inhalation injury and pneumonia on burn mortality. Ann Surg 205(1):82–87
3. Traber DL, Herndon DN, Enkhbaatar P et al (2007) The pathophysiology of inhalation injury. In: Herndon DN (ed) Total burn care, 3rd edn. W.B. Saunders/Elsevier, Philadelphia, PA, pp 248–261
4. Prien T, Traber DL (1988) Toxic smoke compounds and inhalation injury – a review. Burns Incl Therm Inj 14(6):451–460
5. Nugent N, Herndon DN (2007) Diagnosis and treatment of inhalation injury. In: Herndon DN (ed) Total burn care, 3rd edn. W.B. Saunders/Elsevier, Philadelphia, PA, pp 262–272
6. Endorf FW, Gamelli RL (2007) Inhalation injury, pulmonary perturbations, and fluid resuscitation. J Burn Care Res 28(1):80–83

Burn Injury, Primary Wound Excision

ARTHUR SANFORD, RICHARD L. GAMELLI
Stritch School of Medicine, Loyola University Medical Center, Maywood, IL, USA

Synonyms

First-degree burn; Full-thickness burn; Partial thickness burn; Second-degree burn; Thermal injury; Third-degree burn

Definition

Burn wounds can be classified as first, second, or third degree based on surface appearance. First-degree wounds are superficial, painful, and reddened. They do not require surgical intervention and are generally treated with topical moisturizers and avoidance of recurrent injury. This injury is typified by the injury from prolonged sun exposure without blisters. Second-degree burns are deeper, causing a superficial edema deposition between deeper viable tissues and injured tissues that are more superficial. The surface appearance is moist with blisters in various degrees of rupture. Treatment involves debridement of intact blisters at risk for rupture to remove the fluid, which contain high concentrations of thromboxanes and coverage with topical antimicrobial agents or synthetic wound dressings. The deeper elements of the skin remain intact and can regenerate the epithelial layer. Third-degree wounds are deeper and appear whitened, black, or dry, leather like skin. They require surgical debridement and skin grafting if larger than 2 cm. Full-thickness burns destroy all of the dermal elements, hence there are no epidermal cells left to regenerate the injured area. Partial thickness injuries allow epidermal cells to survive in the dermal elements, such as sweat glands or hair follicles, to repopulate the injured area.

In general, partial thickness and second-degree burns are used interchangeably, while full thickness and third degree are synonymous.

Treatment

Treatment begins by removing the victim from the continuing source of injury.

Evacuation from proximity to flame, extinguishing flames, removal of clothing, continued lavage of chemical agent off the patient to the ground, and removal from contact with electrical circuits are used to stop the initial process of a burn. Subsequently, treatment follows the principles of management of airway, breathing, and circulation of trauma care resuscitation. Patients do not expire from undressed wounds during the initial assessment but are at genuine risk from loss of the airway, hypovolemia, and hypothermia.

Ensuring the patency of the airway with intubation or cricothyroidotomy is necessary if there is any possibility of inhalation injury before massive edema develops. Burned facial structures can be suggestive of inhalation injury, stridor, inspiratory grunting, wheezing, or tachypnea signal impending airway loss. Carbon monoxide binds to hemoglobin, falsely elevating measurements with oxygen saturation monitors. Oxygen at 100% is administered from the scene of the accident to increase the rate of dissociation of CO from hemoglobin. Any suggestion of smoke inhalation should be investigated with an arterial blood gas determination.

Fluid resuscitation is aimed at restoring circulating intravascular volume.

Venous access is best obtained via two large bore peripheral IVs, although alternate methods are sometime necessary, such as central access, venous cutdowns, or interosseous infusions. Delay in administration of resuscitation has been shown to have a direct negative correlation with survival. Commonly used resuscitations administer between 2 and 4 cc/kg body weight/% body surface area burned of lactated Ringer's solution. The "Rule of Nines" is used to estimate percentage body surface area (BSA) with major body parts in the adult divided into multiples of nine. The head and neck are 9% body surface area (BSA), the upper extremity is 9% BSA, the anterior and posterior trunk are 18% BSA each, and each leg and thigh are 18% BSA. This estimation predicts the fluid needs over the first 24 h post injury, with half of the budgeted volume administered during the first 8 h and the remainder over the following 16 h, measured from the time of the injury. It cannot be stressed enough that these formulas provide only a "budget" for required fluids, and must be adjusted based on objective parameters, urine output (0.5 cc/kg for adults or 1.0 cc/kg for children) or persistent metabolic acidosis. Young children have different body proportions and a greater percentage body water; hence evaporative losses can be greater, so the needs are estimated using the Galveston formula of 5,000 cc/m^2 BSA burned and 2,000 cc/m^2 total BSA. Another method to account for the differences of the pediatric population is to administer size appropriate maintenance fluid (containing dextrose because of the limited glycogen reserves of this population) and give 4 cc/kg/% BSA burned. The same administration plan as for adults is used, with the first 1/2 of the volume given over 8 h and the remainder over the next 16 h, again with urine output as the ultimate guide to adequacy of resuscitation. Maintenance Dextrose is administered in children less than 2 years of age to prevent hypoglycemia with their relatively diminished glycogen stores. After a burn injury, the ensuing shock results from alterations in microvascular permeability and fluid shifts that result in tissue edema, reaching a maximum at between 8 and 48 h post injury. The use of albumin is not advised in the early post burn resuscitation period when the increased albumin would simply pass out into the tissues and cause greater edema.

Later use of albumin replacement is still undergoing evaluation, but no definite answer has been found.

The need for surgical intervention/debridement depends on the depth of the injury. The experienced burn care provider is able to look at the characteristics of a wound and predict potential for healing, based on presence of surviving dermal buds and hair. Maintained sensation in a burned area, particularly to sharp stimulation, indicates the deeper layers of skin are uninjured and will repopulate the burned area. Efforts to scan the surface of a burn wound, usually with a heated laser probe Doppler have been proposed to evaluate depth of injury without widespread acceptance or consistent success. Absence of these characteristics implies the wound will need grafting. Second-degree or partial thickness wounds are expected to heal spontaneously. As such, the role of protection of the wound bed from infection is paramount. Topical antibiotics can be applied in the form of silver sulfadiazine or surface delivery systems for silver products, such as Acticoat™. Temporary wound coverage can be accomplished with amniotic membrane or Biobrane™ promoting a healing environment for the wound. It is generally accepted that early debridement and grafting of wounds requiring surgery reduces hospital stay and morbidity/mortality. Previously wounds became infected, and through bacterial action, the eschar would separate leaving a granulating bed for skin grafting. The risk of such management is the development of invasive wound infection and sepsis. By early, aggressive surgical debridement, nonviable tissue is removed and hence the wound bed is relatively infection free. Every effort is made to have the burn wound completely excised of nonviable tissue within 1 week of the initial injury. This can be done in one aggressive operation or staged excisions to limit operative time and stress on the patient. The removal of dead tissue has the potential to reduce the generation of chemical mediators that stimulate the inflammatory cascade leading to remote and multisystem organ failure. Complete debridement should proceed at the earliest possible opportunity, even if donor sites are insufficient to provide total wound coverage. In this case, biological dressings (preferably Cadaver allograft or porcine xenograft) should be used to cover the remaining wounds. Excision of burn wounds requires large volumes of blood for transfusion (approximately 1cc/cm^2 to be excised). Blood loss can be minimized by the use of excision to the level of fascia, or tourniquets when performing tangential excisions of the extremities. Tangential excision gives a better cosmetic outcome by leaving subcutaneous fat, but blood loss is greater.

After the eschar has been excised, the wound must be closed. In general, wounds of 30% total body surface area or less can be closed in a single operation with split thickness skin grafts taken from unburned areas. As the size of the injury increases, there is proportionately less donor site for autografting; so alternate techniques are required. Larger expansions of the skin using meshers are available, usually requiring cadaver allograft overgrafting of 4:1 or greater autograft skin expansion. Wounds of greater than 90% may require up to ten operations for coverage, or use of cultured epithelial autografts [1].

Organ dysfunction associated with the systemic inflammatory response syndrome may occur. Renal failure previously complicated cases of inadequate resuscitation, but increased awareness of its causes (i.e., poor renal perfusion and nephrotoxic drugs) have reduced the frequency of this complicating factor. Pulmonary injury from smoke and toxin inhalation can be minimized by use of aerosolized heparin and mucomyst the high-frequency percussive ventilator, minimizing barotraumas, and expeditious removal of the endotracheal tube to allow coughing for pulmonary hygiene. Smoke inhalation injury and multisystem organ failure in association with burns have a mortality as high as 50%.

Patients with severe burns have metabolic rates from 100% to 150% higher than normal.

The support of the hypermetabolic response to burns is accomplished by keeping patient rooms warm (80–90°F) and meeting nutritional needs (1,500 kcal/m² Total BSA and 1,500 kcal/m² burned) in children or 24 kcal/kg body weight and 40 kcal/% Burn BSA for adults. The use of hormonal modulation is also employed, commonly using oxandrolone, propanolol, and recombinant human growth hormone replacement. Without this treatment, increased energy and protein requirements must be met to prevent impaired wound healing, cellular dysfunction, and decreased resistance to infection [2].

Rehabilitation begins with wound coverage to prevent burn scar contracture. Aggressive physical and occupational therapy with exercise and splinting in position of function are key. Use of pressure garments has been shown to organize the collagen of a wound more rapidly, but evaluation of its cosmetic and functional advantages are currently undergoing study. Plastic and reconstructive surgeons should be involved early on in the hospital course so that future need for releases and surgeries can be planned [3].

References

1. Barret JP, Wolf SE et al (2000) Cost-efficacy of cultured epidermal autografts in massive pediatric burns. Ann Surg 231(6):869–876
2. Williams FN, Jeschke MG et al (2009) Modulation of the hypermetabolic response to trauma: temperature, nutrition, and drugs. J Am Coll Surg 208(4):489–502
3. Herndon DN (2007) Total burn care, 3rd edn. W.B. Saunders, London/New York

Burn Injury, Rule of Nines

Manuel Dibildox[1], Marc G. Jeschke[2], David N. Herndon[1]
[1]Department of Surgery, University of Texas Medical Branch and Shriners Hospital for Children, Galveston, TX, USA
[2]Department of Surgery, Division of Plastic Surgery, University of Toronto, Sunnybrook Research Institute, Toronto, ON, Canada

Synonyms

Estimation of burn size; Lund and Browder chart

Definition

Burn injuries represent a severe insult to body homeostasis. An extensive hypermetabolic and inflammatory response occurs as a consequence of thermal tissue damage to more than 40% of the total body surface area (TBSA) and can lead to considerable morbidity and mortality [1]. This response may be so extensive that victims invariably suffer cardiovascular derangements if more than one third of the TBSA is affected. This condition is defined as burn shock [2].

Characteristics

Quantifying the extent of the burn injury is of utmost importance because it allows the physician to provide an adequate and comprehensive treatment that includes fluid resuscitation, nutritional support, pharmacologic agents, wound care, surgical interventions, and rehabilitation.

The current understanding of how the burn size is associated to the inflammatory response and fluid

Adult body Part	% of total BSA
Arm	9%
Head	9%
Neck	1%
Leg	18%
Anterior trunk	18%
Posterior trunk	18%

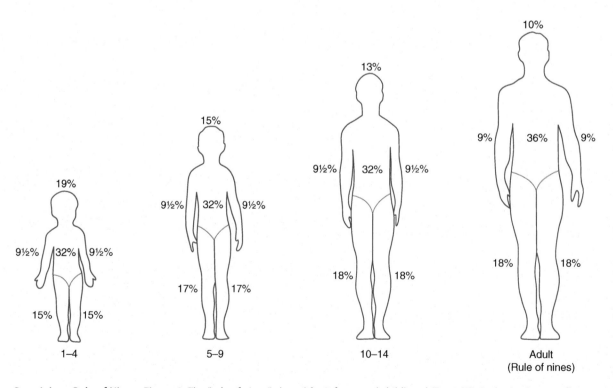

Burn Injury, Rule of Nines. Figure 1 Estimation of burn size in adults using the "rule of nines" (From Advanced Burn Life Support Providers Manual. Chicago, IL: American Burn Association, 2005). Authorization Pending

shifts can be dated back to the studies performed by Frank P. Underhill, who, as a Pharmacology and Toxicology professor at Yale, suggested that burn patient mortality was due to fluid loss and not due to toxins [3]. Work done by Lund and Browder in the 1940s later led to fluid replacement strategies based on the percentage of body surface area burned. Knaysi, Crikelair, and Cosman then proposed the "rule of nines" for calculating the extent of the burn injury [4]. In 1946, Cope and Moore further determined that tissue swelling is due to the shift of fluid into the interstitial space and is proportional to the burn size [5]. They also concluded that this fluid has to be replaced in the first hours after the thermal injury. Moore then developed a formula to calculate the fluid requirements of burn patients based on the extent of body surface area burned [6].

The rule of nines is accurate in determining the extent of body surface area in adults and adolescents. It is important to keep in mind that this rule does not apply to patients younger than 15 years because the surface distribution of body parts between adults and children is different (Fig. 1).

Pediatric patients have a larger cranial surface and a smaller lower extremity surface in relation to the torso

Burn Injury, Rule of Nines. Figure 2 The "rule of nines" altered for infancy and childhood (From [2]) Authorization pending

Age	0–1	1–4	5–9	10–14	15
A – ½ of head	9½%	8½%	6½%	5½%	4½%
B – ½ of one thigh	9½%	8½%	6½%	5½%	4½%
C – ½ of one leg	9½%	8½%	6½%	5½%	4½%

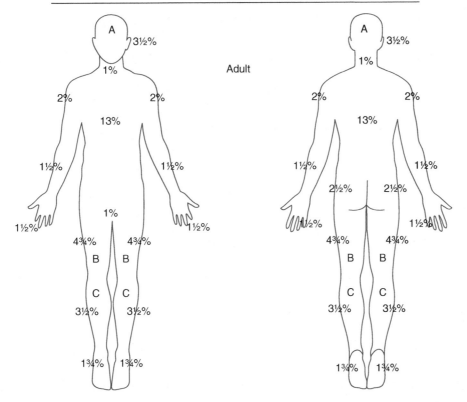

Burn Injury, Rule of Nines. Figure 3 The Lund and Browder chart describes a more detailed distribution of body surface area (From Advanced Burn Life Support Providers Manual. Chicago, IL: American Burn Association, 2005). Authorization pending

than adults. For this patient population, a more accurate assessment can be made by using charts that take into account the anthropomorphic differences in infancy and childhood (Figs. 2 and 3).

In summary, the rule of nines and other detailed charts can be used to accurately quantify the percentage of TBSA burned. This in turn will aid the clinician in providing an appropriate and multidisciplinary treatment plan.

References

1. Jeschke MG, Mlcak RP, Finnerty CC, Norbury WB, Gauglitz GG, Kulp GA, Herndon DN (2007) Burn size determines the inflammatory and hypermetabolic response. Crit Care 11(4):R90
2. Herndon DN (2007) Total burn care, 3rd edn. Elsevier, Philadelphia, PA, p 93
3. Underhill FP (1930) The significance of anhydremia in extensive surface burns. JAMA 95:852
4. Knaysi GA, Crikelair GF, Cosman B (1967) The rule of nines: it's history and accuracy. Presentation at the Am Soc Plast & Reconstruct, New York City, November 6, 1967
5. Blocker TG Jr (October 1, 1981) Lecture given to plastic surgery residents. Galveston, TX (unpublished)
6. Moore FD (1970) The body-weight burn budget. Basic fluid therapy for the early burn. Surg Clin North Am 50(6):1249–1265

Burn Sepsis

▶ Burns Infections

Burn Skin Infection

Kevin S. Akers[1], Clinton K. Murray[2]
[1]Department of Medicine, Brooke Army Medical Center, Fort Sam Houston, TX, USA
[2]Department of Medicine, San Antonio Military Medical Center, Fort Sam Houston, TX, USA

© Springer-Verlag Berlin Heidelberg (outside the USA) 2012

Synonyms

Burn wound cellulitis; Burn wound impetigo; Burn wound infection; Burn wound sepsis

Definition

Burn skin infection refers to an infection in or originating from pathogenic organisms colonizing or infecting a burn wound, typically involving devitalized tissues. Burn skin sepsis can occur when organisms that have colonized the burn eschar invade the bloodstream causing sepsis. Burn wound cellulitis describes the spread of infection from the burn wound into surrounding healthy tissues. Burn wound impetigo is a secondary infection of re-epithelialized skin, such as that healing by secondary intention, or grafted skin. Since treatment of more severe burns involves surgery, surgical site infections may also occur [1].

Epidemiology

Burns are traumatic injuries associated with significant morbidity and mortality. In the United States, there are approximately 500,000 burn injuries treated each year, with 40,000 requiring hospitalization. Sixty percent of hospitalizations occur at specialized burn centers [2]. Fortunately, mortality has improved significantly over the past four decades, with approximately 15,000 deaths annually in the 1970s decreasing to approximately 3,245 non-firefighter deaths in 2006. Whereas in the 1970s, a 30% total body surface area (TBSA) burn was associated with a 50% risk of death, in the modern era this degree of mortality risk requires an 80% TBSA burn. Despite these improvements, the primary predictors of mortality from burn injury remain unchanged: extremes of age, %TBSA, presence of full thickness burns, and inhalational injury [3]. Owing to its prognostic importance, diagrams allowing calculation of %TBSA on the basis of anatomic involvement are readily available in most emergency departments, emergency medicine textbooks, and burn centers.

Pathophysiology and Staging

Cutaneous burns result in a gradient of damage radiating outward from the burn site, with several zones of distinct histologic injury patterns. Nearest the heat source is the zone of coagulation, which includes necrotic and devitalized skin tissue that forms the eschar. Adjacent to this is the zone of stasis, representing viable tissue that is at risk for ischemic necrosis from impaired vascular perfusion. The third area is the zone of hyperemia, in which there is minimal cellular injury and increased blood flow from local vasodilation [1].

Thermal burn injuries are staged on the basis of the depth of injury and the %TBSA involved. First-degree burns involve only the epidermis. Second-degree burns extend below the epidermis to the superficial or deep dermis. Third-degree (full-thickness) burns destroy the overlying dermis and epidermis, down to the level of the subcutaneous tissues. A feature of third-degree burns is the absence of pain due to the complete destruction of cutaneous sensory nerve endings in the dermis [1].

Chemical burns are caused by reactive chemicals such as strong acids or bases, oxidizing agents or corrosive substances [2]. Chemical burns may introduce physiologic concerns unique to the particular agent, such as hypocalcemia with hydrofluoric acid exposure due to the intracellular chelation of calcium. Poison control centers may be a helpful source of information on the care of specific agents causing chemical burns.

Systemic effects of burns generally proceed in two distinct phases, with important implications on pharmacotherapy [3]. The initial 48 hours following injury are characterized by local vasodilation and increased capillary permeability allowing albumin to leak into the interstitial space. Intravascular fluid follows the albumin to maintain neutrality of osmotic forces, and the fluid volume in the interstitial compartment can double. For this reason, burns often cause hypovolemic shock and circulatory failure requiring aggressive fluid resuscitation and secondary organ damage related to hypoperfusion. Thereafter, patients who have been adequately resuscitated with intravenous fluids become hypermetabolic, reflecting the influence of a cascade of inflammatory substances released by dead and dying tissues. Hemodynamic findings can mimic septic shock, with increased cardiac contractility, increased cardiac output, and decreased systemic vascular resistance.

Treatment

Ideally, antibacterial therapies should be selected on the basis of demonstrated antimicrobial susceptibilities and minimal inhibitory concentrations of proven or suspected pathogens isolated in culture, in relation to achievable drug concentrations in burned skin for the selected agent. Empiric therapies should follow the burn unit's antibiogram, which may differ from that of other hospital wards, as intensive care units (ICUs) offer a unique micro-biological niche utilized to great effect by some pathogenic organisms [2]. Empiric therapy should target more viru-lent organisms with established mortality risk, such as *Klebsiella pneumoniae*, *Pseudomonas aeruginosa*, and *Staphylococcus aureus* [3]. Consultation with medical per-sonnel skilled in clinical microbiology and management of infectious diseases may be helpful.

Difficulty in diagnosis of invasive fungal infection can lead to a desire for empiric or preemptive therapy with antifungal agents, such as amphotericin B. *Aspergillus* spp. are generally susceptible to this agent, with the notable exception of *Aspergillus terreus*. Voriconazole has activity against this species, but introduces difficulties with other hepatically metabolized drugs. Amphotericin B has been historically viewed as a nephrotoxic agent, although this toxicity may be reduced with more modern liposomal preparations. Regardless, antifungal therapy may be prob-lematic in patients with renal or hepatic compromise, or who require treatment with other interacting agents.

Systemic Therapy

Conventional antimicrobial doses recommended for non-burned patients may be inadequate for burned patients. This is due to the radical alterations in the physiology of burn patients, as described above. In the initial phase (within 48 hours of injury), the drug distribution is slowed and renal clearance may be reduced if renal function has been compromised [5].

In the hypermetabolic phase (after 48 hours), high cardiac output and low systemic vascular resistance cause blood flow to the liver and kidneys to increase, which in turn may accelerate pharmaceutical clearance. It is well established that aminoglycoside clearance is greatly increased in burn patients, and substantially increased doses are required to achieve target peak levels. Hepatic synthesis of acute-phase reactant proteins is increased, which may decrease the free fraction of protein-bound pharmaceuticals. The pharmacokinetic effects are difficult to predict in burn patients during the hypermetabolic phase, due to the variable individual responses to burn injury. Necessary interventions such as dialysis or limb amputation can further complicate the antimicrobial dose selection [5]. Therefore, drug levels should be uti-lized whenever available. Unfortunately, drug levels are not routinely available in clinical practice for the majority of antimicrobial agents. Furthermore, studies detailing the impact of various dialysis modalities are lacking for many antimicrobial agents in burn patients. Treatment regimens should be considered in the context of anticipated drug–drug interactions with other required therapies.

Topical Agents

Topical antimicrobials have been shown to improve mor-tality in burn patients by decreasing the bacterial burden growing on the eschar [1]. Silver-containing compounds are the most commonly used, with several preparations that differ primarily in their degree of eschar penetration and side effects. Silver atoms interact with thiol groups in key enzymes to poison the biochemical respiratory path-ways of bacteria. Silver compounds can inhibit wound healing through DNA binding, and caution is advised when applying to healing wounds. It is important to note that topical agents can be associated with systemic side effects.

Mafenide (silver sulfamylon) is a topical sulfonamide agent active against Gram negative bacteria, which diffuses freely into the eschar [1]. It is available as a 10% cream, or a 5% solution. The cream is applied twice daily and left uncovered, whereas the solution is applied as a saturated gauze dressing three times daily. It is metabolized to an inhibitor of carbonic anhydrase (*p*-carboxybenzene-sulfonamide), which may cause metabolic acidosis. Appli-cation of mafenide may cause pain.

Silver nitrate is a broad-spectrum bacteriostatic agent with activity against Gram positive and Gram negative bacteria and *Candida* species [1]. Eschar penetration is poor. Drawbacks include oxidation to a black color, which can cause permanent black staining of the patient's imme-diate surroundings. It also obscures visual monitoring of the wound bed for signs of infection, and leaching of cationic electrolytes across the burn wound can cause hyponatremia, hypokalemia, hypocalcemia, and hypo-magnesemia. Electrolytes should therefore be monitored when silver nitrate is used. It is applied in thick layers and covered by mesh gauze to prevent desiccation. Dressings are generally changed twice daily.

Silver sulfadiazine is bactericidal against Gram positive and Gram negative bacteria and *Candida* species [1]. The silver ion binds to nucleic acids, releasing the sulfadi-azine moiety, which interferes with bacterial metabolic pathways. However, its effectiveness may be limited as it does not diffuse beyond the surface epithelium and thus it has poor penetration into the eschar. Leukopenia is the primary side effect of concern, but may not preclude treatment if it develops.

Various nanocrystalline silver dressings are commer-cially available. These dressings are composed of a mesh backing to which crystallized silver coating is applied in a time-release formulation [1]. This provides a longer life span on the wound, reducing the number of dressing changes and the associated mechanical trauma. The silver crystals leach into the wound and become ionic silver.

Their activity is similar to silver nitrate, and the wound is obscured by the dressing and is stained black. However because the silver is adherent to the dressing, it is less likely to stain the surrounding environment. Significant systemic side effects are absent.

Other topical therapies, such as subeschar clysis (direct injection of antimicrobial agents beneath the eschar) date from the pre-escharotomy era, and do not represent standard-of-care practice today. Various antifungal agents are available as topical formulations for direct application onto infected wounds, but data supporting the effectiveness of this approach are lacking.

Surgical Treatments

Surgery is a critical component of burn wound management [2]. The eschar is a moist, avascular, and protein-rich environment that is ideal for the growth of microbes. Without debridement, dead tissue can become a source of persistent and sustained burn wound sepsis. Regional amputation should be considered for extremities harboring deep infections and/or severe vascular compromise limiting the delivery of antimicrobials to infected tissues. Skin grafting and the use of artificial skin materials to cover open burn wounds may reduce infections by reducing the degree of microbial colonization in the wound.

Evaluation and Assessment

Establishing a diagnosis of infection in the burn wound can be exceedingly difficult [2]. If the burn is less severe and localized to a small area surrounded by unaffected skin, the classic signs of inflammation (calor, rubor, dolor, and tumor) developing in the adjacent non-burned skin may be helpful clues. In more severe burns with extensive tissue damage over large areas of the body, the normal physiologic response to cutaneous infection is altered, and these indicators of inflammation may be absent in burned skin.

Inspection of the wound may reveal features concerning for infection: pain, erythema, unexpected change in color, appearance and depth, systemic changes, and premature separation of the burn eschar. _P. aeruginosa_ can produce yellow–green exudates in the wound, but invasive infection with this organism is indicated by purple–black or punched-out areas. Infections with _Candida_ species may produce small purulent papules, and _Aspergillus_ species may look grossly like gray–brown plaques, or whitish fuzz growing on the surface of devitalized skin. In each of these cases, distinguishing colonization from invasive infection is problematic.

Systemic signs of infection such as WBC count, temperature, respiratory rate, and heart rate have poor sensitivity and specificity for detecting infection in burn patients due to the massive metabolic disturbances that occur with higher TBSA and deeper burns [3]. These findings are often present in burned patients in the absence of infection, as cellular damage stimulates the release of pro-inflammatory cytokines, driving the systemic inflammatory response syndrome (SIRS). Inflammatory markers such as C-reactive protein, procalcitonin, and cytokines are not specific for identifying infection in this population. Criteria for diagnosis of wound infection have been established by the American Burn Association (Table 1) [4].

Microbiological investigations include cultures of surface swabs, biopsy specimens, escharotomy specimens, and blood. Surface cultures from swabs or tissue do not discriminate between colonizing and pathogenic organisms, but may be helpful in recovering potential pathogens for antimicrobial susceptibility testing [1]. Wounds typically become colonized with bacteria within 48 hours of injury even in the absence of infection. Colonizing organisms may originate from sweat glands and hair follicles at the time of injury, or may be introduced from the hospital environment or by the hands of health care providers. Quantitative cultures have generally poor predictive

Burn Skin Infection. Table 1 American burn association criteria for diagnosis of burn wound infection

Syndrome	Criteria
Wound colonization	Bacteria on wound surface at low concentration ($<10^5$ bacteria/g tissue); no tissue invasion
Wound infection	Bacteria in the wound and eschar at high concentration ($>10^5$ bacteria/g tissue); no invasive infection
Invasive infection	Pathogens in burn wound at a sufficient concentration (frequently $>10^5$ bacteria/g tissue), depth, and surface area to cause suppurative separation of eschar or graft loss, invasion of adjacent unburned tissue, or sepsis
Cellulitis	Bacteria present in wound and/or wound eschar at high concentration ($>10^5$ bacteria/g tissue) with erythema, induration, warmth, and/or tenderness in surrounding tissue
Necrotizing infection/fasciitis	Aggressive invasive infection with involvement below the skin resulting in tissue necrosis

value for infection and the development of burn wound sepsis.

Blood cultures are more sensitive than surface cultures for invasive infection, but do not distinguish from other anatomic sites of origin, such as the lungs. While clearly desirable, detecting infection once it has reached the bloodstream misses the window of opportunity for early pharmacologic intervention to prevent a progression to sepsis. Invasive burn wound infection may therefore be distinguished from colonization only retrospectively. In addition, some frequent colonizers of wounds, such as *Aspergillus* species, do not readily grow in blood culture even when invasive. Recently, new approaches have been proposed involving surveillance detection of pathogen-specific products, such as 1,3-β-D-glucan produced by replicating fungi or galactomannan (specific for *Aspergillus* species) secreted during fungal replication. Limitations include assay interference by commonly used antimicrobial agents, the fact that not all fungal organisms produce these chemicals, and such markers are lacking for bacterial organisms.

Tissue histology can be used to observe the depth of organisms in the skin layers, with organisms in deeper layers presumed to indicate invasive infection [2]. Tissue depth as a surrogate marker for invasive infection has not been adequately validated, and the reliance of this method on biopsy specimens makes this approach subject to sampling error. With the exception of some fungi, which have pathognomonic appearances, histologic methods are disadvantaged by their inability to provide a definitive identification of the pathogen or aid in selection of an appropriate therapeutic agent. Sample interpretation requires specialized training in dermatopathology, which may not be available at all centers.

Clinical Syndromes

Burn wound sepsis describes the development of sepsis resulting from invasive infection by organisms originating in the devitalized tissues of the burn wound [1]. As noted above, antecedent prediction of and surveillance for the development of invasion is problematic. Traditional parameters of sepsis are insensitive because they are present in many burn patients without sepsis. The American Burn Association has released criteria for sepsis, which add thrombocytopenia, non-diabetic hyperglycemia, and tube feeding intolerance to the traditional parameters of temperature and cardiopulmonary status [4]. Studies validating this approach are limited.

Burn wound cellulitis describes the spread of infection from the burn wound into surrounding healthy tissues [1]. Clinical indications are erythema extending from the perimeter of a burn wound into surrounding non-burned skin. Localized pain, progressive swelling and erythema, and distal lymphangitis along the path of draining lymphatic channels may be present.

Burn wound impetigo is a secondary infection of re-epithelialized skin, such as that healing by secondary intention, or grafted skin [1]. The pathogenic organisms are primarily *Staphylococcus* and *Streptococcus* species, just as in impetigo involving non-burned skin.

Surgical wound infections occur at sites of surgical debridement or escharotomy, similar to other surgical site infections. Erythema in adjacent normal skin, overt culture-positive purulence, and loss of synthetic or autologous overlying skin grafts may be indications of surgical burn wound infection.

Infection Control

ICUs are a unique environmental niche utilized to great effect by some organisms. *Acinetobacter baumannii*, *Enterobacter cloacae*, *Klebsiella pneumoniae*, and *P. aeruginosa* are common Gram negative species that thrive in this environment, and can be associated with disease outbreaks. These organisms have a propensity to develop resistance to multiple antimicrobials, can persist on environmental surfaces for long periods of time, and can be transmitted to uninfected patients on the hands of health care workers or patient care equipment, such as x-ray film cassettes. Strict adherence to infection control measures, such as contact precautions using full gown and gloves with every patient contact, may be necessary to prevent nosocomial infection outbreaks in burn and other ICUs. Unnecessary traffic should be minimized in the burn unit to limit the spread of these organisms to other areas of the hospital. Individual nursing units, isolation rooms, strict hand-washing and use of personal protective equipment, single-patient monitoring equipment, and patient cohorting for nursing care are all strategies that should be considered to limit the spread of pathogens. Surveillance for other resistant pathogens such as MRSA and VRE should be considered as well. Infection control personnel should be involved in monitoring the organisms and antibiograms of pathogens arising from patients in the burn ICU [2, 3].

After-care

Burn injuries can cause prolonged hospitalization and major debility. Physical and occupational rehabilitation are usually required [2]. Reconstructive surgery may be considered on the basis of cosmetic or functional concerns, within the restrictions imposed by the anatomy of affected areas. Burn patients should be screened for psychological sequelae of the inciting traumatic episode, such as the post-traumatic stress disorder, and referred for psychiatric care if appropriate. Physical deformity resulting from burn scars may also heavily impact patients' mental and emotional wellness.

Prognosis

The primary predictors of mortality from burn injury are extremes of age, %TBSA, presence of full thickness burns, and inhalational injury. Mortality has decreased sharply over the past 40 years, attributable to improvements in shock resuscitation, airway and ventilatory management, nutrition, wound care, and infection control practices. The advent of multidrug resistance among more virulent bacteria, such as *Klebsiella* spp., *Enterobacter* spp., and *P. aeruginosa*, has added an additional challenge to the care of the burn patient. Other individual and institutional factors, such as the availability of adequate rehabilitative care, may impact the degree of recovery attainable by the burn patient.

References

1. Church D, Elsayed S, Ried O et al (2006) Burn wound infections. Clin Microbiol Rev 19:403–434
2. Murray CK, Hospenthal DR (2008) Burn wound infections. Emedicine website chapter. http://emedicine.medscape.com. Updated 16 Apr 2008
3. Murray CK (2011) Burns. In: Mandell GL, Bennett JE, Dolin R (eds) Mandell, Douglas and Bennett's principles and practice of infectious diseases, 7th edn. Elsevier, Philadelphia, pp 3905–3909
4. Greenhalgh DG, Saffle JR, Holmes JH et al (2007) American burn association consensus conference to define sepsis and infection in burns. J Burn Care Res 28(6):776–790
5. Blanchet B, Jullien V, Vinsonneau C et al (2008) Influence of pharmacokinetics and pharmacodynamics of drugs used in the care of burn patients. Clin Pharmacokinet 47:635–654

Burn Wound Cellulitis

▶ Burn Skin Infection

Burn Wound Impetigo

▶ Burn Skin Infection

Burn Wound Infection

ARTHUR SANFORD, RICHARD L. GAMELLI
Stritch School of Medicine, Loyola University Medical Center, Maywood, IL, USA

Synonyms

Burn wound sepsis

Definition

Wound colonization is where bacteria are present on the wound surface at low concentrations. There is no invasive infection.

Wound infection is when bacteria are present in the wound and wound eschar at high concentrations. There is no invasive infection.

Invasive burn wound infection occurs when the presence of pathogens in a burn wound is at concentrations sufficient in conjunction with depth, surface area involved and age of patient to cause separation of eschar or graft loss, invasion of adjacent unburned tissue or cause the systemic response of sepsis syndrome. Pathogens are present in the wound at high concentrations. Invasion or destruction of unburned skin/tissue due to an invasive infection may occur with or without sepsis. Many burn wound invasive infections, however, are life threatening and need urgent treatment (usually wound excision).

Cellulitis indicates bacteria present in the wound and/or wound eschar at high concentrations and examination of surrounding tissue reveals advancing erythema, induration, warmth, tenderness. Simple redness around the wound may not require treatment.

Necrotizing soft tissue infection/Necrotizing fasciitis is an aggressive, invasive infection with underlying and aggressive tissue necrosis [1].

Treatment

Effective burn wound management is a combination of excision when appropriate, and minimizing the complications of wounds and the possibility of infection. Infection remains a significant problem until the integrity of the skin, lungs, and gut can be restored and resolution of post burn immunosuppression occurs. Topical antimicrobial therapy is used to control localized infection at the wound site, but will not be effective if significant amounts of devitalized tissue remain. Common topical antimicrobials are listed in Table 1 along with their common side effects.

Burn Wound Infection. Table 1 Common topical antimicrobials

Topical agent	Unique property
Silvadene	Painless to apply, poor penetration of eschar
Sulfamylon	Metabolic acidosis, penetrates eschar
Polymyxin	Control of wound colonization, poor penetration
Silver nitrate	Hyponatremia, surface staining
Nystatin powder	Antifungal
Dakin's solution	Quickly inactivated
Acticoat	Convenient, stable for several days

Evaluation/Assessment

Burn wound sepsis is sometimes difficult to assess in the face of the ongoing hypermetabolism. It is a systemic response to the infected burn wound. The challenge is in determining what the normal hypermetabolic response to a burn is and when the condition is pathologic as in burn wound sepsis. These changes, such as increases in temperature, heart rate, leucocytosis, respiratory rate, and blood pressure, would, by current guidelines to define sepsis, result in the diagnosis in virtually all major burn injuries. The burn sepsis definition must therefore distinguish changes in patient status as the result of infection due to a microbial entity from the alterations secondary to the burn injury itself. Burn wound related sepsis is characterized by five signs: obtundation, hyperventilation, hyperglycemia, thrombocytopenia, and enteral feeding intolerance (as evidenced by diarrhea, ileus, or elevated gastric residuals).

All skin surfaces and wounds have bacteria present. The presence of bacteria alone does not indicate an infection. The patient/bacterial interaction is a more important factor than the presence of bacteria. The wound needs constant surveillance since the major method of detecting an infection is from observing a significant change in the wound appearance. Quantitative wound cultures are useful for surveillance and colony counts of greater than 1×10^5 organisms/gm tissue indicates a wound at risk for invasion. This is best confirmed by histologic examination of a wound biopsy where actual invasion of viable tissue by pathogens is seen. The changes may be subtle but any change should prompt further investigation. The wound may change color, have increased exudate, have increased pain, or appear to increase in depth. The classic definition suggests that there is an early separation of the burn eschar. An eschar is the tough coagulated protein covering a deep burn. Superficial burns develop a dry exudate that forms from fibrin, cellular debris, and the residue of topical antimicrobial agents. These are sometimes called pseudoeschar. The normal process of eschar separation is the result of bacteria digestion of nonviable tissue away from the underlying viable tissue. Today, early separation is rare because most burn surgeons excise a deep burn followed by skin grafting long before bacterial invasion. A frequent burn wound colonizer, *Pseudomonas aeruginosa*, tends to produce a yellow/green exudate. This is not an invasive infection. Invasive *Pseudomonas* is a surgical emergency. This invasive infection produces purple–black and "punched-out" areas of the wound classically described as ecthyma gangrenosum. The invasion frequently destroys both deep and superficial wounds. Split-thickness donor sites and even unwounded skin are sometimes involved. Treatment involves both systemic culture directed antibiotics and injection (clysis) of antibiotics beneath the wound. Most importantly, these wounds need aggressive surgical debridement and excision.

Other pathogens in addition to bacteria can cause disease. Yeast and molds are significant causes of burn wound invasion. In a superficial wound, Candida may present with small papules of purulence. Aspergillus is manifested as gray–brown plaques in a liquefied wound. Herpes simplex is a not uncommon cause of breakdown in a superficial wound where it is characterized by punched-out lesions in normal tissue or in the wound.

Systemic antibiotics are indicated for perioperative coverage of suspected wound pathogens and gut flora and need not be continued after dressings are taken down and healed wounds are exposed. Oral prophylaxis with antifungals has been shown to reduce the incidence of fungal wound infections.

Effectiveness

Early and prompt treatment of the septic wound source can prevent an overwhelming sepsis in the patient. A study by Ramzy et al. [2] demonstrated a better correlation with wound-cultured organisms than central bronchial cultures when post mortem lung abscesses were cultured. The implication is that undertreated wounds lead to a hematogenous spread of organisms.

Pharmacoeconomics

Efficiency of burn care is measured by length of stay, and usually correlated with body surface area burned. The general estimate is for 1 day of hospital stay for each percent body surface area burned (e.g., a 30% total body surface area burn would be expected to remain in hospital for 1 month). This crude estimate does not include correlation with adverse events such as a burn wound infection, although the establishment of a national burn database (TRACS) will provide a means to investigate the cost of this complication.

Prognosis

The presence of a septic wound has been found to increase the incidence of mortality in massively burned children by two to three times [3]. This finding highlights the importance of early recognition and treatment of burn wound infection.

Cross-References

▶ Burns Infections
▶ Burn Skin Infection

References

1. Greenhalgh DG, Saffle JR et al (2007) American Burn Association consensus conference to define sepsis and infection in burns. J Burn Care Res 28(6):776–790
2. Ramzy PI, Jeschke MG et al (2003) Correlation of bronchoalveolar lavage with radiographic evidence of pneumonia in thermally injured children. J Burn Care Rehabil 24(6):382–385
3. Wolf S et al (1997) Enteral feeding intolerance: an indicator of sepsis-associated mortality in burned children. Arch Surg 132 (12):1310–1314

Burn Wound Sepsis

▶ Burn Skin Infection
▶ Burn Wound Infection
▶ Burns, Sepsis

"Burning Hands" Syndrome

▶ Central Spinal Cord Syndrome

Burns Infections

Jessie S. Glasser[1], Clinton K. Murray[2]
[1]Department of Medicine, Brooke Army Medical Center, Fort Sam Houston, TX, USA
[2]Department of Medicine, San Antonio Military Medical Center, Fort Sam Houston, TX, USA

Synonyms

Burn sepsis; Burn wound infection; Ventilator-associated pneumonia

Definition

Any infection that occurs in a burn patient can be defined as a burn infection. However, many reviews focus on burn wound infection and avoid focusing on the entire burn patient. There is clear overlap between the clinical presentation associated with the burn injury itself and the classic parameters used to raise suspicion for a new infection. As a result, burn infections can be more challenging to diagnose than their counterparts in non-burn patients because signs such as fever, tachycardia, and leukocytosis, which are used in the non-burn definition for systemic inflammatory response syndrome (SIRS) and sepsis, are often present in uninfected burn patients due to their extensive wounds, hypermetabolic state, and chronic exposure to inflammatory mediators, but may not always be indicative of an infection in this group [1]. Conversely, infection can occur in the absence of the above signs.

The most common sites of infection are the bloodstream, lungs, wound, and urinary tract [2]. Burn patients are at increased risk of pneumonia with concomitant inhalational injury. Ventilator-associated pneumonia is also common in burn patients and is associated with increased mortality, especially in the setting of inhalational injury. Many of the infections are nosocomial, hence the need for strict infection control in burn centers. Burn units have the highest rates of urinary catheter–associated urinary tract infections, ventilator-associated pneumonias, and central line–associated bloodstream infections as compared to other units. Endocarditis may also occur in burn patients.

Epidemiology

Each year, 450,000 people are treated for burn injuries in the United States, with approximately 3,500 deaths annually from both residential fires and motor vehicle/aircraft crashes and electrical and chemical burns. Nearly 75% of these deaths occur at the scene of the incident or during transport. More than 55% of the 45,000 hospitalizations annually for burns are to the approximately 125 hospitals with specialized burn centers. Thirty-eight percent of admissions exceed 10% total body surface area (TBSA) burned and most include burns of the face, hands, and feet. Seventy percent of patients admitted to burn centers are male and more than half are Caucasian [3].

Mortality has been decreasing with a survival rate of 94% among all admissions to burn centers. Increased mortality risk is associated with TBSA burned, inhalational injury, age, and percentage of full-thickness burns. Improvements in the morbidity and mortality associated with burns can be attributed to advances in burn care including initial resuscitation, nutritional support, ventilator management, burn wound care, and strict infection control strategies [2, 4].

If patients survive the initial burn and resuscitative phase, infections are the cause of mortality in 75% of deaths in patients with more than 40% TBSA burned, with six of the top ten complications also being infectious to include 4.6% of patients with pneumonia, 2.7% with septicemia, 2.6% with cellulitis/traumatic injury, 2.2% with wound infection, 2% other infection, and 1.4% with line infection. Urinary tract infections are more common in older patients. Wound infections and cellulitis are more common in burn injuries related to scalding and contact with hot objects. Patients who sustain burns during military operations are more likely to die from infectious etiologies than those not burned in military operations, who are often older with preexisting comorbidities and are at increased risk for cardiovascular and renal complications in addition to infections [4].

Microbiology

Bacteria, fungi, and viruses can all cause burn infections [2]. They may come from exogenous or endogenous sources. Bacteria that cause burn infections commonly include the gram-negative bacteria *Pseudomonas aeruginosa*, *Klebsiella pneumoniae*, and *Acinetobacter baumannii-calcoaceticus* (ABC) complex, and the gram-positive methicillin-resistant *Staphylococcus aureus* (MRSA) [2]. *K. pneumoniae* and *P. aeruginosa* are associated with increased mortality with *S. aureus* having less impact on mortality. ABC is frequently isolated but has lower virulence than the other commonly isolated gram-negative bacteria. Each individual burn unit has its own resistance pattern, which may differ from other units in the same hospital and from other burn units in different hospitals. Antimicrobial resistance is increasing in burn units, impacting the choice of empiric antibiotic coverage and

making treatment of these organisms more challenging, particularly during prolonged hospitalizations. Use of an individual unit's antibiogram is useful when determining appropriate empiric coverage in an acutely ill burn patient.

Fungal organisms may also cause burn infections, in particular *Candida* species, *Aspergillus* species, and other molds. These organisms contribute to increased mortality in particular in patients with 30–60% TBSA burns [2]. The risk of isolating fungal elements increases over time after the burn injury, with one study stating that fungal invasion was detected on average 16 days after the initial burns. Fungi mainly cause wound infections and pulmonary infections. Burn patients are among the highest risk for invasive fungal infections due to their underlying immune dysfunction, presence of a portal of entry through burn wounds, and use of broad-spectrum antibacterial agents. Urinary catheters, central lines, and total parenteral nutrition are also associated with fungal infections. Fungal pathogens, in particular those with *Aspergillus*-like histology, are responsible for increased mortality in this population. Though *Candida* may be the most common organism cultured, its associated mortality rate is lower than for the molds. A culture from any site positive for mold or *Aspergillus* is strongly predictive of death, increasing the odds ratio nearly 12-fold.

Viruses play an unclear role in burn infections. Viral infections in this population can be due to reactivation or primary infection and are generally due to herpesviruses: cytomegalovirus (CMV), herpes simplex virus (HSV), and varicella-zoster virus (VZV) [2]. Varicella has been described in burned children and may result in wound related complications to include delays in healing as well as varicella pneumonitis. The cases described are of primary varicella after the patient was exposed to an index case highlighting the need for good infection control and isolation of known cases. HSV and CMV have also been described in burned children and are thought to be generally endogenous, likely due to reactivation with the impaired cell-mediated immunity found in large burns. Primary infection with CMV has occurred with blood products and allografted skin. Murine studies have shown that CMV infection may decrease the inflammatory response and consequently decrease resistance to bacterial infection resulting in higher mortality in mice infected with CMV and bacteria than with bacteria alone. Some human studies have demonstrated that CMV infection contributes to a higher rate of episodes of bacterial sepsis; however, currently no increased mortality is associated with CMV infections in burned humans. HSV may be reactivated by fever, which is a common finding in burn patients, as well as due to the depressed cell-mediated immunity in this population. Clinical manifestations include asymptomatic shedding, eruption of vesicles (usually within the margins of healing partial-thickness wounds), prolonged fever, and rarely systemic dissemination. HSV superinfection of burn wounds has been described. Though they may result in delay in wound healing, they do heal spontaneously and otherwise have no effect on outcomes. As with CMV, infection with HSV may predispose to bacterial sepsis, but does not correlate with increased mortality in this group.

Pathophysiology

The skin is the largest organ in the body and is responsible for many vital functions to include serving as the body's first line of defense against infection by acting as a physical barrier. When this barrier is damaged, pathogens can directly enter the body, which may result in infection [5]. In addition, burns suppress both innate and adaptive immune responses. For the innate immune response, natural killer (NK) cells are widely distributed throughout the body and migrate to sites of inflammation. They produce IFN-γ in response to microbial threats but not in response to burn inflammation; thus there is transient IFN-γ deficiency with burns, in effect, a clinical immune paralysis, which may result in the host being more susceptible to infectious complications and sepsis. This deficiency may remain for up to 40 days post burn. T-cell immunity (cell-mediated immunity) is also suppressed after burns, for up to a month after the burn injury. Loss of skin tissue also signals recruitment of polymorphonuclear neutrophils (PMNs) and monocytes initially, also as part of the innate response, and later B-cells and T-cells [5]. The phagocytic cells help in controlling bacterial colonization and preventing invasive wound infections. In full-thickness burns, where keratinocyte progenitors are lost, wound healing will not occur without skin grafting [5]. However in partial-thickness burns, the wound site can heal with help from the phagocytic cells unless there is an infection present to damage the underlying tissue.

Burns result in an inflammatory state with enhanced production of various cytokines and chemokines, which results in fever, leukocytosis, tachypnea, and increased vascular permeability. The hypermetabolic state associated with burns may also result in immunodeficiency which can also result in impaired wound healing and sepsis. Early excision of the burn eschar and closure of the wounds attenuates this response, as does nutritional support.

Risk factors for pneumonia in burn patients include their relative immunosuppression, inhalational injury resulting in dysfunctional ciliary movement which impairs clearance of secretions, acute lung injury resulting in pulmonary inflammatory activation, and leakage of nutrient-rich plasma into the lung parenchyma.

Treatment

Treatment should be focused on the site of infection and causative pathogen. Empiric therapy should be based on the individual burn unit's antibiogram since resistance profiles can vary from other units within the same hospital and from other hospitals. Empiric antibiotics should also be directed at common pathogens with high associated mortality such as *Klebsiella pneumoniae* and *Pseudomonas aeruginosa*. In hospitals with a high rate of extended spectrum beta-lactamase (ESBL)-producing organisms, an antipseudomonal carbapenem is reasonable empiric therapy for the gram-negatives. Vancomycin is often used for empiric coverage for *S. aureus* and other gram-positive bacteria given the high rates of MRSA.

Given the hypermetabolic state of burn patients, pharmacokinetics of antimicrobial agents in burn patients are different from unburned patients [2]. This variability has been noted with vancomycin, aminoglycosides, carbapenems, and cephalosporins. With vancomycin, there is an increase in total clearance with a decreased elimination half-life. Similarly, aminoglycosides are cleared more rapidly in burn patients requiring higher doses than usual to attain goal peaks and troughs. Consequently it is important to check drug levels and closely monitor renal function. In addition, use of hemodialysis including continuous renal replacement therapy needs to be factored in when choosing and dosing antibiotics. Aerosolized antibiotics are sometimes used in burn patients with pneumonia. No clear benefit or harm has been shown from this [2].

The treatment of fungal infections also depends on identifying the causative organism and site of infection. Antifungal options include azoles (such as fluconazole, voriconazole, and posaconazole), echinocandins (such as anidulafungin, micafungin, caspofungin), and amphotericin B (conventional or liposomal). All fungi are not susceptible to amphotericin B, which was the traditional first-line antifungal agent. Currently, selection of antifungal agent depends on the likely fungal pathogen, toxicity, and drug interactions. *Candida glabrata* and *Candida krusei* are resistant to fluconazole. Some burn units have noted the presence of *Aspergillus terreus*, which has inherent resistance to amphotericin B, so voriconazole is often used for empiric coverage of suspected *Aspergillus* infections, despite its many drug–drug interactions. Early antifungal therapy for empiric or preemptive treatment of fungal infections is most beneficial in patients with 30–60% TBSA burned since it is in this population where early therapy may prevent invasive infection and reduce morbidity and mortality [2]. An ophthalmologic exam is necessary for patients with candidemia to evaluate for candidal endophthalmitis since this affects both the outcome and the duration of antifungal therapy.

Surgical treatment is crucial in the prevention and treatment of infections [2]. Early excision of burn eschar, within 5 days of the initial burn injury, is associated with an improved mortality rate since the eschar is an avascular environment ideal for growth of bacteria and difficult for immune cells to reach along with systemic antibiotic therapy. It is also important to cover the burn area with grafts to provide a wound barrier, reduce wound microbial colonization, and prevent evaporative loss, though grafts can also develop infections. Early excision and coverage is also important in the prevention of invasive fungal wound infections especially given the lack of adequate topical antifungal therapies once an invasive fungal wound infection has taken hold.

Topical antimicrobial therapies are generally used in the prevention of burn wound infection and include silver nitrate, silver sulfadiazene, mafenide acetate, and silver-impregnated dressings. Each antimicrobial agent covers a different spectrum of microbes and comes with its own risks and benefits [2].

Acyclovir has been used in children with >20% TBSA burns and VZV infections. Again, the need for strict infection control to prevent cross-infection of other patients is crucial. This isolation should be continued throughout the VZV incubation period of 8–21 days. With more widespread varicella vaccination, herd immunity should increase and fewer children should be at risk. Given the minimal attributable mortality to CMV at this time, there is no specific recommendation for treating with ganciclovir, foscarnet, or cidofovir for CMV-infected burn patients. In CMV seronegative burn patients, consideration of transfusion of seronegative or leukocyte-depleted blood products could be given, though this remains controversial. Topical or systemic acyclovir is generally recommended for HSV infections to avoid a delay in wound healing and to avoid disseminated disease in this immunosuppressed population. Prophylactic acyclovir for seropositive patients at risk for reactivation is not recommended. Surgery should be avoided until the vesicles are dried up and resolving.

Prevention

Strict infection control in burn units is crucial in the prevention of nosocomial infections and reduction in infection-related morbidity and mortality [2]. Individual patient rooms with anterooms or individual doors are necessary and dedicated operating rooms and facilities may help to minimize transmission. Providers should wear full gown and gloves for all patient contact and hand washing must be enforced. Surveillance and aggressive infection control for multidrug-resistant organisms is necessary.

Catheter-related bloodstream infections are associated with the number of lines placed and total number of central line days, but the site of insertion (upper vs. lower) has not been shown to affect infection rates [2]. It is preferable to distance the insertion site from the burned area if possible. It is unknown whether changing a line over a guide-wire is comparable to inserting a new line at a new site. More frequent line changes may be associated with fewer line infections as well. Other invasive measures including endotracheal intubation and urinary catheterization have been shown to be associated with nosocomial infections as well, so use of invasive devices should be avoided as much as possible.

Other burn patient care may also play a role in preventing infections. Selective gut decontamination to decrease pneumonia risk may be effective; further data are needed [2, 4]. The gastrointestinal tract is also involved in the immune response and risk of infection may increase with bacterial translocation in the gut. Enteral nutrition may be helpful in the prevention of bowel complications. Early nutritional support, within 24–72 h after initial resuscitation, may blunt the hypermetabolic response to burn injury [2, 4, 6]. It is unclear at this time whether this actually reduces infection risk. Feeds should be enteral if possible, and are generally continuous. The content of the feeds to include the type of feeds and supplements such as iron, zinc, and vitamins C and E varies from center to center [6]. Medications that may manipulate the hypermetabolic response including beta blockers such as propranolol and metabolic stimulants such as insulin and oxandrolone are often used in burn centers. More data are needed on their effectiveness. Intensive glycemic control is described in the Burn Sepsis chapter.

Evaluation/Assessment

As noted above, the standard definitions of SIRS and sepsis do not apply in burn patients. Patients with extensive burns have baseline tachycardia and tachypnea with baseline temperature reset to 38.5°C even without the presence of infection. Therefore, the term SIRS is not used in burn patients. The American Burn Association (ABA) has defined criteria for sepsis in this population, which can be used to raise concern for the onset of infection and trigger further evaluation (see Burn Sepsis chapter) [1]. Biochemical inflammatory markers including leukocyte count, erythrocyte sedimentation rate, C-reactive protein, and neutrophil count have not been shown to be helpful in distinguishing between septic and non-septic patients in this population [2]. Pro-calcitonin is under evaluation, but at this point does not have a clear role in the clinical management of burn patients.

Bacterial bloodstream infections are diagnosed using the standard analysis of pathogen, clinical syndrome, and number of positive blood cultures [2]. The quantity of blood and type of bottles required is unclear at this time. Blood cultures positive for fungal organisms are predictive of invasive fungal burn wound infections. Fungemia can also be a primary infection, especially when associated with central venous catheters.

Clinical diagnosis of pneumonia may be difficult in burn patients and quantitative cultures from bronchoalveolar lavage are being used more to confirm the diagnosis and avoid unnecessary antibiotic treatment. To diagnose pneumonia, two or more of the following are needed: a new or persistent infiltrate, consolidation, or cavitation on chest x-ray (CXR), sepsis, or a recent change in sputum or purulence in the sputum. The diagnosis is confirmed in patients with the appropriate clinical syndrome plus microbiological confirmation, probable in a patient with the appropriate clinical syndrome without microbiological confirmation, and possible in a patient with an abnormal CXR with low or moderate clinical suspicion but with microbiologic confirmation [1, 2]. Quantitative microbiologic criteria are tracheal aspirate with $\geq 10^5$ organisms, bronchoalveolar lavage with $\geq 10^4$ organisms, or protected bronchial brush with $\geq 10^3$ organisms [1].

Burn patients also experience purulent tracheobronchitis, which consists of fever and increased sputum production without CXR abnormalities or purulent discharge coating the trachea during bronchoscopy. Tracheobronchitis may be associated with increased risk of prolonged mechanical ventilation so may still be treated with antibiotics.

Wound infections are diagnosed by ABA criteria. Concerning findings include changes in the eschar appearance including development of dark brown, black, or violaceous discoloration, edema at the wound margin, or rapid eschar separation [2]. P. aeruginosa colonization can produce yellow-green exudates in the wound but invasive infection presents with purple-black or punched-out areas. Infections with Aspergillus species can look like white fuzz growing on the surface of burned skin or like gray-brown plaques. The yield from cultures from swabs or biopsies is limited since it may not distinguish between colonization and invasive infection. Histology is used

in some burn centers and can help distinguish colonization from invasion into viable tissue, but it does not always correlate with culture results. The use of the galactomannan assay for detection of Aspergillus species and 1,3-β-D-glucan for detection of replicating fungi has not been fully evaluated in this population and may be limited by false positives related to commonly used antimicrobial agents as well as false negatives, since not all fungi produce these chemicals.

Effectiveness
The prolonged hospitalizations required for the treatment of severe burns place patients at risk of recurrent infections. While initial therapy is often effective, it may also select for different pathogens, as illustrated by the later onset of fungal infections, as described above. In addition, it may select for multidrug-resistant pathogens making it more challenging to treat subsequent infections.

Pharmacoeconomics
Long hospital stays with repeated courses of antimicrobials for recurrent infections result not only in direct costs (i.e., the cost of the medications and therapies needed to treat the infections) but also in the indirect costs related to the potential fostering of antimicrobial resistance and selecting for new infections, such as fungal infections. These can lead to further increased costs associated with burn hospital care by necessitating use of novel and often expensive antimicrobial therapy. No systemic measure of these indirect costs has been taken but the cost related to burn infections is likely to be quite high.

After-care
Duration of antimicrobial therapy varies depending on the site of infection and the organism being targeted. Broad-spectrum antibiotic therapy should be tailored to the specific organism(s) isolated when culture and susceptibility results are available. Bacterial infections are generally treated for 10–14 days [2]. Once a bacterial infection has been adequately treated, antibiotics should be discontinued to avoid fostering resistance and prevent unnecessary antibiotic toxicity. Invasive fungal infections are generally treated for longer than bacterial infections. Adequate surgical debridement also affects the duration of antifungal therapy. Patients with severe burns remain at risk for recurrent infections as long as they have uncovered/unhealed burn wounds and until their immunosuppression improves. Continued infection control is necessary. If possible, avoidance of unnecessary invasive devices may also be helpful.

Prognosis

Though overall improvements in survival have been made as a result of advances in burn care including initial resuscitation, airway and ventilator management, wound care, and infection control, mortality is still high. After initial resuscitation, death in a burn patient is most likely to be due to infectious causes. For patients with a burn size greater than 40% TBSA, 75% of all deaths are due to infection. Infections due to *K. pneumoniae, P. aeruginosa,* and invasive fungal infections with *Aspergillus* and other molds carry the worst prognosis while infections due to *Staphylococcus aureus, Candida* species, and herpesviruses play less of a role in mortality in the burn population.

References

1. Greenhalgh DG, Saffle JR, Holmes JH et al (2007) American burn association consensus conference to define sepsis and infection in burns. J Burn Care Rehabil 28:776–790
2. Murray CK (2010) Burns. In: Mandell GL, Bennett JE, Dolin R (eds) Mandell, Douglas, and Bennett's principles and practice of infectious diseases. Churchill Livingstone/Elsevier, Philadelphia, pp 3905–3909
3. American Burn Association [Internet]. Available from http://www.ameriburn.org/resources_factsheet.php. Accessed 7 Mar 2011
4. Gomez R, Murray CK, Hospenthal DR, Cancio LC, Renz EM, Holcomb JB, Wade CE (2009) Causes of mortality by autopsy findings of combat casualties and civilian patients admitted to a burn unit. J Am Coll Surg 208:348–354
5. Shankar R, Melstrom KA, Gamelli RL (2007) Inflammation and sepsis: past, present, and the future. J Burn Care Res 28:566–571
6. Wolf SE (2007) Nutrition and metabolism in burns: state of the science, 2007. J Burn Care Res 28:572–576

Burns, Pneumonia

Carlos M. Luna[1], Abelardo Capdevila[2]
[1]Department of Internal Medicine, Hospital de Clinicas, Universidad de Buenos Aires, Banfield, Buenos Aires, Argentina
[2]French Authority For Health, Haute Autorité de santé, Saint-Denis, La Plaine Cedex, France

Synonyms

Acute Respiratory Distress Syndrome (ARDS); Aspiration pneumonia; Bacterial pneumonia; Bronchopneumonia; Community-Acquired Pneumonia (CAP); Inhalation injury; Pneumonia; Ventilator associated

Introduction

Definition

Pneumonia is defined as an inflammatory illness of the lung; the main cause of pneumonia is infection due to bacteria, viruses, fungi, or parasites. Sometimes noninfectious agents, including physical or chemical injury to the lungs may cause pneumonia. Infectious bacterial pneumonia is a major concern in burn patients, but physical or chemical injuries also occur. Bacterial pneumonia results from the invasion of the lung parenchyma; bacteria cause necrosis of epithelial cells, then these pathogens invade the lungs across the injured epithelium and produce toxins that lead to acute epithelial injury and bacterial dissemination. Inflammatory host's response through the defense mechanisms produces cellular infiltration, parenchymal consolidation, and abnormal alveolar filling with fluid (exudates). The most important syndromes of pneumonia that could be found in burns patients include ► ventilator-associated (VAP) and community-acquired pneumonia (CAP); in patients who sustain burn injury in the setting of risk factors for increased oropharyngeal aspiration, aspiration pneumonia could be the mechanism of acquisition of pneumonia. Inhalation injury can produce similar physiological responses as pneumonia and in fact both, inhalation injury and pneumonia happen usually together in the burned patient. Inhalation injury occurs in approximately 20–35% of burn cases requiring admission; it increases the incidence of pneumonia and mortality. The mortality rate of smoke inhalation victims with burns is 30–50% but without burns is less than 10%.

Pneumonia in burns patients concerns principally VAP, has not been specific to burn patients in the literature, however similar principles of management to those used in non-burn patients should be applied. Pneumonia in burns is a pathologic process that happens in the post-resuscitation period (from 2 days to some weeks post-injury), characterized by a hypermetabolic state and increased risk of infection. Risk of VAP in the intensive care patient is approximately 1% per day but in patients with inhalation injury the risk reaches 40% per day during the first days. A primary admitting diagnosis of burns has been found to be an independent predictor of VAP. Patients with combined thermal and inhalation injury requiring urgent intubation have a high incidence of bacterial bronchial contamination. Inhalation injury creates a damaged tracheobronchial mucosa and early intubation provides a portal for bacterial contamination (Fig. 1, panels B and C). When ► smoke inhalation injury is combined with ► burn injury or pneumonia, the

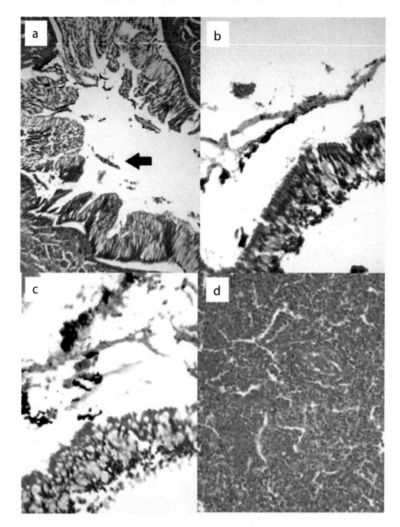

Burns, Pneumonia. Figure 1 Histopathology of the lung and airway of a patient who suffered smoke inhalation injury and developed VAP. **Panel a**: microphotograph of the bronchial wall, the black arrow shows deposits of carbon particles (Montalti sign); **panels b and c**: microphotograph of bronchial mucosa showing partial loss of surface epithelium; **Panel d**: bronchopneumonia: pulmonary alveoli filled with polymorphonuclear leukocyte exudates

physiological responses are different and more severe than those of smoke inhalation injury alone. Treatment strategies should be planned based on these pathophysiological aspects.

Etiology

Most pneumonia in burn patients follows similar patterns to VAP in the non-burn population with early onset pneumonia (≤3 days) more often due to endogenous admission flora; in this setting, gram-positive organisms are the most common causative agents (Table 1). Sometimes this complication follows the pattern of late onset pneumonia; in this setting, pneumonia is more likely due to *Pseudomonas aeruginosa*, Acinetobacter spp, methicillin-resistant

Staphylococcus aureus (MRSA), and enteric gram-negative organisms (Table 1). The distribution of causative organisms and the prevalence of multiple antibiotic resistances may vary between institutions and even within separate units in one institution. The organisms causing bacteremia that exert a species-specific effect on the mortality related to extent of burn injury and patient age have changed in concert with changes in pathogenic flora.

Diagnosis

Pneumonia in burns is defined in the presence of clinical and microbiologic criteria and in the absence or other diagnoses that may mimic pneumonia (ARDS, tracheobronchitis, chest contusion, blast injury, inhalation

Burns, Pneumonia. Table 1 Microbiological data from bronchoalveolar lavage and blood culture from 12 patients that were admitted after smoke inhalation injury showing predominance of gram-positive microorganisms; most of the *Staphylococcus aureus* were methicillin susceptible

| Patient | Bronchoalveolar lavage | | Blood culture |
	Gram stain	Culture ($\geq 10^4$ cfu/mL)	
1	Gram-positive cocci	*Acinetobacter* spp.	Negative
		Streptococcus pyogenes	
		Staphylococcus aureus	
2	Gram-positive cocci	*Staphylococcus aureus*	Negative
3	Negative	*Enterobacter aerogenes*	*Enterobacter aerog,enes,*
			Klebsiella pneumoniae,
			Enterobacter cloacae
4	Negative	No growth	Negative
5	Negative	*Pseudomonsa aeruginosa*	Negative
6	Negative	*Streptococcus pyogenes*	Negative
7	Gram-positive cocci	*Staphylococcus aureus*	Negative
8	Negative	*Staphylococcus aureus*	Negative
9	Gram-positive cocci	*Staphylococcus aureus*	Negative
		Pseudomonas aeruginosa	
10	Negative	No growth	Negative
11	Negative	*Corynebacterium* spp.	Negative
12	Negative	*Acinetobacter* spp.	Negative

injury), but on the other hand, it has to be kept in mind that such conditions could coexist with the presence of pneumonia. The clinical diagnosis of VAP in burn patients is a major challenge due to the low sensitivity of clinical diagnosis including scoring systems, especially in the presence of systemic inflammation and ARDS. The ▶ Clinical Pulmonary Infection Score (CPIS) is considered as a useful tool for the diagnosis of VAP; however, in burn patients its sensitivity is 30% and its specificity of 80% for predicting pneumonia [1]. Due to the poor predictive value of CPIS in VAP in burn patients there exists some consensus that VAP diagnosis should rely on clinical suspicion verified by quantitative culture results of lower respiratory tract specimens. The diagnosis of infection and sepsis following the standard criteria does not apply to burn patients. Burn patients are constantly and chronically exposed to the environment. In response to this exposure, inflammatory mediators that change the baseline metabolic profile of the burn patient are continuously released, the baseline temperature is reset to about 38.5°C, and tachycardia and tachypnea persist for months in patients with extensive burns [2]. Continuous exposure leads to significant changes in the white blood cell (WBC) count, making leukocytosis a poor indicator of sepsis. Clinical diagnosis is defined by at least two of the following: (a) chest x-ray revealing a new and persistent *infiltrate, consolidation, or cavitation*; (b) *sepsis*; and (c) *purulence in the sputum*. Microbiologic definition of pneumonia includes confirmed (clinical + pathogen isolated), probable (clinical without microbiological confirmation), and possible (abnormal chest X-ray with uncertain cause with low or moderate clinical suspicion, but with microbiologic definite criteria met or pathogen identified). Microbiologic confirmation requires that quantitative cultures of tracheal aspirate, bronchoalveolar lavage (BAL), or protected bronchial brush yield $\geq 10^5$; $\geq 10^4$ cfu or $\geq 10^3$ colony forming units (cfu) per ml, respectively, or when positive blood cultures are present.

Treatment

Antimicrobial therapy should be administered empirically for the presence of pneumonia complicating smoke inhalation injury or burn injury. In the presence of pneumonia, the physiological responses are different and more severe than those of smoke inhalation injury alone and treatment strategies should be planned based on these pathophysiological aspects. Early onset VAP is due to microorganisms susceptible to monotherapy with ampicillin-sulbactam, the third-generation cephalosporins cefotaxime or ceftriaxone, ertapenem, or respiratory fluoroquinolones, if they do not have other risk factors for multidrug-resistant microorganisms (Fig. 2, panel a); on the other hand, if there exist conditions favoring the presence of multidrug-resistant microorganisms, the antimicrobial therapy should include the coverage of non-fermentating gram-negatives (*P. aeruginosa* and Acinetobacter spp), enteric bacteria, and MRSA [3]. The use of combination antimicrobial therapy including an anti-pseudomonal beta-lactam + an aminoglycoside or a fluoroquinolone and linezolid or vancomycin, taking into consideration the local epidemiological data could provide appropriate antimicrobial coverage against those microorganisms (Fig. 2, panel b). In some settings, particularly in the presence of *P. aeruginosa* or Acinetobacter spp susceptible only to colistin, nebulized and/or intravenous colistin could be necessary to bring appropriate antimicrobial coverage, newer antimicrobials, and the use of some of the commonly used antibiotics active against those multidrug-resistant non-fermentating gram-negatives administered aerosolized could provide

further coverage but could not be recommended as there are not clinical trials confirming their safety and efficacy (Fig. 2, panel c). Skin infection and colonization may be the starting point for further respiratory tract infection. Non-fermentating microorganisms are frequently found as wound colonizers and may become the pathogens of VAP. Local epidemiological data are essential to prescribe antibiotics in this subset of multidrug-resistant microorganisms.

Brunsvold et al. found in a small series of eight cases of VAP (most of them due to *P. aeruginosa* and *S.* aureus) among 12 critically injured burned patients treated with drotrecogin alpha (recombinant human activated protein C) that the mortality rate was comparable to that of other severe sepsis trials and better than predicted by the SOFA score. Patients in this series tolerated drotrecogin alpha treatment with an acceptable rate of bleeding complications. Also drotrecogin alpha in burn patients significantly attenuates smoke inhalation injury in a dose-dependent manner at 2 h after insult, by preserving microvascular permeability and proinflammatory cytokine IL-1beta (but not TNF-alpha) in bronchoalveolar lavage fluid. More controlled studies are needed, but consideration of its use in appropriate patients may be beneficial in reducing the impact of VAP mortality in these patients.

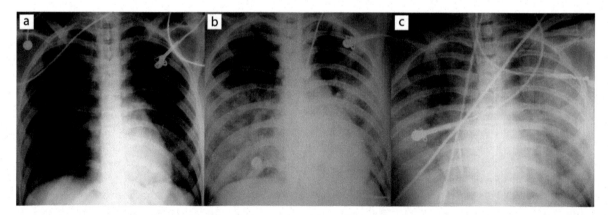

Burns, Pneumonia. Figure 2 A 17-year-old previously healthy female arrived unconscious to the Emergency Room after smoke inhalation during a fire. She was intubated and mechanically ventilated ($FIO_2 = 100\%$). Early bronchoscopy showed inhalation injury (edema, hyperemia, carbon soot) but not burns; temperature 38.5°C, chest X-R: mild opacity at LLL; aspiration pneumonia was suspected (Fig. 1a). Empirical ceftriaxone + clindamycin intravenously were initiated; after 48 h BAL culture result yielded *S. viridans* $>10^4$ cfu/mL, susceptible to the prescribed antimicrobials. Three days later, the infiltrate worsened, superinfection was suspected, and antimicrobials were changed to imipenem + vancomycin (Fig. 1b); BAL culture disclosed *S. maltophilia* (imipenem-resistant) and *A. baumannii* at $>10^4$ cfu/mL. The patient was even worse, $PaO_2/FIO_2 = 120$ mmHg; ARDS in fibroproliferative stage was suspected (Fig. 1c), a new BAL was performed and piperacillin-tazobactam + i.v corticosteroids were added. The BAL culture yielded *A. baumannii* $>10^4$ cfu/mL susceptible only to colistin, iv + inhaled colistin were added, the patient improved and was weaned and extubated 10 days later

Prophylaxis

Nosocomial pneumonia ▶ prophylaxis in burn patients include the usual approach in other critically ill patients based on the recommendations by the Institute for Healthcare Improvement including: to elevate the head of bed to maintain the patient at a semirecumbent position (30–45°), sedation vacation with assessment of extubation readiness, and prevention of peptic ulcer disease and deep vein thrombosis prevention measures. Additionally burn patients should be regularly assessed for aspiration risk; chest physiotherapy and bronchodilators should be used as needed; a rational use of antimicrobials including cessation of antibiotics upon pneumonia resolution together with infection control procedures are also very important.

Infection control procedures, including scheduled surveillance cultures, utilization of cohort patient care methodology, strict enforcement of patient and staff hygiene, and patient monitoring, have been effective in eliminating endemic-resistant microbial strains, preventing the establishment of newly introduced resistant organisms, diagnosing infection in a timely fashion, instituting antibiotic and other necessary therapy in a prompt manner, and documenting the effectiveness of present-day burn patient care and the improved survival of burn patients. Two consecutive, randomized, double-blinded supplementation studies demonstrated that enhancing trace element status and antioxidant defenses by selenium, zinc, and copper supplementation was associated with a decrease of nosocomial pneumonia incidence in critically ill, severely burned patients.

Evaluation/Assessment

Smoke inhalation injury is the injury below the glottis caused by products of combustion; its diagnosis requires the evaluation of the history of exposure to products of combustion and a bronchoscopy revealing carbonaceous material or signs of edema or ulceration. Carboxyhemoglobin levels are used in the evaluation of the burn, when elevated, increase suspicion for smoke inhalation injury, both entities can occur independently of each other. Flame burns to the face may be associated with increased risk for inhalation injury but not all flame burns to the face result in inhalation injury. In burn patients with possible inhalation or thermal injury bronchoscopy should be performed within a few hours after admission for bronchial toilet and to assess the severity of airway injury. Chou's classification is useful to evaluate the airway (Table 2). In those patients with lesions in the airway, bronchoscopy should be repeated each 24–48 h.

Burns, Pneumonia. Table 2 Grading according to depth of mucosal damage estimated by fiberoptic bronchoscopy, as per Chou's classification

Grade	Findings
Grade 0	Negative (no mucosal damage)
Grade b	Positive (mucosal damage) confirmed by biopsy
Grade 1	Mild edema + hyperemia, with or without carbon soot
Grade 2	Severe edema + hyperemia with or without carbon soot
Grade 3	Ulceration, necrosis, no cough reflex or bronchial secretions

Bronchoalveolar lavage should be performed to obtain lower respiratory tract specimens for culture in those patients with possible pneumonia. Scheduled surveillance cultures, diagnosing infection in a timely fashion, documenting the effectiveness of present-day burn patient care and the improved survival of burn patients could be of help. It has been observed that patients intubated before transfer appear to have the greater risk for subsequently developing pneumonia, and this should be taken into account during the initial evaluation.

Prognosis

Advances in burn therapy and the evolution of specialized burn centers have led to improved survival. Pneumonia represents a significant source of morbidity and mortality in the burn population; its contribution to mortality has been reported to be near 80% in patients with combined inhalation injury and pneumonia. Inhalation injury alone increases mortality by approximately 20% and pneumonia by approximately 40%, with a maximum increase of approximately 60% when both are present. The influence on mortality was maximal in the midrange of expected mortality without these complications for any age group. These data indicate that inhalation injury and pneumonia have significant, independent, additive effects on burn mortality and that these effects vary with age and burn size in a predictable manner.

Pneumonia and the ARDS and inhalation injury that may occur simultaneously in the same patient could be responsible for long-term pulmonary dysfunction in burned patients. In one study in Spain it was determined that the etiology of pneumonia or bacteremia is a prognostic factor for death in burn patients, and in a multivariable analysis it was determined that pneumonia and bacteremia were predominantly due to *P. aeruginosa* or Acinetobacter spp among non-fermentative gram-negative bacteria (OR 3.7) and *S. aureus* (OR 2.8). Other microorganisms have no significant association with death.

Pharmacoeconomics

Pneumonia and burn care are associated with increased morbidity, mortality, and costs. VAP increases length of ICU stay from 5 to 7 days, the costs of the diagnostic tests and the cost of antimicrobial therapy indicate that the additional cost of evaluating and treating a patient with VAP would be between $10,019 and $13,647; burn patients could incur in several times higher hospital costs, along with a longer length of stay. Hospital costs related to VAP are strongly influenced by hospital mortality and may not reflect the actual costs of treating patients with VAP due to multidrug-resistant microorganisms. The cost to the health care system in the incremental hospital cost of burn patients who developed pneumonia is about $40,000. Clinicians caring for patients at risk of nosocomial infections, including VAP, should be aware of the local prevalence of infections due multidrug-resistant microorganisms and should develop local strategies aimed at optimizing the delivery of appropriate initial therapy for these high risk infections. Additionally, future research aimed at more rapid and cost-effective identification of bacterial pathogens and their susceptibilities should be pursued [4]. The age of the population of burn patients developing pneumonia is less than the age of non-burn patients developing pneumonia, while severity of illness, complexity of care, recurrence rate is higher and it is likely that the societal burden of pneumonia in burns will increase.

After-care

Unresolving ▶ acute respiratory distress syndrome complicating pneumonia and smoke inhalation injury have been treated with corticosteroids at a narrow optimal time between the acute and late phases in patients with prolonged mechanical ventilation, fever, hypoxemia, and negative cultures. It has been proposed that this therapy improved their outcome [5]. The deleterious effect that the combination of inhalation and thermal injury together with severe pneumonia could produce on the future lung health of patients should be taken into account, evaluation of lung function, administration of inhaled bronchodilator or corticosteroid therapy and prophylactic vaccination should be considered after discharge.

References

1. Pham TN, Neff MJ, Simmons JM, Gibran NS, Heimbach DM, Klein MB (2007) The clinical pulmonary infection score poorly predicts pneumonia in patients with burns. J Burn Care Res 28:76–79
2. Greenhalgh DG, Saffle JR, Holmes JH 4, Gamelli RL, Palmieri TL, Horton JW, Tompkins RG, Traber DL, Mozingo DW, Deitch EA, Goodwin CW, Herndon DN, Gallagher JJ, Sanford AP, Jeng JC, Ahrenholz DH, Neely AN, O'Mara MS, Wolf SE, Purdue GF, Garner WL, Yowler CJ, Latenser BA (2007) American Burn Association consensus conference to define sepsis and infection in burns. J Burn Care Res 28:776–790
3. Niederman MS, Craven DE (co-chaires), Bonten MJ, Chastre J, Craig WA, Fagon J-Y, Hall J, Jacoby GA, Kollef MH, Luna CM, Mandell LA, Torres A, Wunderink RG (2005) Guidelines for the management of adults with hospital-acquired, ventilator-associated, and healthcare-associated pneumonia. Am J Respir Crit Care Med 171:388–416
4. Kollef KE, Schramm GE, Wills AR, Reichley RM, Micek ST, Kollef MH (2008) Predictors of 30-day mortality and hospital costs in patients with ventilator-associated pneumonia attributed to potentially antibiotic-resistant gram-negative bacteria. Chest 134:281–287
5. Irrazabal CL, Capdevila AA, Revich L, Del Bosco CG, Luna CM, Vujacich P, Villa R, Jorge MA (2008) Early and late complications among 15 victims exposed to indoor fire and smoke inhalation. Burns 34:533–538

Burns, Sepsis

Brian K. Hogan, Clinton K. Murray
Department of Medicine, San Antonio Military Medical Center, Fort Sam Houston, TX, USA

© Springer-Verlag Berlin Heidelberg (outside the USA) 2012

Synonyms

Burn wound sepsis; Infection; Septicemia; Systemic inflammatory response

Definition

Sepsis is a systemic inflammatory response secondary to an underlying infectious process. Clinical signs and symptoms may be relatively mild as can be seen in some elderly or immunosuppressed patients. Conversely, they may be quite dramatic. When it occurs in a patient with burn injury, it is referred to as burn sepsis. When clinical signs of "sepsis" develop in a burn patient, it can often be difficult to distinguish between an infectious and noninfectious etiology. Sepsis exists on a continuum of severity based on evidence of end organ dysfunction and the development of shock. "Severe sepsis" refers to sepsis with multiple organ dysfunction syndrome (MODS). This term no longer applies to burn patients, as there is rarely an intermediate phase between sepsis and the development of septic shock. Also, the classification is not useful for clinical trials. MODS is still used but is only applicable after the initial resuscitation (3 days). The Marshall MODS scoring system is currently preferred. With the onset of shock-like hemodynamics, the term septic shock is used [1].

Epidemiology

More than 500,000 burn injuries occur annually in the United States leading to more than 40,000 hospital admissions and 4,000 deaths. For those that survive transport and resuscitation, infection has been estimated to contribute to mortality in 75% of patients. Infection typically precedes the onset of multiple organ dysfunction and sepsis by a median of 4 days. Bloodstream infection with subsequent development of sepsis represents one of the most significant and costly types of infection encountered [2]. The American Burn Association maintains a running repository of burn-related data. Over the preceding 10 years, infections caused seven of the top 10 clinically relevant complications with "septicemia" ranking as the sixth most common.

Microbiology

Burn sepsis can be caused by a wide range of organisms including bacteria, fungi, and viruses. They may be of an exogenous or endogenous source and the relative incidence varies depending upon a number of factors. One factor is the site of underlying infection. Most commonly, this is pneumonia, bloodstream infection (BSI), or invasive wound infection. Bloodstream infections may or may not be catheter related. Urosepsis is less common but does occur. It should also be noted that involved microorganisms can vary over time in a single patient, and so past isolates should be considered but not relied upon when selecting empiric therapy. *Streptococcus* species represented the most commonly involved organisms in burn sepsis, however this is no longer the case. The most common organisms now include *Staphylococcus aureus*, *Pseudomonas aeruginosa*, *Acinetobacter baumannii*, and *Klebsiella pneumoniae* [2].

Antimicrobial resistance has become a significant problem in the current treatment of burn patients. Methicillin resistant *Staphylococcus aureus* (MRSA), vancomycin resistant *Enterococcus* (VRE), and multidrug-resistant (MDR) gram-negative rods (e.g., *Pseudomonas aeruginosa*, *Acinetobacter* species, and *Enterobacteriaceae*) have all been associated with infections in burn patients. Appropriate antibiotic treatment and strict infection control practices are paramount [2].

Nonbacterial causes of systemic infection are increasingly being recognized in burn patients. *Candida* species and *Aspergillus* species are the most commonly isolated fungi, but a number of other fungi have also been reported including *Mucor* and *Fusarium* species [3]. The potential impact of fungal infection on the patient cannot be understated. In a study of attributable mortality of fungal infections in burn patients, *Aspergillus* was found to be a contributing factor in more than 30% of cases when identified on histopathology at the time of autopsy. *Candida* species are frequent colonizers in burn patients but should always be considered a pathogen when isolated from blood culture. Disseminated viral infections are uncommon but do occur. Herpesviruses such as herpes simplex virus and cytomegalovirus have been associated with significant morbidity and mortality [3].

Pathophysiology

The pathophysiology of sepsis involves the interactions between an infecting microorganism, the resulting immune response, and the inflammatory and coagulation cascades. It is further complicated in burn patients given that severe burn injury (i.e., >20% total body surface area or TBSA) leads to metabolic, physiologic, and immunologic alterations. These changes are both more severe and prolonged when compared to other forms of trauma. Understanding these alterations is essential to recognizing a patient with burn sepsis given that patients will often manifest changes in various clinical parameters (e.g., temperature, heart rate, respiratory rate, and white blood cell count). The underlying pathogenesis begins with direct tissue injury and disruption of the body's natural barrier to infection. This leads to activation of the inflammatory and coagulation cascades. A state of systemic inflammation coupled with hypermetabolism ensues. It is generally proportional to the severity of injury. Metabolic alterations include increased energy requirements, altered glucose metabolism, increased lipolysis, and increased proteolysis. Neuroendocrine changes include an increase in catecholamines, decreased growth hormone, and altered thyroid hormone concentrations. The immunologic response is both dynamic and complex. It begins with the initial inflammatory response and involves both innate and adaptive immunity. Activated macrophages play a key role and lead to an increase in cytokines and other inflammatory mediators. The body attempts to maintain homeostasis with what is often referred to as the counter-anti-inflammatory response. A number of host factors serve to mitigate the immune response including hormonal changes, extremes of age, nutritional status, as well as other comorbidities. Additionally, there are a number of pathogen-specific factors that contribute to the ability of pathogens to evade the immune system and cause infection. The end result is an immunosuppressed state leaving the burn patient at risk of infection [4].

Treatment

Treatment of burn sepsis is challenging and requires a multifaceted approach consisting of specific antimicrobial therapy, aggressive resuscitation, and supportive care. This includes early excision of the burn wound, volume resuscitation, aggressive nutritional support, and intensive insulin therapy. Other potential adjunctive therapies have also been considered, including renal replacement therapy, corticosteroids, specific immune modulating therapies, and activated protein C. Preventive measures should emphasize strict infection control practices.

Early initiation of appropriate antibiotic therapy is essential. Studies of sepsis in intensive care unit (ICU) patients have shown increased morbidity and mortality in those not receiving early and adequate antimicrobial therapy. In order to achieve "adequate" therapy, local antibiograms must be utilized when selecting empiric antibiotics. MDR pathogens are prevalent and vary between different burn units. Isolates from burn units are often more resistant compared to those from other ICUs and wards of the same hospital. Risk factors for acquisition of a drug-resistant pathogen include antibiotic use prior to infection, prolonged hospitalization, invasive procedures, and age. Empiric antibiotics generally include coverage for MRSA as well as drug-resistant gram-negative bacteria (i.e., *P. aeruginosa, K. pneumoniae*, etc.). Again, the antibiogram should guide the selection. In facilities with high rates of extended spectrum beta-lactamase producing organisms (ESBL), an antipseudomonal carbapenem might be considered as initial therapy. Empiric antifungal coverage should be chosen based on the site of primary infection and the suspected organism. It will also depend upon the incidence of fungal organisms present in the particular burn unit. Commonly available options include azoles (i.e., fluconazole, voriconazole, and posaconazole), echinocandins (i.e., anidulafungin, micafungin, and caspofungin), and formulations of amphotericin B. Drug selection should be based upon efficacy, toxicity, and drug interactions. Fluconazole-resistant *Candida* species such as *C. krusei* and *C. glabrata* are increasingly being recognized. Resistance to amphotericin B is also seen. Some burn units have reported a relatively high prevalence of *Aspergillus terreus*, which is intrinsically resistant to amphotericin B. Once the organism is known and the patient is stabilized, antimicrobial therapy can be narrowed as appropriate based on susceptibilities. Duration of treatment is typically 10–14 days but may need to be adjusted in some patients [2].

The pharmacokinetics of antimicrobial agents in patients with severe burns varies considerably making it difficult to optimize antimicrobial therapy. Vancomycin exhibits an increased total clearance while the elimination half-life is decreased. Significant pharmacokinetic variability has also been shown for other commonly used antimicrobials in the burn unit including aminoglycosides, carbapenems, and cephalosporins. Complicating matters further is the frequent use of dialysis including the use of continuous renal replacement therapy, which needs to be taken into account when selecting and dosing drugs. Therapeutic drug monitoring should be employed whenever available [2].

Aggressive surgical care of the burn wound includes early excision (within 5 days) and skin grafting. While it has become the standard of care in many nations, this is based on limited evidence. In a recent meta-analysis, decreased mortality rates were found only in patients without inhalation injury [2]. The specific impact early excision has on burn sepsis is unknown.

Supportive treatment aimed at early and aggressive resuscitation to maintain blood volume and adequate tissue perfusion is appropriate. Early goal-directed resuscitation with measurement of oxygen delivery is associated with improved survival in ICU patients with septic shock. However, the appropriateness in burn patients is not clear at this time. This strategy would entail the administration of a significantly greater volume of fluid increasing the risk of abdominal compartment syndrome [1].

Early institution of enteral feedings (e.g., within 24 h of admission) has been shown to have several benefits. There are decreases in catecholamines and glucagon as well as improved caloric intake, increased insulin secretion, and improvement in protein retention. The catabolic response is blunted, leading to an overall decrease in weight loss. In patients who cannot tolerate enteral feedings, centrally administered parenteral feedings are appropriate. Enteral nutrition appears to be superior with regard to preserving gastrointestinal function and mucosal integrity. This leads to a decrease in bacterial translocation, plasma endotoxin, and inflammatory mediators. Regarding specific immune-modifying diets (i.e., glutamine-enriched diets), there is insufficient evidence currently to recommend their use.

Intensive insulin therapy (IIT) (maintaining serum glucose 80–110 mg/dL) has become a common supportive treatment in most burn centers despite relatively limited study in this patient population. The initial report in 2001 of a mortality benefit in surgical ICU patients (only 4% were trauma or burn patients) led to a shift in thinking with regard to the effects of hyperglycemia in the critically ill. IIT in this study was found to be associated with decreased ventilator dependence, less renal replacement therapy, and fewer episodes of sepsis. The mechanisms underlying these benefits are not completely understood. This mortality benefit has also not been demonstrated in other patient populations. Several studies published in the pediatric burn literature have associated hyperglycemia with increased catabolism, bacteremia, fungemia, skin graft loss, and mortality. Experimental models of burn injury have suggested that insulin therapy may counteract hypercatabolism and mitigate decreases in lean body mass. These studies make IIT an attractive adjunctive treatment in the burn ICU. A recent observational study in adult burn patients showed a decreased rate of pneumonia, ventilator-associated pneumonia, and urinary tract infection. The specific impact regarding sepsis in this population is currently unknown. Based largely on the reduction in morbidity (including sepsis rates) and mortality in surgical ICU patients combined with the limited study in burns, IIT has become the standard of care. It should be noted, however, that it is not without side effect (i.e., hypoglycemia) and further study is required regarding the risks and benefits of this therapy.

Application of renal replacement therapy, specifically continuous renal replacement therapy (CRRT) is becoming a more commonly applied supportive treatment in burn ICUs. The diagnosis of acute kidney injury (AKI) in conjunction with both sepsis and severe burn injury carries a poor prognosis. CRRT is associated with a smaller hemodynamic effect than conventional dialysis and thus is useful in burn sepsis. Questions remain regarding the optimal dosing, timing, and immunomodulatory effect of therapy. CRRT has been evaluated in a prospective randomized trial comparing low- and high-volume dosing (20 versus 35 and 45 mL/kg/h). A mortality benefit was seen with both 35 and 45 mL/kg/h, but no difference was seen between the two. Interestingly, subset analysis revealed a mortality benefit in septic patients with the highest volume. High-volume CRRT may provide patients with significant inflammation (e.g., burn sepsis), a benefit not seen in others. Study in burn patients has revealed the ability of CRRT to decrease endotoxin and cytokines (i.e., IL-1, IL-8, and TNFα). Early application of high-volume CRRT has been retrospectively evaluated in septic and non-septic burn patients. It was associated with a decreased 28 day and in-hospital mortality compared to matched controls. Despite the suggestion that earlier initiation of high-volume CRRT may be beneficial in burn sepsis, the clinical data are limited. Overall, studies of CRRT and sepsis have been small and lack adequate power to demonstrate mortality differences. There is insufficient evidence currently to recommend the use of CRRT in burn patients for nonrenal indications.

Low-dose corticosteroid therapy also has potential use in burn sepsis. The basis of this therapy is to treat occult adrenal insufficiency and peripheral glucocorticoid resistance. For those patients with refractory septic shock, increases in vasopressor doses and volume are required, which can lead to impairment of the microcirculation. This can worsen burn-induced necrosis. Corticosteroid use in septic patients in the ICU is controversial and not without side effects, including risk of recurrent or secondary infection, impaired wound healing, myopathy, hyperglycemia, and hypernatremia. Efficacy is seen in catecholamine-dependent patients with septic shock. Results of studies in burn patients are conflicting and the role in this population is unclear at this time. Available evidence is based on a few studies with small sample sizes and methodological flaws. Further randomized prospective studies are needed prior to routine use.

Specific immune-modulating therapies such as cytokine inhibitors and antiendotoxins have also been tried, but have not been efficacious. This may be due to the complexity of the interactions between the various components of the immune system. Therapy directed at a single target may not be adequate for impact. Future research directed at multiple targets may be warranted.

Activated protein C is another potential adjunctive treatment for the most severely ill patients. It has been shown to decrease mortality in ICU patients with severe sepsis and Acute Physiology and Chronic Health Evaluation (APACHE) II scores ≥25. It works by inhibiting the inflammatory and procoagulant responses. While this mechanism suggests there may be some utility in burn sepsis, the therapy carries significant risk. The major side effect is bleeding. The initial studies leading to FDA approval of activated protein C did not include burn patients. For these reasons, despite the potential utility, its use cannot be recommended at this time. Further study is required.

Infection control is a critical component of preventing infection in burn patients. Strict aseptic technique (i.e., sterile gloves, gowns, and masks) is important. Various environmental controls (e.g., contained perimeter, isolation rooms, and cohorting of nursing care) are often used. Surveillance for common hospital-associated infections may help to identify outbreaks when they occur. Antibiograms should be maintained and practices should be adjusted based on resistance trends. Proper infection control requires the cooperation of all members of the health care team [3].

Evaluation/Assessment

Being able to distinguish between the septic and non-septic burn patient is critical. Instituting early and appropriate therapy has been demonstrated in various patient populations to impact mortality. The metabolic, physiologic, and immunologic perturbations associated with severe burn injury make the traditional signs and symptoms of infection and sepsis insensitive, nonspecific, or both. Fever has classically been the most common finding associated with infection. This finding is unreliable with burn injury as patients are often febrile in the absence of infection. Also, patients are often hypothermic or normothermic even in the setting of severe infection. Other clinical and laboratory parameters have been and are being evaluated to determine their association with burn sepsis and mortality [1]. Biochemical inflammatory markers such as total white blood cell count, neutrophil count, erythrocyte sedimentation rate, C-reactive protein, tumor necrosis factor-α, interleukin-6, and procalcitonin have been studied. None reliably distinguish between the septic and non-septic burn patient. Procalcitonin is perhaps the most promising of the biomarkers and is much debated in the literature, but to this point does not have a clear role in the clinical management of the infected burn patient [5].

The systemic inflammatory response syndrome (SIRS) defined in 1992 as part of the American College of Chest Physicians/Society of Critical Care Medicine Consensus Conference is a set of criteria used to identify a state of systemic inflammation that when associated with an underlying infectious process is the basis for a definition of sepsis. Unfortunately, it is not specific in burn patients. Although not systematically evaluated in this population, up to 90% of surgical ICU patients meet the SIRS criteria in some series. It has not helped our understanding that burn injury has been an exclusion criterion for most trials investigating sepsis. To address this and establish standardized definitions regarding burn sepsis, a Consensus Conference to Define Sepsis and Infection in Burns was convened in early 2007 by the American Burn Association. Sepsis was defined as a change in the patient that should "trigger" concern for infection. The trigger is the presence of ≥3 of 6 clinical criteria (Table 1). The criteria include temperature, progressive tachycardia, progressive tachypnea, thrombocytopenia, hyperglycemia, and inability to continue enteral feeds. The selection of these criteria was based upon expert opinion and the limited published data regarding burn sepsis in the adult and pediatric burn literature. The diagnosis of sepsis should always be tied to a documented

Burns, Sepsis. Table 1 American burn association sepsis criteria

The "trigger" is the presence of ≥3 of six clinical criteria
I. Temperature (>39° or <36.5°C)
II. Progressive tachycardia • Adults >110 beats per minute • Children >2 SD above age-specific norms (85% age-adjusted heart rate)
III. Progressive tachypnea • Adults >25 breaths per minute or minute ventilation >12 L/min if ventilated • Children >2 SD above age-specific norms (85% age-adjusted respiratory rate)
IV. Thrombocytopenia (Does not apply until 3 days after the initial resuscitation) • Adults <100,000/mcL • Children >2 SD below age-specific norms
V. Hyperglycemia (Does not apply in diabetics) • Untreated plasma glucose >200 mg/dL Or • Insulin resistance (>7 units/h or >25% increase in insulin requirement over 24 h)
VI. Inability to continue enteral feeds >24 h • Abdominal distension Or • Increased residuals two times the feed rate for adults or >150 mL/h in children Or • Uncontrollable diarrhea (>2,500 mL/day for adults or >400 mL/day for children)

infection. This may be a positive culture, pathologic tissue source, or clinical response to antimicrobials. It should be recognized that there is still significant heterogeneity among burn patients with respect to the inciting focus as well as the involved organism leading to sepsis. While practical, the above criteria serve as a framework for study of a complex process in a complex patient population. These specific criteria have yet to be validated [1].

Once there is concern for sepsis, the patient should immediately be evaluated for the site and source of infection. Major sources of sepsis include invasive wound infection, pneumonia, bloodstream infection and, catheter-related infection. Blood, sputum, and urine cultures should be obtained. Evaluation should include inspection of the entire burn wound. Tissue biopsy of concerning areas should be performed. Not only should histopathology be sent, but also bacterial and fungal cultures should be done. Correlation between histopathology and fungal culture results is variable. Given the prevalence of resistant organisms, identification to the species level is required to guide therapy. When evaluating for ventilator-associated pneumonia, consideration should also be given to use of quantitative bronchoalveolar lavage, which has been shown to increase both sensitivity and specificity. Empiric antibiotic therapy should not be delayed.

Pharmacoeconomics

Burn sepsis is a common clinical syndrome with a high mortality. Surprisingly, there is relatively limited data regarding incidence, cost, and outcome. What is available is incomplete. Considering all patients with sepsis, recent estimates have placed the cost per case at more than $20,000 in adults and more than $40,000 in children, respectively. This translates to annual costs in the billions, in the United States alone. Costs are generally recognized to be greater in ICU and surgical patients and expected to increase annually. Based on this information, sepsis in a burn patient represents a common and costly complication.

After-care

Both treatment and aftercare of burn patients requires a multidisciplinary approach. This involves physicians, nurses, physical and occupational therapists, nutritionists, and social workers. In those whose course is complicated by burn sepsis, emphasis should be placed on the preventive measures discussed above in order to prevent recurrent episodes. Should they occur, they should be approached systematically to avoid misdiagnosis or inadequate treatment. The site of infection, the organism (or its resistance profile), and the patient's clinical status may all be different.

Prognosis

Sepsis is a leading cause of morbidity and mortality in the burn population. While progress is being made, there is still only a 50% survival rate in patients with 80% TBSA [2]. Full thickness burn size, inhalation injury, and extremes of age are risk factors for sepsis and death. For septic patients with evidence of end organ damage, mortality has been estimated in some series at more than 50%. Outcomes may be worse with certain pathogens and with polymicrobial infections. Longitudinal studies have demonstrated an increase in attributable mortality of more than 20% with gram-negative bacteremia and fungemia [3]. There are also reports of gram-negative organisms being associated with a 50% increase in predicted mortality in patients with bacteremia compared to those without. More specifically, *Klebsiella pneumoniae* has been associated with a greater virulence leading to excess mortality when compared to other organisms such as *Acinetobacter baumannii*. *Acinetobacter* spp. demonstrate more resistance but may be less virulent [2]. Further study is needed to better define the relative contribution of sepsis to the overall morbidity and mortality of burn patients.

References

1. Greenhalgh DG, Saffle JR, Holmes JH et al (2007) American burn association consensus conference to define sepsis and infection in burns. J Burn Care Res 28:776–790
2. Murray CK (2010) Burns. In: Mandell GL, Bennett JE, Dolin R (eds) Mandell, Douglas and Bennett's principles and practice of infectious diseases, 7th edn. (Vol 2). Churchill Livingstone, New York, pp 3905–3909
3. Church D, Elsayed S, Reid O et al (2006) Burn wound infections. Clin Microbiol Rev 19:403–434
4. Shankar R, Melstrom KA, Gamelli RL (2007) Inflammation and sepsis: past, present, and the future. J Burn Care Res 28e:566–571
5. Lavrentieva A, Kontakiotis T, Lazaridis L et al (2007) Inflammatory markers in patients with severe burn injury. What is the best indicator of sepsis? Burns 33:189–194

Burst Abdomen

▶ Evisceration

C

C2/C3 Traumatic Spondylolisthesis

▶ Hangman's Fracture

Calcium Channel Antagonist Poisoning

▶ Calcium Channel Blocker Toxicity

Calcium Channel Blocker Toxicity

ADEEL ABBASI, FRANCIS DEROOS
Emergency Medicine, Hospital of the University of
Pennsylvania, Philadelphia, PA, USA

Synonyms

Calcium channel antagonist poisoning

Definition

Calcium channel blockers (CCBs) are widely used throughout the world and are commonly prescribed for the treatment of hypertension as well as dysrhythmias, migraine headaches, Raynaud phenomenon, esophageal spasm, and post-subarachnoid hemorrhage vasospasm. While CCBs are relatively well tolerated therapeutically, in overdose, these agents can lead to significant hemodynamic instability including hypotension and bradycardia. For the most severely poisoned patients, there is no consistently reliable treatment available. Therefore, management decisions must be individualized on a case-by-case basis and the physiologic response to each intervention should be careful monitored and considered while the treatment continues.

All calcium channel blockers act by antagonizing ▶ voltage-sensitive calcium channels (L-type) which are involved in excitation-contraction coupling in both the myocardial and vascular smooth muscle as well as the spontaneous depolarization and conduction within the SA node, the AV node, and the conduction tissue in the myocardium. While these calcium channels are also present on skeletal smooth muscle cells, CCBs have little effect on these tissues function because these cells rely almost exclusively on intracellular calcium stores rather than calcium influx for their contractility needs [1].

In general, CCBs are well absorbed orally and are hepatically metabolized, predominantly by the CYP3A subgroup of the cytochrome P450 enzyme system. This metabolism can by saturated in overdose, potentially prolonging the half-life and duration of activity of these drugs. CCBs are highly protein bound and have relatively large volumes of distribution making it unlikely that hemodialysis or even hemoperfusion would be of any value in treating an overdosed patient [2].

In therapeutic doses, CCBs reduce calcium influx into vascular smooth muscle cells resulting in a decrease in the baseline contractility or tone of the peripheral vascular smooth muscle and, ultimately, a reduction in peripheral vascular resistance and blood pressure. In a typical myocardial cell, this reduction in calcium influx also results in decreased contractility. However, in the specialized conduction cells within the myocardium, this reduction in the influx of positively charged calcium both decreases the rate of spontaneous depolarization (phase 0) of the SA and AV nodes, and it reduces the electrically induced depolarization essential in cardiac conduction (Purkinje tissue). In therapeutic dosing, this reduces the resting heart rate as well as the conduction through the AV node, and may suppress spontaneous depolarizations initiated by abnormal or diseased myocardium as well as their propagation and thereby suppressing dysrhythmias [1].

Effects in Poisoned Patients

In poisoned patients, the physiologic effects that have just been described for therapeutic dosing become exaggerated resulting in hypotension (most common) and

Jean-Louis Vincent & Jesse B. Hall (eds.), *Encyclopedia of Intensive Care Medicine*, DOI 10.1007/978-3-642-00418-6,
© Springer-Verlag Berlin Heidelberg 2012

bradydysrhythmias. The clinical symptoms and presentation of CCB toxicity depends predominantly on the degree of cardiovascular compromise with symptoms ranging from fatigue, dizziness, and postural light-headedness, seen early and in milder cases, to confusion, syncope, and shock, seen later and in more severe cases. Myocardial chronotropy, dromotropy, and inotropy may become impaired with initially causing sinus bradycardia but progressing to AV conduction abnormalities, idioventricular rhythms, or complete heart block [2].

Although in overdose all CCBs are capable of causing severe cardiovascular compromise and death, there are some subtle differences in physiologic manifestations depending on the particular agent. The CCBs with the most significant myocardial effects, verapamil and diltiazem, have the most profound inhibitory effects on the SA and AV node. Because of this, these two agents, especially verapamil, are responsible for the majority of CCB overdose deaths. In contrast, nifedipine and the other dihydropyridines have little myocardial binding. They may initially produce a hypotensive patient with relatively normal or even increased heart rate before progressing into a bradycardic rhythm if the poisoning is severe enough.

Consequences of severe cardiogenic shock such as seizures, cerebral and bowel ischemia, and renal failure are all associated with severe CCB poisoning. Notably, severe CNS depression without cardiogenic shock is uncommon. In fact, any overdose cases involving CCBs in which altered mental status is a predominant feature in the setting of relatively normal vital signs, a coingestant should be strongly considered. In addition, hyperglycemia is often seen in severely poisoned patients which is, in part, due to the impairment of calcium into the β-islet cells and insulin secretion

The degree of toxicity present ultimately depends on multiple factors including which CCB is ingested, the total dose of the ingestion, the product formulation, and the patient's underlying cardiovascular health. The timing of presentation of CCB toxicity can be as early as 2–3 h postingestion but can be significantly delayed for 8–12 h when sustained release products are involved. Sustained release formulations are particularly difficult to manage because of this potential delay in onset of hemodynamic changes combined with the continued and prolonged duration of absorption, and, often, the large amount of the CCB ingested [1].

Treatment

Given the high mortality associated with CCB toxicity, patients presenting with CCB overdose should be started on treatment immediately, starting if applicable, with gastrointestinal decontamination. If the patient is able to cooperate, activated charcoal should be given orally at a recommended dose of 1g/kg to help reduce systemic absorption from the gastrointestinal tract.

Multiple doses of activated charcoal (MDAC), in a reduced dose of 0.5 g/kg and without a cathartic, should be repeated every 1–2 h in ingestions involving sustained release CCBs. This is an attempt to fill the gastrointestinal tract with charcoal in an attempt to rapidly adsorb the CCB as it is slowly, but continuously, released from its formulation. Orogastric lavage should be considered if the ingestion involves a large dose of CCB, if the patient presents within 1–2 h postingestion, or if they are critically ill. Orogastric lavage may increase vagal tone and potentiate any bradydysrhythmias.

▶ Whole bowel irrigation (WBI) with polyethylene glycol in poisonings involving sustained-release formulations should also be strongly considered, even in asymptomatic patients. The dosing is 1–2 L/h via a nasogastric tube in adults and 300–500 mL/h in children and may be the most effective method of removing the large gastrointestinal reservoir of the CCB from the patient before it is systemically absorbed. This should be continued until the rectal effluent is clear. Both MDAC and WBI are important gastrointestinal decontamination methods and should be initiated as early as possible in cases involving sustained-release CCBs, even in well-appearing patients and particularly children, in an attempt to avoid progressive toxicity [3].

Pharmacotherapy should focus on improving and supporting both cardiac output as well as peripheral vascular tone. There is no single drug or regimen that has been consistently effective. A crystalloid bolus of 10–20 mL/kg of normal saline for hypotension and atropine 0.1 mg/kg for bradycardia are reasonable starting points for each manifestation respectively and may be initially stabilizing for mildly poisoned patients but are often inadequate in moderate to severe poisonings where multiple modalities are often needed simultaneously. A reasonable approach to a CCB-poisoned patient, after a fluid bolus and dose of atropine, may be to treat with a calcium bolus as well as a catecholamine infusion while you prepare to administer ▶ hyperinsulinemic euglycemia therapy (HIET). Recently, lipid emulsion therapy has been used successfully and should be strongly considered in significantly poisoned patients [1]. Drugs including glucagon and phosphodiesterase inhibitors may have limited efficacy and should be considered secondary adjuncts in the most critically ill patients.

Calcium

Calcium administration transiently improves myocardial inotropy and chronotropy and reverses the hypotension seen in CCB toxicity, and should be given early in bradycardic or hypotensive patients. It also improves the action of atropine if given concurrently. The exact dosing is unclear but a reasonable initial bolus is approximately 13–25 mEq of Ca^{2+} IV (10–20 mL of 10% calcium chloride or 30–60 mL of 10% calcium gluconate), followed either by repeat boluses every 15–20 min up to 3–4 doses or a continuous infusion of 0.5 mEq/kg/h of Ca^{2+} (0.2–0.4 mL/kg/h of 10% calcium chloride or 0.6–1.2 mL of 10% calcium gluconate). Although there is no difference in the efficacy of calcium chloride or calcium gluconate, the calcium salt administered should be chosen carefully as 1 g of calcium chloride contains 13.4 mEq of calcium, which is more than three times the 4.3 mEq found in 1 g of calcium gluconate. If repeat dosing or continuous infusions of calcium are used, the serum concentrations of calcium and phosphate should be monitored for hypercalcemia or hypophosphatemia. In addition, intravenous calcium may also cause nausea, vomiting, flushing, constipation, confusion, and angina.

Catecholamines

Catecholamines are indicated in any hypotensive CCB-poisoned patient. Mechanistically, it is logical to select an agent, such as norepinephrine, that has both β_1-adrenergic effects and α_1-adrenergic effects as a first line drug. Assessing the patient's cardiac output and systemic vascular resistance will allow more refined catecholamine choices. Dopamine is not recommended as a first-line agent because it is predominantly an indirect acting pressor that acts by stimulating the release of norepinephrine from the distal nerve terminal rather than by direct α- and β-adrenergic receptor stimulation and these presynaptic catecholamines are often depleted in severely stressed patients.

Insulin and Glucose

The use of insulin and glucose, often termed hyperinsulinemic euglycemia (HIEG) therapy, has become the treatment of choice for severe CCB poisonings. The rational for this use is multifactorial and includes CCB poisoning inhibiting insulin release, forcing the normally free fatty acid–dependent myocardial tissue to become predominantly carbohydrate dependent as well as resistant to insulin [4]. In addition, insulin itself has positive inotropic effects. Dosing recommendations, based on published clinical experience, include an initial bolus of 25–50 g of dextrose (0.5–1 g/kg) and 0.1 U/kg of insulin.

Follow this by infusions of dextrose at 0.25–0.5 g/kg/h and insulin at 0.5 u/kg/h. This insulin infusion rate should be increased every 30–60 min if there is no hemodynamic improvement. Serum glucose should be monitored hourly throughout HIEG treatment [4].

Lipid-Emulsion Therapy

Calcium channel blockers are highly lipophilic agents, and lipid emulsion therapy is emerging as a promising new adjunctive therapy for the management of CCB toxicity. The efficacy of this treatment is likely a pharmacokinetic one in that the highly lipophilic drugs are tightly bound to the fat emulsions and thereby lower the free serum drug levels. A recommended initial bolus infusion of a 20% lipid emulsion at 1 mL/kg over 1 min, repeated every 3–5 min to a maximum of 3 mL/kg, should be followed by a drip of 0.25/mL/kg/min [5]. This treatment has gained great favor in the anesthesiology literature for the treatment of iatrogenic bupivacaine poisoning, and many institutions have protocols that can be extrapolated to CCB-poisoned patients.

Adjunctive Hemodynamic Support

In a few cases of severe CCB poisonings, the bradydysrhythmias and severe hypotension can be refractory to any and all pharmacologic therapy, so successful treatment may require more invasive measures such as cardiopulmonary bypass or extracorporeal membrane oxygenation. These modalities are technically demanding and only available at tertiary care centers; however, if implemented appropriately, they have been shown to provide the hemodynamic support needed until the CCB is metabolized and eliminated, and baseline myocardial function is restored. Cardiac pacing may be attempted but is often unhelpful because patients with severe bradydysrhythmias from CCB poisoning are also like to have dramatically impaired cardiac contractility as well. Therefore, even if the heart rate is successfully improved, the cardiac output remains poor

Evaluation and Assessment

Any patient suspected of a CCB overdose should be immediately evaluated, even if there are no symptoms or signs of toxicity at the time of initial presentation. This is paramount given the seriousness and potentially fatal nature of CCB poisoning. Even with early and aggressive management, patients who present asymptomatic can deteriorate rapidly developing cardiogenic shock. This is especially true for pediatric patients who can be poisoned with very small doses [3]. Furthermore, with higher-dose and extended-release preparations available, the clinical presentation of toxicity can be significantly delayed for up to 12–15 h post ingestion.

Intravenous access and continuous electrocardiographic monitoring should be initiated immediately upon arrival of the patient. In patients exhibiting any evidence of cardiovascular compromise, early central venous access and arterial catheterization is strongly recommended to allow for more accurate hemodynamic monitoring and guide therapy. Initial treatment should begin with adequate oxygenation and airway protection as clinically indicated. Given the potential for rapid deterioration of a severely poisoned patient, and the need for aggressive critical therapies, early control of the airway should be obtained.

A 12-lead ECG should be obtained promptly to assess for dysrhythmias and conductional abnormalities, and repeated at least every 1–2 h for the first several hours. If the patient's condition improves over time, ECGs can be repeated at longer intervals.

Careful assessment of the degree of hypoperfusion and its sequelae, if any, may include a chest radiograph, pulse oximetry, serum chemistry analysis for metabolic acidosis and renal function, and monitoring urine output. Assays for various CCB serum concentrations are not routinely available and are not used to manage patients after overdose. If a patient presents with bradycardia of unclear origin, assessing electrolytes, particularly potassium and magnesium, renal function, and a digoxin concentration, is warranted.

All patients who have overdosed with CCBs who manifest any consistent signs or symptoms should be admitted to an intensive care setting. In addition, because of the possibility of significant delayed toxicity, cases involving sustained-release formulations should be admitted for 24 h to a monitored setting, even if they are asymptomatic. This is particularly important for toddlers and small children in whom even one or a few tablets may produce significant toxicity [3]. Only patients with a reliable history involving an immediate release formulation of the CCB, who received appropriate gastrointestinal decontamination, who had a consistently normal ECG over several hours of monitoring and who are asymptomatic, can be safely referred directly for further psychiatric assessment as needed.

After-care

The disposition of patients following treatment of calcium channel blocker toxicity will depend on the extent of their recovery. Patients who sustain any permanent neurologic injury will need appropriate care including rehabilitation. Otherwise, for those who make a complete recovery and

regain their baseline neurologic function, their after-care will be limited to treating any complications from their hospital stay. Myocardial and peripheral vascular function should return to its baseline function. Patients with intentional ingestions, regardless of the degree of toxic manifestations, typically will require formal psychiatric evaluation.

Prognosis

While severe calcium channel blocker toxicity can cause profound cardiogenic collapse and death, if treatment is not delayed and invasive hemodynamic support is available, even severely poisoned patients can be supported for days with subsequent full recoveries. Multiple case reports document severely poisoned patients who were treated with seemingly extraordinary measures such as several days of extracorporeal membrane oxygenation or cardiopulmonary bypass despite minimal neurologic function, who make a complete recovery and regain their baseline cardiac and neurologic function. Many hypothesize that CCBs' unique neuroprotective effects may explain these remarkable results.

References

1. DeRoos F (2010) Calcium-channel blockers. In: Goldfrank's toxicologic emergencies, 9th edn. McGraw-Hill, New York, pp 911–921
2. Kerns W (2007) Management of b-adrenergic blocker and calcium channel antagonist toxicity. Emerg Med Clin North Am 25:309–331
3. Arroyo AM, Kao LW (2009) Calcium channel blocker toxicity. Pediatr Emerg Care 25:532–538
4. Patel NP, Pugh ME, Goldberg S, Eiger G (2007) Hyperinsulinemic euglycemia therapy for verapamil poisoning: a review. Am J Crit Care 16:498–503
5. Jamaty C, Bailey B, Larocque A et al (2010) Lipid emulsions in the treatment of acute poisoning: a systematic review of human and animal studies. Clin Toxicol 48:1–27

Calcium Heparin

▶ Heparin

California Valley Fever

▶ Coccidioidomycosis

Candida Infection

▶ Candidiasis

Candidemia

▶ Candidiasis

Candidiasis

JOSÉ ARTUR PAIVA, J. M. PEREIRA
UAG da Urgência e Cuidados Intensivos, Hospital Sao Joao and Medical School, University of Porto, Porto, Portugal

Synonyms

Candida infection; Candidemia; Invasive candidiasis

Definition

Although there are no strict definitions for non-immunocompromised, critically ill patients, Invasive Candidiasis (▶ IC) encompasses a wide variety of severe or invasive diseases that excludes superficial or less severe diseases, like oropharyngeal and esophageal candidiasis, and includes four overlapping forms: candidemia, acute disseminated candidiasis, chronic disseminated candidiasis, and deep organ candidiasis. Essentially, all forms of IC probably begin as an episode of candidemia, but the clinical presentations of these four forms are different enough to make this classification useful. Therefore: (a) *candidemia* means the isolation of *Candida* from one or more blood specimens; given its high mortality and morbidity, essentially all patients with candidemia, even those with a single culture, should receive therapy; (b) *acute disseminated candidiasis* usually presents as candidemia, but the special feature of this form is that spread to several organs, namely liver, kidney, spleen, eyes, brain, and heart, is apparent; (c) *chronic disseminated candidiasis* (previously hepatosplenic candidiasis) occurs almost exclusively following prolonged episodes of bone marrow dysfunction and neutropenia; the liver, spleen, and sometimes kidney are prominently infected with *Candida*, and blood cultures are rarely positive at this point, although presumably they were positive at the time infection was initiated; (d) *deep organ candidiasis* in which, at the time of presentation, the blood is sterile and focal infection of the specific organ is the only manifestation, although an episode of candidemia must have led to seeding of the affected area.

Treatment

Epidemiology

Candida spp. infections can no longer be considered as rare infections restricted to neutropenic or immunocompromised patients. All types of patients are now concerned, particularly those with severe underlying disease or critical illnesses that need aggressive diagnostic or treatment procedures. Increased survival in patients with severe diseases, more aggressive use of surgery, invasive procedures and immunosuppression, and also increased use of broad spectrum antibacterial agents led to an increasing incidence of candidemia in Europe and in the USA.

Candida species are the most common cause of invasive fungal infections (70–90%) and are generally reported to be the fourth most prevalent pathogen isolated in blood cultures or deep-site infections, although this prevalence varies depending on the population surveyed [1].

▶ ICU candidiasis represents one third of all IC. The incidence of candidemia, although rather variable from unit to unit, ranging from 0,5 to 2,22 per 10,000 patient days, is tenfold higher in the ICU than in the wards, and *Candida* species are responsible for around 10% of all ICU-acquired infections worldwide. In the recent SOAP study, *Candida* spp. accounted for 17% of all sepsis in the ICU and for 20% of all ICU-acquired sepsis.

A marked increase in the proportion of non-albicans *Candida* isolates has been reported in several countries, usually accounting for 40–60% of cases. This observation correlated with the increasing use of azoles for prophylaxis or empirical treatment. However, the association of previous fluconazole use with the isolation of non-albicans strains has been shown in some studies but not proven in many more. The increasing incidence of non-albicans *Candida* species is important, as some studies show that candidemia due to non-albicans species, especially *C. glabrata*, *C. tropicalis* and *C. krusei*, are associated with higher mortality. The fact that *C. glabrata* has reduced susceptibility, and *C. krusei* intrinsic resistance to fluconazole, may have to do with this higher mortality and must be taken into account for the empiric therapeutic choice (Table 1). In fact, Kovacicova et al. found a significantly higher attributable mortality in patients infected with fluconazole-resistant strains [1].

However, there are important geographic and demographic variations in terms of the prevalence of species of *Candida*. For instance, *C. glabrata* is the second most prevalent species, following albicans, in North America and Northern Europe, but not in Southern Europe, Asia, and Latin America, where *C. parapsilosis* occupies that position. This fact may also have therapeutic implications

Candidiasis. Table 1 Epidemiological distribution and common susceptibility patterns of *Candida* species

Species	Frequency (%)	Common susceptibility patterns				
		Amphotericin B	5-FC	Fluconazole and itraconazole	Voriconazole and posaconazole[a]	Echinocandins[b]
C. albicans	40–60	S	S	S	S	S
C. glabrata	20–30	S to I	S	S-DD to R	S to S-DD?	S
C. Krusei	5–10	S to I	I to R	R	S to S-DD?	S
C. lusitaniae	0–5	R	S	S	S	S
C. parapsilosis	10–20	S	S	S	S	S to I?
C. tropicalis	20–30	S	S	S	S	S

5-FC 5-fluorocytosine, *S* susceptible, *I* intermediate, *S-DD* susceptible does-dependent (dose needs to be increased to achieve therapeutic efficacy), *R* resistant

[a]Although voriconazole and posaconazole are active in vitro, in vivo, and in early clinical experience against *C. glabrata* and *C. krusei*, their efficacy against these classically azole-resistant organisms hasn't been clearly established

[b]Minimum inhibitory concentrations of the echinocandins are higher for *C. parapsilosis* than for other *Candida* species

as *C. parapsilosis* may have reduced susceptibility to echinocandins and, therefore, azoles are the preferred agents (Table 1).

Timing

Kumar et al. showed that median time to initiation of effective antimicrobial therapy in septic shock is significantly higher for *Candida* (35.1 h) than for bacteria (5.5 h). He also demonstrated that survival decreased 12% per hour of delay of initiation of adequate antifungal therapy in patients with fungal sepsis and shock [2]. Morrell et al. evaluated the impact of delayed antifungal therapy in mortality. Time to initiation of empiric antifungal therapy was measured in 12-h increments, and a significant mortality benefit was observed when therapy was started within 12 h of the drawing of the first positive blood culture [2, 4]. Garey et al. showed that early – within 24 h – antifungal initiation was associated with significantly less mortality rate and that there was a progressive mortality increase with increasing delays in initiation of therapy [2, 4]. More recently, Parkins et al. found that early adequate empiric antifungal therapy was associated with a significant reduction in mortality [4]. Taur et al. subdivided time from collection of blood cultures to initiation of antifungal therapy in three periods: incubation period (time from collection to positivity), provider notification period (time from blood culture positivity to provider notification), and antifungal initiation period (from provider notification to the administration of the first dose of antifungal). In this study, in cancer patients with candidemia, the incubation period (median 32.1 h) accounted for a significant amount of time compared with the provider notification (median 0.3 h) and antifungal

initiation times (median 7.5 h), and its duration was associated with inhospital mortality. Therefore, as modern blood culture systems still require around 24–48 h of incubation to positivity, new strategies are needed to shorten the incubation time.

Which Antifungal Drug?

"Old" (fluconazole and polyenes) and "new" (second-generation azoles and echinocandins) antifungals for the management of candidemia and other forms of IC differ from each other in terms of spectrum, pharmacokinetics and pharmacodynamics, efficacy, interactions, and side effects. Two main factors should be taken into account in the choice of the antifungal: the species of *Candida* and the host (focus, hemodynamic stability, organ dysfunction, previous use of azoles, concomitant drugs).

Triazoles

Triazoles exert their effects within the fungal cell membrane. The inhibition of cytochrome P450 (CYP)-dependent 14-α-demethylase prevents the conversion of lanosterol to ergosterol. This mechanism results in the accumulation of toxic methylsterols and resultant inhibition of fungal cell growth and replication.

Fluconazole remains one of the most prescribed triazoles because of its excellent bioavailability, tolerability, and side-effect profile. More than 80% of ingested drug is found in the circulation, and its absorption is not affected by food consumption, gastric pH, or disease state. Almost 60–70% is excreted unchanged in the urine; therefore, the dose should be adjusted in patients with a reduced clearance of creatinine. Only 10% is protein bound, and it also exhibits excellent tissue penetration, namely, in the central nervous system, where CSF levels are 80% of matched serum levels [4]. Fluconazole is active (fungistatic) against most *Candida* spp. with the exception of *Candida krusei* (intrinsic resistance because of an altered cytochrome P-450 isoenzyme). *Candida glabrata* can be resistant or dose-dependent susceptible (12 mg/kg/day). For IC, a loading dose of 12 mg/kg followed by a daily dose $\geq$6 mg/kg should be administered since higher doses seem to be associated with a better outcome [3]. Although fluconazole has substantially fewer drug–drug interactions than other triazole compounds, it may increase serum levels of phenytoin, warfarin, rifabutin, benzodiazepines, cyclosporine, glipizide, and glyburide. On the other hand, fluconazole levels are reduced with concomitant use of rifampin [4].

Voriconazole is a low molecular weight water-soluble second-generation triazole with a chemical structure similar to fluconazole. It has a potent fungistatic activity against *Candida* spp. usually with lower MICs compared to fluconazole. Voriconazole is available in intravenous ($\blacktriangleright$ IV) and oral formulations. This last formulation has an excellent bioavailability which is reduced with fatty foods by 80%. Like fluconazole, CSF and vitreous penetration is excellent. In adults weighing more than 40 kg, the recommended oral dosing regimen includes a loading dose of 400 mg twice daily on day 1, followed by 200 mg twice daily. Intravenously, after a loading dose of 6 mg/kg twice daily, a maintenance dose of 3–4 mg/kg IV every 12 h is recommended [3]. In patients with a creatinine clearance lower than 50 ml/min, IV voriconazole should not be used as the risk of accumulation of cyclodextrine, to which the drug is complexed, exists. Oral voriconazole does not require dosage adjustment for renal failure, but it is the only triazole that requires dosage reduction for patients with moderate-to-severe liver failure [3]. In adults, voriconazole presents a nonlinear hepatic metabolism. Polymorphisms within CYP2C19 are responsible for interpatient serum concentrations differences. The unpredictability of patient enzymatic activity has generated an interest in the routine use of voriconazole serum-level determination. During first week of treatment, serum levels should be kept between 1 and 5.5 mg/l, not only to prevent treatment failures, but also to reduce toxicity, mainly neurotoxicity. In IC, its clinical use has been primarily for step-down oral therapy in patients with *C. krusei* and fluconazole-resistant but voriconazole-susceptible *C. glabrata* infections. Voriconazole is typically well tolerated, but some patients experience abnormal vision (up to 23%; usually transient and infusion related, without sequelae), skin rash, and transaminase elevation [5].

Despite having in vitro activity against *Candida* spp. that is similar to voriconazole, posaconazole is not recommended for primary IC therapy. It is currently available only as an oral suspension with high oral bioavailability, especially when given with fatty foods [3].

Polyenes

Amphotericin B and nystatin are the currently available polyenes, but nystatin is limited to topical use. Amphotericin B binds to ergosterol within the fungal cell wall membrane. This process disrupts cell-wall permeability by forming oligodendromes functioning as pores with subsequent efflux of potassium and intracellular molecules causing fungal death. Amphotericin B deoxycholate ($\blacktriangleright$ Amb-d) demonstrates a rapid fungicidal in vitro activity against almost all *Candida* spp. with the exception of *Candida lusitaniae*, but is associated with high toxicity. To avoid amphotericin B deoxycholate–induced nephrotoxicity, several lipid formulations were developed: liposomal amphotericin B ($\blacktriangleright$ L-Amb), amphotericin B lipid complex, and amphotericin B colloidal dispersion. These lipid formulations are generally less toxic but equally effective as Amb-d [5]. The peak serum level to mean inhibitory concentration ratio is the best predictor of outcome. All formulations are highly protein bound, have long half-lives, and are widely distributed into tissues, but exhibit poor CSF penetration. The exact route of elimination of amphotericin B is not known and, despite its nephrotoxicity, no dose adjustment is necessary in patients with renal failure. Renal toxic effects of Amb-d are associated with a sixfold increase in mortality and a significant increase in hospital costs. Infusion-related reactions (fever, chills, hypotension, and hypoxemia) are also frequently observed [3, 5].

For most IC, the usual dosage of Amb-d is 0.5–0.7 mg/kg/day, but dosages as high as 1 mg/kg/day should be considered for infections caused by less susceptible species such as *C. glabrata* or *C. krusei*. The typical dosage for lipid formulations is 3–5 mg/kg/day [3].

Echinocandins

Echinocandins (caspofungin, anidulafungin, micafungin) are the most recently introduced class of antifungals. They inhibit the synthesis of β-1,3 glucan by inhibiting the activity of glucan synthase. This mechanism impairs cell-wall integrity and leads to osmotic lysis. They are fungicidal drugs, active against albicans and non-albicans species, and susceptibility differences between the different agents in this class are minimal. *C. parapsilosis* and *C. guilliermondii* demonstrate less in vitro susceptibility to echinocandins than do most other *Candida* spp. related to amino acid polymorphism in the main subunit of glucan synthase (Fks1). However, association between ▶ MIC and treatment outcome is inconsistent [4]. Considering that echinocandin efficacy is predicted by peak to MIC ratios (five- to tenfold), they are administered once daily. Although echinocandin resistance is uncommon, it may occur during therapy. Several studies reported a decrease in microbial kill at higher doses and supra-MIC concentrations: the paradoxical effect. However, its mechanism and clinical implications are unknown. This class of antifungals is only available in IV formulations due to its poor oral absorption. They are highly protein bound, have long half-lives, and their vitreal and CSF penetration is negligible [4]. Caspofungin is metabolized by both hepatic hydrolysis and N-acetylation, and inactive metabolites are then eliminated in the urine. Micafungin is metabolized by nonoxidative metabolism within the liver, and anidulafungin undergoes unique nonenzimatic degradation. All echinocandins have few side effects (phlebitis, headache, abdominal pain, diarrhea, elevated liver transaminases) and do not need dosage adjustment in patients with renal failure or dialysis. It is recommended to reduce caspofungin dosage in patients with moderate-to-severe hepatic impairment [3, 5]. No significant drug interactions were described for anidulafungin. Caspofungin has several drug interactions with agents metabolized through the cytochrome P450 system. As serum levels are reduced in the presence of rifampin, phenytoin, carbamazepine, and phenobarbital, caspofungin dosage should be increased to 70 mg/day in patients taking these medications. Tacrolimus serum levels may decrease with concomitant administration of this echinocandin [4]. Micafungin may increase levels of sirolimus, nifedipine, and cyclosporine. For IC, a loading dosage for caspofungin (70 mg/day) and anidulafungin (200 mg/day) is necessary. The maintenance dosage for caspofungin, micafungin, and anidulafungin is 50, 100, and 100 mg/day, respectively [3].

Antifungal Therapy: A Patient-Based Approach

All current antifungals have been shown to be either equivalent or non-inferior to each other in several studies that included critically ill patients [3, 4]. In these clinical trials, success of therapy ranged from 60% to 83%. The high incidence of adverse events with polyene led to a higher incidence of therapy discontinuation. Due to this potential for toxicity, several international recommendations considered fluconazole and echinocandins as first-line therapy for IC, leaving polyenes as a valid alternative [2, 3].

The hemodynamic status of the patient is an important criterion for selection of *empiric antifungal therapy*.

In hemodynamically stable patient without organ dysfunction, fluconazole is a safe choice. Alternative drugs are echinocandins or amphotericin B. In contrast, hemodynamically unstable patients with severe sepsis or septic shock should be treated with a fungicidal, broad spectrum agent with a good safety profile and, therefore, an echinocandin is the first choice. Alternatively, a lipid formulation of amphotericin B may be used [2, 3].

The likelihood of a patient being infected with an azole-resistant *Candida* spp. is very difficult to predict but must be taken into account. Colonization by an azole-resistant species, previous exposition to an azole or admission to an ICU with a high prevalence (>15–20%) of these species should lead the physician to prescribe an echinocandin, or as an alternative amphotericin B, and avoid azole [2].

The presence of organ dysfunctions is an important issue. Fluconazole dosage should be reduced in patients with renal dysfunction, and IV voriconazole should not be used in patients with creatinine clearance lower than 50 ml/min. Caspofungin and voriconazole dosages should be adjusted in patients with liver impairment [3].

As azoles and echinocandins, except anidulafungin, have important drug–drug interactions, concomitant therapy should also influence antifungal choice. An adequate penetration of antifungal to the source of infection is crucial. For instance, azoles penetrate well in the CNS and in the eye while echinocandins do not. Higher dosages may be necessary for the treatment of fungal endocarditis if an echinocandin is used [3].

Candida spp. ability to adhere to inert and biological surfaces is associated with virulence. Echinocandins and polyenes are the only classes of antifungals with high capacity to act in *Candida* biofilms. Intravenous catheter removal is strongly recommended for non-neutropenic patients with candidemia. This strategy is associated not only with shorter duration of candidemia but also with reduced mortality [2, 3].

The concept of transition or step-down is also recommended. If the patient is clinically stable and the isolate is azole-susceptible, a switch from an echinocandin or an amphotericin B formulation to fluconazole is indicated. Voriconazole is recommended as step-down oral therapy for selected cases of IC due to *Candida krusei* or voriconazole-susceptible *Candida glabrata* [2, 3].

In the management of *documented IC*, an echinocandin is the preferred agent for the treatment of *C. glabrata* infections. For infection due to *C. parapsilosis*, fluconazole is recommended. Yet, if the patient initially received an echinocandin, is clinically improving, and follow-up cultures are negative, continuing the use of an echinocandin is reasonable. IC by *C. albicans* or *C. tropicalis* may be treated with fluconazole as long as the patient is not in severe sepsis or septic shock [2, 3].

Regarding deep organ candidiasis, namely endocarditis, meningitis, osteomyelitis, and endophtalmitis, amphotericin B with or without 5-flucytosine is the preferred treatment in unstable patients. Fluconazole may be used in stable patients or for step-down therapy in these situations [3, 5].

Combination Therapy

The rationale for the use of combination therapy is based on the hypothesis that efficacy can be improved when drugs with different mechanisms of action are used. The combination of antifungals may be used in forms of deep organ candidiasis as stated above. In a study recently conducted by Rex et al. comparing fluconazole with amphotericin B to fluconazole alone for patients with candidemia, combination therapy resulted in a better response rate (69% vs. 56%), especially in patients with APACHE II score between 10 and 22, and more rapid clearance of Candida from blood, but amphotericin B was associated with significant toxicity [2]. Another study has shown that combination therapy of the antibody to Heat Shock Protein (HSP) 90 with L-Amb is superior to L-Amb in monotherapy [5]. In contrast, the usefulness of adding echinocandins to fluconazole may be limited due to a possible antagonism demonstrated in an in vitro Candida biofilm model [5]. To date, the use of combination antifungal therapy in patients with IC is not recommended, and further studies are required [2].

Duration

In candidemia without obvious metastatic complications, treatment should be continued for 2 weeks after the last positive blood culture and resolution of symptoms. However, the duration of antifungal therapy must be prolonged in endophtalmitis, CNS, and osteoarticular and cardiovascular Candida infections [3].

Evaluation and Assessment

The diagnosis of IC is still a major challenge in the ICU, and it is often made late in the course of the infection. Clinical manifestations are often nonspecific, and, frequently, it is hard to differentiate colonization from infection. The current "gold standard" for the diagnosis of IC is either a positive culture specimen from a sterile site or characteristic histopathology. These two methods have limited sensitivity. Blood cultures are known to be negative for around 50% of patients with IC, and improvements in blood culture technique have increased the sensitivity to 70%, at the best.

The difficulties of clinically recognizing Candida infections together with the paramount importance of early initiation of treatment favored the search for predictive factors of fungal infection on which early empiric antifungal treatment should be based. Recognized risk factors for IC are: severity of illness (APACHE II score), neutropenia, colonization with Candida spp., presence of central venous catheter, parenteral nutrition, ICU length of stay ≥7 days, prior abdominal surgery, previous broad spectrum antibiotherapy, hemodyalisis or renal failure, and cancer chemotherapy [1].

In order to improve the risk factor–driven approach, several authors have focused on combining risk factors to develop predictive algorithms and scoring systems that may help physicians to identify patients who will benefit from early antifungal therapy. Pittet et al. in a prospective cohort study identified two independent risk factors that predicted subsequent invasive Candida infection: the severity of illness assessed by the APACHE II score and the intensity of Candida spp. colonization defined as the colonization index (threshold for intervention set at 0.5). The corrected index (product of the colonization index times the ratio of the number of distinct body sites showing heavy growth to the total of distinct body sites growing Candida spp.) with a threshold of 0.4 was associated with a 100% sensitivity and specificity [1, 4].

In a retrospective cohort analysis with prospective validation, Dupont et al. developed a predictive score for the isolation of yeast from peritoneal fluid in critically ill patients with peritonitis. In patients with three of four independent risk factors (female gender, upper GI tract origin, intraoperative cardiovascular failure, and antimicrobial therapy at least 48 h before onset of peritonitis), the positive and negative predictive values for isolation of yeast were 67% and 72%, respectively. Leon et al. based on a large prospective, cohort, observational, and multicentre study developed the bedside "Candida score": total parenteral nutrition (1 point), surgery (1 point), multifocal colonization (1 point), and severe sepsis/septic shock (2 points). A Candida score ≥3 points was associated with a 7.75-fold increased likelihood of proven IC and accurately predicted (sensitivity 81% and specificity 74%) patients who could benefit from early antifungal therapy and is highly improbable if a Candida colonized non-neutropenic critically ill patient has a Candida score <3 [1, 4, 5].

Ostrosky-Zeichner et al. developed a prediction rule that can be applied to 10% of patients who stay in the ICU ≥4 days. The presence of at least one major risk factor (previous antibiotherapy or presence of central venous catheter) and at least two minor risk factors (total parenteral nutrition, dialysis, any major surgery, pancreatitis, steroids, use of other immunosuppressive agents) was associated with a low sensitivity (34%) but with a high negative predictive value (97%) [1, 4, 5].

At present, no single predictive rule provides a gold standard algorithm for IC, and further prospective validation in a clinical setting is necessary.

New methods to avoid delays in appropriate antifungal therapy are therefore needed. (1,3)-β-D-glucan (▶ BG) is a cell-wall component of most fungi, except *Zygomycetes* and *Cryptococcus*, which is released during tissue invasion. BG test seems to be a promising tool for early diagnosis of IC given its high sensitivity (from 55% to 100%) and specificity (78–100%). Positive results occur not only in patients who have candidiasis, but also in aspergillosis, gastrointestinal colonization with *Candida* spp., endemic mycoses, and *Pneumocystis jiroveci* pneumonia. However, its use in the critically ill patient has two main limitations: it was not yet validated in non-neutropenic patients and there is a significant rate of false positive results (bacteremia, surgical gauze, albumin, hemodyalisis, and antibiotics such as piperacilin) [1, 4]. In addition, the cutoff for positive result is not well defined ranging from 20 to 75 pg/ml.

Leon et al. showed that procalcitonin increased the predictive value of "*Candida* score," as patients with multifocal colonization by *Candida* spp., staying more than 7 days in the ICU, that develop IC showed significantly higher values of this biomarker.

The detection of *Candida* DNA by ▶ PCR holds great promise as a sensitive and potentially rapid diagnostic test, but, unfortunately, methodologies have not been standardized and only limited evaluations have been performed in clinical specimens. McMullan et al. conducted a prospective study of 145 consecutive non-neutropenic patients admitted to a single adult ICU. Serum was drawn twice weekly and fungal DNA amplified using a real-time PCR capable of detecting *Candida* spp. This assay showed a high sensitivity (71–99%) and specificity (99–100%) and an excellent positive (83–100%) and negative (99–100%) predictive value. These data suggest that this assay may perform well for the rapid diagnosis of candidemia in non-neutropenic adults, providing results on the same day [1, 4].

Since both time and distinction between albicans and non-albicans species are important new techniques are necessary. Actually, the rapid identification and differentiation of *Candida albicans* from *Candida glabrata* can be achieved within 3 h using commercial nucleic acid fluorescent in situ hybridization (PNA FISH) technique [4].

After-care

Once a patient has been started on antifungal treatment, it is advisable to repeat blood cultures after 4–5 days to monitor response and breakthrough infections. All patients with candidemia should undergo funduscopic examination within the first week after initiation of therapy to rule out endophtalmitis, which occurs in about 10% of patients with candidemia and impacts on antifungal selection and duration of therapy.

Patients showing suboptimal responses in spite of adequate antifungal therapy should be evaluated for several common causes of therapeutic failure, namely: lack of removal of an intravascular catheter, presence of other vascular niduses (e.g., an infected heart valve or endovascular graft), seeding of a protected site (e.g., endophtalmitis, osteomyelitis, and hepatosplenic disease) or other prosthetic devices (e.g., artificial joints and peritoneal dialysis catheters).

Prognosis

Invasive candidiasis is associated with a crude mortality rate of around 60%. As underlying diseases contribute to mortality, the estimated "attributable" mortality is usually reported as 40–49%. However, attributable mortality varies depending on study design: 20–50% in retrospective case-control studies and 5–7% in prospective clinical trials [4].

Tumbarello et al. in a retrospective analysis, identified three risk factors for mortality: inadequate antifungal therapy, infection with biofilm-forming *Candida* species, and APACHE III score [1]. In the study performed by Morrell et al. APACHE II score prior use of antibiotics and initiation of antifungal therapy more than 12 h after the first positive blood culture were independent determinants of hospital mortality [4].

IC and candidemia are also associated with a high ICU (12.7 days) and hospital stay (15.5 days) and with increased costs [1]. The extra cost of an episode of candidemia in adults has been estimated as 44,000 USD and 16,000€. These data underscore the need for improved means of prevention and treatment of candidemia.

References

1. Guery BP, Arendrup MC, Auzinger G, Azoulay E, Sá MB, Johnson EM, Müller E, Putensen C, Rotstein C, Sganga G, Venditti M, Crespo RZ, Kullberg BJ (2009) Management of invasive candidiasis and candidemia in adult non-neutropenic intensive care unit patients: part I. Epidemiology and diagnosis. Intensive Care Med 35:55–62
2. Guery BP, Arendrup MC, Auzinger G, Azoulay E, Sá MB, Johnson EM, Müller E, Putensen C, Rotstein C, Sganga G, Venditti M, Crespo RZ, Kullberg BJ (2009) Management of invasive candidiasis and candidemia in adult non-neutropenic intensive care unit patients: part II. Treatment. Intensive Care Med 35:206–214

3. Pappas PG, Kauffman CA, Andes D, Benjamin DK Jr, Calandra TF, Edwards JE Jr, Filler SG, Fisher JF, Kullberg BJ, Ostrosky-Zeichner L, Reboli AC, Rex JH, Walsh TJ, Sobel JD (2009) Clinical practice guidelines for the management of candidiasis: 2009 update by the Infectious Diseases Society of America. Clin Infect Dis 48:503–535
4. Playford EG, Eggimann P, Calandra T (2008) Antifungals in the ICU. Curr Opin Infect Dis 21:610–619
5. Hollenbach E (2008) Invasive candidiasis in the ICU: evidence based and on the edge of evidence. Mycoses 51(2):25–45

CAP

Community-acquired pneumonia: Pneumonia occurring in any patient who does not meet the criteria for HCAP, HAP, or VAP.

Capillaries

▶ Microcirculation

Capillary Refill

BRIAN G. HARBRECHT
Department of Surgery, University of Louisville, Louisville, KY, USA

Synonyms

Circulation; Microvascular perfusion; Perfusion

Definition

Capillary refill is a subjective, noninvasive assessment of peripheral cutaneous perfusion used to evaluate the adequacy of the regional or systemic circulation. A test of capillary refill involves manual compression, typically on the nailbed or distal skin of an extremity, to blanch the skin followed by rapid release of the pressure. If it takes <2 s for the skin to return to normal pink coloration, capillary refill is adequate. Delayed return of normal coloration to the area of compression (>2 s) suggests an abnormality in either the regional or systemic circulation.

By definition, capillary refill measures or assesses the status of the perfusion of the skin of an extremity. In clinical practice, it is often used to evaluate the presence or absence of shock. The ability of capillary refill to reflect the adequacy of the systemic circulation is based on the body's compensatory responses to shock [1]. When global tissue hypoperfusion is present due to hypovolemia, cardiac dysfunction, or other causes, increased sympathetic activation leads to α_1-adrenergic-mediated peripheral vasoconstriction. This peripheral vasoconstriction increases peripheral arteriolar resistance and shunts blood from the less essential peripheral vascular beds (skin, splanchnic organs) to more essential visceral organs such as the heart and the brain [1]. Increased sympathetic tone also constricts capacitance vessels in selected vascular beds to increase venous return. These responses contribute to the pale appearance of the skin and its cool, clammy consistency to the touch.

Several environmental and patient factors can introduce variability into assessments of capillary refill [2, 3]. These factors include patient age, gender, and the ambient temperature the patient is exposed to. Much of the variability in capillary refill between individuals, however, appears to be due to factors that are difficult to define. Despite the subjective element in its interpretation and the relative nonspecific nature of the test, assessment of capillary refill remains a commonly performed component of the physical examination of patients. It has been reported to correlate well with hypovolemia in selected populations of patients such as infants. Capillary refill remains a component of the physical assessment of injured patients in the Advanced Trauma Life Support^R course from the American College of Surgeons and is included in guidelines for the assessment of perfusion in critically ill patients [4, 5].

Technical issues can interfere with the accuracy of using capillary refill as an index of systemic perfusion. Severe hypothermia can induce intense peripheral vasoconstriction that can interfere with capillary perfusion of peripheral tissues even though the intravascular volume may be adequate. Adequate illumination is essential to determine when normal coloration returns to the skin after compression. While generally not a problem in the Emergency Department or Intensive Care Unit, this limitation hinders applicability of capillary refill in the prehospital setting, at night, or in austere environments such as military field triage. This limitation can be significant since a technically simple, readily available test to assess perfusion may be most useful in these environments where physical examination is the only tool available to assess the patient. As mentioned above, variability between individuals can also exist independent of the status of the systemic circulation due to patient-specific factors that remain difficult to define. The assessment of capillary refill is particularly useful in the field of orthopedics where casts, splints, and braces may limit access to peripheral pulses to assess perfusion. The examiner should keep in mind, however, that peripheral vascular disease, peripheral vascular injuries, or other disorders of regional blood flow can interfere with the ability of capillary refill to reflect the status of the systemic circulation.

As technology has improved, a variety of modalities have been developed to assess peripheral perfusion. These technologies measure different endpoints in peripheral tissues that reflect distal tissue circulation. Their ability to measure systemic perfusion is based, in part, on the same compensatory physiologic responses that govern capillary refill. These modalities include near-infrared spectroscopy (NIRS) to measure peripheral muscle tissue oxygen saturation (StO_2), microprobes, or transcutaneous sensors to measure arterial pH, arterial oxygen pressure, and arterial carbon dioxide pressure, and laser Doppler flowmetry to measure cutaneous capillary blood flow. Clinical trials on the use of NIRS to monitor StO_2 as an index of the adequacy of shock resuscitation in trauma patients have been performed and the devices are commercially available for clinical use. Laser Doppler flowmetry has also been utilized clinically in selected centers, primarily to monitor microvascular perfusion of flaps in free tissue transfer operations (free flaps). One could even consider sublingual capnometry, gastric tonometry, and oxygen consumption/oxygen delivery-based goal-oriented therapy as extremely sophisticated technologies designed to measure tissue or peripheral perfusion analogous to the capillary refill test [3]. Unfortunately, none of these modalities are universally accepted for assessing the adequacy of the peripheral circulation or as an index of the adequacy of resuscitation from shock in all cases. Several of these technologies continue to undergo active investigation in both the clinical and the basic science environment. Whether these tools will prove to be more useful than simple clinical assessment of the patient remains undetermined.

Differential Diagnosis

When used to assess the adequacy of peripheral perfusion as an index of the systemic circulation, a normal capillary refill test reassures the clinician that the systemic perfusion is adequate enough to perfuse the least essential part of the body. Abnormalities of capillary refill should heighten one's suspicion for inadequate perfusion, but they are fairly nonspecific. Additional parameters of diminished perfusion should be sought such as altered mental status from decreased cerebral perfusion, location and quality of peripheral pulses, character of the skin to palpation (cool and clammy versus warm and dry), and the appropriate clinical setting for a patient in shock. Once shock is suspected, resuscitative maneuvers should be implemented while an etiology is sought. The clinician should keep in mind that the body's compensatory mechanisms to circulatory disturbances will act to restore intravascular volume and maintain perfusion to key visceral systems through increased heart rate, increased contractility, and activation of neuroendocrine responses. Hypotension is a relatively late development when these compensatory mechanisms have been overwhelmed. The presence of shock should not be equated with hypotension since significant hypoperfusion can occur before systemic blood pressure falls.

As previously discussed, the clinician needs to be aware of potential confounders that can result in abnormal capillary refill in the face of adequate intravascular volume. Hypothermia, peripheral vascular disease, age, and poor ambient light can all interfere with the ability of capillary refill to reflect the status of the systemic circulation. One should keep in mind that constricting casts or bandages, proximal peripheral vascular injuries, or proximal vascular thromboses may produce regional abnormalities of perfusion in the face of normal systemic circulation. Assessment of the opposite extremity or a different peripheral vascular bed will prove useful in these cases.

As with many other tests used to evaluate perfusion and shock resuscitation, a single measurement may provide useful information, but serial assessments over time are frequently optimal to gauge the response to therapy. Other parameters to assess perfusion and the systemic circulation are discussed in greater detail in other sections of this work. Repetitive assessment of a number of clinical endpoints (capillary refill, heart rate, urine output, base deficit, etc.) will often help the clinician to determine whether shock persists or homeostasis is being restored.

References

1. Harbrecht BG, Forsythe RM, Peitzman AB (2008) Management of shock. In: Feliciano DV, Mattox KL, Moore EE (eds) Trauma, 6th edn. McGraw-Hill, New York
2. Anderson B, Kelly AM, Kerr D, Clooney M, Astat DJ (2008) Impact of patient and environmental factors on capillary refill time in adults. Am J Emerg Med 26:62–65
3. Lima A, Bakker J (2005) Noninvasive monitoring of peripheral perfusion. Intensive Care Med 31:1316–1326
4. Lima A, Jansen TC, van Bommel J, Ince C, Bakker J (2009) The prognostic value of the subjective assessment of peripheral perfusion in critically ill patients. Crit Care Med 37:934–938
5. Brierley J, Carcillo JA, Choong K et al (2009) Clinical practice parameters for hemodynamic support of pediatric and neonatal septic shock; 2007 update from the American College of Critical Care Medicine. Crit Care Med 37:666–688

Capnograph

▶ End-Tidal CO2

Capnography

▶ End-Tidal CO2
▶ Pulse Oxymetry and CO2 Monitoring

Capnometry

▶ End-Tidal CO2

Capsaicin- 8-methyl-N-vanillyl-6-nonenamide

Capsaicin- 8-methyl-N-vanillyl-6-nonenamide, is the active component of chili peppers, plants which belong to the genus *Capsicum*. It is an irritant for animals and produces a sensation of burning in tissues that it contacts. Capsaicin selectively binds to a protein known as TRPV1 that is located on the membrane of heat and pain sensing neurons. Prolonged activation of these neurons depletes presynaptic substance P, one of the body's neurotransmitters for pain and heat, and the sensation of pain is reduced.

Carbonic Anhydrase Inhibitors

▶ Diuretics for Management of AKI

Cardiac and Endovascular Infections

DONALD P. LEVINE, PATRICIA D. BROWN
Department of Medicine, Wayne State University, Detroit, MI, USA

Synonyms
Bacterial endocarditis; Endocarditis; Fungal endocarditis

Definition
Infective endocarditis (IE) is defined as infection involving the endocardium. Although any part of the endocardial surface may be involved, the heart valves are affected most frequently. Endocarditis may also occur at the site of a septal defect or a site where the endocardium has been disrupted by abnormal flow or intracardiac devices. The term infective endocarditis is now preferred to the older terminology, bacterial endocarditis, as it is recognized that a wide variety of pathogens may cause endocarditis. The pathologic lesion at the site of infection is the vegetation which consists of fibrin, platelets, and the offending microorganism; a paucity of inflammatory cells is present. Injury to the endothelium results either in direct infection by organisms present, even transiently, in the blood stream or may result in the formation of a platelet-fibrin thrombus that may then become secondarily infected.

Treatment
Comprehensive, evidenced based guidelines for the diagnosis and management of IE are published by the American Heart Association (AHA) which were last updated in 2005 [1]. Probably the most important development impacting the initial empiric therapy of suspected IE is the emergence of *Staphylococcus aureus* as the most common etiology of native valve IE in most centers, reflecting the fact that a significant proportion of IE cases are now health care associated infections [2]. Methicillin resistant *S. aureus* (MRSA), both community-acquired and health care associated strains, must be considered a potential etiology of IE, particularly in patients whose severity of illness is sufficient to warrant admission to the intensive care unit. Because receipt of initial empiric therapy that covers the causative organism is an important predictor of favorable outcome in critically ill patients with sepsis, it is anticipated that even patients with suspected IE will receive broad-spectrum antimicrobial therapy initially. Once the diagnosis is confirmed and the causative organism identified, antibiotic therapy should be revised to a regimen known to be effective for the treatment of IE due to the isolated pathogen. The recommendations discussed below are targeted toward patients with native valve IE (NVE); the treatment of prosthetic valve infective endocarditis (PVE) is discussed separately.

Viridans Group Streptococci and *Streptococcus bovis*
The appropriate regimen for IE caused by viridans streptococci and *S. bovis* depends on the minimum inhibitory concentration (MIC) to penicillin for the isolate. Increasing penicillin MICs among these streptococci is

well described; therefore it is imperative that MIC values be available and reviewed before antibiotic therapy is adjusted. Highly susceptible isolates (MIC $\leq$ 0.12 µg/ml) can be treated with aqueous crystalline penicillin G sodium (12–18 million units per day, given by continuous infusion or divided into 4 or 6 equal doses) or ceftriaxone (2 g every 24 h) for 28 days. The duration of therapy may be shortened to 14 days if gentamicin (3 mg/kg every 24 h) is used; however, this "short course" regimen should not be used in patients with cardiac or extra-cardiac complication of IE or in patients at increased risk of aminoglycoside related nephrotoxicity. Vancomycin for 28 days is an alternative in patients with severe penicillin allergy. Clinicians are reminded that the strong association between *S. bovis* IE and colonic lesions (including malignancy) mandates an evaluation of the gastrointestinal tract once the patient's clinical condition has stabilized.

Viridans streptococci and *S. bovis* isolates with penicillin MIC > 0.12 to $\leq$ 0.5 µg/ml should be treated with penicillin or ceftriaxone for 28 days with single daily dose gentamicin for the first 14 days of therapy.

Viridans streptococci with penicillin MIC > 0.5 µg/ml along with *Abiotrophia*, *Granulicatella*, and *Gemella* species should be managed as for enterococcal IE (discussed below). If vancomycin is used, combination with gentamicin is not necessary.

IE due to *S. pyogenes* can be treated with 28 days of penicillin, as outlined above. Cefazolin or ceftriaxone are alternatives; vancomycin should only be utilized in cases of severe B-lactam allergy. IE due to groups B, C, or G streptococci is managed similarly; some experts do recommend the addition of gentamicin to the regimen for the first 14 days of therapy and consideration of a more prolonged (42 day) total course of treatment for these three pathogens.

Although uncommon, *S. pneumoniae* remains an important pathogen in IE. Isolates with penicillin MICs up to 4 can be successfully treated with high dose (up to 24 million units/day) of penicillin; if the patient has concomitant meningitis, cefotaxime or ceftriaxone must be used for isolates with penicillin MICs $\geq$ 0.1 (provided the isolate is susceptible to these agents); penicillin and cephalosporin resistant isolates are generally managed with vancomycin in combination with cefotaxime or ceftriaxone.

Enterococci

Enterococcal isolates suspected of causing IE must undergo testing for penicillin (or ampicillin) and vancomycin MICs as well as testing for the presence of high level resistance to gentamicin and streptomycin. Relative resistance to penicillin (ampicillin) and vancomycin is an intrinsic property of enterococci; therefore serous infections such as IE due to enterococci are optimally managed with the addition of an aminoglycoside for synergy. IE due to strains susceptible to penicillin and gentamicin should be treated with ampicillin (12 g daily, divided into six equal doses) or aqueous crystalline penicillin G sodium (18–30 million units daily, continuously or divided into six equal doses) plus gentamicin 3 mg/kg daily in two or three divided doses (adjusted for peaks of 3–5 µg/ml with a trough of <1 µg/ml). Four weeks of therapy is sufficient for patients whose symptoms have been present less than 3 months; 6 weeks of therapy is recommended for those with symptoms more than 3 months. If the organism is sensitive, vancomycin can be substituted in patients with penicillin allergy; however, these patients should receive 6 weeks of therapy, regardless of the duration of symptoms. Streptomycin should be used for isolates that have high level resistance to gentamicin, but not to streptomycin; 15 mg/kg every 24 h divided into two doses is recommended in patients with normal renal function.

Optimal therapy of isolates that demonstrate susceptibility to penicillin but high level resistance to gentamicin and streptomycin is not well established. Several studies support the use of high dose ampicillin (12 g/day) in combination with ceftriaxone (2 g every 12 h) in these cases; therapy should be given for 6 weeks. This regimen may also be a reasonable alternative for patients with aminoglycoside susceptible isolates who develop progressive nephrotoxicity during therapy.

Optimal therapy for enterococcal isolates that are resistant to penicillins, vancomycin, and aminoglycosides is also unknown. For infections due to *Enterococcus faecium*, the AHA guidelines recommend either linezolid (1,200 mg/day in two divided doses) or quinopristin-dalfopristin (22.5 mg/kg per day divided into three equal doses) for a minimum of 8 weeks. Resistant *E. faecalis* infections may be treated with ceftriaxone plus ampicillin or imipenem-cilastatin plus ampicillin for a minimum of 8 weeks. Surgery should be a strong consideration for the management of these infections for which synergistic antimicrobial therapy is not possible. An increasing number of case reports have documented successful treatment with daptomycin in such cases, although therapeutic failures have also been reported and additional data are clearly needed.

Staphylococci

As discussed above, *S. aureus* is now the most common cause of IE in the developed world and patients critically ill with suspected IE should receive initial empiric therapy that includes coverage for this pathogen, including the possibility of MRSA. Although typically considered important pathogens mainly in early PVE, coagulase-negative staphylococci (CoNS) have emerged as important pathogens in NVE, causing almost 8% of such infections in non-injection drug users with IE in a recent large prospective study. Almost half of NVE due to CoNS is health care associated; medical comorbidities, long-term intravenous catheter use, and recent invasive procedures appear to be risk factors. Among the CoNS, *S. lugdunensis* appears to be particularly virulent, often associated with metastatic infection as well as periannular extension of the infection. Surgical treatment may be required more frequently in patients with IE due to CoNS than in patients with *S. aureus* infections.

Patients with IE due to methicillin-susceptible *S. aureus* (MSSA) should be treated with nafcillin (12 g/day divided into four or six equal doses); cefazolin (6 g/day divided into three equal doses) is an alternative for patients with non-life threatening penicillin allergy. Vancomycin can be used in patients with severe B-lactam allergy. Although clinicians may be tempted to substitute vancomycin for a B-lactam, particularly in patients with reduced renal function because of the convenience of less frequent dosing, vancomycin is inferior to the B-lactams for the treatment of susceptible isolates, therefore this practice is not acceptable. It is very important to note that while the AHA guidelines recommend vancomycin dosing to achieve serum trough concentrations of 10–15 µg/ml, a more recently published consensus review recommends a vancomycin target trough of 15–20 µg/ml for serious infections such as IE [3]. The AHA guidelines list the addition of 3–5 days of gentamicin therapy as optional, noting that a clinical benefit of initial aminoglycoside therapy in *S. aureus* IE has not been proven. Recently, initial low dose gentamicin for *S. aureus* bacteremia and native valve IE was associated with significant risk of nephrotoxicity. Given the lack of data regarding benefit in this setting, we do not recommend it.

Vancomycin is the recommended therapy for IE due to MRSA. However, a growing body of evidence indicates that patients with serious infections due to MRSA whose isolates have vancomycin MICs > 1 µg/ml respond less favorably to vancomycin therapy than those due to isolates with lower MICs. Daptomycin achieved clinical success rates that were non-inferior to vancomycin for bacteremia and right-sided endocarditis due to MRSA; data for the use of daptomycin in the treatment of left-sided IE is derived mainly from observational studies and case reports. There are very limited data to support the use of other agents for MRSA IE. Success has been reported with the use of trimethoprim-sulfamethoxazole, doxycycline,

minocycline, linezolid, and quinopristin-dalfopristin. Clearly, the optimal management of MRSA IE, especially infections due to isolates with higher vancomycin MICs, remains to be defined.

Despite *in vitro* susceptibility, the addition of rifampin to the regimen for the treatment of native valve IE due to *S. aureus* is not recommended.

In general, 6 weeks of therapy is recommended for patients with *S. aureus* IE; patients with uncomplicated infections can be treated with 4 weeks of therapy. Injection drug users (IDUs) with uncomplicated right-sided IE due to MSSA can be successfully managed with a 2 week course of nafcillin in combination with an aminoglycoside; the presence of septic pulmonary emboli does not preclude the use of "short course" therapy in this setting.

NVE due to CoNS should be treated with regimens similar to those outlined above, based on the *in vitro* susceptibility data.

Gram-Negative Pathogens

Native valve IE due to organisms of the HACEK group (Haemophilus, Actinobacillus, Cardiobacterium, Eikenella, and Kingella) should be treated with ceftriaxone (2 g daily); ampicillin-sulbactam and ciprofloxacin are alternatives. A 4 week course of antibiotic therapy is recommended. Non-HACEK Gram-negatives account for less than 2% of cases of NVE. Therapy should be based on *in vitro* susceptibility data; surgery is frequently required for successful management.

Culture Negative Infective Endocarditis

Blood cultures may be negative in patients with IE due to the presence of a fastidious bacterial pathogen, a non-bacterial pathogen or the receipt of antibiotic therapy before blood cultures are obtained. The latter reason is probably most common, particularly among patients who are critically ill on presentation. The importance of assuring that blood cultures are obtained, even in the most critically ill patient, prior to the administration of antibiotics cannot be over emphasized. Options for the empiric therapy of culture negative NVE include ampicillin-sulbactam plus gentamicin or vancomycin plus gentamicin plus ciprofloxacin. A recent case series of patients with culture negative endocarditis underscored the importance of aminoglycoside therapy in the management of this infection; patients who did not receive an aminoglycoside containing regimen had a significantly higher mortality.

Fungal Endocarditis

The majority of cases of fungal IE are due to *Candida* species. *C. albicans* is most common in non-IDUs; non-albicans candida are more common in IDUs. Recommendations for management of fungal endocarditis are based mainly on expert opinion. The most current recommendations can be found in the guidelines for the management of candidiasis from the Infectious Diseases Society of America (available at www.idsociety.org). Initial therapy should consist of amphotericin B, either a standard or a liposomal preparation, with or without five flucytosine, or an echinocandin. Fungal endocarditis remains a strong indication for valve replacement.

Prosthetic Valve Endocarditis

PVE occurs in 1–6% of patients with a prosthetic valve. Mechanical and bioprosthetic valves have similar rates of infection overall; however, mechanical valves have a higher rate of infection during the first 3 months after implantation. S. aureus has emerged as the most common infecting agent, followed by CoNS and streptococci. Initial empiric antibiotic therapy for critically ill patients with suspected PVE will likely include broad-spectrum coverage for both Gram positive and Gram-negative pathogens; the regimen chosen should always include coverage for MRSA. If S. aureus or CoNS are confirmed, nafcillin or vancomycin should be utilized, based on susceptibility results. Rifampin (900 mg daily in three divided doses) and gentamicin should be added, although gentamicin may be discontinued after 2 weeks. Prolonged (at least 6 weeks) therapy will be required. Therapy for viridans streptococci and S. bovis isolates with penicillin MIC ≤ 0.12 µg/ml is the same as that outlined for native valve infections except that short course (2 week) regimens should not be used. The addition of gentamicin (single daily dose) to a B-lactam for the first 2 weeks of therapy is optional and the total duration of therapy should be 6 weeks. PVE due to viridans streptococci and S. bovis isolates with penicillin MIC > 0.12 µg/ml should be treated with penicillin or ceftriaxone plus gentamicin (single daily dose) for 6 weeks; vancomycin should only be utilized for patients with severe B-lactam allergy. The treatment of enterococcal PVE is the same as for native valve infections; all regimens should be given for a minimum of 6 weeks.

Therapy for culture negative PVE depends on whether the onset is early (less than 1 year since valve replacement) or late. Empiric therapy for early culture negative PVE should include vancomycin, gentamicin (3 mg/kg daily in three divided doses), cefepime, and rifampin. For late PVE, the regimens outlined for native valve culture negative IE may be used, with the addition of rifampin.

Anticoagulation

Anticoagulation has not been shown to provide benefit in patients with native valve IE, and active IE is considered a strong contraindication to anticoagulation because of the potential risk of bleeding from unrecognized central nervous system (CNS) mycotic aneurysms. The use of anticoagulation in patients with PVE is much more controversial. The AHA guidelines recommend continuing anticoagulation in patients with PVE, except in patients with S. aureus infections who have experienced a CNS embolic event. Anticoagulation may be cautiously resumed once these patients have completed 2 weeks of appropriate antibiotic treatment.

Surgery

In a recently published multicenter cohort study of IE, almost 50% of patients underwent valvular surgery for the management of their infection. Despite widespread use and the belief that surgery improves outcomes in selected patients, there are virtually no data from randomized controlled clinical trials regarding appropriate indications and timing of surgery. Congestive cardiac failure (CHF) is the most common indication for surgery in IE and the clinical condition of the patient, not the duration of antibiotic therapy, dictates the timing of surgery. Surgical intervention should also be considered for infections due to resistant pathogens for which optimal bactericidal therapy cannot be devised (e.g., vancomycin resistant enterococci) and patients with left-sided IE who remain bacteremic after a week of appropriate antimicrobial therapy, provided that a metastatic focus of infection has been excluded as a cause of persistent bacteremia (4). Other generally accepted indications for surgery include one or more major embolic events in patients with left-sided IE, paravalvular extension of infection, and valve perforation or rupture. Fungal IE has long been considered a strong indication for valve replacement; however, the availability of newer and less toxic antifungal agents and the use of oral azoles for long-term suppressive therapy has resulted in clinical success.

The availability of transesophageal echocardiography (TEE) has resulted in additional recommendations for surgery including persistence of a vegetation after a systemic embolic event, anterior mitral leaflet vegetations (particularly those >10 mm in size), and increase in the size of a vegetation despite appropriate antibiotic therapy.

In addition to the indications listed above, surgical therapy should be considered for PVE due to S. aureus, S. lugdunensis, and early PVE due to other CoNS.

Indications for surgical treatment are likely prevalent among patients with IE who require admission to the intensive care unit. The perception that the patient is "too sick" to undergo surgery often results in a delay of a potentially lifesaving procedure. Decisions regarding surgical intervention must be made with input from the intensivist, cardiologist, infectious diseases specialist, and the surgeon. The timing of surgical intervention in those who have had a CNS embolic event, especially if hemorrhagic, is particularly problematic. In addition to the team outlined above, input from the neurologist or neurosurgeon will be essential to optimize management for these patients.

Evaluation

Although it remains an uncommon infection, advances in medical technology and care have expanded the number of patients who are at risk for IE. As many as 20% of individuals with IE have no recognized preexisting cardiac condition that places them at increased risk for the infection. The diagnosis should be considered in any patient with persistent bacteremia, evidence of a systemic embolic event, or evidence of infection in the setting of a predisposing cardiac lesion. Up to 25% of IE cases are health care associated infections. The presenting features of IE may include stroke and other embolic phenomenon, evidence of metastatic infection such as musculoskeletal infection or splenic abscess, or CHF but most patients have nonspecific manifestations of infection. Elderly patients with IE are more likely to have been hospitalized for an invasive procedure before the onset of infection and have lower rates of embolic events, immune phenomena, and septic complications. Older individuals are likely to present acutely with infection due to virulent pathogens such as *S. aureus*; the classic peripheral stigmata of IE have become far less common as a presenting manifestation of the disease. Nevertheless, meticulous examination of the patient who presents with evidence of sepsis may reveal a conjunctival, retinal, or subungual (splinter) hemorrhage or even Janeway lesions or Osler's nodes, findings that suggest the diagnosis even before blood cultures turn positive or the results of echocardiography are available. The majority (up to 85%) of individuals with IE will have an audible murmur. Mitral valve involvement is more common than aortic valve infection. Tricuspid valve IE is a well-recognized complication of IDU; however, in several recent series left-sided IE was more common than right-sided infections in this patient population. Tricuspid valve IE also occurs in non-IDUs with central venous catheters. Patients with right-sided IE often present with pulmonary manifestations due to septic pulmonary emboli. The possibility of IE should be seriously considered in all patients with *S. aureus* bacteremia. Risk factors for valve infection in these patients include an unknown source of bacteremia, presence of a prosthetic valve, persistent fever, and persistent positive blood cultures. The risk of IE in patients with community-onset enterococcal bacteremia is also high.

Because of the requirement to provide specific pathogen-directed antimicrobial therapy for a prolonged course, the necessity of ensuring that a microbiologic diagnosis is confirmed cannot be overemphasized. Two sets of blood cultures should be obtained prior to the initiation of empiric antimicrobial therapy. One set of blood cultures is defined as a blood sample drawn at a single time from a single site, regardless of how many bottles or tubes are submitted from that sample. In total, 3–4 sets of blood cultures should be obtained during the first 24 h of evaluation. In patients who have no or limited peripheral venous access, cultures may be obtained via an intravascular device; however, a sample obtained in this manner represents a single set of blood cultures, even if obtained from more than one port. At least two sets of blood cultures should be obtained on each subsequent day to document the persistence or clearing of bacteremia.

While blood cultures remain the single most important diagnostic test in the evaluation of patients with suspected IE, echocardiography, particularly TEE, has significantly improved both diagnosis and earlier recognition of complications of IE. The sensitivity of transthoracic echocardiography (TTE) for the diagnosis of IE is 60–65%; the sensitivity of TEE is 90–95%. Both have a specificity of greater than 90%. The superior sensitivity of TEE is even more significant in the evaluation of PVE. In patients at high risk of IE or for whom the clinical suspicion of IE is moderate to high, TEE should be the initial imaging procedure chosen; the procedure can be safely performed even in patients who are critically ill.

Previously, the definite diagnosis of IE required confirmation of infection based on specimens obtained at the time of valve replacement surgery. With the advent of echocardiography, a definite diagnosis can now be made based on a constellation of clinical, microbiologic and echocardiographic findings. The modified Duke criteria are now widely accepted for the diagnosis of IE [4].

Pacemakers and Implantable Cardioverter-Defibrillators

As the number of accepted indications for the use of permanent pacemakers and implantable cardioverter-defibrillators has increased, cardiac device–related infections (CDIs) have become more common. CDIs may be confined to the generator pocket, or may include wire infections complicated by endocarditis. The majority of patients with CDIs present with localized findings of infection at the site of the generator pocket; however, the absence of such findings does not exclude the device as a potential source of sepsis. TTE lacks sufficient sensitivity to evaluate for device-related infection. *S. aureus* is implicated most often; infections due to CoNS, enterococci, Gram-negatives, and candida also occur.

Successful treatment of CDIs in association with positive blood cultures requires complete removal of the device, especially in patients with IE. The mortality rate for device-related IE is as high as 66% without device removal, but is as low as 18% with complete removal and appropriate antimicrobial therapy. Emergent device removal is particularly important in the management of patients with severe sepsis. Baddour and colleagues devised an algorithm for the management of these infections that is a useful guide [5]. The device may not be safely re-implanted until the generator pocket has been adequately debrided and the blood cultures are negative.

Prognosis and After-care

In-hospital mortality for IE is 15–20%; the 1 year mortality may be as high as 40%. Risk factors for in-hospital death include increasing age, CHF, infection due to *S. aureus* or CoNS, the presence of mitral valve vegetations, paravalvular complications, surgery indicated but not performed, and PVE. Surgical treatment for IE and infection due to *S. viridans* is associated with a decreased risk of in-hospital mortality. For right-sided IE, there is tremendous disparity in the risk of mortality based on the risk factor for acquisition. Overall mortality is very low in IDUs, but much higher in patients with right-sided IE due to intravascular devices. IE that is health care associated is an independent predictor of both in-hospital and 1 year mortality from the infection as is IE due to *S. aureus*. In addition, there is a significant difference between the risk of mortality in right-sided vs. left-sided IE in IDUs. A TEE should always be performed, even in patients with clear evidence of right-sided infection (such as septic pulmonary emboli) because concomitant infection of the left-sided valves may also be present.

Because a prior episode of IE is one of the strongest risk factors for subsequent episodes of IE, these patients must receive prophylactic antibiotics as recommended in the AHA guidelines for the prevention of IE.

References

1. Baddour LM, Wilson WR, As B et al (2005) Infective endocarditis: diagnosis, antimicrobial therapy and management of complications: a statement for healthcare professionals from the Committee on Rheumatic Fever, Endocarditis and Kawasaki Disease, Council on Cardiovascular Disease in the Young, and the Councils on Clinical Cardiology, Stroke and Cardiovascular Surgery and Anesthesia, American Heart Association: endorsed by the Infectious Diseases Society of America. Circulation 111:394–434
2. Fowler VG, Miro JM, Hoen B et al (2005) *Staphylococcus aureus* endocarditis: a consequence of medical progress. J Am Med Assoc 293:3012–3021
3. Rybak M, Lomaestro B, Rotschafer JC et al (2009) Therapeutic monitoring of vancomycin in adult patients: a consensus review of the American Society of Health-System Pharmacists, the Infectious Diseases Society of America and the Society of Infectious Diseases Pharmacists. Am J Health Syst Ph 66:82–98
4. Js L, Sexton DJ, Mick N et al (2000) Proposed modifications to the Duke criteria for the diagnosis of infective endocarditis. Clin Infect Dis 30:633–638
5. Sohail MR, Uslan DZ, Khan AH et al (2007) Management and outcome of permanent pacemaker and implantable cardioverter-defibrillator infections. J Am Coll Cardiol 49:1851–1859

Cardiac Contractility

Lara Wijayasiri[1], Andrew Rhodes[2], Maurizio Cecconi[3]
[1]Department of Anaesthesia, St. George's Hospital, London, UK
[2]Department of Intensive Care, St. George's Hospital, London, UK
[3]Department of General Intensive Care, St. George's Hospital, London, UK

Synonyms

Inotropy

Definition

Cardiac contractility can be defined as the tension developed and velocity of shortening (i.e., the "strength" of contraction) of myocardial fibers at a given preload and afterload. It represents a unique and intrinsic ability of cardiac muscle to generate a force that is independent of any load or stretch applied.

Characteristics

Factors increasing cardiac contractility – positive inotropic effect [1]:

- Sympathetic nervous system activation
- Circulating endogenous catecholamines

- Drugs – inotropic agents, digoxin, calcium ions (Ca^{2+})
- Metabolic – hyperthermia, hypercalcaemia
- Heart rate – as heart rate increases (e.g., during exercise), contractility increases (this occurs up to a certain point beyond which the tachycardia impairs normal cardiac function). This phenomenon is known as the Treppe or Bowditch effect. It is thought to be mediated by an increase in cytoplasmic Ca^{2+} due to reduced reuptake by the sarcoplasmic reticulum secondary to a reduction in the diastolic time.

Factors reducing cardiac contractility – negative inotropic effect [1]:

- Parasympathetic nervous system activation (e.g., vagal maneuvres)
- Drugs – β adrenoceptor antagonists
- Metabolic – hypothermia, hypoxia, hypercapnia, hyperkalemia, hypocalcemia
- Pathological states – diastolic and systolic dysfunctions

Assessment

It is very difficult to clinically assess cardiac contractility in vivo. One method involves measuring the rate of change of ventricular pressure with respect to time (dP/dt) and then using the maximum rate of pressure rise (peak dP/dt) to compare contractility of the heart.

Another method involves the use of serial pressure – volume (PV) loops to obtain end-systolic pressure–volume relationship (ESPVR) curves (Fig. 1). These methods are quite invasive and clinically are not practical [2].

Direct, real-time visualization of myocardial wall motion and blood ejection patterns using echocardiography and Doppler allow an assessment of the functional status of the heart to be made. With echocardiography, two useful parameters are ejection fraction and shortening fraction. The left ventricle (LV) ejection fraction (normal range between 55% and 75%) is defined by (LV diastolic volume – LV systolic volume)/LV diastolic volume. The shortening fraction ratio measures the change in diameter of the LV between its contracted and relaxed states (LV end-diastolic diameter – LV end-systolic diameter)/LV end-diastolic diameter. These measurements can give an idea of heart performance, but they cannot provide objective assessments of myocardial contractility.

The concept of contractility can be illustrated using force–velocity curves (where the term "force" represents the afterload to the heart and "velocity" refers to the speed of myocardial muscle shortening) (Figs. 2–4) [3]. A heart with a good contractility responds to volume loading in a different way to a heart with impaired contractility (Fig. 5).

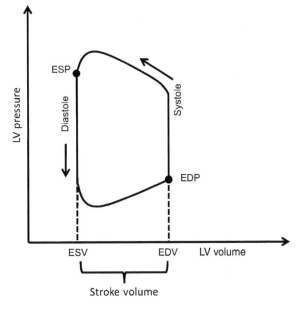

Cardiac Contractility. Figure 1 Pressure volume loop for normal left ventricle. Where: EDP is end-diastolic point (when mitral valve closes), ESP is end-systolic point (when aortic valve closes), ESV is end-systolic volume and EDV is end-diastolic volume. Increasing contractility moves the ESP up and to the left, while decreasing contractility moves it down and to the right

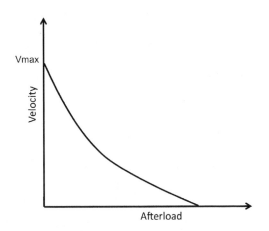

Cardiac Contractility. Figure 2 Force–velocity curve for an isolated myocardial fiber: as the force (afterload) reduces, the velocity of muscle contraction increases until a maximal velocity (Vmax) is achieved at zero afterload (in reality, Vmax cannot be obtained experimentally because the myocardium does not contract in the absence of any load, and therefore this value is obtained by extrapolation)

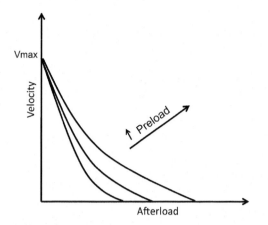

Cardiac Contractility. Figure 3 Effects of increasing preload on force–velocity curve for an isolated myocardial fiber. As preload gradually increases, the isometric tension within the myocardial fiber increases as dictated by the Frank–Starling mechanism of the heart (length–tension relationship). However, Vmax remains unchanged, demonstrating the fact that it does not depend on the length of the muscle fiber (i.e., preload) from which contraction is initiated

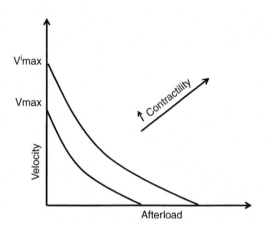

Cardiac Contractility. Figure 4 As contractility increases, the curve is shifted up and to the right with an increase in both Vmax and isometric tension. This increase in Vmax (V'max) is of particular significance as it is a measure of cardiac contractility that is unrelated to changes in preload or afterload

Systolic Dysfunction

Systolic dysfunction, often termed ventricular failure, refers to an impairment in ventricular contractility which results in a reduced stroke volume and hence inadequate cardiac output. If the left ventricle is affected, left ventricular end-diastolic pressures gradually rise which can lead to an increase in left atrial and pulmonary pressures resulting in pulmonary edema. If the right ventricle is

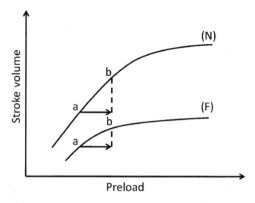

Cardiac Contractility. Figure 5 Modification of Frank–Starling curve. A heart with normal contractility (N) and a failing heart with poor contractility (F) have different abilities to respond to volume loading and hence increase their stroke volumes by different amounts

affected, right ventricular end-diastolic pressures rise which can lead to an increase in right atrial pressures and venous congestion resulting in peripheral edema, ascites, and hepatomegaly. Quite often left-sided systolic dysfunction will eventually cause right-sided systolic dysfunction, and this is commonly termed biventricular failure or congestive cardiac failure.

There are numerous causes of systolic dysfunction including coronary artery disease (myocardial ischemia and infarction), valvular heart disease, dilated cardiomyopathy, myocarditis, amyloidosis, drugs (e.g., ethanol excess and cocaine) and toxins (e.g., sepsis).

References

1. Parrillo JE, Dellinger RP (2008) Critical care medicine: principles of diagnosis and management in the adult, 3rd edn. Mosby Elsevier, Philadelphia, pp 39–52
2. Wigfull J, Cohen AT (2005) Critical assessment of haemodynamic data. CEACCP 5(3):84–88
3. Klabunde RE (2005) Cardiovascular physiology concepts, 1st edn. Lippincott Williams and Wilkins, Philadelphia, pp 81–85

Cardiac Disease

▶ Congenital Heart Disease in Children

Cardiac Doppler

▶ Echocardiography

Cardiac Failure in Children

JONATHAN R. EGAN, MARINO S. FESTA
The Children's Hospital at Westmead, Westmead,
Australia

Definition

Inability of the heart to meet the metabolic needs of the body as a result of an inability to sustain an effective cardiac output.

Characteristics

Cardiac failure can occur as a result of a myriad of cardiogenic causes in the setting of congenital cardiac disease, which can be grouped into four main categories. Cardiac failure resulting from acquired disease is discussed subsequently.

Increased Pulmonary Blood Flow

An atrial, ventricular, or large vessel communication (e.g., patent ductus arteriosus (PDA)) results in shunting of blood and a volume load on the systemic left ventricle. This leads to ventricular failure and pulmonary venous congestion.

Left Ventricular Outflow Obstruction

In the setting of aortic stenosis or coarctation there can be early myocardial failure in the neonatal, infant, or childhood age groups – depending on the degree of obstruction.

Valvular Regurgitation

A volume load on the ventricle leads to forward delivery failure and backward obstruction to venous inflow.

Right Ventricular Failure

Isolated right ventricular failure occurs in the setting of pulmonary embolism, pulmonary hypertension, or chronic respiratory failure.

Management

An A, B, C approach to stabilization is required – it is important to consider the effect of excessive inspired oxygen upon pulmonary vascular resistance, which can exacerbate left-to-right shunting and worsen pulmonary venous congestion. Providing positive end expiratory pressure (PEEP) via a bag and mask, with an initial FiO_2 of 0.3–0.4 maximum should prove both safe and beneficial. A carefully observed trial of noninvasive ventilation may improve oxygenation and the work of breathing. Subsequently intubation can be performed if considered necessary. Intubation of a neonate or child with cardiac failure can be risky and should be undertaken by senior trained intensivists/anesthetists. Induction drugs that can lead to pronounced reductions in systemic vascular resistance and myocardial contractility – such as thiopentone or propofol are best avoided. Ketamine is a good alternative. Apart from optimizing oxygenation and induction drugs, the hemodynamic status of the child should be preemptively stabilized with administration of fluid boluses (5–10 ml/kg of normal saline) and vasopressors (5 mcg/kg/min dopamine). Vasopressor and inodilator therapy can be modified following stabilization, full assessment, and provision of central venous and arterial lines. Initially reducing the systemic vascular resistance with either dobutamine and milrinone or levosimendan infusions – as systemic perfusion pressure permits and then transitioning to captopril will optimize myocardial performance.

It is important to determine the underlying lesion(s) and any contributing factors – viral pneumonitis/bronchiolitis through careful history, examination, echocardiography, and other directed investigations. Management of fluid balance, energy requirements, and expenditure will provide a foundation on which to add diuretic, inotropic, and vasodilator therapy. Surgical repair maybe indicated and the timing of this depends on overall patient stability and local resources.

Cardiac Magnetic Resonance Imaging

CHADWICK D. MILLER[1], DANIEL W. ENTRIKIN[2],
W. GREGORY HUNDLEY[3]
[1]Department of Emergency Medicine, Wake Forest University Baptist Medical Center School of Medicine, Winston-Salem, NC, USA
[2]Department of Radiology and Internal Medicine, Section on Cardiology, Wake Forest University School of Medicine, Winston-Salem, NC, USA
[3]Department of Internal Medicine, Section on Cardiology and Department of Radiology, Wake Forest University School of Medicine, Winston-Salem, NC, USA

Synonyms

Cardiac MR; Cardiac MRI; CMR

Definition

Cardiac magnetic resonance imaging (CMR) is the use of magnetic resonance (MR) techniques to obtain images of the heart. As with all MR technology, tissues are subjected to a strong magnetic field that orients the protons of hydrogen atoms so that they rotate, or "precess," in a uniform manner. These hydrogen atoms are then exposed to a radio signal, commonly referred to as a pulse sequence, which transiently changes their orientation. After the radio signal, the protons revert to their original precession patterns and create a signal that is captured to create images. The time to reversion to their orderly precession is dependent on tissue composition and therefore the resulting signal patterns are specific to the tissue composition. As disease states change tissue composition, the tissues provide a different signal allowing the determination of normal and disease states.

By utilizing ECG-gating, signals obtained from CMR can be processed to create both still and motion images of the heart. Further, imaging can be conducted during rest, or during cardiac stress. Finally, contrast agents can be used to exploit subtle differences in cellular and tissue composition or function.

Pre-existing Condition

Overview

CMR has seen increased use over the past decade. Newer imaging techniques and scanner technologies have greatly enhanced the quality and diagnostic accuracy of CMR. Common indications for CMR are discussed in the section immediately below. However, in the critically ill patient, obtaining CMR testing is associated with several logistical challenges that are discussed in the Application section. Because of these challenges, other imaging modalities are often preferred over CMR. Circumstances when CMR may be strongly considered in the critically ill patient are further discussed under the heading "Clinical circumstances in which CMR would be useful in critically ill patients."

Common Indications and Appropriateness Criteria

Criteria developed by a multidisciplinary panel provide guidance to determine when CMR is considered an appropriate diagnostic test [1]. These appropriate indications are summarized in the paragraphs below.

Evaluation of Acute Chest Pain

CMR in combination with pharmacologic vasodilator (adenosine, Persantine) perfusion imaging or inotropic stimulation (dobutamine) wall motion imaging can be used to detect inducible myocardial ischemia. Multiple studies have demonstrated that stress CMR has equal or higher accuracy compared to other stress testing modalities with sensitivity ranging from 86% to 96% and specificity from 83% to 100% for detecting 50% coronary artery luminal narrowings [2, 3]. Patients unable to exercise or who have ECGs that are not interpretable are particularly well suited for CMR imaging. CMR to evaluate acute chest pain is inappropriate in low risk patients with interpretable ECGs and the ability to exercise, as well as in patients with high pretest probability of CAD combined with positive biomarkers or ST-segment deviation. All uses of MR angiography to evaluate for CAD as a cause of acute chest pain are considered inappropriate.

Evaluation of Cardiac Structure and Function

CMR is well suited to provide information on cardiac anatomy and function. CMR is particularly useful when technically limited echo images have been obtained. CMR can appropriately be used to determine left ventricular function after myocardial infarction (AMI) or in patients with heart failure, assess for congenital heart disease including anomalous coronary arteries, and evaluate native and some prosthetic valves. Furthermore, CMR is useful and appropriate to evaluate for cardiomyopathies, myocarditis, pericardial disease, cardiac thrombus, cardiac masses, and aortic dissection. Although aortic dissection can be detected by cardiac MRI, the aorta is extra-cardiac and is not further discussed in this chapter.

Application

Equipment

CMR exams are commonly performed on commercially manufactured MRI machines with specialized software to obtain cardiac images. 1.5 Tesla machines are widely used, with some institutions adopting machines with stronger magnetic fields. Power injectors are ideal if perfusion imaging is to be performed. Specialized monitoring equipment that is MRI compatible is required.

Policies and Procedures

Policies and procedures must be in place for patient screening and emergency response. Patients must be screened for MRI compatibility. Pacemakers, defibrillators, and ferrous implants are generally not compatible with MRI. Emergency response plans should be well delineated in the event the patient's condition deteriorates during the exam.

Components

CMR consists of several components that must be tailored to the clinical question.

Stress Agents

Stress testing is commonly used to assess acute chest pain. The "stress" component can be either a vasodilator or an inotropic agent such as dobutamine. Vasodilators such as adenosine are used in conjunction with perfusion imaging techniques to capture stress myocardial perfusion images, which can then be compared with similar rest myocardial perfusion images obtained in the absence of the vasodilator and other infarct "delayed enhancement" techniques. By comparison, dobutamine stress examinations rely on the identification of a regional left ventricular wall motion abnormality that occurs when the patient has achieved target heart rate (target heart rate = [220−age] × 0.85) during peak pharmacologic stress. The detection of perfusion defects or wall motion abnormalities during stress is suggestive of significant coronary stenosis.

Use of Gadolinium: Perfusion Imaging and Delayed Enhancement

Gadolinium containing contrast agents are used to enhance the information provided from CMR. The presence of gadolinium contrast agents modifies the signal emanating from nearby protons. By exploiting differences in normal and abnormal gadolinium distribution within the myocardium both perfusion imaging and delayed enhancement imaging can aid in the diagnosis of underlying disease states. For instance, in the normal heart there should be no perceptible difference in the perfusion of

gadolinium through the myocardium during rest or stress perfusion imaging with vasodilators such as adenosine. The presence of a perfusion defect during adenosine stress perfusion is strongly suggestive of inducible ischemia, and the myocardial segments involved are predictive of the vascular territory affected by a high-grade flow-limiting stenosis, as demonstrated in Fig. 1.

Delayed enhancement imaging exploits the fact that various disease states allow abnormal accumulation of gadolinium within myocardial tissue. Because of this, inflammation and cell death from acute myocardial infarction or acute myocarditis, scarring from old myocardial infarction or prior myocarditis, and infiltrative processes that result in myocardial scarring (such as sarcoidosis, amyloidosis, and hypertrophic cardiomyopathy) can all be identified with delayed enhancement imaging. In the setting of acute inflammation as can be seen with myocarditis or acute infarction it is the leaky basement membranes of the myocardial microvasculature, expanded extracellular space related to edema and leaky cell membranes that allow excessive accumulation of gadolinium within affected myocardial territories. In the setting of chronic scarring from prior infarct or prior myocarditis, ventricular remodeling results in the deposition of a fibro-fatty infiltrate in the area of scarring. The collagenous matrix of this infiltrate expands the extracellular space and traps gadolinium in these regions of scarring. And finally, with the various infiltrative cardiomyopathies, there is typically an abnormal accumulation of proteins and/or disordered array of myocytes also associated with regions of fibrosis and scarring that result in accumulation of gadolinium. In all of these settings, delayed enhancement imaging

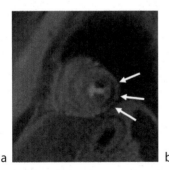 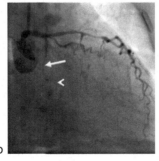 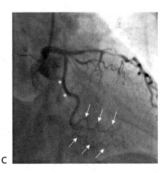

Cardiac Magnetic Resonance Imaging. Figure 1 (**a**) Short axis image obtained through the mid-ventricle during adenosine stress perfusion. The white arrows demonstrate a large region of decreased signal intensity indicative of an area of decreased perfusion involving the lateral wall segments. (**b**) Catheter angiogram demonstrating injection of the left main coronary artery. The *white arrow* demonstrates a critical stenosis of the proximal left circumflex coronary artery, while the *white arrowhead* demonstrates the limited perfusion of a large obtuse marginal branch from the circumflex. (**c**) Repeat angiogram following percutaneous transluminal coronary intervention with stent (*white asterices*) placement in the proximal obtuse marginal branch. Note restoration of normal flow in the distal vessels (*small white arrows*)

sequences allow clear recognition and delineation of disease regions of myocardium when compared with adjacent normal myocardium.

T2-Weighted Images

T2-weighted image sequences are able to detect myocardial edema. Myocardial edema is an early marker of myocardial ischemia or inflammation. The use of T2 weighted images allows the early determination of myocardial infarction, at times before chemical evidence is present in the blood. The combined use of T2-weighted imaging sequences and delayed enhancement imaging sequences can be used to discriminate between several types of myocardial injury including, acute inflammation in the setting of myocarditis, acute injury in the setting of acute myocardial infarction, and chronic scarring in the setting of remote myocardial injury. Figure 2 demonstrates features of a severe left anterior descending (LAD) territory infarction.

Complications

Flying objects – Metallic objects in the room or entering the room will be forcefully attracted to the magnet. This can cause severe injury or death.

Burns – Unrecognized implanted metallic objects can cause tissue heating, neural stimulation, or skin burns.

Implanted device malfunction – Some devices are MRI compatible, such as some ventriculo-peritoneal shunts, but require programming after the scan is completed. Others are not compatible, such as defibrillators, and can cause death if MRI is conducted.

Nephrogenic systemic fibrosis – The use of gadolinium containing contrast agents has been linked to nephrogenic systemic fibrosis, which can be a progressive fatal condition. The relationship between gadolinium containing contrast agents and nephrogenic systemic fibrosis resulted in a boxed warning from the FDA against use in patients with acute or chronic renal insufficiency (glomerular filtration rate <30 ml/min), acute renal insufficiency of any severity due to hepatorenal syndrome, or in the perioperative liver transplant period. Because this is a rapidly evolving area, readers are encouraged to consult the most recent guidance on the risk of nephrogenic systemic fibrosis.

Claustrophobia – MRI is conducted in a closed environment. Therefore it may not be tolerated by patients with severe claustrophobia unless sedation is provided.

Logistical Barriers to CMR Use

Ultrasound or computed tomography is often used for patients in the first 24 h of an acute illness due to their wide availability. Even in some instances where CMR may be the preferred test, CMR is less commonly used due to logistical challenges performing the procedures in critically ill patients.

The logistical challenges associated with CMR include the need to have a scanner capable of CMR imaging, expertise and support to perform these examinations, and skilled readers to provide high quality expert interpretation. Critical illness adds complexity for a multitude

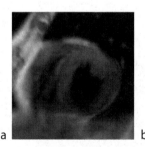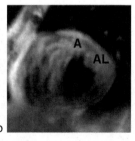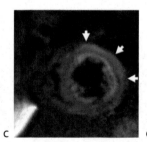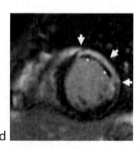

a   b   c   d

Cardiac Magnetic Resonance Imaging. Figure 2 (**a**) Short axis T1-weighted image of the heart at the level of the mid left ventricle before the administration of IV gadolinium. (**b**) Similar T1-weighted image shortly after the administration of gadolinium demonstrates increased signal intensity within the anterior (A) and anterolateral (AL) wall segments, representative of early accumulation of gadolinium within the territory of the LAD coronary artery. (**c**) T2-weighted short axis image at the same level demonstrating increased signal intensity in the same distribution (*small white arrows*) representative of myocardial edema in the LAD territory. (**d**) Delayed enhancement image at the same level demonstrating extensive delayed enhancement in the LAD territory (*small white arrows*) indicative of progressive accumulation of gadolinium in the myocardium related to acute LAD territory infarction. In this particular instance the patient suffered a ST-elevation myocardial infarction (STEMI) secondary to complete occlusion of the LAD resulting in profound ischemia; the black subendocardial regions (*white asterices*) within this distribution are representative of regions of complete microvascular occlusion in the LAD territory

of reasons. First, life-sustaining equipment must be non-ferrous and MRI compatible. Second, imaging times can last 30–60 min, which may be impossible in patients with hemodynamic instability. Third, patients must lie flat during the exam, which can exacerbate some disease processes. Fourth, critically ill patients commonly have renal insufficiency. Renal insufficiency increases the risk of developing nephrogenic systemic fibrosis after administration of gadolinium containing contrast agents that are commonly used in CMR. Finally, CMR may not be available emergently when it is needed.

Clinical Circumstances in Which CMR Would Be Useful in Critically Ill Patients

1. Patients with new onset heart failure of uncertain etiology when echocardiography is unavailable or nondiagnostic.

   CMR will identify myocardial edema, inflammation, wall motion, ventricular function, and can distinguish acute from chronic myocardial infarction. This information can provide supporting or refuting evidence for AMI, myocarditis, cardiomyopathies, cardiotoxic effects of therapy, restrictive pericardial disease, and valvular dysfunction.

2. Concern of AMI or ACS in patients with a non-interpretable ECG and nondiagnostic cardiac markers.

   Patients with bundle branch blocks or other conditions preventing an accurate ECG assessment, or continuous unrelieved symptoms may benefit from CMR imaging. While bedside echo is often used to determine ejection fraction and to assess for regional wall motion abnormalities, CMR may also serve in similar capacity. This may be particularly useful in patients with a complicated revascularization history. CMR can be used to assess for edema, obtain resting wall motion and perfusion, and delayed enhancement. These latter features help to characterize tissue and define the etiology of left or right ventricular wall motion abnormalities. In addition, these imaging strategies have previously been shown to accurately detect MI and can do so before elevation of cardiac markers [4]. Early acquisition of this information may allow early planning of treatment strategies.

3. Clinical history concerning for a cardiac thrombus or mass.

   In patients with suspected intracardiac thrombus, CMR can accurately depict the presence of an intracavitary thrombus within the heart, and commonly offers superior visualization of the apical regions that may improve detection in the setting of apical thrombus. CMR is also capable of identification and characterization of mass lesions intrinsic to the heart, including not only benign lesions but also primary and metastatic neoplasms.

Conclusion

CMR is able to provide a comprehensive evaluation for cardiac disease. CMR exams are able to assess for structural and functional disease of the heart with high accuracy. However, the logistical challenges associated with obtaining a CMR exam in patients with critical illness limits its use in these patients. However, there are several scenarios in which care providers, despite these logistical challenges, may choose to perform CMR imaging over other imaging modalities.

References

1. Hendel RC, Patel MR, Kramer CM, ACCF/ACR/SCCT/SCMR/ASNC/NASCI/SCAI/SIR et al (2006) Appropriateness criteria for cardiac computed tomography and cardiac magnetic resonance imaging: a report of the American College of Cardiology Foundation Quality Strategic Directions Committee Appropriateness Criteria Working Group, American College of Radiology, Society of Cardiovascular Computed Tomography, Society for Cardiovascular Magnetic Resonance, American Society of Nuclear Cardiology, North American Society for Cardiac Imaging, Society for Cardiovascular Angiography and Interventions, and Society of Interventional Radiology. J Am Coll Cardiol 48:1475–1497
2. Ingkanisorn WP, Kwong RY, Bohme NS et al (2006) Prognosis of negative adenosine stress magnetic resonance in patients presenting to an emergency department with chest pain. J Am Coll Cardiol 47:1427–1432
3. Nagel E, Lehmkuhl HB, Bocksch W et al (1999) Noninvasive diagnosis of ischemia-induced wall motion abnormalities with the use of high-dose dobutamine stress MRI: comparison with dobutamine stress echocardiography. Circulation 99:763–770
4. Cury RC, Shash K, Nagurney JT et al (2008) Cardiac magnetic resonance with T2-weighted imaging improves detection of patients with acute coronary syndrome in the emergency department. Circulation 118:837–844

Cardiac Markers for Diagnosing Acute Myocardial Infarction

James McCord
Henry Ford Hospital Center, Detroit, MI, USA

Synonyms

Cardiac troponin I; Cardiac troponin T; Creatine kinase-MB; Myoglobin

Definition

Cardiac markers are proteins that are released from myocardial cells during acute myocardial infarction (AMI).

Characteristics

Cardiac Markers

Creatine Kinase-MB

Prior to the use of cardiac troponin I (cTnI) and cardiac troponin T (cTnT), creatine kinase-MB (CK-MB) was the most common marker used in the evaluation of individuals for possible acute myocardial infarction (AMI). Creatine (CK) is a dimer composed of two subunits, M and B. Skeletal muscle is predominantly composed of CK-MM, and CK-BB is mainly in brain and kidney. CK-MB, which comprises 20–30% of cardiac muscle, is released into the circulation during myocardial injury that occurs during AMI. Although CK-MB is predominantly located in the myocardium, 1–3% of the CK in skeletal tissue is CK-MB; smaller quantities of CK-MB are also located in other tissues such as intestine, diaphragm, uterus, and prostate. The use of CK-MB in the diagnosis of AMI is limited by low specificity in the setting of trauma or renal insufficiency. A relative index has been used, which is a function of the amount of CK-MB relative to total CK. The use of the relative index does improve specificity but decreases sensitivity in the diagnosis of AMI. In the setting of AMI, CK-MB becomes elevated in the circulation 3–6 h after symptom onset, and can remain elevated for 24–36 h.

Cardiac Troponin I and T

The cardiac troponins (cTn) are proteins that modulate the interaction between actin and myosin in myocardial cells. There are isoforms of cTnI and cTnT that are unique to cardiac tissue, which has allowed specific assays to be developed that measure only the cardiac forms. Most of the cTn is bound to the contractile apparatus in the myocardium but 3% of cTnI and 6% of cTnT exist free in the cytoplasm. The initial elevation of cTnI and cTnT is likely due to the free cTn, while the more prolonged elevation is secondary to the degradation of cTn bound to the contractile apparatus. The early release kinetics of cTnI and cTnT are similar becoming elevated 3–6 h after the initiation of an AMI. However, cTnI and cTnT may remain elevated for 4–7 and 10–14 days, respectively. There is a standard assay used for cTnT so there is consistent reporting of values. However, at present there is no such standardization for the different cTnI assays, and cTnI is released in various forms. Different assays detect these forms in varying degrees leading up to a 20-fold difference in measurement for the same cTnI serum concentration. These different cTnI assays, with different cut-points and measured absolute values, can lead to clinical confusion when a patient is transferred from one hospital to another. Also cTnT, as compared to cTnI, is more commonly elevated in patients with renal insufficiency.

In the evaluation of patients for possible AMI, cTnI and cTnT have numerous advantages over CK-MB, and are the recognized preferred cardiac markers to be used in evaluating such patients [1]. In addition to having better specificity, the cTn have higher sensitivity detecting AMI. Patients that previously would have been diagnosed with unstable angina with normal CK-MB values may have minor myocardial necrosis that can be detected by an abnormal cTnI or cTnT. With some of the newer more sensitive assays the number of patients with ACS classified as AMI will increase further. Multiple studies have consistently shown that elevated cTn is associated with adverse events: higher mortality, recurrent MI, and need for urgent revascularization. Even minor cTn elevations are associated with high-risk angiographic findings: extensive atherosclerosis, visible thrombus, complex lesions, and slower coronary flow. Patients with ACS and an elevated cTn benefit from aggressive pharmacologic therapy and revascularization.

The recommended cut-point for an elevated cTn is the 99th percentile of a normal reference population at a precision level of < 10% coefficient of variation [1, 2]. The coefficient of variation is a measure of precision and defined as the standard deviation/mean when a sample is run multiple times on the same assay. In the past cTn assays where not able to meet the precision requirement at low values so only higher levels were reported as abnormal, but newer assays are more precise at low levels and guidelines recommend reporting these low levels as abnormal. Although cTn elevation is very specific for myocardial injury it does not indicate the mechanism of myocardial injury. When cardiac markers have been measured the diagnosis of AMI requires an elevated marker (preferably cTn) and at least one of the following: ischemic electrocardiographic changes, symptoms consistent with myocardial ischemia, or a new wall motion abnormality with cardiac imaging. Many acute conditions may lead to myocardial stress and damage with elevated cTn.

Myoglobin

Myoglobin is a protein that is found in all tissues. Myoglobin is a smaller molecule as compared to CK-MB or cTn, and has been used as an early marker in the identification of AMI as it can be detected 1–2 h after symptom onset. However, the sole use of myoglobin has significant limitations in that the levels may normalize in patients that present > 24 h after symptom onset, and has low specificity for AMI in the setting of renal insufficiency or muscle trauma. Considering its low specificity, and rapid rise and fall, myoglobin has usually been used in combination with either CK-MB or cTn. An elevated myoglobin is also associated with a worse prognosis in both patients with ACS and non-ACS even after adjusting for cTn elevation. The reason for this association is unclear and there is no known specific therapy that should be given to a patient based on an elevated myoglobin.

Serial Measurement of Cardiac Markers

The measurement of cardiac markers at presentation in the Emergency Department is not sufficiently sensitive to exclude AMI, and markers in general need to be measured serially over time. Guidelines recommend that cardiac markers, preferably cTn, should be measured over 6–9 h [1, 2]. Patients that present 8 h after their last symptoms only need one cTn to be measured. In a study of 383 consecutive patients with nondiagnostic electrocardiograms, no high-risk clinical features, and normal CK-MB values at presentation had CK-MB and cTnT measured at 0, 4, 8, and 12 h. All patients that were identified by elevated CK-MB and cTnT at 12 h had elevation of both CK-MB and cTnT at 8 h. Thus, this study suggests that measurement of cardiac markers beyond 8 h does not improve sensitivity. Another study of 773 patients who were evaluated for possible ACS had cTnI measured at presentation and at least 6 h after symptom onset. In this study there was one death and one AMI at 30 days in the 602 patients that had all normal cTnI, yielding an adverse event rate of 0.3%.

Multi-marker Strategies and Dynamic Change in Markers

Studies have taken advantage of the different release kinetics of various cardiac markers to be used in combination to more rapidly exclude MI. A marker that rises early during MI, such as myoglobin, combined with one that becomes elevated later, CK-MB or cTn, enables AMI to be identified earlier, and therefore more rapidly excluded. In a study of 817 patients evaluated in the Emergency Department for possible ACS had CK-MB, cTnI, and myoglobin measured at 0, 1.5, 3, and 9 h. There were 65 patients diagnosed with AMI. The combined sensitivity for myoglobin and cTnI at 90 min was 96.9% with a

negative predictive value of 99.6%. The measurement of CK-MB and sampling at 3 h did not improve sensitivity. In another study the combined sensitivity of CK-MB and myoglobin was 100% at 4 h.

A dynamic change in individual cardiac markers, or a combination of markers, can identify patients with AMI earlier. In a study of 817 patients the combined sensitivity of cTnI, myoglobin, and a change in myoglobin (defined as a > than 20 ng/ml increase) had a combined sensitivity of 97.3% at 90 min. In a study of over 1,000 patients evaluated in the Emergency Department the combined sensitivity of CK-MB, cTnI, and a change in myoglobin (defined as a > 25% increase), had 100% sensitivity at 90 min. In addition, a study of 975 patients demonstrated a change of CK-MB of > 0.7 ng/ml over 2 h and had a higher sensitivity for MI at 93.2%, when compared to a change of myoglobin of > 9.4 ng/ml over the same time period of only 77%. Most institutions employ a simple single point cut-point strategy as opposed to a change in cardiac maker strategy over time, likely because a single cut-point approach is simpler.

Improved Troponin Assays: Sensitivity, Precision, and Implications for CK-MB/Myoglobin

Until recently most cTn assays did not meet the stringent precision recommendation of < 10% coefficient of variation at the 99th percentile as advised in the consensus document the Universal Definition of MI in 2007 [2]. The newer more sensitive and precise assays have implications for the utility of CK-MB and myoglobin measurement, and the required time period for serial testing. Many earlier studies used a CK-MB definition of MI and/or older cTn assays that were less sensitive and precise than assays presently available, which makes protocols based on these studies inapplicable for present practice. There have been some studies that foreshadowed how cardiac markers will be used in the era of these newer cTn assays. In a retrospective study from stored specimens of 258 patients, samples drawn at presentation and then hourly for 6 h in 1996 demonstrated that there was no significant difference between the number of AMIs identified at 3 h compared to 6 h. In a multicenter trial published in 2009, 718 patients had measurement of cardiac cTn by four more contemporary assays at 0, 1, 2, 3, and 6 h [3]. The sensitivity for AMI (using a cTn-based definition) with these four assays at presentation ranged from 85% to 95%. The overall diagnostic utility of all four assays was very high at 3 h with an area under the curve of 0.98 as measured by receiver operator characteristic curve analysis, and was not improved by blood sampling at 6 h. The implication of this study is that with these newer assays sampling is adequate at 3 h and measurement at 6 h is not required. With the introduction of these new cTn assays patients with ACS that were identified as unstable angina will be reclassified as AMI. A study using a research assay that is not commercially available demonstrated that in patients with unstable angina and normal cTnI values using a contemporary cTnI assay, 44% had elevated cTnI at presentation and 82% at 8 h [4].

The advantage of myoglobin has been its early release in the setting of AMI enabling the early identification of myocardial necrosis. Several single center studies have shown that the newer more sensitive cTn assays can identify MI as early as myoglobin. This was confirmed in the Reichlin study where neither myoglobin nor CK-MB measurement improved early diagnostic utility (as measured by area under the curve) when added to sensitive cTn measurement. Presently many institutions use CK-MB in combination with cTnI, although CK-MB does not improve diagnostic accuracy when added to cTn measurement. Even when cTn is used as the sole marker evaluating patient with possible AMI, CK-MB may be helpful in identifying reinfarction in patients that have sustained a definite AMI and have recurrent symptoms several days after presentation when cTn values are still elevated and CK-MB may have normalized. However, newer studies suggest that following a change in cTn after recurrent symptoms may be able to replace CK-MB measurement to identify recurrent MI. The Universal Definition of AMI recommends a change in cTn values greater than 20% over 6 h after recurrence of symptoms to identify recurrent AMI. The role of an early change in either myoglobin or CK-MB needs to be studied further in the context of the new cTn assays, but recent studies suggest there is no use for myoglobin or CK-MB (using an absolute cut-point) in evaluating patients with possible or definite MI.

Although low-level cTn detection by these new assays enable a more rapid detection of myocardial necrosis, and therefore a more rapid exclusion of AMI, these low-level elevations have lower specificity for AMI. Elevation of cTn is specific for myocardial necrosis but does not determine the mechanism of injury. Conditions that are well-known to be associated with cTn elevations with the older cTn assays (such as pulmonary embolism, sepsis, heart failure, hypertensive crisis, and many others) will find a higher frequency of cTn elevations in these conditions with the new assays. Ambulatory, asymptomatic patients with a history of chronic kidney disease, heart failure, left ventricular hypertrophy, or diabetes more commonly have cTnT elevation [5]. In this era of the new ultrasensitive cTn assays historical features, electrocardiographic changes, and cardiac imaging studies will be even more important in determining which patients have suffered an AMI.

References

1. Morrow DA et al (2007) National academy of clinical biochemistry laboratory medicine practice guidelines: clinical characteristics and utilization of biochemical markers in acute coronary syndromes. Circulation 115(13):e356–e375
2. Thygesen K et al (2007) Universal definition of myocardial infarction. Circulation 116(22):2634–2653
3. Reichlin T et al (2009) Early diagnosis of myocardial infarction with sensitive cardiac troponin assays. N Engl J Med 361(9):858–867
4. Wilson SR et al (2009) Detection of myocardial injury in patients with unstable angina using a novel nanoparticle cardiac troponin I assay: observations from the PROTECT-TIMI 30 Trial. Am Heart J 158(3):386–391
5. Wallace TW et al (2006) Prevalence and determinants of troponin T elevation in the general population. Circulation 113(16):1958–1965

Cardiac MR

▶ Cardiac Magnetic Resonance Imaging

Cardiac MRI

▶ Cardiac Magnetic Resonance Imaging

Cardiac Output (CO)

▶ Cardiac Output, Measurements

Cardiac Output Monitor

▶ Esophageal Doppler

Cardiac Output Monitoring

▶ Cardiac Output, Measurements

Cardiac Output, Measurements

Giorgio Della Rocca, Maria Gabriella Costa
Department of Anesthesia and Intensive Care Medicine, Medical School of the University of Udine, University of Udine, Udine, Italy

Synonyms

Arterial Pulse Cardiac Output (APCO); Cardiac Output (CO); Cardiac output monitoring; Continuous Cardiac Output (CCO); Pulse Contour Cardiac Output (PCCO)

Definition

The function of the heart is to transport blood to the cells of the body, deliver oxygen, nutrients and chemicals, and removing cellular wastes in order to ensure their survival and proper function. In certain tissues, the perfusion of blood can have additional important functions. In the kidneys, sufficient blood flow is required for maintaining proper excretory function; in the gastrointestinal tract, it is important for glandular secretion and for nutrient absorption; and in the skin, changes in blood flow play a crucial role in the control of body temperature. Thus, each tissue has a certain requirement for blood flow and the cardiac output (CO) must keep in step with these needs. In human physiology, CO represents the volume of blood expelled by the ventricles per minute. It is calculated as the product of stroke volume (SV) and the heart rate (HR), expressed as liters of blood per minute (CO = SV*HR). In the healthy human adult, resting cardiac output is estimated to be slightly greater than 5 L/min. It may increase with anxiety or exercise and as much as fivefold with exercise.

Pre-existing Condition

The stroke volume of the left ventricle is ultimately determined by the interaction between its preload, the contractile state of the myocardium, and the afterload faced by the ventricle. Unfortunately, there is no simple measure of the "contractile state" and consequently no single equation exists that is able to describe the relationship between these three parameters. The fact that "preload" (or rather the stretch) on myocardial fibers at the end of diastole has a significant effect on the subsequent force of contraction was first recognized by Otto Frank toward the end of the nineteenth century. This fundamental relationship has since been analyzed in great detail and the adjustment of preload by blood volume transfusion or depletion remains one of the most important therapeutic maneuvers in acute cardiovascular medicine. In practice, the adjustment of cardiac preload can be achieved via various approaches:

Circulating blood volume can be increased by the administration of fluid, or reduced by the use of diuretics and/or fluid restriction.

Venous return can be varied by the adoption of a head-down or head-up posture.

Venous capacitance can be altered through the use of vasoconstrictor or vasodilator therapy.

In its strictest sense, the term "contractility" refers to the inotropic state of the myocardium – that is, the force and velocity with which the myocardial fibers contract. This can be easily measured in an isolated muscle preparation under specified loading conditions, but it is notoriously difficult to measure in humans. In clinical practice, various contraction-phase indices are used, such as the velocity of fiber shortening, the peak rate of rise in ventricular pressure and the end-systolic pressure-to-volume ratio, but they are all affected to a greater or lesser degree by loading conditions.

The "chronotropic" or "rate" state of the intact heart should also be incorporated into any clinical definition of "contractility" because variations in the pulse rate can have obvious and important effects upon CO, and manipulation of the pulse rate through the use of positive or negative chronotropes can be an important therapeutic maneuver in sick patients. It is not possible to make any precise measurements of contractility with a pulmonary artery catheter (PAC), although it is possible to make reasonable inferences about the contractile state through the use of ventricular function curves. This concept was developed by Barash and colleagues and they have described the use of a "Hemodynamic Tracking System" which defines the relationship between left ventricular stroke work index (LVSWI) and pulmonary artery occlusion pressures (PAOP) in patients with normal, slightly depressed, or severely depressed ventricular function. Adjustment of both the inotropic and chronotropic state of the heart through the use of inotropic drugs is commonly practised in critically ill medicine.

In physiological terms, afterload can be defined as "the sum of all forces which oppose ventricular muscle shortening during systole" – although in a clinical sense it is probably more useful to consider systemic vascular resistance as a more appropriate definition. In isolated cardiac muscle, an inverse relationship exists between afterload and the initial velocity of muscle shortening. This would suggest a potential dependence of CO afterload. Yet, in the intact human, the output of the normal heart is relatively unaffected by changes in vascular resistance until the point when afterload becomes quite extreme. This is probably because an increase in afterload leads to an almost immediate, secondary increase in preload by the "damming up" of the blood within the left ventricle. In turn, this increases end-diastolic volume and enhances contractility according to the Frank-Starling mechanism. On the contrary, if myocardial function is severely depressed, CO may become crucially afterload-dependent.

Thus, "sick" hearts can be considered as being relatively preload independent and afterload dependent, while the reverse is true for "healthy"' hearts. As a result, "afterload reduction" (reduction of systemic vascular resistance by the use of appropriate vasoactive drugs) is of the great benefit in those whose myocardial function is most depressed.

The role played by blood viscosity and, indirectly, hemoglobin concentration in determining systemic vascular resistance (SVR) is often overlooked. Although hemodilution is not commonly used as a therapeutic maneuver for reducing afterload, inadvertent hemodilution is often concomitant of serious illness. Hematocrit and fibrinogen are the most important determinants of blood viscosity and therefore make a significant contribution towards vascular resistance. As blood is a non-Newtonian fluid, no simple expression relating SVR to hematocrit and fibrinogen levels exists; however, it is easy to demonstrate the completely passive increase in venous return and CO which occur during hemodilution.

Finally, it should not be forgotten that the degree of ventricular interdependence can also influence ventricular performance. The position of the interventricular septum (IVS) can alter the compliance of each ventricle under altered loading conditions with secondary effects on contractility. This effect is not usually important, but it can become so in conditions such as tension pneumothorax, cardiac tamponade, right ventricular infarction, and during mechanical ventilation in critically ill patients.

The measurement of cardiac output, as first described by Fick in 1870 (although only put into practice in 1959), also makes an evaluation of respiratory exchange possible: that is, a measure of the delivery of oxygen to the tissues.

The Fick principle involves calculating the oxygen consumed over a given period of time by measuring the concentration of oxygen in venous blood and in arterial blood. Cardiac output can be calculated from the following measurements: VO_2 consumption per minute, using a spirometer (with the subject rebreathing the same air) and a CO_2 absorber; the concentration of oxygen in blood taken from the pulmonary artery (representing mixed venous blood); the concentration of oxygen in blood taken from a cannula in a peripheral artery (representing arterial blood).

We know that:

$$VO_2 = (CO \times Ca) - (CO \times Cv)$$

where Ca is the concentration of oxygen in arterial blood and Cv is the concentration of oxygen in venous blood.

Thus, rearranging the above, it is also possible to calculate cardiac output:

$$CO = (VO_2/[Ca - Cv]) * 100.$$

Whilst it is considered to be the most accurate method for the measurement of CO, the Fick method is invasive, requires time for analyzing the blood samples and making accurate oxygen consumption measurements is difficult. Moreover, the calculation of the arterial and venous blood oxygen concentrations is a straightforward process. Almost all oxygen in the blood is bound to hemoglobin molecules in the red blood cells. Measuring the content of hemoglobin in the blood and the percentage of saturation of hemoglobin (and therefore the oxygen saturation of the blood) is a simple process that is readily available to physicians. Using the fact that each gram of hemoglobin can carry 1.36 mL of O_2, the concentration of oxygen in the blood (either arterial or venous) can be estimated using the following formula:

$$CaO_2 = (Hb \text{ g/dL}) \times 1.36 \times SatO_2/100 + (0.0032 \times PaO_2 \text{ torr})$$

$$CvO_2 = (Hb \text{ g/dL}) \times 1.36 \times SatO_2/100 + (0.0032 \times PvO_2 \text{ torr})$$

The Fick method is considered to be the "gold standard" for measuring cardiac output, but it is not useful in clinical practice as a bedside technique. In current clinical practice, dilution technology is more commonly used.

The dilution technique method was initially described using an indicator dye and assumes that the rate at which the indicator is diluted reflects the CO. The method measures the concentration of a dye at different points in the circulation. The dye is usually administered via an intravenous injection and the blood subsequently sampled at a downstream site, typically in a systemic artery. The dye dilution cardiac output measurement is based on the Stewart–Hamilton equation; more specifically, the CO is equal to the quantity of indicator dye injected divided by the area under the dilution curve measured downstream:

The indicator method has been further developed with the indicator dye being replaced with cooled fluid and the change in temperature being measured at different sampling sites; this method is known as thermodilution (TD).

The pulmonary artery catheter (PAC) was the first clinical device enabling the bedside measurement of cardiac output using the thermodilution technique and since its introduction in 1970 by Swan, Ganz and colleagues, it has been considered as a "clinical standard" for cardiac output assessment despite there being no true reference technique for the clinical determination of CO. The thermodilution method involves the injection of a small amount (10 mL) of cold saline at a known temperature into the pulmonary artery, the temperature of which is measured using the same catheter. The calculation of CO is again based on the Stewart–Hamilton equation:

$$CO = (V(Tb - Ti)K1K2)/(Tb(t)dt)$$

Where: CO = cardiac output, V = volume of injectate, Tb = blood temperature, Ti = injectate temperature, K1 = catheter constant, K2 = apparatus constant, Tb(t)dt = change in blood temperature over a given time.

The Stewart-Hamilton equation should theoretically be used under conditions of constant flow.

Usually, the measurements are repeated three or five times and then averaged to improve accuracy. Under optimal conditions, the coefficient of variation for repeated bolus TD measurements is less than 10%. There are many sources of inaccuracy in the method: the cardiac output derived from PAC (COpa) is influenced by significant variations in respiration, and hence from the phase of the mechanical breath during which the injection is made. Mechanical ventilation was also shown to cause a high incidence of significant tricuspid insufficiency and mild to severe vena caval backward flow, which, like other valvular regurgitations, may reduce the accuracy of COpa measurements.

The insertion of a PAC is a procedure associated with a number of known complications. Catheter insertion can result in arterial injury, pneumothorax, and arrhythmias. The catheter can be associated with potentially fatal pulmonary artery hemorrhage, thromboembolism, sepsis, and endocardial damage.

Following its introduction into clinical practice and for the following 20 years, intermittent thermodilution was the only device available for measuring CO.

Since the late 1970s, PAC monitoring of CO has expanded rapidly and broadly in clinical practice for its use in several subgroups of patients; the receiving patients include those undergoing cardiac surgery and those with sepsis and acute respiratory distress syndrome (ARDS).

The appropriate indications necessitating PAC monitoring have been debated for many years. The potential benefits of using the device are well known. For example, its use in measuring important hemodynamic indices (e.g., pulmonary artery occlusion pressure, CO, mixed venous oxygen saturation) allows for improved accuracy in the determination of the hemodynamic status of critically ill patients compared to that possible by clinical assessment alone. The additional information it provides can also be important when caring for patients with confusing clinical scenarios in whom errors in fluid management and drug therapy can result in severe consequences. In surgical patients, PAC data often help evaluate hemodynamic changes that may lead to serious perioperative complications. Preoperative PAC data are claimed to be helpful in determining whether or not it is safe for high-risk patients to proceed with surgery. Unfortunately, the impact of PAC monitoring in patients during anesthesia and intensive care upon clinical outcomes remains uncertain.

The American Society of Anesthesiologists (ASA) established the Task Force on Pulmonary Artery Catheterization in 1991 in order to examine the evidence on the benefits and risks arising from the use of PAC in the various settings encountered by anesthesiologists. By the time the Society's guidelines had been ascertained in 1992 and published in 1993, and several groups had issued statements on the appropriate indications and on competency requirements for hemodynamic monitoring. These groups included the American College of Physicians, the American College of Cardiology, the American Heart Association Task Force on Clinical Privileges in Cardiology, a panel established by the Ontario Ministry of Health, and an expert panel from the European Society of Intensive Care Medicine. In 1996, a milestone study performed by Connors and colleagues made clinicians reconsider the invasiveness and utility of PAC. The ASA therefore reconvened the Task Force on Pulmonary Artery Catheterization in 2000 in order to review its 1993 guidelines, consider the evidence and the concerns over the use of PAC that had emerged in the interim and issue an updated guideline that was subsequently published in 2003 [1].

Due to criticisms of PAC and research yielding negative judgments over its use, clinicians have started to move to less invasive, time inexpensive, easy to use, and continuous techniques.

Another dilution technique is the transpulmonary indicator dilution technique (TPID). TPID is a less invasive technique developed in the 1980s and the PiCCO system is the oldest and the most studied less invasive device based on TPID technology. A central venous catheter for the injection of a thermal indicator is required, together with an arterial thermistor-tipped catheter normally placed into the femoral artery. The TPID technique works with 15–20 mL of either cold or room temperature injectate. Intermittent cardiac output is calculated from an arterial thermodilution curve in the usual way using the Stewart-Hamilton equation. Cardiac output by intermittent TPID has been widely validated against the intermittent TD [2]. Since transpulmonary thermodilution is less invasive than pulmonary artery thermodilution, the transpulmonary cardiac output (COart) technique is more often used, particularly when cardiac output monitoring is necessary over a long period of time. The TPID method is not suitable for patients with severe peripheral vascular disease, those undergoing vascular surgery, or those showing other contraindications opposing femoral artery cannulation.

The LiDCO system is also based on the TPID technique and uses lithium as a tracer. The lithium dilution technique is performed using 0.3 mL of lithium injected into either a central or a peripheral vein. The resulting lithium concentration–time curve is recorded by withdrawing blood (4.5 mL/min) through a special disposable sensor, attached to the patient's arterial line, which consists of a lithium-selective electrode in a flow-through cell. The voltage across the lithium-selective membrane is digitized online and recorded via a computer that converts the voltage signal into a lithium concentration. The Stewart-Hamilton curve allows the cardiac output (CO_{Li}) to be measured from the indicator dilution curve.

CO_{Li} is calculated according to the equation:

$$CO_{Li} = LiCl * 60/AUC * (1 - PCV)$$

where LiCl is the concentration of lithium chloride (mmol), AUC is the area under the primary dilution curve and PCV is the packed cell volume, which can be calculated when the patient's hematocrit is known. The lithium dilution technique is of sufficient accuracy when there is constant blood flow, homogeneous mixing of the blood, and when there is no loss of indicator between the site of injection and the detection site [3].

This technique cannot be performed in patients receiving lithium therapy. It is also difficult to use in the operating theatre, where the use of muscle relaxants containing quaternary ammonium ions can interfere with the lithium sensor and therefore the TPID should be performed with adequate time before or after muscle relaxant administration.

An advantage of the lithium indicator dilution cardiac output technique is that no central venous line is

necessary. This is because the indicator bolus can also be applied via a peripheral line even if, to the best of our knowledge, only one clinical study has been performed using a peripheral venous line for lithium injection.

The continuous cardiac output measurement was recently introduced in order to provide a continuous or semicontinuous evaluation of cardiac output.

Continuous CO measurements can be obtained using a modified PAC with an embedded heating filament (Edwards Lifesciences, Irvine, California, USA), which releases small thermal pulses every 30–60 s following a pseudorandom binary sequence. The resulting changes in pulmonary artery temperature are measured via a distal thermistor and matched with the input signal. Cross correlation of input and output signals allows for CO values to be calculated with time from the resulting TD wash-out curve. Every 60 s, a trended continuous CO (CCO) measurement is displayed, which reflects the average course of the CO over the previous 3–6 min. As relatively small quantities of heat are used to calculate CO, sudden changes in temperature or infusion of high quantities of cold infusate can influence the accuracy and reliability of the method. Hyperthermia does not influence the accuracy of CCO monitoring, although a relative increase in bias is reported for measurements taken immediately after a hypothermic cardiopulmonary bypass (CPB). (i.e., for Opti-Q, Abbott, Abbott Park, IL and Vigilance catheters, Edwards LifeSciences, Irvine, CA).

Pulse contour (or wave) analysis is based upon the principle that vascular flow can be predicted by means of the arterial pressure wave form that is itself a result of an interaction between stroke volume and the systemic vascular system. Thus, resistance, compliance, and characteristic impedance at the site of signal detection have to be considered. Different models have been used to address these issues in the various pulse wave analysis devices currently available (PiCCO plus, Pulsion Medical Systems, Munich, Germany; PulseCO, LiDCO Ltd, London, UK; FloTrac/Vigileo, Edwards LifeSiences, Irvine, CA, Most-CareTM, Pressure-recording-analytical-method-PRAM; Vytech HealthTM, Padova, Italy).

Pulse contour analysis initially used an algorithm based on the Wesseling algorithm. Over recent years, this algorithm has been evolved in a number of steps into what is today integrated into the PiCCO monitor. For the calculation of continuous cardiac output (PCCO) the system uses a calibration factor (cal) determined by thermodilution cardiac output measurement and heart rate (HR), as well as the integrated values for the area under the systolic part of the pressure curve (P(t)/SVR), the aortic compliance (C(p)) and the shape of the pressure curve, represented by the change of pressure over time (dP/dt). This algorithm is described as follows:

$$SV = cal^* HR^* \int_{systole} [P(t)/SVR + C_{(p)}dP/dt]dt$$

This algorithm uses the TPID technique to convert the PCCO derived from the algorithm into a more accurate "calibrated" value. The calibrated algorithm is then able to track stroke volume in a continuous manner.

Continuous cardiac output measured using the PiCCO monitor has been studied and compared to the TD from the PAC in different clinical fields, and these comparisons confirm the PCCO system as being accurate and precise [2]. However, it has also been shown to have some limitations, particularly during periods of hemodynamic instability.

The pulse power analysis obtained from the LiDCO System (PulseCO) is different from the classic pulse contour analysis. It is based on the hypothesis that a change in the power in the vascular system (i.e., the arterial tree) during systole is due to the difference between the amount of blood entering the system (stroke volume) and the amount of blood flowing out peripherally. It is based on the principle of conservation of mass/power and the assumption that following the correction for compliance and calibration there is a linear relationship between net power and net flow. This algorithm takes the entire beat into account, thus tackling the problem of the reflected waves, and uses a so-called autocorrelation to define which part of the "change in power" is determined by the stroke volume. Autocorrelation is a mathematical function used to analyze signals that tend to be formed of repeated cycles across time (similar to a Fourier transformation), as is clearly the case for SV in human physiology. In this way, all the curve is analyzed and SV continuously recorded. When SV is established, the CO can be easily calculated by multiplying SV by HR.

Initially, the algorithm transforms the arterial pressure waveform into a standardized volume waveform (in arbitrary units) using the formula:

$$\Delta V/\Delta P = calibration \times 250 \times e^{-k.p}$$

where V = volume, P = blood pressure, k = curve coefficient.

The number 250 represents the saturation value in mL, that is, the maximum additional value above the starting volume, at atmospheric pressure, that the aorta/arterial tree can fill to. Autocorrelation uses the volume waveform and derives the period of the beat plus a net effective beat power factor, proportional to the nominal stroke volume ejected into the aorta. This nominal stroke volume is then calibrated in order to be equalized to a measured SV. Until the calibration is performed the system behaves as if the calibration factor is 1. Following calibration, a calibration factor of the ratio between the arbitrary CO and the measured CO can be derived. In theory, the calibration factor should be constant in the patient unless significant hemodynamic changes occur. The lithium dilution technique measures CO that is then used to calibrate the pulse pressure algorithm: the PulseCO. The continuous cardiac output of LiDCO has been validated in several studies in cardiac surgery, in major surgery and in liver transplant patients. This new algorithm has, so far, proven to be reliable in surgical and intensive care patients [3].

The Vigileo system represents the newest arterial pulse wave analysis device (Arterial Pressure Cardiac Output – APCO). This device does not use a dilution technique to calibrate the algorithm as it is an uncalibrated technique. The algorithm gets all the information it needs to calculate the arterial impedance from the analysis of the arterial pressure waveform together with the patient's demographic (age, sex, height, and weight). The system can use any arterial line already in situ. However, the signal needs to be sampled by a specific transducer, the FloTrac. The FloTrac algorithm analyses the pressure waveform at one hundred times per second over 20 seconds, capturing 2,000 data points for analysis. According to the manufacturer, the algorithm is primarily based on the standard deviation of the pulse pressure waveform, as follows:

$$APCO = f(compliance, resistance) \times \sigma_p \, HR$$

where σ_p is the standard deviation of the arterial pressure, HR is the heart rate, and f (compliance, resistance) is a scaled factor proportional to vascular compliance and peripheral resistance. This function is also referred to as X. The calculation of X in the first version of the software was executed every 10 min, whereas in the second version, the software recalculates X every minute and CO is computed every 20 s. The standard deviation of the arterial pressure waveform is computed on a beat-to-beat basis using the following equation:

$$\sigma p = \sqrt{[1/(N-1) * \Sigma_{(N-1, \, k=0)}(P(k) - Pavg)^2]}$$

where P(k) is kth pulse pressure sample in the current beat, N is the total number of samples, and P_{avg} is the mean arterial pressure.

Compliance and resistance are derived from the analysis of the arterial waveform. The hypothesis retains that the shape of the arterial pressure wave, in terms of its degree of kurtosis or skewness, can be used to calculate the effects of compliance and peripheral resistance upon blood flow. Additional parameters, such as the pressure dependent Windkessel compliance C_w, heart rate and the patient's body surface area (BSA) are also included in order to take other specific patient characteristics into account.

Despite the fact that the Vigileo system represents a revolution in the field of pulse pressure analysis, being a real "plug and play" tool, an assessment of the performance of the algorithms (two versions of the software have already been released in less than 3 years) is still underway. It can already be said, however, that some authors have found good agreement between the Vigileo system and intermittent thermodilution, while others have reported poor limit of agreement [4].

Beat-to-beat values of uncalibrated CO can also be obtained using the pressure recording analytical method (PRAM). This new method is based on the mathematical analysis of the arterial pressure profile changes. It allows for the continuous assessment of SV from the pressure signals recorded in the radial and femoral arteries. Based on the perturbation theory from physics, and applied to this issue of physiology, all the elements determining CO can be taken into consideration simultaneously and in a beat-to-beat manner. Sampled at 1000 Hz, the detected pressure curve it must be submitted to a form of analysis; the result is the calculation of actual (beat-to-beat) stroke volume; with no constant value of impedance and as it is derived from an external calibration neither pre-estimated in vivo nor in vitro data are required. In contrast to the bolus TD technique, PRAM is less invasive, easier to use and provides continuous data. To date, PRAM has been used in volunteers, during vascular and cardiac surgery and in patients with congestive heart failure but there have been no studies comparing PRAM with the TD technique under hyperdynamic clinical conditions.

Non-invasive Techniques

Nowadays, several types of Doppler techniques are commercially available for the estimation of CO by measurement of aortic blood flow (ABF) [5]. An ultrasound beam directed along the ABF is reflected, caused by the moving red blood cells, with a shift in frequency (the Doppler effect) that is proportional to the blood flow velocity according to the equation:

$$Fd \ 1/4 \ 2 \ f \ 0 = C \ V \cos u$$

where Fd is the change in frequency (Doppler shift), f 0 is the transmitted frequency, V is the blood flow velocity, and u is the angle between the direction of the ultrasound beam and the blood flow. CO is estimated by multiplying the blood flow velocity by the cross-sectional area (CSA) of the aorta at the insonation point. The esophageal Doppler probe is introduced either orally or nasally and placed at the level of the descending aorta. This technique has some advantages over the classical suprasternal technique, the most important being a more stable positioning of the probe once the descending aorta is insonated. Three models of esophageal CO monitoring systems are commercially available and differ from each other in some important ways. Two systems use a built-in nomogram to obtain a measurement of the descending aortic diameter (CardioQ, Deltex Medical, Chicester, Sussex, UK; Medicina TECO, Berkshire, UK), whereas the other system uses M-mode echocardiography for this purpose (HemoSonic, Arrow International, Reading, PA). By rotating the esophageal Doppler probe, the best Doppler image possible can be achieved. ABF is calculated by multiplying ABF velocity by the CSA of the descending aorta and the heart rate. The limitations of this technique are turbulent flow, negotiation of blood flow to the upper part of the body, and the angle of insonating the aorta. Moreover, the technique is poorly tolerated in awake, nonintubated patients and cannot be used in patients with an esophageal disorder. Once a Doppler probe is in place, transesophageal echocardiography (TEE) cannot be performed. In summary, esophageal Doppler-derived ABF is a semi-invasive approach, which enables trend monitoring of CO. The statistical limit of agreement of this technique are greater compared to invasive technique. However, in contrast to most other techniques, it has been demonstrated in subsets of patients that hemodynamic treatment according to Doppler-derived CO measurements leads to a decrease in perioperative morbidity and length of stay in intensive care units.

Doppler flow measurements obtained with transthoracic echocardiography (TTE) or TEE can also be used to estimate CO. Their accuracy depends upon image quality, sample site, angle of insonation, the profile of the blood flow velocity distribution, the signal-to-noise ratio of the blood flow velocity, and the possibility of measuring the diameter of the vessel and the shape of the cardiac valve. Most often, measurements of blood flow velocity and CSA are performed by both TTE and TEE at the level of a cardiac valve or the right ventricular (RVOT) or left ventricular outflow tract (LVOT). The best results are usually obtained by the transaortic approach using the triangular shape assumption of aortic valve opening and CO determination at the LVOT. In summary, Doppler echocardiography is technically demanding, time-consuming, and requires a skilled operator. It is a safe, fairly reproducible and reasonably accurate method for measuring CO in selected patients, provided the signal quality is adequate during recording.

The ultrasonic cardiac output monitor (USCOM Pty Ltd., Coffs Harbour, NSW, Australia) is a noninvasive transcutaneous device that provides cardiac output by continuous-wave. It was introduced for clinical use in 2001 and is based on continuous-wave Doppler ultrasound. The flow profile is obtained by using a transducer (2.0 or 3.3 MHz) placed on the patient's chest in either the left parasternal position to measure transpulmonary blood flow or the suprasternal position to measure transaortic blood flow. A standard ultrasound conducting gel is used. This flow profile is presented as a time–velocity spectral display that shows variations of the blood flow velocity against time. Once the optimal flow profile is obtained, the trace is frozen. The CO is then calculated from the equation:

$$CO = HR \cdot SV$$

where the stroke volume is the product of the velocity time integral (VTI) and the cross-sectional area (CSA) of the chosen valve. The VTI represents the distance that a column of blood travels with each stroke and is calculated from the peak velocity detected. In the USCOM monitor, this is performed using a unique TouchPoint semiautomated flow profile trace which requires the operator to mark out the flow trace for a chosen stroke of the heart. This device simultaneously measures the patient's heart rate. The CSA of the chosen valve is determined by applying height-indexed regression equations that are incorporated into the USCOM device or by using another imaging method (e.g., two-dimensional echocardiography). The regression equation used to calculate the aortic valve area is that proposed by Nidorf and colleagues. The pulmonary valve area is calculated by a separate regression equation derived from the Nidorf equation.

The NICO system (Novametrix Medical Systems, Wallingford, CT, USA) uses Fick's principle applied to carbon dioxide (CO_2) for the measurement of CO. For CO_2 analysis, a mainstream infrared and airflow sensor is used. CO_2 production is calculated as the product of CO_2 concentration and air flow during a breathing cycle and arterial CO_2 content is derived from end-tidal CO_2 and the CO_2 dissociation curve. A disposable rebreathing loop allows an intermittent partial rebreathing state to be determined in cycles of 3 min. The rebreathing cycle induces an increase of end-tidal CO_2 and mimics a drop of CO_2 production. The obtained differences of these values are then used to calculate CO. Validation studies with conflicting results have been published over recent years. Fairly good CO determination was observed as long as the NICO system was applied to intubated and mechanically ventilated patients with minor lung abnormalities and fixed ventilatory settings. However, variations in ventilatory modes, mechanically assisted spontaneous breathing or the use of this technique in patients with lung pathologies (increased shunt fraction) resulted in a decrease of CO accuracy. Thus, good accuracy can only be obtained using the partial CO_2 rebreathing technique when applied in a precisely defined clinical setting to mechanically ventilated patients.

Bioimpedance cardiography is based on the application of a high-frequency, low-alternating electrical current to the thorax (thoracic electrical bioimpedance). Changes in bioimpedance to this current are related to cardiac events and blood flow in the thorax. Using a mathematical conversion, changes in bioimpedance can be transformed into an estimate of stroke volume. Recently, electrical velocimetry was introduced as a new bioimpedance technique using a new algorithm: the Bernstein–Osypka equation (Aesculon, Osypka Medical, Berlin, Germany). The accuracy and reliability of the majority of thoracic bioimpedance devices have been evaluated with conflicting results. It is therefore possible that their use could lead to inappropriate clinical interventions. Common cylinder and cone-based models for bioimpedance stroke volume calculation represent oversimplifications of the complex electrical events that occur inside the thorax during the cardiac cycle; this is also the case when only the intrathoracic blood volume is used as a model. Consequently, bioimpedance CO is not currently accepted as a valid and reproducible method in clinical practice. Although some results do seem promising, this technique requires further investigation.

Bioreactance technology (NICOM system, Cheetah Medical Inc., Portland, OR, USA) is the analysis of the variations in the frequency of a delivered oscillating current that occurs when the current traverses the thoracic cavity, as opposed to traditional bioimpedance that purely relies upon the analysis of changes in signal amplitude. To our knowledge, three validation studies have been conducted that compared bioreactance to intermittent (COpa) and continuous cardiac output (CCO), obtained from PAC, and to PCCO and APCO obtained respectively form PiCCO and Vigileo Systems. In each case bioreactance was found to give results comparable to those arising from the other techniques. More recently, bioreactance was also tested against intermittent and continuous CO obtained from the PiCCO System in 20 cardiac surgical patients during the postoperative period. The authors concluded that although occasional discordance may occur in CO values assessed by transthoracic bioreactance and pulse contour arterial wave analysis, the level of precision was acceptable.

Applications

CO is nowadays monitored in critically ill patients to assess cardiac function with the primary aim of maintaining tissue perfusion (Table 1).

In addition to measurement of CO, modifications of the original PAC have allowed for continuous measurement of mixed venous oxygen saturation (SvO_2), right ventricular function (RVEF), and right ventricular end-diastolic volume (RVEDV); however, the use of PAC can also cause complications. Several reports have described intrinsic morbidity and mortality arising from the use of PAC; thus its application should be restricted to highly selected patient populations. The selective use of the PAC can only be justified in patients with right ventricular failure and patients with increased pulmonary vascular resistance requiring vasodilator therapy. The use of the PAC in low-risk cardiac surgery, vascular surgery and major abdominal, orthopedic or neurosurgical procedures

should not be recommended. Advocates of the PAC suggest that it is crucially important that physicians and nursing staff are familiar with the PAC technology, including the procedure of inserting, positioning and maintaining the PAC. The use of PAC requires training and education as misinterpretation of data obtained with this apparatus is common. Finally, due to its invasiveness, PAC used for the purpose of CO monitoring is no longer justified.

Calibrated vs. uncalibrated wave analysis. The two available CO measurement systems, PiCCOplus and LiDCOplus, require calibration prior to the measurement of continuous CO based on the assumption that the systolic part of the arterial pressure waveform represents stroke volume. The PiCCO system requires transpulmonary thermodilution for the calibration procedure, whereas LiDCO can be calibrated using lithium dilution. Recalibration is also necessary after profound changes in arterial compliance (e.g., sepsis following CPB) and/or hemodynamics in order for subsequent measurements of CO with continuous pulse contour CO to be

Cardiac Output, Measurements. Table 1 Cardiac output monitoring, different tools and clinical applications

OR	OR/ICU	OR/ICU
*Unexpected low CO	*Cardiac patients undergoing major non-cardiac surgery	*Heart failure
Cardiac patients undergoing minor surgery	Hyperdynamic CV status	Patients with PHP and RV dysfunction
Major orthopedic surgery	Intraoperative time in Ltx	Liver transplantation
	HD monitoring for ICU stay (long time)	Lung transplantation
	ARDS/Septic shock/Heart failure	Cardiac surgery
		ARDS/Septic shock
Baseline approach		
Arterial Line	Arterial Line (radial/femoral)	Arterial Line
Peripheral venous line or CVC	CVC	PAC
Devices		
ED	ED	PAC
Vigileo	PiCCOplus	Advanced PAC (Vigilance)
LiDCOplus	LiDCOplus	
Limitations		
Arrhythmias (Vigileo)	Vascular surgery (PiCCO)	PAC related complication
Arterial signal quality (Vigileo)	Esophageal surgery (ED)	Time limited insertion
Esophageal surgery (ED)	Arterial signal quality (PiCCO/LiDCO)	

*If available and you are familiar with, first check the CV status with a TTE and or a TEE
OR: operating room; ICU: intensive care unit; CO: cardiac output; Ltx: liver transplant; HD: hemodynamic; PHP: pulmonary hypertension; RV: right ventricle; CVC: central venous catheter; PAC: pulmonary artery catheter; ED: esophageal Doppler; CV: cardiovascular; TTE: transthoracic echocardiography; TEE: transesophageal echocardiography

carried out with the usual accuracy. This prerequisite is mainly due to resulting changes in vasomotor tone. When these criteria are fulfilled, the accuracy of both techniques is sufficient for clinical purposes.

Moreover, the PiCCO System (based on TPID technique) allows the estimation of preload index as intrathoracic blood volume index (ITBVI) and a "lung edema" index as extravascular lung water index (EVLWI). The ITBVI has been extensively investigated as a static preload index in critically ill and surgical patients (cardiac surgery, liver, and lung transplant surgery). These studies have shown that the ITBVI can predict preload better than filling pressure, particularly during the intraoperative period. The EVLWI positively correlated with survival and seems to be an independent predictor of prognosis in critically ill patients, especially in septic patients. It seems reasonable that fluid management based on EVLWI measurements can be beneficial to the critically ill. Indeed, it has been shown that fluid restriction and keeping a low EVLWI improves oxygenation, reduces the length of time that mechanical ventilation is required, and may also improve survival rates. Unfortunately no definitive data have been published so far on EVLWI and its clinical applications. Moreover, stroke volume variation (SVV) and pulse pressure variation (PPV) experimentally and clinically validated fluid responsiveness indexes in controlled mechanically ventilated patients are also continuously monitored with PiCCOplus.

Together with CO, the LiDCOplus system provides information about a series of derived variables including oxygen delivery (Hb values and SaO$_2$ need to be inserted manually) and fluid responsiveness indices such as PPV, SVV, and Systolic Pressure Variation (SPV). Recently, a protocol targeting DO$_2$I of 600 mL/m^2 in high-risk surgical patients, using the LiDCO system was proven to improve patient outcome, reduce morbidity, and length of hospital stay. Good accuracy and precision between the intermittent and continuous data obtained from LiDCO and PAC were also detected in hyperdynamic patients in the postoperative period following liver transplantation procedures.

The uncalibrated Vigileo technique showed conflicting results even when the last generation algorithm was used; particularly in the hyperdynamic setting (liver transplant and septic shock patients). Together with CO, the monitor gives other derived variables such as oxygen delivery (Hb values and SaO$_2$ together with PaO$_2$ are inserted manually) and dynamic indices of fluid responsiveness. Based on actual references, Vigileo monitoring seems to be useful in patients with a low or normal CO level, that is, for intraoperative goal-directed therapy

(GTD). At present, its use in septic shock, liver transplant, and arrhythmic patients should not be encouraged.

Doppler flow measurements for CO estimation can be performed in the descending aorta using probes that are smaller than conventional TEE probes; their correct insertion is crucial requiring highly skilled operators. Initially the esophageal Doppler technique was serially utilized in multiple prospective, randomized, controlled perioperative trials to guide hemodynamic management and it consistently demonstrated a reduction in complications and lengths of hospital stay. It has been used intraoperatively in cardiac surgical, femoral neck repair, and abdominal surgical patients, as well as postoperatively following cardiac surgery and multiple trauma; the control group in each study was randomized to standard practice either with or without the use of a central venous catheter. More recent clinical trials have, however, shown conflicting results.

Limited accuracy may result from signal detection problems, the assumption of fixed regional blood flow or the use of nomograms to determine aortic cross-sectional area. The *HemoSonic 100* device was developed to eliminate the latter by echocardiographic aortic diameter measurement, but optimal adjustment of both the Doppler technique and the ultrasonic signal can be challenging. Therefore, the value of the esophageal Doppler technique is limited in clinical practice. However, Doppler devices may be used in specific situations by skilled observers. Based on the ability to reliably track CO changes over time, early goal directed therapy in the intraoperative setting may be a typical indication, since different studies have demonstrated improved outcomes when using this concept.

Until now, tools for continuous CO monitoring have been validated as if they were tools for snapshot measurements. Most authors have compared variations in CO between two time-points and have used Bland–Altman representations to describe the statistical agreement between these variations. The impact of time and repetitive measurements over time have not been taken into consideration. Recently Squara and coworkers proposed a conceptual framework for the validation of CO monitoring devices [6]. Four quality criteria were suggested and studied: accuracy (with a small bias), precision (with a small random error in measurements), a short response time, and an accurate amplitude response. As an amount of deviation in each of these four criteria is admitted, the authors proposed to add, as a fifth criterion, the ability to detect significant cardiac output directional changes. Other important issues regarding the designing of studies to validate cardiac output monitoring tools were also underscored: the choice of patient population to be studied, choice of reference method, the method of data acquisition, data acceptability checking, data segmentation, and the final evaluation of reliability. The application of this framework underlines the importance of precision and time response for the clinical acceptance of monitoring tools.

References

1. Practice Guidelines for Pulmonary Artery Catheterization (2003) An Update Report by the American Society of Anesthesiologists Task Force on Pulmonary artery Catheterization. Anesthesiology 99:988–1014
2. Della Rocca G, Costa MG, Pompei L, Coccia C, Pietropaoli P (2002) Continuous and intermittent cardiac output measurement: pulmonary artery catheter versus aortic transpulmonary technique. Br J Anaesth 88:350–356
3. Costa MG, Della Rocca G, Chiarandini P, Mattelig S, Pompei L, Barriga MS, Reynolds T, Cecconi M, Pietropaoli P (2008) Continuous and intermittent cardiac output measurement in hyperdynamic conditions: pulmonary artery catheter vs. lithium dilution technique. Intensive Care Med 34(2):257–263
4. McGee WT, Horswell JL, Calderon J, Janvier G, Van Severen T, Van den Berghe G, Kozikowski L (2007) Validation of a continuous, arterial pressure-based cardiac output measurement: a multicenter, prospective clinical trial. Crit Care 11:R105
5. Singer M (2009) Oesophagela doppler. Curr Opin Crit Care 15(3):244–248
6. Squara P, Cecconi M, Rhodes A, Singer M, Chiche JD. Intensive Care Med 2009; Jul 11 Epub ahead of print

Cardiac Steroids and Glycoside Toxicity

NIMA MAJLESI, DIANE P. CALELLO, RICHARD D. SHIH
Department of Emergency Medicine, Morristown Memorial Hospital, Morristown, NJ, USA

Synonyms

Digoxin toxicity; Foxglove toxicity; Oleander toxicity

Definition

Cardioactive steroids are a class of animal and plant-derived compounds with a steroid nucleus and a specific inotropic, chronotropic, and dromotropic effect. The term *cardiac glycoside* refers to a subgroup of cardioactive steroids that also contain sugar residues and include digoxin, digitalis, and ouabain. In the United States, the most common source of cardioactive steroid exposure is pharmaceutical digoxin. Plant sources include oleander

(*Nerium oleander*), foxglove (*Digitalis spp.*), lily of the valley (*Convallaria majalis*), and red squill (*Urginea maritima*), a rodenticide of historical significance. The dried secretions of the *Bufo* toad, a purported aphrodisiac when topically applied, contain a cardioactive steroid and have also caused toxicity when ingested.

Pathophysiology

Ingested cardioactive steroids (CAS) are approximately 80% bioavailable. However, toxicokinetics depends on multiple factors, including electrolyte abnormalities, medication interactions, renal dysfunction, and disruption of gastrointestinal flora. Hypokalemia, in particular, results in excessive sensitivity to CAS as less binding to skeletal Na+-K+ ATPase may result in increased effects on the myocardium. Hypomagnesemia and hypercalcemia may also potentiate CAS toxicity. Drug interactions are unfortunately common with other cardiovascular medications. Amiodarone, spironolactone, furosemide, diltiazem, carvedilol, and verapamil can all interfere with the kinetics of CAS through alteration of protein binding, inactivation of P-glycoprotein, and decreased renal perfusion.

Cardioactive steroids inhibit the Na+-K+ ATPase on the membrane of the cardiac myocyte, thereby raising the intracellular Na+ content, which then prevents the Na+-Ca2+ antiporter from expelling Ca2+ in exchange for Na+. This results in an increase in intracellular Ca2+ within the myocyte and calcium-mediated Ca2+ release from the sarcoplasmic reticulum. Positive inotropy is achieved by increased available calcium to bind troponin, actin, and myosin. CAS also can affect the parasympathetic nervous system through increase of acetylcholine from the vagus nerve.

The resultant effect on cardiac conduction and electrophysiology is variable. Therapeutically, CAS cause a decreased rate of depolarization and conduction through both the sinoatrial and atrioventricular nodes. A higher resting membrane potential also leads to shortened repolarization and increased automaticity of the atria and ventricles. The common ECG finding in patients on therapeutic CAS is referred to as "digitalis effect." Digitalis effect is characterized by PR interval prolongation, QT shortening, and the ST-segment forces opposite in direction from the QRS. This is a reflection of therapeutic effect in contrast to the ECG findings in CAS toxicity.

Presentation

It is important to distinguish between those patients with acute and chronic CAS toxicity as clinical manifestations and management differ significantly. An assessment of the serum digoxin concentration, serum electrolytes, especially potassium and magnesium, renal function, and electrocardiogram are essential in determining the severity of toxicity and the need for treatment. In the case of plant-derived CAS exposure, the serum digoxin immunoassay exhibits some cross-reactivity with these compounds and will provide qualitative assessment. These cases should be managed more by the clinical picture than the actual serum level. Digoxin toxicity, however, typically requires a concentration greater than 2 ng/mL.

In acute toxicity, early nausea and vomiting are nearly universal; extracardiac manifestations may include confusion and lethargy. ECG findings vary widely, and essentially any rhythm is possible in CAS toxicity with the notable exception of rapidly conducted supraventricular tachydysrhythmias. Biventricular tachycardia, while pathognomonic, is rarely seen. The most commonly observed findings are premature ventricular contractions and atrial fibrillation or flutter with atrioventricular block [1]. Digitalis effect is not the result of CAS toxicity and represents normal therapeutic effect as mentioned earlier.

An elevated serum potassium concentration as a result of Na+-K+ ATPase pump inhibition has been shown to be prognostic in adults with acute ingestion. A large observational cohort study performed before the development of digoxin-specific antibodies demonstrated a strong correlation between serum potassium and mortality [2]. A potassium concentration between 5.0 and 5.5 mEq/L was associated with a 50% mortality, and a serum potassium concentrations greater than 5.5 mEq/L was associated with 100% mortality. Though hyperkalemia may exacerbate the toxicity due to CAS, it is more a marker of severity in adults with acute ingestion rather than the primary etiology.

Chronic CAS toxicity is more challenging both to diagnose and to manage. Systemic symptoms are often present, including malaise, GI symptoms, weakness, confusion, delirium, and various visual disturbances. These often include decreased visual acuity and visual color changes (xanthopsia).

Unlike acute CAS toxicity, chronic toxicity is often complicated by hypokalemia due to concomitant diuretic use which as mentioned may potentiate toxicity. Hypomagnesemia, when present, will enhance the myocardial irritability these patients exhibit. However, hyperkalemia and hypermagnesemia may also be present, most commonly in the setting of new onset renal failure or insufficiency.

Similar bradydysrhythmias and ventricular tachydysrhythmias which occur in acute toxicity are more common in patients presenting with chronic CAS toxicity.

Treatment

Digoxin-specific antibody fragments have revolutionized the treatment of CAS toxicity. The decision to administer is multifactorial and should consider the amount ingested, serum level, clinical evidence of toxicity, as well as the patient's underlying conditions which may be exacerbated by complete removal of digoxin where clinically needed. In general, digoxin-specific Fab should be given to patients with:

1. CAS-related dysrhythmias
2. Acute ingestion with potassium greater than 5 mEq/L
3. Chronic toxicity presenting with dysrhythmias, CNS findings, or gastrointestinal symptoms
4. Serum digoxin concentration greater than 15 ng/mL at any time or greater than 10 ng/mL 6 h post-ingestion regardless of symptoms in an acute ingestion
5. Poisoning with a non-digoxin CAS

The optimal dosing of digoxin-specific Fab can be determined based on the serum concentration, amount ingested, or clinical presentation [3].

1. If the serum digoxin concentration is known, the dose is calculated as:

$$\text{\# of vials} = [\text{serum digoxin concentration (ng/mL)} \times \text{weight}]/100$$

2. If the amount ingested is known and the ingestion is acute, the dose is calculated as:

$$\text{\# of vials} = [\text{amounted ingested (mg)}/0.5 \text{ (mg/vial)} \times 0.8 \text{ (represents 80\% bioavailability)}$$

3. In the patient presenting with life-threatening toxicity requiring immediate treatment before the serum concentration can be obtained, with an unknown amount ingested, the recommended empiric dose is 10–20 vials in acute poisoning, and 5 vials in chronic poisoning.

Gastrointestinal decontamination should be considered in patients with acute ingestions especially for those with non-digoxin CAS ingestions. Multiple dose–activated charcoal may be effective due to enterohepatic recirculation of CAS. Gastric lavage and emesis should be limited to the very few presenting early with non-digoxin CAS ingestions.

Replacement of potassium and magnesium should occur prior to administration of digoxin-specific antibody fragments as correction often leads to abatement of the presenting cardiac dysrhythmia, and Fab administration may decrease the potassium further. In contrast, correction of hyperkalemia should begin with administration of digoxin specific antibody fragments followed by intravenous insulin, dextrose, and sodium bicarbonate, being careful not to cause hypokalemia. Intravenous calcium administration is contraindicated due to the relative intracellular hypercalcemia which exists in CAS-poisoned patients. Administration has been associated with cardiac dysfunction and arrest.

Transvenous and external pacing is contraindicated in patients with CAS poisoning due to increased adverse outcomes associated with delay in digoxin-specific Fab administration and conversion to unstable ventricular dysrhythmias [4]. However, cardioversion and defibrillation is indicated in those with hemodynamic instability and ventricular dysrhythmias.

Prognosis

The prognosis of CAS-poisoned patients is dependent upon the complications of CAS toxicity that develop.

After-care

After management of acute medical consequences, patients with intentional overdoses should be referred for counseling. Patients with chronic CAS toxicity should be evaluated for alternative treatment of the underlying disorders so that unintentional toxicity will be less likely to recur.

References

1. Bismuth C, Gaultier M, Conso F, Efthymiou ML (1973) Hyperkalemia in acute digitalis poisoning: prognostic significance and therapeutic implications. Clin Toxicol 6(2):153–162
2. Ma G, Brady WJ, Pollack M, Chan TC (2001) Electrocardiographic manifestations: digitalis toxicity. J Emerg Med 20(2):145–152
3. Antman EM, Wenger TL, Butler VP Jr, Haber E, Smith TW (1990) Treatment of 150 cases of life-threatening digitalis intoxication with digoxin-specific Fab antibody fragments. Final report of a multicenter study. Circulation 81(6):1744–1752
4. Taboulet P, Baud FJ, Bismuth C, Vicaut E (1993) Acute digitalis intoxication–is pacing still appropriate? J Toxicol Clin Toxicol 31(2):261–273

Cardiac Tamponade

Dominic W. K. Spray
Anaesthetics and Intensive Care, St. George's Hospital, London, UK

Synonyms

Pericardial tamponade

Definition

Cardiac Tamponade describes the hemodynamic sequelae resulting from compression of the cardiac chambers due to accumulation of fluid (or gas) within the pericardium.

Pathophysiology [1, 2]

An understanding of the underlying pathophysiology is essential to fully grasp the clinical findings associated with tamponade. The pericardial sac is relatively inelastic. It can stretch to accommodate a limited volume (pericardial reserve volume) before any further increase in pericardial contents causes increased pericardial pressure and competition between the extracardiac contents and the contents of the cardiac chambers for the finite available space. As tamponade develops, the cardiac chambers are compressed and their compliance is reduced. This imposes a constraint on cardiac filling, reduces stroke volume and ultimately leads to a decrease in cardiac output.

The compliance of the pericardium and the rate of fluid accumulation determine the likelihood of tamponade occurring (Fig. 1). Rapid accumulation of fluid (e.g., traumatic intrapericardial hemorrhage) will rapidly result in tamponade. Conversely, with slow fluid accumulation (e.g., as a result of inflammation), up to 2 l of fluid may be present before causing tamponade.

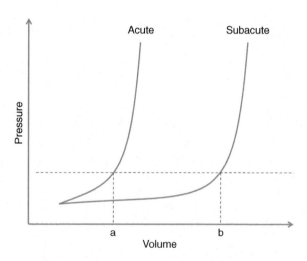

Cardiac Tamponade. **Figure 1** The effect of rapid accumulation of pericardial fluid compared to gradual accumulation. In acute tamponade, very little volume (*point a*) is needed before pericardial reserve volume is exhausted and a critical pressure reached. With gradual accumulation, compensatory mechanisms allow more volume (*point b*) to be accommodated before this critical pressure is reached. In both cases, small increments in pericardial fluid beyond this point result in rapid pressure rises

Chronic changes in pericardial compliance allow the pericardium to accommodate this extra fluid. Compensatory mechanisms based on sympathetic stimulation (tachycardia, increased peripheral vascular resistance and increased ejection fraction due to increased contractility) with increased blood volume (upregulation of the renin-angiotensin system) act to delay the decrease in cardiac output.

In all cases, at the critical inflection point, very little extra fluid needs to accumulate to substantially raise pericardial pressure and cause tamponade (likewise, great benefit is seen from the initial removal of fluid during pericardiocentesis). As tamponade increases, eventually the diastolic pressures in all cardiac chambers equalize at a level similar to the pericardial pressure (15–30 mmHg).

Pneumopericardium is rare but may occur after trauma, due to iatrogenic causes or secondary to gas-forming infections. It can present in a similar way to fluid tamponade and is similarly a medical emergency.

Hemodynamic Sequelae

Venous Return

Venous return usually has two peaks – one during early diastole and one during ventricular systole. Progressive tamponade causes increased pericardial pressure throughout the cardiac cycle. Since the heart chambers in total are fullest during diastole (and diastolic pressure is increased) there is effectively no space for extra blood to flow into. In contrast, the stroke volume leaving during ventricular systole makes room for venous return. Filling is therefore progressively shifted towards systole and diastolic filling diminishes. Jugular venous distension is present and the x descent of the central venous pressure trace is lost, but the y descent remains. Once tamponade is advanced enough, filling also drops during systole leading to a further fall in total venous return and cardiac output.

Ventricular Interdependence and Pulsus Paradoxus

Changes in pleural pressure are still transmitted to the heart during tamponade. Therefore, in spontaneous inspiration, systemic venous return increases due to the fall in intrathoracic pressure. Since the RV free wall is constricted by the pericardial effusion, the extra volume can only be accommodated by shifting the interventricular septum leftward at the expense of left ventricular volume. Therefore, during spontaneous inspiration, left ventricular cardiac output drops, manifested by an exaggerated decrease in systolic blood pressure (>10 mmHg), a phenomenon known as pulsus paradoxus (Fig. 2). Increased LV

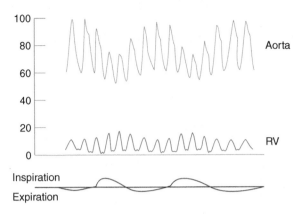

Cardiac Tamponade. Figure 2 Pulsus paradoxus. Note the decreased aortic systolic pressure and narrowing of pulse pressure during spontaneous inspiration and rise again during expiration. Timings are reversed in the RV pressure trace

afterload due to the decreased intrathoracic pressure may also contribute to this decrease in left ventricular stroke volume.

Right ventricular output will increase during inspiration secondary to the increased venous return. Since the ventricles are in series, a few beats later, this also contributes to an increased left ventricular stroke volume during expiration. Thus the effects of ventilation during tamponade are to produce right and left sided stroke volume and pressure changes which are 180° out of phase.

Note that with intermittent positive pressure ventilation (IPPV), the above findings will be reversed as intrathoracic pressure is at its highest during inspiration and decreases during expiration.

Decreased Cardiac Output

The end-result of the effects of tamponade is a decrease in cardiac output. The decrease in systemic venous return and reduction in end diastolic chamber volumes are the primary reasons for the low cardiac output state. End systolic volume does also decrease due to increased contractility secondary to sympathetic activation. However, this is not sufficient to maintain stroke volume, hence the reliance on tachycardia to maintain adequate cardiac output.

The effects of IPPV itself on cardiac output are complicated and variable, but on the whole, IPPV tends to reduce venous return and consequently cardiac output. Therefore, IPPV should be avoided in patients who are not intubated at presentation. Corrective treatment by rapid pericardiocentesis should be the aim as this will reverse most indications for ventilation.

Etiology and Subtypes of Tamponade

Classical Tamponade

This presents with a spectrum of severity, from a simple effusion with few symptoms to a life-threatening emergency. It is sometimes divided on the basis of duration into acute and sub-acute. Acute tamponade is usually due to trauma, cardiovascular rupture (e.g., retrograde flow from type A aortic dissection) or iatrogenic causes (e.g., cardiac catheterization). Sub-acute tamponade develops more insidiously, usually as a result of an inflammatory process (e.g., infection, neoplasm, autoimmune, radiation or drug-induced) but sometimes due to a non-inflammatory process (e.g., hypothyroidism, amyloidosis) in which the underlying pathogenesis of the effusion remains unclear. Idiopathic pericardial effusion is also seen, often presenting with large volumes of pericardial fluid. Whatever the cause, it is important to treat any decompensation as a medical emergency and institute the appropriate management.

Low Pressure Tamponade

It is the trend towards pressure equalization between pericardial pressure and intracardiac pressure that gives rise to tamponade. Therefore in patients who are severely hypovolemic for whatever reason (e.g., hemorrhage, hemodialysis), with low intracardiac pressures, tamponade has been demonstrated with pericardial pressures in the range of 6–12 mmHg. Echocardiographic features are similar to patients with classic tamponade (effusion size, chamber collapse, exaggerated respiratory variation in transvalvular flow), but clinical signs such as tachycardia, jugular venous distension and pulsus paradoxus are less prevalent.

Regional Tamponade

Loculated or localized effusions or hematoma can occur, commonly after cardiac surgery. The hemodynamic effects of these vary widely depending on the affected chambers and the typical features of classical tamponade are often missing. Although the presentation may mimic that of heart failure, it is difficult to generalize about clinical findings and detailed imaging is often necessary to establish the diagnosis. A high index of suspicion should prevail if there is a possibility of regional tamponade given the clinical findings and a suggestive history.

Evaluation and Assessment

As mentioned above, tamponade manifests a continuum of symptoms with a range of clinical severity. Presentation may also include many non-specific signs and symptoms. Ultimately, the presentation will be that of cardiogenic shock and the differential diagnosis should include other causes for this.

History

In cases of suspected tamponade, the usual history should be taken and predisposing factors should be sought. This may be more relevant on the ICU where patients may not be able to communicate.

Symptoms

Symptoms tend to relate to the degree of impairment in cardiac output. Patients may complain of tachycardia, dyspnea and fatigue as well as a central chest discomfort, often relieved by sitting forward.

Clinical Signs

These become all the more relevant in sedated intensive care patients who are unable to give a history or describe their symptoms. Sympathetic upregulation resulting in tachycardia is seen in virtually all cases, with exceptions being those patients in whom their underlying disease manifests bradycardia (e.g., hypothyroidism).

Cardiac sounds may be muffled and the apex beat difficult to palpate in the presence of a large effusion. A pericardial rub may be present if pericarditis is the underlying etiology. Elevated jugular venous pressure is seen, with the y descent often attenuated or absent due to the absence of diastolic filling as discussed above. The x descent is usually preserved. This is usually more easily appreciated on a central venous pressure trace than by clinical examination.

Pulsus paradoxus can be demonstrated in most cases of tamponade. The sphygmomanometer cuff is deflated slowly. Initially, the first Korotkoff sounds are only audible during spontaneous expiration (or IPPV inspiration), but as the cuff is deflated further, sounds are heard throughout the respiratory cycle. The difference in pressure between these two events quantifies the degree of pulsus paradoxus. There are situations in which tamponade does not give rise to pulsus paradoxus. These include any pre-existing condition where left ventricular diastolic pressure or volume are already raised (e.g., atrial septal defects, severe aortic regurgitation, chronic renal failure). Pulsus paradoxus may also occur outside the context of tamponade. It is seen in severe asthma or COPD, pulmonary embolism and in up to one third of cases of constrictive pericarditis.

In intensive care patients, tamponade must always be amongst the differential diagnosis of any patient who manifests cardiogenic shock. The usual symptoms of hypotension, diaphoresis, shut down extremities and oliguria may also be used as a crude indicator of progression

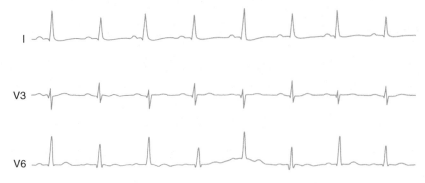

Cardiac Tamponade. Figure 3 Electrical alternans. Note the changing size of sequential QRS complexes possibly due to the heart "swinging" in the pericardial effusion

of tamponade over time and the need to perform pericardiocentesis.

Investigations

Tamponade remains a clinical diagnosis, but certain investigations are useful to confirm suspicions.

Electrocardiography

This usually demonstrates tachycardia and may be of lower voltage than usual, although this is a non-specific finding. It may be possible that this finding is limited to tamponade alone rather than effusion per se. Patterns associated with acute pericarditis may also present. Electrical alternans (Fig. 3) is very specific, but insensitive for tamponade. There is a beat to beat variation in the size of electrical complexes, often, but not necessarily, restricted to the QRS. This is thought to be possibly due to the heart "swinging" in the pericardial fluid although the exact mechanism is poorly understood.

Chest Radiography

At least a moderate pericardial effusion (approx. 200 ml) is required before the cardiac silhouette begins to enlarge to a characteristic, round, "flask-shaped" appearance. A lateral view may show a pericardial fat pad due to separation of pericardial fat from epicardium by the pericardial fluid. Chest radiographs typically appear normal in acute tamponade, except that the lung fields usually appear oligemic.

Echocardiography [3]

Echocardiography remains the standard for non-invasive assessment of pericardial effusion and its hemodynamic consequences. There is a class 1 recommendation for its use in assessment of patients with suspected pericardial disease (American College of Cardiology/American Heart Association/American Society of Echocardiography

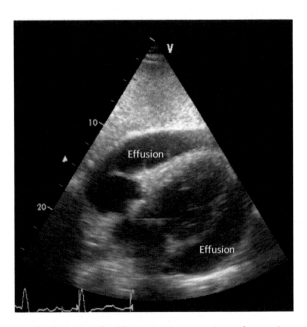

Cardiac Tamponade. Figure 4 Large anterior and posterior effusion containing fibrin strands

guidelines 2003). The presence of pulmonary hypertension may mask echocardiographic findings in tamponade.

Typical echocardiographic findings associated with tamponade include:

- Effusion

Effusion is usually well visualized (Fig. 4). It normally needs to be circumferential for classical tamponade to occur, but regional tamponade may present with loculated or localized effusions.

- Diastolic chamber collapse

During atrial relaxation, the pressure in the RA is at its lowest and pericardial pressure at its highest leading

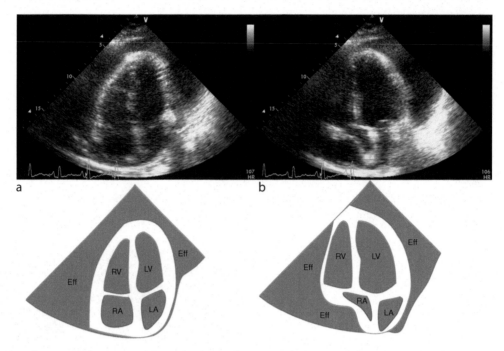

Cardiac Tamponade. Figure 5 Right atrial collapse as a result of tamponade. In mid diastole, the RA is seen to be full (**a**). After end diastole the RA collapses – this has persisted into early systole (**b**). Note the free wall of the RV and the LA are not well visualized in **b**. Eff,Effusion; RA, Right Atrium; RV, Right Ventricle; LA, Left Atrium; LV, Left Ventricle

to atrial collapse (Fig. 5). If this persists for more than one third of the cardiac cycle, it is highly specific and sensitive for tamponade. Brief collapse may occur for other reasons.

RV collapse occurs in early diastole when the RV is still empty (Fig. 6). This is a less sensitive, but more specific finding for tamponade than RA collapse and may not occur when diastolic pressure is raised, there is raised RV afterload, or there is RV hypertrophy (since the RV becomes less compliant).

Left sided collapse occurs less often. LV collapse occurs very rarely since the wall is more muscular. LA collapse when found is very specific for tamponade.

● Ventricular interdependence and septal shift

As discussed earlier, changes in right sided filling with spontaneous inspiration result in the interventricular septum shifting into the LV (Fig. 7), the cause of pulsus paradoxus.

Respiratory variation in trans-mitral and trans-tricuspid flow is also a result of the respiratory influence on filling and ventricular interdependence. During spontaneous inspiration (or IPPV expiration), right-sided filling increases and trans-tricuspid flow is increased relative to that during spontaneous expiration

(or IPPV inspiration). The reverse is true for trans-mitral flow. Therefore the respiratory variation in flow across the atrio-ventricular valves is 180° out of phase (Fig. 8).

The presence of pulmonary hypertension can mask some of the echocardiographic signs of tamponade.

● Venous hemodynamics

A plethoric IVC is often seen due to the raised central venous pressure, which may also manifest a reduced reduction in IVC diameter (<50%) during spontaneous inspiration (Fig. 9) despite the transmission of intrathoracic pressure to the RA. Doppler patterns of atrial filling will also reflect the shift towards systolic filling and the loss of the diastolic component.

CT/MRI [4]
These should not be used in unstable patients, but may have a role in situations where the diagnosis is unclear and the patient is relatively stable (e.g., suspected regional tamponade). Pericardial effusion may also be an incidental finding on CT. Findings suggestive of tamponade include large sized effusions, systemic venous distension, chamber deformity and interventricular shift as seen on echocardiography. Cine MRI is also capable of

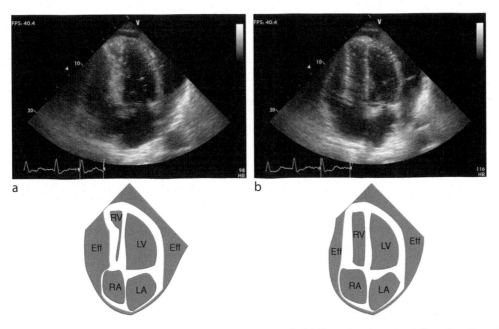

Cardiac Tamponade. Figure 6 RV collapse in diastole due to tamponade (**a**). Note that the RV end diastolic volume is also reduced (**b**), contributing to the low cardiac output state. Eff, Effusion; RA, Right Atrium; RV, Right Ventricle; LA, Left Atrium; LV, Left Ventricle

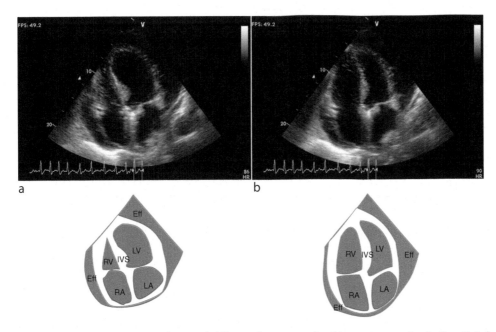

Cardiac Tamponade. Figure 7 Interventricular septal shift seen in tamponade with spontaneous inspiration. Note both frames are taken at the same point of the electrocardiogram. In (**a**), during spontaneous expiration, a normal anatomical relationship exists. In (**b**), the patient has inhaled, resulting in increased filling of the right side and bowing of the interventricular septum into the left ventricle as the only way to accommodate the extra RV volume. Eff, Effusion; RA, Right Atrium; RV, Right Ventricle; LA, Left Atrium; LV, Left Ventricle

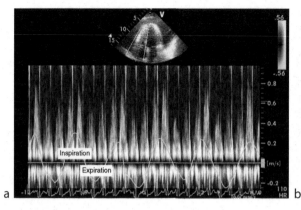 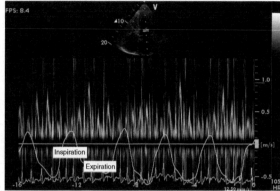

Cardiac Tamponade. Figure 8 The effect of spontaneous ventilation on atrio-ventricular valve flow velocities in tamponade. Trans-tricuspid flow (**a**) increases during spontaneous inspiration due to the increased systemic venous return, and decreases during expiration. During inspiration, trans-mitral flow (**b**) is impaired due to reduced LA filling and increased LV pressure as a result of ventricular interdependence. The reverse is true during expiration

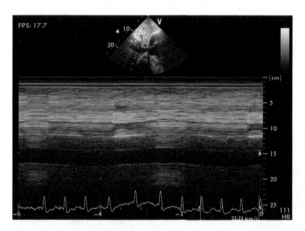

Cardiac Tamponade. Figure 9 M-mode echocardiography of the inferior vena cava during tamponade, showing a plethoric IVC with very little respiratory variation in size

demonstrating all findings seen by echocardiography. Underlying pericardial pathology is better assessed by CT than echocardiography.

Invasive Pressure Measurement

A pulmonary artery catheter will show equalization of diastolic pressure across cardiac chambers and the respiratory changes in right and left sided pressures responsible for pulsus paradoxus. It is also useful to monitor the effects of treatment – filling pressures that remain elevated after pericardiocentesis may indicate underlying pericardial pathology. Monitoring after pericardiocentesis can help in early detection of any reaccumulation of fluid and pressure changes indicating impending tamponade.

Treatment

This depends on the severity of the hemodynamic disturbance. Early tamponade with minimal hemodynamic disturbance and no significant loss in cardiac output may be treated conservatively, especially since the risks associated with pericardiocentesis are increased with small effusions. Treatment should be aimed at the underlying cause (e.g., steroids for autoimmune disease, correction of clotting etc.) and monitoring must be commensurate with the clinical picture. Invasive monitoring (including consideration of a pulmonary artery catheter) is indicated and these patients should be nursed in a high dependency setting. Serial assessment is needed to ascertain the likelihood of worsening tamponade and the patient watched carefully for evidence of end organ dysfunction due to any decrease in cardiac output (e.g., oliguria, altered mental state).

In patients with idiopathic effusion alone, but no tamponade, opinion is divided as to treatment. Removal of fluid should only be undertaken for treatment of possible tamponade, and not for routine diagnosis. There is conflicting evidence as to the rate of progression to tamponade, but an effusion measuring greater than 20 mm on echocardiography should be considered for drainage. This may also reduce recurrence in the future.

Patients with overt tamponade represent a clinical emergency and require definitive treatment by removal of the pericardial fluid. Intravenous fluids have been used as a temporizing measure, with best effects seen in patients with a systolic blood pressure of <100 mmHg. Hydration raises pericardial pressure as well as RA pressure and LV end diastolic pressure which may explain why some patients do not benefit. Positive inotropes with or without vasodilators are of limited efficacy, probably because of the maximal endogenous sympathetic drive seen in most cases.

Pericardiocentesis and Pericardectomy [4]

Pericardial fluid is usually removed either percutaneously or by surgical pericardectomy, although balloon pericardectomy has been described in neoplastic effusions.

Echocardiography allows the optimum site for pericardiocentesis to be located (the shortest route to the pericardial fluid via an intercostal approach). Echocardiography also reduces the risk of myocardial puncture and allows visualization of fluid removal and consequent hemodynamic effects. Under full asepsis, a needle is advanced into the pericardial fluid. Agitated saline may be used to confirm needle position (easily seen on echocardiography). Up to 150 ml of fluid should be removed through the needle to ameliorate the worst of the tamponade (as discussed earlier, removal of only a small volume of pericardial fluid may have great benefit). A guidewire is fed through the needle and a pigtail catheter passed over this and secured in place. This procedure in the Mayo Clinic had a success rate of 97% with complication rates of 3.5% (minor) and 1.2% (major) respectively. Complications include perforation of myocardium or coronary vessels, arrhythmias, pneumothorax, air embolism, and abdominal trauma. Pericardiocentesis should be done in the cardiac catheter laboratory unless the patient is too unwell to be moved.

Fluoroscopy may be used if echocardiography is unavailable, with the sub-xiphoid route being commonest, the needle being directed towards the left shoulder. Once pericardial fluid is aspirated, a small amount of contrast is injected to confirm position and the guidewire introduced. The guidewire position is checked in two planes and the pigtail catheter passed over it.

In emergency situations (e.g., during a pulseless electrical activity arrest), a sub-xiphoid entry point is used and the needle directed toward the patient's shoulder.

Aortic dissection is a major contraindication to pericardiocentesis and coagulopathy a relative one. A surgical approach is preferred where there are loculated effusions, small effusions (<1 cm) or where there is evidence of clot or adhesions. Recurrent tamponade (especially due to neoplasm) is also often best managed surgically. Pericardectomy is usually performed via a sub-xiphoid approach under general anesthesia since a small window is usually sufficient to relieve tamponade (whereas removal of the entire pericardial sac via an anterior approach is used in constrictive pericarditis).

Balloon pericardectomy allows drainage from the pericardium into the pleural cavity. The risks of general anesthesia are increased in tamponade and even partial drainage by pericardiocentesis prior to induction may help to decrease risk.

Pericardial fluid samples should be sent to the laboratory for staining and culture (including mycobacteria), plus differential white cell count, specific gravity, hematocrit and protein content if the diagnosis is not known beforehand. Adenosine deaminase levels should also be requested if tuberculous effusion is a possibility.

After Care and Prognosis

A pericardial drain usually stays in place until drainage is less than 25 ml/day. During this time, the patient should remain fully monitored for recurrence of tamponade or possible complications. Mortality and morbidity are very low since the advent of echocardiography guided procedures, with recent studies estimating the major complication rate to be between 1.2% and 1.6%. Patients with pre-existing pulmonary hypertension complicated by tamponade seem to be at higher risk of death.

Comparison between Cardiac Tamponade and Constrictive Pericarditis [5]

There are some important similarities and differences between constrictive pericarditis and cardiac tamponade. Constrictive pericarditis also results in increased intracardiac pressure and equalization of left and right filling pressures. The fibrotic, scarred pericardium prevents changes in intrathoracic pressure being transmitted to the cardiac chambers (unlike tamponade). These changes are still transmitted to the pulmonary circulation. On spontaneous inspiration, the gradient from pulmonary veins to left atrium is therefore reduced and left-sided filling is impaired. This allows an increase in right sided filling during spontaneous inspiration (the same ventricular interdependence which occurs in tamponade occurs in constrictive pericarditis). The opposite occurs with spontaneous expiration. Therefore, although the mechanism is different to tamponade, pulsus paradoxus can occur in constrictive pericarditis, so cannot reliably be used to distinguish between the two (although it is more common in tamponade). Changes in transmitral and transtricuspid flows are similar between the two.

In constrictive pericarditis, atrial filling occurs primarily in diastole due to raised atrial pressures driving flow. This stops abruptly around mid-diastole when the noncompliant ventricle reaches its volume limit (due to pericardial constriction). This results in the so called "square root sign" – the right ventricular pressure trace shows an initial dip followed by an acute rise in early diastole and then a subsequent plateau during which no more filling occurs. This is not seen in tamponade.

The JVP in constrictive pericarditis is raised (also in tamponade) but contains both an x descent and a prominent, collapsing y descent (unlike tamponade where the y descent is attenuated or may be missing). Since inspiratory pressures are not transmitted to the RA, the usual increase in right heart return does not occur and so systemic venous pressure increases (or at least does not drop) during spontaneous inspiration (Kussmaul sign). The Kussmaul sign does not occur in tamponade.

Pericardial effusion leading to tamponade does occur in patients with pre-existing constrictive pericarditis (effusive constrictive pericarditis). Echocardiographic findings may initially be intermediate, but pericardiocentesis unmasks the typical findings associated with constrictive pericarditis.

References

1. Spodick DH (2003) Acute cardiac tamponade. N Engl J Med 349:684–690
2. Zipes DP, Libby P, Bonow RO, Braunwald E (eds) (2005) Braunwald's heart disease: a textbook of cardiovascular medicine, 7th edn. Elsevier Saunders, Philadelphia, pp 1762–1769
3. Wann S, Passen E (2008) Echocardiography in pericardial disease. J Am Soc Echocadiogr 21:7–13
4. Restrepo CS, Lemos DF, Lemos JA et al (2007) Imaging findings in cardiac tamponade with emphasis on CT. Radiographics 27:1595–1610
5. Maisch B, Seferovic PM, Ristic AD et al (2004) Guidelines on the diagnosis and management of pericardial diseases. executive summary. The task force on the diagnosis and management of pericardial diseases of the European society of cardiology. Eur Heart J 25:587–610

Cardiac Troponin I

▶ Cardiac Markers for Diagnosing Acute Myocardial Infarction

Cardiac Troponin T

▶ Cardiac Markers for Diagnosing Acute Myocardial Infarction

Cardiac Ultrasound

▶ Echocardiography

Cardiogenic Pulmonary Edema

▶ Heart Failure, Acute
▶ Ventricular Dysfunction and Failure

Cardiogenic Shock

▶ Acute Heart Failure: Risk Stratification
▶ Heart Failure, Acute
▶ Ventricular Dysfunction and Failure

Cardiomyopathy in Children

JONATHAN R. EGAN, MARINO S. FESTA
The Children's Hospital at Westmead, Westmead, Australia

Definition

A disease of the heart muscle in children is typically the result of inherited conditions (consider genetic and metabolic disorders) or viral myocarditis that has become indolent – characterized by cardiogenic failure.

Characteristics

It is useful to categorize pediatric cardiomyopathy into the following four groups, the majority of which present prior to 12 months of age [1]:

Hypertrophic Cardiomyopathy (HCOM)
Caused as a result of hypertrophic expansion either of the left ventricular septum alone or in combination with free wall hypertrophy. This disease leads to impingement on the left ventricle cavity, impaired ventricular filling, and variable left ventricular outflow obstruction. Most commonly, this is an inherited condition and there is a strong association with Noonan's syndrome, it is characterized by shortness of breath or syncope on exertion. It is an important cause of sudden death in young people.

Dilated Cardiomyopathy (DCMP)

Typically as the result of burnt out viral myocarditis (40%) or idiopathic in origin. There is reduced systolic performance and global cardiac dilatation. This has a poor prognosis and apart from supportive therapies will require heart transplant where feasible and appropriate. As a result of the dilatation and resulting arrhythmic propensity there is also a risk of mural thrombus formation. Selenium deficiency also results in a dilated cardiomyopathy.

Restrictive Cardiomyopathy (RCMP)

RCMP is not common and results from infiltrative conditions such as hemochromatosis, amyloidosis, and glycogen storage diseases. It is increasingly prevalent with increasing age and diastolic function is primarily compromised.

Arrhythmogenic Right Ventricular Dysplasia and Left Ventricular Noncompaction

Right ventricular dysplasia is an inherited condition in which the right ventricle is replaced by fibrous-fatty tissue. Patients typically present with arrhythmias in early adulthood. Left ventricular noncompaction is variably inherited and associated with systemic disorders. There are coarse trabeculations of the ventricular apex, which can affect both systolic and diastolic performance of the systemic ventricle.

Management

Patients with HCOM have restrictions on physical activity and typically receive beta blockade prophylaxis. Partial septal myomectomy can also be considered. Given the generally guarded prognosis of the cardiomyopathies it is important to determine any (rarely) reversible causes – in particular deficiencies of thiamine, selenium or carnitine, endocrinopathies (thyroid and growth hormone abnormalities as well as phaeochromocytoma) need to be considered. Anticoagulation should be considered and maintained in those with dilated cardiomyopathy. Subsequently, supportive medical and mechanical therapies maybe indicated together with heart transplant depending on the underlying cause and overall condition of the patient. Initial supportive measures are similar to those outlined in the *cardiac failure* section, but about half of pediatric heart transplants are for cardiomyopathies [6].

References

1. Nugent AW, Daubeney PE, Chondros P, Carlin JB, Cheung M, Wilkinson LC, Davis AM, Kahler SG, Chow CW, Wilkinson JL, Weintraub RG (2003) The epidemiology of childhood cardiomyopathy in Australia. N Engl J Med 348(17):1639–1646

Cardioparacentesis

▶ Periocardiocentesis

Cardiopulmonary Resuscitation

Raghu R. Seethala[1], Benjamin S. Abella[2]
[1]Department of Anesthesiology, Perioperative and Pain Medicine, Brigham and Women's Hospital, Boston, MA, USA
[2]Department of Emergency Medicine and Department of Medicine, Pulmonary, Allergy, and Critical Care Division, Hospital of the University of Pennsylvania, Philadelphia, PA, USA

Synonyms

Basic life support (BLS); Chest compression (CC)

Definition

Cardiopulmonary resuscitation (CPR) is a method of providing artificial (externally-generated) circulation and ventilation during cardiac arrest to achieve the return of spontaneous circulation (ROSC). The main actions performed during CPR are delivery of chest compressions (CC) and rescue breaths. In a newer form of the therapy specifically for lay public providers ("hands-only" CPR), only CCs are delivered without the provision of rescue breaths.

Role of CPR

Indication

Cardiac arrest (CA), defined as the abrupt cessation of cardiac output usually due to sudden arrhythmia, is an exquisitely time-sensitive condition common in intensive care environments. In-hospital CA has a survival to hospital discharge rate of approximately 20%. It is critical to perform CPR as promptly as possible in all patients suspected of suffering from CA that do not have advanced directives stating a preference to eschew resuscitation efforts. It can be difficult to determine if a patient is truly in CA. Generally speaking, international resuscitation guidelines put forth by the International Liaison Committee on Resuscitation (ILCOR) recommend that rescuers begin CPR in any victim who becomes suddenly unconscious with absent or markedly abnormal (gasping) respirations [1]. This definition was primarily designed for recognition of out-of-hospital CA; for in-hospital skilled providers, CA can be identified by the lack of a palpable pulse and/or measurable blood pressure. It is important to remember that CPR does not represent definitive therapy, in that correction of the underlying cause of CA must be addressed to reverse the condition (see Table 1).

Epidemiology

Each year over one million people in Europe and North America are afflicted with CA. Survival rates vary greatly depending on initial cardiac rhythm, location of arrest (in-hospital versus out-of-hospital, for example), and a number of other factors. Including all initial rhythms, survival rates have been documented below 10% for out-of-hospital CA, and approximately 20% for in-hospital CA. During out-of-hospital CA, bystander CPR has been shown to more than double the survival rate. Unfortunately, the prevalence of CPR performed by bystanders has been documented to be as low as 25% [2].

Cardiopulmonary Resuscitation. Table 1 Potential underlying causes of cardiac arrest

Category	Specific etiology
Cardiac	Myocardial ischemia
	Primary arrhythmia
	Secondary arrhythmia from myocardial scar
	Cardiac tamponade
Pulmonary	Pulmonary embolism
	Hypoxic respiratory failure
Metabolic	Hyperkalemia
	Acidemia
	Hypothermia
Toxins	Carbon monoxide
	Opioid toxicity
Hemorrhage	Cerebral hemorrhage
	Gastrointestinal bleeding
Other	Drowning
	Hanging
	Penetrating or blunt trauma

Common etiologies of cardiac arrest are represented here; this list is not intended to be comprehensive. Readers are encouraged to consult with reference [1] for further information

Application

CPR is designed to maintain coronary and cerebral perfusion as well as oxygenation during CA until definitive therapy, such as defibrillation or reversal of underlying CA pathophysiology, can be performed to achieve ROSC. The commonly used acronym ABC (airway, breathing, circulation) describes the main principles that are highlighted during CPR. It must be noted that the ensuing description most aptly applies to the general case of an out-of-hospital (non-intubated) patient. For patients already in intensive-care environments, the approach to CC remains the same although clearly airway and breathing approaches will vary. See Table 2 for summary of CPR delivery recommendations.

Airway and Breathing

Technique

The initial step in evaluating the unresponsive patient is to establish an open airway. This can be accomplished by the head-tilt, chin-lift maneuver. If obstructing material (food, emesis) is visible in the oropharynx, then the rescuer may perform a finger sweep in an attempt to clear the airway. Additionally, if airway obstruction with a foreign body is suspected, then chest thrusts, back blows, or abdominal thrusts should be performed in order to relieve the obstruction. Once an open airway has been established, and the patient is still not breathing, rescue breaths should be given. Current resuscitation guidelines recommend administering two rescue breaths for every 30 CCs for adult victims of SCA [1]. Once advanced medical support is available, endotracheal intubation should be performed. Endotracheal intubation is considered the definitive airway management in CA patients.

Cardiopulmonary Resuscitation. Table 2 Summary of CPR recommendations

Characteristic	Parameters
Chest compressions (CCs)	Rate of 100 per min
	Depth of 5+ cm
	Complete recoil between CCs
	Minimize interruptions in CCs
Ventilations	Rate of 8–10 per min
	Volume of 400–800 cc for most adults
	Employ F_iO_2 of 1.0
Other	Call for assistance from others
	Obtain defibrillator

Once this has been established, then a ventilation rate of 8–10 per minute is recommended, and should be performed in parallel to ongoing CCs [1].

Traditionally, performing rescue breaths was considered as important a procedure as providing CCs. The purpose of ventilation during cardiac arrest is to provide oxygenation, decrease hypercapnia, and reduce acidosis. However, recent evidence has demonstrated the detrimental effects of hyperventilation and prolonged pauses in CCs while providing ventilation. Hyperventilation increases intrathoracic pressure, thereby causing decreased venous return to the heart. This ultimately results in decreased coronary and cerebral perfusion. Additionally, interruptions in CCs to provide ventilation (in the non-intubated patient) result in decreased blood flow to the heart and brain.

Circulation
The most important action during CPR is to provide high quality CCs, which generate blood flow and perfusion to the brain and heart. Indeed, a more recently explored form of resuscitation care for the lay public, "hands-only" CPR, consists solely of CC delivery without rescue breaths, until the arrival of trained health-care personnel.

Technique
The patient should be supine on a hard surface. If the patient is on a soft surface (e.g., a mattress), a backboard should be placed under the patient. The proper technique for performing CCs in adults is to place the heel of one hand in the center of the chest over the lower portion of the sternum, with the other hand on top of the first. The rescuer should keep the elbows straight and push firmly and quickly. The sternum should be compressed to a depth of 4 to 5 cm at a rate of 100 compressions per minute. After reaching maximum depth, the chest wall should be allowed to fully recoil before the next CC is delivered [1].

Physiology of CC
Currently, two models of the mechanism of blood flow during CC exist. The "cardiac pump model" postulates that the heart is compressed between the sternum and vertebra generating an artificial systole with forward blood flow from the ventricles; then during the decompression phase, the heart passively fills [3]. The "thoracic pump model" argues that direct compression of the heart is not responsible for the forward blood flow. This model suggests that CCs cause an increase in intrathoracic pressure, which creates a pressure differential for blood to flow to the lower-pressure extrathoracic arteries. During

decompression, the intrathoracic pressure falls, resulting in passive refilling of the heart [3]. It is likely that this latter model more accurately represents the action of CPR.

CPR Quality
CA outcomes are dependent on the quality of CPR. The key components of CPR quality are CC rate, CC depth, chest-wall recoil, ventilation rate, and CC pauses. Higher CC rates have been associated with higher rates of ROSC. Increased depth of CC has been associated with greater defibrillation success for ventricular tachycardia/ventricular fibrillation. In addition, decreased interruptions in CC have been linked to improved survival. Incomplete chest-wall recoil increases intrathoracic pressure, thereby decreasing the preload of the heart and decreasing coronary and cerebral blood flow.

Adjunct CPR Techniques and Devices
Despite evidence demonstrating that high-quality CPR positively impacts outcomes from SCA, studies have documented that overall CPR performance is poor, both during out-of-hospital and in-hospital CA. As a result, there have been a variety of adjunctive techniques and devices developed with this in mind.

Active Compression-Decompression CPR (ACD-CPR)
In this method of resuscitation, CPR is performed with a suction cup compression device that is attached to the middle of the sternum. The purpose of this suction cup is to convert the passive decompression phase of CC into an active decompression phase. This in turn produces a greater negative intrathoracic pressure between compressions, which enhances venous return to the heart, subsequently increasing blood flow from the heart. Evidence supporting ACD-CPR has been conflicting. While some animal and human investigations have demonstrated that ACD-CPR is capable of producing higher perfusion pressures compared to standard CPR, most have shown no overall survival benefit [3].

Mechanical CPR Devices
It has been well documented in the literature that CCs are not performed to a quality consistent with guideline recommendations, partly due to rescuer fatigue. This has led to the introduction of mechanical devices that are able to deliver CCs at a consistent rate and depth. Furthermore, these devices are able to liberate rescuers from the function of CC delivery so that they can perform other important resuscitation tasks.

Two types of these tools are the mechanical piston device and the load-distributing band (LDB) device. The mechanical piston device compresses the sternum via a plunger mounted on a backboard. This mechanical adjunct has been shown to improve perfusion parameters like mean arterial pressure and end-tidal CO_2 in both in and out-of-hospital settings [4].

The LDB uses a load-distributing compression band that is placed circumferentially around the chest and attached to a small backboard. It compresses the entire anterior chest wall resulting in increased intrathoracic pressure at a specified rate. Use of this device has shown to improve mean aortic pressure as well as coronary perfusion pressure. In 2006, two studies were published comparing an LDB device with standard CPR that yielded conflicting results. One study showed an improvement in survival to discharge with the LDB compared to standard CPR. The other study showed no improvement in survival and actually reported a significant decrease in patients with good neurological outcome. One common criticism of all mechanical CPR devices is that using these devices may lead to a clinically significant delay in the initiation of CPR. Currently, evidence supporting the use of mechanical CPR devices in lieu of standard CPR remains inconclusive but suggestive of benefit.

Impedance Threshold Device (ITD)
The ITD is a valve that attaches between the endotracheal tube and resuscitation ventilation bag or mechanical ventilator. It limits the flow of air into the thoracic cavity during the decompression phase of CC. In doing so, intrathoracic pressure is reduced allowing for improved venous return to the heart. Studies have suggested that the use of an ITD improves early outcome in patients with out-of-hospital SCA. As of yet, no study has shown an improvement in the victim's long-term outcome [4].

Monitoring and Feedback Devices
In an effort to improve the quality of CPR, defibrillators have been developed with CPR-sensing capabilities and the ability to provide automated feedback. In this fashion, CPR parameters such as CC rate, depth and ventilation performance can be "coached" via an automated system. Such devices still require provider action to modify errors in CPR delivery. Recent investigations in both the in-hospital and out-of-hospital setting have suggested that the use of CPR-sensing defibrillators can improve both CPR delivery and initial survival rates, although these devices have not been tested in randomized controlled

trials at this time. CPR-sensing and recording defibrillators may also serve an important educational role, allowing for detailed debriefing after CA events where rescuers can be shown their individual CPR performance characteristics.

Cardiocerebral Resuscitation (CCR)
Recent evidence has shown that interruptions in CCs during CPR results in poor hemodynamic consequence and are associated with poor outcomes. These observations have led investigators to study an alternative strategy to resuscitation, known as cardiocerebral resuscitation or CCR. This resuscitation approach involves providing a greater number of uninterrupted CCs to optimize cardiac and cerebral perfusion. One such protocol was instituted by investigators in Arizona with promising results. This protocol entailed initially providing 200 uninterrupted CCs before defibrillating a shockable cardiac rhythm, followed by 200 uninterrupted CC post-defibrillation. Further minimization of interruptions in CCs was accomplished by delaying endotracheal intubation and positive pressure ventilation by initially providing passive oxygen insufflation via an oral pharyngeal airway and non-rebreather face mask. This study demonstrated a significant improvement in survival to discharge for OHCA from 1.8% before the CCR protocol to 5.4% after the protocol [5].

Continuous Chest Compression (CCC)-CPR or "Hands-Only" CPR
Recently, there has been a parallel trend in bystander CPR questioning the necessity of ventilations early during CA-resuscitation care. Some resuscitation experts have even called for the abandonment of ventilations altogether in bystander CPR for out-of-hospital CA victims. One of the major arguments for CCC-CPR is that bystanders are more likely to perform CCC-CPR than standard CPR. Also, in CA from sudden arrhythmia early ventilations are unnecessary as blood is likely to be adequately oxygenated. In fact, ventilations require pauses in CCs which decrease coronary and cerebral perfusion. CCC-CPR is also easier to learn and teach. Several animal investigations have demonstrated improved hemodynamics and outcome comparing CCC-CPR to standard CPR. Several non-randomized clinical studies have shown that there is no difference in outcome when comparing CPR with rescue breathing to CCC-CPR. In fact, one study showed that CCC-CPR led to better neurological outcome in certain population subsets. The American Heart Association issued an advisory statement in 2008 that encouraged CCC-CPR in witnessed CA, when untrained bystanders or bystanders are not willing to perform rescue breathing [2].

Complications

Complications from CPR can result from providing ventilation or CCs. Victims of CA may suffer tracheal or other airway injuries during intubation attempts. Inadvertent esophageal intubation may result in increased intragastric pressures leading to vomiting and aspiration. Rib fractures and sternal fractures are uncommon but recognized complications from receiving CCs. The incidence of these fracture complications is not known; recent work has suggested that they are both uncommon, and when they do occur, they are of small clinical consequence.

References

1. 2005 international consensus on cardiopulmonary resuscitation (CPR) and emergency cardiovascular care (ECC) science with treatment recommendations, part 2: adult basic life support. *Circulation* 112(suppl):III-5–III-16
2. Sayre MR, Berg RA, Cave DM, Page RL, Potts J, White RD (2008) Hands-only (compression-only) cardiopulmonary resuscitation: a call to action for bystander response to adults who experience out-of-hospital sudden cardiac arrest: a science advisory for the public from the American Heart Association Emergency Cardiovascular Care Committee. Circulation 117:2162–2167
3. Ornato JP, Peberdy MA (eds) (2005) Cardiopulmonary resuscitation. Humana Press Inc., Totowa, NJ
4. 2005 international consensus on cardiopulmonary resuscitation (CPR) and emergency cardiovascular care (ECC) science with treatment recommendations, part 6: CPR Techniques and Devices. *Circulation* 112(suppl):IV-47–IV-50
5. Bobrow BJ, Clark LL, Ewy GA et al (2008) Minimally interrupted cardiac resuscitation by emergency medical services for out-of-hospital cardiac arrest. J Am Med Assoc 299:1158–1165

Cardiopulmonary Resuscitation (CPR)

Is a constellation of maneuvers provided by bystander(s) to a person who has lost spontaneous respiration and circulation. Described by the American Heart Association (AHA), it is designed to temporarily sustain life while awaiting definitive medical care and typically involves rhythmic external compression of the chest and rescue breathing ("mouth-to-mouth").

CardioQ

▶ Esophageal Doppler

Cardiorenal Syndrome

Claudio Ronco[1], Mikko Haapio[2], Nagesh S. Anavekar[3], Andrew A. House[4], Rinaldo Bellomo[5]
[1]Department of Nephrology, St. Bortolo Hospital, Vicenza, Italy
[2]Division of Nephrology, HUCH Meilahti Hospital, Helsinki, Finland
[3]Department of Cardiology, The Northern Hospital, Melbourne, Australia
[4]Division of Nephrology, London Health Sciences Centre, London, Canada
[5]Department of Intensive Care, Austin Hospital, Melbourne, Australia

Synonyms

Heart–kidney interaction

Definition

Although generally defined as a condition characterized by the initiation and/or progression of renal insufficiency secondary to heart failure, the term cardiorenal syndrome is also often used to describe the negative effects of reduced renal function on the heart and circulation (more appropriately named ▶ reno-cardiac syndrome) (Fig. 1, Tables 1 and 2) [1–4].

A major problem with the previous terminology is that it does not allow clinicians or investigators to identify and fully characterize the relevant pathophysiological interactions. This is important because such interactions differ according to the type of combined heart/kidney disorder. For example, while a diseased heart has numerous negative effects on kidney function, renal insufficiency can also significantly impair cardiac function. Thus, a large number of direct and indirect effects of each organ dysfunction can initiate and perpetuate the combined disorder of the two organs through a complex combination of neurohumoral feedback mechanisms. For this reason a subdivision into different subtypes seems to provide a more concise and logically correct approach to this condition. We will use such a subdivision to discuss several issues of importance in relation to this syndrome.

Evaluation

Cardiorenal Syndrome Type I (Acute Cardiorenal Syndrome)

Type I CRS or Acute Cardiorenal Syndrome (ACRS) is characterized by a rapid worsening of cardiac function,

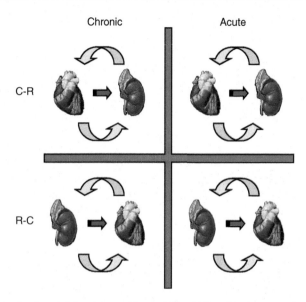

Cardiorenal Syndrome. Figure 1 The bidirectional nature of the cardiorenal syndrome and the acute or chronic temporal characteristics of the syndrome

Cardiorenal Syndrome. Table 1 Heart and kidney interactions

	• CKD secondary to HF
	• AKI secondary to contrast induced nephropathy (CIN)
	• AKI secondary to cardiopulmonary bypass (CPB)
	• AKI secondary to heart valve replacement
	• AKI secondary to HF
	• Cardiovascular mortality increased by end stage kidney disease (ESKD)
	• Cardiovascular risk increased by kidney dysfunction

	• Chronic HF progression due to kidney dysfunction
	  • Uremia-related HF
	  • Volume-related HF

	• HF due to acute kidney dysfunction
	  • Volume/uremia-induced HF
	  • Renal ischemia-induced HF
	  • Sepsis/cytokine induced HF

Cardiorenal Syndrome. Table 2 Proposed definition of cardiorenal syndromes

Cardiorenal syndrome (CRS) general definition	A pathophysiologic disorder of the heart and kidneys whereby acute or chronic dysfunction in one organ may induce acute or chronic dysfunction in the other organ.
CRS type I (acute cardiorenal syndrome)	Abrupt worsening of cardiac function (e.g., acute cardiogenic shock or decompensated congestive heart failure) leading to acute kidney injury.
CRS type II (chronic cardiorenal syndrome)	Chronic abnormalities in cardiac function (e.g., chronic congestive heart failure) causing progressive and permanent chronic kidney disease.
CRS type III (acute reno-cardiac syndrome)	Abrupt worsening of renal function (e.g., acute kidney ischemia or glomerulonephritis) causing acute cardiac disorder (e.g., heart failure, arrhythmia, ischemia).
CRS type IV (chronic reno-cardiac syndrome)	Chronic kidney disease (e.g., chronic glomerular disease) contributing to decreased cardiac function, cardiac hypertrophy, and/or increased risk of adverse cardiovascular events.
CRS type V (secondary cardiorenal syndrome)	Systemic condition (e.g., diabetes mellitus, sepsis) causing both cardiac and renal dysfunction.

which leads to acute kidney injury (Fig. 2). Acute heart failure may then be divided into four main subtypes (hypertensive pulmonary edema with preserved LV systolic function, acute decompensated chronic heart failure, cardiogenic shock, and predominant right ventricular failure). Type I cardiorenal syndrome (CRS) is common. More than one million patients in the USA alone are admitted to hospital every year with either de novo acute heart failure (AHF) or with an acute decompensation of chronic heart failure (ADCHF) [2]. Among patients with ADCHF or de novo acute heart failure (AHF), premorbid chronic renal dysfunction is common and predisposes to acute kidney injury (AKI). The mechanisms by which the onset to AHF or ADCHF leads to AKI are multiple and complex. They are broadly described in previous

Cardiorenal Syndrome: Type I

Cardiorenal Syndrome. **Figure 2** Diagram illustrating and summarizing the major pathophysiological interactions between heart and kidney in type I cardiorenal syndrome

publication [1]. The clinical importance of each of these mechanisms is likely to vary from patient to patient (e.g., acute cardiogenic shock vs. hypertensive pulmonary edema) and situation to situation (AHF secondary to perforation of a mitral valve leaflet from acute bacterial endocarditis vs. worsening right heart failure secondary to noncompliance with diuretic therapy). In AHF, AKI seems to be more severe in patients with impaired left ventricular ejection fraction (LVEF) compared to those with preserved LVEF and increasingly worse when LVEF is further impaired. AKI achieves an incidence >70% in patients with cardiogenic shock. Furthermore, impaired renal function is consistently found as an independent risk factor for 1-year mortality in AHF patients with ST-elevation myocardial infarction. A plausible reason for this independent effect might be that an acute decline in renal function does not simply act as a marker of illness severity but also carries an associated acceleration in cardiovascular pathobiology leading to a higher rate of cardiovascular (CV) events, both acutely and chronically, possibly through the activation of inflammatory pathways.

Cardiorenal Syndrome Type II (Chronic Cardiorenal Syndrome)

Type II CRS or chronic Cardiorenal syndrome (CCRS) is characterized by chronic abnormalities in cardiac function

(e.g., chronic congestive heart failure) causing progressive chronic kidney insufficiency (Fig. 3).

Worsening renal function (WRF) in the context of heart failure (HF) is associated with significantly increased adverse outcomes and prolonged hospitalizations. The prevalence of renal dysfunction in chronic heart failure (CHF) has been reported to be approximately 25%. Even limited decreases in estimated GFR of >9 ml/min appears to confer a significantly increased mortality risk. Some researchers have considered WRF a marker of severity of generalized vascular disease. Independent predictors of WRF include: old age, hypertension, diabetes mellitus, and acute coronary syndromes.

The mechanisms underlying WRF likely differ based on acute versus chronic HF. Chronic HF is characterized by a relatively stable long-term situation of probably reduced renal perfusion, often predisposed by both micro- and macrovascular disease in the context of the same vascular risk factors associated with cardiovascular disease. However, although a greater proportion of patients with low estimated GFR have a worse NYHA class, no evidence of association between LVEF and estimated GFR can be consistently demonstrated. Thus, patients with chronic heart failure and preserved LVEF appear to have similar estimated GFR than patients with impaired LVEF (<45%). Neurohormonal abnormalities are present with excessive production of vasoconstrictive

Cardiorenal Syndrome: Type II

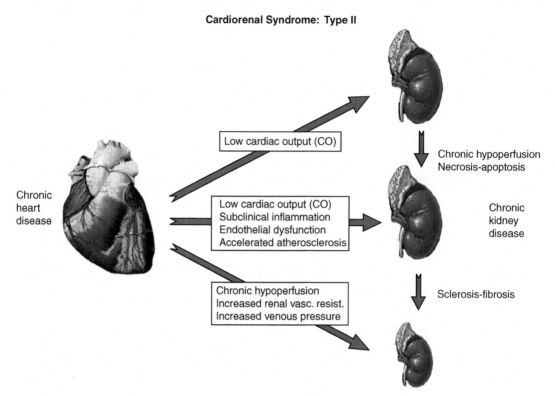

Low cardiac output (CO)

Chronic hypoperfusion
Necrosis-apoptosis

Chronic
heart
disease

Low cardiac output (CO)
Subclinical inflammation
Endothelial dysfunction
Accelerated atherosclerosis

Chronic
kidney
disease

Chronic hypoperfusion
Increased renal vasc. resist.
Increased venous pressure

Sclerosis-fibrosis

Cardiorenal Syndrome. Figure 3 Diagram illustrating and summarizing the major pathophysiological interactions between heart and kidney in type II cardiorenal syndrome

mediators (epinephrine, angiotensin, endothelin) and altered sensitivity and/or release of endogenous vasodilatory factors (natriuretic peptides, nitric oxide).

Cardiorenal Syndrome Type III (Acute Reno-Cardiac Syndrome)

Type III CRS or acute reno-cardiac syndrome (ARCS) is characterized by an abrupt and primary worsening of renal function (e.g., acute kidney injury, ischemia, or glomerulonephritis), which then causes or contributes to acute cardiac dysfunction (e.g., heart failure, arrhythmia, ischemia). The pathophysiological aspects are summarized in Fig. 4.

The development of AKI as a primary event leading to cardiac dysfunction (Type III CRS) is considered less common than type I CRS. This is partly because, unlike Type I CRS, it has not been systematically considered or studied. However, AKI is a condition with a growing incidence in hospital and ICU patients. Using the recent RIFLE consensus definitions and its Injury and Failure categories, AKI has been identified in close to 9% of hospital patients and, in a large ICU database, AKI was observed in more than 35% of critically ill patients. AKI

can affect the heart through several pathways whose hierarchy is not yet established. Fluid overload can contribute to the development of pulmonary edema. Hyperkalemia can contribute to arrhythmias and may cause cardiac arrest. Untreated uremia affects myocardial contractility through the accumulation of myocardial depressant factors and can cause pericarditis. Partially corrected or uncorrected acidemia produces pulmonary vasoconstriction, which, in some patients, can significantly contribute to right-sided heart failure. Acidemia appears to have a negative inotropic effect and may, together with electrolyte imbalances, contribute to an increased risk of arrhythmias. Finally, as discussed above, renal ischemia itself may precipitate activation of inflammation and apoptosis at cardiac level.

Cardiorenal Syndrome Type IV (Chronic Reno-Cardiac Syndrome)

Type IV CRS or chronic reno-cardiac syndrome (CRCS) is characterized by primary chronic kidney disease (CKD) (e.g., diabetes or chronic glomerular disease) contributing to decreased cardiac function, ventricular hypertrophy, diastolic dysfunction, and/or increased risk of adverse cardiovascular events (Fig. 5). The National Kidney

Cardiorenal Syndrome: Type III

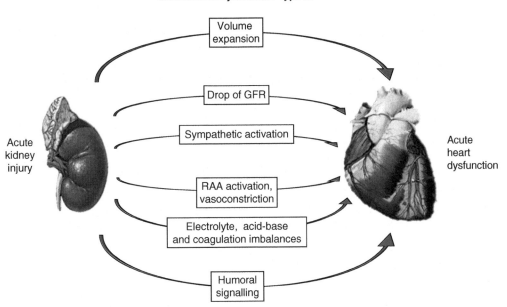

Cardiorenal Syndrome. Figure 4 Diagram illustrating and summarizing major pathophysiological interactions between heart and kidney in type III cardiorenal syndrome

Cardiorenal Syndrome: Type IV

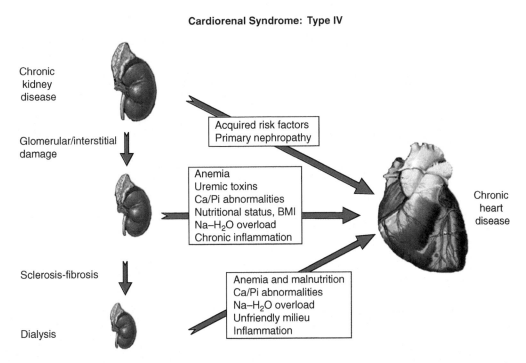

Cardiorenal Syndrome. Figure 5 Diagram illustrating and summarizing the major pathophysiological interactions between heart and kidney in type IV cardiorenal syndrome

Foundation divides CKD into five stages based on a combination of severity of kidney damage and GFR. Individuals with CKD, particularly those receiving renal replacement therapies are at extremely high cardiovascular risk. Greater than 50% of deaths in CKD stage V cohorts are attributed to CV disease, namely, coronary artery disease (CAD) and its associated complications. The 2-year mortality rate following myocardial infarction (MI) in patients with CKD stage V is high and estimated to be 50%. In comparison, the 10-year mortality rate post MI for the general population is 25%. Type IV cardiorenal syndrome is becoming a major public health problem. A large population of individuals entering the transition phase towards end stage kidney disease (ESKD) is emerging. National Kidney Foundation guidelines define these individuals as having CKD. CKD, which also encompasses ESKD, is defined as persistent kidney damage (confirmed by renal biopsy or markers of kidney damage) and/or glomerular filtration rate (GFR) $<$60 ml/min/1.73 m^2 over 3 months. This translates into a serum creatinine level of $\geq$1.3 mg/dl, which would ordinarily be dismissed as not being representative of significant renal dysfunction. Using these criteria, current estimates of CKD account for at least 11 million individuals and rising. The association between increased CV risk and renal dysfunction originally stemmed from data arising from ESKD or stage V CKD cohorts. The leading cause of death ($>$40%) in such patients is cardiovascular event-related. This observation is supported by Australian and New Zealand Dialysis and Transplant Registry (ANZDATA), United States Renal Data System (USRDS), and the Wave 2 Dialysis Morbidity and Mortality Study. Based on these findings, it is now well established that CKD is a significant risk factor for cardiovascular disease, such that individuals with evidence of CKD have from 10- to 20-fold increased risk for cardiac death compared to age- and sex-matched controls without CKD. As discussed, part of this problem may be related to the fact that such individuals are also less likely to receive risk modifying interventions compared to their non-CKD counterparts. Less severe forms of CKD also appear to be associated with significant cardiovascular risk. Evidence for increasing CV morbidity and mortality tracking with mild to moderate renal dysfunction, has mainly stemmed from community-based studies [5]. All these studies documented an inverse relationship between renal function and adverse cardiovascular outcomes. In particular, the association between reduced renal function and CV risk appears to consistently occur at estimated GFR levels below 60 ml/min/1.73 m^2, the principal GFR criterion used to define CKD. Among high CV risk cohorts, baseline creatinine clearance is a significant and independent predictor of short-term outcomes (180 days follow-up), namely, death and myocardial infarction. Similar findings were also noted among patients presenting with ST-elevation myocardial infarction, an effect independent of the Thrombolysis in Myocardial Infarction (TIMI) risk score. Other large-scale studies that have examined the relationship between renal function and cardiovascular outcomes among high CV risk cohorts with left ventricular dysfunction have included the Studies of Left Ventricular Dysfunction (SOLVD), Trandolapril Cardiac Evaluation (TRACE), Survival and Ventricular Enlargement (SAVE), and Valsartan in Acute Myocardial Infarction (VALIANT) trials. These studies excluded individuals with baseline serum creatinine of $\geq$2.5 mg/dl. In all these studies, reduced renal function was associated with significantly higher mortality and adverse CV event rates.

Renal insufficiency is highly prevalent among patients with heart failure and is an independent prognostic factor in both diastolic and systolic ventricular dysfunction. It is an established negative prognostic indicator in patients with severe heart failure.

Cardiorenal Syndrome Type V (Secondary Cardiorenal Syndrome)

Type V CRS or secondary cardiorenal syndrome (SCRS) is characterized by the presence of combined cardiac and renal dysfunction due to systemic disorders (Fig. 6). There is limited systematic information on type V CRS, where both kidneys and heart are affected by other systemic processes. Although there is an appreciation that, as more organs fail, mortality increases in critical illness, there is limited insight into how combined renal and cardiovascular failure may differently affect such an outcome compared to, for example, combined pulmonary and renal failure. Nonetheless, it is clear that several acute and chronic diseases can affect both organs simultaneously and that the disease induced in one can affect the other and vice versa. Several chronic conditions such as diabetes and hypertension are discussed as part of type II and type IV CRS.

In the acute setting, severe sepsis represents the most common and serious condition, which can affect both organs. It can induce AKI while leading to profound myocardial depression. The mechanisms responsible for such changes are poorly understood but may involve the effect of tumor necrosis factor on both organs. The onset of myocardial functional depression and a state of inadequate cardiac output can further decrease renal function as discussed in type I CRS and the development of AKI can affect cardiac function as described in type III CRS. Renal

Cardiorenal Syndrome: Type V

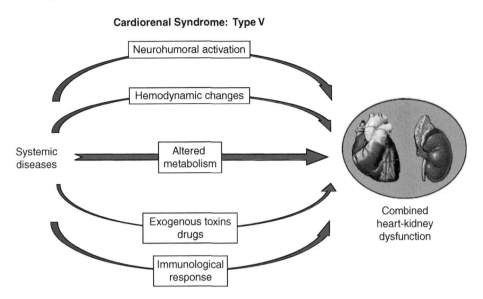

Cardiorenal Syndrome. **Figure 6** Diagram illustrating and summarizing the major pathophysiological interactions between heart and kidney in type V cardiorenal syndrome

ischemia may then induce further myocardial injury in a vicious cycle, which is injurious to both organs.

Treatment

Cardiorenal Syndrome Type I

The salient clinical issues of type I CRS relate to how the onset of AKI (de novo or in the setting of chronic renal impairment) induced by primary cardiac dysfunction impacts on diagnosis, therapy, and prognosis and how its presence can modify the general approach to the treatment of AHF or ADCHF. The first important clinical principle is that the onset of AKI in the setting of AHF or ADCHF implies inadequate renal perfusion until proven otherwise. This should prompt clinicians to consider the diagnosis of a low cardiac output state and/or marked increase in venous pressure leading to kidney congestion and take the necessary diagnostic steps to either confirm or exclude them (careful physical examination looking for ancillary signs and laboratory findings of a low cardiac output state such as absolute or relative hypotension, cold extremities, poor post compressive capillary refill, confusion, persistent oliguria, distended jugular veins, and elevated or rising lactate). The second important consequence of the development of type I CRS is that it may decrease diuretic responsiveness. In a congestive state (peripheral edema, increased body weight, pulmonary edema, elevated central venous pressure), decreased response to diuretics can lead to failure to

achieve the desired clinical goals. The physiological phenomena of *diuretic breaking* (diminished diuretic effectiveness secondary to post-diuretic sodium retention) and *post-diuretic sodium retention* may also play an enhanced part in this setting. In addition, concerns of aggravating AKI by the administration of diuretics at higher doses or in combination are common among clinicians. Such concerns can also act as an additional, iatrogenic mechanism equivalent in its effect to that of diuretic resistance (less sodium removal). Accordingly, diuretics may best be given in AHF patients with evidence of systemic fluid overload with the goal of achieving a gradual diuresis. Furosemide can be titrated according to renal function, systolic blood pressure, and history of chronic diuretic use. High doses are not recommended and a continuous diuretic infusion might be helpful. In parallel, measurement of cardiac output and venous pressure may also help ensure continued and targeted diuretic therapy. Accurate estimation of cardiac output can now be easily achieved by means of arterial pressure monitoring combined with pulse contour analysis or by Doppler ultrasound. Knowledge of cardiac output allows physicians to develop a physiologically safer and more logical approach to the simultaneous treatment of AHF or ADCHF and AKI. If diuretic-resistant fluid overload exists despite an optimized cardiac output, removal of isotonic fluid can be achieved by ultrafiltration (Fig. 7). This approach can be efficacious and clinically beneficial. The presence of AKI with or without concomitant hyperkalemia may also affect patient outcome by

Extracorporeal Ultrafiltration

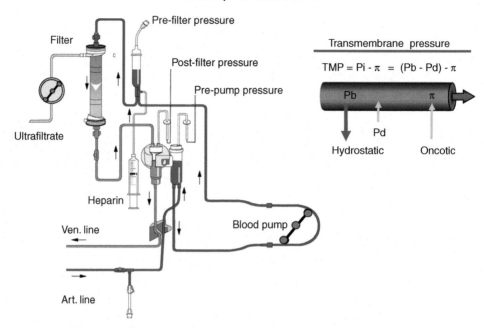

Pre-filter pressure

Filter

Post-filter pressure

Pre-pump pressure

Ultrafiltrate

Heparin

Ven. line

Blood pump

Art. line

Transmembrane pressure

$$TMP = Pi - \pi = (Pb - Pd) - \pi$$

Pb

π

Pd

Hydrostatic   Oncotic

Cardiorenal Syndrome. Figure 7 Diagram presenting the technical features of ultrafiltration as applicable to patients with acute heart failure and diuretic-resistant fluid overload

inhibiting the prescription of ACE inhibitors and aldosterone inhibitors (drugs that have been shown in large randomized controlled trials to increase survival in the setting of heart failure and myocardial infarction). This is unfortunate because, provided there is close monitoring of renal function and potassium levels, the potential benefits of these interventions likely outweigh their risks even in these patients.

The acute administration of beta-blockers in the setting of type I CRS is generally not advised. Such therapy should wait until the patient has stabilized physiologically and concerns about a low cardiac output syndrome have been resolved. In some patients, stroke volume cannot be increased and relative or absolute tachycardia sustains the adequacy of cardiac output. Blockade of such compensatory tachycardia and sympathetic system-dependent inotropic compensation can precipitate cardiogenic shock and can be lethal. Particular concern applies to beta-blockers excreted by the kidney such as atenolol or sotalol, especially if combined with calcium antagonists. These considerations should not inhibit the slow, careful, and titrated introduction of appropriate treatment with beta-blockers later on, once patients are hemodynamically stable.

This aspect of treatment is particularly relevant in patients with the cardiorenal syndrome where evidence suggests that undertreatment after myocardial infarction

is common. Attention should be paid to preserving renal function, perhaps as much attention as is paid to preserving myocardial muscle. Worsening renal function during admission for ST-elevation myocardial infarction is a powerful and independent predictor of in-hospital and 1-year mortality. In a study involving 1,826 patients who received percutaneous coronary intervention, even a transient rise in serum creatinine (>25% compared to baseline) was associated with increased hospital stay and mortality. Similar findings have also been shown among coronary artery bypass graft cohorts. In this context, creatinine rise is not simply a marker of illness severity but it rather represents a causative factor for cardiovascular injury acceleration through the activation of hormonal, immunological, and inflammatory pathways. Given that the presence of type I CRS defines a population with high mortality, a prompt, careful, systematic, multidisciplinary approach involving invasive cardiologists, nephrologists, critical care physicians, and cardiac surgeons is both logical and desirable.

Cardiorenal Syndrome Type II

Pharmacotherapies used in the management of HF have been touted as contributing to WRF. Diuresis-associated hypovolemia, early introduction of renin-angiotensin-aldosterone system blockade, and drug-induced hypotension, have all been suggested as contributing factors. However, their role remains highly speculative. More recently, there has been increasing interest in the pathogenetic role of relative or absolute erythropoietin (EPO) deficiency contributing to a more pronounced anemia in these patients than might be expected for renal failure alone. EPO receptor activation in the heart may be protective from apoptosis, fibrosis, and inflammation. In keeping with such experimental data, preliminary clinical studies show that EPO administration in patients with chronic heart failure, chronic renal insufficiency, and anemia leads to improved cardiac function, reduction in left ventricular size, and lowering of B-type natriuretic peptide. Patients with type 2 CRS are more likely to receive loop diuretics and vasodilators and also to receive higher doses of such drugs compared to those with stable renal function. Treatment with these drugs may participate in the development of renal injury. However, such therapies may simply identify patients with severe hemodynamic compromise and thus a predisposition to renal dysfunction rather than being responsible for worsening renal dysfunction. Regardless of the cause, reductions in renal function in the context of heart failure are associated with increased risk for adverse outcomes.

Cardiorenal Syndrome Type III

The development of AKI, especially in the setting of chronic renal failure can affect the use of medications that normally would maintain clinical stability in patients with chronic heart failure. For example, an increase in serum creatinine from 1.5 mg/dl (130 µmol/l) to 2 mg/dl (177 µmol/l), with diuretic therapy and ACE inhibitors, may provoke some clinicians to decrease or even stop diuretic prescription; they may also decrease or even temporarily stop ACE inhibitors. In some, maybe many cases, this may not help the patient. An acute decompensation of CHF may occur because of such changes in medications. When this happens the patient may be unnecessarily exposed to an increased risk of acute pulmonary edema or other serious complications of undertreatment.

Finally, if AKI is severe and renal replacement therapy is necessary, cardiovascular instability generated by rapid fluid and electrolyte shifts secondary to conventional dialysis can induce hypotension, arrhythmias, and myocardial ischemia. Continuous techniques of renal replacement, which minimize such cardiovascular instability, appear physiologically safer and more logical in this setting.

Cardiorenal Syndrome Type IV

The logical practical implications of the plethora of data linking CKD with CV disease is that more attention needs to be paid to reducing risk factors and optimizing medications in these patients, and that undertreatment due to concerns about pharmacodynamics in this setting may have lethal consequences at individual level and huge potential adverse consequences at public health level. Nonetheless, it is also equally important to acknowledge that clinicians looking after these patients are often faced with competing therapeutic choices and that, with the exception of MERIT-HF, large randomized controlled trials that have shaped the treatment of chronic heart failure in the last two decades have consistently excluded patients with significant renal disease. Such lack of CKD population-specific treatment effect data makes therapeutic choices particularly challenging. In particular, in patients with advanced CKD, the initiation or increased dosage of ACE inhibitors can precipitate clinically significant worsening of renal function or marked hyperkalemia. The latter may be dangerously exacerbated by the use of aldosterone antagonists. Such patients, if aggressively treated, become exposed to a significant risk of developing dialysis dependence or life-threatening hyperkalemic arrhythmias. If too cautiously treated they may develop equally life-threatening cardiovascular complications. In these patients, the judicious use of all options while taking into account patient preferences, social circumstances, other comorbidities, and applying a multidisciplinary approach to care seems to be the best approach.

Cardiorenal Syndrome Type V

Treatment is directed at the prompt identification, eradication, and management of the source of infection while supporting organ function with invasively guided fluid resuscitation and inotropic and vasopressor drug support. In this setting, all the principles discussed for type I and type III CRS apply. In these septic patients, preliminary data using more intensive renal replacement technology suggest that blood purification may have a role in improving myocardial performance while providing optimal small solute clearance. Despite the emergence of consensus definitions and many studies, no therapies have yet emerged to prevent or attenuate AKI in critically ill patients. On the other hand, clear evidence of the injurious effects of pentastarch fluid resuscitation in septic AKI has recently emerged. Such therapy should, therefore, be avoided in septic patients.

After-care

The proportion of individuals with CKD receiving appropriate risk factor modification and/or interventional strategies is lower than in the general population, a concept termed "therapeutic nihilism." Many databases and registries have repeatedly shown that these therapeutic choices seem to parallel worsening renal function. In patients with CKD stage V, who are known to be at extreme risk, less than 50% are on the combination of aspirin, β blocker, ACE inhibitors, and statins. In a cohort involving over 140,000 patients, 1,025 with documented ESKD were less likely to receive aspirin, β blockade, or ACE inhibition post MI. Yet those ESKD patients who did receive the aspirin, β blocker, and ACE inhibitor combination had similar risk reductions in 30-day mortality when compared to non-ESKD patients who had received conventional therapy. This failure to treat is not just limited to ESKD patients. Patients with less severe forms of CKD are also less likely to receive risk modifying medications following myocardial infarction compared to their normal renal function counterparts.

Potential reasons for this therapeutic failure include concerns about worsening existing renal function, and/or therapy-related toxic effects due to low clearance rates. Bleeding concerns with the use of platelet inhibitors and anticoagulants are especially important with reduced renal function and appear to contribute to the decreased likelihood of patients with severe CKD receiving aspirin and/or clopidrogrel despite the fact that such bleeding is typically minor and the benefits sustained in these patients. However, several studies have shown that when appropriately titrated and monitored, cardiovascular medications used in the general population can be safely administered to those with renal impairment and with similar benefits.

Newer approaches to the treatment of cardiac failure such as cardiac resynchronization therapy (CRT) have not yet been studied in terms of their renal functional effects, although preserved renal function after CRT may predict a more favorable outcome. Vasopressin V2-receptor blockers have been reported to decrease body weight and edema in patients with chronic heart failure, but their effects in patients with the cardiorenal syndrome have not been systematically studied and a recent large randomized controlled trial showed no evidence of a survival benefit with these agents.

Prognosis

Considering that the presence of any type CRS defines a population with high mortality, a multidisciplinary approach involving cardiologists, nephrologists, critical care physicians, and cardiac surgeons is recommended. In both chronic and acute situations, an appreciation of the interaction between heart and kidney during dysfunction of each or both organs has practical clinical implications. The depth of knowledge and complexity of care necessary to offer best therapy to these patients demands a multidisciplinary approach. In addition, by using an agreed definition of each type of cardiorenal syndrome, physicians can describe treatments and interventions, which are focused and pathophysiologically logical. They can also conduct and compare epidemiological studies in different countries and more easily identify aspects of each syndrome, which carry a priority for improvement and further research. Randomized controlled trials can then be designed to target interventions aimed at decreasing morbidity and mortality in these increasingly common conditions. Increasing awareness, ability to identify and define, and physiological understanding will help improve the outcome of these complex patients.

Acknowledgments

We thank Drs. Alexandre Mebazaa, Alan Cass, and Martin Gallagher for their useful advice in the development of this manuscript.

References

1. Ronco C (2008) Cardiorenal and reno-cardiac syndromes: clinical disorders in search of a systematic definition. Int J Artif Organs 31:1–2
2. Liang KV, Williams AW, Greene EL, Redfield MM (2008) Acute decompensated heart failure and the cardio-renal syndrome. Crit Care Med 36(Suppl):S75–S88
3. Ronco C, House AA, Haapio M (2008) Cardio-renal syndrome: refining the definition of a complex symbiosis gone wrong. Intensive Care Med 34(5):957–962
4. Ronco C, Haapio M, House AA, Anavekar N, Bellomo R (2008) Cardiorenal syndrome. J Am Coll Cardiol 52(19):1527–1539
5. Go AS, Chertow GM, Fan D et al (2004) Chronic kidney disease and the risks of death, cardiovascular events, and hospitalization. N Engl J Med 351:1296–1305

Carukia barnesi

▶ Jellyfish Envenomation

Carybdeid Jellyfish

▶ Jellyfish Envenomation

Catabolism

▶ Metabolic Disorders, Other

Catheter and Line/Tubing/Administration Sets Change

▶ Change

Catheter Port Allocation

▶ Port Designation

Catheter-Associated Bloodstream Infection

▶ Catheter-Related Bloodstream Infection

Catheter-Associated Urinary Tract Infection

ANDREW M. MORRIS
Mount Sinai Hospital and University Health Network, University of Toronto, Toronto, ON, Canada

Synonyms

Foley-catheter infection; Pyelonephritis; Urinary catheter sepsis; Urosepsis

Definition

Catheter-associated urinary tract infection (CAUTI) is generally defined in the medical literature as bacteriuria or funguria (of at least 10^3 cfu/mL) in association with a urinary catheter. The definition has remained problematic, as it ignores a central tenet in the management of infections: differentiating colonization from infection. In patients without urinary catheters, pyuria is strongly associated with urinary tract infection, but some have contested using such a criterion for CAUTI. A preferred definition would be the symptoms and signs of urinary tract infection accompanied by pyuria and greater than 10^3 cfu/mL microorganisms in association with an urinary catheter.

Epidemiology

The epidemiology of CAUTI is poorly understood, owing to the problematic definition used in the literature, but CAUTI appears to affect approximately 9% of all patients in the ICU, with a rate of 12.0 per 1,000 catheter-days. Risk factors include female sex, duration of catheterization, and duration of ICU stay. Outside of the ICU, failure to use a closed collection system has also been associated with CAUTI. Antibiotic use appears protective, but this may be because of confounding. Gram-negative bacilli and enterococci are the most common isolates, although candida species are frequently isolated in patients with prolonged ICU stay (usually in patients receiving prolonged and/or repeated courses of broad-spectrum antimicrobials).

Prevention

Avoiding urinary catheters and removing them when unnecessary are the best means of preventing CAUTI. Condom catheters for men have been shown to reduce CAUTI with acceptable tolerability; in-and-out catheterization is also well tolerated. Nevertheless, neither of these methods has been widely adopted in ICUs to prevent CAUTI. Use of antimicrobial catheters may reduce bacteriuria, but have not been shown to prevent CAUTI or other meaningful outcomes [1].

Treatment

There are few randomized trials evaluating management of CAUTI. A small trial of catheter-associated bacteriuria in women (not in the ICU) demonstrated that asymptomatic bacteriuria frequently progressed to symptomatic CAUTI that single-dose antibiotic treatment was equivalent to a 10-day course of therapy. Another recent trial compared short-course (3 days) antibiotics and catheter change with standard care (i.e., no change, no antibiotics) for patients with asymptomatic catheter-associated bacteriuria and found no difference in meaningful outcomes, including development of pyelonephritis. Similarly, treatment of candiduria with fluconazole in immunocompetent patients temporarily eradicated the candidura, but failed to offer any long-term benefit.

Evaluation

As mentioned above, evaluation is problematic. At present, routine urinalyses cannot be advocated. In catheterized patients, pyuria (greater than 10 white blood cells/mL) is specific but insensitive for the presence of bacteriuria. Because it is unclear if treatment of asymptomatic patients with bacteriuria is warranted, routine cultures are also not warranted. Investigation of fever of unknown origin should include, however, urinalysis and urine culture.

Prognosis

When adjusted for confounding factors, CAUTI does not appear to be associated with increased mortality in critically ill patients.

Economics

The attributable patient cost of CAUTI in the USA ranges from $862 to $1, 007, costing US hospitals $0.39 to $0.45 billion annually [2].

References

1. Lo E, Nicolle L, Classen D, Arias KM, Podgorny K, Anderson DJ et al (2008 Oct) Strategies to prevent catheter-associated urinary tract infections in acute care hospitals. Infect Control Hosp Epidemiol 29(Suppl 1):S41–50
2. Scott II RD (2009) The direct medical costs of healthcare-associated infections in U.S. hospitals and the benefits of prevention. In: Department of Health and Human Services, Centers for Disease Control and Prevention, 2009

Catheter-Related Bloodstream Infection

ANDREW M. MORRIS
Mount Sinai Hospital and University Health Network, University of Toronto, Toronto, ON, Canada

Synonyms

Catheter-associated bloodstream infection; Catheter-related infection; Central line infection; Central venous catheter infection; Line sepsis; Vascular catheter infection

Definition

Catheter-related bloodstream infection (CRBI) is bacteraemia or fungaemia that originate from an intravascular catheter. For the purpose of this chapter, CRBI will be limited to catheters that are usually inserted and removed in intensive care units and will not include tunneled catheters or other long-term catheters. CRBI most commonly originates from the skin-insertion site, with microorganisms traveling along the course of the vascular catheter into the bloodstream. Less often, organisms contaminate the catheter hub and travel intraluminally. Some organisms, primarily coagulase-negative staphylococci, elaborate a protective multilayered biofilm matrix preventing immune system effectors and antimicrobials from reaching the organisms. Although localized infection may occur at the site of insertion (often termed "exit site infection"), such infections are easy to diagnose, do not generally cause systemic illness, and are beyond the scope of discussion here. The study of CRBI has been complicated by the lack of a definition that is both sensitive and specific. Fever and other clinical criteria are sensitive but nonspecific, whereas repeatedly positive blood cultures drawn from the periphery and vascular catheter with identical organisms in the presence of clinical signs of infection without other primary foci are specific but insensitive. For this reason, catheter-*associated* bloodstream infection is often measured, which identifies bacteraemia in the presence of a vascular catheter, but may not be caused by the catheter.

Epidemiology

The epidemiology of CRBI is not well known, although the reported rate of CRBI in the province of Ontario, Canada (population 13 million), is 1.4 per 1,000 catheter-days. The National Nosocomial Infection Surveillance system of the CDC estimates the rate to be 1.8–5.2 per 1,000 catheter-days. There are an estimated 92,011 cases of CRBI annually in the USA [1]. Coagulase-negative staphylococci are the most common organisms responsible for CRBI, followed by (in decreasing order) *Staphylococcus aureus*, *Candida* species, and gram-negative bacilli.

Prevention

The Centers for Disease Control recommend five procedures that are likely to have the greatest impact on reducing CRBI with the lowest barriers to implementation: hand washing, using full-barrier precautions during the insertion of central venous catheters, cleaning the skin with chlorhexidine, avoiding the femoral site if possible, and removing unnecessary catheters. Using these very same procedures resulted in dramatic reductions across 103 ICUs in Michigan, reducing median rates of CRBI from 2.7 per 1,000 catheter-days to zero [2].

Hand Washing

The evidence supporting hand-washing in preventing CRBI is not strong but is it low-cost, theoretically appealing, and, when bundled with full-barrier precautions, is proven to be effective in reducing CRBI.

Full-Barrier Precautions During Insertion

Sterile gloves, long-sleeved sterile gown, mask, cap, and large sterile sheet drape during insertion have been shown to dramatically reduce CRBI.

Cutaneous Antisepsis

Although povidone–iodine remains the most widely used skin antiseptic in hospitals, there is strong evidence that chlorhexidine is superior to povidone–iodine. Tincture of iodine also appears to be superior to povidone–iodine, but is less well studied.

Site of Insertion
The femoral site is unequivocally inferior to the subclavian site vis à vis infection risk. However, preference between internal jugular and subclavian veins is less clear, with colonization being greater for internal jugular venous catheters compared with subclavian venous catheters, but there is no evidence showing lower rates of CRBI with the subclavian site.

Routine Changing of Lines
Although most teaching (including that of the CDC) states that routine changing of lines is not advised, it is based on little evidence. One study from 1981 looked at routine changing of haemodialysis catheters in 90 patients, and showed no difference between routine changes over a wire at 7 days rather than at a new site. Another study from 1990 compared no routine changes with routine changes over a wire and routine changes at a new puncture site, and showed no difference.

Treatment
Treatment of CRBI begins with removal of the vascular catheter when infection is suspected. In many cases, this proves curative, with fever abating and leukocytosis resolving without the need for antimicrobials. Clearly, however, this requires further study. Optimal treatment of documented CRBI requires (a) removal of the catheter (where feasible) and (b) antimicrobial therapy [3].

Catheter Removal
Catheter removal for CRBI is always preferred; however, situations do occur when this is not feasible or desired. In such situations, an option includes *antibiotic lock therapy*, whereby an aliquot of antibiotic is left in the catheter hub and tubing continuously. This is only likely to be beneficial for patients whose CRBI is due to an intraluminal infection, and is not supported by high-quality trials. Some experts recommend retaining the vascular catheter for CRBI due to coagulase-negative staphylococci, but the recurrence risk is high.

Antimicrobial Therapy

Empiric Therapy
Treatment, as with all nosocomial infections, should be based on the likely organism coupled with severity of illness. For many such infections, patients will be haemodynamically stable, and treatment of the most likely pathogens (usually staphylococci) will suffice. In centers with a high prevalence of methicillin-resistant *S. aureus*, vancomycin is likely an appropriate empiric therapy. However, it may be reasonable to consider a methicillin-like penicillin (e.g., cloxacillin) or first-generation cephalosporin in stable patients.

Pathogen-Specific Therapy
Coagulase-negative staphylococci: Removal of the catheter is often sufficient, but many authorities recommend 5–7 days therapy, unless there is no other medical hardware *in situ*, the vascular catheter has been removed, the patient is haemodynamically stable, and repeated blood cultures are negative. No approach has been formally evaluated with randomized controlled trials. *S. lugdunensis* is a coagulase-negative staphylococcus that should be treated as *S. aureus*.

S. aureus: Treatment should be based on susceptibilities. The most effective therapy for methicillin-susceptible *S. aureus* is a β-lactam. However, in cases of severe allergy or resistance, vancomycin is a preferred agent. Recently, concerns have been raised regarding the effectiveness and safety of vancomycin, especially with the emergence of strains that are either resistant to or have reduced susceptibility to vancomycin. However, a recent open-label non-inferiority trial comparing linezolid with vancomycin for CRBI showed a trend favoring vancomycin in intention-to-treat analysis. Optimal duration of therapy for *S. aureus* CRBI is unclear. Although teaching for many years has maintained the axiom "treat for 2 weeks if a removal focus of infection, and it has been removed," recent studies have questioned this wisdom with the recognition that (a) infective endocarditis may complicate up to 13% of catheter-associated bacteraemia and (b) infective endocarditis and other complications may be seen in approximately 6% of cases of *S. aureus* CRBI treated with 2 weeks therapy (compared with 4 weeks). I prefer 4 weeks of therapy unless a trans-esophageal echocardiogram is performed and is negative (making endocarditis highly unlikely), which is largely consistent with recent recommendations [3].

Enterococci: The optimal treatment of enterococci is ampicillin; if unable to use ampicillin because of resistance or allergy, then vancomycin is the preferred agent. Linezolid or daptomycin are options when ampicillin or vancomycin cannot be used, although there is limited experience with these agents. The duration of treatment for enterococcal bacteraemia is unclear, although 7–14 days is usually sufficient. The risk of subsequent infective endocarditis is quite low, estimated at around 1%.

Gram-negative bacilli: The optimal treatment of Gram-negative bacilli (GNB) is dependent on local susceptibilities. Empiric choices prior to speciation should cover the majority of possibilities, and may include combination therapy (especially if the patient is neutropaenic, severely ill, or known to be colonized with multidrug-resistant organisms). However, there is weak evidence supporting combination therapy once susceptibility is known, including therapy for non-lactose-fermenting agents such as *Pseudomonas aeruginosa*. The optimal duration of therapy is also unknown, although 7–14 days is usually sufficient.

Candida species: Candidaemia is a frequent cause of CRBI in patients who have been receiving prolonged broad-spectrum antibacterial agents, as well as patients receiving total parenteral nutrition, or who have received solid organ or stem cell transplantation. Empiric therapy should be based on local data, but may include amphotericin B, fluconazole, or an echinocandin. These appear to be equally efficacious, although azole resistance has been rising in centers with high azole use. For this reason, many have recommended echinocandin therapy to be first-line treatment. Candidaemia is generally treated with 2 weeks of effective therapy, with the first negative blood culture being considered day 1.

Evaluation

Diagnosis is primarily a microbiological one following clinical suspicion. Where possible, cultures should come from both peripheral blood and the catheter lumen prior to antimicrobial therapy. Catheter tip cultures (using a 5 cm segment and using either a roll-plate method or sonification) are also advised; however, positive tip cultures reflect colonization, not CRBI.

CRBI can be confidently diagnosed when:

(a) Peripheral and catheter-drawn blood cultures are positive with the same isolate, and the catheter-drawn culture grew more quickly (i.e., with a differential time-to-positivity, or DTP, of at least 2 h)

(b) A catheter-drawn blood culture and a catheter-tip culture are positive with the same isolate

(c) Both peripheral and catheter-drawn blood cultures are positive, but the colony-count is threefold higher in the culture growing from the venous catheter.

Prognosis

CRBI has an attributable mortality of approximately 12–25%.

Economics

The attributable patient cost of catheter-associated bloodstream infection (not CRBI) in the USA ranges from $7,288 to $29,156, costing US hospitals $0.67–2.68 billion annually [1].

References

1. Scott II RD (2009) The direct medical costs of healthcare-associated infections in U.S. hospitals and the benefits of prevention. In: Department of Health and Human Services, Centers for Disease Control and Prevention, 2009
2. Pronovost P, Needham D, Berenholtz S, Sinopoli D, Chu H, Cosgrove S et al (2006 Dec 28) An intervention to decrease catheter-related bloodstream infections in the ICU. N Engl J Med 355(26):2725–2732
3. Mermel LA, Allon M, Bouza E, Craven DE, Flynn P, O'Grady NP et al (2009 Jul 1) Clinical practice guidelines for the diagnosis and management of intravascular catheter-related infection: 2009 Update by the Infectious Diseases Society of America. Clin Infect Dis 49(1):1–45

Catheter-Related Infection

▶ Catheter-Related Bloodstream Infection

Cauda Equina Syndrome

Scott E. Bell[1], Kathryn M. Beauchamp[2]
[1]Department of Neurosurgery, School of Medicine, University of Colorado Health Sciences Center, Denver, CO, USA
[2]Department of Neurosurgery, Denver Health Medical Center, University of Colorado School of Medicine, Denver, CO, USA

Definition

Cauda equina syndrome is a clinical condition arising from acute, subacute, or chronic dysfunction of nerve roots that comprise the structure known as the "cauda equina." It is considered a spine emergency during the acute stages of neurologic deterioration from compressive lesions. Anatomically, the spinal cord ends at approximately the first to second lumbar vertebrae in normal adults. The dural sac continues as a fluid-filled structure to approximately the second sacral vertebrae. Within this sac, between levels L2 to S2, are contained the nerve roots that have emanated from the spinal cord. These nerve roots are collectively referred to as the "cauda equina," as they exist prior to exiting the dural sac and spinal canal in pairs, through the neural foramina at each level.

A variety of lesions can serve as the etiology for cauda equina syndrome, including herniated intervertebral disks, intradural, or extradural tumors, traumatic fractures, hematoma, abscess, and non-compressive causes such as neuropathy or ankylosing spondylitis [1].

The incidence of cauda equina syndrome (CES) as a true clinicopathologic entity is extremely rare; however, it is frequently over-diagnosed on initial evaluation of patients with signs and symptoms from spine or nerve dysfunction in the lower extremities. This is likely due to two reasons, (1) the highly generalized symptoms that are found at presentation, and (2) the consequences of permanent functional impairment with under-diagnosis. Because of its rarity, epidemiologic data is sparse, but historic reports place its prevalence at 1–3: 100,000 population. In patients with low back pain, the occurrence of CES is 4: 10,000. The most common etiology is herniated nucleus pulposis (HNP), still presenting as only 1–2% of those HNP cases requiring surgery [1].

Clinical Presentation

The classic symptomatology of cauda equina syndrome includes perineal anesthesia, urinary or fecal retention and/or incontinence, low back and/or radicular pain, numbness in the lower extremities, weak rectal tone, or weakness in the lower extremities and associated reflexes [1]. While none of these symptoms are specific for CES individually, their presence in various combinations, frequently accompanied by certain anatomic hallmarks, can be highly sensitive for cauda equina dysfunction. The symptom with the greatest sensitivity for CES is urinary retention, found to be 90% sensitive in multiple series [2]. Without this, only 1:1,000 cases of suspected CES will be true [1]. Likewise, "saddle anesthesia," which is absent sensation in the perineal region, has a sensitivity of 75% for CES. In the astute patient who presents early, rapid progression of clinical findings can also be an indication of CES. However, patients frequently fail to recognize the severity of their symptoms until they are more advanced.

Shi et al. created a classification system to categorize severity of CES [2]. Patients fell into preclinical, early, middle, or late categorization, with no determination as to temporal progression of symptoms. The preclinical patient was considered to show only electrophysiologic changes in pudendal reflexes with imaging signs of compression; the early CES patient was considered to show slight saddle sensory disturbances and sciatica; the middle CES patients were considered to show severe saddle sensory disturbances, some bowel or bladder dysfunction, and lower extremity weakness; and late CES patients were considered to show no saddle sensation, severe bladder

and bowel dysfunction, severe sexual dysfunction. It is an important concept to attempt a categorization of severity for CES patients, as a differential response to surgery based on severity is well recognized throughout the literature [2]. The severity at presentation is as important for prognostication as timing of intervention for many patients [3]. This confounder is difficult to account for, and sometimes the distinction is minimized or ignored in level II and III analyses focusing on timing of intervention.

Recognizing the difference between cauda equina dysfunction and spinal cord/conus medullaris dysfunction is important for diagnosis of CES. Asymmetry of sensory or motor disturbances can be an important finding that distinguishes cauda equina dysfunction from higher lesions affecting the spinal cord or conus medullaris [2]. For example, saddle anesthesia or lower extremity weakness can be a unilateral process in CES, but is frequently bilateral and symmetric in conus medullaris lesions. Another distinguishing finding of the saddle anesthesia resulting from CES is its lack of sensory dissociation, which is often found in spinal cord pathology. Pain can sometimes distinguish a cauda equina lesion from a spinal cord lesion. While not as sensitive for CES, if present, pain is frequently the symptom that will bring the patient to seek medical attention early. Pain from CES will be in the lumbar region or radicular in nature, radiating to lower extremities or the perineal region. The pain from CES may be quite prominent, while spinal cord lesions will usually cause only local pain (above L1 level), or little to no pain in the case of conus medullaris lesions [1]. Because of the anatomic relationship between the autonomic nervous system (ANS) and the cauda equina, symptoms relating to the function of the ANS are frequently encountered late in the course of CES, while they may be encountered relatively early with spinal cord or conus lesions due to their second degree neurons' intramedullary location [2]. These ANS symptoms include bladder dysfunction, impotence, and sphincter disturbances.

Cauda equina syndrome is considered a clinical diagnosis that is usually, but not always, accompanied by imaging findings suggesting compressive pathology. When the above-mentioned symptomatology is linked with compressive anatomic findings, urgent to emergent surgical remediation may be warranted. However, caution in diagnosis should be applied as there are many instances when imaging studies convey a compressive structural abnormality in the lumbar spine, while the patient experiences little or no symptoms. Without symptomatology, there is no indication for a diagnosis of CES. This is an important distinction when deciding if emergent surgery is needed for treatment.

Evaluation

Treatment is dictated by accompanying findings on full clinical evaluation. A thorough history and physical examination are paramount as a guide for proper decision-making in diagnosis and treatment. An appropriate physical exam will consist of the standardized format for a full neurologic examination, which consists of (1) mental status and executive function evaluation, (2) cranial nerve evaluation, (3) sensory exam, (4) motor exam, (5) central and peripheral reflex exam, (6) coordination evaluation, (7) gait evaluation.

For the purpose of this discussion, focus will be placed on examination of peripheral function, i.e., sensory, motor, reflex, coordination, and gait examination, of the lower extremities. The elements of a thorough sensory exam include the dermatomal distribution of light touch, sharp-dull distinction, pain, and temperature, as well as non-segmental proprioception. Figure 1 shows the generally accepted distribution of segmental nerve root

innervation for cutaneous sensation, described by Foerster in 1933 [4]. With specific nerve root impingement, one expects to find derangement in those dermatomes served by its respective lumbosacral segmental level. Frequently in CES, there is impingement of multiple roots producing a regional derangement of sensory function, which usually includes the lower sacral dermatomes, producing the saddle anesthesia in addition to more distal sensory changes.

Motor function, likewise, has been well characterized with respect to the segmental innervation of the lower extremity musculature, termed myotomes. It follows a similar pattern as the innervation of cutaneous sensation. It is most valuable to describe any motor derangements by the function that is impaired or absent. The myotome served by L1 nerve roots causes hip flexion, L2-3 causes knee extension, L4 causes hip adduction, L5 causes foot inversion, eversion and dorsiflexion. The sacral nerves cause plantar flexion and knee flexion (S1-2). Strength is described as a gradient from 0 (no movement

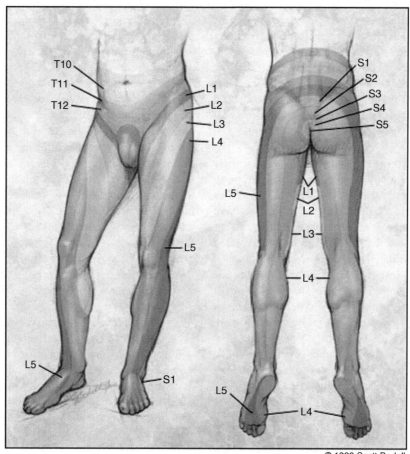

© 1999 Scott Bodell

Cauda Equina Syndrome. Figure 1 Lower extremity dermatomes (Adapted from aafp.org)

or muscle contraction) to 5 (full strength). Cauda equina syndrome may cause weakness along any point of the strength spectrum with lower motor neuron findings, which include atrophy from trophic influences, decreased tone, and reflex arc interruption. The degree of weakness found along the strength spectrum tells the story of the severity of the cauda equina lesion. Coordination and gait disturbances will occur in so much as the patient has weakness of the lower extremities. The degree of weakness will dictate the success or failure of the measures of multiple muscle coordination, such as gait. Lower sacral nerve impairment will cause weakness of rectal tone; this is always an important test to perform when evaluating for spinal cord or spinal nerve injury.

Deep tendon reflexes are another element of the physical examination that will inform the examiner of the extent of injury. Reflexes become diminished in CES due to interruption of the reflex arc at the level of the lower motor neuron. It is usually the knee jerk and ankle jerk that are affected. The neurons serve an arc that communicates tendon stretch directly with alpha motor neurons and inhibitory interneurons. Interruption of this arc will cause a diminution or absence of the reflex for its respective myotome. This may be noticeable at multiple levels, reflecting the common multi-neuronal dysfunction within the cauda equina during the process of CES.

In the acute stages of the disease, imaging is an important modality to help guide the clinician toward surgical treatment if appropriate pathology is seen. If trauma is suspected, initial imaging should include lumbar roentgenography or computed tomography (CT) scans, if available. The sensitivity and specificity of lumbar CT scan have been shown to be 97% and 95%, respectively, compared with 86% and 58%, respectively, for lumbar roentgenograms (9). A CT scan has better resolution for fractures, and their relationships with the spinal canal and neural foramina can be viewed in sagittal, coronal, and axial planes. While harder to interpret due to its 2-dimensional, monoplanar depiction, roentgenograms are frequently used as a screening tool to guide decision algorithms for subsequent diagnostic maneuvers, especially in those patients in whom CT scan is contraindicated or impractical due to habitus, availability, etc.

For better representation of soft tissue structures including neural elements, a magnetic resonance image (MRI) of the lumbar spine may be important in determining the nature and anatomic location of compressive pathology if surgical considerations are being made. Figure 2 shows a representation of lumbar stenosis causing neural compression. No contrast is needed in any imaging modality on evaluation of an acute process, as the diagnostic value is not improved. However, if tumor or infection is suspected, either iodinated contrast for CT scans, or gadolinium for MRI scans, is an important addition for diagnostic considerations.

Another important factor in consideration of the traumatic etiology of CES is to recognize an unstable lumbar spine. With or without ongoing neural compression, treatment considerations will shift to a multimodal approach. If ongoing compressive pathology exists, surgical plans may include decompression as well as stabilization procedures. On the other hand, if CES is the result of a transient compression of neural elements that underwent closed reduction, then conservative treatment of the CES symptoms, in conjunction with a surgical stabilization procedure, may be appropriate.

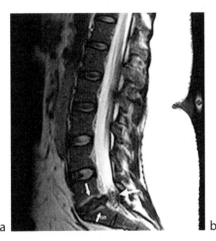 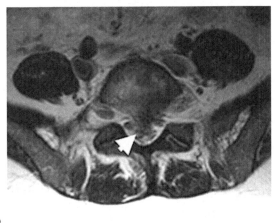

Cauda Equina Syndrome. Figure 2 (**a** and **b**) MRI in sagittal (**a**) and axial (**b**) planes showing a herniated disc causing cauda equine syndrome (Adapted from Chou et al. *Orthopedics* 2008[13])

Treatment

The timing of when to address a surgical lesion in CES is the most controversial aspect of this syndrome. It is commonly accepted as a surgical emergency. Once recognized, if appropriate compressive signs are found on imaging, surgery should be performed within 48 h from the onset of CES symptoms [3]. Some surgeons argue that evidence supports a time frame within 24 h from symptom onset. Shaprio [3] analyzed 39 cases of documented CES and described that cases operated within 24 h showed better functional recovery of lower extremity strength than cases operated within 48 h, which showed better functional recovery than cases operated after delay (two groups with mean delays of 3.4 and 9 days). Likewise, for pudendal symptoms, 24 h proved better than 48 h for urinary, bowel, and sexual function recovery, and delayed surgery showed no return of function. However, the differences in post-surgical recovery between surgery timed at <24 h versus <48 h were determined from $n=2$. In patients presenting after 48 h from onset of symptoms, especially if symptoms include urinary retention or incontinence, and saddle sensory changes, functional recovery is poor with or without surgery.

The Shapiro study only grouped patients by timing of surgery, and did not address analysis by severity of symptoms at presentation. In a meta-analysis, Ahn et al. found that there was multivariate significance in improvement among patients presenting with CES – that based on surgery <48 h and that based on a lower degree of symptom severity at presentation. Those with worse symptom severity, including chronic low back pain, urinary symptoms, saddle anesthesia, and rectal dysfunction on presentation, tended to show worse prognosis for improvement postoperatively, even in patients operated within 48 h. Those patients with less severe symptoms, for instance, lower extremity weakness and saddle hypoesthesia, had greater chance of improvement with surgery <48 h from onset compared with surgery >48 h from onset.

Other factors found to contribute to results from surgery include acuity of symptoms. Those with more acute symptom onset tend to have a better chance at improvement after surgery compared with those showing a more insidious, chronic onset. Time to recovery of symptoms has been shown to vary in small level II and III analyses [5]. Usually full extent of recovery is found within 2 years, but gradual recovery of some function has been observed for up to 5 years.

The type of surgery performed also varies widely in the literature. It is a consensus that minimally invasive lesionectomy, such as semi-hemilaminotomy and microdiscectomy, is inadequate to decompress the nerve roots from the offending lesion once CES has developed. Among the procedures that produce adequate decompression exist high variability in approach. Hemilaminectomy, bilateral foraminal decompression with wide laminectomy, as well as one study that purported the need for transdural disk exploration in up to 18% of cases, have all been shown to be effective in treating CES. Rationale for the latter procedure is that it reduces the traction on injured nerves during surgery, thus improving the chances for recovery of function.

When ankylosing spondylitis (AS) is found to be the etiology of CES, the pathophysiologic mechanism is not entirely clear. It is thought to be a progressive ectasia of the dura. The effectiveness of either conservative or surgical treatments has been called into question. There are some studies that advocate medical management is superior, while others that endorse surgical treatment is the most effective. This problem is classically treated conservatively, but in the last decade, a variety of surgical approaches have been employed including lumbar decompression and durotomy, and even cerebrospinal fluid shunting, to treat the ectatic lumbar dura.

When there is clear lack of compressive pathology in CES, conservative management focuses on the presumed inflammatory process causing the nerve injury, similar to CES in ankylosing spondylitis. The treatment of choice for acute peripheral nerve injuries is high-dose intravenous steroids, and pain control [1]. Physical therapy early in the process of recovery, whether after conservative or operative treatment, is an important aspect of convalescence.

Summary

Cauda equina syndrome is a dangerous, but uncommon entity in spine pathology. If acute onset and progression are confirmed clinically, surgery should be performed without delay, within 24–48 h. While compression is the most common etiology, some inflammatory processes are found to be the cause, warranting conservative management. The prognosis for functional recovery is poor when the onset is insidious, or the presentation severe. But, under the correct circumstances, with acute onset and early symptoms, prognosis for recovery is good when treated emergently. Surgical approaches vary, but it is generally accepted that wide decompression and removal of the offending lesion are the best treatment for compressive causes of CES. Further studies, accounting for both severity on presentation and timing of treatment, are warranted to establish the best management for maximizing the patients' ability to overcome this illness.

References

1. Greenberg MS (ed) (2010) Handbook of neurosurgery, 7th edn. Thieme Medical Publications, New York
2. Shi J, Jia L, Yuan W, Shi GD, Ma B, Wang B, JianFeng W (2010) Clinical classification of cauda equina syndrome for proper treatment: A retrospective analysis of 39 patients. Acta Orthopedica 81 (3):391–395
3. Shapiro S (2000) Medical realities of cauda equina syndrome secondary to lumbar disc herniation. Spine 25(3):348–352
4. Foerster O (1933) The dermatomes in man. Brain 56:1
5. Ahn UM, Ahn NU, Buchowski JM, Garrett ES, Seiber AN, Kostuik JP (2000) Cauda equina syndrome secondary to lumbar disc herniation: a meta-analysis of surgical outcomes. Spine 25(12):1515–1522

C-Collar

This is the cervical collar that is used for stabilizing the neck in the neutral position.

CCS

▶ Central Spinal Cord Syndrome

Celiotomy

▶ Laparotomy

Central Cord Injury Syndrome

▶ Central Spinal Cord Syndrome

Central Cord Syndrome

▶ Spinal Cord Injury Syndromes

Central Line Infection

▶ Catheter-Related Bloodstream Infection

Central Spinal Cord Syndrome

SARAH E. PINSKI[1], ARIANNE BOYLAN[2], JENS-PETER WITT[3], TODD F. VANDERHEIDEN[4], PHILIP F. STAHEL[5]
[1]Department of Orthopaedic Surgery, Denver, CO, USA
[2]Department of Neurosurgery, University of Colorado Denver, School of Medicine, Denver, CO, USA
[3]Neuro Spine Program, Department of Neurosurgery, University of Colorado Hospital, Colorado, CO, USA
[4]Department of Orthopaedic Surgery, Center for Complex Fractures and Limb Restoration, Denver Health Medical Center, University of Colorado School of Medicine, Denver, CO, USA
[5]Department of Orthopaedic Surgery and Department of Neurosurgery, Denver Health Medical Center, University of Colorado School of Medicine, Denver, CO, USA

Synonyms

"Burning Hands" syndrome; CCS; Central cord injury syndrome

Definition

A syndrome associated with ischemia, hemorrhage, or necrosis involving the central portions of the spinal cord due to traumatic injury sustained in the cervical or upper thoracic regions of the spine, characterized by weakness in the arms with relative sparing of the leg strength associated with variable sensory loss.

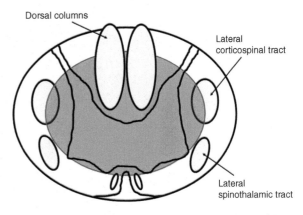

Central Spinal Cord Syndrome. Figure 1 Illustration of the affected area (*red color*) of central cord syndrome (CCS) in a schematic axial drawing through the spinal cord. Note that the sacral structures are more peripheral in the dorsal columns and the lateral corticospinal tract. These structures are therefore preferentially spared in patients with CCS

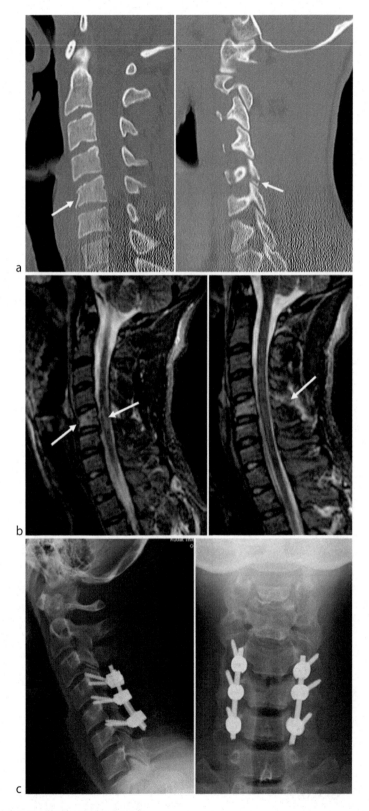

Central Spinal Cord Syndrome. Figure 2 (Continued)

Anatomy

The main descending motor pathway is the lateral corticospinal tract. The tract is arranged with the cervical (cranial) nerve paths more centrally located and the sacral (caudal) nerve paths more peripherally located. The major ascending sensory pathway is the dorsal column (fasciculus gracilis, fasciculus cuneatus). Similar to the lateral corticospinal tract, the dorsal columns are arranged such that cervical structures are centrally located and sacral structures are more peripherally located (Fig. 1) [1]. Central cord syndrome (CCS) originates from a vascular compromise in the distribution area of the anterior spinal artery, which supplies the central portions of the spinal cord.

Epidemiology

CCS is the most common type of incomplete spinal cord injury (SCI), comprising 15–25% of all cases [1]. The "classic" mechanism leading to CCS is represented in elderly patients with underlying degenerative spinal changes, who sustain a hyperextension injury the cervical spine (C-spine), with or without evidence of acute spinal injury on plain X-rays. Susceptibility to CCS is represented by a preexisting narrowing of the cervical spinal canal due to spondylosis, osteophyte formation, stenosis and ossification of the posterior longitudinal ligament. The cervical cord may be injured by direct compression from buckling of the ligamentum flavum into a narrowed, stenotic spinal canal [1]. CCS may also occur in younger individuals sustaining high-energy trauma that results in unstable spinal fractures, ligamentous instability, or fracture-dislocations [2]. Young patients with congenital cervical stenosis are also at particular risk for sustaining a CCS after trauma. This entity presents with a wide spectrum of neurological symptoms, ranging from preserved sensation with burning dysesthesia and allodynia in the hands, to motor weakness to the upper extremities, to a complete quadriparesis with sacral sparing. As a general rule, the upper extremities are more affected than the lower extremities. The classic paradigm is represented by a patient who walks around but can't move the arms. Return of motor function follows a characteristic pattern, with the lower extremities recovering first, bladder function next, and the proximal upper extremities and hands last [3].

Application

Diagnosis is made based upon clinical and radiographic examination. Initial radiographic evaluation consists of anteroposterior, lateral, and open-mouth odontoid X-rays. CT scans may also be obtained to gain a better understanding of fractures and dislocations. The MRI represents the "gold standard" for evaluating injuries to the soft tissues (discs, ligaments), to quantify the extent of spinal stenosis and cord compression, and to asses for presence of epidural hematoma, spinal edema, and spinal contusions. At the time of initial evaluation, sacral sparing may be the only neurologic function present to differentiate incomplete from complete SCI. Most cases of CCS are successfully managed non-operatively, with the likelihood of considerable neurologic recovery [1, 3]. Medical management of CCS consists of admission to intensive care for close monitoring of neurologic status and hemodynamics. Maintenance of blood pressure (mean arterial pressure of >85 mmHg) by volume resuscitation supplemented by vasopressors, if needed, has been shown to improve neurologic outcome by presumably maximizing spinal cord perfusion and limiting secondary injury [1, 3]. Intravenous methylprednisolone is the most commonly used pharmacologic treatment for SCI. The established standard dosing is 30 mg/kg bolus followed by 5.4 mg/kg/h for 24 h if the infusion is started within 3 h of injury, and for 48 h if the infusion is started between 3 and 8 h from the time of injury. This is a controversial treatment that recent literature reviews showed no evidence for the use of corticosteroids as a neuroprotective agent. Additionally, corticosteroids may adversely affect patient outcome due to the side effects related to immunosuppression, including pulmonary infections [4].

Any patient with suspected CCS should be immobilized in a hard cervical orthosis to prevent further motion and potential injury. The cervical collar is typically used for an additional 6 weeks or until neck pain has resolved and neurologic improvement is noted. Once the patient is medically stable, early mobilization and

---

Central Spinal Cord Syndrome. Figure 2 Case example of a 21-year old man who sustained a fall while snowboarding. He presented with bilateral upper extremity motor weakness and subjectively "burning" hands. Imaging with plain X-rays, CT scan, and MRI reveals an unstable C5/C6 flexion/distraction injury with a three-column fracture at C5, and a spinal cord contusion on MRI (*arrows* in panels A and B). This patient was managed surgically by posterior fusion due to the inherent instability of the injury (panel C). No decompression was performed. The patient recovered well within 3 months of surgery, with a full resolution of dysethestesia and allodynia and improved upper extremity function. The patient was able to return to work without restrictions as a pizza delivery courier

rehabilitation with physical and occupational therapy is essential. Gait and hand function training are the main goals. Surgery is indicated in those cases with spinal instability [2, 5], as outlined in the case example shown in Fig. 2. Surgical intervention for CCS without spinal instability is controversial. However, in the setting of persistent cord compression, failure of motor recovery, or neurologic decline, surgical intervention may be warranted. These symptoms may be due to a herniated disk, an epidural hematoma, or bony fragments in the spinal canal. In such cases, the early spinal decompression may prevent the progression of neurologic impairment and may lead to improved recovery and function [1, 5].

References

1. Nowak DD, Lee JK, Gelb DE, Poelstra KA, Ludwig SC (2009) Central Cord Syndrome. J Am Acad Orthop Surg 17:756–765
2. Stahel PF, Flierl MA, Matava B (2011) Traumatic spondylolisthesis. In: Vincent JL, Hall J (eds) Encyclopedia of intensive care medicine. Springer, Heidelberg
3. Aarabi B, Alexander M, Mirvis SE, Shanmuganathan K, Chesler D, Maulucci C, Iguchi M, Aresco C, Blacklock T (2011) Predictors of outcome in acute traumatic central cord syndrome due to spinal stenosis. J Neurosurg Spine 14:122–130
4. Hurlbert RJ, Hamilton MG (2008) Methylprednisolone for acute spinal cord injury: 5-year practice reversal. Can J Neurol Sci 35:41–45
5. Fehlings MG, Rabin D, Sears W, Cadotte DW, Aarabi B (2010) Current practice in the timing of surgical intervention in spinal cord injury. Spine 35(suppl 21):S166–S173

Central Venous Access Catheter (CVC)

▶ Vascular Access for RRT

Central Venous Catheter Infection

▶ Catheter-Related Bloodstream Infection

Central Venous Pressure

GORAZD VOGA
Medical ICU, General Hospital Celje, Celje, Slovenia

Synonyms
Right atrial pressure

Definition
Central venous pressure (CVP) is the pressure of blood in the thoracic vena cava at the point where the superior vena cava meets the inferior vena cava prior to entry into the right atrium (RA) of the heart.

Characteristics
Normal values of CVP in spontaneously breathing patients are 5–10 cm of water and can be up to 5 cm of water higher in patients mechanically ventilated with positive inspiratory pressure. The normal CVP waveform consists of three upward deflections ("a", "c", "v" waves) and two downward deflections ("x" and "y" descents) (Fig. 1). The "a" wave reflects right atrial contraction and occurs just after the "P" wave on the ECG. It is followed by "c" wave, which is the result of tricuspid valve bulging into RA during isovolumic ventricular contraction. The third positive deflection is "v" wave and represents the filling of the RA during late ventricular systole. The "x" descent occurs during right ventricular ejection when the tricuspid valve is pulled away from the atrium and the "y" descent represents rapid blood flow from the RA into right ventricle (RV) during early diastole.

Clinical Estimation of CVP
Physical assessment of jugular venous distension and pressure in patients sitting up at 45–60% angle allows CVP estimation. The level of internal jugular veins filling can be determined and pulsations can be clearly seen. The vertical distance from the filling level and sternal angle is measured. Five centimeters (the approximate distance from sternal angle and RA) is added to the measured distance in order to get the CVP estimation. The external jugular veins are observed in the 20° angle of the upper part of the body against horizontal line. In patients with normal CVP values, the veins are filled to one third of the distance

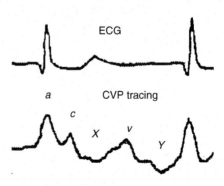

Central Venous Pressure. Figure 1 Simultaneous ECG and CVP tracing between clavicle and mandible. Unfortunately, considerable disagreement and inaccuracy exists in the clinical assessment of CVP in critically ill patients and therefore measurement is mandatory.

Invasive CVP Measurement

The CVP is usually measured by placing a catheter in one of the veins and then threading it to the superior vena cava. Internal jugular and subclavian veins are most suitable for cannulation, since the catheter is easily advanced to the proper position. Antecubital veins can be also used, if catheter is long enough to reach the superior vena cava. The CVP is measured using a manometer filled with intravenous fluid and attached to the central venous catheter. Zero point, approximately the mid-axillary line in the fourth intercostal space in supine position, must be determined. Catheter should not be blocked or kinked to allow free flow of the fluid. The manometer is filled with fluid and then three-way stopcock is open to the catheter. Fluid level steadily drops to the level of the CVP, which is measured in centimeters of water. Fluid level should fluctuate slightly with breathing and may slightly pulsate. On the other hand, prominent pulsations are due to significant tricuspid regurgitation or improper position of the catheter tip in the right ventricle, which usually requires reposition of the catheter. In the ICU setting, catheters are usually connected with transducers, and the CVP waveform is continuously displayed in the monitor. Transducers also have to be zeroing and put at the standard reference level for hemodynamic measurements, which is usually 5 cm below the sternal angle. The electronically measured values are displayed in the monitor and expressed in mmHg (10 cm H_2O is 7.5 mm Hg).

Besides proper levelling and zeroing, changes of intrathoracic pressure should be considered in the interpretation of CVP values. Increased intrathoracic pressure is commonly seen in patients with high levels of PEEP or forced expiration, on the other hand, highly negative intrathoracic pressure frequently results from vigorous inspiratory efforts. Both conditions can markedly change CVP. Therefore, CVP waveform should be always observed in order to assess proper CVP values. Factors that affect CVP measurement are summarized in the table (Table 1).

Nonivasive CVP Estimation

Nonivasive estimation of CVP is possible by transthoracic echocardiography. In the subcostal view, inferior vena cava (IVC) is visualized and the diameter during inspiration and expiration is measured. The IVC collapsibility index (IVCCI) is defined as difference between maximum

Central Venous Pressure. Table 1 Factors affecting CVP measurement

| Zeroing and reference level of the transducer |
| Central venous blood volume |
| Venous return |
| Blood volume |
| Vascular tone |
| Right ventricular compliance |
| Intrathoracic pressure |
| Tricuspid regurgitation and stenosis |

Central Venous Pressure. Table 2 Estimation of CVP from measurement and respiratory variation of IVC diameter

IVC diameter (cm)	Inspiratory decrease	Estimated CVP (mm Hg)
<1.5	Collapse	<5
1.5–2.5	>50%	5–10
>2.5	<50%	10–15
>2.5	No	>20

and minimum IVC diameter, expressed in percent. The estimation of CVP by IVC measurement is showed in the table and is reliable in the spontaneously breathing patients (Table 2). The IVC size of 2 cm and the IVC collapsibility of 40% discriminates CVP below or above 10 mm Hg with 73% sensitivity and 85% specificity [1].

Clinical Value of CVP

CVP is a static pressure variable, which is frequently used for preload assessment. CVP measurement is the essential part of hemodynamic assessment in critically ill patients and is frequently performed during surgery to estimate cardiac preload and circulating blood volume, also. CVP reflects the amount of blood returning to the heart and the ability of the heart to pump the blood into the arterial system. Measurement of the "c" wave value at the end expiration reflects end-diastolic pressure in the right ventricle and can be used as an index RV preload. At the same time CVP represents the back pressure for venous return and gives an estimate of the intravascular volume status. It predominantly depends on circulating blood volume, venous tone, and right ventricular function. In patients with normal cardiac function increased venous return is associated with increased cardiac output, without major change in CVP. On the other hand, CVP is elevated in patients with poor right ventricular contractility and/or obstruction to the inflow in right atrium (tamponade, tension pneumothorax) or to the outflow in pulmonary circulation (pulmonary embolism).

Unfortunately, CVP poorly reflects left ventricular preload and is of little value for hemodynamic assessment in patients with heart failure and cardiogenic shock. Very poor relationship between CVP and blood volume and poor prediction of CVP changes for fluid responsiveness was found [2]. CVP values lower than 5 mm Hg have only 47% positive predictive value for fluid responsiveness in mechanically ventilated septic patients [3]. Nevertheless, CVP values in septic shock are significantly different in survivors and nonsurvivors 6–48 h after admission and CVP values 8–12 mm Hg are proposed as an early resuscitation goal of the initial hemodynamic stabilization in patients with septic shock [4].

CVP is only a part of hemodynamic assessment and must be interpreted together with other hemodynamic variables and clinical state of patient. It is clear that very high and low CVP values must be considered as abnormal, but they are not conclusive for any specific hemodynamic situation. Therefore, such findings require further diagnostic workup. Normal CVP values also can be associated with different hemodynamic disturbances in critically ill patients.

Examination of the CVP waveforms gives some additional information regarding tricuspid regurgitation, cardiac tamponade, cardiac restriction, decreased thoracic compliance, and arrhythmias. Patients with tricuspid regurgitation have prominent "v" waves, on the other hand restrictive RV filling is associated with large and deep "y" descent. In patients with cardiac tamponade "x" and "y" descent usually disappear. Large inspiratory rise in the CVP during mechanical ventilation suggests decreased thoracic wall compliance. In patients with atrial fibrillation "a" wave is absent, and in presence of atrioventricular dissociation high and tall (cannon) "a" wave can be seen due to atrial contraction against closed tricuspid valve [5].

References

1. Brennan JM, Blair JE, Goonewardena S, Ronan A, Shah D, Vasaiwala S, Kirkpatrick JN (2007) Spencer KT reappraisal of the use of inferior vena cava for estimating right atrial pressure. J Am Soc Echocardiogr 20:857–861
2. Marik PE, Baram M, Vahid B (2008) Does central venous pressure predict fluid responsiveness? A systematic review of the literature and the tale of seven mares. Chest 134:172–178
3. Osman D, Ridel C, Ray P, Monnet X, Anguel N, Richard C, Teboul JL (2007) Cardiac filling pressures are not appropriate to predict hemodynamic response to volume challenge. Crit Care Med 35:64–68
4. Dellinger RP, Levy MM, Carlet JM et al (2008) Surviving Sepsis Campaign: International guidelines for management of severe sepsis and septic shock. Crit Care Med 36:296–327
5. Magder S (2006) Central venous pressure monitoring. Curr Opin Crit Care 12:219–227

Central Venous, Arterial, and PA Catheters

José Rodolfo Rocco
Clementino Fraga Filho University Hospital, Federal University of Rio de Janeiro, Rio de Janeiro, Brazil

Introduction

Vascular cannulation is an essential tool for fluid and drug administration, accurate monitoring of hemodynamic parameters, and blood sampling in critically ill patients. Preparation, indications, contraindications, clinical utility, and techniques for vascular cannulation are reviewed in this chapter. The sites of catheterization and complications of arterial, central venous, and pulmonary artery catheterization are also presented.

Central Venous Catheterization

The main indications for central venous catheterization (CVC) are: (1) monitoring of hemodynamic and tecidual perfusion, and (2) therapeutic (Table 1).

Central Venous, Arterial, and PA Catheters. Table 1 Indications for central venous catheterization

1 – Monitoring of hemodynamic and tecidual perfusion
1.1 – Measurement of central venous pressure
1.2 – Placement of pulmonary (Swan-Ganz) catheter and Presep®
1.3 – Placement of jugular bulb catheter
2 – Therapeutic
2.1 – Fluid therapy in general
2.2 – Fluid therapy of irritant solutions (concentrated potassium chloride, parenteral nutrition, hypertonic saline) and vasopressor amines
2.3 – Hemodyalisis and plamapheresis
2.4 – Placement of transvenous pacemaker
2.5 – When peripherical venous access is impossible

Volemic resuscitation is not an indication for CVC. However, in a hypovolemic patient if the peripheral vein cannulation is difficult, it would be necessary to access a central vein.

During cardiac arrest, there is an urgency to access a vein (peripheral or central) for drug administration. In this case, femoral vein is the first option. Cannulation of femoral vein can be done without stopping the cardiac massage.

Sites of Catheterization

In general, the site of catheterization is selected based on doctor's experience. However, for some procedures, there are preferential sites (Table 2).

If the patient had a pleural catheter, the venous cannulation must be done at the same side of the thoracic drain.

Preparation

Patient and operator preparation is a crucial component of the vascular cannulation procedure.

If possible, it is advisable to obtain informed consent from the patient or surrogate whenever an invasive procedure is to be performed.

Hand washing is mandatory (and often overlooked) before the insertion of vascular devices. Scrubbing with antimicrobial cleansing solutions does not reduce the

incidence of catheter-related sepsis, so a simple soap-and-water scrub is sufficient.

A CVC is a sterile procedure. If there is a contamination, the procedure must be interrupted and the contaminated material must be replaced. If a patient is cannulated in an emergency situation (e.g., during cardiac arrest), the venous catheter must be replaced as soon as possible.

The insertion site is prepped and povidone-iodine or alcoholic solution of chlorhexidine is most commonly used, although chlorexidine appears to be more efficient. After skin preparation, the insertion site should be draped with a sterile field. The sterile field must be big enough to cover the head and the body of the patient (maximum barrier). This procedure reduced the incidence of catheter-related sepsis six times compared to the use of sterile gloves and a small camp (Fig. 1).

To avoid patient discomfort, local anesthesia, analgesia, and/or sedation need to be performed. Most vascular cannulations are done percutaneously because of the facility to insert the catheter and reduced risk of infection. Cannulation over direct vision through a surgical cut down may be performed in very difficult situations.

Most of the central venous and arterial catheters are inserted passing a guidewire through the needle (the Seldinger technique) (Fig. 2).

In Fig. 3, steps of the right internal jugular vein cannulation are depicted.

Central Venous, Arterial, and PA Catheters. Table 2 Sites of catheterization in diverse clinical conditions

Indication	First choice	Second choice	Third choice
Venous access in general	SCV	IJV or EJV	FV
Placement of (Swan-Ganz) catheter	RIJV	LSCV	LIJV or RSCV
Coagulopathy	EJV	IJV	FV
Pulmonary disease or elevated PEEP	RIJV	LIJV	EJV
Total parenteral nutrition	SCV	IJV	–
Hemodyalisis/plasmapheresis	IJV	FV	SCV
Cardiac arrest	FV	SCV	IJV
Transvenous pacemaker	RIJV	SCV	–
Hypovolemic patient	SCV or FV	IJV	–
Urgent access to airway	FV	SCV	IJV
Monitoring of venous saturation	SCV	IJV	EJV
CVP monitoring	IJV	EJV	SCV

SCV – subclavian vein; IJV – internal jugular vein; EJV – external jugular vein; FV – femoral vein; RIJV – right internal jugular vein; LSCV – left subclavian vein; LIJV – left internal jugular vein; RSCV – right subclavian vein; PEEP – positive end expiratory pressure; CVP central venous pressure

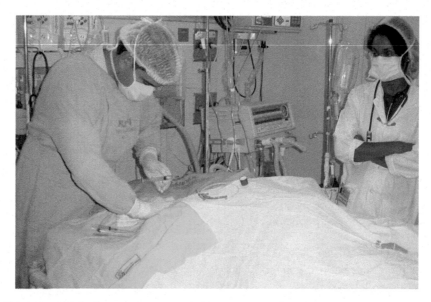

Central Venous, Arterial, and PA Catheters. Figure 1 Vascular cannulation of right internal jugular vein in an intensive care unit setting. Note the use of sterile field covering the face and body of patient (maximum barrier)

The use of Doppler or ultrasound-guided vascular access increase the success of cannulation, reducing the risk of complications related to the insertion. In the future, the use of ultrasound equipment associated with a trained team will improve this technique. Figure 4 demonstrate the collapse sign, useful to differentiate arterial from venous vessels.

Catheter Tip Position

After cannulation, the catheter placement in jugular or subclavian veins must be checked with a thoracic radiography. Ideally, the tip of the catheter need to be positioned 3–5 cm above the junction of the superior vena cava and right atrium or 1 cm below the right tracheobronchial angle (never below the main carina) or outside cardiac silhouette (Fig. 5). The catheter length position must be 16–18 cm at right-side cannulation and 19–21 cm at the left-side cannulation, independently of the gender or patient biotype.

Subclavian Vein Catheterization

The access to the subclavian vein may be gained by the supraclavicular or infraclavicular approach. The angle of insertion for all infraclavicular approaches is parallel to the coronal plane. Initially, the patient is positioned in Trendelenburg (15–30°) in order to increase venous return (~37%) with a small rolled towel between the scapulae to increase the distance between the clavicle and

the first rib. However, Trendelenburg position is not well tolerated in cardiac patients. In these cases, legs are elevated to increase venous return filling subclavian vein, facilitating the cannulation. The head is slightly rotated to the opposite side and the arms are located along the body. After skin preparation and local anesthesia with lidocaine (1% or 2%), the needle is advanced 2–3 cm caudal to clavicle in the delto-peitoral angle. The insertion point can be performed lateral to the midclavicular line at the junction of the lateral and middle thirds of the clavicle, in the mid-clavicle, or at the junction of the middle and medial thirds of the clavicle (Fig. 6).

When blood comes into the syringe (because a slight negative pressure is applied), the needle is fixed with fingers and the syringe is removed, and the guidewire is introduced 15 cm with the J-tip turned lower. If resistance is met when advancing the guidewire, both the guidewire and needle should be withdrawn simultaneously. It is always important to control the guidewire. The tip of guidewire is flexible to avoid vascular lesion (J-tip) during the introduction. Never try to introduce the other tip because of the risk of vascular lesion. The catheter should be introduced over the guidewire without resistance.

This approach has a success rate of 70–99% and is easier to maintain, and is preferably used when airway control is necessary. Disadvantages include difficulty in controlling bleeding, higher risk of pneumothorax, and

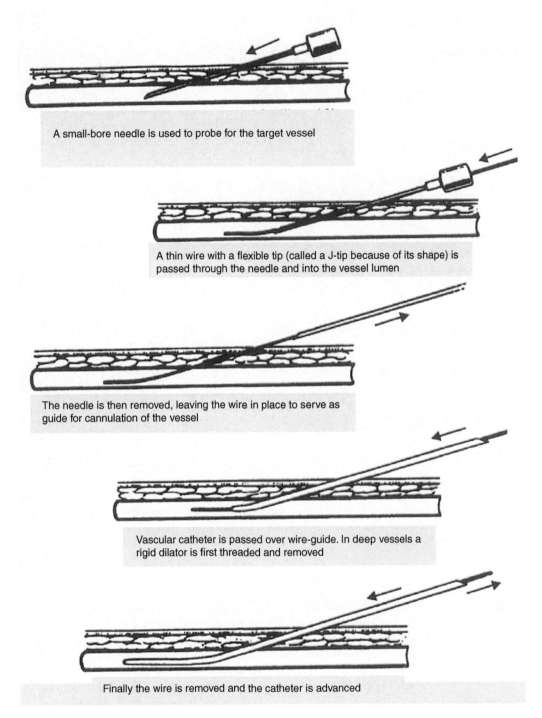

A small-bore needle is used to probe for the target vessel

A thin wire with a flexible tip (called a J-tip because of its shape) is passed through the needle and into the vessel lumen

The needle is then removed, leaving the wire in place to serve as guide for cannulation of the vessel

Vascular catheter is passed over wire-guide. In deep vessels a rigid dilator is first threaded and removed

Finally the wire is removed and the catheter is advanced

Central Venous, Arterial, and PA Catheters. Figure 2 Vascular cannulation with a guidewire (the Seldinger technique)

interference with chest compressions during cardiopulmonary resuscitation.

One study shows that the strongest predictor of a complication is a failed catheterization attempt. Many clinicians feel that three attempts are enough, and then it is time to ask another clinician to attempt catheterization from another site.

The use of Doppler guidance to reduce the complications related to subclavian vein catheterization needs to be better elucidated.

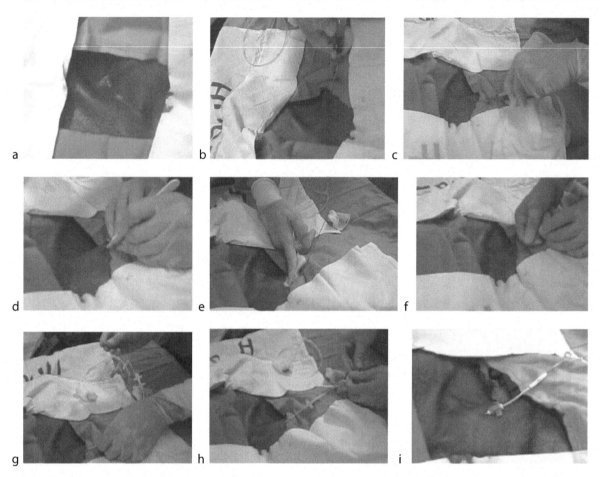

Central Venous, Arterial, and PA Catheters. Figure 3 Steps for right internal jugular vein cannulation: (**a**) preparation of skin with chlorexidine and collocation of fields, (**b**) local anesthesia, (**c**) needle vein cannulation and guidewire is advanced through needle, (**d**) cutdown the skin with a blade (to facilitate the introduction of catheter), (**e**) the guidewire in place and compression of the site to avoid bleeding, (**f**) introduction of dilator, (**g**) introduction of vascular catheter is passed over guidewire, (**h**) the guidewire is retired, and (**i**) the catheter is fixed

Internal Jugular Vein Catheterization

The internal jugular vein has been cannulated with success rate similar to that of the subclavian vein (58–99% success rate). Three different approaches have been described (Fig. 7): (a) anterior to the sternocleidomatoid (SCM); (b) central between the two heads of the SCM, and (c) posterior to the SCM.

The carotid artery lies posterior and medial to the vein. The operator must maintain a minimum pressure in internal carotid artery with the left hand and using the (b) technique previously described (Fig. 7), the vessel is cannulated at an angle of 45° pointing the needle to the ipsilateral nipple. The puncture is achieved by introducing the needle at about 1–5 cm. The rest of the procedure is same as that of a cannulation of subclavian vein.

Internal jugular vein catheterization has a lower risk of pneumothorax and is easier to compress the insertion site if bleeding occurs. However, it may be more difficult to cannulate in patients with volume depletion or shock. Dressing and maintaining are also difficult.

External Jugular Vein Catheterization

The cannulation of the external jugular vein has reduced incidence of complications, but a higher incidence of failure (60–90% success rate). The patient is placed in the Trendelenburg position with the head turned away

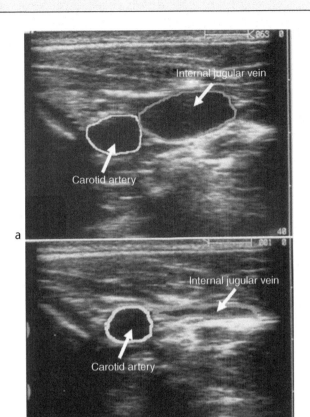

Central Venous, Arterial, and PA Catheters. Figure 4
Transversal axis ultrasound view of cervical region. In (**a**)
carotid artery is located at the left side (smaller circle) and
internal jugular vein is at the right side (larger circle). In (**b**)
there is a collapse of internal jugular vein with transducer
compression

from the insertion site. If necessary, the vein can be
occluded just above the clavicle (with forefinger of the
nondominant hand) to engorge the entry side.
The recommended insertion point is midway between
the angle of the jaw and the clavicle.

The external jugular vein has little support from the
surrounding structures, thus the vein should be anchored
between the thumb and forefinger when the needle is
inserted. Sometimes it is difficult to advance the guidewire
or the catheter. If the catheter does not advance easily, do
not force it, as this may result in vascular perforation.
However, as many as 15% of patients do not have an
identifiable external jugular vein.

It is ideal for coagulopathy patients, because any significant bleeding can be easily recognized and treated with
local pressure. The risk of pneumothorax is also avoided.

Because catheters inserted through the neck are more
difficult to dress and maintain than those in other sites,
this approach is not suitable for prolonged venous access.

Femoral Vein Catheterization

The femoral vein is the easiest, large vein to be cannulated
and does not lead to pneumothorax. The vein is located
just medial to the femoral artery 2 cm below the inguinal
ligament. The needle is directed cephalad at a 45° angle.
The distal tip of needle should not traverse the inguinal
ligament to minimize the risk of retroperitoneal hematoma. The risk of infection and thrombosis limit its general acceptance for long-term use in critically ill patients.
Other disadvantages associated with this route are the
femoral artery puncture (5%) and limited ability to flex
the hip (which can be bothersome for awake patients).
Figure 8 shows the anatomy of the femoral sheath.

Table 3 shows the advantages, disadvantages, and main
contraindications of central vein cannulation.

Complications Related to Vein Catheterization

Complications occurring during catheter placement
include catheter malposition, arrhythmias, embolization, and vascular, cardiac, pleural, mediastinal, and neurologic injuries. Pneumothorax is the most frequently
reported immediate complication of subclavian vein
catheterization, and arterial (carotid) puncture is the
most common immediate complication of internal jugular vein cannulation.

When a carotid artery puncture is performed (2–10%
of attempted cannulations), the needle should be removed
and pressure should be applied to the site for at least 5 min
(10 min if the patient has coagulopathy). If the carotid
artery has been inadvertently cannulated, the catheter
should not be removed, as this could provoke serious
hemorrhage. In this situation, a vascular surgeon should
be consulted immediately.

Pneumothorax can be detected in the postinsertion
chest films in upright position and during expiration (if
possible). Expiratory films facilitate the detection of small
pneumothoraxes because expiration decreases the volume
of air in the lungs, but not the volume of air in the pleural
space. Pneumothorax can be life threatening in ventilated
patients. In minutes, the patient can develop hypertensive
pneumothorax and evolution to cardiopulmonary arrest.
Sometimes the physical examination (hyperresonance at
thoracic percussion) can be the tip for diagnosis.

Pneumothorax may not be radiographically evident
until 24–48 h after central venous cannulation

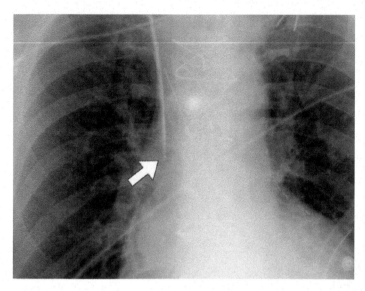

Central Venous, Arterial, and PA Catheters. Figure 5 Thoracic radiography showing the correct placement of catheter tip (*arrow*)

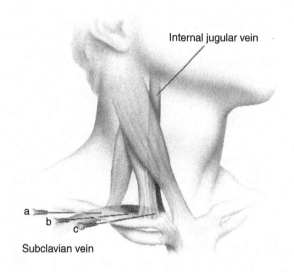

Central Venous, Arterial, and PA Catheters. Figure 6 Three approaches for infraclavicular access to the subclavian vein. a – Junction of the lateral and medial thirds of the clavicle; b – mid-clavicle; c – junction of the middle and medial thirds of the clavicle

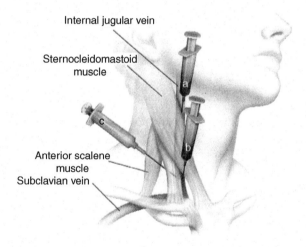

Central Venous, Arterial, and PA Catheters. Figure 7 Three approaches to access the internal jugular vein. a – Anterior to the sternocleidomastoid; b – central between the clavicular and sternal heads of sternocleidomastoid, and c – posterior to the sternocleidomastoid

(delayed pneumothorax). Therefore, the absence of a pneumothorax on an immediate postinsertion chest film does not absolutely exclude the possibility of a catheter-induced pneumothorax. This is an important consideration in patients who develop dyspnea or other signs of pneumothorax in the first few days after central venous cannulation.

Venous air embolism is one of the most feared complications of central venous cannulation. Prevention is the hallmark of reducing the morbidity and mortality of venous air embolism. Placing patient in Trendelenburg position with the head 15° below the horizontal plane

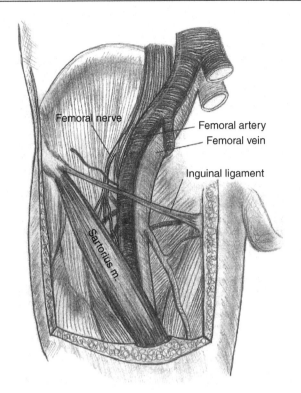

Central Venous, Arterial, and PA Catheters. **Figure 8** The anatomy of the femoral sheath

Central Venous, Arterial, and PA Catheters. Table 3
Advantages, disadvantages, and main contraindications of central vein cannulation

Vein	Advantages	Disadvantages	Contraindications
EJV	Secure	Difficult access in obese or short neck patients	Previous surgery, difficult view
IJV	Low risk of pneumothorax	Difficult view in obese and skin flaccidity. High risk of infection	Coagulopathy, previous surgery, short neck, or obese patients
SCV	Constant anatomy	More risk of pneumothorax, difficult to compress	Coagulopathy, clavicle deformity, low functional respiratory reserve, cifoescoliosis
FV	No interference of thoracic masses	Difficult to progress the guidewire in ascitis patients, difficult hygiene, more risk of infection	Obese, urinary incontinence, infection, or local venous thrombosis

EJV – external jugular vein; IJV – internal jugular vein; SCV – subclavian vein; FV – femoral vein

can facilitate the elevation of venous pressure above the atmospheric pressure. Special care must be employed during changing connections in a central venous line.

Long-term complications related to the length of time that the catheter remains in place include infection and thrombosis. Surface-modified central venous catheters have been developed to reduce catheter-related infection (e.g., minocycline and rifampin impregnated cook spectrum glide® central venous catheter).

The complications observed in a study of over 4,000 cannulations of central veins are shown in Table 4.

Swan-Ganz Catheter

The use of Swan-Ganz (pulmonary artery) catheter is not just important for the specialty of critical care, but it is also responsible for the specialty of critical care. This catheter is so much a part of patient care that it is impossible to function properly in the ICU without a clear understanding of this catheter and the information it provides. It is indicated whenever the data obtained improves therapeutic decision making. Although no carefully designed study has definitely established the benefit of hemodynamic monitoring to the individual patient, it is reasonable to

Central Venous, Arterial, and PA Catheters. Table 4
Comparison between the incidence of complication in SCV and IJV

	SCV (%)	IJV (%)
Risk of arterial puncture	0.5	3.0
Catheter malposition	9.3	5.0
Hemo- or pneumothorax	1.3	1.5
Bloodstream infection	4.0	8.6
Vessel occlusion/thrombosis	1.2	0

SCV – subclavian vein; IJV – internal jugular vein

assume that more precise bedside knowledge of cardiovascular parameters would allow earlier diagnosis and guide therapy. Table 5 shows the indications for pulmonary artery catheterization most often noted in the literature.

The Swan-Ganz catheter is a multilumen catheter 110 cm long and has an outside diameter of 2.3 mm

(7 French gauge). There are two internal channels: proximal (right atrium) and distal (pulmonary artery). The tip of the catheter is equipped with a balloon with 1.5 mL capacity. Finally, there is a thermistor (i.e., a transducer device that senses changes in temperature) located on the outer surface of the catheter 4 cm from the catheter tip. The thermistor measures the flow of a cold fluid that is injected through the proximal port of the catheter, and this flow rate is equivalent to the cardiac output. An example of this catheter is illustrated in Fig. 9.

Other accessories are available on specially designed Swan-Ganz catheter: (1) an extra channel that can be used as infusion channel or for passing temporary pacemaker that leads into the right ventricule; (2) a fiberoptic system that allows continuous monitoring of mixed venous oxygen saturation; (3) a rapid-response thermistor that can measure the ejection fraction of right ventricle, and (4) a thermal filament that generates low-energy heat pulses and allow continuous thermodilution measurement of the cardiac output.

It is essential to prepare the electronic equipment and test the catheter component before insertion. The access to central venous circulation for insertion of Swan-Ganz catheter is the same for placement of a central venous catheter in subclavian or internal jugular positions.

The procedure has been facilitated by the use of introducer assemblies. Once an introducer sheath is in place, the pulmonary catheter is inserted and advanced until the tip reaches an intrathoracic vein (as evidenced by respiratory variations on the pressure tracing). The balloon is then inflated with 1.5 mL of air and the catheter is advanced while the pressure waveform and

Central Venous, Arterial, and PA Catheters. Table 5
Recommendations of pulmonary artery catheterization

I. Surgical
Perioperative management of high-risk patients undergoing extensive surgical procedures
Postoperative cardiovascular complications
Multisystem trauma
Severe burns
Shock despite perceived adequate fluid therapy
Oliguria despite perceived adequate fluid therapy
II. Cardiac
Myocardial infarction complicated with pump failure
Congestive heart failure unresponsive to conventional therapy
Pulmonary hypertension (for diagnosis and monitoring during acute drug therapy)
III. Pulmonary
To differentiate noncardiogenic (acute respiratory distress syndrome) from cardiogenic pulmonary edema
To evaluate effects of high levels of ventilatory support on cardiovascular status

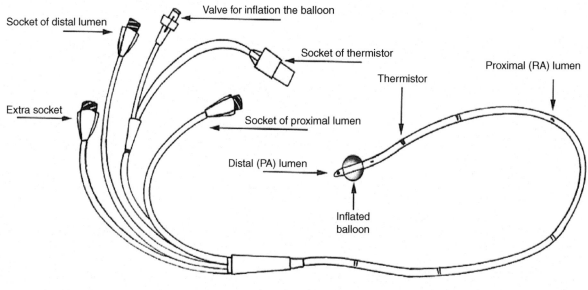

Swan-Ganz Catheter

Central Venous, Arterial, and PA Catheters. Figure 9 The Swan-Ganz catheter. PA – pulmonary artery; RA – right atrium

the electrocardiogram tracing are monitored. The catheter is advanced through the right atrium and into right ventricle where a sudden increase in the systolic pressure appears on the tracing. The catheter is subsequently advanced through pulmonic valve and into the pulmonary artery where a sudden increase in the diastolic pressure is recorded. The catheter is gently advanced until a pulmonary artery occlusion or "wedge" tracing is obtained (Fig. 10). The balloon is deflated, a pulmonary artery tracing is confirmed, the catheter is secured, and a chest radiograph is obtained (Fig. 11).

Data Collected for Swan-Ganz Catheter

The Swan-Ganz catheter provides a significant amount of physiologic information that can guide therapy in critically ill patients. This information includes central venous pressure; pulmonary artery: diastolic, systolic, and mean pressures; pulmonary artery occlusion "wedge" pressure, cardiac output by bolus or continuous thermodilution techniques; mixed venous blood gasses by intermittent sampling; and continuous mixed venous oximetry. A multitude of derived parameters can also be obtained.

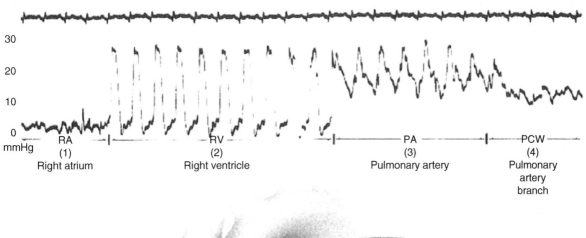

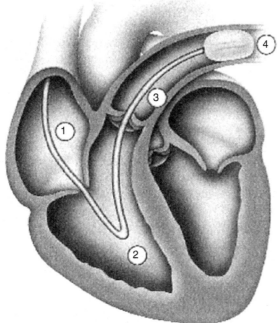

Central Venous, Arterial, and PA Catheters. Figure 10 Pressure tracing recordings with corresponding locations as the pulmonary catheter is passed into the "wedge" position

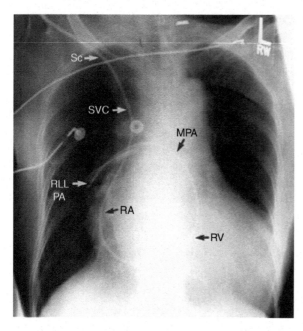

Central Venous, Arterial, and PA Catheters. Figure 11
Normal course of a Swan-Ganz catheter. A Swan-Ganz catheter inserted on the right goes into the subclavian vein (Sc), into the superior vena cava (SVC), right atrium (RA), right ventricle (RV), main pulmonary artery (MPA), and in this case, the right lower lobe pulmonary artery (RLL PA)

Hemodynamic variables are often expressed in relation to body size. A simple equation can replace the use of normograms: BSA (m^2) = [Ht(cm) + Wt(kg) − 60]/100

The parameters of cardiovascular performance directly measured (and normal values) are shown below:

Central venous pressure (CVP) = 1–6 mmHg

CVP is equal to pressure in right atrium. The right atrium pressure (RAP) should be equivalent to right-ventricular end-diastolic pressure (RVEDP); then

CVP = RAP = RVEDP

Pulmonary capillary wedge pressure (PCWP) = 6–12 mmHg

PCWP should be the same as the left-atrial pressure (LAP). The LAP should also be equivalent to the left-ventricular end-diastolic pressure (LVEDP) when there is no obstruction between left atrium and ventricle.

PCWP = LAP = LVEDP

Cardiac index (CI) = 2.4–4.0 L/min/m^2

CI = cardiac output/BSA

Stroke volume index (SVI) = CI/heart rate (HR) (N = 40–70 mL/beat/m^2)

Right ventricular ejection fraction (RVEF) = SV/RVEDP (= CVP) (N = 46–50%)

Right ventricular end-diastolic volume (RVEDV) = SV/RVEF (N = 80–150 mL/m^2)

Left ventricular stroke work index (LVSWI) = (MAP − PCWP) × SVI (× 0.0136) (N = 40–60 g.m/m^2) where MAP = medium arterial pressure and 0.0136 is the factor that converts pressure and volume to units to work

Right ventricular stroke work index (RVSWI) = (PAP − CVP) × SVI (× 0.0136) (N = 4–8 g.m/m^2) where PAP = medium pulmonary arterial pressure

Systemic vascular resistance index (SVRI) = (MAP − RAP) × 80/CI (N = 1,600–2,400 dynes.s.m^2/cm^5)

Pulmonary vascular resistance index (PVRI) = (PAP − PCWP) × 80/CI (N = 200–400 dynes.s.m^2/cm^5)

The parameters of systemic oxygen transport are shown below (Hb = hemoglobin).

Mixed venous oxygen saturation (SvO_2) = 70–75%

Oxygen delivery (DO_2) = CI × 13.4 × Hb × SaO_2 (N = 520–570 mL/min.m^2)

Oxygen uptake (VO_2) = CI × 13.4 × Hb × (SaO_2 − SvO_2) (N = 110–160 mL/min.m^2)

Oxygen extraction ratio (O_2ER) = VO_2/DO_2 (× 100) (N = 20–30%)

Complications of Swan-Ganz Catheter

The most common complication during the passage of pulmonary catheter is the development of arrhythmias. If an arrhythmia is noted, withdraw the catheter into the vena cava, and the arrhythmia should disappear. Rarely, treatment of arrhythmias is necessary, except complete heart block (which should be treated with a temporary transvenous pacemaker) and sustained ventricular tachycardia (which should be treated with lidocaine or other suitable antiarrhythmic agent).

Coiling, looping, or knotting in the right ventricle may occur during catheter insertion. This can be avoided if no more than 10 cm of catheter is inserted after a ventricular tracing is visualized and before a pulmonary artery tracing appears. Aberrant catheter locations such pleural, pericardial, peritoneal, aortic, vertebral artery, renal vein, and inferior vena cava have also been reported.

After catheter insertion, the complications include infection, thromboembolism, pulmonary infarction, pulmonary artery rupture, hemorrhage, pseudo aneurysm formation, thrombocytopenia, cardiac valve injuries, catheter fracture, and balloon rupture.

Finally, complications can result from delay in treatment because of time-consuming insertion problems and from inappropriate treatment based on erroneous information or erroneous data interpretation.

Arterial Catheterization

Arterial catheterization is indicated whenever continuous monitoring of blood pressure or frequent sampling of arterial blood is required. Patients with shock, hypertensive crisis, major surgical interventions, and high levels of respiratory support require precise and continuous blood pressure monitoring, particularly when vasoactive or inotropic drugs are being administered. In shock patients, the difference between direct blood pressure and cuff blood pressure could be more than 30 mmHg in 50% of patients.

The radial, ulnar, axillary, brachial, femoral, dorsalis pedis, and superficial temporal arteries have been used to access the arterial circulation for continuous monitoring. The radial artery of nondominant hand should be attempted first. The dual blood supply to the hand and the superficial location of the vessel make the radial artery the most commonly used site for arterial catheterization. The Allen test is frequently used to test the adequacy of collateral circulation before cannulation (Fig. 12). Ultrasonic Doppler technique, plethysmography, and pulse oximetry have also been used to assess the adequacy of the collateral arterial supply.

The puncture site is slightly proximal (2 cm) to the flexion skin fold with a small catheter at 30–45° angle to the skin. For cannulation in the direct threading technique, the anterior wall of the artery is penetrated (A). When blood return is noted (B), the catheter is advanced farther up the arterial lumen as the needle is withdrawn (C) (Fig. 13). The cannula is then connected to a pressure monitoring system.

The axillary artery has been recommended for long-term direct arterial pressure monitoring because of its larger size, freedom for the patient's hand, and close proximity to the central circulation. Pulsation and pressure are maintained even in the presence of shock with marked vasoconstriction. Thrombosis does not result in compromised flow in the distal arm because of the extensive collateral circulation. The major disadvantages are its low accessibility, visibility, and location within the neurovascular sheath, which may increase the risk of neurologic compromise if a hematoma develops.

The major advantages of using femoral artery are its superficial location and large size, which allow easier localization and cannulation when the pulses are absent over more distal vessels. The major disadvantages are the decreased mobility of the patient, contamination from ostomies or draining abdominal wounds, and the possibility of occult bleeding into the abdomen or thigh.

Both axillary and femoral arteries are cannulated by using the modified Seldinger technique.

The dorsalis pedis artery may be absent in up to 12% of feet. Assessment of collateral flow to the remainder of the foot through the posterior tibial artery should precede cannulation. This can be done by occluding the dorsalis pedis artery, blanching the great toe by compressing the toenail for several seconds, and then releasing the toenail while observing the return of color.

The major disadvantages of using the dorsalis pedis artery are its relatively small size and overestimation of systolic pressure (5–20 mmHg higher than the radial artery).

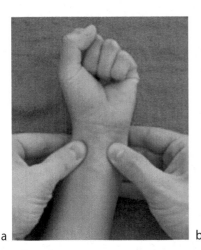 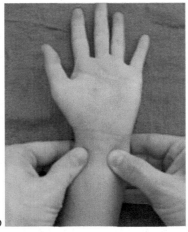 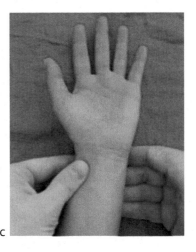

a   b   c

Central Venous, Arterial, and PA Catheters. Figure 12 Allen test: In (**a**) occlusion of both ulnar and radial arteries while patient makes a fist; (**b**) radial and ulnar arteries occluded after hand is opened; and (**c**) release of pressure on ulnar artery and observation for color return to hand within 5–10 s. This is a demonstration of patency of ulnar artery

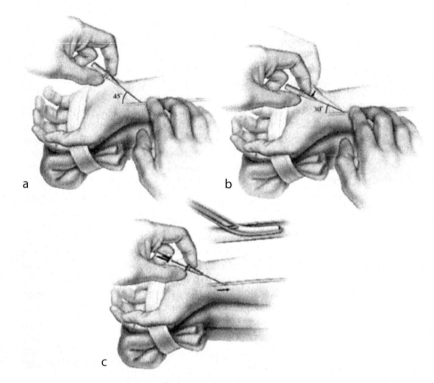

Central Venous, Arterial, and PA Catheters. Figure 13 Direct approach to cannulation of the radial artery

The superficial temporal artery has been extensively used in infants and in some adults for continuous pressure monitoring. Because of its small size and tortuousity, surgical exposure is required for cannulation. A small incidence of neurologic complications resulting from cerebral embolization has been reported in infants.

The brachial artery is not used often because of high complication rate associated with arteriography. Although this artery has been successfully used for short-term monitoring, there are little data to support prolonged brachial artery monitoring, and its use has been discouraged. Disadvantages include difficulty in maintaining the site and the possibility of hematoma formation in anticoagulated patients. The latter may lead to median nerve compression neuropathy and Volkmann's contracture. Compartment syndrome of the forearm and hand has also been reported.

Complications of Arterial Catheterization

Major complications for all sites of arterial line insertion include: bleeding, ischemia, distal embolization, sepsis, neuropathy, arteriovenous fistula, and pseudoaneurysm formation. Inadvertent injection of vasoactive drugs or other agents into an artery can cause severe pain, distal ischemia, and tissue necrosis. Minor complications are: thrombosis, skin ischemia and local inflammation, infection, and hematoma. Infections are more frequent: (a) after 4 days of catheter placement, (b) when insertion is made by surgical cut down, and (c) presence of local inflammation.

References

1. Irwin RS, Rippe JM (eds) (2007) Intensive care medicine, 6th edn. Wolkers Kluwer/Lippincott, Williams & Wilkins, Philadelphia, PA
2. Marino PL (1998) The ICU book, 2nd edn. Williams & Wilkins, Baltimore, MD
3. O'Donnell JM, Nácul FE (eds) (2001) Surgical intensive care medicine. Kluwer, Boston, MA/Dordrecht/London

Cerebral Abscess

▶ Post-neurosurgical Brain Abscess and Subdural Empyema

Cerebral Concussion

Daniel B. Craig[1], Kathryn M. Beauchamp[2]
[1]Denver, CO, USA
[2]Department of Neurosurgery, Denver Health Medical Center, University of Colorado School of Medicine, Denver, CO, USA

Synonyms

The term "cerebral concussion" is often used interchangeably with "minor traumatic brain injury" or MTBI. Other less common synonyms are: mild head injury, minor head trauma, mild brain injury.

Definition

Cerebral concussion can be defined as a post-traumatic, immediate, and transient change in neural function. The roots of "concussion" come from two Latin words – concutere (to shake violently) and concussus (the act of striking together). It is the most common type of head injury and has been recognized as a group of symptoms for centuries. The diagnosis of concussion is almost entirely clinical, and the range of symptoms is broad. The specific clinical definition of concussion has been contested over the years. The Vienna conference in 2001 set out to offer a comprehensive current definition resulting in a broad definition with highlights including: "*an impulsive force transmitted to the head...rapid onset of short-lived impairment...resolves spontaneously...symptoms largely reflect a functional disturbance rather than structural injury...may or may not involve loss of consciousness...sequential resolution of symptoms...associated with grossly normal structural imaging studies.*"

The Debate

Concussion amongst athletes is increasingly common and therefore it is important to have a common definition amongst practitioners from which to guide treatment. Many consider loss of consciousness at the time of injury or some minimal period of peri-traumatic amnesia as necessary symptoms. Others have searched for a clear structural brain injury – especially as imaging modalities improved to complement the physiological definition. In general, neurological and cognitive concussion symptoms are *immediate, transient,* caused by *blunt-force trauma,* and generally exist *without a clear structural anatomic lesion.*

Historically, several evaluation systems evolved to categorize injuries based on initial symptoms, and many recovery guidelines still use this grading system to determine return to activity protocol. At the Prague International Conference on Concussion in Sport (2004) [1], the authors supported the trend toward abandoning the classic concussion grading scale as true severity of injury has shown limited correlation to the number and duration of acute concussion signs/symptoms. Instead, they argued for a division based on management needs into simple or complex concussion. Progressive resolution of symptoms within 7–10 days defines simple concussion and represents the vast majority of injuries without the need for formal intervention or extensive neuropsychological screening. Complex concussion indicates persistent symptoms, prolonged loss of consciousness (>1 min), or prolonged cognitive impairment and requires more formal medical management with consideration of imaging, and multi-disciplinary follow-up.

One final area of current debate is that of concussion being a linear spectrum of severity or a group of distinct subtypes. The spectrum ideology has been the classic model, but the variations in clinical outcome with the same impact force suggest discreet differences in pathology. This complements the progress in understanding the mechanism of injury, and may help explain why a clear common pathway in concussion remains somewhat elusive.

Mechanism

The blunt forward or oblique force with impact causes a rapid acceleration/deceleration of the head and a resulting anterior/posterior movement of the brain within the cranial vault. Several theories about the resulting neuronal dysfunction involve ionic shifts, altered metabolism, impaired connectivity, and changes in neurotransmission. Reticular theory suggests a temporary paralyzation of the brainstem reticular formation. Centripetal hypothesis involves a mechanical disruption of neuronal tracts. The pontine cholinergic scheme describes an activation of cholinergic neurons causing a suppressed behavioral response. The convulsive response theory is based on induction of generalized neuronal firing. No conclusive human studies have confirmed a specific mechanism, and the underlying pathophysiology is likely multifactorial.

Giza and Hovda [2] describe in an animal model a train of biochemical activity in response to blunt trauma. The initial insult causes a neurochemical cascade and membrane/axon dysfunction leading to: increased extracellular potassium → depolarization → excitatory neurotransmitter release → neurotransmitter storm → generalized post-storm suppression. This series ultimately causes increased glucose use and lactate production, decreased cerebral blood flow, NMDA receptor activation, calcium influx, and impaired oxidative metabolism. This theory is limited with respect to neuro/cognitive evaluation in an animal model, but it does offer a hypothesis on the biochemical basis of the generalized post-concussion syndrome.

Overall, concussion can be viewed as a combination of mechanical changes from shearing or torsional forces in addition to a related cascade of neurochemical events. This is characterized in an animal model by massive initial depolarization and ultimate decrease in cerebral perfusion leading to metabolic depression. The real-time progression of physiologic events helps explain the later onset of some symptoms of concussion, and the cascade has been shown to render brain tissue more vulnerable to further injury. Recent studies have shown persistent metabolic alterations long after initial injury, and further studies may one day explain or even predict long-term post-concussion syndrome.

Presentation

The injured patient will present after a non-penetrating blunt impact to the head with a range of neurologic and cognitive symptoms. Common presentations include: brief loss of consciousness, period of retro and anterograde amnesia, visual disturbances, and disorientation. He or she may also experience dizziness, nausea and vomiting, balance problems, emotional lability, sleep disturbances, sensitivity to light or sound, fatigue, numbness/tingling, and loss of concentration. Autonomic signs include pallor, bradycardia, mild hypotension, and sluggish pupillary reaction. Less common are brief convulsions and specific neurologic deficits.

Assessment of these symptoms may depend on witnesses to the event (loss of consciousness may be very brief and often missed), and availability of immediate evaluation (symptoms may be transient). This need for rapid assessment of mental status and neurologic changes encourages the use and standardization of the initial survey by the first responder (coach, trainer, doctor, EMT).

Treatment

In the majority of cases, the symptoms of concussion resolve spontaneously – usually in 7–10 days. Thorough serial neurologic examinations are crucial to monitor resolution of symptoms and to rule out more serious injury. At a molecular and anatomic level, the pathophysiology of the brain injury and its progression remains loosely defined and thus resists development of medical/surgical intervention to hasten recovery. As our ability to evaluate

concussion has grown, the need for and length of hospitalization has decreased. Several overlapping and competing theories for the proper rehabilitative steps to return to play will be discussed in more detail later.

A handful of studies have examined the importance of intentional supervised rehabilitation post concussion. Original trials in the late 1970s showed the benefit of early ambulation, activity, and education [3]. More recently, there is focus on outpatient rehab as hospital stays decrease. A randomized controlled trial in 2007 showed that early active rehabilitation did not change the outcomes of post-concussive symptom resolution and life satisfaction after 1 year between intervention and control groups [4]. Treatment is primarily tailored to the individual while determining the extent of injury. One of the most important factors in recovery remains the time from the initial injury.

The pharmacologic management of the specific symptoms of concussion lacks high-level evidence. Antidepressants are the most commonly prescribed treatment for post-concussion syndrome, specifically SSRI's and newer heterocyclics. Trazodone can be an effective choice for insomnia, although its anticholinergic side effect profile may limit its use. Acetylcholinesterase inhibitors (physostigmine, donepezil), and choline precursors (lecithin, CDP-choline) have been shown to improve neuropsychological test performance, but are limited by short half-life, side effects, and route of administration.

Evaluation

At the Scene

Initial survey at the scene of the head injury is crucial. Primary trauma survey should be the first step (airway, breathing, circulation, disability, exposure). After vital signs have been stabilized, a more detailed examination may be performed. A neurologic exam assessing cranial nerves, coordination, motor function, and cognitive function should be performed based on the severity of injury. Questionnaires such as the mini-mental-status exam and the Maddocks questions can be quite useful for quick evaluation of a patient's cognition and orientation and can be learned and used effectively by nonmedical personnel.

At the Hospital

Patient's arriving at the hospital after concussion should be evaluated similar to the initial screen but with more thorough neurologic exam. A non-contrast head CT may be considered. Indications of a more serious injury include: focal neurologic deficit; seizures; prolonged altered level of consciousness; oto-rhinorrhea; diplopia; anisocoria; and progressive symptoms. Concussion is classically characterized as *immediate* onset of symptoms, but this is not always the case. Symptoms may arise up to hours after the initial injury. However, progressive worsening of an established symptom is a red flag for possible structural injury and indicates the need for further workup.

Patients presenting with a mild concussion generally do not require hospital admission, but it is important to verify that they go home with another adult capable of following their symptoms. For outpatient treatment of pain, acetaminophen is the drug of choice and narcotics and NSAIDS should be avoided due to the risks of increased intra-cranial pressure and hemorrhage respectively.

If the presence of a more serious injury is suspected based on previously mentioned criteria, a more thorough evaluation is warranted. These patients should be admitted for close observation. In these instances, CT or MRI imaging is useful to rule out epidural/subdural hematoma, cerebral contusion, or possible skull fracture. Length of inpatient stay depends on individual recovery and diagnosis of more serious injury.

The Acute Concussion Evaluation (ACE) provides a thorough initial medical evaluation of the patient presenting with concussion. This questionnaire evaluates the specifics of the injury and assessment of symptoms and risk factors. The Sport Concussion Assessment Tool (SCAT) developed by the Prague International Conference in 2004 is another tool for thorough graded assessment combining elements of the sideline tests with more exhaustive neuro-physical exam. The use of a standardized form is especially helpful to provide a baseline for future evaluations. It can also be an effective means of standardizing communication between various levels of medical personnel (PA, EMT, nurse, trainer, MD).

Role of Imaging

Indications for CT and MRI to rule out more serious injury have classically been controversial and subjective, and there have been efforts to standardize these practices (Canadian Head CT Rule, New Orleans Criteria). In addition to ruling out anatomic injury, the role of imaging in evaluation of concussion has progressed significantly with the advent of more sophisticated techniques. Thus far, studies have demonstrated inability to correlate post-concussive MRI findings with symptoms or long-term outcome. Positron emission tomography (PET) scans

consistently demonstrate frontal and/or temporal hypometabolism following concussion both at rest and during tasks, but have had limited clinical applicability. Several newer modalities show promise in both diagnosis and assessment of recovery, specifically functional MRI (fMRI), event-related potentials (ERP's), and magnetic source imaging (MSI) [5].

fMRI studies demonstrate increased overall brain activation during memory and sensorimotor tasks in post-concussion patients, and note a discernible difference in prefrontal cortex usage between injured and non-injured subjects with an inverse relationship between prefrontal working memory area (mid-dorsolateral) usage and symptom severity. The symptomatic subjects included in these studies had no abnormalities on T2 MRI, thus functional impairment can be observed in the absence of clinical imaging abnormalities. ERP's represent the average electroencephalogram (EEG) signal in response to stimulus, and response time and amplitude have both proven to consistently vary with symptom severity where EEG and evoked potential (EP) testing results have been largely mixed and inconclusive. MSI integrates MRI anatomic data with magnetoencephalography which measures electrical signal parallel to skull surface detecting real-time brain activity without distortion from tissue connectivity variance between brain, bone, and skin. MSI sensitivity surpasses that of MRI or EEG alone. The clinical utility of these more complex imaging techniques is in its infancy, but they show potential for a quantifiable method of diagnosis, assessment of recovery, and further explanation of underlying pathophysiology [5].

Effectiveness

The effectiveness of mTBI evaluation is best measured by the ability to rule out more serious injury and ensure safe return to normal activity. As discussed in the previous section, consistent clinical exams, proper use of imaging, and patience ensure high sensitivity and specificity of diagnosis.

Tolerance

The cautious approach to returning to high risk activity comes in large part from the vulnerability of the post-concussion patient to a second injury more severe than the first. The Second Impact Syndrome (SIS) is a controversial term introduced in the 1980s describing repeat head injury within a few weeks of a concussion causing diffuse cerebral swelling, brain herniation, and death. Controversy stems from the paucity of case data with most examples coming from disputed cases primarily in children [6].

Despite the low incidence, the extreme morbidity of SIS makes it hard to ignore and encourages lengthening recovery time especially in children.

While the SIS debate continues, the increased risk for subsequent traumatic brain injury (TBI) in patients who have sustained at least one previous TBI is much less contested. The significance of this increased risk encompasses more than just multiple mTBI recoveries as a history of repeated concussions over an extended period of months to years can result in cumulative neurologic and cognitive deficits. This has been studied especially in boxers and football players and is a major concern regarding long-term management. This cumulative risk as well as the fear of SIS explains the previous concussion as a factor in return to play guidelines.

Pharmacoeconomics

The CDC estimates the incidence of mTBI at 1.1 million per year including 300,000 sports-related concussions. This translates to roughly $17 billion spent on concussion evaluation and treatment each year. These figures likely underestimate actual disease burden due to variance in assessment and reporting. Costs include both direct evaluation and treatment and time lost at work or on the field.

After-care

At Home

Patients sent home with a mild concussion require observation and frequent reassessment, noting any continuation and/or deterioration of symptoms. Mental status changes and potential amnesia in the patient make it important to clearly explain red flag symptoms and serial evaluation instructions to the accompanying adult as well as the patient. There has been no documented evidence regarding the common practice of waking the patient every 3–4 h to assess, but in patients experiencing loss of consciousness, prolonged amnesia, or other persistent significant symptoms this is still recommended. Decisions regarding day to day activities such as driving and return to work or school should reflect the individual patient's rate of recovery. A follow-up visit to and outpatient provider is appropriate to confirm symptom resolution.

Return to Play

Many sets of guidelines offer rational and clinical approaches for return to activity, and it is important to clearly communicate these recommendations amongst patients, families, and providers. In 1991, the Colorado Medical Society Guidelines (CMSG) emerged in response to several deaths due to head injury, and, along with algorithms by Cantu (1986), the American Academy of Neurology (AAN) and others, their structure reflects the initial symptom milieu of the injury (specifically presence and duration of loss of consciousness and amnesia) and number of previous concussions. These guidelines express the need for longer asymptomatic waiting periods based on injury severity.

The Vienna Summary and Agreement Statement from 2001 emphasizes a medically supervised, *stepwise* process for return to play, moving from no activity to light aerobic exercise, sport-specific training, non-contact drills, full-contact training, and finally game play with minimum stage duration of 24 h. This system depends first on the complete lack of symptoms before starting any activity. These two schools of thought lend themselves to a combination approach with the guidelines of the CMSG, Cantu, AAN et al. determining when to begin activity and the Vienna statement clarifying a stepwise method of return to full-speed, full-contact participation.

Prognosis

Most concussions fall into the "simple" category as outlined earlier. In these cases the prognosis is very good, with symptoms resolving completely in 7–10 days in 90% of cases. In more complex injuries, the duration and severity of symptoms increase, but a full recovery is common. Up to one-third of patients report increased headaches 1 year after trauma. Multiple concussions over time increase the risk of permanent neurologic damage, and up to 15% of patients may experience long-term symptoms after a single event.

References

1. McCrory P, Johnston K, Meeuwisse W et al (2005) Summary and agreement statement of the 2nd international conference on concussion in sport. Clin J Sport Med 15(2):48–55
2. Giza C, Hovda D (2001) The neurometabolic cascade of concussion. J Athletic Train 36(3):228–235
3. Relander M, Troupp H, Bjorkesten G (1972) Controlled trial of treatment of cerebral concussion. Br Med J 4:777–779
4. Andersson E, Emanuelson I, Bjorklund R et al (2007) Mild traumatic brain injuries: the impact of early intervention on late sequelae, a randomized control trial. Acta Neurochir 149(2):151–160
5. Mendez C, Hurley R, Lassonde M et al (2005) Mild traumatic brain injury: neuroimaging of sports-related concussion. J Neuropsychiatry Clin Neurosci 17:297–303
6. McCrory P (2001) Does second impact syndrome exist? Clin J Sport Med 11(3):144–149
7. Aubry M, Cantu R, Dvorak J et al (2001) Summary and agreement statement of the first international conference on concussion in sport, Vienna 2002. Br J Sports Med 36:6–7

Cerebral Malaria

SUZANNE M. SHEPHERD, WILLIAM H. SHOFF
Department of Emergency Medicine, Hospital of the
University of Pennsylvania, Philadelphia, PA, USA

Synonyms
Paludism

Definition
Cerebral malaria has been strictly defined by the World
Health Organization (WHO, 2000) as a patient with
confirmed plasmodium infection, usually P.falciparum,
who is unarousable (Glasgow Coma Scale score $</= 9$),
and has had other potential causes of coma excluded.
Many metabolic and infectious processes may cause the
types of neurologic signs and symptoms associated with
malaria, and the presence of malaria parasite may be
incidental in endemic areas. This rather strict definition
was developed for research, as such many individuals
with cerebral malaria have less severe impairment of
consciousness. In practice, the diagnosis of cerebral
malaria is difficult with a high sensitivity but a low specificity. The diagnosis of falciparum malaria should be
considered in any patient with a febrile illness including
neurological symptoms, who has visited or lived in
a malaria-endemic area in the past 3 months. Cerebral
malaria is an acute, widespread infection of the brain
with features of diffuse encephalopathy. The neurological
manifestations of malaria develop rapidly and include
acute severe headache, irritability, agitation, delirium,
psychosis, seizures, and the hallmarks of impaired consciousness and coma. Cerebral malaria is the most serious complication of falciparum infection and the most
common cause of death. Cerebral malaria is also reported
in individuals infected with P.vivax and more recently P.
knowlesi.

Treatment
If left untreated, cerebral malaria is fatal within days of
infection. Severe malaria is considered a medical emergency and institution of immediate treatment is crucial.
Patients should be managed at the highest level of care at
the best available health care facility. ICU facilities are
limited in malarial areas; therefore, patient triage to these
scarce resources must identify those at greatest risk of
complications. Misra et al. developed a simple but
specific triage tool for adults, the malaria severity
assessment (MSA) score; however, this tool requires
information that is not available at the time of hospitalization. Hanson et al., using logistic regression, developed a five-point scoring system which was validated in
patient series from Vietnam and Bangladesh. The level of
acidosis (base deficit) and the Glasgow Coma Scale were
the two main independent predictors of outcome and the
coma acidosis malaria (CAM) score was derived from
these variables. Mortality was found to increase with
increasing score. A CAM score <2 predicted survival
(PPV 95.8%, CI 93–97.7%) and safe treatment on
a general ward if renal function could be carefully monitored [1].

Treatment involves administration of parenteral
antimalarials, close patient monitoring to ensure early
recognition and management of common complications, and the use of adjunctive treatment measures.
Common complications include hypoglycemia, seizures,
fluid and electrolyte imbalances, anemia, coagulation
disorders, acidosis and respiratory distress and renal
dysfunction. Serum glucose, sodium, lactate, urine output, and renal function should be monitored frequently.
Hypoglycemia may occur with minimal to no clinical
signs; therefore, serum glucose should be monitored at
frequent intervals.

Pharmacologic Management
Use of antimalarials is the only treatment that clearly
reduces mortality. Antimalarials are administered intravenously for 48 h and then orally if the patient is able to take
oral medications. Even fast acting antimalarials often
require 12–18 h to kill plasmodia. Treatment response
is assessed by daily parasite count until clearance of all
P.falciparum trophozoites is achieved from the blood.
Parasitemia may increase during the initial 12–24 h
because available antimalarials do not inhibit schizont
rupture with release of merozoites. Rising parasitemia
beyond 36–48 h after the initiation of antimalarials indicates treatment failure, usually because of high-level drug
resistance. Because nonimmune hosts may have a high
pretreatment total parasite burden ($\approx$1,000 parasites), it
may take up to 6 days to achieve complete elimination.
Treatment duration depends on the sensitivity of the parasite and parasite burden, but usually lasts 7 days. Parenteral quinine has been the traditional treatment of choice
for cerebral malaria, as patients with severe malaria are
assumed to have chloroquine resistance. Artemisinin
derivatives are now recommended by the World Health
Organization (WHO) as the drugs of choice for severe
malaria. Both drugs are used in combination with other

antimalarial drugs, such as doxycycline (100 mg bid PO or IV x7d) with quinine, to shorten therapy duration and prevent the emergence of resistance.

Quinine is one of four main alkaloids derived from the bark of the Cinchona tree. Quinine kills plasmodia in the late stages of their erythrocyte cycle via inhibition of hemazoin biocrystallization, facilitating aggregation of cytotoxic heme products. A loading dose of quinine is recommended to rapidly develop anti-parasitic levels. 20 mg/kg body weight (salt), in normal saline or dextrose saline solution, is infused over 4 hours, preferably via infusion pump. Maintenance dosing is 10 mg/kg body weight (salt) infused every 8 h until the patient is able to take oral medication. Quinine has a narrow therapeutic window. Quinine can produce hypoglycemia via promotion of insulin secretion. Quinine causes hypotension with rapid intravenous infusion. It slows ventricular repolarization, with resultant QT prolongation. Quinine also produces cinchonism and dizziness. Quinidine has been used preferentially in the USA, given in a loading dose of 6.25 mg/kg base (=10 mg/kg salt) infused intravenously over 1–2 h, and then as a continuous infusion of 0.0125 mg/kg/min base (=0.02 mg/kg/min base). If continuous infusion is not feasible, 15 mg/kg base (=24 mg/kg salt) loading dose is infused intravenously over 4 hrs, then 7.5 mg/kg base (=12 mg/kg salt) infused over 4 h every 8 h, beginning 8 h after the loading dose. Cinchonism is a symptom complex characterized by tinnitus, hearing impairment, postural hypotension and vertigo or dizziness that occurs in a high percentage of individuals treated with quinine for malaria.

Newer studies demonstrate artemisinin derivative superiority in both rapidity of parasite clearance and fever defervescence, but they have not demonstrated improved effect on mortality rates [2]. Currently, two derivatives, artesunate and artemether, are the most widely used due to efficacy and low cost. Artemisinin, was developed as a traditional treatment for fever and malaria in China (Qinghaosu). Artemisinin is a sesquiterpene lactone derived from the sweet wormwood, Artemesia annua. Artemisinin derivatives kill all stages of the parasite within the erythrocyte and also kill gametocytes. Artemisinin derivatives can also be administered intramuscularly or rectally and have few local or systemic adverse effects. Artesunate is given as two 2.4 mg/kg doses intravenously 12 h apart on day 1, and then is administered as 2.4 mg/kg daily for 6 days or given orally if the patient is awake and able to swallow. Artesunate is used in combination with Amodiaquine 10 mg/kg once a day for 3 days. These derivatives are not fully licensed in many countries; however, intravenous artesunate is available as an investigational new drug in the USA for management of severe malaria.

A number of adjunctive treatments have been studied in cerebral malaria. Fluid balance is critical. Children are often hypovolemic and require fluid administration; however, there is no consensus with regard to the optimal type and amount of fluid replacement. In patients with cerebral malaria who have elevated intracranial pressure maintenance of cerebral perfusion, pressure is necessary and it has been suggested that fluid management be optimized; however, no guidelines have been developed. Adults with severe malaria may develop pulmonary edema and severe renal impairment, in these instances fluid may need to be restricted. Albumin has been studied, as it is suggested to improve microcirculatory flow and treat hypovolemia. Initial data from Phase II Clinical trials in children with malaria suggest that 4% albumin improves mortality compared with saline, particularly in those children with coma. Albumin is currently under investigation in a large study of children with sepsis and malaria. Other colloidal agents, including hetastarch and dextran 70, are also currently under investigation.

Acetaminophen (paracetamol) may be used to reduce fever. It remains unclear if reduction in core temperature benefits cerebral consequences.

Phenobarbital sodium, phenytoin, or benzodiazepines are utilized for seizure management. Benzodiazepines may have reduced efficacy as malarial infection appears to downregulate γ-aminobutyric acid (GABA) receptors. Both phenytoin and phenobarbital have been used successfully to terminate prolonged seizures. Prophylactic anticonvulsant use has also been studied. Prophylactic administration of a single dose of phenobarbital reduced seizure frequency in studies of both Indian and Thai adults and Kenyan children with cerebral malaria; however, it was associated with an increased rate of death, probably due to depression of hyperpnea that compensated for metabolic acidosis in these unventilated patients.

Standard treatment regimens have been used to manage hypoglycemia. Both the administration of glucose solutions and the administration of longer acting somatostatin analogs have been utilized successfully to manage hypoglycemia, the later in patients receiving quinine therapy. Theoretical concern has been raised whether the correction of hypoglycemia in the presence of tissue hypoxia may worsen brain tissue acidosis.

A number of other adjunctive treatments have been studied. None have shown clear-cut improvement in clinical trials. Most were studied in conjunction with quinine treatment; as such their efficacy in combination with artemisinin derivatives remains undetermined. None are recommended as standard management at this time.

Corticosteroids were the initial agents studied in randomized controlled trials, as they were felt to have promise in reducing intracranial pressure and inflammatory response. Two randomized trials in Southeast Asian adults and a smaller study in Indonesian children did not demonstrate any benefit. In fact, in one trial dexamethasone demonstrated an increased rate of significant complications, including sepsis, gastrointestinal bleeding and prolonged recovery time from coma.

Anti-inflammatory drugs, mannitol, urea, iron chelators (deferoxamine), low-molecular-weight dextran, heparin, pentoxyfylline (reduces cytokine secretion, prevents rosetting and reduce cytoadherence), hyperimmune globulin, dichloroacetate, and hyperbaric oxygen have shown either mixed results or no value. Monoclonal antibodies against TNF-α have been found to shorten fever duration but have shown no impact on mortality, and may actually increase morbidity from neurologic sequellae. N-acetylcysteine, another antioxidant which improves erythrocyte deformability and reduces TNF release is currently under trial. Erythropoietin is also currently being investigated, based on human and animal studies that suggest a neuroprotective effect with reduction in inflammatory response and apoptosis in the brain [3, 4].

Blood transfusions are indicated for severe anemia, with the amount and rapidity of transfusion different for children and adults. In children, fresh whole blood (10–20 ml/kg) is often transfused. In adults, small quantities of blood are administered over a more prolonged period due to concerns about fluid overload. The role of exchange transfusion in severe malaria is controversial. Exchange transfusion has been utilized when the level of parasitemia exceeds 10–20% of circulating erythrocytes. The WHO currently recommends that individuals with severe malaria receive exchange transfusion with a parasitemia >20%. Exchange transfusion also allows correction of severe anemia without the risk of fluid overload. Exchange transfusion is expensive. No data from well-conducted clinical trials demonstrate improved outcomes with exchange transfusion.

Epidemiology

Malaria is felt to be the most deadly vector-borne disease globally. An estimated 2.4 billion individuals live in malaria-endemic areas worldwide, with 300–500 million clinical episodes and approximately two million deaths reported annually. 10% of admissions and 80% of deaths are due to central nervous system involvement. *Plasmodium falciparum* causes most cases of severe malaria and approximately 35–43% of all cases of malaria globally. More than 70% of falciparum malaria infections occur in children living in sub-Saharan Africa, although individuals of any age may become infected. Males and females are equally affected, but malaria, especially falciparum, can be devastating in pregnancy to both the mother and fetus. Malaria is seen increasingly in non-endemic countries due to individuals traveling to endemic areas for business and pleasure and infected individuals emigrating or traveling from endemic areas. Occasionally, malaria is seen in individuals who have traveled to an endemic area more than one year previously, during relapse in those previously infected, or in individuals in non-endemic areas who have been bitten by local mosquito populations which have become infected after biting a parasitemic individual, or in individuals who live near airports. Malaria is infrequently transmitted congenitally, in those who needle share, or in those who have received blood transfusions or organ transplant. More than 1,500 cases are diagnosed in the USA each year, most of which were acquired internationally.

Malaria is transmitted via the bite of an infected female *Anopheles spp* mosquito obtaining a human blood meal. Anopheles mosquitoes predominantly bite between dusk and dawn. Malaria usually occurs below elevations of 1,000 m (3,282 ft). At risk areas include more than 100 countries, including portions of Central America, South America, the Caribbean, the Middle East, sub-Saharan Africa, Southeast Asia, the Indian Subcontinent and Oceania. Malaria, due to intense vector control efforts, ceased to be endemic in the USA in 1947.

After malarial sporozoites are injected into the bloodstream by an infected mosquito, parasites develop in an asymptomatic hepatic stage. Infected hepatocytes burst, releasing merozoites which enter erythrocytes. *P. falciparum* is able to infect a red cell during any stage of its development. As such, *P. falciparum* cause asynchronous cycles of schizont lysis. This asynchronous release of trophozoites and hemazoin and other toxic metabolites does not necessarily produce the classically described cyclical paroxysms of fever, chills, and rigors. In late stages of infection, infected erythrocytes adhere to the capillary and venule endothelial cells, becoming sequestered in many areas of the body. The brain appears to be preferentially targeted. Parasites are metabolically active, consuming glucose and producing increased amounts of lactate via anaerobic glycolysis.

Current estimates suggest that nearly half of all children admitted to the hospital with falciparum malaria exhibit neurological signs and symptoms. In endemic areas, adults and children develop cerebral disease in similar proportions. The incidence of cerebral malaria in adults is higher in low and moderate transmission areas and areas of varying endemicity than in hyper- and holoendemic areas. In travelers, cerebral malaria occurs in approximately 2.4% of those documented with falciparum malaria infection.

The pathophysiology of cerebral malaria is not completely understood, but appears to be multifactorial. First, sequestration of parasitized red blood cells produces mechanical clogging of the cerebral microvasculature. Infected red blood cells develop parasite-mediated changes in cytoadherent properties due to specific interaction between *P. falciparum* erythrocyte membrane protein (PfEMP-1) and ligands on endothelial cells, such as ICAM-1 or E-selectin. Parasitized cells and nonparasitized red blood cells selectively adhere to each other and to venule and capillary endothelium, termed rosetting. Decreased deformability of infected cells increases obstruction. Platelet microparticles also mediate clumping. Obstruction of the microcirculation leads to a critical reduction in oxygen supply and increase in lactic acidosis locally. Hemazoin is found in cerebral blood vessels on autopsy, suggesting that rupture of sequestered infected erythrocytes may produce local inflammation.

Parasite and host immune response also contribute significantly to the pathophysiology of cerebral malaria. P.falciparum infection and RBC lysis releases both parasite toxins and host intracellular molecules. These are recognized by pattern recognition receptors on immune surveillance cells that promote the activation and release of both pro-inflammatory and anti-inflammatory cytokines from monocytes and neutrophils and upregulation of the expression of adhesion molecules and metabolic changes in endothelial cells. It is thought that this inflammatory response is initially beneficial to the host by reducing parasite growth and activating pathways to eliminate parasites and parasite and host toxins. At later stages, uncontrolled, this inflammatory response causes host damage directly and elimination pathways are inadequate to remove generated toxins. Increased amounts of macrophage-released TNF-α, IL-1, IL-6, IL-10, and other pro-inflammatory cytokines have been documented in murine models and patients with cerebral malaria. Several pediatric studies suggest an association between elevated levels of IL-1 receptor antagonist and severe malaria, while high levels of vascular endothelial growth factor have been found to be protective against death in patients with cerebral malaria. Nitric oxide (NO) has been suggested as a key effector for TNF in malaria pathogenesis. Cytokines upregulate nitric oxide synthase in leukocytes, vascular smooth muscle, microglia, and brain endothelial cells. One theory suggests that uncontrolled amounts of nitric oxide diffuse easily through the injured blood brain barrier. NO may change blood flow and decrease glutamate uptake, producing neuro-excitation. As a potent inhibitor of synaptic neurotransmission, NO also reduces the level of consciousness rapidly and reversibly, similar to that caused by general anesthetics and alcohol. This would explain reversible coma without residual neurological deficits. Apoptosis has been documented in the brainstems of adults who died from cerebral malaria; however, the level of caspase staining was not significantly higher than that in control individuals without malaria.

The blood brain barrier is impaired in patients with cerebral malaria and vascular permeability is increased. T cells have been shown in murine models of cerebral malaria to impair endothelial cell function by perforin-mediated mechanisms leading to blood brain barrier leakage. Postmortem analysis of individuals with cerebral malaria show widespread disruption of vascular cell junctional proteins (occludin and viculin). Diffuse brain swelling is demonstrated on imaging studies and autopsy materials. This swelling is not associated with vasogenic edema. Brain swelling is probably attributable to increased blood volume that occurs secondary to sequestration and increased cerebral blood flow. Greater than 80% of children with cerebral malaria develop elevated ICP and some develop severe intracranial hypertension, and herniation is more common in children. Intracranial hypertension is not seen as frequently in adults.

Risk Factors

A number of factors are associated with poor outcome in cerebral malaria. Historical factors include pretreatment at home with antimalarials and chronic malnutrition. Clinical factors include an abnormal respiratory pattern, hyperpyrexia, hypoperfusion with cool extremities, tachycardia, jaundice, prolonged seizures, and the absence of corneal reflexes or a coma score of 0 or 1. Laboratory factors include hyperparasitemia (>500,000/μL), leukocytosis (>10,000/μL), hypoglycemia, abnormal AST, and elevated lactate and urea levels.

Mortality risk is very high in children less than 5 years of age. Young women during their first pregnancy are at increased risk. Malaria complications in pregnancy are thought to be mediated by placental sequestration of plasmodia and pregnancy-associated anemia and decreases in immune function. Fetal complications include premature birth and low birth weight, severe anemia and death. Nonimmune individuals are also at increased risk. Individuals who live in malaria-endemic areas develop partial immunity to infection after repeated exposure; as such they experience less severe infections.

Individuals with HIV coinfection are at increased risk for worsened clinical outcomes in both infections. Malaria and intestinal helminths often coexist in the same poor populations globally; as such increasing attention is being paid to the interaction between these organisms in coinfected individuals. Data from some recent field studies suggest that helminth coinfection may play a protective role in cerebral malaria, via Th2 response and the interaction between nitric oxide and the low affinity immunoglobulin E binding receptor CD23 [5].

Individuals with sickle cell trait (Hemoglobin S), and less so with Hemoglobin C, thalassemias, glucose-6-phosphate-dehydrogenase deficiency (G6PD) are protected against infection and death from falciparum malaria. Individuals with Hemoglobin E may be protected against vivax malaria. Individuals of West African ancestry lacking RBC Duffy antigen are completely protected against *P. vivax* infection. Several TNF gene-promoter polymorphisms have been shown to be associated with an increased risk of cerebral malaria, neurological sequelae and death. Plasma levels of inducible TNF receptor proteins have been suggested as potential biomarkers of cerebral malaria severity and mortality risk.

Evaluation and Assessment

Almost all patients will have fever, rigors, and chills. Altered sensorium may be present initially or may develop over the course of 24–72 h. Coma usually develops rapidly in children, often after seizure activity. If seizure activity has occurred, the patient should remain unresponsive for more than 30 min to 1 h after active seizure activity to suggest the diagnosis of cerebral malaria rather than postictal state. Approximately 15–20% of adults demonstrate seizure activity. Most seizures appear generalized, but on EEG many are documented to have a focal origin. In adults, coma tends to develop more slowly and may not be associated with seizure activity. Mild neck stiffness may be present, but true meningismus is usually absent. Photophobia is rare. Malarial retinopathy has been demonstrated to be more specific than any other clinical or laboratory feature in distinguishing coma due to malaria from other etiologies. Malarial retinopathy consists of vessel changes, retinal pallor, hemorrhages, and less commonly papilledema. Retinal hemorrhages occur in approximately 15% of cases and may have a white center. Pupils are normally reactive. Transient dysconjugate gaze may be seen. Motor examination usually demonstrates symmetrical upper motor neuron dysfunction, although muscle tone may be decreased. Bilateral extensor plantar reflexes may be seen in comatose patients. Pout reflex, bruxism, jaw spasm, opisthotonos, and decorticate and decerebrate posturing may be present, more commonly in children. Corneal reflexes are preserved except in deep coma. Patients often exhibit a change in diurnal rhythm, with excessive sleepiness during the day and difficulty sleeping at night. Patients may exhibit somnambulism.

The criterion standard diagnostic test for malaria is the microscopic examination of Giemsa-stained blood smears by an appropriately trained individual, including a thin smear to determine the level of parasitemia and a thin smear to speciate the organism(s) present. Three negative sets of smears at 8–12 h intervals are required to rule out malaria. More than one species of malarial organism may be present. Microhematocrit centrifugation and Fluorescent dye Quantitative Buffy Coat staining may also be utilized; however, these do not allow speciation.

Rapid testing (RDT) for *P. falciparum* and *P. vivax* has assumed a more prominent role in the last several years. RDTs are based on antibody recognition of histidine-rich protein 2 (HRP-2) parasite antigens. In most cases, they have been found to be as specific as microscopy, although they are not as reliable when parasite levels are <100 parasites/ml blood. A false positive may occur up 2 weeks post treatment due to the persistence of circulating antigen after parasite death. A list of currently available RDTs, and technical information, can be found at the WHO/WRPO site Malaria Rapid Diagnostic Tests (http://www.wpro.who.int/sites/rdt).

PCR for parasite mRNA or DNA is specific, and more sensitive than microscopy; as such it will detect organisms at very low levels of parasitemia. It is more expensive, requires specific equipment, and does not provide an estimate of the parasite load.

A number of factors globally, including a lack of diagnostic materials and of trained technicians to perform blood smears and rapid testing, low sensitivity of rapid tests in patients with low-level parasitemia, the inability of some treatment centers and hospitals to exclude other diagnoses, lack of severe symptoms in some individuals in endemic areas, a low specificity of the clinical features of the disease, and the concomitant occurrence of other organ dysfunctions and metabolic changes present in severe malaria contribute to both misdiagnosis and overdiagnosis of cerebral malaria. Overdiagnosis leads to unnecessary treatment with potentially dangerous drugs, insufficient investigation of other potentially deadly causes, high mortality rates, and the development of resistance.

Patients will have variable degrees of anemia, thrombocytopenia, and may have jaundice, hepatosplenomegaly, and renal dysfunction. It is important to determine if the patient is pregnant.

A number of factors may contribute to neurological symptoms and signs in malaria. Coinfection may be present, and other causes of fever, such as bacterial meningitis/meningoencephalitis and viral encephalitis, must be considered and ruled out with lumbar puncture and CSF analysis. In malaria, CSF opening pressure is normal to elevated, fluid is clear, protein and lactate levels are elevated to varying degrees, and a mild pleocytosis is present with a white blood cell count less than 10/μL. Fever alone may cause impairment of consciousness, delerium and febrile seizures. Hypoglycemia due to cerebral infection or the use of antimalarials such as quinine may also produce altered mental status, neurological deficits or seizure activity. Hypoglycemia is most common in very young children and pregnant patients. Antimalarial drugs, including chloroquine, quinine, mefloquine and halofantrine may cause neuropsychiatric symptoms, including altered behavior, hallucinations, psychosis, and delerium and seizures. Hyponatremia in elderly patients, due to repeated vomiting, or secondary to injudicious fluid administration may lead to altered mental status and seizures. Severe anemia and hypoxemia may lead to altered mental status. Focal neurological deficits are rare in falciparum malaria and should suggest another cause.

An EEG may be helpful in delineating ongoing seizure activity in the comatose individual. EEG may show a number of nonspecific abnormalities.

Neuroimaging may demonstrate edema, cortical infarcts, hemorrhage, and white matter changes; however, these changes are non-diagnostic for cerebral malaria. MRI may show hemorrhagic lesions and infarction.

After-care

Thin and thick smears should be obtained weekly for at least one month after the patient is discharged to ensure resolution of parasitemia. Individuals with residual neurological issues should be followed to determine resolution or possibly provide additional rehabilitation in those with permanent disability.

Prognosis

Cerebral malaria carries a mortality of approximately 15% in children and 20% in adults. A common cause of death is acute respiratory arrest, which may be due to brain stem herniation. Prolonged duration and deeper level of coma, recurrent episodes of hypoglycemia, severe anemia, renal dysfunction, repeated seizures, and higher cerebral fluid lactate levels are predictors of a worsened prognosis.

Cerebellar ataxia may occur without impaired consciousness and may occur up to 3–4 weeks after an attack of malaria. This usually recovers completely after 1–2 weeks. Other late neurological complications include the post-malaria neurological syndrome (PMNS), acute inflammatory demyelinating polyneuropathy (AIDP) and acute disseminated encephalomyelitis (ADEM). Malaria, and certain antimalarials such as mefloquine, can exacerbate preexisting psychiatric illness. Depression, paranoia, delusions, and personality changes also may develop during convalescence from cases of otherwise uncomplicated malaria. The prevalence of neuropsychiatric deficits ranges between 6% and 29% at the time of discharge from the hospital. Residual deficits are unusual in adults (<3%). Neurologic defects may improve rapidly over weeks to months or may occasionally persist following cerebral malaria, especially in children (10%). Individuals may experience long-term cognitive impairments in speech, language, memory and attention, ataxias, palsies, speech disturbances, deafness, and blindness. In one prospective study of Ugandan children aged 5–12 years, cognitive impairment, most prominently in attention, was present in 26.3% of children with cerebral malaria at 2-year follow-up [6].

Economics

Cerebral malaria is one of the most life-threatening complications of malaria, with an annual incidence of 1.12 cases per 1,000 children, and a 7–18.6% mortality rate, often in the initial 24 h, despite rapid treatment. It accounts for 10% of pediatric admissions in some sub-Saharan hospitals. In 2004, the Disease Control Priorities in Developing Countries project estimated the global burden of malaria, expressed in disability adjusted life years (DALYs), as 42,280,000.

References

1. Hanson J, Lee SJ, Mohanty S et al (2010) A simple score to predict the outcome of severe malaria in adults. Clin Infect Dis 50 (1):679–685
2. Dondorp A, Nosten F, Stepniewska K et al (2005) Artesunate versus quinine for treatment of severe falciparum malaria: a randomized trial. Lancet 366:717–725
3. Enwere GA (2005) A review of the quality of randomized clinical trials of adjunctive therapy for the treatment of cerebral malaria. Trop Med Int Health 10:1171–1175

4. Mishra SJ, Newton CRJC (2009) Diagnosis and management of the neurological complications of falciparum malaria. Nature Rev Neurol 5:189–198

5. Basavaraju SV, Schantz P (2006) Soil-transmitted Helminths and Plasmodium falciparum Malaria: Epidemiology, clinical manifestations, and the role of nitric oxide in Malaria and geo-helminth co-infection. Do worms have a protective role in P.falciparum infection? Mt Sinai J Med 73(8):1098–1105

6. John CC, Bangirana P, Byarugaba J et al (2008) Cerebral malaria in children is associated with long-term cognitive impairment. J Pediatr 122(1):e92–e99

Cerebral Perfusion Pressure

SAMUEL WALLER[1], KATHRYN M. BEAUCHAMP[2]
[1]Department of Neurological Surgery, University of Colorado School of Medicine, Denver, CO, USA
[2]Department of Neurosurgery, Denver Health Medical Center, University of Colorado School of Medicine, Denver, CO, USA

Synonyms
CPP

Definition

Cerebral perfusion pressure (CPP) is the pressure at which the brain receives blood flow. Conceptually speaking, CPP is pressure at which the blood can force its way into the closed box that is the cranial vault and overcome the cranial vault's intrinsic pressure. Clinically, CPP can be derived by taking the difference between the mean arterial pressure and the intracranial pressure (CPP = MAP − ICP). One cannot consider CPP without thinking about cerebral blood flow (CBF) as it is only intuitive that the pressure allows for the tissue to receive its required blood flow. Tissue requires adequate blood flow in order to maintain normal physiologic functioning. CBF is a difficult to measure and derive clinically without specialized equipment. Therefore, CPP is often utilized.

Clinically, CBF is the CPP divided by the cerebral vascular resistance (CVR): CBF = CPP/CVR. It is well known that CBF rates of less than 20 mL per 100 g tissue/min lead to ischemia and, if prolonged, will lead to cell death [1]. In order to conceptualize cerebral blood flow, we then must think about cerebral vascular resistance.

Cerebral vascular resistance is affected by the patient's $PaCO_2$ and CPP. That is to say that in the ranges of $PaCO_2$ 20–80 mmHg, there is a linear increase in CBF for an increase in $PaCO_2$. Similarly, there is a linear relationship between CVR and CPP in the ranges of CPP ∼50–150 mmHg CPP. These variances together are called cerebral autoregulation and exist in order to maintain a near-constant cerebral blood flow.

Normal CPP is >50 mmHg. The critical threshold below which CBF diminishes and ischemia is produced varies per individual but normally is in the range of 50–60 mmHg; hence, it is a typical goal to maintain CPP >60 mmHg [2].

Clinical Relevance

Typically, parameters such as cerebral blood flow and cerebral perfusion pressure matter in settings where an injury such as a stroke, hematoma, intracranial mass lesion, hydrocephalus or similar has occurred. In these settings, neurologic deterioration may be impending and interventions must be implemented in order to preserve brain tissue through preservation of cerebral blood flow. In these settings, again CBF is a difficult clinical number to assess at the bedside in order to help guide therapies but CPP can be derived relatively easily through monitoring of the patient's intracranial pressure.

Intracranial pressure monitoring is generally indicated in any patient whose Glascow Coma Score (GCS) is <9 and who has an abnormal brain imaging study or who has risk factors for intracranial hypertension (age >40, SBP <90, or decerebrate/decorticate posturing on motor examination). Other indications for intracranial pressure monitoring include patients with multiple system injuries requiring therapies that may be deleterious to cerebral blood flow and intracranial pressure such as high levels of positive end-expiratory pressure ventilator settings, high volumes of fluid required for resuscitation, or the need for heavy sedation. Relative contraindications to intracranial pressure monitoring include: (1) the awake patient, as they have a neurologic exam to follow, (2) coagulopathic patients in whom the risk of placing a monitor and causing an acute intracranial mass lesion (hemorrhage) is high, and (3) patients with an exam consistent with brain death who do not respond quickly to empiric therapies to lower intracranial pressure.

Types of intracranial pressure monitoring include: intraventricular catheters, intraparenchymal monitors, subarachnoid screws, subdural monitors, epidural monitors, or in infants fontanometry. Of these, intraventricular catheters and intraparenchymal monitors are the most common.

Means of treating intracranial pressure elevations in order to preserve cerebral perfusion pressure include the following [2]:

1. Elevate the head of the bed to 30°–45° in order to increase venous drainage of the brain
2. Keep the neck inline in order to prevent restriction of jugular venous outflow
3. Avoid tight trach or endotracheal tube taping in order to prevent restriction of jugular venous outflow
4. Avoid hypotension (SBP <90) by ensuring intravascular volume is normalized, use pressors if needed; this ensures cerebral perfusion is not compromised
5. Control hypertension in order to prevent cerebrovascular constriction
6. Avoid hypoxemia (pO_2 <60 mmHg) in order to prevent further ischemic injury and cerebrovascular vasodilation, which increases intracranial pressure
7. Ventilate the patient to normocarbia; hyperventilation is useful as an adjunct for short-term control of intracranial hypertension but long term can worsen ischemic injuries
8. Light sedation

More aggressive measures to control elevations in intracranial pressure include [2]:

1. Heavy sedation and/or paralysis, which reduces sympathetic tone and hypertension caused by movement and tensing abdominal vasculature
2. Drain 3–5 mL of cerebrospinal fluid (if an intraventricular catheter is present), which reduces intracranial volume and therefore the related pressure
3. Mannitol or similar osmotic therapy in order to draw fluid out of the brain parenchyma and possibly improve blood rheology
4. Hypertonic saline, bolus with 10–20 mL of 23.4% saline; when the serum osmolarity is less than 320, some patients refractory to osmotic diuretics will respond to hypertonic saline
5. Hyperventilate to a pCO_2 near 30, which decreases cerebral blood flow and the related intracranial pressure
6. Continued refractory intracranial pressure may require more aggressive therapy and should prompt one to:
   a. Check a noncontrasted head CT in order to ensure there is not a new surgical intracranial lesion
   b. Barbiturate coma (thiopental or pentobarbital), which sedates, treats seizures, and reduces cerebral metabolism and thereby cerebral blood flow without risking further ischemic injury; one must be cautious of the myocardial depressant effect of barbiturates
   c. Decompressive craniectomy, which opens the intracranial vault and physically creates more volume for the brain to expand into
   d. Hypothermia, again reduces cerebral metabolism but has multiple side effects including increased risk for infections, decline in cardiac index, pancreatitis, elevated creatinine clearance, and shivering, which can cause elevations in intracranial pressure [3]

Goals of treatment of intracranial pressure include the following:

1. Intracranial pressure < 20 mmHg [4]
2. Cerebral perfusion pressure >60 mmHg

Cerebral perfusion pressure critical threshold varies by the individual but is in the range of 50–60 mmHg before ischemic injury is encountered. Therefore, goals of treatment should be to maintain a CPP of 60 or greater, thereby ensuring that dips in CPP to levels where ischemia occurs are avoided.

In summary, CPP is the clinical measure whereby physicians can ensure the brain receives the blood flow needed in order to prevent ischemic injury. This is accomplished by measures and treatments of intracranial pressure and monitoring of hemodynamics.

References

1. Astrup J, Siesjo BK, Symon L (1981) Thresholds in cerebral ischemia – the ischemic -penumbra. Stroke 12:723–725
2. Greenburg M (2006) Handbook of neurosurgery, 6th edn. Thieme Medical Publishers, New York
3. Bratton SL, Chestnut RM, Ghajar J et al (2007a) Guidelines for the Management of Severe Traumatic Brain Injury. Journal of Neurotrauma. 24, supplement 1, 31–36
4. Bratton SL, Chestnut RM, Ghajar J et al (2007b) Guidelines for the Management of Severe Traumatic Brain Injury. Journal of Neurotrauma. 24, supplement 1, 65–68

Cerebral Perfusion Pressure (CPP)

Defined as the difference between the mean arterial pressure (MAP) and the intracranial pressure (ICP); CPP = MAP – ICP. The target CPP in the setting of severe TBI is greater than or equal to 60 mmHg.

Cerebral Trauma

▶ Traumatic Brain Injury, Initial Management

Cerebrospinal Fluid Pressure Monitoring

▶ ICP Monitoring

Cervical Rib Syndrome

▶ Thoracic Outlet

Cervicobrachial Syndrome

▶ Thoracic Outlet

Change

Sonia Labeau[1], Dominique Vandijck[1], Stijn Blot[2]
[1]Faculty of Medicine and Health Sciences,
Ghent University, Ghent, Belgium
[2]Department of General Internal Medicine & Infectious Diseases, Ghent University Hospital, Ghent, Belgium

Synonyms

Catheter and line/tubing/administration sets change; Replacement of vascular access devices and line/tubing/ administration sets

Definition

Catheter change is defined as the replacement of a catheter in situ and its administration set(s) by a new catheter and administration set(s).

Administration sets are defined as the area from the spike of tubing entering the fluid container to the hub of the vascular access device. However, a short extension tube might be connected to the catheter and might be considered a portion of the catheter to facilitate aseptic technique when changing administration sets [1].

Rationale

Bloodstream infections associated with the insertion and maintenance of vascular access devices are among the most dangerous complications associated with health care. They have been shown to be associated with increases in patient morbidity and mortality and with a prolonged intensive care unit and hospital stay. Moreover, catheter-related bloodstream infection is associated with high costs of care [2]. The method and frequency of changing catheters and catheter lines can influence the risk of infection.

Methods of Central Venous Catheter Replacement

Central venous catheters can be replaced by percutaneously inserting a new catheter at another body site or by placing a new catheter over a guide wire at the existing site.

Percutaneous Insertion

A catheter's insertion site directly influences the subsequent risk for infection. The density of skin flora at the insertion site is a major risk factor. After insertion, certain sites are easier to maintain clean and dry.

Catheters inserted into an internal jugular vein are associated with a higher risk for infection than those inserted into a subclavian vein. For infection control purposes, the subclavian site is generally recommended. However, this recommendation must be balanced against individual patient-related and noninfectious issues such as patient comfort and mobility and the risk of mechanical complications. In adults, it is strongly recommended to avoid use of the femoral vein for central venous access due to a greater risk of infection and deep venous thrombosis. In children, the increased infection risk has not been demonstrated [3].

Other aspects of catheter insertion, such as the use of maximal sterile barriers, skin antisepsis, use of a checklist and insertion cart, selection of catheter type, and technical insertion issues, are beyond the scope of the current procedure.

Guide Wire Insertion

Guide wire insertion has become an established method to replace a malfunctioning catheter or to exchange a pulmonary artery catheter for a central venous device when invasive monitoring had become superfluous.

The technique offers a better patient comfort and causes a significantly lower rate of mechanical complications as compared to percutaneous insertion at a new body site [2].

Guide wire-assisted catheter exchange to replace a malfunctioning catheter or to exchange an existing catheter is only recommended in the absence of evidence of infection at the catheter site or proven catheter-related bloodstream infection. Suspicion of catheter infection without evidence of infection at the catheter site should lead to removal of the catheter in situ and insertion of a new catheter over a guide wire; if subsequent tests demonstrate catheter-related infection, the newly inserted catheter should be removed and, if still required, another new catheter inserted at a different body site.

In patients with catheter-related infection, replacement of catheters over a guide wire is not recommended. If continued vascular access is required in these patients, the concerned catheter is to be removed and to be replaced with another catheter at a different insertion site [2].

Frequency of Catheter Replacement

In central venous catheters, including peripherally inserted central catheters and hemodialysis catheters, routine catheter replacement without clinical indication has been shown not to reduce the rate of catheter colonization, nor the rate of catheter-related bloodstream infection [2]. The most recent SHEA/IDSA evidence-based recommendations to prevent central line-associated bloodstream infections in acute care hospitals strongly recommend catheter replacement on an as-needed basis only. Routine catheter replacement is not recommended, neither percutaneously nor over a guide wire [3].

In adults, peripheral artery catheters should not be replaced routinely to prevent catheter-related infection [1, 3], while in pediatric patients no recommendation for the frequency of catheter replacement is currently available [1]. Similarly, it is recommended not to replace pulmonary artery catheters to prevent catheter-related infection [1].

Frequency of Replacing Intravenous Tubing and Add-On Devices

In central venous catheters intravenous sets not used for the administration of blood, blood products, or lipids should be replaced at intervals not longer than 96 h [3]. All tubing used to administer blood products or lipid emulsions should be replaced within 24 h of initiating the infusion [1, 4]. Moreover, all fluid administration tubing and connectors should be replaced when the central venous access device is replaced [2].

The above recommendations also pertain to the administration sets of pulmonary artery catheters [1]. In peripheral arterial catheters transducers are to be replaced at 96 h intervals. Continuous flush devices and intravenous tubing are to be replaced at the time the transducer is replaced [1].

Pre-existing Condition
This procedure applies to adult patients with a central venous, pulmonary arterial or peripheral arterial intravascular device in place.

Application
The application described below only pertains to the change in administration sets of central venous catheters. Change in tubing of other vascular access devices can be extrapolated from this description.

The procedure pertaining to the insertion of a catheter percutaneously or by guide wire assistance is beyond the scope of this procedure.

Data Collection
Collect patient and catheter data.
Inform about the need to continue catheterization.

Preparation of Work Area
Restrict activities around bed.
Assure patient privacy and safety.
Make room at the bedside area.
Ensure good visibility.
Adjust the bed height.

Preparation of Material
Clean catheter cart surface.
Ensure all needed material is present.
Apply appropriate hand hygiene.
Open sterile field and dressing packs and prepare using aseptic technique.
Hang new intravenous solution as ordered by physician in reach.
Spike new solution bag with new administration set, protecting distal end from contamination.
Prime intravenous line with appropriate solution to remove all air and clamp administration set with roller clamp.

Preparation of Patient
If possible, explain procedure to patient.

Assist/place patient into backrest position that is both comfortable and convenient for the procedure.

Clear space around the insertion site of clothes and blankets.

Procedure

Take cart to bedside.

Apply appropriate hand hygiene and put on nonsterile gloves.

Place bed protection.

Loosen and remove dressing.

Observe dressing.

Remove gloves and discard gloves and dressing.

Apply appropriate hand hygiene.

Observe and inspect catheter site.

Take culture, if appropriate.

Assess which type of dressing to use.

Peel open dressing packet and open sterile field.

Apply aseptic technique by no-touch technique.

In case of dried blood or drainage at the insertion site, cleanse with sterile NaCl 0.9%.

Disinfect the insertion site with a 2% chlorhexidine-based solution.

Allow the insertion site to air dry.

On the catheter tubing being changed, stop the infusion pump if applicable, and clamp the intravenous line with the roller clamp.

Put on sterile gloves.

Thoroughly swab catheter pigtail and line being changed 5 cm on both sides of port connection with 2% chlorhexidine-based solution and allow to air dry.

According to the type of catheter in situ, clamp off the line of the catheter pigtail being changed with the blue slide clamp or close the catheter lock.

Disconnect cleaned IV line from cleaned catheter pigtail.

Connect new line to catheter pigtail.

Remove blue slide clamp from pigtail or open catheter lock.

Observe for adequate infusion flow.

Observe for leakage or blood back up from catheter pigtail connection site.

Apply appropriate dressing using aseptic technique and fix, avoiding traction and pressure, and bearing patient comfort and mobility in mind.

Place new administration set and solution into infusion pump.

Apply appropriate hand hygiene.

Post-Procedure Care

Install the patient comfortably.

Label IV administration set with time and date of change.

Adjust the bed height.

Remove trolley from bedside area.

Dispose of waste according to the institutional instructions.

Clean the cart surfaces and dry well.

Documentation

Document the lines that have been changed and site assessment in medical record and/or flow sheet.

Record date and time of next line change on flow chart.

Inform physician of signs of infection.

References

1. O'Grady NP, Alexander M, Dellinger EP, Gerberding JL, Heard SO, Maki DG, Masur H, McCormick RD, Mermel LA, Pearson ML, Raad II, Randolph A, Weinstein RA (2002) Guidelines for the prevention of intravascular catheter-related infections. MMWR 51:1–29
2. Pratt RJ, Petlowe CM, Wilson JA, Loveday HP, Harper PJ, Jones S, McDougall C, Wilcox MH (2007) EPIC2: national evidence-based guidelines for preventing healthcare-associated infections in NHS hospitals in England. J Hosp Infect 65:S1–S64
3. Marschall J, Mermel LA, Classen D, Arias KM, Podgorny K, Anderson DJ, Burstin H, Calfee DP, Coffin SE, Dubberke ER, Fraser V, Gerding DN, Griffin FA, Gross P, Kaye KS, Klompas M, Lo E, Nicolle L, Pegues DA, Perl TM, Saint S, Salgado CD, Weinstein RA, Wise R, Yokoe DS (2008) Strategies to prevent central line-associated bloodstream infections in acute care hospitals. Infect Control Hosp Epidemiol 29:S22–30
4. Labeau S, Vandijck D, Lizy C, Piette A, Verschraegen G, Vogelaers D, Blot S (2009) Replacement of administration sets used to administer blood, blood products, or lipid emulsions for the prevention of central line-associated bloodstream infection. Infect Control Hosp Epidemiol 30:494

Chelator

A **chelator** is a chemical compound capable of sequestering a substrate atom, often a metal, via two or more chemical bonds.

Chemical and Physical Forces

They are involved in adsorption including Van der Waals forces generated by atomic and molecular interactions, ionic bonds generated by electrostatic forces and finally hydrophobic bonds.

Chest Bleeding

▶ Hemothorax

Chest Compression (CC)

▶ Cardiopulmonary Resuscitation

Chest Discomfort

▶ Chest Pain: Differential Diagnosis

Chest Infection

▶ Mediastinitis, Postoperative

Chest Pain: Differential Diagnosis

JOHN TOBIAS NAGURNEY
Department of Emergency Medicine, Massachussets
General Hospital, Harvard Medical School, Boston,
MA, USA

Synonyms
Ache; Chest discomfort; Heaviness

Definition
As the name implies, the term "chest pain" refers to "pain," an uncomfortable or unpleasant body sensation that a patient experiences in the "chest" area. The chest is the area of the body located between the neck and the abdomen, and more formally as the area below the clavicles but above the inferior borders of the rib cage. It contains the lungs, the heart, and part of the aorta. The walls of the chest are supported by the dorsal vertebrae, the ribs, and the sternum. This definition represents a good starting point to think about the diseases that cause pain in this area, but is somewhat misleading for two reasons.

The "pain" may represent little more than a vague discomfort or sensation of heaviness all the way to the more classic description of "elephant sitting on my chest." Furthermore, while the chest as an anatomic entity is clearly defined, many of the diseases that cause "chest pain" can present with pain outside the chest as well. An example would be the shoulder or epigastric pain presentation of ▶ acute coronary syndrome. Moreover, many of these diseases can present with non-pain symptoms. Unexplained shortness of breath is a common presentation of acute coronary syndrome in the elderly or of ▶ pulmonary embolism in patients of all ages. As a practical issue, providers learn the differential diagnosis of all of the diseases that can present with chest pain and then learn the alternate presentations of these diseases.

Pathophysiology
Afferent visceral nerve fibers from the intrathoracic organs traverse sympathetic ganglia en route to thoracic dorsal nerve roots and dorsal ganglia. Somatic afferent nerve fibers synapse in the same dorsal ganglia. This complex neurologic configuration leads to visceral pain that is often poorly localized, vague, and capable of radiation to other anatomic areas.

Differential Diagnosis
The ability for the clinician to distinguish among the many diseases presenting with chest pain is truly important. Chest pain is the second most common presenting complaint among emergency department (ED) patients in the USA. The diagnoses of ▶ acute myocardial infarction or unstable angina pectoris are missed in EDs in 2–8% of patients. The missed diagnosis of myocardial infarction represents an estimated 20% of total dollars spent for medical malpractice claims. Because of these among other reasons, most ED providers are relatively conservative in their evaluation and admission practices for patients who present with chest pain. As a result, it is estimated that only a small percent of patients admitted to an observation or in-patient service to rule-out acute coronary syndromes turn out to have that disease.

Chest pain represents a series of syndromes that are both common and difficult to diagnose. The difficulty in diagnosis occurs for a number of reasons. The first is that over 30 diseases or syndromes are scattered among the six different organ systems (lungs and pleura, heart and great vessels, gastroesophageal, nervous system, musculoskeletal system, and others, e.g., psychiatric) that are represented in the chest (Table 1) [1].

A second reason is that many of the diseases which present with chest pain are not easily identified by a single highly sensitive and specific diagnostic study or

Chest Pain: Differential Diagnosis. Table 1 Diseases presenting with chest pain (Adapted from [1])

Organ system	Emergent diagnoses	Urgent but not critical diagnoses	Nonemergent
Cardiovascular	Acute MI Unstable angina Aortic dissection Aortic aneurysm Cardiac tamponade	Pericarditis Myocarditis Severe aortic stenosis	Cardiomyopathy Mitral valve prolapse Noncritical valvular disease
Pulmonary	Pulmonary embolus Tension pneumothorax	Pneumothorax Mediastinitis	Pneumonia Pleuritis Cancer Pneumomediastinum Bronchitis
Gastrointestinal	Esophageal rupture	Cholecystitis Acute pancreatitis	Esophageal spasm Esophageal reflux Peptic ulcer disease Biliary colic Hiatal hernia
Musculoskeletal			Muscle strain Rib fracture Arthritis Tumor Costochondritis
Neurological			Spinal root compression Thoracic outlet syndrome
Other			Herpes zoster Post herpetic neuralgia Hyperventilation Panic attack

procedure. For example, while an ▶ aortic dissection can usually be identified or excluded by an aortic dissection computerized axial tomography, magnetic resonance imaging, a trans-esophageal echocardiogram or an angiogram, pain from musculoskeletal origin is usually a diagnosis of exclusion. There is no single diagnostic test that definitively diagnoses an acute coronary syndrome. This diagnosis is made by a combination of the clinical presentation, electrocardiograms, cardiac biomarkers, and usually an anatomic or physiologic risk stratification test. When the data elements conflict, the definitive final diagnosis often remains in doubt and the term "non-cardiac chest pain" becomes the final diagnosis [2].

Given the fact that diagnosing the cause of chest pain in individual patients can be extremely challenging, the question becomes: what is the most reasonable approach when caring for such a patient? The establishment of the differential diagnosis is largely achieved through a consideration of the patient's demographic data (age and sex), their past medical history, a consideration of risk factors for specific diseases, and the nuances of their chest pain story. The context of the chest pain is important. Chest pain that occurs after trauma has a different differential diagnosis than nontraumatic chest pain. Typically, the provider begins by addressing diseases in the differential diagnosis that, if undiagnosed and untreated, can potentially lead to death within minutes. Classically, these diseases include aortic dissection, massive pulmonary embolism, and acute coronary syndrome. Some authors include tension pneumothorax or pericardial tamponade as well [3]. A second set of diseases can cause potential mortality and significant morbidity, although usually less acutely than this highly lethal group. Examples of diseases in this second category include ▶ pneumonia and multiple rib fractures. The third set of diseases, far more common than the others, include diseases that cause pain, anxiety, and morbidity to patients but usually do not result in loss of life or limb. Examples of diseases in this category include gastroesophageal reflux disease, musculoskeletal chest pain, viral pleurodynia, and herpes zoster. Typically, the patient remains under relatively intensive observation and monitoring until potentially life-threatening diseases are excluded. Once this has been accomplished, potential other diagnoses can be pursued during that hospitalization or as an outpatient. In summary, the primary goal in caring for a patient presenting with chest pain is to perform a brief but accurate risk stratification so that life-threatening diseases can be intervened upon [4].

Most diseases which present with chest pain occur within relatively characteristic age and sex strata. For example, acute coronary syndrome becomes more common with advancing age and is rarely seen in premenopausal women. Conversely, pulmonary embolism is commonly seen in patients of all ages. Young women are at risk because many have risk factors such as pregnancy. After consideration of age and sex, most providers consider the patient's risk factors for particular diseases. For acute coronary syndrome, aortic dissection, and pulmonary embolism these risk factors are relatively well defined. Unfortunately, none are hard-and-fast. For example, approximately 10–20% of patients presenting with acute myocardial infarction lack all five of the classic risk factors for that disease. For many diseases, a history of having had that disease previously represents an important risk factor. In the context of a presentation with acute chest pain, patients with a history of myocardial infarction or pulmonary embolism are more likely to have these respective diseases when compared to patients without such a history. Finally, establishing the differential diagnosis often requires that providers obtain an accurate and complete history of the patient's chest pain story. Unfortunately, many elements of the chest pain story lack sensitivity, specificity, or both [5, 6]. Restated, the chest pain story allows the clinician to establish prior probabilities to be refined by diagnostic testing but these probabilities are at best approximate (Table 2).

Pain Location

The chest pain story begins with pain location. For practical purposes, pain that is substernal or left-sided is equivalent. Pain in these locations is consistent with fatal diseases such as acute coronary syndrome as well as non life-threatening diseases such as gastroesophageal reflux disease and ▶ pericarditis. Pain in the periphery of the chest is more consistent with a disease of pleural, pulmonary, or musculoskeletal origin. Associated with location is the concept of radiation, or extension of the pain into other areas of the body. Again, certain diseases have classic radiations. Examples include the pain of aortic dissection which typically radiates to the back or

Chest Pain: Differential Diagnosis. Table 2 Elements of the chest pain story

Element	Specific details	Comment
Timing		
	Average duration	Seconds, minutes, or hours?
	Frequency	Only once or multiple occurrences?
	Time of onset	First time ever that the pain occurred?
	Time of most recent episode	Within the past 6 h, 24 h, or longer?
Location		Right or left chest, upper or lower, central or peripheral?
Radiation		Where?
Quality		Best descriptive adjective for the pain?
Precipitating factors		Eating, breathing, exertion?
Relieving factors		Resting, nitroglycerin, antacids?
Associated symptoms		Diaphoresis, nausea, shortness of breath?

that of acute myocardial infarction which often radiates to the left shoulder.

Quality and Intensity

The quality and intensity of the pain are the next characteristics that are usually considered. Both of them are, in general, nondiscriminating. The pain of acute myocardial infarction may be described as "pressure," "heaviness," "burning," "aching," or "discomfort." The intensity of the pain is usually also nondiscriminating as well. For example, the intensity of pain in patients presenting with acute myocardial infarction or of acute aortic dissection is usually severe but can be mild or even nonexistent. Conversely, the pain from gastroesophageal reflux or musculoskeletal origin is usually mild but may be extremely severe.

Timing of Pain

The timing of the chest pain is probably the most difficult element of the chest pain story to capture. The concept of timing includes when the pain originally began, its typical duration, the frequency with which it occurs, and the onset of the most recent episode. While no hard-and-fast rules apply, some general principles are useful. One such principle is that pain that has been going on for weeks or months does not usually cause major morbidity or mortality. Conversely, for a patient presenting with an acute myocardial infarction, the average interval between the onset of pain and presentation to an emergency department is between 3 and 9 h. The duration of chest pain from pulmonary, pleural, musculoskeletal, and gastrointestinal sources can be hours without interruption. The number of times per day or week that the pain occurs can be helpful as well. In general, pain that occurs frequently is usually less worrisome than pain that occurs occasionally. Finally, the time of the most recent occurrence can be used to determine the value of certain diagnostic tests such as cardiac biomarkers.

Relieving and Precipitating Factors

Cardiac pain is typically precipitated by exertion and relieved by rest. It is often relieved by stopping a strenuous activity. Chest pain from pleural, pulmonary, or musculoskeletal sources is often worsened by coughing or deep breathing. Examples include the pains of viral pleuritis, pulmonary embolism, pneumonia, or intercostal muscle strain.

Associated Symptoms

Symptoms that typically accompany the chest pain can increase the probability of certain diseases. For example, nausea and diaphoresis are common accompaniments to chest pain in patients presenting with acute coronary syndrome. A sour taste in a patient's mouth during episodes of chest pain increases the possibility of gastroesophageal reflux disease. And acute neurologic symptoms accompanying chest pain increase the probability that the chest pain is caused by an aortic dissection.

Cross-Reference to Disease

▶ Acute Coronary Syndrome
▶ Acute Myocardial Infarction
▶ Aortic Dissection
▶ Aortic Stenosis
▶ Pericarditis
▶ Pneumonia
▶ Pneumothorax, Tension Pneumothorax
▶ Pulmonary Embolism

References

1. Brown JE, Hamilton GC (2010) "Chest pain." Rosen's emergency medicine: concepts and clinical practice, 7th edn. Mosby Elsevier, Philadelphia, pp 132–141
2. Lenfant C (2010) Chest pain of cardiac and noncardiac origin. Metabolism 59(Suppl 1):S41–S46
3. Jones ID, Slovis CM (2001) Emergency department evaluation of the chest pain patient. Emerg Med Clin North Am 19:269–282
4. Jesse RL, Kontos MC (1997) Evaluation of chest pain in the emergency department. Curr Probl Cardiol 22:149–236
5. Goodacre S, Locker T, Morris F, Campbell S (2002) How useful are clinical features in the diagnosis of acute, undifferentiated chest pain? Acad Emerg Med 9:203–208
6. Swap CJ, Nagurney JT (2005) Value and limitations of chest pain history in the evaluation of patients with suspected acute coronary syndromes. JAMA 294(20):2623–2629

Chest Tube: Chest Drain or Thoracostomy Tube

▶ Thoracocentesis and Chest Tubes

Chest Wall Stabilization

Donald D. Trunkey[1], John C. Mayberry[2]
[1]Department of Surgery, Oregon Health & Science University, Portland, OR, USA
[2]Trauma/Critical Care, Oregon Health & Science University, Portland, OR, USA

Synonyms

Fixation or repair; Flail chest stabilization; Rib and/or sternal fracture operative reduction and internal fixation (ORIF)

Definition

Chest wall stabilization is a surgical procedure in which rib and/or sternal fractures are reduced (i.e., the fracture ends are realigned and brought into proximity) and the fractures are fixated with a plating system.

Pre-existing Condition

Chest wall injury syndromes for which operative intervention may be indicated are listed in Table 1. Category recommendations are based upon review of literature and upon the authors' experience.

Flail chest is defined by three or more ribs fractured in two or more places. Paradoxical motion of the chest wall (i.e., flail motion) may or may not be visible. If the patient has already been endotracheally intubated and mechanically ventilated, the flail segment will not be externally

Chest Wall Stabilization. Table 1 Recommendations for chest wall stabilization for each indication

Chest wall injury	Category recommendation
Flail chest	II
Chest wall implosion syndrome	II
Chest wall defect/pulmonary herniation	I
Intractable acute pain with displaced fractures	III
Thoracotomy for other ("on the way out")	III
Displaced or comminuted acute sternal fracture	III
Rib or sternal fracture nonunion (pseudoarthrosis)	III

apparent. The diagnosis is established by CT scan. Two small, single center randomized trials and cohort comparison studies have demonstrated several benefits of early flail chest ORIF including decreased intensive care length of stay, less pneumonia, early return to work, and improved forced vital capacity (FVC) [1, 2].

Chest wall implosion syndrome is characterized by multiple, displaced rib fractures along the medial edge of the scapula, a clavicle fracture/dislocation, and often a scapular fracture. Although this injury does not meet the anatomic definition of flail chest, these patients are physiologically similar to patients with anterolateral flail chest, i.e., nearly all will require mechanical ventilation for respiratory failure [3].

Chest wall defect or acute pulmonary herniation is a rare injury where a portion of the chest wall is traumatically missing or the lung herniates through the chest wall, e.g., through an intercostal muscle tear with associated rib fractures. Operative repair is indicated to debride severely damaged tissue and to restore pulmonary mechanical integrity. A bioprosthesis such as acellular human or porcine dermis may be necessary to cover the tissue defect. Serial operations with staged repair are recommended for more severe tissue defects. Operative intervention is the standard of care based on the lack of an acceptable alternative to surgical repair [4].

An occasional patient with significant displacement including overriding of the fractured ribs will complain of intractable pain with attempts at mobilization which defies the usual attempts at pain control including epidural catheter infusion. This indication has not been studied, but in the authors' experience ORIF of the displaced rib

fractures can result in a dramatic improvement in pain and allow the patient to recuperate and return to normal function more rapidly.

Thoracotomy for other indications or "on the way out" indicates a patient with rib fractures who requires a thoracotomy for a traumatic indication such as retained hemothorax, pulmonary laceration, ruptured diaphragm, or even aortic injury. As the surgeon is closing the thoracotomy it may be reasonable, depending on the nature of the rib fractures and the condition of the patient, to take extra time to include rib fracture ORIF with the intent of preventing future disability. This indication also applies to non-traumatic situations where ribs are fractured or purposely cut during thoracotomy exposure for elective surgery. Rib fracture ORIF for this indication can be considered safe in select patients but has not been studied for efficacy.

Sternal fractures are occasionally acutely repaired when they are completely displaced or comminuted. The literature describing the operative techniques and results are case series only and include no comparison groups [5]. Acute sternal fracture ORIF is therefore an acceptable option in select patients and can be considered safe, but warrants a Category III recommendation only.

Rib or sternal fracture nonunions (pseudoarthroses) occur in 1–5% of patients and can be a source of persistent pain and disability. Resection of the pseudocapsule and margins of the bony defect to reinitiate osteosynthesis in conjunction with internal fixation has been reported as successful and efficacious in case series [5]. The successful use of bone grafting techniques in situations of bone loss for both rib and sternal fracture nonunions has also been described. Neither indication has been studied in a controlled fashion and, therefore, warrants a Category III recommendation only.

Four different levels of recommendations exist:

- Category I. Operative intervention is standard of care.
- Category II. Operative intervention is acceptable in selected patients based on the results of single-center randomized trials and case-control series.
- Category III. Operative intervention is not clearly indicated based on insufficient evidence.
- Category IV. Operative intervention has been demonstrated to have a lack of efficacy.

Application
Several plating systems have been used but none has proven superior to another. Both metal and absorbable plates have been used successfully [3]. Ribs are classified as membranous bone because of their relatively thin cortex

compared to their inner marrow and are not expected to hold a plate and/or screws as reliably as cortical or cancellous bone. Efficacious plating systems must also take into account the curvature of ribs and the constant stress of respiratory effort of the patient during the several weeks of healing process.

References

1. Tanaka H, Yukioka T, Yamaguti Y, et al (2002) Surgical stabilization of internal pneumatic stabilization? A prospective randomized study of management of severe flail chest patients. J Trauma 52 (4):727–732; discussion 32
2. Marasco S, Cooper J, Pick A, Kossmann T (2009) Pilot study of operative fixation of fractured ribs in patients with flail chest. ANZ J Surg 79(11):804–808
3. Solberg BD, Moon CN, Nissim AA, Wilson MT, Margulies DR (2009) Treatment of chest wall implosion injuries without thoracotomy: technique and clinical outcomes. J Trauma 67(1):8–13; discussion
4. Mayberry JC, Ham LB, Schipper PH, Ellis TJ, Mullins RJ (2009) Surveyed opinion of American trauma, orthopedic, and thoracic surgeons on rib and sternal fracture repair. J Trauma 66:875–879
5. Richardson JD, Franklin GA, Heffley S, Seligson D (2007) Operative fixation of chest wall fractures: an underused procedure? Am Surg 73(6):591–596; discussion 6–7

Chicago Disease

▶ Blastomycosis

Childbed Fever

▶ Puerperal Sepsis

Child-Pugh

Also known as Child-Turcotte-Pugh is a prognostic scoring system used in patients with cirrhosis which consists of five components, namely, bilirubin, albumin, INR, ascites, and hepatic encephalopathy. Based on the levels of each of these parameters, a score of 1–3 is awarded for each component with a composite score of 6 or less equating to Child-Pugh A, 7–9 to Child-Pugh B, and 10 or more to Child-Pugh C disease. Prognosis worsens as an individual moves from Child-Pugh A through to Child-Pugh C cirrhosis.

Chirodropid Jellyfish

▶ Jellyfish Envenomation

Chironex fleckerfi

▶ Jellyfish Envenomation

Choice of Catheter Lumen

▶ Port Designation

Cholangiopathy

▶ HIV-Related Cholecystitis

Cholecystitis

CHRISTOPHER M. WATSON[1], ROBERT G. SAWYER[2]
[1]Division of Trauma and Acute Care Surgery, Palmetto Health, Columbia, SC, USA
[2]Department of Surgery, University of Virginia Health System, Charlottesville, VA, USA

Synonyms

Acute acalculous cholecystitis; Acute calculous cholecystitis; Acute cholecystitis

Definition

Cholecystitis is defined as inflammation of the gallbladder. The disease can present acutely without prior symptoms but more commonly after episodes of biliary colic, associated with or without gallstones, in which case the descriptor calculous or acalculous is added, respectively. In either case, it is believed that stasis of bile and gallbladder ischemia occur leading to inflammation of the gallbladder wall and eventually to surrounding structures as well resulting in a localized peritonitis. It was originally thought that the disease was solely attributable to infection. Later, in the early 1940s, studies on animals demonstrated that stasis was a primary pathologic condition that was necessary but not sufficient for cholecystitis to develop.

With further work, it became clearer that ischemia was also an important part of the pathogenesis. Since acute calculous cholecystitis develops as a result of impaction of a gallstone in the cystic duct, two conditions are met: bile stasis and localized ischemia from distension of the gallbladder wall.

In acute acalculous cholecystitis (AAC), ischemia and stasis are also present although with distinct mechanisms. A generalized ischemic insult, whether from trauma, surgery, or a condition such as septic shock or vasopressor use, is thought to precede inflammation. Stasis is due to decreased gallbladder contraction secondary to starvation or the severe disease state itself. Traditionally, postoperative states or trauma were most commonly associated with the development of AAC, but a review of patients undergoing cholecystectomy for AAC found that infection was the most common admission diagnosis, with postoperative state and trauma in only 33% [1]. In the general medical and surgical population, patients with AAC tend to be sicker with higher Sequential Organ Failure Assessment (SOFA) scores [1], whereas in the trauma population other markers of severity, such as Injury Severity Score, number of units of packed red blood cells transfused, and tachycardia, are associated with AAC [2]. Although prolonged nil per os (NPO) status has been associated with this disease, the same study found 56% had received mainly enteral nutrition, while the remainder received mainly parenteral nutrition [1]. More indirect evidence seems to contradict this observation. A randomized controlled trial of postoperative patients receiving either enteral nutrition or intravenous saline infusion showed that gallbladder volume was lower with the former treatment thus indicating less stasis of bile [3]. There was no discussion of the proportion of patients developing AAC in either group.

The role of bacteria in cholecystitis is still being defined. Matsushiro et al. evaluated 52 patients presenting with acute cholecystitis for the presence of bacteria in the gallbladder at the time of cholecystectomy [4]. They found bacteria present in 52% of those gallbladders with stones and 33% of those without stones, although the generally agreed upon culture positivity rate in acute cholecystitis is in the 60–80% range. Of those with stones, those gallbladders with impacted stones more likely had bacteria present. Time to surgery did not show significantly different bacteria in this study, although in other studies, patients undergoing cholecystectomy earlier than 72 h after symptoms began were less likely to have bacteria in their gallbladder. Also, infected bile seems to be more common with age. Further complicating the picture is the finding that the region of gallbladder cultured may also determine whether bacteria are recovered [5].

Specific organisms differ somewhat regionally, but enteric gram-negative aerobes, especially *Escherichia coli* and *Klebsiella* species, and *Streptococcus (Enterococcus) faecalis* predominated in the Matsushiro review. Other reviews demonstrated more anaerobes, accounting for as much as 25% of bacterial isolates [6].

Diagnosis

Traditionally, clinical indicators of infection or inflammation and right upper quadrant abdominal pain, coupled with data from specific imaging modalities, have been used to diagnose both acute cholecystitis and AAC. Although fever and an abnormal white blood cell count (WBC) may be present, they are not invariably so. The Tokyo Guidelines require both local and systemic signs of inflammation to suspect cholecystitis, and typical imaging findings to confirm cholecystitis (Table 1) [7]. In AAC,

Cholecystitis. Table 1 Tokyo guideline grading system for acute cholecystitis

Mild (grade I) acute cholecystitis	• Does not meet the criteria for moderate (grade II) or severe (grade III) cholecystitis • Also defined as a healthy patient with no organ dysfunction and mild local inflammation making cholecystectomy a low-risk procedure
Moderate (grade II) cholecystitis – any one of the following	• WBC > 18,000/mm^3 • Palpable, tender, RUQ mass • Duration of complaints >72 h • Marked local inflammation (biliary peritonitis, pericholecystic abscess, hepatic abscess, gangrenous cholecystitis, emphysematous cholecystitis)
Severe (grade III) cholecystitis – organ system dysfunction	• Cardiovascular dysfunction (requiring vasopressors or inotropes) • Neurologic (depressed level of consciousness) • Respiratory (P:F < 300) • Renal dysfunction (oliguria, creatinine > 2.0 mg/dl) • Hepatic (PT-INR > 1.5) • Hematologic (platelet count <100,000/mm^3)

Source: Adapted from [21].

fever may be present in only 13% and leukocytosis in only 54% [1]. Unlike acute appendicitis, where right lower quadrant pain and a correlative history may lead directly to the operating room without further study, imaging should always be included in the work-up of presumed acute cholecystitis. This is because no examination finding alone has been found sufficiently accurate to justify cholecystectomy, and associated findings, such as the presence of stones or dilated common bile duct, may change the procedure to include an intraoperative cholangiogram or common bile duct exploration. Also, signs of gangrenous, emphysematous, or perforated cholecystitis will affect prognosis and the likelihood of conversion to an open procedure. The most important imaging studies are focused ultrasonography (US) or scintigraphy (HIDA, Hepatobiliary iminodiacetic Acid), and computed tomography (CT) with intravenous contrast. More recently, modifications of these modalities have been introduced and may increase accuracy but have not penetrated the mainstream. Magnetic resonance imaging (MRI) may also have a role in the diagnosis of cholecystitis in difficult cases, but especially for possible malignancy or evaluation for CBD stones.

Ultrasound

US findings consistent with cholecystitis include gallstones, especially incarcerated, or debris echo; a positive sonographic Murphy's sign; wall thickening (>4 mm); gallbladder distention (long axis >8 cm, short axis >4 cm); and pericholecystic fluid. Of these findings, the first three are considered the most specific [8], especially when considered together. For example, the findings of gallstones with a sonographic Murphy's sign or wall thickening has a positive predictive value for cholecystitis of 92% and 95%, respectively [9]. But, sensitivity for the diagnosis of cholecystitis is, as with all US studies, operator dependent. In a later study, sensitivity of US diagnosis of cholecystitis compared with histology was only 48% [10], but a meta-analysis by Shea et al. reported a sensitivity of 94% for the diagnosis of acute cholecystitis [11]. Recently studies have evaluated surgeon-performed US as a modality for diagnosis of cholecystitis. These studies show that resident surgeons with minimal training could detect gallstones and cholecystitis as well as consultant radiologists [12].

Ultrasound also has a poor sensitivity when used alone for the detection of AAC. In a study of critically ill patients undergoing open cholecystectomy for presumed AAC, only 80% had an abnormal US prior to surgery [1]. Similarly, in a trauma ICU population, US had a sensitivity of 30% and specificity of 93% [13]. However, in another study of trauma patients, all patients with thickening and layering of the gallbladder wall or necrotic degeneration, edema of the surrounding tissue, and/or impending rupture coupled with major clinical symptoms (pain and/or abdominal distention, hemodynamic instability requiring increasing amounts of vasopressors and/or fluid resuscitation and organ failure) were found to have AAC.

Scintigraphy

Hepatobiliary scintigraphy evaluates the biliary uptake of Tc-99 m-labeled iminodiacetic acid agents (Tc-99 m IDA) and has a high sensitivity and specificity for the diagnosis of acute cholecystitis. A study that does not show filling of the gallbladder with contrast within 60 min is considered positive for cholecystitis. Another sign that is suspicious for cholecystitis is a "rim sign," defined as augmentation of radioactivity around the gallbladder fossa. After its introduction, scintigraphy was suggested as a first-line test in patients with presumed cholecystitis. Sensitivity and accuracy were 91% and 93% in an early study [14]. Specificity, however, was lacking. This led early investigators to suggest that a positive result indicated cholecystitis only when serum bilirubin was less than 5 mg/dl while in patients with bilirubin higher than 5 mg/dl the test was considered indeterminate. A negative test was considered reliable. However, an evaluation done a decade later found a similar sensitivity (94%), but a specificity of only 36% [15]. This low specificity led these later investigators to suggest HIDA be eliminated as a first-line study. Confounding the issue even more was a study comparing US, HIDA, and combined US/HIDA. HIDA was found to be more sensitive than US and again the recommendation was made to use HIDA as a first-line study, only using US when stones are suspected in order to evaluate for common bile duct dilation or obstructing stones [10, 16]. With better contrast agents and patient selection, specificity has improved. Also, morphine can be given to increase the tone of the sphincter of Oddi. Filling of the GB within 30 min is considered a negative test with a false-negative rate of only 0.5%. Filling between 30 min and 4 h increases the false-negative rate to 15–20% [17]. However, in a corroborating study, morphine cholescintigraphy had a sensitivity of 99%, a specificity of 91%, a positive predictive value of 0.9, a negative predictive value of 0.99, and an overall accuracy of 94%. This study detected both calculous and acalculous cholecystitis [18].

Computed Tomography

Although not required in all cases of presumed cholecystitis, CT is often used when HIDA scintigraphy and US are indeterminate or to evaluate for associated pathology such as gangrenous or emphysematous cholecystitis. Both of these latter findings carry a higher mortality than uncomplicated acute cholecystitis and require conversion to open procedure more often. The presence of these signs may lead to more urgent surgery and a more prolonged antibiotic course postoperatively. Findings consistent with acute cholecystitis are much the same as US, absent the sonographic Murphy's sign of course. The detection of stones is also limited, such that only 75% of stones are seen on CT. As such, the most specific sign of cholecystitis is pericholecystic inflammatory changes. Overall sensitivity, specificity, and accuracy of CT for the diagnosis of cholecystitis in one study was 92%, 99%, and 94%, respectively [19], and in another directly comparing US with CT, was 100% accurate, sensitive, and specific for the diagnosis of acute cholecystitis [20].

For AAC, CT has a variable sensitivity. In a study by Laurila et al., only 58% of patients had CT signs of AAC prior to operation but in another study, CT was used to correctly diagnose AAC in six of seven patients with one false positive finding. CT may have an adjunctive role in patients with indeterminate US studies though [2].

Magnetic Resonance Imaging (MRI) and Other Imaging Modalities

In a comparison of MRI with US, there was no difference in the diagnosis of acute cholecystitis with a sensitivity of 50% for both and specificities of 89% and 86% for US and MRI, respectively [21]. The authors suggested that limited MRI may be indicated for "sonographically challenging" patients. This likely means patients with large amounts of bowel gas or other anatomically hidden gallbladders and/or ductal structures. Cost-effectiveness was not evaluated, however. Another modality currently being investigated for both diagnosis and treatment of cholecystitis in the critically ill patient is bedside laparoscopy.

Conclusion

In conclusion, US should be performed as a first-line study for presumed cholecystitis because of its broad availability and ability to be performed at bedside. If in a patient with a clinical picture of acute cholecystitis and an US that shows stones and either a thickened GB wall or a sonographic Murphy's sign, then the patient should be treated for cholecystitis. If the US is indeterminate, and clinical suspicion is low, morphine-HIDA scintigraphy should be used to rule-out the diagnosis. If, however, the clinical suspicion is high, CT scanning should be performed to try to rule-in the diagnosis. CT is also indicated for patients with known cholecystitis that may have emphysematous or gangrenous cholecystitis who

would otherwise have been treated conservatively, since these signs indicate the need for urgent surgery. If on any of the imaging studies the patient has distal CBD dilation, an MRCP may be useful to evaluate for obstructing CBD stones unless the surgeon is experienced with CBD exploration.

Treatment

Controversy exists over the optimal treatment of acute cholecystitis. In an attempt to better define the categories of severity of cholecystitis and thus guide treatment, The Tokyo Guidelines were developed [7]. Experts in the fields of cholecystitis and cholangitis convened to develop standardized diagnostic criteria, a severity grading system, and a treatment guideline based on this grading system (Table 1). The categories were based on factors increasing the likelihood of conversion to an open procedure and the possibility of complications during surgery. Certain high-risk situations may increase the likelihood of conversion to an open procedure, such as a white-cell count of more than 18,000 cells/mm^3 at the time of presentation, duration of symptoms of greater than 72–96 h, and an age over 60 years, all of which are indicators of a more advanced disease and increased likelihood of perforation or emphysematous changes [22]. These guidelines have not gained widespread acceptance yet and need to be validated in well-constructed trials.

Patients with mild cholecystitis should be treated with antibiotics with or without early laparoscopic cholecystectomy, depending on the patient's operative risk. Those with moderate cholecystitis are the most difficult to draw firm conclusions regarding treatment. These patients can also be treated with early laparoscopic cholecystectomy, especially if symptoms have been present for less than 96 h. In a prospective cohort study of laparoscopic versus open cholecystectomy for gangrenous cholecystitis, patients having a cholecystectomy completed laparoscopically had significantly shorter ICU stays, less ileus, but more abscess formation [23]. Bile leaks were more common in the laparoscopic group (12% versus 6% in the open group) but this did not reach statistical significance. Since conversion to open cholecystectomy is higher in this group, attempts at laparoscopic surgery should only be made in those that could tolerate an open surgical procedure and by an experienced laparoscopic surgeon. A Cochrane Review was performed evaluating studies of timing of cholecystectomy for acute cholecystitis. The authors noted that early laparoscopic cholecystectomy was feasible and preferred in some select patients as long as an experienced laparoscopic surgeon performed the procedure. This recommendation was based on the observation that 17.5% of patients undergoing delayed treatment had recurrent cholecystitis requiring operation and of those undergoing laparoscopic surgery, 45% required conversion to an open procedure [24]. Because of the small size of the included studies, conclusions could not be made regarding the more rare complications, such as bile duct injury. Large population studies seem to imply a higher rate of bile duct injury in the early group. If these patients are poor operative risks, percutaneous cholecystostomy drainage is an alternative. In the most severe patients with organ failure, percutaneous drainage is preferred, but in the rare situation in which this cannot be accomplished, laparoscopic cholecystectomy should be performed if possible, with early conversion to open surgery if needed. Whether cholecystostomy should be followed by interval surgery or endoscopic sphincterotomy is also debated. In a study of patients in the ICU that had interval surgery during the same admission, the conversion rate was 14% compared to the hospital-wide conversion rate of 1.4% [25]. In another study of patients with Grade II or III cholecystitis in the ICU treated with percutaneous cholecystostomy tube placement only two of 21 patients at a mean of 17.5 months follow-up presented with recurrent cholecystitis, and both of these were successfully treated by conservative means [26].

The use of antibiotics in patients with acute cholecystitis is not controversial but the length of treatment continues to be a source of debate. In patients undergoing early cholecystectomy (<72 h from the onset of symptoms), standard perioperative (<24 h) antibiotics should be administered. In patients that are very ill from cholecystitis, had a delay in treatment >72 h, are immunosuppressed, are > 60 years old, or have concomitant cholangitis, a prolonged course of treatment, usually no longer than 7 days, is indicated. Although the Tokyo Guidelines do not comment on antibiotic length of treatment it can be extrapolated that patients with Grade I or II cholecystitis can have perioperative dosing lasting less than 24 h, while those with Grade III should likely receive a 7–14 day course. If infected with a resistant pathogen or associated bacteremia is noted, antibiotics may need to be continued for 14 days.

The choice of antibiotic should include coverage for gram-negative enteric pathogens, as well as anaerobic bacteria. Enterococcal species need not be covered. In community acquired infections that are mild, ampicillin/sulbactam, ticarcillin/clavulinate, or ertapenem may be selected. In high-risk patients, and those with recent hospitalization or antibiotic use of more broadspectrum agents, such as pipericillin/tazobactam or meropenem.

After-care

Most patients that have cholecystitis treated adequately require no special aftercare. Patients can expect to spend between 1 and 7 days in the hospital depending on the severity of the cholecystitis, whether the surgery was laparoscopic or open, and whether prolonged antibiotics are administered. Patients are allowed to resume a regular diet as soon as ileus resolves which again is dependent on the type of surgery. Some patients may experience early fatty meal intolerance but this is expected to resolve within a few weeks as the patient alters their diet to compensate.

Patients treated with percutaneous drain placement do require special care. The patient will be discharged with the tube in place. Most will have had the tube clamped prior to discharge and are educated about tube care and what symptoms should prompt resumption of drainage. If the tube was placed for calculous disease, a contrast study is performed to evaluate for remaining stones. If stones remain, a decision to remove these is made in conjunction with a surgeon, endoscopist, and interventional radiologist. If the patient is an operative candidate, cholecystectomy can be performed. In older more debilitated patients an endoscopic sphincterotomy can be performed with the expectation of good results. An alternative is exchange of the percutaneous cholecystostomy tube using a guidewire to a larger bore tube followed by stone extraction. When it has been verified that all stones are cleared and the common bile duct is patent, the tube can be removed.

Prognosis

Prognosis after cholecystectomy is excellent. If performed by an experienced laparoscopic surgeon the rate of complications is very low. Most studies comparing early to late cholecystectomy show that delayed surgery results in a relatively large number of patients presenting with recurrent cholecystitis requiring urgent operation prior to the planned cholecystectomy. A large number of these patients will need open surgery. From other studies that evaluate interval cholecystectomy, it appears that conversion rates are lower in those that actually make it to planned operation.

References

1. Laurila J, Syrja LA, Laurila PA, Ala-Kokko TI (2004) Acute acalculous cholecystitis in critically ill patients. Acta Anaesthesiol Scand 48:986–991
2. Pelinka LE, Schmidhammer R, Hamid L et al (2003) Acute acalculous cholecystitis after trauma: a prospective study. J Trauma 55:323–329
3. Sustic A, Krznaric Z, Naravic M et al (2000) Infuence on gallbladder volume of early postoperative gastric supply of nutrients. Clin Nutr 19(6):413–416

4. Matsushiro T, Sato T, Umezawa A et al (1997) Pathogenesis and the role of bacteria in acute cholecystitis. J Hepatobiliary Pancreat Surg 4:91–94

5. Manolis EN, Filippou DK, Papadopoulos VP, Kaklamanos I, Katostaras T, Christianakis E, Bonatsos G, Tsakris A (2008) The culture site of the gallbladder affects recovery of bacteria in symptomatic cholelithiasis. J Gastrointest Liver Dis 17(2):179–182

6. Claesson B, Holmlund D, Mätzsch T (1984) Biliary microflora in acute cholecystitis and the clinical implications. Acta Chir Scand 150:229–237

7. Mayumi T, Takada T, Kawarada Y, Nimura Y, Yoshida M et al (2007) Results of the Tokyo consensus meeting Tokyo guidelines. J Hepatobiliary Pancreat Surg 14:114–121

8. Bennett GL, Balthazar EJ (2003) Ultrasound and CT evaluation of emergent gallbladder pathology. Radiol Clin North Am 41 (6):1203–1216

9. Ralls PW, Colletti PM, Lapin SA et al (1985) Real-time sonography in suspected acute cholecystitis: prospective evaluation of primary and secondary signs. Radiology 155:767–771

10. Kalimi R, Gecelter GR, Caplin D, Brickman M, Tronco GT, Love C, Yao J, Simms HH, Marini CP (2001) Diagnosis of acute cholecystitis: sensitivity of sonography, cholescintigraphy, and combined sonography-cholescintigraphy. J Am Coll Surg 193 (6):609–613

11. Shea JA, Berlin JA, Escarce JJ, Clarke JR, Kinosian BP, Cabana MD, Tsai WW, Horangic N, Malet PF, Schwartz JS et al (1994) Revised estimates of diagnostic test sensitivity and specificity in suspected biliary tract disease. Arch Intern Med 154(22): 2573–2581

12. Eiberg JP, Grantcharov TP, Eriksen JR, Boel T, Buhl C, Jensen D, Pedersen JF, Schulze S (2008) Ultrasound of the acute abdomen performed by surgeons in training. Minerva Chir 63(1):17–22

13. Puc MM, Tran HS, Wry PW, Ross SE (2002) Ultrasound is not a useful screening tool for acute acalculous cholecystitis in critically ill trauma patients. Am Surg 68(1):65–69

14. Bennett MT, Sheldon MI, dos Remedios LV, Weber PM (1981) Diagnosis of acute cholecystitis using hepatobiliary scan with technetium-99 m PIPIDA. Am J Surg 142(3):338–343

15. Johnson H Jr, Cooper B (1995) The value of HIDA scans in the initial evaluation of patients for cholecystitis. J Natl Med Assoc 87 (1):27–32

16. Alobaidi M, Gupta R, Jafri SZ, Fink-Bennet DM (2004) Current trends in imaging evaluation of acute cholecystitis. Emerg Radiol 10(5):256–258, Epub 2004 Mar 17

17. Hicks RJ, Kelly MJ, Kalff V (1990) Association between false negative hepatobiliary scans and initial gallbladder visualization after 30 min. Eur J Nucl Med 16:747–753

18. Flancbaum L, Choban PS, Sinha R, Jonasson O (1994) Morphine cholescintigraphy in the evaluation of hospitalized patients with suspected acute cholecystitis. Ann Surg 220(1):25–31

19. Bennett GL, Rusinek H, Lisi V, Israel GM, Krinsky GA, Slywotzky CM et al (2002) CT findings in acute gangrenous cholecystitis. AJR Am J Roentgenol 178:275–281

20. De Vargas Macclucca M, Lanciotti S, De Cicco ML, Bertini L, Colalacomo MC, Gualdi G (2006) Imaging of simple and complicated acute cholecystitis. Clin Ter 157(5):435–442

21. Oh KY, Gilfeather M, Kennedy A, Glastonbury C, Green D, Brant W, Yoon HC (2003) Limited abdominal MRI in the evaluation of acute right upper quadrant pain. Abdom Imaging 28(5):643–651

22. Strasberg SM (2008) Acute calculous cholecystitis. N Engl J Med 358 (26):2804–2811

23. Stefanidis D, Bingener J, Richards M et al (2005) Gangrenous cholecystitis in the decade before and after the introduction of laparoscopic cholecystectomy. JSLS 9:169–173

24. Gurusamy KS, Samraj K, Fusai G, Davidson BR (2008) Early versus delayed laparoscopic cholecystectomy for biliary colic. Cochrane Database Syst Rev 8(4):CD007196

25. Spira RM, Nissan A, Zamir O, Cohen T, Fields SI, Freund HR (2002) Percutaneous transhepatic cholecystectomy and delayed laparoscopic cholecystectomy in critically ill patients with acute calculous cholecystitis. Am J Surg 183:62–66

26. Griniatsos J, Petrou A, Pappas P et al (2008) Percutaneous cholecystostomy without interval cholecystectomy as definitive treatment of acute cholecystitis in elderly and critically ill patients. South Med J 101(6):586–590

Chronic Bronchial Sepsis

▶ Bronchitis and Bronchiectasis

Chronic Bronchitis

▶ Decompensated Chronic Obstructive Pulmonary Disease

Chronic Kidney Disease (CKD)

▶ Decreased Estimated Glomerular Filtration Rate (eGFR): Interpretation in Acute and Chronic Kidney Disease

Chronic Lung Disease

▶ Decompensated Chronic Obstructive Pulmonary Disease

Chronic Obstructive Airway Disease

▶ Decompensated Chronic Obstructive Pulmonary Disease

Chronic Salicylate Toxicity

▶ Salicylate Overdose

Churg–Strauss Syndrome

▶ Pulmonary-Renal Syndrome

Chylothorax

LAURA J. MOORE
Department of Surgery, The Methodist Hospital Research
Institute, Houston, TX, USA

Synonyms
Chylous pleural effusion

Definition
Chylothorax is defined as the presence of chyle in the
thoracic cavity. This typically occurs when chyle leaks
from the thoracic duct or one of its major branches into
the pleural space. This leakage of chyle can be due to
congenital abnormalities, traumatic injury of the thoracic
duct, invasion of the thoracic duct by a tumor or malignancy, infection, or thrombosis of the venous system.

Chyle is lymphatic fluid that is typically laden with free
fatty acids, cholesterol and phospholipids resulting in
a milky color to the fluid. The predominant cell type
within chyle is lymphocytes. The concentration of free
fatty acids, cholesterol and phospholipids varies
depending upon absorption of these products from the
small intestine. The ingestion of triglycerides and phospholipids results in their absorption by the intestinal epithelium. Upon absorption, those triglycerides that contain
fatty acids of 12 carbons or less are absorbed directly into
the blood stream. These are termed medium-chain triglycerides. Triglycerides composed of fatty acids that are
longer than 12 carbons (long-chain triglycerides) are not
directly absorbed into the bloodstream. Instead, long-
chain triglycerides are complexed with cholesterol, phospholipids, and binding proteins to form lipoproteins.
Once assembled, the lipoproteins are transported through
the lymphatic system, eventually arriving in the thoracic
duct. Once in the thoracic duct, lipoproteins are emptied

into the venous blood near the junction of the left jugular
and left subclavian veins. Therefore, in the event that
a patient has not had any recent oral intake, the appearance of the chyle may actually be clear. The diagnosis of
a chylothorax is confirmed by the presence of chylomicrons in the pleural fluid.

The thoracic duct is the final common channel
through which all lymphatic fluid in the body reenters
the blood stream. The thoracic duct originates at the
cysterna chyli, typically between the third lumbar vertebrae and the tenth thoracic vertebrae. It then ascends
along the anterior surface of the vertebral bodies, lying
between the aorta and the azygos vein. At the level of the
fifth thoracic vertebrae (T5), the thoracic duct crosses over
from right to left and continues its ascent posterior to the
aortic arch. Finally, it courses through the thoracic inlet
where it ultimately empties into the venous system some-
where near the junction of the left internal jugular vein
and left subclavian vein. While anatomic variations of the
thoracic duct do exist, this is the most common course.
Therefore, a thoracic duct injury below T5 will produce
a right sided chylothorax but an injury above T5 will
produce a left sided chylothorax.

Evaluation
Patients with a chylothorax may have symptoms that are
commonly associated with any type of pleural effusion
including shortness of breath, fatigue, chest discomfort,
and cough. The presence of chyle in the pleural space does
not cause any irritation of the pleura. Therefore, patients
will not typically complain of pleuritic chest pain if their
effusion is secondary to a chylothorax. Patients with
chylothorax will have evidence of a pleural effusion on
plain radiographs and/or computed tomography (CT) of
the chest. However, radiographic imaging alone cannot
distinguish chylothorax from other causes of pleural effusions. Definitive diagnosis of a chylothorax requires sampling of the pleural fluid. While the classic description of
a chylothorax is the return of milky white fluid, this is not
always present and the return of clear fluid from the
pleural space does not exclude chylothorax. The presence
of chylomicrons in the pleural fluid is the gold standard
for diagnosing a chylothorax.

Once the diagnosis of chylothorax has been made, the
etiology of the chyle leak must be further investigated. The
etiology of a chylothorax typically falls into one of three
categories: congenital, traumatic, or neoplastic. By far the
two most common causes of chylothorax are trauma and
neoplasms [1]. Obtaining a thorough history will often
elucidate the cause. Common surgical procedures associated with the development of a chylothorax include

esophagectomy, pneumonectomy, repair of aortic aneurysm, radical lymph node dissections of the neck, chest, or abdomen, and surgery for the removal of mediastinal tumors. In addition, blunt or penetrating trauma can result in injury to the thoracic duct with subsequent development of a chylothorax. Obstruction of the thoracic duct by tumor is the most common cause for non-traumatic chylothorax. Lymphoma is the by far the most common malignancy seen in non-traumatic cases of chylothorax, accounting for 70% of the cases. Other potential but uncommon causes include congenital atresia of the thoracic duct, mediastinal radiation, and transdiaphragmatic passage of chylous ascitic fluid in patients with cirrhosis [1].

In the event that the etiology of the chylothorax remains unclear, diagnostic imaging may be helpful. CT scan of the chest may reveal underlying tumor or mediastinal lymphadenopathy that had been previously undiagnosed. If available, lymphangiography or lymphoscintigraphy can be utilized to define lymphatic anatomy and identify the source of the leak [2]. This can be potentially useful for operative planning purposes.

Treatment

Having a basic understanding of lipid metabolism and thoracic duct anatomy is helpful in understanding the role of various therapies in the management of chylothorax (see above). The treatment plan should be individualized for each patient and should take into account the underlying etiology, duration, symptoms, nutritional status, and other co morbid conditions. Treatment options can be broadly categorized into nonoperative and operative therapies. Most clinicians would favor an initial trial of nonoperative therapy for a period of 1–2 weeks. However, in those patients this may be associated with longer hospital stays and an increased risk of complications. Therefore, the risk versus benefit of nonoperative therapy must be critically evaluated on a patient by patient basis.

Nonoperative Management

The initial step in the nonoperative management of chylothorax is placement of a tube thoracostomy to drain the pleural space and allow for re-expansion of the lung. Tube thoracostomy is preferred over repeated thoracentesis because it allows for apposition of the pleural surface which may promote sealing of the site of the leak and because thoracentesis alone rarely results in complete drainage of the effusion. In addition, repeated thoracentesis unnecessarily exposes the patient to the risk of pneumothorax or hemothorax.

A key component of the nonoperative management of chylothorax is an assessment of the patient's nutritional status. Because chyle is rich with triglycerides, proteins, and electrolytes the ongoing loss of these substances can result is significant malnutrition and electrolyte abnormalities. Hyponatremia and hypocalcemia are the most commonly encountered electrolyte disturbances. The severity of these derangements is dependent upon the volume and duration of the chyle leak. Monitoring the patient's nutritional status through weekly weights, serum prealbumin and transferrin levels, and nitrogen balance is critical. Manipulation of a patient's enteral intake can decrease the volume of chyle generated and therefore increase the chances of the leak sealing with nonoperative management. As mentioned above, long-chain triglycerides are unable to be absorbed directly into the blood stream by the enterocytes. Therefore, they must be packaged as lipoproteins and travel through the thoracic duct before re-entering the blood stream. By removing long-chain triglycerides from the diet, the volume of chyle transported through the thoracic duct can be significantly decreased. Instituting a low fat, medium-chain triglyceride diet will result in closure of the leak in 50% of cases [3]. Total parenteral nutrition may be utilized in the event that dietary modification is unsuccessful and surgical management is not an option.

In those patients with chylothorax due to malignancy, therapies targeted the primary malignancy may be of benefit but the results are inconsistent [1]. Chemical pleurodesis may be useful in patients that are not surgical candidates that have failed chemotherapy and radiation therapy. Talc, tetracycline, and bleomycin have all been used successfully for chemical pleurodesis. In addition, somatostatin has been shown to reduce the production of intestinal chyle with results decrease in chyle leak [6].

Operative Management

The surgical treatment of chylothorax involves ligation of the thoracic duct. Surgical treatment should be considered first line therapy in those patients with post surgical chylothorax. This is because conservative management of post surgical chylothorax has been associated with increased mortality when compared with surgical treatment [4, 5]. Patients that have failed a trial of nonoperative therapy should also be managed surgically. As a general rule of thumb, two groups of patients will likely fail conservative management; (1) those patients with a chyle leak of greater than 1.5 L/day and (2) those patients with a sustained chyle leak of 1 L/day for 5 consecutive days. In these patients, surgical intervention should be considered, as it will likely result in better outcomes.

Once the decision to pursue operative intervention has been made, there are several techniques that can be utilized to ligate the thoracic duct. Operative approaches include open and thoracoscopic. In general, operating on the same side as the effusion is preferred. Selective ligation of the thoracic duct at the site of the leak may be performed if the leak can be identified. Methylene blue may be mixed with a fat source such as olive oil or cream and administered enterally to help visualize the site of the leak. Once the leak is identified, the thoracic duct is ligated above and below the site of the leak. In the event that the leak cannot be easily identified, further dissection around the thoracic duct to identify the leak is discouraged, as this may lead to further injury to the thoracic duct and its tributaries. Instead, mass ligation of the soft tissues lying between the aorta, spine, esophagus, and pericardium should be performed just above the diaphragmatic hiatus in the right chest.

After-care
The main focus following resolution of a chylothorax is to ensure correction of any nutritional, immunologic, or electrolyte abnormalities that may have occurred. This can include weekly assessments of nutritional status, monitoring for evidence of immunosuppression, and electrolyte replacement.

Prognosis
The prognosis for patients with chylothorax is highly variable and dependent upon the underlying etiology. With more aggressive management, there has been a decrease in the morbidity and mortality associated with this condition. Patients with iatrogenic or traumatic chylothorax have the best prognosis for recovery. Those patients with malignant chylothorax tend to have a worse prognosis.

Cross Reference
▶ Pleural Disease and Pneumothorax

References
1. Nair SK, Petko M, Hayward MP (2007) Aetiology and management of chylothorax in adults. Eur J Cardiothorac Surg 32(2):362–369
2. Ngan H, Fok M, Wong J (1988) The role of lymphography in chylothorax following thoracic surgery. Br J Radiol 61(731):1032–1036
3. Fernández Alvarez JR, Kalache KD, Graüel EL (1999) Management of spontaneous congenital chylothorax: oral medium-chain triglycerides versus total parenteral nutrition. Am J Perinatol 16(8):415–420
4. Al-Zubairy SA, Al-Jazairi AS (2003) Octreotide as a therapeutic option for management of chylothorax. Ann Pharmacother 37(5):679–682
5. Orringer MB, Bluett M, Deeb GM (1988) Aggressive treatment of chylothorax complicating transhiatal esophagectomy without thoracotomy. Surgery 104(4):720–726

Chylous Pleural Effusion
▶ Chylothorax

Circulation
▶ Capillary Refill

Circulatory Assist Devices

ARES KRISHNA MENON[1], RÜDIGER AUTSCHBACH[2]
[1]Klinik f. Thorax-, Herz-, Gefäßchirurgie, Klinikum der RWTH, Aachen, Germany
[2]Clinic for THG Surgery, University of Aachen, Aachen, Germany

Synonyms
Biventricular Assist Device (BVAD); Left Ventricular Assist Device (LVAD); Left Ventricular Assist System (LVAS); Mechanical Circulatory Assist; Mechanical Circulatory Support (MCS); Right Ventricular Assist Device (RVAD); Ventricular Assist Device (VAD)

Definition and History
After the first use of cardio pulmonary bypass (CPB) in the 1950s and the increasing number of cardiac procedures, the need for extended circulatory assistance in patients who could not be weaned from CBP was obvious. After the first experimental use of ventricular assist devices (VAD) in 1963 De Bakey introduced the first clinical use of a VAD in a patient after aortic valve replacement. Only a few months later the group of Denton Cooley presented their first successful use of an assisted circulation as a bridge to transplantation (BTT). During these pioneering works two different systems were surveyed: Pneumatically driven rubber-tube or sac pumps which offer a pulsatile flow and continuous flow devices like, for example, centrifugal pumps.

As recorded in the recommendations of the National Heart Advisory Group the importance of mechanical support was recognized by the National Institute of Health in the USA in 1964. The former initial goal was to develop a total artificial heart (TAH). While the first TAH program was abandoned in 1991due to the enormous rate of severe complications, the National Heart and Lung Institute meanwhile put its effort in the development and evaluation of left ventricular assist devices (LVADs). This led to the Food and Drug Administration (FDA) approval of LVAD for BTT use in 1994. Thus, under high volume sponsored research during the last 20 years, two different types of devices became available: Pulsatile VADs as well as the newer and smaller continuous flow pumps. Both systems are usable for intracorporeal and paracorporeal implantation. According to the degree of individual disease, more or less all appliances can be used as a univentricular support for LVAD, as a right ventricular assist device (RVAD), or as a biventricular assist device (BVAD).

Pre-existing Condition

The treatment of heart failure is of tremendous growing interest even at the intensive and intermediate care units in our hospitals.

In heart failure or even in cardiogenic shock patients the caring physician has to decide whether to treat the patient with medication only or to use circulatory support to stabilize hemodynamics and preserve organ function. The so-called Intention to Treat (ITT) in the rising use of VADs for mechanical cardiac support is the key issue and has essential influence on the choice of the individual device: Whether as for Bridge to Recovery (BTR), Bridge to Transplantation (BTT), or for long-term circulatory support as the so-called Destination Therapy (DT). Other patients fall in the category of Bridge to Candidacy (BTC). These are patients who at the time of an urgent device implantation are either critically ill and have not been completely evaluated for OHT or are bearing a major or relative contraindication to transplantation. Furthermore, the type of the support needed has to be considered: Is an univentricular assist device sufficient? or is the use of a biventricular device (BVAD) crucial?.

Indications for Assisted Circulation

Usually, the use of a VAD is indicated in case of severe heart failure which is refractory to the conservative treatment options. If the patient is not able to offer adequate systemic oxygen delivery to maintain normal end-organ function despite maximal medical therapy, mechanical support is indicated. The common hemodynamic criteria for device implantation include a systolic blood pressure less than 80 mmHg, mean arterial pressure less than 65 mmHg, cardiac index less than 2.0 L/min/m^2, pulmonary capillary wedge pressure greater than 20 mmHg, and a systemic vascular resistance greater than 2100 dyn-s/cm [1].

The large variety of diseases treated with assisted circulation devices includes both acute and chronic forms of heart failure.

The acute cardiogenic shock is one of the main reasons for treating the patient in an emergency ward or chest pain unit. There are several reasons for cardiogenic shock. Acute myocardial infarction, for example, complicated by cardiogenic shock has a very high mortality rate. A trend towards early intervention reached a better outcome by early and more aggressive coronary reperfusion strategies such as percutaneous intervention, coronary bypass surgery, or aortic counterpulsation. Moreover, up to 6% of patients after heart operation are still suffering from low output syndrome, the post-cardiotomy shock, especially after complex surgical procedures like heart transplantation, multivalve replacement, or treatment of severely impaired left ventricular function. Depending on the age of patients who require assisted circulation, there are some other typical indications. Myocarditis or dilated cardiomyopathy (DCM) affects the younger patient group with an often unpredictable outcome. The global dilatation of both, the left and right ventricle, often leads to a biventricular heart failure and therefore requires an adequate biventricular support. Moreover, a rare indication for VAD therapy is a complex ventricular arrhythmia, if refractory to medical treatment.

The second and also large cohort of patients which is considered for AC is the chronic heart failure group. An estimated 2–5 million patients are suffering from heart failure worldwide [2]. The continued aging of mankind leads to a growing number of patients. The incidence and prevalence of this disease is obviously age dependant: On an average 2–5% of the population aged 65–70 years and about 10% in the group of persons aged more than 70 years are affected, and around 500,000 new cases per year are registered. In spite of all advances in medical treatment of severe heart failure the prognosis of the patients is poor. In patients with severe heart failure more than 50% die within 1 year.

These patients have to be divided in two groups: Those who are eligible for orthotopic heart transplantation (OHT), and those, who are not. OHT is the only treatment that provides substantial individual benefit, but with fewer than 4,000 donors available per year worldwide its impact is epidemiologically trivial. Additionally, we find a growing number of patients who are ineligible for cardiac transplantation because of advanced age, presence of diabetes mellitus with end-organ damage, chronic renal failure, or pulmonary hypertension. Therefore, the limitations of cardiac transplantation procedures have stimulated the development of alternative approaches to the treatment of severe heart failure.

For these reasons within the chronic heart failure group of patients assisted circulation is exercisable as a BTT or as destination therapy.

Device Selection

Due to the above-mentioned circumstances the treating physician has to decide, which specific blood pump would be the appropriate tool for the individual patient. The operative risk of the implantation procedure has to be weighed against the potential lifestyle and survival benefit with mechanical support, the already stated intention to treat.

Application

Short-Term Circulatory Support

A large variety of technical devices do exist to support the failing heart for a short time period. These devices have the advantage of an easy implantation technique based on the hope of an early cardiac recovery or bridging the patient to use a more permanent ventricular device.

Intra-Aortic Balloon Pump (IAPB)

Kantrowicz and coworkers presented the first clinical use of an Intra Aortic Balloon Pump (IABP) for the treatment of cardiogenic shock after myocardial infarction in 1968. Once percutaneously placed in the descending aorta, its diastolic pulsation and systolic deflation is triggered by ECG or arterial pressure, resulting in reduction of afterload and improvement of coronary perfusion. The application of IABP is widespread because of its uncomplicated use and improved outcome in the treatment of myocardial infarction, postcardiotomy shock, postinfarction VSD, or acute mitral valve regurgitation caused by posterior wall infarction [3]. Critical limp perfusion is a rare, but severe complication, and therefore IABP use has to be considered deliberatively in case of peripheral vascular disease.

Centrifugal Pumps

Originally used for CPB, centrifugal pumps were thereafter in many cases also applied for assisted circulation because of the low costs, uncomplicated implantation techniques, and easy handling. The Biomedicus Bio-Pump (Medtronic Inc., Minneapolis MN, USA), the Sarns centrifugal pump (3-M Health Care, Ann Arbor, Michigan, USA), and the newer Centrimag (Levitronix Inc.) are the most common pumps in this field. Placed paracorporeally, the implantation could either be achieved via cannulation of the groin vessels or – in case of postcardiotomy shock – via connection to the cannulas of the CBP intraoperatively. In case of a collateral respiratory failure, the connection to an oxygenator is possible, resulting in an extra corporeal membrane oxygenation system (ECMO). Especially in the pediatric field of assisted circulation, the ECMO is widespread and leads to a remarkable improvement in survival rates of these high-risk cases.

The very new Tandem Heart paracorporeal centrifugal pump (CardiacAssist, Inc., Pittsburgh, Penn., USA) can easily be implanted via percutaneous insertion of the groin vessels without a surgical procedure. In doing so, the inflow cannula is brought up the femoral vein and through the atrial septum into the left atrium percutaneously.

Axial Flow Pumps

The microaxial blood pump Impella Recover Device (Impella CardioSystems AG, Aachen, Germany) is a newer short-term support system for up to 7 days. Brought through the aortic valve inside the left ventricle percutaneously, this pump generates flow up to 5 L/min. Therefore, it can be used as an ideal tool for postcardiotomy support or myocardial infarction with cardiac shock to establish a rapid unloading of the failing left ventricle. Since last year a paracardiac right-ventricular device (RVMBP) of the Impella family was available until the product was withdrawn from the European market.

Pulsatile Short-Term Pumps

A dual chamber polyurethane blood sac pump, the Abiomed BVS 5000i (Abiomed Cardiovascular, Inc., Danvers, Mass. USA) is a passively filled, pulsatile short-term assist device for the use after postcardiotomy shock. This device can be used for univentricular as well as for biventricular support generating flows up to 6 L/min. Its cost-effectiveness and the ease of implantation have lead to a widespread use, especially for the BTR short term, or a bridging to another, more permanent system, the bridge to bridge (BTB). The same company introduced another, more complex pulsatile, paracorporeal, fully automated device with pneumatically driven full-to-empty mode: the AB 5000. Similar to the older paracorporeal long-term devices, such as Berlin Heart Excor (Berlin Heart Inc. Berlin, Germany) or the Thoratec PVAD (Thoratec Inc., California, USA), the AB 5000 is able to reach a complete unloading of the failing left or right ventricle and, got FDA approval for 30 days in the USA, so far.

All of these short-term devices have the advantage of a more or less easy implantation and application. The main disadvantage of almost every short-term pump is the impossible mobilization of the patient. Only the newer, more costly devices such as the Centrimag or the AB 5000 do allow for a better mobilization of the individual patient. However, they touch the boarder of the permanent VADs not only clinically, but financially in particular.

Long-Term Circulatory Support

Pulsatile Devices

The first generation of LVADs are electromechanically or pneumatically controlled mechanical assist systems. They are used for BTT or DT and generate pulsatile blood flow up to 10 L/min. Some examples for the permanent use of VADs are the paracorporeal systems Excor (Berlin Heart, Germany) (Fig. 1), Thoratec PVAD (Thoratec, California, USA), and the Medos HIA (Medos Inc., Aachen Germany). The pump chambers of the Excor and HIA are offered in different sizes so that pediatric use is possible. Patients treated with these large, bulky devices are difficult to mobilize, also because of the risk of kinking the grafts and the large control units. The following, implantable pulsatile devices are brought into a huge preperitoneal pocket connected to a percutaneous driveline. The HeartMate XVE (Thoratec Inc.) is the most used implantable VAD with more than 4,000 implantations worldwide. The peculiarity of the HeartMate XVE is its structured inner surface, leading to a neointima formation to reduce the risk of thrombus formation. Because this device has biological valves, anticoagulation is not necessary. A large amount of clinical experience has been gained with the Heartmate LVAD. The pioneering REMATCH trial [4] was established by using this device for DT.

Historically, it is necessary to mention two other systems which were withdrawn from the market in 2005 and 2008 respectively: The LionHeart 2000 LVAD (Arrow International, PA, USA) and the Novacor LVAS(Baxter Healthcare/Worldheart Inc.) devices. The Novacor is implanted in the same approach as the Heartmate VXE, including the typical connection to a console by a percutaneous driveline. The fully implantable Lion Heart was powered by transcutaneous energy transfer, thereby obviating the need for external lines, which is a common course of infection in LVAD recipients. A pump controller was implanted as well regulating the external power supply. The external power pack with rechargeable and replaceable batteries could be removed from the transcutaneous site maximal 30 min. The inside of this system achieves unidirectional blood flow by mechanical heart valves and therefore necessitates Warfarin or Heparin treatment. The system was licensed for trials in Europe and the USA for long-term support in patients with end-stage-heart failure. Because of some major technical failures, for example, fatal fracture of the blood sac, the device was displaced from the market in 2005. The Novacor device was developed in the 1970s. Its regulatory approval in Europe and the USA for BTT came in the 1994 and 1998, respectively, followed by a regulatory approval for long-term support in Europe. More than 1,800 implantations could be accomplished worldwide. It carries biological valves for achievement of unidirectional flow, although because of the inner structure of this device systemic anticoagulation is mandatory as well in the LionHeart. Here, similar to the technical failures of the LionHeart, the durability was obviously very limited and consequently the Novacor LVAD was withdrawn from the market in 2008.

Continuous Flow Devices

One of the most promising advances in the field of circulatory assist devices is the development of axial flow pumps, like the HeartMate II (Thoratec) (Fig. 2), the Micromed DeBakey (MicroMedTechnology Inc., Houston , TX, USA), the Incor (Berlin Heart), and the Jarvik 2000 (Jarvik Heart Inc., NY, USA) (Table 1). These devices, the so-called second generation of VADs, generate continuous flow via a very small electromagnetically actuated impeller that rotates at high speeds and are able to provide up to 10 L/min flow. Moreover, in the implantable pulsatile devices the particular inflow cannula is connected to the LV apex, the outflow graft to the ascending aorta. The remarkably small size of these devices allows

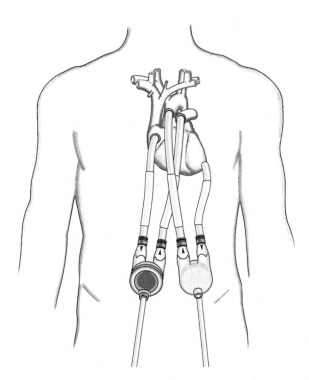

Circulatory Assist Devices. Figure 1 Excor

of 10 L/min at 10,000 rpm, but usually is initiated at 8,000 rpm, resulting in a 5–6 L flow per minute. It carries a special ultrasonic flow probe at the outflow graft site, which allows for exact flow measurements. The HeartMate II (Fig. 3) is a newer device and obtained its approval in Europe a few years ago and FDA approval for BTT was obtained in 2009. Fabricated with titanium, it operates at speeds between 6,000 and 12,000 rpm resulting in a flow up to 10 L/min in a fixed or automatic operating mode (http://www.thoratec.com/about-us/media-room/videos.aspx). An overview is shown in Table 1.

The recently developed implantable centrifugal circulatory assist devices represent the so-called third generation of implantable LVADs. Examples are the VentrAssist (Ventracor Inc., Australia), the HVAD (Hardware Inc., USA), and the DuraHeart (Terumo Inc., Japan). These devices use the magnetic technology in which rotating blades or an impeller is magnetically suspended within a column of blood, obviating the need for contact-bearing moving parts.

The DuraHeart is a magnetically suspended centrifugal pump with impeller blades, magnetic bearing, and a direct motor. Its relatively large volume (200 mL) requires an implantation pocket, which is clearly bigger than the ones needed for axial pumps. The DuraHeart works with speeds of 2,000–3,000 rpm and creates a flow between 5–6 L/min. The VentrAssist device is a smaller titanium centrifugal pump with a carbon coating at its inner surface. It was implanted worldwide in more than 200 patients as a LVAD in CE marked use-and-pilot trials, but the company became bankrupt in spring 2009. The HVAD system was introduced recently and has just gained CE approval. It has a volume of only 50 mL and is directly implanted at the surface of the LV apex, allowing an intrapericardial pocket. The speed range of 2,000–3,000 rpm creates a flow up to 8–10 L/min. All centrifugal VADs require systemic anticoagulation.

The Total Artificial Heart

Severe failure of both the left and right ventricle of the human heart necessitates sometimes even more than the implantation of a paracorporeal BVAD. In selected cases like structural heart diseases, for example, hypertrophic cardiomyopathy or complex congenital cardiac diseases after a large number of operations with mechanical valve prosthesis inside, the orthotopic positioning of a totally implantable artificial heart (TAH) is required. The CradioWest (Syn Cardia Inc., Tucson, AZ, USA) is a pneumatically driven orthotopic, implantable biventricular assist system and at present the only available TAH. Its rigid pump housing contains dual spherical

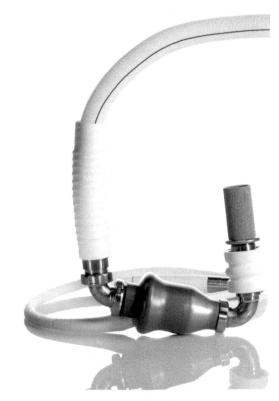
Circulatory Assist Devices. **Figure 2** HeartMate II

for enormous reduction in surgical trauma caused by a diminishment of the preperitoneal or even intrapericardial pump pocket. This is why the use for patients with a small body surface area is now possible, resulting in FDA approval for pediatric use for the MicoMed device. The other systems are now under trial for this indication. Moreover, these axial pumps are generating no relevant noise. Permanent anticoagulation therapy is necessary, but after early experiences are initiated and not until a minimum 12–24 h after implantation. The unique design of the Jarvik consists of an impeller, which is placed in the LV apex directly as a sort of inflow cannula housing the pump. Therefore, less invasive implantation is possible via a lateral thoracotomie leading the outflow graft to the descending aorta, in case a sternotomy should be avoided. This device operates at fixed rate motor speeds that are set by the controller at between 8,000 and 12,000 rpm with an average capacity of 5–7 L/min. Another implantation feature of this small pump is a titanium pedestal screwed into the very well-vascularized skull with a transcutaneous connector that attaches to the power cord. The MicroMed DeBakey AD is a titanium electromagnetically actuated axial flow pump with a maximum flow capacity

Circulatory Assist Devices. Table 1 Characteristics of the most common continuous flow left ventricular assist devices (LVAD). Status: June 30, 2009

	Thoratec HeartMate II	BerlinHeart Incor	Ventracor VentrAssist[a]	Terumo DuraHeart	Heartware HVAD	Jarvik Heart Jarvik 2000	MicroMed De Bakey HeartAssist
System	Axial	Axial	Centrifugal	Centrifugal	Centrifugal	Axial	centrifugal
Weight gr.	280	200	298[a]	590	145	90	92
Size mm	81 × 43	120 × 43	~40 × 60	~73 × 46 × 85	Volume ~50 mL	Volume ~30 mL	71 × 31
Max. flow	5–10	5–10	5–10	5–10	5–10	~5–7	~5–10
Implantations	~2900	~500		~100	100	~200	~300
CE	Yes	Yes	Yes[a]	Yes	Yes	Yes	No
FDA-adult	Yes	Under investigation	No	Under investigation	Under investigation	under investigation	Yes
FDA-pediatric	No	Under investigation	No	No	No	No	Yes

[a]Company went bankrupt 2009

polyurethane chambers. The inflow and outflow conduits are made of Dacron and carry mechanical valve prosthesis (Medtronic Inc. USA). The stroke volume is about 70 mL and the CardioWest is able to generate a maximum flow of 10 L/min. The condition of insufficient space inside the patients' thorax is a major problem. It requires a minimum BSA of 1.7 m^2 or ventricular volumes of the native heart from more than 1.5 L. In Europe the pneumatic drivelines are connected to a smaller console, which allows for a better mobilization of the patient. The CW got the CE and FDA approval for BTT use.

Implantation Technique

A very large variety of surgical implantation techniques are necessary to accommodate an appropriate function of the specific device. In most cases cardiac support systems are implanted for left heart failure, since isolated insufficiency of the right ventricle is rare. Whereas in the short-term devices mostly an access to the groin vessels is sufficient; the devices for permanent support require a median sternotomy or another adequate access to the left ventricle and the aorta. The fully heparinized patient is put on CPB and the apex of the left ventricle is exposed for the insertion of the inflow cannula of the VAD, which is usually done by beating the heart on pump without cardioplegic arrest. After having prepared the device pocket in the preperitoneal or intrapericardial position, the driveline is tunneled and brought out of the skin in the right upper quadrant. The correct position of the LV apex is cut with a special core knife, the myocardium is removed, and the

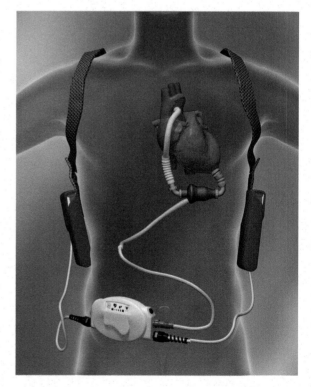

Circulatory Assist Devices. Figure 3 External equipment

LV is accurately inspected. The thrombi have to be removed carefully and trabecular structures have to be excised in case they might hinder the free flow to the inflow cannula. The apex cannula is then fixed to the left ventricle by 2-0 polypropylene sutures reinforced by felt pledges. The device once brought in correct position is then connected and the outflow graft, a Dacron vascular prosthesis, is sutured into an end-to-side anastomosis to the aorta followed by the careful de-airing of the device. Subsequently, the patient is weaned from CPB while the VAD is initiated. In this context, the correct position of the inflow cannula has to be monitored carefully by transesophageal echocardiography (TEE) to ensure an unrestricted blood flow to the assist device. In LVAD implantation particular interest is then given to the right ventricle and the right atrium to safeguard the adequate systolic function and to obviate a persistent PFO, which might have been hidden by an assumed high left atrium pressure before a LVAD implantation due to low cardiac output. Protamine is admitted and meticulous hemostasis is established before chest drains are placed and the sternum is closed with permanent wires. To minimize trauma of the device or the outflow graft, a Gore-Tex surgical membrane can be used to cover these delicate structures before the sternum is closed. The use of phosphodiesterase inhibitors, inhaled nitric oxide and aggressive inotropic support of the right ventricle in case of any impaired systolic right ventricular function should be applied very liberally. Again, the TEE is an ideal and essential tool for the effective treatment of a patient after LVAD implantation beside the information from the measurements of the pulmonary artery catheter. After having reached stable conditions in the operating theatre a seamless constant treatment of these patients should always be the main goal. Such is the postoperative care at the ICU. Decent monitoring of a stable right heart hemodynamic, excellent oxygenation, and proper function of the device to guarantee a sufficient perfusion of all organs is the main target of the intensive care doctor, who then should always be very alert to the drain blood loss and the urine output. Well-dosed substitution of blood products like plasma or platelets should be applied whenever it is needed. Antibiotics should be given minimum 48 h postoperatively for prophylactic use.

Outcome of Circulatory Assist Device Treatment

Randomized Evaluation of Mechanical assistance for the Treatment of Congestive Heart Failure (REMATCH) trail is a landmark in the history of clinical trials in heart failure [4]. The study included end-stage heart failure patients who were ineligible for cardiac transplantation and randomized them to either surgical therapy (implantation of a HeartMate XVE LVAD) or optimal medical treatment. All patients were classified in NYHA class IV, LV EF <25%, and either peak oxygen consumption < 12–14 mL/KG/min or dependence on inotropes. Within the cohort of these critically ill the 1- and 2-year survival rates of 52% and 23% in LVAD recipients were significantly better than the 25% and 8% survival observed in patients treated with maximum medical therapy [4]. Despite more adverse events in the LVAD group the survival rate and quality of life were better in these patients. Later on, this tendency continued resulting in an improvement of the 2-year survival of 37% in the LVAD group versus 12% in the medical group (Late REMATCH). Bleeding, infection, and multiorgan failure were the major cause of early mortality after LVAD implantation. Long-term mortality was mostly related to device dysfunction and infectious complications. Sepsis and local infections were the most common cause of morbidity and mortality in LVAD recipients and account for 25% of deaths. In the post-Rematch area, the 1-year survival increased to 56% with an in-hospital mortality of 27% after LVAD surgery [5]. Again the main causes for death were sepsis, right heart failure, and multiorgan failure. The Interagency Registry for Mechanically assisted Circulatory support (INTERMACS) database, funded by the US National Heart, Lung and Blood Institute (NHLBI), is a new registry for patients who receive durable FDA-approved mechanical circulatory support devices for the treatment of advanced heart failure [6]. The patients' clinical status before VAD implantation was classified into seven different INTERMACS levels, grated from 1, representing the sickest patients in severe cardiogenic shock, to 7, representing an advanced NYHA level III. The first report presented in 2008 gives a further positive tendency in the development of VAD treatment in more than 400 patients. Included were BTT, as well as DT, or BTR patients. The overall survival rate was 56% after 1 year, but with a close look at the extent of support, LVAD recipients had a much better survival rate (67%), than the BVAD cohort (<40%). The main causes of death were central neurologic events (18% of all deaths), multiorgan failure (16%), right ventricular failure and arrhythmias (15%), and infections (8%). By multivariable analysis the risk factors for early death were INTERMACS level 1, older age, ascites at the time of implant, higher bilirubin level, and placement of a BVAD or Total Artificial Heart. The results of an early European study on the axial flow HeatMate II device for LVAD proved far better than the early experiences with pulsatile devices [7]. After 1 year a comparable survival was observed in both, the DT (69%), and the BTT (63%) group of patients. Main causes of death in this multicentre trial were multiorgan failure and cerebrovascular accidents. The survival remained stable in this cohort of LVAD recipients even after 6 months.

This correlates to the findings of the first studies with axial flow devices in the USA.

Adverse Events (AE)

In the Rematch trial, non-neurologic bleedings, neurologic events, and perioperative bleeding were the most common complications [4]. Recently, the INTERMACS data analysis showed comparable results, with bleeding and infection as the most common adverse events in the early and late postoperative period [6]. Neurologic events were most likely in the first 1–2 months after implant. Device malfunction, formerly the second most frequent cause of death (Rematch), was relatively uncommon during the duration of follow-up, with 84% freedom at 6 months. Moreover, malfunction of the newer axial flow devices was totally absent in the European HeartMate II study. The most common adverse events in this trial were bleeding requiring surgery (21% of all AE), cardiac arrhythmias (19%), and sepsis (11%) which occurred mainly without exception in the early postoperative period (<90 days), whereas the driveline and local infections were the most common AE of the late period [7]. A remarkable reduction of neurologic events was also notable in the newer data analysis. Right heart failure, one of the most common AE after LVAD implantation in the earlier studies, seems to play a cumulatively minor role in last examinations. Coming out of an incidence of 20%, the right heart failure after LVAD implantation is clearly reduced to less than 10% as well in the INTERMACS data base, as well in the European HeartMate II study.

Conclusions

Circulatory assist devices have become a major therapeutic option in treatment of either acute or chronic heart failure patients. In the last years, long-term circulatory support has made a great deal of progress, and the trends towards better device durability and reduced complication rates will most likely continue to improve through the development of more innovative ventricular assist devices.

References

1. Pagani FD, Aaronson KD (2003) Mechanical devices for temporary support. In: Franco KL, Verrier ED (eds) Advanced therapy in cardiac surgery, 2nd vol. BC Decker, Hamilton, Ontario
2. Hunt SA, Abraham WT, Chin MH et al (2005) ACC/AHA 2005 Guideline update for the diagnosis and management of chronic heart failure in the adult—summary article. Circulation 112:1825
3. Aggarwal S, Cheema F, Oz M, Naka Y (2008) Long-term mechanical circulatory support. In: Cohn LH (ed) Cardiac Surgery in the Adult. McGraw-Hill, New York, pp 1609–1628
4. Rose EA, Gelijns AC, Moskowitz AJ, Moskowitz AJ, Heijan DF, Stevenson LW, Dembitsky W, Long JW, Ascheim DD, Tierney AR, Levitan RG, Watson JT, Meier P (2001) Randomized Evaluation of Mechanical Assistance for the Treatment of Congestive Heart Failure (REMATCH) Study Group. Long-term mechanical left ventricular assistance for end-stage heart failure. N Engl J Med 345:1435–1443
5. Lietz K, Long JW, Kfoury AG, Slaughter MS et al (2007) Outcomes of left ventricular Assist Device Implantation as Destination Therapy in the post-REMATCH Era-Implications for Patient Selection. Circulation 116:497–505
6. Kirklin JK, Naftel DC, Stevenson LW, Kormos RL, Pagani FD, Miller MA, Ulisney K, Young JB (2008) INTERMACS Database for Durable Devices for Circulatory Support: First Annual Report. J Heart Lung Transplant 27:1065–1072
7. Stüber M, Sander K, Lahpor J, Ahn H, Litzler PY, Drakos SG, Musumeci F, Schlensak Ch, Friedrich I, Gustaffson R, Oertel F, Leprince P (2008) HeartMate II Left Ventricular Assist Device, early European experience. Eur J Cardiothorac Surg 34:289–294

Circulatory Collapse

▶ Shock, Ultrasound Assessment

Cl $_{H2O}$

▶ Free-Water Clearance

Classification of Pulmonary Hypertension

Functional classification of pulmonary hypertension modified after the New York heart association functional classification according to the World Health Organization 1998. Class I: No limitation of physical activity. Ordinary physical activity does not cause undue dyspnea or fatigue, chest pain or near syncope. Class II: Slight limitation of physical activity. They are comfortable at rest. Ordinary physical activity causes undue dyspnea or fatigue, chest pain or near syncope. Class III: Marked limitation of physical activity. They are comfortable at rest. Less than ordinary physical activity causes undue dyspnea or fatigue, chest pain or near syncope. Class IV: Inability to carry out any physical activity without symptoms. These patients manifest signs of right heart failure. Dyspnea and/or fatigue may even be present at rest. Discomfort is increased by any physical activity.

Clearance

The volume of blood that is cleared from a given solute in the time unit.

▶ eGFR, Concept of

Clenched-Fist Injury

▶ Bite Injuries

Clinical Pulmonary Infection Score (CPIS)

Clinical score suggested for the diagnosis of VAP composed of the severity of infiltrate, body temperature, tracheal secretions, oxygenation derangement, positivity of endotracheal aspirate cultures, and white blood cell response.

Closed Forequarter Amputation

▶ Scapulothoracic Dissociation

Closed Head Injury (CHI)

▶ Traumatic Brain Injury-Fluid Management

Clostridium botulinum

▶ Biological Terrorism, Botulinum Toxin

Clostridium difficile Diarrhea

▶ Clostridium difficile-Associated Diarrhea

Clostridium difficile Infection

▶ Clostridium difficile-Associated Diarrhea

Clostridium difficile-Associated Diarrhea

ANDREW M. MORRIS
Mount Sinai Hospital and University Health Network, University of Toronto, Toronto, ON, Canada

Synonyms

Antibiotic-associated diarrhea; Clostridium difficile-associated disease; Clostridium difficile infection; Clostridium difficile diarrhea; Pseudomembranous colitis

Definition

Clostridium difficile-associated diarrhea (CDAD) is a colonic infection caused by the overgrowth of the anaerobic Gram-positive bacillus, *C. difficile*. Patients may be asymptomatically colonized, but CDAD severity ranges from mild watery diarrhea to severe diarrhea with pseudomembranous colitis. Although *C. difficile* has various virulent factors, two pro-inflammatory exotoxins (Toxins A and B) appear to contribute most to the watery diarrhea [1].

Epidemiology

CDAD is an emerging infectious disease in most healthcare institutions worldwide. Recently, a more virulent fluoroquinolone-resistant strain, known as the ribotype 027 (BI/NAP1) strain, has emerged. The prevalence of *C. difficile* colonization ranges from 7–11% in acutely ill hospitalized patients to 1–2% in the general population. An estimated 178,000 cases of nosocomial CDAD occur in the USA annually, reflecting an incidence of roughly 50 per 1,000 patient-days or 5 per 1,000 admissions, although there is wide variability in reported rates, which are rising worldwide. Data on incidence in critical care units outside an outbreak setting are unclear, although one study reported a rate of 3.2 per 1,000 patient-days. Transmission is via *C. difficile* spores, which can remain on surfaces for prolonged periods and can also be transmitted directly person-to-person. However, CDAD usually requires altered fecal flora, which is most commonly caused by antibiotic use but can also be altered by chemotherapy, radiation, proton-pump inhibitors, anti-peristaltic agents, stool softeners, enemas, and naso-gastric feeds or drainage.

Prevention

The only effective method of prevention is avoiding (or minimizing) antimicrobial use. Most antimicrobials reduce the concentration of healthy fecal flora, allowing overgrowth of *C. difficile*. Infection control measures such as hand washing and barrier precautions clearly reduce transmission from index cases and can avert or halt outbreaks.

Treatment

The most important first step in managing CDAD is to remove predisposing factors such as antimicrobials, proton-pump inhibitors, etc. Many cases of mild disease can be effectively managed with metronidazole 500mg po (preferred over iv) tid for 10–14 days. More severe or refractory cases often require vancomycin 125mg qid enterally (oral, nasogastric, or via enema). General surgeons should be consulted rather early in the course of illness in moderate to severe cases: undoubtedly, deaths may occur because of delayed surgery. Relapses occur in 5–10% of cases; management of relapses is beyond the scope of this text.

Evaluation

CDAD should be considered in all patients with new, unexplained watery diarrhea. In the ICU, certain feeds (especially high-osmotic feeds) and bowel regimens may be the underlying cause of diarrhea, but they may also be contributing factors to CDAD. Diagnosis of CDAD is challenging because of the lack of a highly sensitive and specific test. CDAD is unlikely in patients with fewer than three bowel movements per day, and testing is therefore not advised. When testing is indicated, the best test (>90% sensitive, and >97% specific) is a quantitative PCR (qPCR) which gives results in hours. The *C. difficile* qPCR tests for a gene that codes for toxin B or its regulators, although most laboratories do not perform this test. The more common enzyme immunoassays test for either toxin A or toxins A and B; they are only about 70% sensitive although specificity and turnaround time are comparable to qPCR. Tissue culture cytotoxicity assay has similar diagnostic characteristics to qPCR, but results are only available after about 48 h and so it is falling out of favor.

Prognosis

CDAD carries overall 1–2% mortality, although there is a wide variability of reported mortality, depending on the site of care. Mortality in the ICU setting has recently been reported to be 37%. Population-based mortality of CDAD appears to be rising, with associated mortality in the USA of 5.7 per million population in 1999 and 23.7 per million in 2004. Whether this is due to a higher case fatality, an increasing incidence of disease, or both is uncertain.

Economics

The attributable patient cost of CDAD in the USA ranges from $6.408 to $9.124, costing US hospitals $1.14 to $1.62 billion annually [2].

References

1. Poutanen SM, Simor AE (2004 Jul 6) *Clostridium difficile*-associated diarrhea in adults. CMAJ 171(1):51–58
2. Scott II RD (2009) The direct medical costs of healthcare-associated infections in U.S. hospitals and the benefits of prevention. Department of Health and Human Services, Centers for Disease Control and Prevention

Clostridium difficile-Associated Disease

▶ Clostridium difficile-Associated Diarrhea

Closure Time (PFA)

The closure time, or platelet function analyzer, is an in vitro test of primary hemostasis. The assay measures the time necessary for whole blood to occlude a ring coated with collagen and adenosine diphosphate (ADP) or collagen and epinephrine while circulated through a cartridge at high shear flow.

CMR

▶ Cardiac Magnetic Resonance Imaging

Cnidaria

▶ Jellyfish Envenomation

CO (Cardiac Output)

▶ MostCare Monitor

Coagulation, Monitoring at the Bedside

WERNER BAULIG, DONAT R. SPAHN, MICHAEL T. GANTER
Institute of Anesthesiology, University Hospital Zurich,
Zurich, Switzerland

Definition

Bedside coagulation monitoring is useful and essential in assessing patients' hemostatic status with minimal time delays. The primary goal of therapeutic interventions in the coagulation system is to keep the optimal and individual balance between sufficient hemostasis and prevention of thrombosis. In severely bleeding patients, early evidence suggests that treatment directed at aggressive and targeted hemostatic resuscitation can lead to dramatic reductions in mortality. For example, by specific and goal-directed treatment guided by transfusion algorithms, coagulopathic patients may be optimized readily, thereby minimizing exposure to blood products, reducing costs and improving patients' outcome.

Pre-existing Condition

Point of care (POC) monitoring of blood coagulation at the patient's bedside is becoming increasingly important in the perioperative period to guide both pro- and anticoagulant therapies. This monitoring, for example, allows diagnosing potential causes of hemorrhage, to guide hemostatic therapies, to predict the risk of bleeding during consecutive surgical procedures, and to identify patients at risk for thrombotic events [1].

Routine laboratory-based coagulation tests (e.g., PT/INR, aPTT, Fibrinogen) measure clotting times and factors in recalcified plasma after activation with different coagulation activators. Platelet numbers are given to complete overall coagulation assessment. Although accurate, standardized, and used for a long time, the value obtained by routing coagulation testing has been questioned in the perioperative setting because values are measured in plasma, no information on platelet function (PF) is available, and there is a time delay of at least 45–60 min from sampling to obtaining the results. POC coagulation monitoring may overcome several limitations of routine coagulation testing. Blood is analyzed bedside close to the patient and not necessarily in the central laboratory. The coagulation status is assessed in whole blood, better describing the physiological clot development by letting the plasmatic coagulation system interact with platelets and red cells. Furthermore, results are available earlier and clot development can be visually displayed real-time using certain devices.

According to their main objective and function, POC coagulation analyzers can be categorized into (i) techniques analyzing combined plasmatic coagulation, platelet function, and fibrinolytic system, i.e., viscoelastic techniques, (ii) instruments assessing therapeutic anticoagulation like the activated clotting time (ACT) or heparin management devices, and (iii) specific ▶ platelet function analyzers.

Viscoelastic Coagulation Monitoring

Thrombelastography (TEG®), Rotational Thrombelastometry (ROTEM®)

Thrombelastography is a method to assess the overall coagulation function and was first described by Hartert in 1948. Because the thrombelastograph measures the shear elasticity of the blood sample, thrombelastography is sensitive to all interacting cellular and plasmatic components such as coagulation and fibrinolysis. The thrombelastograph measures and graphically displays the time until initial fibrin formation, the kinetics of fibrin formation and clot development, and the ultimate strength and stability of the fibrin clot as well as fibrinolysis. In the earlier literature, the terms thrombelastography, thrombelastograph, and TEG have been used generically. However, in 1996, thrombelastograph and TEG® became a registered trademark of the Haemoscope Corporation (Niles, IL, USA) and from that time onwards these terms have been employed to describe the assay performed using hemoscope instrumentation only. Alternatively, Pentapharm GmbH (Munich, Germany) markets a modified instrumentation using the terminology rotational thrombelastometry, ROTEM®.

The TEG® (Haemonetics Corp., formerly Haemoscope Corp, Niles, IL, USA) measures the clot's physical property by the use of a stationary cylindrical cup that holds the blood sample and is oscillated through an angle of 4°45′. Each rotation cycle lasts 10 s. A pin is suspended in the blood by a torsion wire and is monitored for motion (Fig. 1, TEG®). The torque of the rotation cup is transmitted to the immersed pin only after fibrin–platelet bonding has linked the cup and pin together. The strength of these fibrin–platelet bonds affects the magnitude of the pin motion. Thus, the output is directly related to the strength of the formed clot. As the clot retracts or lyses, these bonds are broken and the transfer of cup motion is again diminished. The rotation movement of the pin is converted by a mechanical-electrical transducer to an electrical signal finally being displayed as the typical TEG® tracing (Fig. 2, TEG®). The ROTEM® (tem International GMBH, formerly Pentapharm GmbH, Munich, Germany) technology avoids some limitations of traditional instruments for thrombelastography, especially the susceptibility to mechanical shocks. Signal transmission of the pin suspended in the blood sample is carried out via an optical detector system, not by a torsion wire and the movement is initiated from the pin, not from the cup. Furthermore,

the instrument is equipped with an electronic pipette (Fig. 1, ROTEM®).

▶ TEG®/ROTEM® both measure and graphically display the changes in viscoelasticity at all stages of the developing and resolving clot (Fig. 2, TEG®/ROTEM®), i.e., the time until initial fibrin formation (TEG® reaction time [R]; ROTEM® clotting time [CT]), the kinetics of fibrin formation and clot development (TEG® kinetics [K], alpha angle [α]; ROTEM® clot formation time [CFT], alpha angle [α]), the ultimate strength and stability of the fibrin clot (TEG® maximum amplitude [MA]; ROTEM® maximum clot firmness [MCF]), and clot lysis (fibrinolysis). TEG®/ROTEM® are fibrinolysis-sensitive assays and allow for diagnosis of hyperfibrinolysis in bleeding patients. To determine the fibrinogen influence,

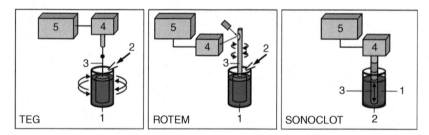

Coagulation, Monitoring at the Bedside. Figure 1 Working principles of viscoelastic point of care (POC) coagulation devices. **TEG®**. rotating cup with blood sample (1), coagulation activator (2), pin and torsion wire (3), electromechanical transducer (4), data processing (5). **ROTEM®**. Cuvette with blood (1), activator added by pipetting (2), pin and rotating axis (3), electromechanical signal detection via light source and mirror mounted on axis (4), data© processing (5). **SONOCLOT®**. Blood sample in cuvette (1), containing activator (2), disposable plastic probe (3), oscillating in blood sample mounted on electromechanical transducer head (4), data processing (5)

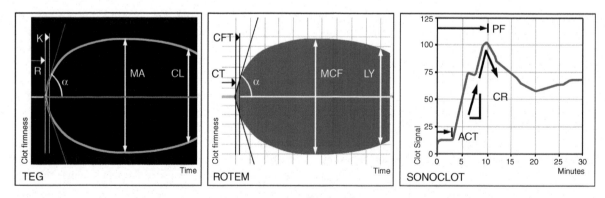

Coagulation, Monitoring at the Bedside. Figure 2 Typical TEG®/ROTEM® tracing and Sonoclot Signature. **TEG®**. R = reaction time, K = kinetics, α = slope between R and K, MA = maximum amplitude, CL = clot lysis. **ROTEM®**. CT = clotting time, CFT = clot formation time, α = slope of tangent at 2 mm amplitude, MCF = maximal clot firmness, LY = Lysis. **SONOCLOT®**. ACT = activated clotting time, CR = clot rate, PF = platelet function

tests can be performed eliminating platelet function by a GPIIb/IIIa inhibitor (e.g., fib-TEM). This concept has been proven to work and a good correlation of this modified MA/MCF with fibrinogen levels determined by Clauss method has been shown. Most common tests for both technologies are listed in Table 1. The repeatability of measurements by both devices has shown to be acceptable, provided they are performed exactly as outlined in the user's manuals.

Sonoclot Coagulation and Platelet Function Analyzer (Sonoclot®)

The Sonoclot Analyzer® (Sienco Inc., Arvada, CO) has been introduced in 1975 by von Kaulla et al. The Sonoclot® measurements are based on the detection of

viscoelastic changes of a whole blood or plasma sample. A hollow probe is immersed into the blood sample and oscillates vertically in the sample (Fig. 1, Sonoclot®). The changes in impedance to movement imposed by the developing clot are measured. Different cuvettes with different coagulation activators/inhibitors are commercially available (Table 1). Normal values for tests run by the ▶ Sonoclot® Analyzer depend largely on the type of sample (whole blood vs plasma, native vs citrated sample) and cuvette used.

The Sonoclot® Analyzer provides information on the entire hemostasis process both in a qualitative graph, known as the Sonoclot® Signature (Fig. 2, Sonoclot®) and as quantitative results: the activated clotting time (ACT), the clot rate (CR), and the platelet function (PF).

Coagulation, Monitoring at the Bedside. Table 1 Commercially available tests for viscoelastic point of care coagulation devices (Modified according to [1])

Assay	Activator inhibitor	Proposed indication
Thrombelastograph hemostasis system (TEG®)		
Kaolin	Kaolin	Overall coagulation assessment including platelet function
Heparinase	Kaolin + heparinase	Specific detection of heparin effect (modified kaolin test adding heparinase to inactivate present heparin)
Platelet mapping	ADP arachidonic acid	Platelet function, monitoring anti-platelet therapy (aspirin, ADP-, GPIIb/IIIa inhibitors)
Native	None	Nonactivated assay
		Also used to run custom hemostasis tests
Rotational thrombelastometry (ROTEM®)		
ex-TEM	TF	Extrinsic pathway; fast assessment of clot formation and fibrinolysis
in-TEM	Contact activator	Intrinsic pathway; assessment of clot formation and fibrin polymerization
fib-TEM	TF + GPIIb/IIIa antagonist	Qualitative assessment of fibrinogen function
ap-TEM	TF + Aprotinin	Fibrinolytic pathway; fast detection of fibrinolysis when used together with ex-TEM
hep-TEM	Contact activator + heparinase	Specific detection of heparin (modified in-TEM test adding heparinase to inactivate present heparin)
na-TEM	None	Nonactivated assay
		Also used to run custom hemostasis tests
Sonoclot® coagulation and platelet function analyzer		
SonACT	Celite	High-dose heparin management
kACT	Kaolin	High-dose heparin management
gbACT+	Glass beads	Overall coagulation and platelet function assessment
H-gbACT+	Glass beads + heparinase	Overall coagulation and platelet function assessment in presence of heparin; detection of heparin
Native	None	Nonactivated assay
		Also used to run custom hemostasis tests

ACT = activated clotting time, TF = tissue factor, ADP = adenosine diposphate, GPIIb/IIIa = glycoprotein IIb/IIIa receptor

The ACT is the time in seconds from the activation of the sample until the beginning of a fibrin formation. This onset of clot formation is defined as a certain upward deflection of the Sonoclot® Signature and is detected automatically by the machine. Sonoclot®'s ACT corresponds to the conventional ACT measurement (see below), provided that cuvettes containing a high concentration of typical activators (celite, kaolin) are being used. The CR, expressed in units/min, is the maximum slope of the Sonoclot® Signature during initial fibrin polymerization and clot development. PF is reflected by the timing and quality of the clot retraction. PF is a calculated value, derived by using an automated numeric integration of changes in the Sonoclot® Signature after fibrin formation has completed (see manufacturer's reference). In order to obtain reliable results for PF, cuvettes containing glass beads for specific platelet activation (gbACT+) should be used. The nominal range of values for the PF goes from 0, representing no PF (no clot retraction and flat Sonoclot® Signature after fibrin formation), to approximately 5, representing strong PF (clot retraction occurs sooner and is very strong, with clearly defined, sharp peaks in the Sonoclot® Signature after fibrin formation).

Bedside Monitoring of Anticoagulation

Activated Clotting Time
The ACT is a functional test of the intrinsic clotting pathway and has been developed for guiding unfractioned heparin-induced anticoagulation at the bedside, particularly during cardiac surgery, extracorporeal membrane oxygenation (ECMO), and coronary interventions. Originally described by Hattersley in 1966, ACT reflects the amount of time to form a clot by contact activation of the coagulation cascade.

Several ACT instruments are commercially available and ACT measurements can be performed using different coagulation activators, each with unique characteristics and various interactions. Results from different ACT tests cannot be used interchangeably. This variability highlights the importance of establishing appropriate instrument-specific reference values for monitoring anticoagulation.

ACT monitoring of heparinization is not without limitations, and its use has been criticized because of significant variability and the poor correlation with plasma heparin concentrations during cardiopulmonary bypass (CPB). It has been suggested that many factors – patient, operator, and equipment – can alter ACT. Therefore, ACT prolongation during CPB is not necessarily caused by heparin administration alone and may be associated with patient hypothermia, inadequacy of specimen warming, hemodilution, quantitative and qualitative platelet abnormalities, or aprotinin infusion. Furthermore, low factor XII levels, which are found in patients with sepsis and patients undergoing renal replacement therapy may lead to falsely high ACT values.

Heparin Concentration Measurement
Because of the limitations of ACT estimating plasma levels of heparin, POC devices have been developed to more accurately measure heparin concentration. The most studied device is the Hepcon HMS Plus Hemostasis Management System (Medtronic, Minneapolis, MN). It calculates heparin doses before initiation of CPB by performing a heparin dose response, measuring heparin concentrations, and calculating protamine doses based on residual heparin levels. A number of clinical studies report that Hepcon guided anticoagulation results in higher total heparin but lower protamine doses than conventional management and may thereby decrease activation of the coagulation and inflammatory cascade [2]. Results are provided readily, however, higher costs, more complex handling, greater dimensions compared to a conventional ACT device, and lack of large studies showing benefit on patient's outcome limited its widespread use so far.

Monitoring Oral Anticoagulants
Several POC coagulation devices have been developed to measure the effects of oral anticoagulants (warfarin therapy) and to provide modified prothrombin time (PT)/INR values. The last-generation devices include the Harmony (Lifescan Inc./Johnson & Johnson, Milpitas, CA) and the INRatio (Hemosense, Inc., Milpitas, CA). Harmony uses thromboplastin as coagulation activator and detects clot formation by light transmission; INRatio uses electrochemical detection of changes in impedance in the blood sample. Results are available immediately in both devices and correlation with PT/INR performed by conventional laboratory coagulation analyzers was good ($R > 0.9$). No vein puncture is required and test results are readily available for clinical use, particularly during phases of rapid changes in the coagulation state [1].

Platelet Function Monitoring
Currently, an increasing number of patients are on antiplatelet medication, such as cyclooxygenase-1 (COX-1) inhibitors, adenosine diphosphate (ADP) antagonists, and glycoprotein (GP) IIb/IIIa inhibitors. In these patients, knowledge of residual platelet function (PF) is highly warranted in order to maintain an optimal and individual balance between platelet function and

inhibition, i.e., bleeding and thrombosis. Traditional assays, such as turbidimetric platelet aggregometry, are still considered clinical standards of PF testing. Turbidimetric platelet aggregometry is one of the most widely used tests to identify and diagnose PF defects. However, conventional platelet aggregometry is labor intensive, costly, time-consuming, and requires a high degree of experience and expertise to perform and interpret. Another important limitation of this technique is that platelets are tested under relatively low shear conditions and in free solution within platelet-rich plasma conditions that do not accurately simulate primary hemostasis. Because of these disadvantages of conventional platelet aggregometry, new automated technologies have been developed to measure PF and several techniques can be used at the bedside [3].

Whole Blood Impedance Platelet Aggregometry

The novel impedance aggregometer ▶ Multiplate® (Dynabyte, Munich, Germany) represents a significant progress in platelet aggregometry and avoids several methodological problems of the original turbidimetric platelet aggregometry, especially by using whole blood, disposable test cuvettes, standardized commercially available test reagents, an automated pipetting system, and rapidly available results. Furthermore, this assay has a high sensitivity in detecting effects of acetylsalicylic acid, thienopyridines, and GPIIb/IIIa inhibitors on platelets.

The principle of Multiplate® impedance platelet aggregometry is based on two silver-coated conductive copper electrodes immersed into whole blood and the ability of activated platelets to adhere to the electrode surface. The instrument continuously measures the change of electrical resistance, which is proportional to the amount of platelets attached to the electrodes. The measured impedance values are transformed to arbitrary aggregation units (AU), which are plotted against the time (Fig. 3). Three parameters are provided: aggregation units (AU), velocity (AU/min), and area under the aggregation curve (AUC), where AUC has the highest diagnostic power. The device has five channels, therefore, parallel testing of five blood samples with different platelet activators at the same time is possible.

Multiplate® has some limitations: it requires high sample volumes, test results are not independent of the actual platelet number, and running the tests is time-consuming and expensive. Additionally, as with other platelet function tests, a resting time of 30 min after blood sampling is recommended before running the tests, which may impede immediate detection of platelet dysfunction intraoperatively.

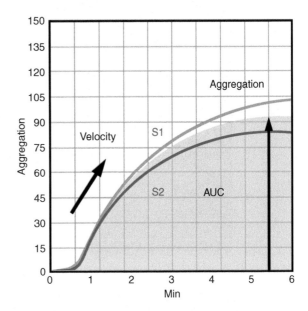

Coagulation, Monitoring at the Bedside. **Figure 3** Whole blood impedance platelet aggregometry: Mulitplate® tracing. The measured impedance values are transformed to arbitrary aggregation units (AU), which are plotted against the time. Measurements are performed in duplicates (S1, S2) and averaged against each other. Velocity (AU/min), aggregation (AU), and area under the aggregation curve (AUC) (Modified according to [5])

VerifyNow™/Ultegra

The ▶ VerifyNow™ Analyzer (Accumetrics, San Diego, CA) incorporates the technique of optical platelet aggregometry. Initially, this technique was distributed as Ultegra Rapid Platelet Function Analyzer (RPFA). The original RPFA assay measured agglutination of fibrinogen-coated beads in response to platelet stimulation. Activated platelets stick to the beads with a consecutive increase in light transmission (Fig. 4). Variation of light absorbance over time is displayed as platelet aggregation units. Early clinical investigations yielded conflicting results and the assay has been modified to the VerifyNow™ assay, now detecting effects of acetylsalicylic acid, ADP-, and GPIIb/IIIa antagonists. This assay has been used, for example, to determine clopidogrel response in clinical trials and its results correlated well with those of platelet aggregometry.

VerifyNow™ tests are easy to perform, and only small sample volumes without necessity of pipetting are required. The absence of flow conditions and the scarce consistency over time in the identification of aspirin-resistant individuals are the limitations of this assay.

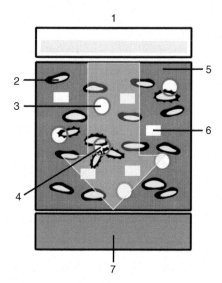

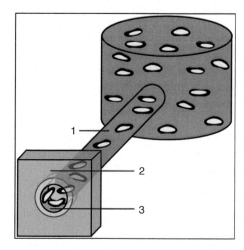

Coagulation, Monitoring at the Bedside. Figure 5 Platelet function analyzer PFA-100®. Citrated whole blood is aspirated at high shear rates through a capillary (1) with a membrane coated microaperture (2). The membrane may be coated with collagen and epinephrine (COL-EPI), or collagen and adenosine diphosphate (COL-ADP) to activate platelets (3). The closure time of PFA-100® is the time taken for activated platelets to occlude the membrane

Coagulation, Monitoring at the Bedside. Figure 4 Working principle of the VerifyNow™/Ultegra device. The VerifyNow™ assay uses platelet agonists (arachidonic acid [aspirin assay], adenosine diphoshate [P2Y12 assay], or thrombin receptor agonist peptide [IIb/IIIa assay]) to activate platelets. As the platelets are activated and start to aggregate with the fibrinogen-coated beads light transmission increases, which will be measured by the light detector. Light source (1), platelet (2), fibrinogen-coated beads (3), activated platelets attached to beads (4), whole blood (5), platelet agonist (6), light detector measuring light transmission (7)

Platelet Function Analyzer (PFA-100®)

The PFA-100® assay (Dade Behring, Schwalbach, Germany) has been clinically introduced in 1985 by Katzer and Born as a screening test for inherent and acquired platelet disorders, as well as von Willebrand's disease. Citrated whole blood is aspirated at high shear rates through a capillary with a membrane-coated microaperture (collagen and either epinephrine [COL-EPI] or ADP [COL-ADP]). Both shear stress and platelet agonists lead to attachment, activation, and aggregation of platelets forming a plug and occluding this microaperture (Fig. 5). The time taken to occlude the aperture is known as closure time (CT) and is a function of platelet number and reactivity, von Willebrand factor activity, and hematocrit. The main advantages of this assay are that it does not require fibrin formation, provides rapid results, and is particularly useful in the diagnosis of von Willebrand's disease and overall platelet dysfunction. However, to get valid results a hematocrit $\geq$30% and platelet counts $\geq$100 $\times$ 10^3/L are required. Additionally, citrate concentration, blood type, and leukocyte count may interfere

with its accuracy. While early reports suggested a high sensitivity for detection of acetylsalicylic acid by prolonged PFA-100® COL-EPI closure time in association with normal values for COL-ADP, more recent investigations cannot confirm these results.

Modified Thrombelastography: Platelet Mapping

Since conventional TEG®/ROTEM® are not sensitive to targeted pharmacological platelet inhibition, a more sophisticated test has been recently developed for the TEG® to specifically determine platelet function in presence of anti-platelet therapy (modified TEG®, Platelet Mapping). Briefly, the maximal hemostatic activity of the blood specimen is first measured by a kaolin-activated whole blood sample. Then, further measurements are performed in presence of heparin to eliminate thrombin activity: reptilase and Factor XIII (Activator F) generate a cross-linked fibrin clot to isolate the fibrin contribution to the clot strength. The contribution of the ADP or TxA2 receptors to the clot formation is provided by the addition of the appropriate agonists, ADP, or arachidonic acid. The results from these different tests are then compared to each other and the platelet function is calculated.

Platelet mapping seems to be a suitable procedure for the assessment of all three classes of anti-platelet agents, but at present the sensitivity and specificity compared to laboratory platelet aggregometry has not been determined in detail. Additionally, the reagents are expensive, multiple channels are required to run the tests, and well-trained personnel are required for optimal performance, limiting its use as POC procedure.

Platelet-Activated Clotting Time

Platelet-activated clotting time (PACT; HemoSTATUS, MedtronicHemoTec, Inc., Parker, CA) is a modified whole blood-activated clotting time test (ACT) adjoining platelet activation factor (PAF) to the reagent mixture for detection of platelet responsiveness by shortening the kaolin-activated clotting time in whole blood samples. Until now, only two studies investigating the correlation to clinical bleeding in patients undergoing cardiac surgery have been performed and their results were controversial.

ICHOR/Plateletworks System

This platelet count ratio assay from Helena Laboratories (Beaumont, TX) simply compares whole blood platelet count in a control EDTA blood sample with the platelet count in a similar sample that has been exposed to a platelet activator. In patients without platelet dysfunction or anti-platelet drug treatment, the presence of the agonist reduces platelet counts close to zero, due to aggregation of most of the platelets. The findings of recent studies indicate that adding the agonist ADP to the test sample appears useful for the assessment of both P2Y12 inhibitors (clopidogrel) and GPIIb/IIIa antagonists. Minimal sample preparation and whole blood processing are advantages of this assay. The main disadvantage, however, is the lack of sufficient investigations.

Impact Cone and Plate(Let) Analyzer

The Impact Cone and Plate(let) Analyzer (CPA, DiaMed, Israel) tests whole blood platelet adhesion and aggregation under artificial flow conditions. A small amount of whole blood is exposed to a uniform shear in a spinning cone and platelet adhesion to the polystyrene wells is automatically analyzed by an inbuilt microscope. The quantity of moistening the surface of the plates (surface covering) depends on platelet function, fibrinogen, von Willebrand's factor levels, and the bioavailability of GPIb and GPIIa/IIIa receptors. Test duration accounts less than 6 min. The addition of arachidonic acid and ADP to the test specimens may assess the effect of acetylsalicylic acid and ADP antagonists on platelets. The Impact Analyzer is a simple and rapid whole blood platelet analyzer requiring small sample volumes. Test results are however dependent on platelet count and hematocrit. Furthermore, only limited published data are available on its clinical performance so far.

Applications

In patients sustaining severe trauma or undergoing major surgery, such as cardiac, aortic, and hepatic surgery, maintaining an adequate coagulation status is essential besides preserving sufficient blood volume and oxygen carrying capacity. These patients require sophisticated and real-time coagulation monitoring to adequately assess and treat hemostasis based on the underlying cause of bleeding (e.g., metabolic disorders, hypothermia, lack of clotting factors, dilutional coagulopathy, platelet dysfunction, hypo-, or hyperfibrinolytic state).

Monitoring Pro-coagulant Therapy

Modern practice of coagulation management is based on the concept of specific component therapy and requires rapid diagnosis and monitoring of the pro-coagulant therapy (i.e., clotting times, clot kinetics, and clot strengthening). Fibrinogen is a key coagulation factor (substrate to form a clot). Fibrinogen levels can be assessed by measuring clot strength (MCF/MA) in the presence of platelet inhibition by a GPIIb/IIIa inhibitor (e.g., fib-TEM) or by assessing Sonoclot®'s CR. Fibrinogen substitution should be considered in a bleeding patient, if MCF levels are lower than 9 mm in a fib-TEM test. Factor XIII is needed for cross-linking fibrin, therefore stabilizing the clot, increasing clot strength and resistance to fibrinolysis. There are reports on patients with unexplained intraoperative bleeding due to decreased factor XIII and subsequent stabilization after substitution.

In order to study thrombin generation, modified TEG®/ROTEM® parameters (based on the original tracing) have been introduced recently: maximum velocity of clot formation (maximum rate of thrombus generation, MaxVel), time to reach MaxVel (time to maximum thrombus generation, tMaxVel), and total thrombus generation (area under the curve, TTG). These parameters are supposed to be more sensitive to rVIIa than standard TEG®/ROTEM® parameters and dilute tissue factor should be used as coagulation activator for best sensitivity.

Antifibrinolytic drugs (e.g., tranexamic and epsilon aminocaproic acid) are used to treat hyperfibrinolysis and to reduce bleeding and transfusion requirements in complex surgical procedures. Antifibrinolytic therapy may be predicted in vitro in TEG®/ROTEM® with certain tests already containing an antifibrinolytic agent (e.g., ap-TEM). Ap-TEM predictive for a good patient response would then show a significantly improved initiation/propagation phase compared to ex-TEM and or disappearance of signs of hyperfibrinolysis. There are no conclusive studies on monitoring desmopressin (DDAVP) therapy so far.

During hepatic surgery and particularly orthotopic liver transplantation (OLT) large derangement in the coagulation status makes POC coagulation monitoring highly desirable. Decreased synthesis and clearance of clotting factors and platelet defects lead to impaired hemostasis and hyperfibrinolysis [5]. Systemic inflammatory response syndrome (SIRS), sepsis, and disseminated intravascular coagulation (DIC) may further complicate a preexisting coagulopathy. Finally, dramatic hyperfibrinolysis may occur during the anhepatic phase of OLT and immediately following organ reperfusion, resulting from accumulation of tissue plasminogen activator due to inadequate hepatic clearance, a release of exogenous heparin, and endogenous heparin-like substances, as well as an overt activation of the complement system. In addition to the hemorrhagic risk associated with hepatic surgery and OLT, hypercoagulability and thrombotic complication have been described in the postoperative period and this can adequately be assessed with TEG®/ROTEM®.

Monitoring Anticoagulant Therapy

The complex process of anticoagulation with heparin for cardiopulmonary bypass (CPB), antagonism with protamine, and postoperative hemostasis therapy in patients undergoing cardiac surgery cannot be performed without careful and accurate bedside coagulation monitoring.

ACT and Sonoclot® Analyzer have been used to guide heparin management for CPB measuring the activated clotting time (ACT) and its accuracy and performance have been shown to be comparable. Furthermore, the Sonoclot® Analyzer has been shown to reliably detect pharmacological GPIIb/IIIa inhibition and successfully used to assess the coagulation status and platelet function successfully in patients undergoing cardiac surgery [6].

Viscoelastic POC coagulation devices have been applied, with limited success, to predict excessive bleeding after CPB. However, large prospective and retrospective studies have demonstrated a significant decrease in perioperative and overall transfusion requirement if hemostasis management was guided by TEG®/ROTEM®-based algorithms.

To detect non-heparin-related hemostatic problems even in presence of large amounts of heparin during CPB, tests with heparinase have been developed for each instrument (Table 1) and algorithms based on heparinase-modified TEG® resulted in a significant reduction of hemostatic products.

Additionally, perioperative administration of drugs with specific anti-platelet activity theoretically requires specific platelet function monitoring at the bedside to guarantee optimal hemostatic management. However, the current commercially available platelet function POC devices are of limited use since these devices often require frequent quality controls and well-trained personnel to run the tests accurately, are time consuming, and expensive. Furthermore, large studies showing the reliability and clinical usability are lacking for most of these POC platelet analyzers.

Monitoring Hypercoagulability and Thrombosis

Recognized risk factors for thrombosis are generally related to one or more elements of Virchow's triad (stasis, vessel injury, and hypercoagulability). Major surgery has been shown to induce a hypercoagulable state in the postoperative period and this hypercoagulability has been implicated in the pathogenesis of postoperative thrombotic complications, including deep vein thrombosis (DVT), pulmonary embolism (PE), myocardial infarction (MI), ischemic stroke, and vascular graft thrombosis.

Identifying hypercoagulability with conventional non-viscoelastic laboratory tests is difficult unless the fibrinogen concentration or platelet count is markedly increased. However, hypercoagulability is readily being diagnosed by viscoelastic POC coagulation analyzers and TEG®/ROTEM® have been increasingly used in the assessment of postoperative hypercoagulability for a variety of surgical procedures. Hypercoagulability is being diagnosed if the R/CT time is short and the MA/MCF is increased (exceeding 65–70 mm) [1].

References

1. Ganter MT, Hofer CK (2008) Coagulation monitoring: current techniques and clinical use of viscoelastic point-of-care coagulation devices. Anesth Analg 106:1366–1375
2. Aziz KA, Masood O, Hoschtitzky JA, Ronald A (2006) Does use of the Hepcon point-of-care coagulation monitor to optimise heparin and protamine dosage for cardiopulmonary bypass decrease bleeding and blood and blood product requirements in adult patients undergoing cardiac surgery? Interact Cardiovasc Thorac Surg 5:469–482
3. Michelson AD (2009) Methods for the measurement of platelet function. Am J Cardiol 103:20A–26A
4. Heindl B, Spannagl M (2008) Gerinnunsmanagement beim perioperativen Blutungsnotfall. Uni-Med Verlag Bremen, 1-Auflage, p 57
5. Dickinson KJ, Troxler M, Homer-Vanniasinkam S (2008) The surgical application of point-of-care haemostasis and platelet function testing. Br J Surg 95:1317–1330
6. Gibbs NM (2009) Point-of-care assessment of anti platelet agents in the perioperative period: a review. Anaesth Intensive Care 37:354–369

Coagulopathy

Jeffry L. Kashuk
Division of Trauma, Acute Care and Critical Care Surgery
and Section of Acute Care Surgery, Penn State Hershey
Medical Center, Hershey, PA, USA

Synonyms

Acute coagulopathy of trauma; posttraumatic DIC

Definition

Hemorrhagic shock leading to postinjury coagulopathy
accounts for approximately half of deaths worldwide of
patients arriving at the hospital with acute injury. This
death rate has improved only marginally over the past
25 years despite the widespread adoption of damage control techniques. Accordingly, postinjury coagulopathy,
defined as continued hemorrhage and ooze despite appropriate surgical control of the bleeding site, remains the
main challenge for improved outcome in this critically
injured cohort.

Previous studies have shown that among patients
presenting with massive acute blood loss, the majority
succumb to refractory coagulopathy despite surgical control of their bleeding. Although the entity has been recognized for over 40 years, the pathogenesis of associated
coagulation abnormalities and appropriate treatment
has remained a matter of debate. Contributing factors
to the "bloody vicious cycle," proposed by our group
over 25 years ago [1], focused on acidosis, hypothermia,
and dilutional effects from excess crystalloid.

Recent evidence, however, suggests that coagulopathy
exists very early after injury and that the condition is
initially independent of clotting factor deficiency, as over
one third of multiply injured patients are coagulopathic by
conventional laboratory assessment on arrival to the emergency department. The fact that this subset of patients also
has an increased incidence of subsequent multiple organ
failure (MOF) and death underscores the importance of
understanding the pathogenesis of early postinjury
coagulopathy. Brohi and Cohen [2] have suggested that
the mechanism of acute endogenous coagulopathy is
mediated by the thrombomodulin pathway via activated
protein C, leading to increased fibrinolysis. Such a process
may be teleologically protective by inducing an "auto-
anticoagulation" state that could potentially protect critical tissue beds in the circulation from thrombosis in the
face of an activated coagulation system responding to
systemic shock and tissue factor release.

Treatment

A uniform approach to management of postinjury
coagulopathy remains a substantial challenge, due to the
fact that hemostasis represents a fusion of multiple
dynamic reactions with complex interactions of thrombin,
fibrinogen, platelets, other protein clotting factors, Ca^{2+},
and endothelium. Furthermore, the contributions of tissue factor release modified by hypothermia and acidosis in
the development of early acute coagulopathy appear
important, and this process may be initiated by either
endothelial-based tissue factor or collagen pathways in
the setting of systemic shock[3]. Our updated "bloody
vicious cycle" [4] emphasizes the fact that early postinjury
coagulopathy ("acute endogenous coagulopathy") occurs
very soon after injury and is unrelated to clotting factor
deficiency and thus resistant to factor replacement.

Rather, this injury complex is triggered by cellular
ischemia and exposed tissue factor, activating endothelium well before clotting factor depletion occurs. However,
with continued blood loss and clot formation in tissue,
factor depletion ultimately occurs, leading to a "systemic
coagulopathy," which unquestionably requires factor repletion to restore coagulation homeostasis. Regardless of the
mechanisms involved, current clinical massive transfusion
protocols promoting "damage control resuscitation"; i.e.,
pre-emptive transfusion of plasma, platelets, and fibrinogen, appropriately represent an initial attempt to replete
substrate for the coagulation system. But appropriate continued use of these expensive, limited resources with potential untoward effects mandates rapid assessment of the
patient's response to the administration of blood components via real-time assessment of coagulation function.

Strategies for Blood Component Replacement

Traditionally, fresh frozen plasma (FFP) is prepared by
isolating the plasma from the cellular components, via
centrifugation of whole blood within 6–8 h of collection.
However, with the advent of apheresis methods little plate-
let-poor plasma is made and most FFP is platelet-rich
plasma, which is then frozen. Some plasma (especially
AB plasma) is collected by apheresis and many centers
use thawed plasma, often referred to as FP24. Regardless
of the plasma source, the hemostatic activity of the various
coagulation factors can be maintained for long periods of
time when frozen; however, upon thawing the concentrations of the various components decrease with the most
significant factors being V and VIII. In the injured patient
requiring factor replacement, the conversion of prothrombin to thrombin requires the coagulation factors XII,
XI, IX, and VIII, along with activated factors X and V.

Thus, the initial management of postinjury coagulopathy requires the administration of thawed fresh frozen plasma (FFP), which contains the above-mentioned coagulation factors and up to 400 mg of fibrinogen. Red blood cell concentrates contain minimal amounts of plasma and coagulation factors.

Consequently, isolated administration of RBC transfusion in the absence of plasma will further potentiate postinjury coagulopathy because of its limited hemostatic potential. The exact dosing and timing of FFP administration is one of the most widely debated topics in trauma.

The "evidence-based" European guidelines for the management of bleeding in major trauma recommends a dose of 10–15 mg/kg of FFP in patients with massive bleeding complicated with coagulopathy, defined as INR >1.5, although these guidelines readily recognize a lack of prospective data. A significant drawback of this approach is the time discrepancy related to the assessment of coagulation parameters and the coagulation status at the time when laboratory values become available. Based on this notion, current US protocols have recommended the pre-emptive substitution of plasma by a standardized ratio of FFP to RBC.

We noted that >85% of transfusions were accomplished within 6 h postinjury [4]. Accordingly, we have focused on this narrower time frame for assessing the effects of resuscitation strategies. Furthermore, our results suggested that the survival threshold appeared to be in the range of 1:2–1:3 of FFP to RBC.

Platelet concentrates have been traditionally prepared from pooling platelets obtained through centrifugation via individual units of whole blood. Currently, apheresis or "single-donor" collections result in fewer donor exposures for a given dose of platelets. Furthermore, apheresis platelets contain between 210 and 250 mL of donor plasma, although clotting factors that are present will diminish rapidly at typical storage temperatures (20–24°C). Clearly, the lack of an accurate assessment of platelet function, as opposed to platelet count, appears to be a significant limiting factor. Thus, the relationship of platelet count to hemostasis and the contribution of the platelet to formation of a stable clot in the injured patient remain largely unknown. The complex relationship of thrombin generation to platelet activation requires dynamic evaluation of clot function, as opposed to static measurements of platelet count, or older methods of clot assessment, such as the bleeding time, which is of no use in the trauma setting. Accordingly, there is no direct evidence to support an absolute trigger for platelet transfusions in trauma.

While the "classic" threshold for platelet transfusion has been 50 K/mm^3, a higher target level at 100 K/mm^3 has been suggested for multiply injured patients and patients with massive hemorrhage. A pool of four to eight platelet concentrates, or one single-donor platelet apheresis unit, have been suggested to provide adequate hemostasis related to thrombocytopenia in bleeding patients, increasing the platelet count by 30–50 K/mm^3. Similar to plasma and packed red cell administration, platelet transfusion is also associated with immunological complications, with a reported incidence of >200 per 100,000 transfused patients. Based on the fact that platelet counts >100 × 109/L are unlikely to contribute to coagulopathy, routine platelet administration in this patient cohort appears unjustified at this time.

Cryoprecipitate is the cold insoluble fraction formed when FFP is thawed at 4°C. "Cryo" is rich in factors VIII, XIII, VWF, and fibrinogen. Generally, fibrinogen levels greater than 50 mg/dL have been considered sufficient to support physiologic hemostasis. Although recent reports have suggested that fibrinogen should be replaced early in coagulopathic trauma patients with hypofibrinogenemia, none have recommended pre-emptive administration.

Many guidelines recommend a replacement threshold for plasma fibrinogen levels <100 mg/dL (1 g/L), using either fibrinogen concentrate (3–4 g) or cryoprecipitate (50 mg/kg or 15–20 units). It is often underappreciated, however, that FFP, pooled platelets, and even packed red blood cells contain fibrinogen. Accordingly, evaluation of plasma fibrinogen levels after administration of component therapy with FFP and platelets during massive resuscitation may avoid unnecessary use of cryoprecipitate. Four units of FFP contain approximately 1,500 mg of fibrinogen, equivalent to one pooled cryoprecipitate pack (1,400 mg). A pooled ten pack of platelets contains approximately 300 mg of fibrinogen. Currently there is no scientific evidence available to support pre-emptive fibrinogen replacement in patients at risk for postinjury coagulopathy.

Thrombelastography

The complexity of the coagulation process and the current evolving understanding of the fundamental mechanisms driving postinjury coagulopathy underscore the lack of available evidence-based studies linking coagulation with mortality. Rapid, real-time functional assessment of coagulation function appears imperative to guide goal-directed therapy of specifically identified coagulation abnormalities.

Recent experience with thrombelastography in our institution [5] suggests that this technology may provide a real-time viscoelastic analysis of the blood clotting process, and could serve as the template for clinical applications of the cell-based model of coagulation. Subsequent treatment protocols could then be tailored based on specific evaluation of clot formation as a representative assay of the coagulation process.

Whole blood (0.35 mL) is placed in a rotating metal cuvette heated to 37°C. A piston is suspended in the sample, and the rotational motion is transferred to the piston as fibrin strands form between the wall of the cuvette and the piston. An electronic amplification system allows for the characteristic tracing to be recorded (see Fig. 1).

Thrombelastography (TEG) assesses clot strength from the time of initial fibrin formation, to clot retraction, ending in fibrinolysis. Of significance, TEG is the only single test that can provide information on the balance between two important and opposing components of coagulation, namely thrombosis and lysis, while the battery of traditional coagulation tests, which include bleeding time, prothrombin time (PT), partial thromboplastin time (PTT), thrombin time, fibrinogen levels, factor assays, platelet counts, and functional assays are based on isolated, static end points. Furthermore, TEG takes into account the interaction of the entire clotting cascade and platelet function in whole blood. The PT is limited as a measure of only the extrinsic clotting system, which includes activation of factor VIIa, Xa, and IIa, while the PTT test is limited by enzymatic reactions in the intrinsic system, including the activation of factor XIIa, XIa, IXa, and IIa. Furthermore, it is well known that hypothermia affects various aspects of the coagulation process and leads to functional coagulation abnormalities. Platelet dysfunction is directly influenced by concentrations of thrombin and fibrinogen, and previous work in our laboratory and by others has demonstrated platelet dysfunction related to hypothermia, acidosis, and hypocalcemia.

Rapid thromboelastography (r-TEG) differs from conventional TEG because tissue factor is added to the whole blood specimen, resulting in a rapid reaction and subsequent analysis. Given the importance of rapid, real-time assessment of coagulation function in trauma, r-TEG appears to be ideal for this purpose. Our recent studies with this technique suggest that a reduction of blood product use may be accomplished [5]. Furthermore, an important aspect of such monitoring is that the results are available point of care (POC), transmitted directly to the operating room computer screens within minutes, enabling prompt resuscitation strategies based on the r-TEG results.

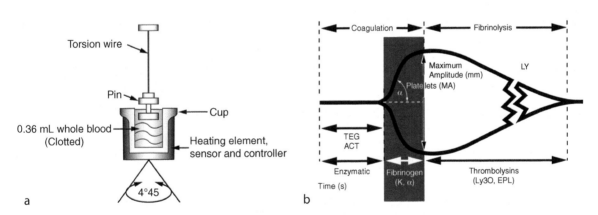

Coagulopathy. Figure 1 Technique of Thrombelastography (reprinted with permission from Hemoscope Corporation, Niles, IL). (**a**) A torsion wire suspending a pin is immersed in a cuvette filled with blood. A clot forms while the cuvette is rotated 45 degrees, causing the pin to rotate depending on the clot strength. A signal is then discharged to the transducer that reflects the continuity of the clotting process. The subsequent tracing (**b**) corresponds to the entire coagulation process from thrombin generation to fibrinolysis. The R value, which is recorded as TEG-ACT in the rapid TEG specimen, is a reflection of enzymatic clotting factor activation. The K value is the interval from the TEG-ACT to a fixed level of clot firmness, reflecting thrombin's cleavage of soluble fibrinogen. The α is the angle between the tangent line drawn from the horizontal base line to the beginning of the cross-linking process. The MA, or maximum amplitude, measures the end result of maximal platelet-fibrin interaction, and the LY 30 is the percent lysis which occurs at 30 minutes from the initiation of the process, which is also calculated as the EPL, or estimated percent lysis

The various components of the r-TEG tracing are depicted in Fig. 1. The r value represents initial thrombin generation and is a reflection of enzymatic clotting factor activation. It is recorded as TEG-ACT for the r-TEG assay, which includes tissue factor.

K is the interval measured from the TEG-ACT to a fixed level of clot firmness or the point that the amplitude of the tracing reaches 20 mm; this reflects thrombin's ability to cleave soluble fibrinogen. The α is the angle between the tangent line drawn from the base horizontal line to the beginning of the cross-linking process, measured in degrees, and is affected primarily by the rate of thrombin generation, which directly influences the conversion of fibrinogen to fibrin; thus the higher the angle, the greater the rate of clot formation. The maximum amplitude (MA) measures the maximum amplitude, and is the end result of maximal platelet–fibrin interaction via the GPIIb-IIIa receptors, which simulates the end product of coagulation via the platelet plug. G is a computer-generated value reflecting the complete strength of the clot from the initial fibrin burst through fibrinolysis and is calculated from A (amplitude), which begins at the bifurcation of the tracing. This is based on a curvilinear relationship: $G = (5000 \times A)/(100 - A)$.

Conceptually, G is the best measure of clot strength because it reflects the contributions of the enzymatic and platelet components of hemostasis. Normal coagulability is defined as G between 5.3 and 12.4 dynes/cm^2 (Haemoscope Corporation, Niles, IL). The r-TEG tracing represents a global analysis of hemostatic function from initial thrombin generation to clot lysis.

Component Blood Product Therapy Guided by Rapid(r) TEG

Transfusion therapy guided by r-TEG has become an integral part of resuscitation in our institution. Using this technology, a variety of coagulation abnormalities have been noted, which in the past would have been overlooked. The various r-TEG values, being derived from a single measurement of whole blood coagulation, are not independent measurements, but a continuum of blood coagulation with interactions between all components. For instance, thrombin liberates fibrinopeptides from fibrinogen, allowing association with other fibrinogen molecules for "soluble fibrin" and subsequently thrombin-activated factor XIII converts "soluble" into "cross-linked" fibrin. Furthermore, thrombin affects platelet function due to combined effects with factor VIII and von-Willibrand factor. In contrast, routine laboratory coagulation tests represent variables that cannot always be compared to r-TEG by simple linear association. Our current protocol of component transfusion therapy emphasizes goal-directed treatment based on r-TEG findings, with the rapid availability of sufficient FFP to provide a final ratio in the range of 1:2–1:3 of FFP to packed red blood cells. Goal-directed therapy enables accurate, stepwise correction of coagulation dysfunction by comparative assessment of the r-TEG tracings generated. Primary fibrinolysis has a distinctive tracing, which should prompt treatment with epsilonaminocaproic acid (Amicar), a lysine analogue which binds reversibly to the kringle domain of the enzymogen plasminogen, preventing its activation to plasmin, which can therefore not split fibrin. Furthermore, we have observed post-fibrinolysis consumptive coagulopathy, which represents diffuse clotting factor deficiency secondary to massive consumption of factors after fibrinolysis. This severe deficit of thrombin may be an indication for r-VIIa, and we have noted rapid improvement with normalization of r-TEG patterns after such treatment. Platelet dysfunction is evident by narrowed maximum amplitude (MA), and decreased clot strength (G value), and the impact of fibrinogen are readily detected on r-TEG as expressed by the angle and K value. r-TEG may allow for improved resuscitation based on real-time coagulation monitoring. The potential benefits of such an approach include (1) reduction of transfusion volumes via specific, goal-directed treatment of identifiable coagulation abnormalities, (2) earlier correction of coagulation abnormalities with more efficient restoration of physiological homeostasis, (3) improved survival in the acute hemorrhagic phase due to improved hemostasis from correction of coagulopathy, and (4) improved outcomes in the later phase due to attenuation of immunoinflammatory complications, including adult respiratory distress syndrome (ARDS) and multiple organ dysfunction (MOF).

References

1. Kashuk J, Moore EE, Milikan JS et al (1982) Major abdominal vascular trauma – a unified approach. J Trauma 22:672
2. Brohi K, Cohen MJ, Ganter MT et al (2008) Acute coagulopathy of trauma: hypoperfusion induces systemic anticoagulation and hyperfibrinolysis. J Trauma 64:1211–1121
3. Furie B, Furie BL (2008) Mechanisms of thrombus formation. N Engl J Med 359:938–949
4. Kashuk JL, Moore EE, Johnson JL et al (2008) Postinjury life threatening coagulopathy: is 1:1 fresh frozen plasma: packed red blood cells the answer? J Trauma 65:261–270
5. Kashuk JL, Moore EE, Wohlauer M et al (2009) Point of care rapid thrombelatography improves management of life threatening postinjury coagulopathy J Trauma (in press)

Cocaine

Judd E. Hollander
Department of Emergency Medicine, University of
Pennsylvania, Philadelphia, PA, USA

Synonyms

Cocaine toxicity; Stimulant toxicity

Definition

Medical complications temporally associated with cocaine
use may occur in many different organ systems.

Most severe cocaine-related toxicity and deaths
follow intense sympathetic stimulation (e.g., tachycardia,
hypertension, dilated pupils, and increased psychomotor
activity). Increased psychomotor activity generates heat
production, which can lead to severe hyperthermia and
rhabdomyolysis.

Cocaine-associated cardiovascular effects are common. Myocardial infarction (MI) due to cocaine occurs
in approximately 6% of patients presenting with cocaine-
associated chest pain [1] and is increased 24-fold in the
hour after cocaine use. In patients aged 18–45 years, 25%
of MIs are attributed to cocaine use and is most common
in patients without large cocaine exposures. Cardiac
conduction disturbances (e.g., prolonged QRS and QTc)
and cardiac dysrhythmias (e.g., sinus tachycardia,
atrial fibrillation/flutter, supraventricular tachycardias,
idioventricular rhythms, ventricular tachycardia, and
ventricular fibrillation) may occur after cocaine use.

The neurologic effects are varied. Altered mental status
and seizures are typically short lived and without serious
sequelae but serious conditions such as cerebral infarction,
intracerebral bleeding, subarachnoid hemorrhage, transient ischemic attacks, and spinal infarction also occur.
Cocaine is associated with a sevenfold increased risk of
stroke in women.

Pulmonary complications of cocaine include asthma
exacerbation, pneumothorax, pneumomediastinum,
noncardiogenic pulmonary edema, alveolar hemorrhage,
pulmonary infarction, pulmonary artery hypertrophy,
and acute respiratory failure. The inhalation of cocaine
is typically associated with deep Valsalva maneuvers
to maximize drug delivery and can cause pneumothorax,
pneumomediastinum, and noncardiogenic pulmonary
edema.

The intestinal vascular system is particularly sensitive
to cocaine effects because the intestinal walls have a wide
distribution of alpha-adrenergic receptors with resulting
acute intestinal infarction.

Patients who present after ingesting packets filled
with cocaine are "body packers" or "body stuffers." Body
packers swallow carefully prepared condom or latex
packets filled with large quantities of highly purified
cocaine to smuggle it into the country. Body stuffers are
typically smaller time drug dealers who swallow packets of
cocaine while avoiding police. Toxicity occurs when
cocaine leaks from the ingested packets. The most severe
manifestations of cocaine toxicity are seen in body packers
carrying large quantities of cocaine who have dehiscence
of a package with a large amount of cocaine.

Chronic cocaine use can predispose patients to other
medical conditions. Chronic users develop left ventricular
hypertrophy that can lead eventually to a dilated cardiomyopathy and heart failure. This is in contrast to the acute
cardiomyopathy from cocaine that appears to have
a reversible component after cessation of cocaine use.

Chronic severe cocaine users can present with lethargy
and a depressed mental status that is a diagnosis of exclusion (cocaine washout syndrome). This self-limited syndrome usually abates within 24 h but can last for several
days and is thought to result from excessive cocaine usage
that depletes essential neurotransmitters.

Treatment

The initial management of cocaine-toxic patients should
focus on airway, breathing, and circulation. Treatments
are directed at a specific sign, symptom, or organ system
affected and are summarized in Table 1.

Sympathomimetic Toxidrome/Agitation

Patients with sympathetic excess and psychomotor agitation are at risk for hyperthermia and rhabdomyolysis.
Management focuses on lowering body temperature, halting further muscle damage and heat production, and
ensuring good urinary output. The primary agents used
for muscle relaxation and control of agitation are benzodiazepines. Doses beyond those typically used for patients
without cocaine intoxication may be required. Antipsy-
chotic agents are useful in mild cases, but their safety in
severe cocaine-induced agitation is not clear. Elevations in
core body temperatures should be treated aggressively
with iced water baths or cool water mist with fans.
Some cases of severe muscle overactivity may require
general anesthesia with nondepolarizing neuromuscular
blockade. Nondepolarizing agents are preferred over succinylcholine, because succinylcholine may increase the
risk of hyperkalemia in patients with cocaine-induced

Cocaine. Table 1 Treatment summary for cocaine-related medical conditions

Medical condition	Treatments
Cardiovascular	
Dysrhythmias	
Sinus tachycardia	Observation
	Oxygen
	Diazepam or lorazepam
Supraventricular tachycardia	Oxygen
	Diazepam or lorazepam
	Consider diltiazem, verapamil, or adenosine
	If hemodynamically unstable: cardioversion
Ventricular dysrhythmias	Oxygen
	Diazepam or lorazepam
	Consider Sodium bicarbonate and/or lidocaine or amiodarone
	If hemodynamically unstable: defibrillation
Acute coronary syndrome	Oxygen
	Aspirin
	Diazepam or lorazepam
	Nitroglycerin
	Heparin
	For ST-segment elevation (STEMI): Percutaneous intervention (angioplasty and stent placement) preferred. Consider fibrinolytic therapy.
	Consider morphine sulfate, phentolamine, verapamil, or glycoprotein IIb/IIIa inhibitors
Hypertension	Observation
	Diazepam or lorazepam
	Consider nitroglycerin, phentolamine, and nitroprusside
Pulmonary edema	Furosemide
	Nitroglycerin
	Consider morphine sulfate or phentolamine
Hyperthermia	Diazepam or lorazepam
	Cooling methods
	If agitated, consider paralysis and intubation
Neuropsychiatric	
Anxiety and agitation	Diazepam or lorazepam
Seizures	Diazepam or lorazepam
	Consider Phenobarbital
Intracranial hemorrhage	Surgical consultation
Cocaine washout syndrome	Supportive care
Rhabdomyolysis	IV hydration
	Consider sodium bicarbonate or mannitol
	If in acute renal failure: hemodialysis
Body packers	Activated charcoal
	Whole-bowel irrigation
	Laparotomy or endoscopic retrieval

rhabdomyolysis. Plasma cholinesterase metabolizes both succinylcholine and cocaine; therefore, prolonged clinical effects of either or both agents might occur when both are used.

Hypertension
Patients with severe hypertension can usually be safely treated with benzodiazepines. When benzodiazepines alone are not effective, nitroglycerin, nitroprusside, or phentolamine can be used. Beta-blockers are contraindicated because in the setting of cocaine intoxication, they cause unopposed alpha-adrenergic stimulation with subsequent exacerbation of hypertension.

Myocardial Ischemia or Infarction
Patients with cocaine-associated myocardial ischemia or infarction should be treated with aspirin, benzodiazepines, and nitroglycerin as first-line agents. Benzodiazepines decrease the central stimulatory effects of cocaine, thereby indirectly reducing its cardiovascular toxicity. Benzodiazepines have a comparable and possibly an additive effect to nitroglycerin with respect to chest pain resolution and hemodynamic parameters for patients with chest pain. Weight-based unfractionated heparin or enoxaparin, as well as clopidogrel are reasonable to use in patients with documented ischemia. Patients who do not respond to these initial therapies can be treated with phentolamine or calcium channel-blocking agents. In the acute setting, beta-blockers are contraindicated, as they can exacerbate cocaine-induced coronary artery vasoconstriction [1, 2].

When patients have ST-segment elevation and require reperfusion, primary percutaneous coronary intervention (PCI) is preferred over fibrinolytic therapy due to a high rate of false-positive ST-segment elevations in patients with cocaine-associated chest pain, even in the absence of acute myocardial infarction (AMI), as well as the possibility of an increased rate of cerebral complications in patients with repetitive cocaine use [2].

Dysrhythmias
Supraventricular dysrhythmias may be difficult to treat. Initially, benzodiazepines should be administered. Adenosine can be given, but its effects may be temporary. The use of calcium channel blockers in association with benzodiazepines appears to be most beneficial. Beta-blockers should be avoided.

Ventricular dysrhythmias can be managed with benzodiazepines, lidocaine, or sodium bicarbonate. Bicarbonate is preferred in patients with QRS widening and ventricular dysrhythmias that occur soon after cocaine use, since these dysrhythmias are presumably related to sodium channel-blocking effects of cocaine. Lidocaine can be used when dysrhythmias appear to be related to cocaine-induced ischemia.

Seizures
Benzodiazepines and phenobarbital are the first- and second-line drugs, respectively. Phenytoin is not recommended in cases associated with cocaine. Although no studies have compared barbiturates to phenytoin for control of cocaine-induced seizures, barbiturates are theoretically preferable because they also produce central nervous system (CNS) sedation and are generally more effective for toxin-induced convulsions. Newer agents have not been well studied in the setting of cocaine intoxication.

Cerebrovascular Infarction
Cocaine can lead to both ischemic and hemorrhagic strokes. Most of these patients should be managed similarly to patients with non-cocaine-associated cerebrovascular infarctions with two exceptions: The utility of tPA in patients with recent cocaine-associated cerebrovascular events is unknown; blood pressure management should follow the recommendations that are mentioned above.

Aortic Dissection
Cocaine use can lead to aortic dissection. Various studies have found that 1–37% of aortic dissections may be due to cocaine. Treatment is similar to other patients with aortic dissection but medical management should be adjusted to try avoid beta-blockade.

Body Stuffers and Packers
Body stuffers who manifest clinical signs of toxicity should be treated similarly to other cocaine-intoxicated patients. Gastrointestinal decontamination with activated charcoal should be performed. Assessment for unruptured cocaine packages should be considered. In some cases, whole bowel may be necessary.

Body packers are typically asymptomatic at the time of detention when passing immigration. In patients who present with symptoms or develop symptoms of cocaine toxicity or rapidly deteriorate because of exposure to huge doses of cocaine, immediate surgical removal of the ruptured packages may be necessary.

Evaluation/Assessment
Patients manifesting cocaine toxicity should have a complete evaluation focusing on the history of cocaine use, signs, and symptoms of sympathetic nervous system excess, and evaluation of specific organ system complaints.

It is important to determine whether signs and symptoms are due to cocaine itself, underlying structural abnormalities, or cocaine-induced structural abnormalities.

Laboratory Tests

Since some patients may deny cocaine use, urine testing may be helpful. If the patient manifests moderate or severe toxicity, laboratory evaluation may include a complete blood cell count, serum electrolytes, glucose, blood urea nitrogen, creatinine, creatine kinase (CK), cardiac marker determinations, arterial blood gas analysis, and urinalysis. Hyperglycemia and hypokalemia may result from sympathetic excess. Rhabdomyolysis can be diagnosed by an elevation in CK. Cardiac troponin I or T should be used to identify acute MI in symptomatic patients with cocaine use.

Imaging and Other Tests

Chest radiography and electrocardiography should be obtained in patients with potential cardiopulmonary complaints. Computerized tomography (CT) of the head can be used to evaluate seizure or stroke. Patients with concurrent headache, suspected subarachnoid hemorrhage, or other neurologic manifestations may necessitate lumbar puncture after head CT to rule out other CNS pathology.

After-care

The appropriate diagnostic evaluation should follow general principles for the specific complication that occurred. For risk stratification in patients who presented with potential coronary artery disease, it is recommended that most patients receive imaging with some form of stress testing or CT coronary angiography.

Prognosis

Patient prognosis is dependent upon the type of complication the patient had from cocaine use. Continued cocaine usage, however, is associated with an increased likelihood of recurrent symptoms, and therefore, aggressive drug rehabilitation may be useful.

Cessation of cocaine is the hallmark of secondary prevention. Recurrent chest pain is less common and MI and death are rare in patients who discontinue cocaine [2–4]. Aggressive risk factor modification is indicated in patients with MI or with evidence of premature atherosclerosis, coronary artery aneurysm, or ectasia. This includes smoking cessation, hypertension control, diabetes control, and aggressive lipid-lowering therapy. While these strategies have not been tested specifically for patients with cocaine, they are standard of care for patients with underlying coronary artery disease.

Patients with evidence of atherosclerosis may be candidates for long-term antiplatelet therapy with aspirin with or without clopidogrel for patients who received stent placement. The role of nitrates and calcium channel blockers remains speculative and should be used for symptomatic relief. The use of beta-adrenergic antagonists, although useful in patients with previous MI and cardiomyopathy needs special consideration in the setting of cocaine abuse. Since recidivism is high in patients with cocaine-associated chest pain (60% admit to cocaine use in the next year), beta-blocker therapy should probably be avoided in many of these patients.

References

1. McCord J, Jneid H, Hollander JE, de Lemos JA, Cercek B, Hsue P, Gibler WB, Ohman EM, Drew B, Philippides G, Newby LK (2008) Management of cocaine-associated chest pain and myocardial infarction a scientific statement from the American Heart Association Acute Cardiac Care Committee of the Council on Clinical Cardiology. Circulation 117:1897–1907
2. Hollander JE (1995) Management of cocaine associated myocardial ischemia. N Engl J Med 333:1267–1272
3. Hollander JE, Hoffman RS, Burstein J, Shih RD, Thode HC, the Cocaine Associated Myocardial Infarction Study (CAMI) Group (1995) Cocaine associated myocardial infarction. Mortality and complications. Arch Intern Med 155:1081–1086
4. Weber JE, Shofer FS, Larkin GL, Kalaria AS, Hollander JE (2003) Validation of a brief observation period for patients with cocaine associated chest pain. N Engl J Med 348:510–517

Cocaine Toxicity

▶ Cocaine

Coccidioidomycosis

Julie P. Chou[1], Tom Lim[1], Andrew G. Lee[2],
Christopher H. Mody[3]
[1]Department of Internal Medicine, University of Calgary, Calgary, AB, Canada
[2]Department of Radiology, University of Calgary, Calgary, AB, Canada
[3]Departments of Internal Medicine and Microbiology, Immunology and Infectious Disease, University of Calgary, Calgary, AB, Canada

Synonyms

California valley fever; Desert fever; San Joaquin valley fever; Valley fever

Definition

Coccidioidomycosis is an infection caused by the dimorphic fungi of the genus *Coccidioides*. *Coccidioides* species are endemic to semiarid regions of the western hemisphere, including the San Joaquin Valley of California, the south-central region of Arizona, and northwestern Mexico. They can also be found in parts of Central and South America.

Infection is generally acquired through inhalation, whereby infectious arthroconidia reach the lower respiratory tract. Only a small proportion of infected individuals will come to medical attention, as the majority of infections are subclinical. Although a wide spectrum of manifestations is possible, the majority of primary infections present with symptoms and signs comparable to community-acquired pneumonia or an upper respiratory tract infection. In addition to nonspecific symptoms such as chest pain, cough, and fever, other presenting complaints may include marked fatigue, arthralgias, erythema nodosum, and erythema multiforme. Peripheral eosinophilia and an elevated erythrocyte sedimentation rate can be observed. A pulmonary infiltrate with or without hilar adenopathy can be evident on chest x-ray or CT scan (Fig. 1).

In immunocompetent hosts, primary pulmonary coccidiodomycosis is usually a self-limiting disease. However, patients with suppressed cellular immunity, such as those with HIV infection, solid organ transplant recipients, or individuals receiving chronic corticosteroid treatment, are predisposed to disseminated disease. African-American, Hispanic men, and pregnancy, place individuals at increased risk for disseminated disease. Extrapulmonary infection can be found in any organ system, but most commonly affects skin, bones, joints, and meninges. CSF analysis should be performed in patients with primary coccidioidomycosis presenting with CNS symptoms, and in patients who are severely ill warranting intensive care unit admission, or patients that may find it difficult to be followed by a physician.

Others at risk include patients who are receiving TNF-alpha inhibitor therapy. They are more likely to develop symptoms when infected. Preexisting diabetes mellitus is associated with a higher likelihood of developing chronic pulmonary coccidioidomycosis, in particular cavitary disease. Because of the concern for hemoptysis from cavities, these patients require close monitoring.

Treatment

Immunocompetent Patients

Immunocompetent patients are unlikely to present to the intensive care unit and treatment is usually not required in

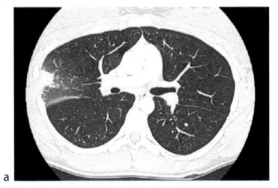
a
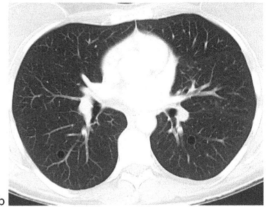
b

Coccidioidomycosis. Figure 1 Coccidioidomycosis in two different patients. (**a**) A peripheral pulmonary infiltrate on computed tomography. (**b**) Thin-walled cavities as a late sequela of coccidioidomycosis

primary pulmonary coccidioidomycosis. However, if the symptoms persist for greater than 6 weeks, therapy should be considered.

Immunosuppressed Patients

Patients with risk factors for disseminated disease are offered treatment when they present with primary pulmonary coccidioidomycosis. All forms of disseminated coccidioidomycosis require antifungal therapy.

First-line therapy for treating chronic coccidioidomycosis is an oral azole. Ketoconazole, fluconazole, and itraconazole have all been well studied. Itraconazole may be superior in treating bone and join disease than fluconazole. Amphotericin B is reserved for the most severe cases of coccidioidomycosis or for those who fail to respond to azoles. Although the evidence is lacking for superiority in treatment using liposomal amphotericin B, it should be considered for therapy in individuals with underlying renal disease.

The duration of therapy is generally prolonged for chronic coccidioidomycosis, with a minimum course of 12–18 months. A longer course might be considered in immunocompromised patients. Moreover, if the meninges are involved, lifelong azole antifungal therapy is required because of a high relapse rate. Although intravenous amphotericin B lacks efficacy in the treatment of *Coccidioides* meningitis, intrathecal amphotericin B can be used in cases refractory to azole therapy, or in situations when a more rapid response is desired.

As for other classes of antifungal agents, the echinocandins have yet to be adequately assessed in coccidioidomycosis. By contrast, there are small series and case reports suggesting efficacy of voriconazole and posaconazole when used as salvage therapy. However, no definitive recommendation can be made at this time.

Evaluation/Assessment

The diagnosis can be established by detecting the presence of anticoccidioidal antibody in the serum via a variety of techniques including ELISA, immunodiffusion, tube precipitin, and complement fixation assays. It should be remembered; however, that critically ill patients may not mount an effective antibody response and thus, may have false negative serology. Alternatively, the diagnosis can also be confirmed by identifying coccidioidal spherules in tissue or by culturing the organism from a clinical specimen.

In the future, polymerase chain reaction (PCR) and real-time PCR may play a greater role in diagnostics. However, no commercial methods are currently available for direct detection of *C. immitis* from patient specimens.

After-care

For patients with severe infection, immunosuppression or other risk factors for dissemination, lifelong follow-up may be required. In milder cases, patients require close monitoring of their disease every 2–4 weeks following initial diagnosis. After noting improvement of their symptoms, clinic visits may be extended to intervals of every 3–6 months, for up to 2 years. Changes in complement fixation serologic titers can be useful, as a rise in titer is usually associated with disease progression. Radiographic abnormalities should be reexamined on a periodic basis.

Prognosis

For patients that have had a critical illness with disseminated disease, the outlook depends on the anatomic site of infection and the underlying immune status of the patient.

Relapses are common in this population of patients. While the prognosis is good for most people with pulmonary coccidioidomycosis, many patients have protracted fatigue after resolution of pulmonary symptoms.

References

1. Dewsnup DH, Galgiani JN, Graybill JR, Diaz M, Rendon A, Cloud GA, Stevens DA (1996) Is it ever safe to stop azole therapy for *Coccidioides immitis* meningitis? Ann Intern Med 124:305–310

Coelenterata

▶ Jellyfish Envenomation

Coelenterate

▶ Jellyfish Envenomation

Cold Sore

▶ Herpes Simplex

Collapse

▶ Syncope

Collapsed Lung

▶ Pneumothorax

Colloid Challenge

▶ Fluid Challenge

Colloids

Lewis J. Kaplan, Roselle Crombie, Gina Luckianow
Department of Surgery, Yale University School of
Medicine, New Haven, CT, USA

Synonyms

Plasma volume expander (PVE); Synthetic colloid (as
opposed to biologically active colloids such as fresh frozen
plasma and human albumin)

Trade Names

As the number of colloid products is legion, a complete
listing of all manufactured colloids available throughout
the world is beyond the scope of this chapter. A partial
listing of commonly utilized colloids is presented in
Table 1.

Class and Category

All colloids belong to the class of drugs known as plasma
volume expanders. The category of different colloids
relates to the specific composition of each colloid. Nonetheless, unique differences within each category explain
the differing efficacies and plasma half-lives, and often
frequency of use. Following is a general categorization of
commonly utilized colloids for plasma volume expansion.
Of note, hypertonic saline preparations are not colloids
even though they are used for plasma volume expansion
and will not be further discussed within this chapter.

General Principles of Colloids [1]

Colloids are defined as a preparation of a homogenous
noncrystalline substance that is dispersed throughout
another substance that is usually a water-based solution
(for medical use). The colloid may be large macromolecules or microparticles, which do not settle and are not
separable from their suspending solution by filtration or
centrifugation. Colloids are generally polydispersed,
representing a span of molecular sizes that characterize
a single preparation. Molecular weight (MW) which is
generally constant may be described in two different
fashions:

1. Weight-averaged MW: (# molecules at each weight
   X particle weight)/total weight of all molecules
2. Number-averaged MW: mean of all particle weights

Furthermore, the weight distribution pattern may be
assessed by the colloid oncotic pressure ratio, a ratio that
reflects the osmotic activity to a colloid solution across
membranes with different pore sizes.

In general practice, the size, persistence, efficacy at
plasma volume expansion, side effect profile, and, of
course, product approval by regulatory agencies, tend to
govern clinician product selection. The clinician should
remain acutely aware that the colloid preparations contribute very little free water to the patient's system and
therefore, should always be utilized with maintenance
solutions to avoid inadvertently creating a hyperoncotic
state (see Adverse Reactions below).

Starches [1]

Starches are synthetic colloid preparations derived from
amylopectin extracted from either maize or sorghum.
Amylopectin is a D-glucose polymer that is synthetically
modified with hydroxyethyl substitutions at the second
carbon (C2) as well as the sixth carbon (C6) with rather
few substitutions occurring at the third carbon (C3);
hydroxylation retards the rate of hydrolysis by plasma
nonspecific α-amylases. Starches are characterized by
their average molecular weight and average molecular
size as they exist as a polydispersed preparation of different molecular weight and sizes. Thus, starches may be
further classified by their average molecular weight into
high MW (>450 kDa), medium MW (~200 kDa), and
low MW (70–130 kDa). Furthermore, they are characterized by the C2/C6 substitution ratio; the greater the ratio,
the slower the degradation. The number of hydroxyethyl
groups per 100 glucose groups is known as the degree of
substitution (DS) or substitution ratio (MS); ratios are
expressed as a number spanning 0–1. In a fashion similar
to the C2/C6 substitution ratio, the greater the DS or MS,
the longer the half-life ($t_{1/2}$).

By way of example, Hextend is a commercially available starch used in the USA. It may be characterized as
a large MW starch (670 kDa) with a high degree of
substitution (0.7). The last two characteristics are the
concentration of the prepration and the diluent in
which the colloid is prepared. Hextend is a 6% starch
preparation is a balanced salt solution. Changing the
diluent may change important consequences of administration rendering the product functionally different.
For instance, Hextend's predecessor, Hespan, is the identical starch in every way but was prepared in a saline
base. Hespan contains a FDA black box warning with
regard to volume of administration and induced bleeding
risk; no such black box exists for Hextend. Table 1 presents commonly utilized colloid preparations and their
characteristics.

Colloids. Table 1 Common starch-based colloids used for resuscitation

Colloid	MW/DS	Concentration	Diluent	C2/C6
Voluven[a]	HES 130/0.4	6% 10%	NSS	9:1
Volulyte	HES130/0.4	6%	Balanced solution	6:1
Pentastarch	HES 200/0.5	6% 10%	NSS	5:1
Hextend[a]	HES 670/0.7	6%	Balanced solution	4.5:1
Hespan[a]	HES 670/0.7	6%	NSS	4.5:1

HES = hydroxyethyl starch
NSS = 0.9% normal saline solution
MW = molecular weight in kiloDaltons (kDa)
DS = degree of substitution
Note: not all colloids are available in the US Food and Drug Administration; approved colloids are indicated by ([a])

Gelatins [1]

Gelatins are preparations created from the hydrolysis of bovine collagen and then further modified by either succinylation (polygeline; Gelofusine) of urea linkage (Hemaccel). Succinylation results in no change in MW but a significant increase in molecular size; no such changes occur with urea linkage. The diluents are different between the two products with only Hemaccel being prepared with calcium and potassium. It is important to note that the only cases of prion-related disease derived from cattle involve food-based disease transmission, not pharmaceutical preparations.

Dextrans [1]

Dextrans are fairly homogenous preparations of D-glucose polymers principally joined by α-1,6 bonds creating linear macromolecules that are characterized by their concentration into two commercially available preparations, Dexran 40 (MW avg = 40 kDa) and Dextran 70 (MW avg = 70 kDa). The glucose moieties are derived from enzymatic cleavage of sucrose generated by *Leuconostoc* bacteria utilizing the enzyme dextran sucrase yielding high molecular weight detrains that are modified into the final product using acid hydrolysis and ethanol-based fractionation processes.

Clearance is proportional to MW with 50–55 kDa molecules being readily renally filtered and excreted unchanged in the urine such that 70% of a Dextran 40 dose is excreted unchanged over a 24-h period. Molecules with a larger MW undergo GI clearance or cleavage within the reticuloendothelial system via extant dextranases. Only

Dextran 40 appears to have clinical use at present due to issues with allergic reaction and bleeding with Dextran 70.

Combination Preparations

Combinations of hypertonic saline and hyperoncotic starch are available as well. These preparations rely on starch plasma volume expansion and the concentration-dependent movement of water from the extravascular space to the intravascular domain on the basis of creating a hyperoncotic plasma space. Their efficacy or outcome advantage over other colloid solutions has yet to be demonstrated.

Indications [2, 3]

Colloids are indicated for the treatment of suspected or proven hypovolemia that requires plasma volume expansion. However, as there is increasing evidence that hyperchloremic metabolic acidosis (HCMA) deleteriously impacts outcomes, likely through activation of inflammatory pathways, colloid administration may have a selective advantage. In general, one needs to administer much less colloid than crystalloid to achieve equivalent plasma volume expansion, and therefore, one delivers much less chloride to the patient's system. Thus, plasma volume expansion with colloids reduces the likelihood of creating a HCMA when large volume plasma volume expansion is required for the restoration of appropriate perfusion.

Dosage

Dosage of different preparations varies with local geography as a reflection of different regulatory bodies' approval process. However, certain commonalities may be articulated. The general goal of a plasma volume expansion challenge is to provide 5% plasma volume expansion (PVE) for those with hypovolemia but no hypotension, and to provide 10% PVE for those with hypotension as an initial bolus. Thus, based on the properties of Hextend, 250 cc of the solution is appropriate for hypovolemia, but 500 cc is ideal for hypotension. Given the properties of the smaller MW starch Voluven, the same volumes would be used in identical scenarios. However, the dose of Voluven would need to be repeated more frequently based on its shorter $t_{1/2}$ than Hextend. The reader should be aware that more frequent dosing is not a deleterious property, but rather reflects the biologic behavior of the colloid, and may be advantageous in certain circumstances (see Contraindications below).

Preparation/Composition

The preparation and composition of many of the commercially available colloid solutions are presented in Table 1. The reader should be aware that new products and preparations are in development and therefore, the listing in Table 1 should be viewed as only a partial presentation.

Contraindications

The main contraindications for synthetic colloid administration are allergy or intolerance to the colloid or its diluent. A further contraindication is hypervolemia in a patient with dialysis-dependent renal failure as if one induces heart failure or pulmonary edema, starch is not dialyzable and one must wait for enzymatic degradation. Along similar lines, chronic renal insufficiency (although not dialysis dependent) as well as evolving acute renal failure are relative contraindications for long half-life starches. The need for >20 cc/kg bw in 24 h is a contraindication for Hespan specifically, although not for Hextend according to the US Food and Drug Administration. Some authors have advanced the notion that sepsis is a contraindication for starch-based colloid administration but the authors of this chapter do not believe that such a claim is justified (see below).

Adverse Reactions

Allergic reaction is exceedingly rare with starch or gelatin products, but appears to be a limiting factor with large MW Dextrans. Perhaps the most notable adverse reaction is that of suspected renal dysfunction presenting as acute kidney injury or acute renal failure in patients who have undergone PVE using starch-based synthetic colloids in the setting of sepsis. The reader is encouraged to critically review this literature as there are several key features that call the conclusions into serious question.

A review of actual practice in 3,147 patients in 198 European Union ICUs during 2 weeks in May 2002 identified that colloid administration was often a combination of different colloids, and not limited to a single colloid [4]. Furthermore, in clinical practice, there was no difference in any measured or derived index of renal function, or the need for renal replacement therapy, with regard to colloid administration of any variety including hyper- or hypooncotic albumin, starches, gelatin, and dextran; approximately 15% of ICUs used more than one colloid at the same time on a given patient.

The reader should recall that since there are a multitude of colloid preparations, comparing across multiple studies is exceptionally difficult as the preparations differ in MW, DS, diluent, volume, whether or not there was a fluid administration protocol, when in the clinical course did the patient receive colloid, and whether there was a pressure or flow-based monitoring system guiding therapy. Furthermore, delays prior to presentation, persistence of shock, timing of pressor use, specific pressors used, rapidity of resuscitation (before or after the vigorous volume expansion popularized by the Early Goal-Directed Therapy trial), the rapidity of source control, and the number of hypotensive episodes all influence renal perfusion. None of the trials are controlled for the presence of hyperchlormic metabolic acidosis, an entity known to reduce renal perfusion in an independent fashion. Furthermore, the definitions utilized for renal failure all differ, and many studies were performed prior to the recognition of acute kidney injury as a distinct entity. Additionally, the indications for renal replacement therapy are not uniform and some studies use the need for RRT as the definition of renal failure. Thus, drawing any conclusion from the case reports, case series, and few large but heterogenous trials that claim starch-based PVE indices renal injury and failure is problematic at best.

Furthermore, trials such as the VISEP study comparing pentastarch to lactated Ringers solution either over-resuscitate the pentastarch group or under-resuscitate the LR group depending on your perspective as both groups received identical volumes of fluid [5]. This ignores the basic concept underpinning colloid-based PVE – colloid are better retained in the plasma space and therefore, one administers a smaller volume. It is little surprising that the pentastarch group evidences a higher CVP and a lower hemoglobin than the LR group based on unequal fluid administration. Also, there was an unequal distribution of patients requiring emergency operative undertakings to the pentastarch group – the at-risk group for acute tubular necrosis, AKI, and ARF!

Perhaps equally important is the unreported presence or absence of concomitant maintenance fluid in trials addressing colloid administration versus crystalloid-based plasma volume expansion regimens. An important trial evaluated several different fluids for PVE in the treatment of shock, but categorized the fluids based on whether the fluid was hyper- or hypo-oncotic and determined the occurrence of renally relevant events [6]. Crystalloids were compared to hypo-oncotic albumin and gelatin versus hyperoncotic starch versus hyperoncotic albumin. Importantly, *all* of the renally relevant events including the need for renal replacement therapy occurred in the hyperoncotic groups. Unfortunately, the definition of ARF used in this trial was a doubling of baseline creatinine, or the need for dialysis. This study underscores the need to avoid creating an inadvertent hyperoncotic state when using hyperoncotic PVEs at least in patients with shock. It is likely that this observation may be extended to those with hypovolemia without shock as well, but the decreased effective circulating volume that characterizes septic and hypovolemic shock places this patient population at particular risk for hyperoncoticity when the principle administerd fluid is a hyperoncotic colloid.

Current bias has begun to focus on the use of low MW and lesser substituted starch-based colloids such as Voluven (6% HES, 130/0.4 prepared in saline) and its counterpart agent, Volu-Lyte that is prepared in a balanced salt solution in a fashion similar to that of Hespan and Hextend. Since the lower MW and less substituted compounds have a shorter half-life, it is expected that renal accumulation will occur less frequently and present a reduced risk of AKI and ARF as a consequence of starch administration in sepsis. However, the concerns articulated above may not support such notions, and there are other elements that remain unidentified. For instance, since starch has been identified in the renal tubular cells of those with ARF who have received starch-based PVE, we do not know if the starch presence is causative or simply coincident and of no functional consequence. Data are conflicting even in the renal transplantation patient population. Moreover, since one does not biopsy normal kidneys, one does not know if a patient who received a starch-based PVE regimen and who did not change their creatinine also had starch molecules accumulate in their renal tubular cells. While there is much bias and speculation, the medical community appears to be divided into those who have already lost their clinical equipoise with regard to starch and renal injury and those who are awaiting data.

Drug Interactions

There are no significant drug interactions noted for colloid preparations. There is some concern, although unfounded, that calcium containing colloids may not be administered through the same IV line as blood products for fear of clotting. In clinical practice, given the rapid rate of administration of each agent, clotting is not clinically identified.

Mechanisms of Action

Colloids serve to expand plasma volume by exerting osmotic activity and having synthetic modification to retard the rate of degradation or filtration, thus preserving their plasma half-life. Incidental modification of rheology is also noted with colloid administration that is mediated in part by altering RBC flexibility through small-diameter vessels, and in part through reductions in viscosity [7]. As a result, some observations identify colloid-based support of microcirculatory delivery of oxygen as judged by muscle tissue oximetry compared to non-colloid-based PVE regimens when fluids and blood products were administered on protocol and titrated to a CVP measurement.

Cross-References

▶ Intravenous Fluids

References

1. Grocott M, Mythen M, Gan TJ (2005) Perioperative fluid management and outcomes in adults. Anesth Analg 100:1093–1106
2. Mike James review of colloids
3. Boldt J (2002) Hydroxyethyl starch as a risk factor for acute renal failure: Is a change of practice indicated? Drug Saf 25(12):837–846
4. Sakr Y, Payen D, Reinhart K et al (2007) Effects of hydroxyethyl starch administration on renal function in critically ill patients. Br J Anaesth 98(2):216–224
5. Brunkhorst FM, Engel C, Bloos F et al (2008) Intensive insulin therapy and pentastarch resuscitation in severe sepsis. N Engl J Med 358:125–139
6. Schortgen F, Girou E, Deye N et al (2008) The risk associated with hyperoncotic colloids in patients with shock. Inten Care Med 34(12):2157–2168
7. Neff TA, Fischler L, Mark M et al (2005) The influence of two different hydroxyethyl starch solutions (6% HES 130/0.4 and 200/0.5) on blood viscosity. Anesth Analg 100:1773–1780

Colonization

The process whereby microorganisms inhabit a specific body site (such as the skin, bowel, or chronic ulcers) without causing a detectable host immune response, cellular damage, or clinical signs and symptoms. It involves adherence of organisms to epithelial cells, proliferation, and persistence at the site of attachment. The presence of the microorganism may be of varying duration and may become a potential source of transmission.

Colonoscopy

▶ Gastrointestinal Endoscopy

Coma

DERRICK SUN, KATHRYN M. BEAUCHAMP
Department of Neurosurgery, Denver Health Medical Center, University of Colorado School of Medicine, Denver, CO, USA

Synonyms

Blackout; Encephalopathy; Stupor; Unconsciousness; Vegetative state

Definition

Coma is defined as the state of profound unconsciousness, from which the patient cannot be aroused to respond appropriately to external stimuli. It originates from the Greek word meaning "deep sleep or trance." It represents an acute and life-threatening emergency, requiring rapid diagnosis and intervention in order to preserve brain function and life.

Coma lies on a spectrum of terms used to describe varying degrees of alteration of consciousness, including lethargy, stupor, and obtundation. The Glasgow Coma Scale (GCS) is a simple and objective scoring system used by health-care professionals to quickly assess the severity of brain dysfunction, composed of three tests: eye-opening response, verbal response, and motor response. Eye opening is graded from 1 to 4. Verbal response is graded from 1 to 5. In intubated patients, a score of "1" is given for verbal response with a modifier of "T." Motor response is graded from 1 to 6. The GCS score, a sum of all three components, ranges from 3 (deep coma or death) to 15 (fully awake person). GCS score of 8 or less is generally accepted as operational definition for coma.

Consciousness is defined as the state of awareness of oneself and one's surrounding environment. Consciousness has two major interconnected components: wakefulness (i.e., arousal) and awareness. Both components are necessary to maintain consciousness. Wakefulness is dependent on a network of neurons called the ascending reticular activating system (ARAS), originating in the midbrain and rostral pontine tegmentum and projecting to the diencephalon (hypothalamus and midline and intralaminar nuclei of the thalamus). From there, widespread projections are sent to bilateral cerebral cortex. Damage to the ARAS would result in impairment of wakefulness. Awareness, sometimes referred to as the "content" of consciousness, represents the sum of all functions mediated by cerebral cortical neurons and their reciprocal projections to and from subcortical structures [1]. These functions include sensation and perception, attention, memory, executive function, and motivation. Awareness requires wakefulness, but wakefulness may be observed in the absence of awareness, as in the case of vegetative state.

The vegetative state describes a state of wakefulness without awareness. The vegetative patient exhibits sleep–wake cycles, evident by "eyes-open" periods, without evidence of awareness of self or environment. The term *persistent vegetative state* is reserved for patients who remain in the vegetative state for at least 30 days.

The minimally conscious state (MCS) is a condition defined by severely impaired consciousness with minimal but definite behavioral evidence of self or environmental awareness [2]. Like the vegetative state, MCS may be a transitional state during recovery from coma, or progression of worsening neurologic disease.

Another condition worth recognizing is the locked-in syndrome, in which the patient has complete paralysis of all four limbs and the lower cranial nerves. The locked-in syndrome is not a disorder of consciousness, as the patient retains awareness. The most common cause is a lesion in the base and tegmentum of the midpons, interrupting the descending cortical motor fibers responsible for limb movement, while preserving vertical eye movement and eye opening. A high level of suspicion on the part of the clinician is required to make this diagnosis.

Psychogenic unresponsiveness may mimic coma, and is characterized by normal neurologic exam, including normal oculocephalic and oculovestibular reflexes. Patient may sometimes forcibly close the eyelids. If psychogenic etiology is suspected, an electroencephalogram (EEG) may be helpful to aid in diagnosis. In more challenging cases, Amytal interview can be used, wherein the patient is slowly injected with an anxiolytic drug while repeated neurologic exam is performed. Patients with psychogenic unresponsiveness should exhibit improvement in function.

Brain death is defined as the irreversible cessation of all functions of the entire brain, such that the brain is no longer capable of maintaining respiratory or cardiovascular function.

Etiology and Pathophysiology

Coma could be caused by focal or "structural" conditions that lead to disruption of the ARAS anywhere in the brain stem, bilateral diencephalon, or diffuse bilateral cerebral cortex. On the other hand, systemic or "metabolic" disorders that interfere with the normal metabolism of the brain and disturb normal neuronal activity could also lead to coma.

Structural Etiology

Structural causes of coma can be categorized into "compressive" or "destructive" lesions. Compressive lesions (e.g., intracranial hemorrhage or tumor) may cause impairment of consciousness by several mechanisms: (1) by directly distorting the ARAS or its projection, (2) by increasing ICP and thus impairing cerebral blood flow, (3) by distorting and displacing normal brain tissue, (4) by causing edema and further distortion of brain, or (5) by causing herniation [2].

Compressive lesion such as epidural hematoma classically results from traumatic fracture of the skull that lacerates a meningeal vessel branch. Blood accumulates between the skull and the dura, causing brain compression and shift. Some patients exhibit a period of lucid interval after trauma, until the expanding hematoma grows large enough to cause displacement of the diencephalon and brain stem, leading to impaired consciousness. Subdural hematoma usually results from tearing of bridging cerebral veins. They are more commonly seen in elderly or alcoholic patients with cerebral atrophy, or patients who are anticoagulated with warfarin, clopidogrel, or aspirin. Acute subdural hematoma has a high mortality rate due to high association with other injuries, such as brain contusions.

Subarachnoid hemorrhage, when due to rupture of aneurysm, has high rates of mortality and morbidity. As the blood in the subarachnoid space breaks down, inflammatory reaction is incited, resulting in cerebral vasospasm. Delayed brain ischemia and infarction can occur. Hydrocephalus can also complicate subarachnoid hemorrhage due to impairment of cerebrospinal fluid absorption, leading to elevated intracranial pressure (ICP) and impairment of consciousness.

Brain tumors often present with headaches, focal neurologic deficits, or seizures. They may present with impaired consciousness due to compression or infiltration of the diencephalon or due to herniation.

Destructive lesions (e.g., cerebral infarct) cause coma by directly damaging the ARAS or its projections. Bilateral cortical or subcortical infarcts, due to cardioembolism or severe bilateral carotid stenosis, could result in coma. Although impairment of consciousness rarely occurs due to unilateral cerebral hemispheric infarct, it may occur in delayed fashion secondary to edema of infarcted tissue causing compression of the other hemisphere and diencephalon. Occlusion of the thalamo-perforators branches of the basilar artery can lead to infarcts of bilateral thalami, causing coma or hypersomnolence [2]. Pontine hemorrhage, usually due to uncontrolled hypertension, is characterized by sudden onset of coma, pinpoint pupils, breathing irregularity, and ophthalmoplegia. Cerebellar hemorrhage, another possible consequence of uncontrolled hypertension, presents with occipital headache, nausea and vomiting, unsteadiness, and ataxia. Early diagnosis and treatment is crucial, as once the patient is comatose, surgical intervention is often futile.

Traumatic brain injury (TBI) is another common cause of coma. Mechanism of loss of consciousness in TBI may be due to shearing forces applied to the ARAS. Diffuse axonal injury (DAI) is associated with severe TBI, and portends a poor prognosis.

Herniation Syndromes

The Monro–Kellie doctrine hypothesizes that the central nervous system and its accompanying fluids are enclosed in a rigid container, and the sum of the volume of the brain, cerebrospinal fluid (CSF), and intracranial blood remains constant. An increase in volume of one component (e.g., a growing mass lesion) can be compensated to a degree by the displacement of an equal volume of another component (e.g., CSF). When this compensatory mechanism is overwhelmed, even a small increase in volume will lead to a large increase in pressure. The differential pressure gradient between adjacent intracranial compartments leads to herniation.

Several herniation syndromes are commonly described. Uncal herniation occurs when a mass lesion in a lateral cerebral hemisphere pushes the uncus, or medial temporal lobe, medially and inferiorly over the tentorial edge. Uncal herniation causes stretching of ipsilateral oculomotor nerve, which leads to fixed and dilated pupil. Hemiparesis, either contralateral or ipsilateral, could result from compression of the cerebral peduncles. The posterior cerebral artery runs along the tentorial notch, and its compression could lead to ischemia of ipsilateral occipital lobe, leading to visual field deficit. In central herniation, or transtentorial herniation, pressure from expanding supratentorial mass lesion displaces the diencephalon caudally. In addition to distorting the ARAS, branches of the basilar artery are also stretched, leading to brainstem hemorrhage. Tonsillar herniation results when the cerebellar tonsils are pushed caudally down the foramen magnum, causing direct compression of the medulla; fourth ventricular CSF outflow is closed off, leading to further increase in intracranial pressure. Subfalcine herniation, or cingulate herniation, occurs when one cerebral hemisphere pushes medially under the rigid falx cerebri, causing displacement of the cingulate gyrus. Branches of the anterior cerebral artery are sometimes pushed against the falx, leading to ischemia of medial cerebral hemispheres.

Metabolic Etiology

Diffuse, multifocal, and metabolic diseases cause stupor and coma due to interruption in delivery of oxygen or substrates (e.g., hypoxia, ischemia, hypoglycemia), alterations in neuronal excitability and signaling (e.g., drug toxicity, acid–base imbalance), or changes in brain volume (e.g., hypernatremia, hyponatremia) [3].

Hypoxia and ischemia can lead to impairment of consciousness. The brain has one of the highest metabolic rates of any organ and requires a constant supply of oxygen, glucose, and cofactors to generate energy, synthesize proteins, and carry out electrical and chemical reactions. The brain lacks reserves of its essential substrates, and therefore it is vulnerable to even temporary cessation of substrates or blood flow [2]. Cerebral autoregulation maintains cerebral blood flow at a relatively constant rate over a range of systemic blood pressure. When autoregulation fails in the extremes of systemic blood pressure, cerebral blood flow decreases and lactic acid builds up, leading to a decrease in pH and impairment in ATP generation. Neuronal cell death could occur due to calcium influx and free radical formation [2].

Glucose is a major substrate for brain metabolism. Profound hypoglycemia causes damage to the cerebral hemispheres, producing laminar or pseudolaminar necrosis in severe cases [2]. Hypoglycemia could present as delirium, stroke, or coma; therefore, finger-stick glucose should be checked on all patients presenting with impaired consciousness.

Wernicke's encephalopathy is a syndrome caused by thiamine deficiency, with classic symptoms of confusion, ataxia, and ophthalmoplegia. If left untreated, Wernicke's encephalopathy could progress to Korsakoff's syndrome, an irreversible syndrome characterized by amnesia and confabulation.

Acute liver failure causes increased permeability of blood-brain barrier, leading to cerebral edema and elevated ICP. Elevated ICP is a major cause of death in patients with acute liver failure [2]. Elevated ammonia level is implicated in hepatic encephalopathy, although direct correlation between ammonia level and degree of clinical impairment is lacking. Clinical presentation varies from delirium to obtundation. Hyperventilation with respiratory alkalosis is common. Nystagmus, dysconjugate eye movement, and muscle spasticity have been described. Decorticate or decerebrate posturing is possible with deep coma.

Renal failure may lead to uremic encephalopathy. The precise pathophysiology of uremic encephalopathy is not clear. Furthermore, treatment of uremia by hemodialysis may cause rapid change in osmolarity, leading to rapid water shifts and cerebral edema, which could result in coma.

Endocrinopathies such as panhypopituitarism, adrenal insufficiency, hypothyroidism, and hyperthyroidism have all been implicated as causes of coma. Patients with diabetes may present with nonketotic hyperglycemic hyperosmolar coma or coma from diabetic ketoacidosis.

Many drugs can cause coma. Sedative drugs such as benzodiazepines and barbiturates, opioids, and ethanol can cause impairment of consciousness, as can psychotropic drugs such as tricyclic antidepressants, lithium, and selective serotonin reuptake inhibitors; anticholinergic drugs, amphetamines, and illicit drugs all can cause delirium and coma.

Acid–base imbalance, especially respiratory acidosis, and electrolyte derangements such as hyper- and hyponatremia, hyper- and hypocalcemia, and hypophophatemia can result in delirium, stupor, and coma.

Infectious and inflammatory diseases of the central nervous system, including meningitis, encephalitis, and cerebral vasculitis could present with impaired consciousness.

Seizures and postictal states can also present as coma. In one series of comatose patients without overt clinical seizure activity, EEG demonstrated nonconvulsive status epilepticus in 8% of patients [2]. Seizure produces an increase in cerebral metabolic demand, and sustained seizures can lead to hypoxic-ischemic brain damage if untreated.

Treatment

When presented with the unconscious patient, basic principles of life support apply. Check airway, ensure breathing and oxygenation, and maintain circulation. Intubate the patient if GCS $\leq$ 8. The PaO_2 should be maintained above 100 mmHg and the pCO_2 kept ideally between 35 and 40 mmHg. The mean arterial pressure (MAP) should be maintained above 70 mmHg to ensure adequate brain perfusion. Intravascular volume depletion should be corrected, and vasopressors may need to be used to maintain systemic pressure. Hypertension should be treated cautiously, keeping in mind that for patients with chronic hypertension, a sudden drop in blood pressure may lead to relative hypoperfusion of the brain.

Finger-stick glucose should be checked, and both hyperglycemia and hypoglycemia should be treated. Glucose should be administered along with thiamine to avoid precipitating Wernicke's encephalopathy.

If narcotic overdose is suspected, naloxone can be given intravenously and repeated as necessary. Keep in mind that, while naloxone has duration of action of 2–3 h, some narcotics have a much longer half-life. Thus, close observation is needed for patients who recover after naloxone administration. If benzodiazepine overdose is suspected, flumazenil, a benzodiazepine antagonist, is sometimes used. Gastric lavage with activated charcoal is sometimes utilized for suspected drug ingestion.

If the stuporous or comatose patient is relatively stable, an emergency CT scan should be obtained. However, if elevated ICP is suspected, or if impending or active herniation is suspected, intracranial hypertension needs to be treated first. Hyperventilation to $PaCO_2$ between 25 and 30 mmHg will transiently lower ICP while other therapeutic measures take effect. Mannitol, a hyperosmolar agent, may be given as a bolus to draw water from the brain, thus lowering ICP. Mannitol is also reported to lower blood viscosity and thus improve cerebral perfusion. Alternatively, hypertonic saline can be given either as a bolus of 23.4% solution or as a continuous drip of 3% solution to lower ICP.

Seizures must be quickly diagnosed and treated, as repeated or continuous seizures (i.e., status epilepticus) could cause secondary brain injury. Lorazepam should be administered to stop generalized seizures, followed by a loading dose of phenytoin or valproic acid. When these measures fail, general anesthesia with propofol or pentobarbital may be necessary.

If meningitis or encephalitis is suspected, broad spectrum antimicrobials should be instituted after blood cultures are obtained. A CT scan should be obtained to rule out a mass lesion prior to lumbar puncture, although treatment should not be delayed while waiting for culture results. Steroid is used as an adjunct to antibiotics in bacterial meningitis to decrease inflammatory response. Additional therapy should be tailored toward specific etiology.

Evaluation and Assessment

The prompt diagnosis and treatment of patient in coma is crucial to outcome. Coma caused by some metabolic derangements, such as hypoglycemia, is reversible if appropriate and timely therapy is instituted. Coma due to compression from subdural hematoma or epidural hematoma could be reversible if promptly diagnosed and surgically evacuated. Therefore, the evaluation and assessment of the unconscious patient ought to proceed in a rapid, systematic, and focused manner, sometimes simultaneously with treatment.

When possible, history should be obtained from patient's relatives, friends, paramedics, or police. The onset and progression of coma sometimes could give clues to the etiology. General physical exam looking for signs of trauma or systemic medical illness should be performed. Periorbital ecchymosis (raccoon eyes), drainage of clear or bloody fluid from the ears or nose, and skull base ecchymosis (Battle's sign) are all signs of trauma.

A quick neurologic exam should be performed, assessing verbal response, eye opening, and motor response. Brainstem reflexes such as pupillary light reflex, oculocephalic reflex, oculovestibular reflex, and corneal reflex should be tested. Deep tendon reflexes and skeletal muscle tone should also be assessed.

Respiratory pattern should be noted as regular, periodic, or ataxic, or combination of these. Cheyne–Stokes respiration is a pattern of periodic breathing with phases of hyperpnea alternating with apnea. The depth of respiration waxes and wanes in a crescendo–decrescendo manner. It is generally seen in patients with diffuse forebrain lesions, uremia, hepatic failure, or heart failure. Sustained hyperventilation is sometimes seen in patients with hepatic coma, sepsis, diabetic ketoacidosis, meningitis, or pulmonary edema. True central neurogenic hyperventilation is rare, and may be due to midbrain or pons lesions. Apneustic breathing is characterized by prolonged pause at full inspiration, and it usually reflects lesion in the pons, as seen in patients with brainstem strokes from basilar artery occlusion. Ataxic breathing, or irregular, gasping respiration, implies damage to the medullary respiratory center. Cluster breathing is characterized by periods of rapid irregular respiration, followed by apneic spells, and is indicative of lesion in the medulla.

Emergency laboratory tests for evaluation of coma should include complete blood count, electrolyte panel, coagulation studies, ammonia, arterial blood gas, cerebrospinal fluid studies, and electrocardiogram. Additional studies, such as liver function test, thyroid and adrenal function tests, blood culture, urine culture, and toxicology screen should be considered.

After-care

The cost of caring for a patient in the comatose state carries beyond the acute intensive care setting. Coma is often a transient stage; few patients remain in eyes-closed coma for more than 10–14 days [4]. Patients ultimately will die, recover, or transition to vegetative state. The comatose and vegetative patients have shortened life expectancy due to several factors, often succumbing to respiratory or urinary tract infections, multisystem organ failure, and respiratory failure [5].

Survival of these patients depends, to some degree, on the quality and intensity of medical treatment and nursing care. Proper skin care, such as frequent turning and repositioning, helps reduce incidence of decubitus ulcers. Daily passive range of motion exercise helps reduce limb contractures. Tracheostomy and percutaneous gastric feeding tube are often necessary for maintaining airway and providing nutrition and hydration [5].

Prognosis

The prognosis for coma is variable and largely dependent on the etiology, location, and severity of brain damage. The Glasgow Outcome Scale (GOS) is often used to grade the level of functional recovery from coma: Grade 5 indicates recovery to previous level of function; Grade 4 describes patients who recover with moderate disability but remains independent; Grade 3 indicates recovery with severe disability with dependence on others for daily support; Grade 2 indicates recovery to vegetative state, and Grade 1 indicates no recovery.

In one series of 500 patients with nontraumatic coma, 16% led an independent life at some point within the first year (GOS grade 4 or 5), while 11% regained consciousness but was dependent on others for activities of daily living, 12% never improved beyond the vegetative state, and 61% died without recovery from coma [4]. Patients who survived nontraumatic coma made most of their recovery within the first month. Longer duration of coma was associated with worse chance of functional recovery. Among different disease processes, subarachnoid hemorrhage had the worst outcome, while hepatic encephalopathy and other metabolic causes had the best. Lack of verbal response, eye opening, motor response, pupillary light reflex, corneal reflex, oculocephalic response, oculovestibular response, or spontaneous eye movements were all independently associated with lack of recovery to independent function.

Coma arising from TBI portends better prognosis than nontraumatic coma [2]. A comprehensive review by the Brain Trauma Foundation listed several factors with class I prognostic evidence. Advanced age was predictive of poor outcome, with 56% of patients younger than 20 and only 5% of patients older than 60 able to achieve GOS of 4 or 5. Each lower GCS score was associated in a stepwise fashion with progressively worse outcome. Absent pupillary light reflex or oculocephalic response at any point in the illness predicts an outcome of less than 4 on the GOS. Hypotension and hypoxia were also independent predictors of poor outcome. Abnormal neuroimaging findings such as compression of basal cisterns or midline shift of brain structures, indicative of elevated ICP, were predictive of poor outcome.

While EEG is useful in identifying nonconvulsive status epilepticus in the comatose patient, it has not been shown to be predictive of outcome. Somatosensory-evoked potentials (SSEPs), on the other hand, are a better predictor. In several studies, bilateral absence of cortical SSEPs predicted death or vegetative state in almost all patients [2].

Cross-References

▶ Encephalopathy and Delirium

References

1. Young GB, Pigott SE (1999) Neurobiological basis of consciousness. Arch Neurol 56:153–157
2. Posner JB, Saper CB et al (2007) Plum and Posner's diagnosis of stupor and coma. Contemporary Neurology Series 71, 4th edn. Oxford University Press, New York
3. Stevens RD, Bhardwaj A (2006) Approach to the comatose patient. Crit Care Med 34(1):31–41
4. Levy DE, Bates D, Caronna JJ et al (1981) Prognosis of nontraumatic coma. Ann Intern Med 94:293–301
5. The Multi-Society task Force on PVS (1994) Medical aspects of the persistent vegetative state – second of two parts. N Engl J Med 330:1572–1579

Coma depasse

▶ Brain Death
▶ Death by Neurologic Criteria

Community-Acquired Pneumonia (CAP)

▶ Burns, Pneumonia
▶ Pneumonia, Empiric Management

Compliance

Ratio between the change in volume determined by a change in pressure ($C_{rs} = \Delta V/\Delta P$), depending on the elastic properties of the respiratory system.

Complicated Intra-abdominal Infections

▶ Abdominal Cavity Infections

Complicated Parapneumonic Effusion

Fluid in the pleural space that does not resolve spontaneously with treatment of the underlying infection, and requires drainage with therapeutic thoracentesis or placement of a chest tube.

▶ Empyema

Computed Tomography

▶ Imaging for Acute Abdominal Pain

Confirmed STSS

Clinical case definition+isolation of GAS from a normally sterile site.

Confusion

▶ Septic Encephalopathy

Congenital Heart Disease in Children

JONATHAN R. EGAN, MARINO S. FESTA
The Children's Hospital at Westmead, Westmead, Australia

Synonyms
Cardiac disease; Heart disease

Definition
Malformation of the heart present at birth.

Characteristics
It is estimated that 4–10 liveborn infants per 1,000 are diagnosed with congenital heart disease (CHD), with approximately 40% diagnosed in the first year of life and the remainder some time in childhood or adulthood [1]. The majority of lesions are amenable to surgical repair or palliation and it has been estimated that the prevalence of adults with CHD in the USA is increasing by approximately 5% per annum [2].

CHD may present in the newborn period or later in childhood, usually with heart failure, central cyanosis, episodic collapse, or as an incidental finding of a heart murmur:

Heart Failure
Tachypnea, worse with exertion or feeding in an infant, is a common sign of heart failure in CHD. This is most common in conditions that allow blood to shunt from left to right (i.e., from the systemic to pulmonary circulation), or in conditions that obstruction to flow through the heart at the level of the valves, pulmonary veins, or either ventricular outflow tract causing pulmonary venous congestion.

In the infant, sweating with feeds and hepatomegaly are commonly seen, and though dependent edema may occur, pitting edema of the peripheries is much less common than in adults. Severe heart failure may manifest at the time of spontaneous closure of the patent ductus arteriosus at or around 1 week of age in a previously asymptomatic neonate with an obstructive lesion of the left heart such as critical aortic stenosis, hypoplastic left heart syndrome (HLHS), interrupted aortic arch, or severe coarctation of the aorta.

In later infancy and early childhood, undiagnosed CHD leading to increased pulmonary blood flow or obstruction to pulmonary venous drainage (e.g., ventricular septal defect, atrioventricular septal defect, patent ductus arteriosus, anomalous pulmonary venous drainage) may cause chronic heart failure leading to impaired growth and failure to thrive.

A chest X-ray will usually show cardiomegaly and increased pulmonary vascular markings, with the notable exception of obstructed total anomalous pulmonary venous drainage of the infradiaphragmatic type where marked pulmonary congestion is present in the absence of cardiomegaly.

The normal fall in pulmonary vascular resistance in the postnatal period may lead to increasing left-to-right shunt and pulmonary blood flow in the first week of life. Similarly, increased inspired oxygen or respiratory alkalosis may both decrease pulmonary vascular resistance and lead to worsening heart failure.

Central Cyanosis

Cyanosis of the lips and tongue in the newborn infant is indicative of desaturation of arterial hemoglobin and may be readily identified by direct comparison with the mother. Typically the baby with cyanotic congenital heart disease looks otherwise well with little or no respiratory difficulty. An arterial blood sample pO_2 taken in maximal inspired oxygen will not exceed 100 mmHg.

The most common cause of cyanotic heart disease in the newborn period is transposition of the great arteries where separation of the pulmonary and systemic circulation requires mixing either at the level of the atrium via the patent foramen ovale, or via a patent ductus arteriosus or sometimes via a ventricular septal defect, to allow oxygenated blood to cross the systemic circulation.

Other CHD resulting in decreased pulmonary blood flow (e.g., pulmonary atresia with an intact ventricular septum, tetralogy of Fallot, tricuspid atresia, Ebstein's anomaly) or anomolous to pulmonary venous return to the right atrium (e.g., total anomalous pulmonary venous drainage with or without obstruction to the pulmonary venous blood flow) may present with central cyanosis commonly in the newborn period, or later in infancy or childhood.

Incidental Murmur

It remains common for less severe forms of CHD to be diagnosed in childhood by detection of a significant murmur on routine or coincidental examination.

Significant murmurs may be caused by turbulent flow across abnormal structures (e.g., patent ductus arteriosus, pulmonary stenosis) or connections (e.g., ventricular septal defect) or due to increased flow across normal structures (e.g., atrial septal defect causing left-to-right shunt and a pulmonary flow murmur).

Episodic Collapse

Infants and children may have episodes of extreme tachycardia or bradycardia associated with alteration of consciousness, pallor, and sometimes collapse. Signs of heart failure may initially be absent, especially in infants, and develop over several hours if the abnormal rhythm persists.

Supraventricular tachycardia is a rapid tachyarrhythmia with a rate usually over 220 bpm that may present de novo in infants and older children. The electrocardiograph (ECG) is characterized by the absence of P waves and absolutely regular R–R interval. Up to a third of cases have an underlying structural heart abnormality and a proportion of the remainder have a short PR interval with a delta wave on electrocardiograph (ECG) during normal sinus rhythm implying early excitation via an accessory pathway (Wolf–Parkinson–White syndrome).

Recurrent ventricular tachycardia is a recognized cause of sudden death in childhood and may be associated with a family history of sudden death. Prolonged QT syndromes (e.g., Romano-Ward syndrome or if associated with sensorineural deafness Jervell and Lange-Nielsen syndrome) due to inherited defects in myocardial potassium channel function that allow early repolarization typically present with episodes of torsades de point causing sudden collapse or death. Inherited defects of myocardial sodium channels (e.g., Brugada syndrome) may present with sudden onset of ventricular arrhythmia in older children and young adults [3].

Congenital complete heart block may present with heart failure in the prenatal (hydrops fetalis) or postnatal period and may be associated with maternal anticardiolipin syndrome.

Management

Fetal Screening

An effective antenatal screening program may help improve prenatal detection of life-threatening CHD. This allows parents the choice of termination of pregnancy and the chance of improved outcomes by avoiding unanticipated postnatal collapse and the careful planning of perinatal care [4].

Postnatal Stabilization

Stabilization of the newborn with CHD depends on detailed knowledge of the cardiac anatomy and assessment of the changing physiology in the postnatal period. This can only be achieved by a multidisciplinary approach to care. Transthoracic echocardiography with Doppler measurement and color flow mapping is essential to confirm diagnosis based on prenatal ultrasound or clinical examination and to rule out additional lesions. Cardiac catheterization is usually reserved for complex cases or if an interventional procedure is indicated.

Full history and examination for associated abnormalities or syndromes should be undertaken. A systematic approach to stabilization of the airway and breathing is required in the initial postnatal period prior to cardiac assessment. This may include intubation and ventilation to normalize lung volumes and reduce left ventricular wall stress in some cases. In cases of suspected or known duct-dependent CHD (e.g., transposition of the great arteries with intact ventricular septal defect (VSD), hypoplastic left heart syndrome, interrupted aortic arch), the neonate should be commenced on an intravenous infusion of epoprostenol (Prostacyclin) in order to maintain the duct open (usual dose 5–25 ng/kg/min). Care should be taken to ensure that the baby maintains an adequate preload after starting the infusion as systemic vascular resistance and cardiac filling pressures are likely to fall. The self-ventilating neonate should also be closely observed for apnea at this time as this is known to be associated with commencement of epoprostenol infusion.

Babies with single ventricle anatomy and physiology, in which a single ventricle effectively supplies pulmonary and systemic blood flow (e.g., hypoplastic left heart syndrome, pulmonary atresia) are sensitive to changes to systemic and pulmonary vascular resistance, which will influence the relative flow to the two circuits. Hence, in addition to maintaining good cardiac output by attention to adequate preload and myocardial contractility, manipulation of factors to influence the vascular resistance in the systemic and pulmonary circulations should be used to allow adequate systemic blood flow. Avoidance of noxious stimuli, maintenance of normothermia and appropriate analgesia are important, in addition to pharmacological manipulation by systemic vasodilators, in order to avoid a situation of increased systemic vascular resistance leading to excess pulmonary flow and decreased systemic oxygen delivery. This situation may be exacerbated by the normal fall in pulmonary vascular resistance in the postnatal period, or by use of high inspired oxygen or hyperventilation, both of which should be avoided.

Babies born with separated pulmonary and systemic circulations (e.g., transposition of the great arteries) are dependent on communications between the atria, ventricles, or at the level of the patent ductus arteriosus to allow adequate mixing of oxygenated and desaturated blood. This may need to be augmented at the level of the atrial connection by a balloon atrial septostomy following femoral or umbilical vein catheterization soon after birth in babies where low systemic arterial oxygen saturation of hemoglobin (usually below 70–75%) is significantly contributing to decreased systemic oxygen delivery. Preductal pulseoximetry saturations should be monitored, usually in the right hand, in order to monitor saturation of blood reaching the brain and myocardium.

Cardiac Surgery and Cardiopulmonary Bypass

Surgery, if required, may be in the neonatal period, or early or late childhood. The aim of surgery may be corrective or palliative, and surgery may need to be conducted on more than one occasion in a staged approach. In a significant proportion of cases, cardiopulmonary bypass (CPB) and some degree of cooling is required to allow adequate oxygenation of vital organs during surgery, which requires an empty heart and usually a period of cardiac standstill. Occasionally, a short period of low-flow CPB or of complete hypothermic circulatory arrest may be required to allow a relatively bloodless field during complex surgery on the aorta. Clearly, this is a time of high risk with potential for embolic or ischemic damage and the prospect of disturbed physiology in the postoperative period following myocardial and end-organ reperfusion.

Advances in the care of newborns with CHD have meant that neonatal reparative surgery is increasingly possible. Though complex and challenging, early repair offers significant advantages. These include early elimination of cyanosis and of congestive heart failure, optimal circulation for growth and development, and reduced anatomic distortion from palliative procedures.

Palliative cardiac surgery remains the only option in infants with an anatomical single ventricle (e.g., hypoplastic left heart syndrome). This usually requires a three-staged approach. Firstly, pulmonary blood flow is secured via a systemic to pulmonary arterial shunt. Later, in infants without elevated pulmonary vascular resistance and with adequate atrioventricular valve and diastolic ventricular function, a cavopulmonary anastamosis is created so that systemic venous return is directed directly into the pulmonary arteries. This is done in two stages, firstly by directing return from the superior vena cava to the pulmonary arteries via a bidirectional cavopulmonary

(Glenn) anastamosis and later by the additional redirection of the inferior vena cava flow, either via a lateral tunnel through the atrium or via an extra-cardiac conduit, to create a complete cavopulmonary (Fontan) circulation. Rearrangement of the systemic and pulmonary circulation to operate "in series" in this way leads to correction of cyanosis. However, given the paucity of long-term outcome data, total cavopulmonary circulation remains viewed as a palliative rather than a curative procedure.

Care of the postoperative cardiac surgical patient is complex and requires knowledge of the underlying anatomy and physiology and details of the surgery and intraoperative course. A progressive low cardiac output state, not attributable to any residual or undiagnosed cardiac lesion, which reaches its nadir usually by 12-h postoperatively, occurs in a significant proportion of patients [5]. This complexity is managed by mechanical ventilation and pharmacological support to optimize myocardial function, pulmonary and systemic afterload, and supportive intensive care therapy.

Lesions with increased pulmonary blood flow or increased pulmonary venous pressure may predispose to increased postoperative pulmonary artery pressures and increased reactivity of the pulmonary vasculature in the postoperative period, necessitating the use of inhaled nitric oxide as a selective pulmonary vasodilator in some cases.

A small number of patients require extracorporeal mechanical oxygenation (ECMO) support to allow myocardial rest and adequate time for recovery following cardiac surgery.

Early postoperative extubation may be of benefit in some patients, particularly in those with cavopulmonary anastamosis, and should be considered in any patient known to have had a smooth intraoperative course and without signs of excessive bleeding, hypoxemia, or low cardiac output state in the early postoperative period.

After-care

Medical management usually involves diuretic therapy with or without ACE inhibitors in the weeks and months following surgery. Regular assessment for late surgical complications including wound infection, chylothorax, postcardiotomy immune pericarditis (Dressler's syndrome), and for residual lesions is undertaken before gradual tapering of medical follow-up. In the case of more complex lesions where further operative interventions or transplant may be required, ongoing follow-up through to adulthood is mandatory and these patients should be transitioned to adult congenital heart disease programs. In addition to echocardiographic and cardiac catheter assessments, cardiac magnetic resonance imaging may also be useful in the assessment of cardiac function in some patients.

In infants following Stage 1 palliation of HLHS, significant interstage mortality may be reduced by careful monitoring of saturations and weight gain either in hospital or at home.

Orthotopic heart transplantation should be considered in infants and children with severe intractable forms of CHD.

Prognosis

CHD is responsible for the most deaths in the first year of life of any other birth defect. While most CHD occurs as an isolated congenital malformation, CHD is more common in several genetic conditions, including Trisomy 21 (Down syndrome), Noonan syndrome, Marfan syndrome, Trisomy 13 (Patau syndrome), and DiGeorge syndrome, and prognosis depends on the type of CHD, as well as any underlying condition.

Advances in perfusion practice, surgical techniques, and postoperative care have all led to overall decreased perioperative mortality. Long-term morbidity, including abnormal neurodevelopmental outcomes, particularly in patients with single ventricle physiology or following prolonged postoperative recovery has been noted and is the topic of ongoing research.

References

1. Hoffman JI (1990) Congenital heart disease: incidence and inheritance. Pediatr Clin North Am 37:25–43
2. Brickner ME, Hillis LD, Lange RA (2000) Congenital heart disease in adults: first of two parts. N Engl J Med 342:256–263
3. Towbin JA (2004) Molecular genetic basis of sudden cardiac death. Pediatr Clin North Am 51(5):1229–1255
4. Khoshnood B, De Vigan C, Vodovar V, Goujard J, Lhomme A, Bonnet D, Goffinet F (2005) Trends in prenatal diagnosis, pregnancy termination, and perinatal mortality of newborns with congenital heart disease in France, 1983–2000: a population based evaluation. Pediatrics 115(1):95–101
5. Wernovsky G, Wypij D, Jonas RA, Mayer JE Jr, Hanley FL, Hickey PR, Walsh AZ, Cahng AC, Castaneda AR, Newburger JW, Wessel DL (1995) Postoperative course and hemodynamic profile after the arterial switch operation in neonates and infants. Circulation 92(8):2226–2235
6. Nugent AW, Daubeney PE, Chondros P, Carlin JB, Cheung M, Wilkinson LC, Davis AM, Kahler SG, Chow CW, Wilkinson JL, Weintraub RG (2003) The epidemiology of childhood cardiomyopathy in Australia. N Engl J Med 348(17):1639–1646

Congestive Heart Failure

▶ Heart Failure, Biomarkers
▶ Heart Failure Syndromes, Treatment

Conscious Sedation

JOHN H. BURTON
Department of Emergency Medicine, Carilion Clinic
Virginia Tech Carilion School of Medicine,
Roanoke, VA, USA

Synonyms

Deep sedation; Procedural sedation; Sedation

Definition

The phrase "conscious sedation" has historically been applied to the administration of sedative or analgesic medications for suppression of a patient's level of consciousness in preparation for, and during, a painful or anxiety-provoking medical procedure.

Conscious sedation as applied to many modern procedures is a misnomer, particularly in the intensive care unit (ICU) or emergency department (ED) setting. In these practice environments, a depth of patient relaxation and sedation well below "conscious" is frequently intended. Many providers attempt to be more descriptive in the depth of intended sedation by adding the descriptors "mild," "moderate," or "deep" for any encounter. Others have been proponents for the terms "procedural sedation" or "procedural sedation and analgesia" in an attempt to emphasize a depth of sedation and analgesia that will be consistent with the one best suited for the intended procedure.

Regardless of the terminology used, the practice of conscious sedation is an essential component of sedation and/or analgesia for many procedural interventions. The proper use of conscious sedation will confer significant benefits to both the patient and the medical provider. For patients, relief of pain, anxiety, and amnesia to the procedure event are obvious desirable outcomes. Similarly, more relaxed and comfortable patients will translate to an improved experience for medical providers with enhanced patient safety, improved procedure success, and less angst for the pain and suffering inflicted on the patient on behalf of the medical procedure [1].

Depth of Conscious Sedation

The depth of intended patient sedation and relaxation can be broadly characterized as mild, moderate, and deep levels of suppressed consciousness. These categorizations exist along a broad spectrum for the depth of patient sedation intended for the procedure. A state of general anesthesia completes the spectrum and describes a depth of sedation characterized by unresponsiveness to all stimuli and the absence of airway protective reflexes.

Minimal sedation typically describes a patient with a near-baseline level of alertness. This level of sedation does not impair the ability to follow commands or respond to verbal stimuli. Under a state of minimal sedation, cardiovascular and ventilatory functions are not threatened or impaired.

Moderate sedation describes a depth of consciousness characterized by many or all of the following: eyelid ptosis, slurred speech, and delayed or altered responses to verbal stimuli. Event amnesia will frequently occur under moderate sedation levels. The patient airway should be minimally threatened by apnea or ventilatory suppression under moderate sedation depths. Similarly, while the likelihood of cardiovascular embarrassment is small, monitoring of cardiovascular status is appropriate for changes in patient oxygenation, blood pressure, and heart rate.

Deep sedation renders the patient level of consciousness unresponsive to most verbal commands with preservation of airway protective reflexes and noxious, painful stimuli. Event amnesia is typical of deep levels of sedation. Monitoring for deep sedation encounters should emphasize the significant potential for reduction in ventilation and cardiovascular complications including changes to heart rate, heart rhythm, and blood pressure. The potential for apnea should also prompt the consideration for more sensitive ventilation monitoring techniques, including exhaled, end-tidal carbon dioxide levels.

Pre-existing Condition

Minimal, moderate, and deep sedation have all been described in the medical literature for conditions that invoke pain, anxiety, and complex medical procedures that may require minimal patient movement and optimized muscle relaxation.

In the ICU setting, conscious sedation should be distinguished conceptually from continuous sedation. The former would be employed toward procedures or events requiring sedation or relaxation, while the latter would imply the use of sedative agents for continuous sedation for patient comfort during periods of mechanical ventilation or to supplement ongoing medical treatment and stabilization. For example, an intubated ICU patient may be treated with a propofol infusion for continuous sedation. This patient may require a procedure, such as tube thoracostomy, that may provoke consideration of a plan for increased sedation and/or analgesia to address the pain associated with this procedure. In most other settings, including emergency or gastroenterology procedures, for example, the likelihood that the patient will be under any form of continuous sedation is much smaller and therefore, a treatment plan for conscious sedation will be initiated from a normal level of patient consciousness.

Conscious Sedation Procedures

Common procedures in which conscious sedation will be utilized in the ICU or emergency setting are listed in Table 1. Procedures such as electrical cardioversion or sedation for radiological imaging may be viewed as events where the addition of an analgesic agent is of limited benefit given the limited amount or complete absence of pain prior to or following the procedure. In these events, the conscious sedation plan may be simplified to emphasize a sedation strategy with minimal or no analgesic considerations.

Procedures such as orthopedic fracture or dislocation reduction are typical of encounters where both patient relaxation and analgesia should be considered in the sedation plan. These patients will have analgesic requirements prior to, during, and following the treatment procedure. These patients should have a conscious sedation plan that incorporates a baseline analgesic treatment plan in addition to the planned sedation.

Pre-sedation Considerations

Preexisting medical illnesses should be considered in the formulation of any conscious sedation treatment plan. Acute or chronic illnesses may render a patient to be at elevated risk for adverse events during conscious sedation,

Conscious Sedation. Table 1 Common procedures in the ICU or emergency setting where conscious sedation should be considered

ICU
Chest tube thoracostomy
Abscess incision and debridement
Ventriculostomy placement
Central venous or arterial line placement
Complex wound management, e.g., burn wound care
Emergency
Orthopedic fracture or dislocation reduction
Complex laceration repair
Abscess incision and debridement
Foreign body removal
Central venous line placement
Electrical cardioversion
Lumbar puncture
Radiological imaging

specifically cardiovascular or ventilatory embarrassment. The contemplation of the use of sedation or analgesic agents should then incorporate these risks into both the decision to use conscious sedation or the selection of specific treatment agents. Conditions such as hemorrhagic shock or sepsis may render a significant degree of cardiovascular instability or risk with conscious sedation. Similarly, traumatic facial injuries, or morbid obesity may render challenges to assisted ventilation in the case of respiratory suppression. At a minimum, preparatory considerations prior to conscious sedation should include a history of present illness, past medical history, and focused physical examination directed toward airway and cardiovascular assessment.

The oral intake of fluids or solids prior to sedation, NPO status, remains a subject of debate among physicians caring for conscious sedation patients [2]. More brief periods of suppressed consciousness as well as lighter depths of sedation during conscious sedation render limited analogies to the operating room patient experience and NPO requirements in that setting. There have been exceptionally few reports in the medical literature of adverse outcomes related to NPO status for conscious sedation patients. Additionally, there are many large series of patients undergoing deep sedation levels with no aspiration or ingested solids/fluids complications. These observations further support the position that the application of operative patient anesthesia principles is of limited utility to the typical conscious sedation patient. Finally, the emergent or critical nature of many procedures in the emergency or ICU setting prompts consideration of a risk/benefit paradigm for any patient requiring a medical procedure and conscious sedation. Taken in summary, the risks of aspiration or obstruction from recent solid or fluid intake must be balanced with the benefits derived from an immediate or timelier sedation intervention [3].

Application

Planned Depth of Sedation and Procedure

Minimal or light conscious sedation is usually performed for procedures that are less painful, particularly with the use of local anesthesia, and require light levels of patient relaxation. Typical light sedation encounters include procedures such as lumbar puncture, radiological studies, simple fracture reductions in combination with local anesthesia, and abscess incision and drainage. Agents and combinations typically utilized for light sedation include fentanyl, midazolam, and low-dose ketamine (Tables 2 and 3).

Moderate and deep conscious sedation is usually performed for procedures that require greater degrees of

Conscious Sedation. Table 2 Agents commonly utilized for conscious sedation

Analgesia agents
Fentanyl
Morphine sulfate
Hydromorphone
Sedation agents
Benzodiazepines, e.g., midazolam
Barbiturates, e.g., methohexital
Propofol
Etomidate
Ketamine[a]

[a]Ketamine has both analgesic and sedation properties

Conscious Sedation. Table 3 Common agents, dosing, and depth of sedation associated with each agent for patient conscious sedation

Agent	Initial dose (mg/kg)	Repeat dose[a] (mg/kg)	Depth of sedation
Midazolam	0.03	0.03	Titrate to desired depth
Etomidate	0.15–0.20	0.1	Deep sedation only
Propofol	0.5–1.0	0.5	Deep sedation only
Methohexital	1.0	0.5	Deep sedation only
Ketamine	1.0	0.5	Moderate and deep sedation

[a]Some providers may prefer a continuous drip infusion to a repeat-bolus dosing strategy

patient relaxation. These procedures often have greater associated levels of pain and anxiety. Common moderate or deep sedation encounters include procedures such as complex orthopedic fracture or dislocation reductions, tube thoracostomy, and more complex wound and debridement procedures including burn dressing changes or large abscess incision and drainage. Agents utilized for moderate or deep sedation include higher dose ketamine, etomidate, methohexital, and propofol as single agents or in combination with an analgesic agent (Table 3).

Monitoring the depth of conscious sedation is best performed with the use and documentation of a standardized sedation assessment scale. Examples of this include the Ramsay Scale (Table 4) or the modified Aldrete-Parr Scale. Each of these scales, and other similar patient assessment tools, utilize a standard set of predicted impairment assessment in a number of body systems or categories. Given that the most clinically relevant complications associated with conscious sedation encounters are adverse respiratory events, patient depth of sedation monitoring should emphasize respiratory assessment in addition to depth of awareness.

Selection of Conscious Sedation Agents

With the exception of ketamine, the most substantial pharmacologic effects of sedation medications impact patient levels of consciousness with minimal to no analgesic effects [4]. Given that the majority of sedation procedures will involve pain, most conscious sedation encounters should incorporate an analgesic approach to augment the planned sedation depth.

The dosing of analgesic and sedative agents should be standardized in a weight-based fashion. Selection of a specific analgesic, sedative, or combination should take

Conscious Sedation. Table 4 Ramsey sedation scale

Score	Responsiveness
1	Patient is anxious and agitated or restless, or both
2	Patient is cooperative, oriented, and tranquil
3	Patient responds to commands only
4	Patient exhibits brisk response to light glabellar tap or loud auditory stimulus
5	Patient exhibits a sluggish response to light glabellar tap or loud auditory stimulus
6	Patient exhibits no response

into consideration the patient's prior experience with sedation as well as the desired duration of clinical affects. The use of short-acting agents such as propofol and etomidate has gained wide-spread acceptance. Brief-acting sedative agents confer shorter periods of impaired levels of consciousness and subsequently less risk for adverse respiratory events. An additional benefit to shorter periods of impaired consciousness is reduced monitoring times that allow for reduced allocations of intense patient monitoring by medical staff.

Conscious sedation agents are typically dosed in weight-based bolus increments in the emergency setting (Table 3). In the ICU setting, the use of continuous infusions following an initial bolus is more commonplace given the frequent use of continuous drip infusions from these providers. Patients who require longer periods of analgesia, such as those with fractures, will benefit from strategies emphasizing longer-acting analgesic agents, such as morphine or hydromorphone, coordinated with sedative dosing.

A combination of agents is a common practice for conscious sedation agent selection. The combination of midazolam and fentanyl has historically been a strategy used in many settings. Recently, the combination of ketamine and propofol ("ketofol") has gained a degree of interest. This combination, typically with bolus dosages less than those employed with the use of propofol or ketamine alone, 0.5–0.75 mg/kg for each agent, has been argued to ameliorate the adverse risks associated with ketamine or propofol alone while also capitalizing on the benefits of each drug: a risk/benefit balance for each agent in combination.

There remains a great deal of variation in the selection of sedation and dosing regimens for conscious sedation between medical providers and medical settings. Provider experience as well as institution or medical consultant preferences may substantially influence individual approaches. A great deal of research has been performed addressing comparative considerations for agent selection, dosing, and patient procedures for conscious sedation principles. Any institutional or medical provider approach toward conscious sedation should be built upon a foundation derived from the extensive findings in the medical literature.

References

1. Miner JR, Burton JH (2007) Clinical practice advisory: emergency department procedural sedation with propofol. Ann Emerg Med 50:182–187
2. Green SM, Roback MG, Miner JR, Burton JH, Krauss B (2007) Fasting and emergency department procedural sedation and analgesia: a consensus-based clinical practice advisory. Ann Emerg Med 49:454–461
3. Miner JR, Martel ML, Meyer M, Reardon R, Biros MH (2005) Procedural sedation of critically ill patients in the emergency department. Acad Emerg Med 12(2):124–128
4. American Society of Anesthesiologists (2002) Task force on sedation and analgesia by non-anesthesiologists: practice guidelines for sedation and analgesia by non-anesthesiologists. Anesthesiology 96:1004–1017

Consumption Coagulopathy

▶ Disseminated Intravascular Coagulation

Contact Precautions

A set of practices used to prevent patient-to-patient transmission of infectious agents that are spread by direct or indirect contact with the patient. Health-care workers caring for patients on contact precautions wear a gown and gloves for interactions that may involve contact with the patient or patient's environment. In addition, patients are placed in a single room or shared room with other patients on contact precautions for the same indication.

Continuous Arterio-venous Hemofiltration (CAVHF)

▶ Hemofiltration in the ICU

Continuous Cardiac Output (CCO)

▶ Cardiac Output, Measurements

Continuous Hemodialysis (CVVHD)

▶ Hemofiltration in the ICU

Continuous Positive Airway Pressure (CPAP)

▶ Noninvasive Ventilation

Continuous Renal Replacement Therapy (CRRT)

▶ Hemofiltration in the ICU

Continuous Veno-venous Hemodiafiltration (CVVHDF)

▶ Hemofiltration in the ICU

Continuous Veno-venous Hemofiltration (CVVHF)

▶ Hemofiltration in the ICU

Contrast Medium-Induced Nephropathy

▶ Contrast Nephropathy

Contrast Nephropathy

ERIC A. J. HOSTE
Department of Internal Medicine, Ghent University
Hospital, Ghent, Belgium

Synonyms

Contrast medium-induced nephropathy; Contrast-associated acute kidney injury; Contrast-induced nephropathy

Definition

Several definitions for contrast-induced acute kidney injury (CI-AKI) have been used in medical literature. CI-AKI is typically defined as an increase of serum creatinine of 0.5 mg/dL or 25% or more within 2 days following contrast medium administration [3]. Multiple variations on this definition are used: some use only the absolute increase and others only the relative increase of serum creatinine, the observation period may be increased up to 5 days, and some use the more specific cut off of an absolute increase of 1 mg/dL. The European Society of Urogenital Radiology defines CI-AKI by an increase of serum creatinine of 0.5 mg/dL or 25% or greater within 3 days following intravascular administration of radio contrast medium, without an alternative etiology.

Recently the Acute Kidney Injury Network (AKIN) proposed a consensus definition where AKI is defined as an increase of 0.3 mg/dL or 50% or greater occurring within a 48 h time period [4].

Treatment

The treatment of established CI-AKI is not different from other types of AKI and consists of prevention of hypotension and hypovolemia and stop administration of potential nephrotoxic agents. For a more detailed discussion on the treatment of AKI we refer to the specific chapters on this in this textbook.

Prevention

Established risk factors for development of CI-AKI include an estimated glomerular filtration rate (eGFR) <60 mL/min/1.73 m^2, diabetes mellitus, volume depletion, nephrotoxic drugs, anemia, and hemodynamic instability [5]. ICU patients have often one or more of these risk factors, and are therefore at greater risk for development of CI-AKI. Also intra-arterial administration of radio contrast medium, high volume of contrast medium, and contrast medium with high osmolality are associated with higher risk for CI-AKI.

Preventive measures for CI-AKI can be categorized into four groups: withdrawal of nephrotoxic drugs, volume expansion, pharmacologic therapies, and hemofiltration or hemodialysis. We will discuss these in detail.

Withdrawal of Nephrotoxic Drugs

All nephrotoxic drugs should be withdrawn >24 h before contrast administration in patients at risk for CI-AKI (GFR<60 mL/min) [5].

Volume Expansion

Volume expansion with crystalloids at a rate of 1–1.5 mL/kg for 1–12 h before the procedure, and continued for 6 to 12 h afterwards, has an established role in reducing the risk for CI-AKI. Isotonic saline 0.9% was in one trial superior to half isotonic saline 0.45% in prevention of CI-AKI. Isotonic sodium bicarbonate (3 mL/kg/h for 1 h before the procedure and at 1 mL/kg/h for 6 h after the procedure) was superior to isotonic saline in prevention of CI-AKI, in a number of smaller studies and in meta-analyses [1]. Although, the number of patients studied, and heterogeneity of the studies, preclude a firm conclusion.

Pharmacological Therapy

No adjunct pharmacological therapy to date has been proven efficacious for reducing the risk for CI-AKI [5].

The CIN Consensus Working Panel has divided the drugs that have been evaluated into three categories based on their results [5].

Positive Results

These drugs are potentially beneficial, but need further evaluation.

- Theophylline/aminophyllin

  These adenosine antagonists block the potent intrarenal vasoconstrictor adenosine, which also is a mediator of tubulo-glomerular feedback. A meta-analysis including seven trials and 480 patients demonstrated a significant decline in serum creatinine after contrast administration.

- Statins

  Retrospective data from large databases demonstrated that patients who were treated with statins had a lower incidence of CI-AKI. This can be explained because statins have beneficial effects on endothelial function, maintain nitric oxide production, and reduce oxidative stress. A prospective randomized study published after the recommendations, in 304 patients undergoing coronary angiography, could not demonstrate a beneficial effect when 80 mg atorvastatin was administered daily, 48 h before and after the contrast procedure.

- Ascorbic acid

  A small prospective randomized study in 231 patients undergoing cardiac catheterization demonstrated a lower incidence for patients treated with oral ascorbic acid (3 g before and two times 2 g after the procedure).

- Prostaglandin E1

  Two small studies including 130 and 125 patients found that the vasodilator prostaglandin E1 and its synthetic analogue misoprostol were effective in reducing the risk for CI-AKI.

Neutral

- N-acetylcysteine (NAC)

  Although NAC is often administered for prevention of CI-AKI, the evidence supporting its use is weak. Over 27 prospective randomized studies and meta-analyses found conflicting results regarding the potential beneficial effects of NAC on CI-AKI. The majority of studies were in patients undergoing non-coronary or coronary angiography with intra-arterial administration of contrast medium. Studies were heterogeneous as several dosing regimes were evaluated, in different cohorts, and different outcomes were assessed.

A study in volunteers suggested that the beneficial effects of NAC could be attributed to an effect on serum creatinine concentration, and not on glomerular filtration rate. However, recent data could not confirm this.

- Fenoldopam/dopamine

  Three small studies and one uncontrolled study suggested that renal dose dopamine could prevent CI-AKI. This could not be confirmed in a prospective randomized study.

  Fenoldopam, a selective dopamine-A1 receptor agonist, was beneficial in several uncontrolled studies, but not in two prospective randomized studies.

- Calcium channel blockers

  Several small studies evaluated the effects of amlodipine, nifedipine, nitrendipine, and felodipine on risk for CI-AKI, but found no consistent effect.

- Atrial natriuretic peptide (ANP)

  Two small studies could not demonstrate a beneficial effect of ANP on the occurrence of CI-AKI.

Negative Effects

- Furosemide, mannitol, and dual endothelin receptor antagonist

  These drugs were evaluated in small studies with conflicting and negative results on prevention of CI-AKI.

Hemofiltration or Hemodialysis

Hemodialysis can effectively remove contrast media. However, even when administered within 1 h after contrast administration, hemodialysis was not effective in reducing the incidence of CI-AKI.

The CIN Consensus Working Panel agreed that in patients with severe renal impairment (GFR <20 mL/kg/min), hemodialysis should be planned in case CI-AKI occurs [5].

Hemofiltration was beneficial in preventing CI-AKI in two studies, when administered 4–6 h before the procedure, and continued for 18–24 h afterwards. These studies were flawed as the primary endpoint CI-AKI, defined by a 25% increase of serum creatinine, is affected by hemofiltration. Secondary endpoints, such as in-hospital and 1-year mortality, were also positively affected by the intervention. Further data are therefore needed.

Evaluation/Assessment

It is important to identify risk factors for CI-AKI in patients who will undergo a contrast procedure. After the procedure it is recommended to monitor serum creatinine concentration for 3–5 days in order to diagnose occurrence of CI-AKI.

After-care

The therapy for CI-AKI is similar to other forms of AKI in ICU patients, and consists of optimization of volume status, and withdrawal of nephrotoxic drugs. Further, one needs to monitor and tread for consequences of CI-AKI such as hyperkalemia and other electrolyte abnormalities, volume overload, and acidosis.

Prognosis

Patients who develop CI-AKI are at greater risk for in-hospital mortality and 1-year mortality [3]. Levy et al. found a 5.5-fold increased risk of hospital death, even after correction for other comorbidities [2]. Risk of death is greater in patients with need for treatment with renal replacement therapy, and in patients with chronic kidney disease before the procedure.

The risk for developing need for dialysis is currently estimated as <1% in patients with CI-AKI in low risk patients. Data in ICU patients are scarce; one study found that 3.5% of 486 ICU patients needed treatment with dialysis after contrast administration. Another study in 139 ICU patients found a nonsignificant higher incidence of dialysis in patients with CI-AKI (19% versus 6%, $p = 0.091$).

CI-AKI is also associated with other adverse cardiovascular outcomes such as myocardial infarction, bypass surgery, pulmonary edema, cardiogenic shock, bleeding requiring transfusion, and vascular complications. Also, length of hospital stay is longer in patients who have CI-AKI.

References

1. Hoste EA, De Waele JJ, Gevaert SA, Uchino S, Kellum JA (2010) Sodium bicarbonate for prevention of contrast-induced acute kidney injury: a systematic review and meta-analysis. Nephrol Dial Transplant 25:747–758
2. Levy EM, Viscoli CM, Horwitz RI (1996) The effect of acute renal failure on mortality. A cohort analysis. JAMA 275:1489–1494
3. McCullough PA, Adam A, Becker CR et al (2006) Epidemiology and prognostic implications of contrast-induced nephropathy. Am J Cardiol 98:5–13
4. Mehta RL, Kellum JA, Shah SV et al (2007) Acute kidney injury network: report of an initiative to improve outcomes in acute kidney injury. Crit Care 11:R31
5. Stacul F, Adam A, Becker CR et al (2006) Strategies to reduce the risk of contrast-induced nephropathy. Am J Cardiol 98:59–77

Contrast-Associated Acute Kidney Injury

▶ Contrast Nephropathy

Contrast-Induced Nephropathy

▶ Contrast Nephropathy

Conus Medullaris Syndrome

Scott E. Bell[1], Kathryn M. Beauchamp[2]
[1]Department of Neurosurgery, School of Medicine, University of Colorado Health Sciences Center, Denver, CO, USA
[2]Department of Neurosurgery, Denver Health Medical Center, University of Colorado School of Medicine, Denver, CO, USA

Definition

Conus medullaris syndrome (CMS) arises from a spectrum of clinicopathologic entities representing dysfunction of the lowest level of the spinal cord, termed the conus medullaris, which consists of the sacral segments. There is a subset of spinal cord injuries referred to as spinal cord injury syndromes, to which conus medullaris syndrome belongs, that are grouped by their respective symptomatology, including central cord syndrome, Brown-Sequard syndrome, anterior cord syndrome, posterior cord syndrome, and cauda equina syndrome. While CMS is classically associated with pathophysiologic disruption isolated to the conus medullaris, it may also be associated with a widespread spinal cord process that includes the conus medullaris, which leads to the generalized syndromic symptoms. By nature of its anatomy, this is an illness characterized by both upper motor and lower motor neuron signs and symptoms that manifest in the perineal region and lower extremities.

The spinal cord ends at the level of the last thoracic to second lumbar vertebrae in a normal adult, with the remainder of the spinal canal being occupied by the cauda equina. This corresponds to the level of the thoracolumbar junction. It is an important concept to recall that the vertebral column level deviates from the spinal cord level starting in the cervical spine. A depiction of this relationship is seen in Fig. 1. In general, the spinal cord level is considered to reside roughly one to two levels above its corresponding vertebral level (at which the nerve root exits) for most of the cervical and upper thoracic spinal cord, three to four levels above for the lower thoracic and lumbar spinal cord, and five or more levels above for the sacral spinal cord. With this relationship in mind, it is to

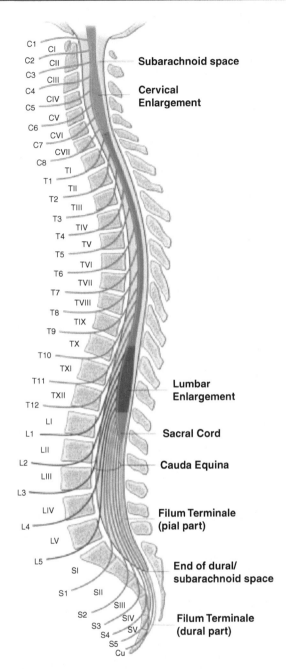

C1
CI
C2
CII
C3
CIII
C4
CIV
C5
CV
C6
CVI
C7
CVII
C8
TI
T1
TII
T2
TIII
T3
TIV
T4
TV
T5
TVI
T6
TVII
T7
TVIII
T8
TIX
T9
TX
T10
TXI
T11
TXII
T12
LI
L1
LII
L2
LIII
L3
LIV
L4
LV
L5
SI
S1   SII
S2   SIII
S3   SIV
S4   SV
S5
Cu

Subarachnoid space

Cervical
Enlargement

Lumbar
Enlargement

Sacral Cord

Cauda Equina

Filum Terminale
(pial part)

End of dural/
subarachnoid space

Filum Terminale
(dural part)

Conus Medullaris Syndrome. Figure 1 Relationship of
spinal cord and nerve roots to vertebral level (Adapted from
Drake et al. 2008)

say that a conus medullaris lesion occurs at the vertebral
level approximately L1, but affects the lower sacral segments of the spinal cord.

Spinal cord injury occurs at a reported annual incidence of 40 per million population, with 11,000 new
cases each year in the United States. Epidemiology of
nontraumatic causes of spinal cord disease is more difficult due to its rarity and the lack of consensus and consistency in reporting. Conus medullaris syndrome as a whole
is quite a rare process, with a diverse array of etiologies
(Table 1). Definitive epidemiologic information about
CMS is sparse. In a series of 839 patients reviewed retrospectively of spinal cord injury (SCI) rehabilitation admissions from 1992 to 2004 at an urban tertiary care center,
1.7% had CMS [1]. A European study reported an average
annual incidence of conus medullaris syndrome at 1.5 per
million population, and prevalence of 4.5 per 100,000
population, over the study period 1996–2004 from etiologies of all types [2].

Etiology

The most common causes of CMS are reported as compression from herniated intervertebral disc, and vertebral
fracture at the thoracolumbar junction [2]. The mechanisms at the root of CMS specifically, underlying these
etiologies, are multimodal. The acute or primary mechanism
involves ischemia and direct injury to neuropil and neuronal
cells at that location by compression, traction, contusion,
and/or laceration. The secondary mechanism involves
a complex cascade of chemical signals and inflammatory
mediators, ion conduction and matrix derangements, cellular respiratory insults, and cytotoxic neurotransmitters that
results in the propagation of irreversible injury. Other etiologies of conus medullaris syndrome includes any lesion that
disrupts the grey and/or white matter of the spinal cord at
that level. Such lesions may include infiltrative, compressive,
demyelinating, ischemic, or inflammatory processes produced by tumors, trauma, infections, or autoimmune and
metabolic diseases. Varying combinations of primary and
secondary mechanisms of spinal cord injury are responsible
for the spectrum of conus medullaris syndrome seen in all
etiologies of this disease.

Tumors of the spine cause damage to the conus
medullaris by compressive and infiltrative mechanisms.
The most common intramedullary tumor of the conus
medullaris is ependymoma [3]. They develop from the
ependymal cells lining the filum terminale, and less
often the ependymal cells of the ventriculus terminalis.
This structure is an ependymal-lined termination of the
central canal, residing at the transition from conus
medullaris to filum terminale. Less frequently encountered intramedullary tumors at the conus include low-
grade astrocytomas and rarely glioblastoma multiforme.
This later form has been shown to occur at the conus as
either primary occurrence or as identified in holocord
disease. The most common extramedullary tumors at the
conus medullaris are peripheral nerve sheath tumors,

Conus Medullaris Syndrome. Table 1 Reported etiologies of conus medullaris syndrome

Inflammatory	Tumor	Infection	Non-tumor	Trauma
Transverse myelitis	Ependymoma	Staphylococcus	Sarcoidosis	HNP
Longitudinal myelitis	Astrocytoma	Tuberculosis	Cavernoma	Burst
Neuromyelitis optica	GBM	Schistosomiasis	AVF/AVM	Fracture
Lupus erythematosus	Ganglioglioma	Cysticercosis	Amyloid angiopathy	Fracture dislocation
Parainfectious myelitis	Meningioma			
	PNET		Ventriculus terminus cyst	Spinal stenosis
	Teratoma			
	Hemangioblastoma		Tethered cord	
	Metastases		Infarct	
	Chordoma		Dermoid cyst	
	Peripheral nerve sheath tumor		Epidermoid cyst	

GBM glioblastoma multiforme, *PNET* primitive neuroectodermal tumor, *AVF* arteriovenous fistula, *AVM* arteriovenous malformation, *HNP* herniated nucleus pulposus

meningioma, and metastases. In contrast to the brain, intramedullary metastases occur much less commonly, likely owing to the difference in blood flow between the brain and spine [3].

Epidermoid and dermoid cysts may be congenital or acquired, and can occur at the conus medullaris. They arise from retained integument within the spinal canal, with or without a sinus tract to the surface. These lesions are due to one of two mechanisms [3]. They may be associated with developmental malformative rests, as well as being acquired by lumbar puncture or after surgery to close myelomeningocele early in life. They can be the source of recurrent infections, and may expand to compress the conus, or cause local vascular derangement producing CMS. Teratomas are congenital, and likewise arise from rests of misplaced tissue. There is debate whether these arise from a migratory problem during development, or from a dysembryogenic-type mechanism. At the conus, they are frequently associated with dysembryogenic defects such as split cord and myelomeningocele.

Inflammatory diseases are rarely associated with conus medullaris syndrome, precluding analysis as a series. However, reports of inflammatory demyelinating diseases that are either isolated to the conus or involving the conus in holocord-type fashion are reported as case reports in the literature. The most common entities showing CMS symptoms include transverse myelitis, NMO, and longitudinal myelitis. Their occurrences have been described in cases where the mechanism is likely autoimmune response after systemic infection or vaccine [4]. Likewise, other systemic inflammatory diseases, such as lupus erythematosus, have been identified in cases where initial presentation of the disease was by way of CMS [5]. Thus far, due to the rarity of these entities, no known specific pathophysiologic process has been described for these causes of CMS.

While tethered cord syndrome is considered as a distinct entity, it may be considered within the spectrum of CMS. This process exerts its deleterious effect on the medullary conus by placing tension on the spinal vessels, and cord itself. This ultimately leads to ischemia by a variety of pathophysiologic mechanisms. One such mechanism of dysfunction as a result of tethered cord includes metabolic derangements leading to increased reduction states of certain oxidase systems in the mitochondria of nerve cells, which appears to be related to ischemia in this area. Mild-to-moderate redox derangements have been reversed with surgical untethering; however, severe cases are more refractory.

Indeed, there have been reports of conus medullaris syndrome after spinal meningitis. Other infectious processes that have been reported affecting the conus medullaris include epidural or intramedullary abscesses from staphylococcus, tuberculosis, as well as schistosomiasis and neurocystercircosis. It is generally accepted that these infections seed via hematogenous route through the valveless system of vascular plexuses around the thoracolumbar junction, or by local phlegmon formation.

Holocord processes may present with conus medullaris syndrome signs and symptoms, in conjunction with other neurologic deficits related to its associated spinal cord pathophysiology. The term "holocord" is used to define diffuse

Conus Medullaris Syndrome. Table 2 Conus medullaris syndrome vs cauda equina syndrome

C

	Conus medullaris syndrome	Cauda Equina syndrome
Presentation	Sudden (inflammatory lesions), insidious (tumors), bilateral	Acute (trauma), gradual (stenosis), may be unilateral
Reflexes	Hyperreflexia; knee jerk preserved, ankle jerk affected	Hyporeflexia; knee jerk and ankle jerk both affected
Radicular pain	Less severe	More severe
Low back pain	Local low back pain only; rarely radiation to perineum	Low back pain with dermatomal radiation
Sensory symptoms/signs	Perianal localization to sensory disturbance; symmetric and bilateral; sensory dissociation present	Stereotypic "saddle anesthesia;" asymmetric and unilateral disturbance possible; no sensory dissociation; possible dermatomal sensory disturbances possible with parasthesias
Motor strength	Usually symmetric; spastic paraparesis, less pronounced; fasciculations possible	Asymmetric and unilateral motor weakness possible; areflexic paraparesis; atrophy common
Impotence	Frequent	Less frequent; erectile dysfunction including inability to maintain erection, inability to ejaculate
Sphincter dysfunction	Urinary retention and atonic anal sphincter causes overflow incontinence; presents early	Urinary retention; presents late

Source: Adapted from Dawodu et al. (2009)

involvement of multiple, or all, regions of the spinal cord in a disease process. This has been seen in as diverse an array of pathologies as there are focal disruptions of the conus itself. Some of the more common holocord processes include infiltrative tumors with widespread dissemination; syringomyelia from compressive pathologies; and neuromyelitis optica, which shows "longitudinal myelitis" type imaging and clinical findings.

Another etiology worth mention is that of ischemic injury or infarction of the conus medullaris. This occurs through a variety of mechanisms, and is thought to represent approximately 1% of stroke cases. Embolism has been described from sickle cell anemia, epidural steroid injection, antiphospholipid antibodies, and abdominal surgical procedures. Other mechanisms include vascular malformations producing a blood flow "steal" phenomenon whereby blood flow bypasses the arteriole and capillary level by arteriovenous shunting.

Clinical Presentation

The symptoms of conus medullaris syndrome may present acutely or insidiously, depending upon the etiology. These symptoms will show mixed upper motor and lower motor neuron signs of the perineum and distal lower extremities, with an emphasis on UMN. Lower motor neuron deficits are due to the presence of lumbar nerve roots present within the thecal sac prior to exit at their respective vertebral level. Due to the anatomic relationship between the conus medullaris and the cauda equina, CMS may be easily confused with cauda equina syndrome to the complacent observer. One must take careful measure to distinguish these disease processes during the evaluation of bowel and bladder, and lower extremity dysfunction. Both syndromes produce weakness and sensory dysfunction of the saddle region as well as variable parts of the lower extremities. Some distinguishing characteristics are outlined in Table 2 . Local back pain, if present, is typically an early symptom, followed by bowel and bladder retention. The pain will be more aching in nature, rather than the sharp, sudden pain associated with cauda equina syndrome. Motor dysfunction is typically a late sign in conus medullaris syndrome. A common sign of severe spinal cord dysfunction includes diminished or absent bulbocavernosus and anal sphincter reflexes. This is likewise represented in conus medullaris syndrome.

Once distinguished from the differentials, attention can be turned to narrowing the list of possible etiologies of the problem. The acuity of onset and history lends to the distinction between surgical lesions and medical lesions. Tumors, vascular malformations, and other surgically remediable lesions tend to present with a more insidious onset. Exceptions to this are those acute processes, such as injury, visibly expansile lesions, hemorrhages, etc., which may require immediate decompression to save neural tissue. Otherwise, acute onset symptomatology tends to occur in those nonsurgical processes, such as autoimmune and inflammatory etiologies, which are more amenable to medical treatments.

Imaging studies are an important adjunct for any diagnostic workup. Of particular importance will be an MRI with and without gadolinium of the entire spine to examine the neural axis for findings. Cystic lesions will be isointense with CSF on both T1W and T2W images. Tumors may show rim-enhancement or varying degrees of homogeneous or heterogeneous lesion enhancement, depending upon the type of tumor. Inflammatory or demyelinating processes may show rim-enhancement as well. The distinguishing characteristic is that tumors typically have an expansile quality identifiable at the conus, while inflammatory processes usually do not. However, this must be taken in the context of the clinical picture. In the absence of acute symptoms and an expansile lesion, tumor is more likely; whereas acute symptoms and an expansile mass may be a harbinger for hemorrhage, for example. Computed tomography of the spine for bony involvement is important for surgical planning and prognosticating, but would not supplant the use of MRI. The diagnostic value of a contrast-enhancing MRI outweighs that of CT scan, and would preclude its usefulness in the later.

Electrophysiologic studies, such as electromyography and nerve conduction velocities, can be useful in distinguishing central from peripheral nervous system processes of duration longer than 2–4 weeks. They are useless in providing information on the nature of symptoms of shorter duration due to the pathophysiology underlying acute denervation, demyelination, and neuromuscular conduction defects.

Treatment

Treatment for conus medullaris syndrome varies based on etiology. As previously mentioned, discrete lesions within the conus identifiable on imaging should be approached with microsurgical technique for biopsy, debulking, and rarely radical resection if curable etiology is known. If traumatic injuries are present with conus medullaris compression, decompression and stabilization at the earliest possible juncture in the patient's acute stages of illness has been argued to be important for optimal convalescence. When to operate under these circumstances depends upon many factors, including hemodynamic instability and associated injuries of a more critical nature. The debate of when spinal cord injuries should be operated has led to much discord in the surgical literature of the traumatized spine.

Whether due to a trauma or nontraumatic causes, the rationale for treading lightly in this region of the spinal cord lies in the functional forgiveness of the location. Once definitively injured, those neuronal elements responsible for bowel, bladder, and sexual function rarely recover.

This is directly opposed to those elements at other locations in the spinal cord responsible for somatic sensory and motor function, which carry a good prognosis with rehabilitation, after incomplete injury. However, there are circumstances, as in the case of ependymoma, where gross total resection will likely lead to cure. In these cases, it is imperative to use meticulous surgical technique in order to minimize the potential for permanent disability.

If it is determined that a nonsurgical lesion is present, the medical treatment depends upon the nature of the lesion. If infection is suspected, antibiotic therapy is initiated only after an organism is identified, either through blood cultures or image-guided aspiration. Then dual agent, IV antibiotics must be initiated for long-term therapy. This treatment for intramedullary and epidural infections can be very successful. In those refractory cases, or cases of acute worsening, surgical debridement may be necessary in addition. If an inflammatory process is suspected, high-dose steroid therapy is the gold standard. Multiple cases of inflammatory conus medullaris syndrome have been shown to be quickly responsive to these treatments, sometimes leading to complete remission of symptoms. More frequently, partial recovery occurs, with gradual improvement to only some disability in weeks to months. In some cases, it is useful or necessary to synergize with other immune modulators, such as IV-IG, cyclophosphamide, and azathioprine.

Prognosis

Often the prognosis for conus medullaris syndrome is more related to the etiology than to the syndrome itself. If the underlying cause is a malignant process, this is far and away the more decisive factor in prognostication than the presence of CMS. However, if CMS is due to a lesion affecting the conus in isolation, then prognosis is related to the degree of neuronal tissue damage. Frequently, with today's techniques of intensive rehabilitation and targeted medical therapy, lesions isolated to the conus medullaris causing CMS will improve to acceptable functional levels, if not full recovery. In rare cases, isolated CMS leads to permanent paraplegia and pelvic sphincter dysfunction.

References

1. McKinley W, Santos K, Meade M, Brooke K (2007) Incidence and outcomes of spinal cord injury clinical syndromes. J Spinal Cord Med 30:215–224
2. Podnar S (2007) Epidemiology of cauda equina and conus medullaris lesions. Muscle Nerve 35:529–531
3. Ebner FH, Roser F, Acioly MA, Schoeber W, Tatagiba M (2009) Intramedullary lesions of the conus medullaris: differential diagnosis and surgical management. Neurosurg Rev 32:287–301

4. Pradhan S, Gupta RK, Kapoor R, Shashank S, Kathuria MK (1998) Parainfectious conus myelitis. J Neurol Sci 161:156–162
5. Katramados AM, Rabah R, Adams MD, Huq AH, Mitsias PD (2008) Longitudinal myelitis, aseptic meningitis, and conus medullaris infarction as presenting manifestations of pediatric systemic lupus erythematosus. Lupus 17:332–336

Convection

The physical mechanism by which a solute is dragged across a semipermeable membrane in association with ultrafiltered plasma water. This water and solute shift is secondary to a pressure gradient across the membrane.

Convective Clearance

Zhongping Huang[1], William R. Clark[2,3], Claudio Ronco[4]
[1]Department of Mechanical Engineering, Widener University, Chester, PA, USA
[2]Gambro Renal Products, Lakewood, CO, USA
[3]Nephrology Division, Indiana University School of Medicine, Indianapolis, IN, USA
[4]Department of Nephrology, St. Bortolo Hospital, Vicenza, Italy

Synonyms

Solvent drag; Ultrafiltration

Definition

The mechanism of ▶ convection may be described as solvent drag: if a pressure gradient exists between the two sides of a semipermeable (porous) membrane, when the molecular dimensions of a solute are such that passage through the membrane is possible, the solute is swept ("dragged") across the membrane in association with ultrafiltered plasma water.

Pre-existing Condition

Although conventional hemodialysis (HD) remains the most commonly used treatment modality for the management of patients with acute kidney injury (AKI), continuous renal replacement therapy (CRRT) is used increasingly in this setting. The removal of low-molecular weight (MW) nitrogenous waste products is very effective with HD. However, ▶ clearance of larger molecules is limited due to HD's primarily diffusive nature. In clinical practice, HD therapy prescription is driven largely by factors influencing urea clearance. On the other hand, convective modalities, namely, ▶ hemofiltration and hemodiafiltration, are capable of removing solutes over a wider MW array than can HD. In AKI, these therapies typically are provided on an extended basis as continuous venovenous hemofiltration (CVVH) and continuous venovenous hemodiafiltration (CVVHDF), being part of the CRRT spectrum.

In a study employing CVVH, Ronco and colleagues [1] reported a direct relationship between daily ultrafiltrate volume and survival in critically ill AKI patients. A normalized ultrafiltration rate of 35 mL/kg/h or more (on average) was associated with a mortality of approximately 45% while a more standard ultrafiltrate rate (mean, 20 mL/kg/h) was associated with a mortality of approximately 65%. Although subsequent studies in which convection has contributed relatively less to total solute clearance have produced mixed results [2], the Ronco study remains the "gold standard" with respect to convective solute removal in AKI.

This chapter provides a review of the determinants of convective solute removal. This is followed by an overview of the manner in which CVVH and CVVHDF are applied clinically.

Application

Convective Clearance

The determinants of convective clearance differ significantly from those of diffusion, which is primarily a concentration gradient-driven process. On the other hand, convective solute removal is determined primarily by the sieving properties of the filter membrane used and the ultrafiltration rate. The mechanism by which convection occurs is termed solvent drag. If the molecular dimensions of a solute are such that transmembrane passage to some extent occurs, the solute is swept ("dragged") across the membrane in association with ultrafiltered plasma water. Thus, the rate of convective solute removal can be modified either by changes in the rate of solvent (plasma water) flow or by changes in the mean effective pore size of the membrane. As discussed below, the blood concentration of a particular solute is an important determinant of its convective removal rate.

Both the water and solute permeability of an ultrafiltration membrane are influenced by the phenomena of secondary membrane formation and concentration polarization. The exposure of an artificial surface to plasma results in the nonspecific, instantaneous adsorption of a layer of proteins, the composition of which generally reflects that of the plasma itself. This layer of proteins, by serving as an additional resistance to mass transfer, effectively reduces both the water and solute permeability of an extracorporeal membrane. Evidence of this is found in comparisons of solute sieving coefficients determined before and after exposure of a membrane to plasma or other protein-containing solution.

Although concentration polarization primarily pertains to plasma proteins, it is distinct from secondary membrane formation. Concentration polarization specifically relates to ultrafiltration-based processes and applies to the kinetic behavior of an individual solute. Accumulation of a solute that is predominantly or completely rejected by a membrane used for ultrafiltration of plasma occurs at the blood compartment membrane surface. This surface accumulation causes the solute concentration just adjacent to the membrane surface (i.e., the submembranous concentration) to be higher than the bulk (plasma) concentration. By definition, concentration polarization is applicable in clinical situations in which relatively high ultrafiltration rates are used. Conditions that promote the process are high ultrafiltration rate (high rate of convective transport), low blood flow rate (low shear rate or membrane "sweeping" effect), and the use of ▶ post-dilution (rather than ▶ pre-dilution) replacement fluids (increased local solute concentrations).

Post-dilution CRRT

The location of replacement fluid delivery in the extracorporeal circuit during CRRT has a significant impact on solute removal and therapy requirements. (For the purpose of the rest of this chapter, CRRT refers either to CVVH or CVVHDF.) Replacement fluid can be delivered to the arterial blood line prior to the hemofilter (pre-dilution mode) or to the venous line after the hemofilter (post-dilution mode). In post-dilution CRRT, the relationship between solute clearance and ultrafiltration rate is relatively straightforward. In this situation, solute clearance is determined primarily by and related directly to the solute's sieving coefficient and the ultrafiltration rate. (Sieving coefficient is defined as the ratio of the solute concentration in the filtrate to the simultaneous plasma concentration.) For a given solute, the extent to which it partitions from the plasma water into the red blood cell mass and the rate at which it is transported across red blood cell membranes also influences clearance. For example, the volume of distribution of both urea and creatinine

includes the red blood cell water. However, while urea movement across red blood cell membranes is very fast, the movement of creatinine is significantly less rapid. Furthermore, red blood cell membranes are completely impermeable to many uremic toxins. A prominent example of this is the low MW protein toxin class, for which the volume of distribution is the extracellular fluid. These observations lead to the obvious conclusion that hematocrit also influences solute clearance in CRRT. Finally, through its effect on secondary membrane formation and concentration polarization (see above), plasma total protein concentration is also a determinant of solute clearance in CRRT.

For a given volume of replacement fluid over the entire MW spectrum of uremic toxins, post-dilution CRRT provides higher solute clearance than does pre-dilution CRRT. As discussed below, the relative inefficiency of the latter mode is related to the dilution-related reduction in solute concentrations, which decreases the driving force for convective mass transfer. Despite its superior efficiency with respect to replacement fluid utilization, post-dilution CRRT is limited inherently by the attainable blood flow rate. More specifically, the ratio of the ultrafiltration rate to the plasma flow rate delivered to the filter, termed the filtration fraction, is the limiting factor. In general, a maximal filtration fraction of approximately 25% usually guides prescription in post-dilution CRRT. At filtration fractions beyond these values, concentration polarization and secondary membrane effects become prominent and may impair hemofilter performance.

The blood flow limitations imposed by the use of temporary catheters for CRRT accentuate the filtration fraction-related constraints on maximally attainable ultrafiltration rate in the post-dilution mode. Therefore, the ultrafiltrate volumes shown by Ronco and colleagues to improve survival can usually be achieved only in the pre-dilution mode. As discussed below, efficient utilization of replacement fluid in acute pre-dilution CRRT is an important consideration.

Pre-dilution HF

From a mass transfer perspective, the use of pre-dilution has several potential advantages over post-dilution. First, both hematocrit and blood total protein concentration are reduced significantly prior to the entry of blood into the hemofilter. This effective reduction in the red cell and protein content of the blood attenuates the secondary membrane and concentration polarization phenomena described above, resulting in improved mass transfer. Pre-dilution also favorably impacts mass transfer due to augmented flow in the blood compartment, because pre-filter mixing of blood and replacement fluid occurs. This achieves a relatively high membrane shear rate, which also reduces solute-membrane interactions. Finally, pre-dilution may also enhance mass transfer for some compounds by creating concentration gradients that induce solute movement out of red blood cells.

The above mass transfer benefits must be weighed against the predictable dilution-induced reduction in plasma solute concentrations, one of the driving forces for convective solute removal. The extent to which this reduction occurs is determined mainly by the ratio of the replacement fluid rate to the blood flow rate. Indeed, a frequently overlooked consideration is the important influence of blood flow rate on solute clearance. For small solutes, which are distributed in the blood water (BW) component within the blood passing through the hemofilter, the operative clearance equation in pre-dilution CRRT is:

$$K = Q_F \cdot S \cdot [Q_{BW}/(Q_{BW} + Q_S)] \qquad (1)$$

where K is solute clearance, Q_{BW} is blood water flow rate, Q_F is ultrafiltration rate, S is sieving coefficient, and Q_S is the substitution (replacement) fluid rate. At a given Q_F value, pre-dilution CVVH is always less efficient than post-dilution CVVH with respect to fluid utilization, as discussed above. A sieving coefficient of 1.0 implies equivalence of blood water and ultrafiltrate concentrations, resulting in small solute clearances that are effectively equal to Q_F in post-dilution CVVH. As Eq. 1 indicates, the larger Q_S is relative to Q_{BW}, the smaller is the entire fraction represented by the third term on the right-hand side. In turn, the smaller is this term, the greater is the loss of efficiency (relative to post-dilution) due to dilution. Since employing a relatively low Q_S is not an option in high-dose CVVH due to the direct relationship that exists between Q_F and Q_S, attention needs to be focused on achieving blood flow rates that are significantly higher than what have been used traditionally in CRRT (i.e., 150 mL/min or less). In fact, widespread attainment of doses consistent with the intermediate and high-dose arms in the study performed by Ronco and colleagues (35–45 mL/h/kg) cannot occur unless blood flow rates of approximately 250 mL/min or more become routine in pre-dilution CVVH.

Evidence supporting the critical importance of Q_B in pre-dilution CVVH appears in Fig. 1 [3]. For this single-pool modeling analysis, a dose equivalent to 35 mL/h/kg in post-dilution is targeted. In addition, a filter operation of 20 h per day is assumed to account for differences in prescribed versus delivered therapy time. For patients of varying body weight, the substitution fluid requirements to attain the above dose are shown as a function of Q_B. For low blood flow rates (= 150 mL/min), these data suggest that substitution fluid rates required to achieve this dose are impractically high in the majority of patients (>70 kg) due to a "chasing the tail" phenomenon. To achieve the

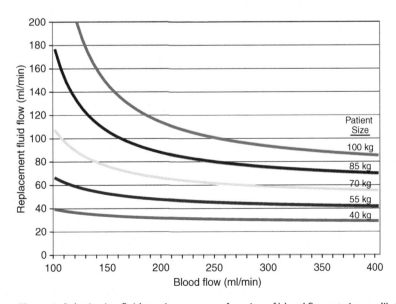

Convective Clearance. Figure 1 Substitution fluid requirements as a function of blood flow rate in pre-dilution CVVH (Reprinted from [3]. With permission from Elsevier)

C

dose target, a high ultrafiltration rate is required. However, the concomitant requirement of a similarly high substitution fluid rate has a relatively substantial dilutive effect on solute concentrations at low Q_B. On the other hand, for Q_B values greater than 250 mL/min, the dilutive effect of the substitution fluid is attenuated significantly and with the resultant improvement in fluid efficiency, the target dose can be delivered practically to a broad range of patients.

The operating principle of CVVHDF is that total clearance can be augmented by combining diffusion and convection. Due to the relatively low flow rates used for these therapies, changes in solute concentrations within the filter are also relatively small. This allows total solute clearance to be estimated by simply adding the diffusive and convective components. In other words, no interaction between the two mass transfer processes occurs.

Practical Considerations

At least until recently, the ultrafiltration rate (Q_F) in CVVH has typically been in the 1–2 L/h range. However, in response to outcome data published by Ronco and colleagues, prescription of significantly higher Q_F values is occurring. In post-dilution CVVH, the mode employed in the Ronco study, the relationship between solute clearance and Q_F is quite straightforward, as mentioned previously. For reasons also described above, the relationship between clearance and Q_F may not be as predictable in pre-dilution, relative to the case of post-dilution. Consequently, the claim that Q_F is a dose surrogate in pre-dilution CVVH needs to be demonstrated. To this end, Huang and colleagues have investigated the effect of Q_F on solute removal parameters in pre-dilution CVVH [4]. For a blood flow rate of 200 mL/min, removal parameters were measured at Q_F values of 20, 40, and 60 mL/min, corresponding to 17, 34, and 51 mL/h/kg for a 70 kg patient. These parameters are measured for solutes of varying MW.

The relationship between solute clearance and Q_F for urea, creatinine, vancomycin, and inulin appears in Fig. 2. Overall, these data are consistent with a convective therapy for two reasons. First, for each solute, the clearance-Q_F relationship is linear, confirming a direct relationship between these two parameters. Second, for a given Q_F over the solute MW range investigated, clearance is not strongly dependent on molecular weight, at least in comparison to hemodialysis. Specifically, very little difference in clearance is observed between the two small solutes and between the two middle molecule surrogates as a function of Q_F. On the other hand, reflecting its diffusive basis, HD is associated with much larger differences in clearance over

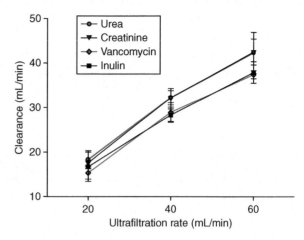

Convective Clearance. Figure 2 Solute clearance (mL/min) as a function of ultrafiltration rate (mL/min) in pre-dilution CVVH (Reprinted from [4]. With permission from Elsevier)

the same MW range. The authors concluded that, because an orderly relationship exists between Q_F and solute clearance, Q_F is a reasonable dose surrogate in pre-dilution CVVH, as has been suggested for post-dilution CVVH and for CVVHDF. Overall, these data seem to validate the use of effluent-based dosing, which has been employed in two recent international trials evaluating the relationship between CRRT dose and outcome [5].

References

1. Ronco C, Bellomo R, Hommel P, Brendolan A, Dan M, Piccinni P, LaGreca G (2000) Effects of different doses in continuous veno-venous hemofiltration on outcomes in acute renal failure: a prospective, randomized trial. Lancet 355:26–30
2. Saudan P, Niederberger M, De Seigneux S et al (2006) Adding a dialysis dose to continuous hemofiltration increases survival in patients with acute renal failure. Kidney Int 70:1312–1317
3. Clark WR, Turk JE, Kraus MA, Gao D (2003) Dose determinants in continuous renal replacement therapy. Artif Organs 27:815–820
4. Huang ZP, Letteri JJ, Clark WR, Zhang W, Gao D, Ronco C (2007) Ultrafiltration rate as a dose surrogate in pre-dilution hemofiltration. Int J Artif Organs 30:124–132
5. Huang Z, Letteri JJ, Clark WR, Ronco C (2008) Operational characteristics of continuous renal replacement therapy modalities used for critically ill patients with acute kidney injury. Int J Artif Organs 31:525–534

Corlopam®

▶ Fenoldopam

Coronary Computerized Tomographic Angiography

JUDD E. HOLLANDER[1], HAROLD LITT[2]
[1]Department of Emergency Medicine, University of Pennsylvania, Philadelphia, PA, USA
[2]Department of Radiology, University of Pennsylvania, Philadelphia, PA, USA

Synonyms

Coronary CTA; CT coronary angiography

Definition

A computed tomography examination of the heart acquired with ECG-synchronization during the arterial phase of intravenous contrast enhancement designed to visualize native coronary arteries and/or bypass grafts.

Pre-existing Condition

Coronary Artery Disease

Coronary CTA is primarily used to evaluate the presence or absence of coronary artery disease. It has a high degree of diagnostic accuracy when compared to cardiac catheterization as the criterion standard. In a meta-analysis of 2,515 patients from 41 studies, the subset imaged on a 64-slice scanner had a per patient sensitivity of 98% with a specificity of 92% for detection of significant coronary artery disease [1]. Newer generation scanners have even greater diagnostic performance.

Potential Acute Coronary Syndrome

Of the nearly eight million patients presenting annually to US emergency departments for evaluation of chest pain, 80–85% are not ultimately found to have a cardiac cause for their symptoms. However, given the prevalence and clinical significance of coronary artery disease, excluding a cardiac cause of chest pain remains a challenging clinical problem and often mandates extensive testing. Although clinical algorithms can successfully risk stratify patients, they have not typically been considered useful in identifying the group of patients who can be discharged safely from the emergency department without requiring an inpatient evaluation.

It is well established that patients without coronary artery disease are at very low risk for adverse cardiovascular events, even when they have symptoms that would otherwise be consistent with a potential acute coronary syndrome. Recent cardiac catheterization with normal or minimally diseased vessels is known to be useful to "rule out" an acute coronary syndrome in such patients. Coronary CTA, as a noninvasive surrogate for catheterization, can be used to risk stratify patients with respect to coronary artery disease and subsequently ACS immediately after onset of symptoms, thus avoiding hospitalization.

Application

Coronary CTA has several promising clinical applications at the present time, including: (1) identifying patients who present with a potential acute coronary syndrome (often in the ED) who may safely be discharged; (2) to evaluate patients for coronary artery disease, either as a first test or after indeterminate or suspected false positive stress test, avoiding unnecessary invasive cardiac catheterization; and (3) to evaluate stent or bypass graft patency and location in patients with symptoms after percutaneous coronary intervention (PCI) or bypass graft surgery (CABG).

Coronary CTA to "Rule Out" Acute Coronary Syndrome

Coronary CTA has high diagnostic accuracy (Fig. 1). Janne d'Othee et al. [1] found a sensitivity of 98% and specificity of 92% relative to cardiac catheterization using 64 slice scanners. Based upon this high diagnostic accuracy, centers with experience in coronary CTA have developed clinical pathways that allow for rapid disposition of patients who present with potential acute coronary syndromes found not to have coronary artery disease. This strategy is based upon the observation noted above that patients without coronary disease at cardiac catheterization are considered to be at low risk for adverse cardiovascular events.

Coronary CTA performs at least as well as myocardial perfusion imaging in identifying patients at low risk for cardiovascular events. Observational studies of symptomatic patients presenting to the ED have found that patients with normal coronary CTA results are at low risk for adverse events over varying time periods of up to one year.

Many small studies (35–103 subjects) have followed patients up to 15 months and have uniformly found that low- to intermediate-risk patients without coronary disease do well during this time period. One study of 568 patients in which coronary CTA was used for clinical decision making demonstrated that patients discharged from the ED following a negative study were at very low risk of 30-day cardiovascular events [2]. In a group of 481 patients with a TIMI score of less than or equal to two without a stenosis of 50% or more who were followed for

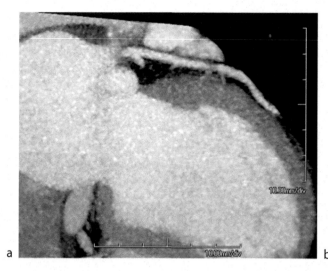
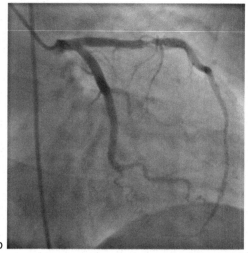

Coronary Computerized Tomographic Angiography. Figure 1 Forty-three-year-old male who presented to the ED with chest pain who was found to have an 80% stenosis in the proximal LAD. (**a**) CCTA demonstrates that the lesion is caused by non-calcified plaque and (**b**) corresponding catheter angiography performed prior to stenting lesion

up to 1 year, there were no patients who had definite cardiovascular events [3].

A coronary CTA based strategy to evaluate low- to intermediate-risk patients in the ED is cost effective. Chang et al. [4] found that immediate coronary CTA was more cost effective in the short term and was associated with a shorter length of stay than observation unit management with coronary CTA, observation unit management with stress test and admission with hospitalist directed care in a cohort of patients similar to this study. Short term benefits occur due to the reduced length of stay and lower cost of coronary CTA relative to single photon emission computed tomography (SPECT) imaging. Coronary CTA has also been associated with reduced utilization of coronary angiography, reduced revisit and readmission rate in other studies.

Clinical Utility to Diagnose or "Rule Out" Coronary Artery Disease

Given the high diagnostic accuracy of coronary CTA compared to cardiac catheterization, several groups have evaluated whether coronary CTA can reduce equivocal test results from stress nuclear imaging as well as the likelihood of receiving an invasive diagnostic procedure like cardiac catheterization.

Weustink et al. [5] compared the accuracy and clinical utility of stress testing and coronary CTA for identifying patients who require invasive coronary angiography (cardiac catheterization). They found that stress testing was not as accurate as coronary CTA. In low-risk patients

(<20% pretest probability of disease), a negative stress test or a negative coronary CTA confirmed no need for invasive angiography. On the other hand, a positive stress test only yielded a positive predictive value of 50%, meaning half the tests were false positive. In patients with an intermediate (20–80%) pretest probability of disease, a positive coronary CTA predicted need for invasive angiography (93% post-test probability of disease) and a negative result confirmed lack of need for further testing (<1% post test probability).

Population-based data from Canada has found that the rate of normal invasive coronary angiograms was relatively reduced by 15% (absolute reduction of 5%) in an institution that implemented coronary CTA.

Thus, it appears that use of coronary CTA can reduce confusion from false positive and false negative stress tests and lead to more appropriate use of invasive coronary angiography.

Evaluation of Symptomatic Patients after PCI or CABG Surgery

In patients who have previously undergone revascularization, recurrent chest pain may be caused by a variety of factors including progression of native vessel disease, stent or bypass graft stenosis or occlusion, and sternotomy or pericardiotomy complications (Fig. 2). For those patients in whom the chest pain is not clearly anginal, coronary CT may allow discrimination among these conditions. If repeat sternotomy is contemplated, whether for repeat CABG, valve replacement, or other reason, CT can

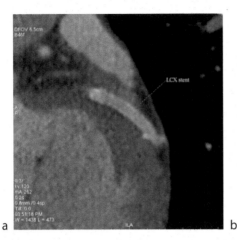 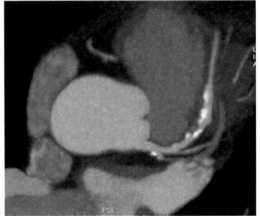

Coronary Computerized Tomographic Angiography. Figure 2 Seventy-two-year-old male with recurrent chest pain one year after PCI. (**a**) CCTA shows patent stent in the circumflex artery, but progression of disease in the LAD (**b**), with up to 70% stenosis caused by calcified and non-calcified plaque

demonstrate the course and position of bypass grafts relative to the sternum, decreasing operative complications. Coronary CT can also identify the course of the internal mammary arteries and location of target vessels for minimally invasive "keyhole" CABG surgery.

Additional Uses

Selection for CT coronary arteriography may also include patients with unexplained or atypical chest pain when an aberrant origin of the coronary artery is considered possible; concerns such as pulmonary embolism or aortic dissection; evaluation of an ischemic etiology for a newly diagnosed cardiomyopathy and/or heart failure; preoperative or preprocedural evaluation of the coronary arteries, cardiac structures, and thoracic anatomy; and evaluation of cardiac and/or coronary artery anomalies.

Indications in patients who have previously undergone CABG and/or percutaneous coronary intervention (PCI) include patients with new or recurrent symptoms of chest pain to confirm graft/stent patency or detect graft/stent stenoses or other complications; and for patients who are scheduled for additional cardiac surgery (e.g., aortic valve replacement or bypass graft revision) when preoperative definition of anatomic detail, including the bypass grafts, is critical.

Difficulties with Interpretation

Anatomy Versus Function

Although coronary CTA is usually performed to evaluate the coronary arteries, sometimes the interpretation of the results or the findings can be difficult. Coronary CTA provides information regarding anatomy. Anatomical abnormalities will not always be the explanation for clinical complaints. In some patients, a "noncritical" stenosis of 60% might be impeding flow to explain the symptoms while in another patient, a typically "critical" stenosis of 90% may not be causing the symptoms. In some situations, a functional test will be required to determine whether the anatomical abnormality explains the symptoms. A wall motion abnormality in the distribution of the stenosis may confirm that the stenosis is clinically relevant. Decreased myocardial perfusion, as evidenced by nuclear imaging, magnetic resonance imaging or contrast perfusion study will similar demonstrate clinical relevance of the stenosis.

Myocardial Bridging

Myocardial bridging is a congenital abnormality where a portion of a major coronary artery has an intramyocardial segment. Although usually not clinically significant, myocardial bridging has also been linked to clinical complications such as ischemia, spasm, dysrhythmias and sudden death. In some series, coronary CTA has identified myocardial bridging in as many as 50% of patients, although dynamic compression occurs in only about a quarter of these patients. Whether or not myocardial bridging detected on coronary CTA is associated with adverse events in patients who are otherwise at low risk is not known.

Incidental Findings

Coronary CTA will often include images of the thorax and the upper abdomen. As a result, abnormalities of other structures within these spaces can be observed. The rate of incidental findings reported in the literature is near 40%. Some incidental findings are clinically relevant and might explain the symptoms leading to the test (e.g., pulmonary embolism, aortic dissection, and malignancies). Others are incidental findings that can lead to further diagnostic evaluation, which may or may not have been otherwise necessary, potentially increasing costs. The most cost-effective approach to incidental findings remains to be determined.

Artifacts and Study Quality

Factors that result in decreased study quality include patient obesity, elevated heart rate, dysrhythmia, and coronary artery calcification. A heart rate of less than 70 is generally desirable for coronary CTA, although newer technologies are loosening this restriction. Oral or intravenous beta blockers are most commonly used for heart rate control when necessary. Sublingual nitroglycerin, administered at the time of the scan, may improve coronary visualization through vasodilation. Coronary CTA study quality may be compromised in patients with atrial fibrillation, as well as those with frequent premature ectopic beats. The presence of a large amount of coronary calcium may obscure the adjacent coronary lumen, and result in overestimation of the degree of stenosis, though this issue is ameliorated by recent technological advances in image acquisition, reconstruction, and post-processing.

Radiation Risk

As with all x-ray imaging studies, there is radiation exposure. For coronary CTA the radiation exposure varies widely between institutions and patients. It is dependent upon patient-related factors such as the weight of the patient (larger patients have more exposure) and the rhythm (sinus rhythm has less exposure). With respect to institutional and scanner-related factors, shorter scan lengths, electrocardiographic, controlled tube modulation, 100-kV tube voltage, sequential ECG-triggered scanning techniques, and experience in cardiac CTA are all associated with lower radiation doses without associated decreases in image quality. The long-term consequences of radiation exposure from medical imaging are not well known. They are based upon modeling rather than actual data, but it seems prudent to limit the radiation exposure when possible. Although dependent upon institutional protocol, myocardial perfusion imaging often has more radiation exposure than coronary CTA, and newer CT techniques result in doses similar to or lower than cardiac catheterization. CT may also decrease dose by reducing the need for additional testing.

References

1. Janne d'Othee B, Siebert W, Cury R, Jadvar H, Dunn EJ, Hoffman U (2008) A systematic review on diagnostic accuracy of CT based detection of significant coronary artery disease. Eur J Radiol 65:449–461
2. Hollander JE, Chang AM, Shofer FS, McCusker CM, Baxt WG, Litt HI (2009) Coronary computerized tomographic angiography for rapid discharge of low risk chest patients with potential acute coronary syndromes. Ann Emerg Med 53:295–304
3. Hollander JE, Chang AM, Shofer FS, Collin MJ, Walsh KM, McCusker CM, Baxt WG, Litt HI (2009) One year outcomes following coronary computerized tomographic angiography for evaluation of emergency department patients with potential acute coronary syndrome. Acad Emerg Med 16:693–698
4. Chang AM, Shofer FS, Weiner MG, Synnestvedt MB, Litt HI, Baxt WG, Hollander JE (2008) Actual financial comparison of four strategies to evaluate patients with potential acute coronary syndromes. Acad Emerg Med 15:649–655
5. Weustink AC, Mollet NR, Neefjes LA et al (2010) Diagnostic accuracy and clinical utility of noninvasive testing for coronary artery disease. Ann Intern Med 152:630–639

Coronary CTA

▶ Coronary Computerized Tomographic Angiography

Coronary Syndromes, Acute

JEREMY CORDINGLEY
Adult Intensive Care Unit, Royal Brompton Hospital, London, UK

Synonyms

Acute myocardial infarction (MI); Non-ST elevation myocardial infarction (NSTEMI); ST elevation myocardial infarction (STEMI); Unstable angina (UA)

Definition

Acute coronary syndromes (ACS) are a spectrum of illness caused by reduction in blood flow to the myocardium because of atherosclerotic disease of one or more coronary arteries and defined by clinical presentation, ECG findings, and biochemical markers of myocardial cell damage. An ACS occurs when blood supply to an area of myocardium is acutely reduced by sudden narrowing or obstruction of the vascular lumen by acute intravascular thrombosis on an atherosclerotic plaque through damaged endothelium. Blood supply becomes insufficient to meet metabolic demands resulting in myocardial ischemia.

The main clinical ACS syndromes that occur are unstable angina, non-ST elevation myocardial infarction (NSTEMI), and ST elevation myocardial infarction (STEMI) [1].

Unstable angina – Clinical presentation is of ischemic chest pain that does not resolve rapidly with sublingual glyceryl trinitrate and is not associated with ECG changes of ST elevation or increased serum concentration of biochemical markers of myocardial necrosis.

NSTEMI – Clinical presentation of myocardial ischemia associated with increased serum concentration of biochemical markers of myocardial necrosis but no ECG ST elevation.

STEMI – Clinical presentation of myocardial ischemia with ECG changes that should include the presence of one of: greater than 2 mm ST elevation in two adjacent chest leads, greater than 1 mm ST elevation in two limb leads (adjacent) or new bundle branch block and is associated with an increased serum concentration of biochemical markers of myocardial necrosis.

Since the widespread availability of highly sensitive biochemical markers of myocardial cell necrosis (troponin I and T), many patients previously classified as having unstable angina now fall into the category of NSTEMI. In practice, decision making about the need for emergency myocardial reperfusion therapy (thrombolytic drugs or percutaneous coronary intervention (PCI)) is based on the presence or absence of new ST elevation. The 2007 ESC (European Society of Cardiology) guidelines therefore classify patients into two categories based on the implications for patient management:

- ST elevation ACS (STE-ACS): Chest pain and ST elevation (STE) for greater than 20 min – immediate goal is to rapidly reestablish coronary flow by primary coronary intervention (PCI) or pharmacological thrombolysis.
- Non-ST elevation ACS (NSTE-ACS): Chest pain without ST elevation for greater than 20 min – immediate management is to treat myocardial ischemia. Serial ECG monitoring and measurements of biochemical markers of myocardial necrosis will guide further management.

Evaluation/Assessment

History

Most patients have chest pain that typically feels like pressure on the chest and may radiate to the left arm, neck, or jaw. The pain may be intermittent or continuous, and there may be associated symptoms including nausea and abdominal pain. Chest pain may be atypical or may be absent (more common in patients with diabetes mellitus). Some patients may have had increasing frequency and severity of chest pain over days or weeks (crescendo angina). Symptoms are not helpful in differentiating STE- and NSTE-ACS.

There may be a history or family history of coronary artery disease or conditions known to be associated with increased incidence such as diabetes mellitus, hyperlipidemia, peripheral or cerebrovascular disease, hypertension, and smoking.

Physical Examination

Full physical examination should be carried out but is often normal. There may be evidence of previous cardiovascular interventions, or signs of heart failure. Specific complications of myocardial infarction with physical signs include pericarditis, mitral regurgitation, and ventricular septal rupture. Physical signs of other potential diagnoses, for example, pneumothorax, should be sought.

Investigations

ECG – 12-lead ECG should be carried out as soon as possible after presentation and repeated after 6 and 24 h and compared, if possible, to previous recordings. Presence of new ST elevation as defined in STEMI (above) leads to a diagnosis of STE-ACS and immediate revascularization therapy. ST depression of at least 0.5 mm in two adjacent leads is seen in patients with NSTE-ACS, with a poorer prognosis associated with deeper ST segment depression. T wave inversion may also occur, but in a small proportion of patients with NSTE-ACS the ECG is normal. Use of right and extended left chest electrode positions may be helpful in identifying right and posterior ischemia. Stress ECG testing is indicated for risk assessment in asymptomatic patients, without diagnostic resting ECG changes or elevated troponin concentrations, prior to hospital discharge.

Biochemical markers of myocardial cell necrosis – Elevated serum troponin T or I concentrations are the most sensitive and specific markers of myocardial cell death and useful as prognostic markers and therefore used to determine management of patients with NSTE-ACS. However, troponin concentrations may not start to rise above reference concentration for at least 3 h after the ACS has started, and in NSTE-ACS this time may be considerably longer. Further troponin measurements should be carried out 6–12 h after episodes of chest pain. Elevated troponin concentrations are found in conditions unrelated to ACS including sepsis, renal failure, cardiac failure, and acute aortic dissection, and therefore troponin concentrations need to be interpreted in the clinical context and in conjunction with other investigations.

Chest X-ray – There may be evidence of an enlarged heart or pulmonary edema. May be required to exclude differential diagnoses.

Echocardiography – Transthoracic echocardiography (TTE) should ideally be carried out in assessment of ACS and may be useful in assessing ischemia-induced regional myocardial motion abnormalities, assessing potential complications of myocardial infarction such as ischemic mitral regurgitation and excluding differential diagnoses. Rapid, focused TTE assessment of severely ill patients by non-cardiologists is being promoted by courses such as FEER-Germany and FEEL-UK in order to increase patient access to emergency echocardiography and allow faster recognition of life-threatening complications.

Coronary angiography – The current gold standard for imaging of coronary arteries and carries rare but serious risks of CVA, arrhythmia, pericardial hemorrhage, arterial dissection and/or obstruction, renal failure, and anaphylaxis. This technique also facilitates reperfusion therapy using angioplasty with or without coronary artery stenting.

Differential Diagnosis of Chest Pain/ACS

Aortic dissection – May present with chest pain and can cause ACS if dissection involves coronary arteries. Other vascular diagnoses that can mimic ACS include aortic aneurysm and aortic coarctation.

Esophageal spasm
Gastric ulceration or perforation, cholecystitis, pancreatitis
Chest wall pain
Pleural pain, pneumonia, pulmonary embolism, and infarction
Pericardial disease
Other types of heart disease, e.g., myocarditis, valvular (e.g., aortic stenosis)

Treatment

The treatment of ACS is an area in which evidence relating to new physical and drug treatments becomes available frequently and there are often changes to best practice. Readers should consult the latest guidelines from the ESC and ACC/AHA (American College of Cardiology/American Heart Association) [2, 3, 4, 5].

General

Presentation

All patients presenting with suspected ACS should be assessed rapidly using a standard ABCDE approach.

Patients with an oxygen saturation <90% should receive supplemental oxygen and an intravenous cannula placed, with blood simultaneously sampled for measurement of troponin, creatinine, glucose, and full blood count. Pain not responding to sublingual nitrate should be managed with intravenous nitrate infusion and morphine with an antiemetic. Basic observations should be recorded, continuous ECG monitoring attached, and 12-lead ECG recorded. Cardiac arrest should be managed with standards ALS protocols. Management will be determined by classification into NSTE-ACS, STE-ACS, or low likelihood of ACS.

NSTE-ACS

Management is based on risk assessment of the likelihood of further coronary events and death with high-risk patients being managed with earlier coronary angiography and revascularization and lower risk patients managed with medical treatment alone.

Risk Stratification

Factors associated with an increased risk of death in patients with ACS include previous coronary artery disease, main stem or three vessel disease, persistent chest pain, diabetes mellitus, increasing age, heart rate, creatinine, Kilip class [6] (Table 1), concentration of biomarkers of myocardial necrosis, ST segment changes, decreasing systolic blood pressure, and occurrence of cardiac arrest. A number of risk scoring systems have been developed to calculate both risks of in-hospital death and mortality over longer time periods. Examples of risk scoring systems include GRACE [7] (Global Registry of Acute Coronary Events) TIMI, FRISC, and PURSUIT.

Medical Therapy

Antiplatelet drugs
- Aspirin
  All patients, without contraindications, should receive standard uncoated oral aspirin 160–325 mg (chewed) on presentation with an ACS and continued at 75–100 mg daily.
- Clopidogrel

Coronary Syndromes, Acute. Table 1 Kilip classification

1. No evidence of heart failure
2. Elevated JVP/crackles on lung auscultation
3. Acute pulmonary edema
4. Cardiogenic shock

All patients, without contraindications, should receive oral clopidogrel 300 mg, followed by 75 mg daily, and continued for 12 months. A dose of 600 mg should be considered in patients about to undergo PCI. Patients receiving clopidogrel and requiring urgent CABG should stop it 5 days prior to surgery if this is clinically possible.

- Glycoprotein IIb/IIIa inhibitors

  Tirofiban or eptifibatide treatment, in addition to aspirin and clopidogrel, is indicated for patients who are at high risk of continued coronary events, and should be used in combination with an anticoagulant. For patients that have not received either and undergo PCI, abciximab should be used.

- Careful assessment of the relative risks of hemorrhagic complications versus further coronary thrombosis should be made prior to administering these drugs.

Anticoagulants

All patients presenting with NSTE-ACS should receive anticoagulants in addition to antiplatelet drugs. Choice of agent will depend on the clinical scenario, risk assessment of further coronary events, and potential hemorrhagic complications.

- Heparin

  Low molecular weight heparins (LMWH) have advantages over unfractionated heparin (UH) in being easier to administer, require less monitoring, and are associated with a lower incidence of heparin induced thrombocytopenia (HIT).

- Fondaparinux (Factor Xa inhibitor)

  Alternative to heparin for patients not undergoing urgent angiography and PCI and associated with a lower incidence of hemorrhagic complications.

- Bivalarudin and other direct thrombin inhibitors

  Alternative to heparin with fewer hemorrhagic complications.

Antianginal Agents

- Nitrates – If sublingual GTN is ineffective in relieving ischemic chest pain, intravenous infusion should be used, but may cause hypotension and is contraindicated in patients taking PDE-5 inhibitors (e.g., sildenafil).

- Beta-blockers – If there are no contraindications, beta-blocking drugs should be administered with a target heart rate of 50–60 bpm. Care should be taken in patients with evidence of AV conduction block or significant left ventricular dysfunction.

- Calcium channel blockers – Indicated for the treatment of angina secondary to coronary vasospasm, particularly dihydropiridines (e.g., nifedipine). In other situations, calcium channel antagonists may be used as alternatives in patients who are unable to take or in addition to beta-blockers. Dihydropyridines should not be used without combination with a beta-blocker in patients with non-vasospastic angina.

Revascularization

High-risk patients should have urgent coronary angiography followed by revascularization particularly when there is continuing or unresolving chest pain with dynamic ST segment changes, hemodynamic instability, heart failure, or life-threatening arrhythmias.

Patients in a medium- to high-risk group, without life-threatening complications, should have coronary angiography performed within 72 h and revascularization (PCI or CABG) if indicated.

Low-risk patients should undergo a noninvasive test of inducible ischemia while in hospital and undergo coronary angiography if positive.

STE-ACS

Following initial assessment and management (as above), patients with STE-ACS presenting within 12 h of symptom require urgent coronary reperfusion therapy using either PCI or thrombolytic drugs. Risk assessment can be carried out using one of the established systems (e.g., TIMI risk score for STEMI).

Aspirin should be given to all patients without contraindications (as for NSTE-ACS). Patients undergoing PCI should have clopridogrel loading dose (300 or 600 mg). During PCI, heparin (UH) is given to reduce thrombotic complications; bivaluridin may be used as an alternative. The GP IIb/IIIa inhibitor abciximab has been shown to improve outcome post PCI and may be commenced during the procedure and infused intravenously for 12 h afterward. ACEI should be started in the first 24 h in high-risk patients and continued. Beta-blockers are useful in decreasing further ischemia but should be avoided in patients with unstable hemodynamics, AV conduction block, or asthma.

Reperfusion Therapy

- PCI – Is indicated urgently for patients with STE-ACS within 12 h of onset of symptoms. Patients presenting after 12 h from the onset of symptoms with continuing evidence of ischemia should also be managed with urgent angiography and PCI.

Longer time to coronary reperfusion is associated with increased mortality. ESC guidelines recommend that the time from first medical contact to intracoronary balloon inflation should be less than 2 h in all patients and less than 90 min in those with a large area of myocardial infarction and low risk of hemorrhage. Primary PCI should be used, where available in preference to pharmacological thrombolysis in all patients but particularly in patients with cardiogenic shock or heart failure and in patients with contraindications to fibrinolytic drugs.

- Fibrinolytic therapy – Is indicated in circumstances when PCI cannot be performed within recommended times or is contraindicated. Pre-hospital administration is associated with improved outcomes compared to in-hospital. Fibrinolysis is associated with 1% risk of intracranial hemorrhage which is more common in women, hypertensives, increasing age, and patients with known cerebrovascular disease. In addition, there is approximately 10% risk of other serious hemorrhage. Because of these risks, fibrinolytic therapy is contraindicated in patients with a previous history of hemorrhagic stroke (or unknown etiology) and within 6 months of an ischemic stroke. Other absolute contraindications are: known bleeding disorder, central nervous system tumors or trauma, head injury, major trauma or surgery within the last 3 weeks, gastrointestinal hemorrhage within the previous month, aortic dissection, and puncture sites that are not compressible. Relative contraindications to thrombolytic therapy are: oral anticoagulants, TIA in the last 6 months, severe hypertension, pregnancy including up to 1 week postpartum, active peptic ulceration, advanced liver disease, infective endocarditis, and failure to respond to cardiopulmonary resuscitation.

Streptokinase should not be readministered because antibody generation reduces its activity and can increase the risk of allergic reactions.

In the event of evidence of failure of pharmacological thrombolysis (approximately 20% patients) or re-infarction (approximately 10% patients), urgent coronary angiography and PCI are indicated. If this is not possible, a second dose of antifibrinolytic agent may be given (not streptokinase if already administered).

Patients presenting after 12 h from initial symptoms should be treated with aspirin, clopidogrel, and an antithrombin drug.

Complications of ACS

Arrhythmia
These are common following STE-ACS and are managed using standard algorithms.

Cardiogenic Shock
Patients have a low cardiac output state usually associated with hypotension and elevated left atrial pressure. Early revascularization is indicated with appropriate supportive therapy which may include mechanical circulatory support with an intra-aortic balloon pump or ventricular assist device.

Mitral Regurgitation
May occur because of annular dilatation or papillary muscle dysfunction or rupture. Clinical features are of mitral regurgitation which may be severe and require support with an intra-aortic balloon pump and afterload reduction. Treatment is early surgical valve repair or replacement.

Ventricular Rupture
- Ventricular septal rupture – Diagnosis suspected because of deteriorating clinical condition with new systolic murmur, increase in oxygen saturation of a catheter moved from the right atrium to ventricle, and appearances on echocardiography. Management is stabilization followed by surgical repair, though small lesions have been closed with percutaneous devices.
- Free wall rupture – Diagnosis suspected because of rapidly deteriorating condition with clinical features of tamponade, confirmed on echocardiography. Treatment is surgical.

RV and Posterior Infarction
Acute right ventricular failure may present with the findings of low cardiac output, ST elevation in inferior and right sided chest leads associated with elevated JVP but no evidence of pulmonary edema. Right ventricular failure is difficult to manage, and it is important to ensure adequate left ventricular preload and maintain coronary perfusion pressure. Early coronary reperfusion should be undertaken.

After-care
All patients with coronary artery disease should be advised about secondary prevention of further disease including

smoking cessation, weight loss, healthy diet, and exercise. Blood pressure should be controlled and diabetes excluded. All patients without contraindications should have lipid lowering therapy with a statin.

Patients with reduced left ventricular function should receive long-term beta-blocking drugs and angiotensin-converting enzyme inhibitors (ACEI) or angiotensin receptor antagonists. ACEI should be considered for all patients with CAD as a preventative therapy but particularly in diabetics, hypertensives, and patients with chronic renal disease. Aldosterone antagonists should be considered for patients, without contraindications, with reduced left ventricular function and evidence of heart failure or diabetes.

Ideally all patients with NSTE-ACS should have a noninvasive assessment of ischemia inducibility 1–2 months post hospital discharge to inform further management and rate of resumption of physical activities.

Patients with poor ventricular function may benefit from resynchronization pacing or an implantable defibrillator.

Prognosis

ACS has a mortality rate of approximately 50% within the first month after initial clinical presentation with half of these deaths occurring within the initial 2 h. Mortality of patients reaching hospital alive after initial presentation has improved markedly (to less than 20%) over recent years following the introduction of rapid reperfusion therapy. Approximately 10% patients with STE-ACS have a further infarction within 1 year.

References

1. Thygesen K, Alpert JS, White HD (2007) Universal definition of myocardial infarction. Joint ESC/ACCF/AHA/WHF task force for the redefinition of myocardial infarction. Circulation 116:2634–2653
2. Anderson JL, Adams CD, Antman EM et al (2007) ACC/AHA 2007 guidelines for the management of patients with unstable angina/non-ST-elevation myocardial infarction. J Am Coll Cardiol 50:654–729
3. Bassand JP, Hamm CW, Ardissino D et al (2007) Guidelines for the diagnosis and treatment of non-ST-segment elevation acute coronary syndromes. Task force for diagnosis and treatment of non-ST-segment elevation acute coronary syndromes of European Society of Cardiology. Eur Heart J 2813:1598–1660
4. Kushner FG, Hand M, Smith SC et al (2009) 2009 focused updates: ACC/AHA guidelines for the management of patients with ST-elevation myocardial infarction (updating the 2004 guideline and 2007 focused update) and ACC/AHA/SCAI guidelines on percutaneous coronary intervention (updating the 2005 guideline and 2007 focused update). Circulation 120:2271–2306
5. Van de Werf F, Bax J, Betriu A et al (2008) Management of acute myocardial infarction in patients presenting with persistent ST-segment elevation: the task force on the management of ST-segment elevation acute myocardial infarction of the European Society of Cardiology. Eur Heart J 23:2909–2945
6. Killip T, Kimball JT (1967) Treatment of myocardial infarction in a coronary care unit. A two year experience with 250 patients. Am J Cardiol 20:457–464
7. Global Registry of Acute Coronary Events. http://www.outcomes-umassmed.org/grace/

Coronavirus

These viruses belong to the family Coronaviridae and are enveloped viruses with a positive-sense single-stranded RNA genome and a helical symmetry. Under electron microscopy, the virus has a characteristic crowned appearance (hence the name "corona"), caused by a ring of large, distinctive spikes in the envelope. Coronaviruses cause a wide range of disease in animals and humans and cause a significant percentage of cases of the common cold.

Correction of Burn Shock

▶ Burn Fluid Resuscitation

Corticosteroid Insufficiency

▶ Adrenal Conditions, Insufficiency/Failure

Counteracting Anticoagulation

▶ Reversing Anticoagulant Treatment in ICU Patients

Coxiella burnetii

THOMAS J. MARRIE
Department of Medicine, University of Alberta, Edmonton, AB, Canada

Synonyms

Coxiellosis; Q fever

Definition

Coxiella burnetii is the etiological agent of the infectious disease in humans known as Q fever. In animals it is termed *coxiellosis*. It is a cocco-bacillus with a gram-negative cell wall measuring 0.2 by 0.7 μm. It is an obligate intracellular pathogen that does not stain with Gram's stain but does with Giminez stain. Within the host cell, it develops in the phagolyzosome, where the acid pH activates its enzymes. It has both large and small cell variants and forms spores. Spore formation is why *C. burnetii* is so successful as a pathogen. It can survive for more than 1 month on meat in cold storage, and for more than 40 months in skim milk at room temperature.

It can also survive in free-living amoebae. Although it is destroyed by 2% formaldehyde, the organism has been isolated from infected tissues stored in formaldehyde for up to 4–5 months. It has also been isolated from fixed "paraffinized" tissues. Either 1% Lysol or 5% hydrogen peroxide kills *C. burnetii*.

Coxiella burnetii undergoes phase variation akin to the smooth-to-rough transition of lipopolysaccharides of Gram-negative bacteria. In nature and in laboratory animals, it is in the phase I state. Phase I organisms react with late convalescent-phase (45 days) guinea pig sera and only slightly with early-convalescent-phase (21 days) sera. After many passages in cell culture or embryonated eggs, truncation of the lipopolysaccharide occurs resulting in phase II cell [1].

Coxiella burnetii is a Centers for Disease Control and Prevention (CDC) category B bioterrorism agent. Agents in this category have the potential for large-scale dissemination but generally cause less illness and death than category A agents. As a biological warfare agent, *C. burnetii* can be easily dispersed as an aerosol with a high infectivity rate, and pneumonia is the major manifestation of infection in this setting. It has been calculated that a concentration of 100 cells/m^3 and an exposure time of 30–60 min can deposit more than one cell in the lung.

Infections with *C. burnetii* can be divided into two groups – acute and chronic. Acute Q fever can manifest as inapparent infection, self-limited febrile illness, pneumonia, hepatitis, or a variety of organ-specific manifestations such as meningitis, encephalitis, pericarditis, pancreatitis, priapism [1]. Chronic Q fever almost always means endocarditis or infection of abdominal aortic aneurysms but occasionally osteomyelitis occurs [1]. Q fever in pregnancy should also be considered as a form of chronic Q fever.

Treatment

Coxiella burnetii is resistant to beta-lactams and aminoglycosides and susceptible to rifampin, co-trimoxazole,

tetracyclines, and quinolones. Many, but not all, isolates are susceptible to macrolides. Quinolone resistance has been reported but seems to be uncommon at present. Acute Q fever is generally adequately treated with 7–10 days of a tetracycline or a quinolone. Most of our knowledge about the treatment of Q fever comes from observational studies. Investigators from Basque Country, Spain, carried out a prospective, randomized double-blind study of doxycycline and erythromycin in the treatment of pneumonia presumed to be due to Q fever [2]. Subsequently, 48 patients were proven by serologic studies to have Q fever, 23 of whom received 100 mg doxycycline twice daily, and 25 received erythromycin (500 mg every 6 h) for 10 days. Fever resolution was faster in the doxycycline-treated group (3 ± 1.6 days vs. 4.3 ± 2 days for erythromycin-treated patients; p = 0.05). By day 40, the chest radiograph was normal in 47 of the 48 patients.

Patients with acute Q fever and coexisting valvular heart disease should be treated for 1 year with doxycycline and hydroxychloroquine as described for the treatment of chronic Q fever. Alternatively, these patients can be followed with Q fever titers every 3 months and treated if the serological profile becomes that of chronic Q fever.

Q fever during pregnancy should be treated with co-trimoxazole for the duration of the pregnancy. In one retrospective study, this approach reduced obstetrical complications from 81% to 44%. There were no intrauterine fetal deaths in the co-trimoxazole-treated group [3]. Patients with a "chronic Q fever serological profile" should be treated with doxycycline and hydroxychloroquine for 1 year following delivery.

Treatment of chronic Q fever is complex. Q fever endocarditis is treated for at least 18 months of therapy with doxycycline 100 mg b.i.d, and hydroxychroroquine 200 mg t.i.d. Plasma levels of doxycycline should be maintained at or above 4.8 μg/mL. Hydroxychloroquine levels should be about 1 μg/mL. The response to treatment is assessed by measuring antibody levels to phase I and phase II antigens. Therapy can be discontinued when the anti-phase I IgG titer by immunofluorescence assay is less than 1:400 and the anti-phase I IgA titer is undetectable.

Pharmacologic Management

The ability to measure serum levels of doxycycline and hydroxychloroquine is very helpful in the management of patients with chronic Q fever, especially for those who are failing therapy or in whom there is a reason to suspect impaired observation of doxycycline. An example of the latter is a patient who is receiving concomitant treatment with blockers of gastric acid secretion and doxycycline.

Vaccination offers the promise of controlling Q fever by immunizing livestock in endemic areas. Those in high risk occupations such as abbatoir workers and veterinarians should also be immunized. A heat inactivate vaccine made from heat inactivated phase I cells is available in Australia. A Q fever vaccine can be obtained from the Centers for Disease Control and Prevention.

Epidemiology

Q fever is an zoonosis and as such the epidemiology is that of its animal reservoirs and those who are in contact with them. Cattle, sheep, and goats are most commonly infected, although cats play an important role in the epidemiology of Q fever in some localized geographic areas such as Nova Scotia, Canada. *Coxiella burnetii* localizes to the endometrium and to the mammary glands in female animals. The organism reaches very high concentrations in the placenta, and at the time of parturition it is shed into the environment and aerosolized. Susceptible hosts who inhale the organisms develop Q fever. Q fever is present throughout the world with the exception of New Zealand and Antarctica.

Q fever is not common in the USA with an average of 51 cases per year from 2000 to 2004.

When a case of Q fever is identified, the source of an outbreak of Q fever may not be apparent, as the organism can be spread up to 11 km from an area with contaminated soil during windstorms [4]. Finding the source of the infection can often be challenging; as in outbreaks due to straw that was used to insulate buildings and when the straw was disturbed during renovations, Q fever occurred. Washing contaminated clothing can also result in Q fever.

Risk Factors

Association with infected animals is an obvious risk factor. For those who work on farms, smoking cigarettes is also a risk factor, presumably because of hand to mouth transmission. It is noteworthy that oral transmission of Q fever has been difficult to prove in an experimental setting. There is a dose response curve in that those who clean up infected products of conception have the shortest incubation period and the most severe disease.

Evaluation and Assessment

A history of exposure to parturient animals within 2 weeks of development of fever and/or pneumonia is suggestive of Q fever. There are no characteristic clinical features of Q fever. Single or multiple rounded opacities on chest radiography in the absence of right-sided endocarditis is very indicative of Q fever. The diagnosis is confirmed by demonstrating a fourfold rise in antibody titers to phase II *C. burnetii* antigen between acute and convalescent serum samples. The convalescent sample should be drawn 2 or more weeks after the acute phase sample.

The diagnosis of chronic Q fever is confirmed by a very high phase I IgG antibody titer – usually >1:800. In chronic Q fever, the phase I titer is higher than the phase II titer, while the reverse is true in acute Q fever.

Patients in whom chronic Q fever is suspected should have a transesophageal echocardiogram to detect vegetations on cardiac valves.

After Care

Some patients with acute Q fever develop chronic fatigue post infection. Patients with acute Q fever who have valvular heart disease should have careful follow-up with serial antibody measurements to detect development of chronic Q fever. Alternatively, the patients can have pre-emptive therapy with 1 year of treatment with doxycycline and hydroxychloroquine. Patients with chronic Q fever require assessment every 3–6 months until cured and frequency of follow-up thereafter dictated by severity of valvular heart disease.

Prognosis

The prognosis for acute Q fever is excellent. Mortality is low at <1% in most series. Chronic Q fever has considerable mortality and morbidity. The problem is usually a delay in diagnosis. Many patients with chronic Q fever will require cardiac valve replacement; however, the decision to do this should be based on hemodynamic factors.

Economics

In Australia, it is estimated that Q fever costs $1 million per year and loss of 1,700 weeks of work [5].

References

1. Raoult D, Marrie TJ, Mege JL (2005) Natural history and pathophysiology of Q fever. Lancet 5:219–226
2. Sobradillo V, Zalacain R, Capebastegui A et al (1992) Antibiotic treatment in pneumonia due to Q fever. Thorax 47:276–278
3. Carcopino X, Raoult D, Bretelle F et al (2007) Managing Q fever during pregnancy: the benefits of long-term cotrimoxazole therapy. Clin Infect Dis 45:548–555
4. Tissot-Dupont H, Amadei MA, Nezri M et al (2004) Wind in november, Q fever in december. Emerg Infect Dis 10:1264–1269
5. Garner MG, Longbottom HM, Cannon RM (1997) A review of Q fever in Australia 1991–1994. Aust N Z J Public Health 21:722–773

Coxiellosis

▶ Coxiella burnetii

CPP

▶ Cerebral Perfusion Pressure

Craniectomy

▶ Emergency Burr Holes

Craniectomy for Intracranial Pressure (ICP) Control

▶ Decompressive Craniectomy

Craniocervical Dislocation

▶ Occipitocervical Dissociation

Craniocervical Dissociation

▶ Occipitocervical Dissociation

Craniocervical Vertical Displacement

▶ Occipitocervical Dissociation

Craniocervical Vertical Distraction Injury

▶ Occipitocervical Dissociation

Craniospinal Dislocation

▶ Occipitocervical Dissociation

Craniospinal Dissociation

▶ Occipitocervical Dissociation

Craniotomy

LUCIDO L. PONCE, CLAUDIA S. ROBERTSON
Department of Neurosurgery, Baylor College of Medicine, Houston, TX, USA

Synonyms
Although not strictly acceptable as a synonym, "crani" is commonly used among healthcare professionals to refer to craniotomy. The term "brain surgery" is widely utilized by the general population and by patients who have undergone a craniotomy.

Definition
Craniotomy is a surgical procedure where a portion of the skull, known as the *bone flap*, is separated from the rest of the cranium in order to access its enclosed structures (i.e., brain, dura, vessels, nerves, etc.). Some authors have proposed that burr holes or key holes are also a form of small craniotomies. Once the surgery goal has been achieved, the bone flap is replaced. When the bone flap is not replaced, *craniectomy* is a more precise name for the procedure. When the intention of the craniectomy is to relieve intracranial pressure caused by brain swelling, then it is called *decompressive craniectomy* (hemicraniectomy or bifrontal). Craniotomies are also named by the bone or region being removed (i.e., parietal, temporal, fronto-parietal, etc.) [1]. "Awake craniotomy" is used when the procedure is performed under local anesthesia with the subject fully conscious to increase the chances of preserving eloquent areas of the brain or when general anesthesia is not an option. "Complex craniotomy" usually refers to skull base surgery where the aim is to expose or reach the most caudal portions of the brain and generally a higher grade of neurosurgeon expertise is required.

Although craniotomy is considered a highly invasive procedure and less invasive endoscopic and intravascular techniques have gained popularity and effectiveness for some neurosurgical problems, a role of craniotomy in neurosurgery will remain for a number of indications, including neurotrauma.

Pre-existing Condition

Virtually any intracranial condition may be surgically approached through the bone defect left by the craniotomy. As with any other surgical operations, careful assessment of the "benefit" versus "risk and/or futility" is always needed from the neurological surgeon.

Craniotomy might be used for diagnosis, therapy, or both. Burr holes (1–3 cm) are used for minimally invasive procedures to introduce an endoscope to remove small tumors or clip aneurysms, to drain a hematoma (stereotactic aspiration), to perform a biopsy, placement of intracranial monitoring devices (i.e., intracranial pressure, brain tissue oxygen pressure, or microdialysis catheter), insertion of an external ventricular drainage (EVD, also called "ventriculostomy"), introduction of a deep brain stimulator (for treatment of Parkinson disease), and placement of penetrating depth electrodes (for epilepsy diagnosis and treatment). Large craniotomies are preferred for larger lesions such as tumors, aneurysms or arteriovenous malformations, evacuation of large hematomas (subdural hematoma or epidural hematoma), large coalescent contused brain areas causing mass effect, or abscesses, and brain debridement after a gunshot wound. Indications for surgery for specific pathologies are discussed elsewhere.

The medical conditions that require craniotomy vary depending on the neurosurgical pathology and the underlying health of the patient. Individual patient characteristics can range from an otherwise healthy patient with a relatively benign intracranial pathology to a critically ill patient with several serious comorbid conditions who is being treated for an independent serious intracranial disease. For elective neurosurgical cases, preoperative care can be appropriately met. However, because some neurosurgical conditions require emergency surgical intervention, there will also be cases where little information regarding patient's general health status is available immediately before a life-saving craniotomy is performed.

Whenever possible, preoperative medical status should be carefully assessed and for those cases where the urgency of surgery overrides extensive preoperative evaluation, subsequent medical assessment must be undertaken at a later time period. The use of preoperative checklists may decrease surgical morbidity and mortality. Preoperative laboratory tests should be ordered based on individualized history and physical examination rather than a standardized battery screening tests. The need for premedication should be evaluated, especially for antibiotic and anticonvulsant prophylaxis, which will vary depending on the neurosurgical procedure. At the beginning of the procedure, the appropriate choice of anesthetic agents has to be determined. This determination will involve factors such as whether preservation of consciousness is desired, if special intraoperative monitoring such as evoked potential monitoring is to be performed, or if a rapid wake up from anesthesia is desired. If the case allows obtaining informed consent, it is important to depict all possible postoperative scenarios that both, patient and family might face as well as the potential intensive care unit course. The neurological surgeon's most essential ally in accomplishing a successful postoperative outcome is a well-informed patient [2].

Application

Complete information regarding the side and site of the pathological lesion, positioning of the patient, as well as the necessary equipment should be appropriately discussed in advance before the arrival of the patient to the operating room. Special requests of unusual equipment, such as fluoroscopy, must also be listed beforehand. Agreement should be obtained with nursing and anesthesiology teams regarding the perioperative administration of osmotic agents, steroids and lumbar or ventricular drainage, prophylaxis for phlebitis, and thromboembolic events such as pneumatic stocking, urinary catheter placement, venous air emboli monitoring, etc. Operating rooms dedicated exclusively to neurosurgical procedures are helpful as are anesthesiology and nursing teams experienced with neurosurgery cases who are thoroughly knowledgeable about the equipment and procedures.

The majority of craniotomies are executed with the patient in the supine, three-quarter prone (lateral-oblique), or fully prone position. The supine position is preferred for procedures in the frontal, temporal, and anterior parietal areas and some cranial base approaches with or without turning the patient's head and shoulder elevation. For exposure of occipital and suboccipital areas the prone position is preferred. Prone or semi-sitting position is advised for surgical approaches involving posterior fossa and cervical region. Extremes of turning the head and neck should be avoided since this condition could potentially impair venous drainage from the head increasing intracranial pressure. Tilting the operating table to elevate the head is recommended as well. Use of head fixation devices allows precise maintenance of the tightly fixed skull. Pinion headholders give some advantages over the padded headrests, including allowing repositioning during surgery, not obscuring the face, which facilitates intraoperative monitoring (i.e., evoked potentials), and are commonly the site for brain retractor systems attachment. Better quality imaging for intraoperative fluoroscopy may be obtained if the pinion headholder is made of radiolucent materials.

During the surgical procedure, the anesthesiologist is usually positioned close to patient's head and chest. Whenever possible, having the anesthesiologist facing toward the patient's face is ideal, giving him easy access to endotracheal tube and intravascular lines. The scrub nurse is preferably positioned on the other side of the patient, in front of the anesthesiologist. Shaving the entire head, limited hair removal (1–2 cm beyond the margin of the incision), and not shaving at all are accepted, although removing hair from the site of the surgery may allow outlining several helpful anatomical landmarks such as sutures, approximation of fissures, pterion, or temporal line before sterile draping. Of esthetic importance is avoiding surgical incisions going beyond the hairline.

A typical supratentorial craniotomy and its general considerations are described as follows:

1. The patient is placed in the supine position (a roll is placed under the back and shoulder to facilitate maintaining of the position) and the head turned to the appropriate side and positioned either on a doughnut or using the head fixation device.
2. A scalp flap is appropriately outlined. This flap will be proportional in length with the size of the craniotomy, which in turn is planned in relation to the intracranial lesion being approached. Scalp flaps should have a broad base in order to preserve adequate blood supply. As a general rule, the pedicle should not be narrower than the width of the flap. Otherwise, the flap edges may become ischemic endangering not just a prompt healing, but also predisposing to scalp, bone flap, and intracranial infections. When there is some uncertainty as the precise type and extent of the intracranial pathology, such as with head trauma, larger bone flaps are preferred since a good exposure is priceless. The skin is incised with a sharp blade.

Two of the largest scalp flaps are the reverse question mark incision for ample exposure of the hemicranium and the bicoronal incision for bifrontal exposure. Both incisions start anterior to the ear at the zygoma level, and attempt to avoid the facial nerve branch that passes through the zygoma ~1.5 cm anterior to the tragus. If it is not possible to avoid this area, the layers of the scalp in which the nerve courses must be protected. The superficial temporal and occipital arteries should be also preserved whenever possible. This is mandatory if an extracranial–intracranial arterial anastomosis might be needed.

During elevation of the scalp, control of bleeding is achieved with pressure of the surgeon's and assistant's fingers against the skin on each side of the incision, followed by the hemostatic clipping or clamping placement along the flap edges, or with dilute epinephrine injected preoperatively along the planned line of incision. Deeper muscle and fasciae layers can be incised with a cutting electrocautery at its upper insertion, but its use should be avoided during elevation of the muscle from the bone. Instead, an accurate dissection with a sharp periosteal elevator should be performed to preserve the bulk and viability of the temporalis muscle. Both the vascular and nerve supplies of the temporalis muscle course tightly along the fascial attachments of the muscle to the bone, and are easily damaged with electrocautery use. If the situation requires rapid opening of the cranium, the quickest method involves dividing and reflecting the scalp flap and muscle as a single unit downward. When the scalp flap base is opposed to or not coincident with the temporalis muscle insertion, then the scalp flap can be elevated as needed and the temporalis muscle reflected downward, preserving its neurovascular unit.

3. An appropriate number of burr holes are made with a manual or a high-speed air or electric drill along the planned margins of the bone flap stripping the underlying dura away. Then a saw provided with a foot plate that protects the dura is placed through one of the burr holes and used to cut the bone as it is directed toward an adjacent burr hole. All of the burr holes are connected in this manner creating the bone flap. Extremely long cuts should be avoided, especially if they extend across an internal bony prominence, such as the pterion, or across a mayor venous sinus. Reducing the risk of injuring the brain or scratching the dura is achieved by drilling several burr holes and making short cuts. If cutting across a venous sinus is required then a burr hole is created on each side of the venous sinus and then the two burr holes are connected with the saw while protecting the dura, which has been carefully stripped from the bone. The Gigli or wire saw along with the dura protector is currently less used. After elevating the bone flap bleeding from bone edges is stopped by applying bone wax. The bone flap may be stored until closure in a sponge moistened with saline or antibiotic solution.

Bipolar coagulation is preferred for scalp, dura, and intracranial sites to control bleeding. At the sites where bipolar coagulation could damage neural structures, the use of hemostatic gelatinous or alternative materials is attempted. If metallic clips are necessary for bleeding control, nonmagnetic alloy or titanium clips are preferred because they will not hamper postoperative computed tomographic scan imaging.

C

4. Tack-up sutures are placed by making small holes near the bone edge with the drill bit, then stitching the dura and holding it against the bony margins with a 3–0 silk suture brought through the dura and then through the small drill holes. Such tack-up sutures are a common practice after elevation of the bone flap; however, when the circumstances are compelling, this step can be skipped. If the brain is initially pressed tightly against the dura, tack-up sutures can be placed after the relief of the pressure when the sutures can be placed with direct visualization of the deep surface of the dura

5. Opening the dura is usually performed initially with a #15 scalpel blade while carefully lifting the dura off the underlying cortex. Then the rest of the dural opening is completed with shielded Metzenbaum or tenotomy scissors, elevating the dura away from the cortex with Penfield or Cushing forceps and cauterizing and dividing any small bridging veins. The dural opening can be along the bony margins (horseshoe-shaped) or in a cruciate (X or Y) fashion. Reflection of the dural flap via small hemostats suspended from sutures placed through the corners of the flap can then be performed.

6. Once the intracranial part of the surgery is completed, the dura is closed with 3-0 silk running or interrupted sutures. When shrinkage of the dura occurs, then soft tissue (fat or muscle) can be sutured over small openings. However, when approaching both dural ends

leaves larger dural defects or considerable tension of the dura, a duroplasty with cadaveric dura, temporalis fascia, or pericranium can be performed.

The bone flap will be held in place tightly with heavy sutures such as nonmagnetic plates with screws, small metal discs or burr hole covers, or fine wire. The remaining defects of the bone surface are usually covered up with bone wax, methylmethacrylate, or other bone substitute. Irrigation with antibiotic solution has proved to help in decreasing extracranial infection, but not intracranial ones.

Deep muscles and fascia are typically closed with 1–0, the temporalis muscle and fascia with 2–0, and the galea with 3–0 absorbable sutures. The scalp is closed either with metallic staples or 3–0 nylon reinforcing sutures. Staples are associated with less tissue reaction than other forms of closure [3].

Postoperative care must be performed in a specialized neurosurgical intensive care unit and will consist of neuromonitoring, neurological examinations, antibiotics, anticonvulsive therapy, thromboembolic prophylaxis, pain control, laxatives, and/or drug level monitoring. Nursing and medical staff should tend to adequate surgical wound care, teaching family and patient about what care should be provided. At least daily inspection of the surgical wound is advised. Wound dressings are usually kept for 24 h, and skin sutures are removed in 7–14 days.

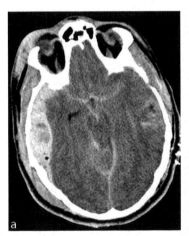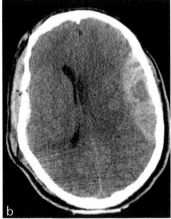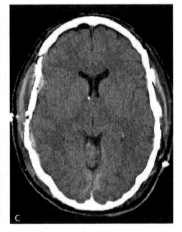

Craniotomy. Figure 1 (a) Axial CT scan with an epidural hematoma visible on the right and a right-to-left midline shift upon hospital admission after severe traumatic brain injury. (b) After undergoing craniotomy for right EDH evacuation CT scan shows an epidural on the left remote from the side of the craniotomy and a left-to-right midline shift. (c) Axial CT scan after second craniotomy for left EDH evacuation shows no midline shift

The most common serious acute complications of a craniotomy are bleeding and infections (intracranial and extracranial). Most series report the incidence of intracranial infections following craniotomy to be <2%. However, 80% of all nosocomial meningitis cases have a history of craniotomy, shunt, or ventriculostomy. Other complications include wound dehiscence, cerebrospinal leak, increased intracranial pressure due to swelling, nerve or vascular damage, hyponatremia due to syndrome of inappropriate antidiuretic hormone secretion, hypernatremia due to diabetes insipidus, and seizures. A postoperative intracranial hematoma is an uncommon but life-threatening complication [4] (see Fig. 1).

Long-term complications of a craniotomy include subdural hygroma formation (30–50%), the majority of which are asymptomatic or can be managed conservatively, bone flap resorption, and late infections. Other rare late complications include late cerebrospinal fluid leak, seizures, hydrocephalus, and pituitary insufficiency. Risk factors associated with development of postoperative infections are male sex, preoperative diagnosis, no antibiotic prophylaxis, long course of cerebrospinal fluid leak, early reoperation, and duration of the surgery [5].

On discharge from the hospital, the patient and family should be instructed to reduce the activity level including driving, weight lifting (<5 lb), avoid walking long distances, constipation, and housework and yard work. Such activities should gradually increase as recovery occurs. The patient should be advised clearly about conditions such as fever, signs of wound infection, focal neurologic signs, decreased alertness, intractable headaches, vomiting, neck pain, etc. which should prompt their seeking care prior to their next scheduled appointment.

Cross-References
▶ Emergency Burr Holes

References
1. Blumenfeld H (2002) Cranium, ventricles, and meninges. In: Neuroanatomy through Clinical Cases. Sinauer, Sunderland, MA, p 163
2. Samuels A (April 2005) The duty to warn the patient. Br J Neurosurg 19(2):117–119
3. Rhoton AL Jr (October 2003) Operative technique and instrumentation for neurosurgery. Rhoton cranial anatomy and surgical approaches. Neurosurgery 53(1):1–6
4. Dimitrov DF, Turner DA (2005) Perioperative care of the neurosurgical patient. In: Rengachary SS, Ellenbogen RG (eds) Principles of neurosurgery, 2nd edn. Mosby, St. Louis, MO, pp 91–98
5. Korinek AM, Goldmard JL, Elcheik A, Bismuth R, van Effenterre R, Coriat P, Puybasset L (April 2005) Risk factors for neurosurgical site infections after craniotomy: a critical reappraisal of antibiotic prophylaxis on 4578 patients. Br J Neurosurg 19(2):155–162

Creatine Kinase-MB
▶ Cardiac Markers for Diagnosing Acute Myocardial Infarction

Creatinine and Creatinine Clearance in Children

CARLA NESTER[1], PATRICK D. BROPHY[2]
[1]Department of Pediatrics, Division of Pediatric Nephrology, Dialysis & Transplantation, University of Iowa Children's Hospital, Carver College of Medicine, Iowa City, IA, USA
[2]Department of Pediatrics, University of Iowa Children's Hospital Carver College of Medicine, Iowa City, IA, USA

Synonyms
Glomerular filtration rate

Other Important Terms
Iohexol; Iothalamate; Nuclear Medicine; Schwartz Equation

Definition
Determining the level of renal function in the intensive care setting can be critical to the management of the child with a serious illness. An understanding of renal function facilitates proper fluid and electrolyte management and safe dosing of medications, and allows for timely intervention and treatment of morbidities when a declining renal function is recognized.

Quantifying renal function in children is not an easy task. Pediatric norms can vary widely and are influenced by age as well as size and body habitus. Rough estimates of renal function are available as "bedside" assessments; however, they are of limited accuracy. More precise measurements often require radioisotopes or cumbersome techniques not always practical in the intensive care unit. Nonetheless, establishing the level of renal function is key to state-of-the-art care in the critically ill patient.

The determination of renal function requires an assessment of the glomerular filtration rate (GFR). The GFR is the volume of plasma ultrafiltrate filtered by the kidney per unit time and represents the functional renal mass. Glomerular filtration is routinely measured indirectly through the concept of clearance. Clearance (C_x) is defined as the volume of plasma from which a substance would have to be totally removed to account for its rate of excretion in urine per unit of time. Clearance is calculated by dividing the excretion rate of a substance by its plasma concentration $(C_x = U_x V/P_x)$ where U_x and P_x are urine and plasma concentrations, respectively, of substance x, and V is urine flow rate in milliliters per minute (ml/min). Any substance that is freely filtered by the kidney is not protein bound (therefore not restricted from filtration), and not reabsorbed, secreted, or metabolized by the kidney tubules once filtered into the urinary space would suffice for this calculation. By determining the clearance of a substance under these circumstances, the glomerular filtration rate is inferred $(C_x = GFR)$ [1–3].

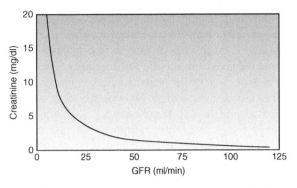

Creatinine and Creatinine Clearance in Children. Figure 1 The relationship between plasma creatinine and GFR is an inverse relationship that is nonlinear

Characteristics

Inulin is the classic substance used for this calculation. Since inulin is not secreted or absorbed it appears in the urine based solely on the filtering capacity (GFR) of the kidneys. Its use can be technically challenging and it is therefore infrequently used for GFR assessment at this time. It is mentioned here primarily because it is considered the gold standard for measurement of GFR [1].

In practice, creatinine is the plasma substance that is used for GFR calculations and is in fact the roughest estimate available of renal function. It is this substance that is more readily available for assessment in the intensive care setting. Creatinine is a product of muscle catabolism and appears to be fairly constantly produced by the body and uniformly handled by the normal kidney on a day-to-day basis. This permits following the plasma level of creatinine as a useful measure of renal function. One important exception exists. When renal failure is advanced, creatinine is relatively more secreted, and therefore when used in calculations can result in an overestimation of GFR [1–3]. The fact that creatinine can be secreted results in a nonlinear relationship between creatinine and GFR (Fig. 1).

Limitations

Small changes in creatinine clearance may go unnoticed due to this relative increase in secretion of creatinine masking loss of renal function. Other limitations exist in utilizing creatinine as a useful measure of renal function. Creatinine rises only after renal injury, therefore limiting preemptive measures to preserve renal function. Furthermore, some medications interfere with creatinine secretion (i.e., trimethoprim/sulfamethoxazole) causing a falsely elevated creatinine, mimicking worsening filtration function. Despite these limitations, creatinine measurements are readily available in most standard laboratories and therefore are the current standard for assessing renal function.

Prior to making renal function calculations based on creatinine, one important caveat must be considered when attempting to estimate GFR; the patient's renal function must be at *steady state*. If the patient's renal function is changing as occurs with renal injury, the use of the creatinine to determine GFR becomes invalid.

If the renal function is stable and the creatinine is not changing, the creatinine may be used to estimate GFR. There are currently two commonly used options for a bedside *estimation* of GFR: the Schwartz formula in children under 18 and the Cockroft–Gault equation in children 12–18. These are both creatinine-based estimates [1–3].

The most commonly used bedside formula is the Schwartz formula: eGFR $= \kappa \bullet L/$Scr; where eGFR is estimated GFR in milliliters per minute per 1.73 square meters, κ is a constant determined empirically by Schwartz and associates [3], L is height in centimeters, and Scr is serum creatinine in milligrams per deciliter. The value of κ is 0.45 for term infants during the first year of life, 0.55 for children and adolescent girls, and 0.7 for adolescent boys. This formula provides a good approximation of GFR when compared with inulin clearance data though in general this formula tends to overestimate GFR. There have been multiple attempts to redefine κ to better account for modern creatinine testing methods and to more accurately represent GFR, however this particular set of κ values continues in general use. The Cockcroft–Gault equation, which is used to estimate GFR in adults, can also be used in children over 12 years of age: eGFR $=$ $(140 - \text{age})$ (body weight in kg)$/(72 \times \text{Scr})$, where eGFR is the estimated GFR in males. In females, a correction factor of 0.85 is used [1–3].

In order to improve the estimates of GFR, other plasma agents have been evaluated for their usefulness. Cystatin C is an enzyme protein that is produced at a relatively constant rate and this constancy appears not to be influenced by the presence of inflammatory conditions, muscle mass, gender, body composition, and age (after 12 months) [4]. Blood cystatin C level is approximately 1 mg/l in healthy individuals. Because cystatin C is catabolized and almost completely reabsorbed by renal proximal tubular cells with little appearing in the urine, standard clearance formulas cannot be used to determine GFR. Nevertheless, serum cystatin can be used to estimate GFR in milliliters per minute per 1.73 square meters according to the following formula: $\log 10\ (GFR) = 1.962 + [1.123 \times \log 10\ (1/cysC)]$, where cysC is serum cystatin C [4]. While cystatin C is not a conventional marker of GFR, reciprocal values of serum cystatin C levels are reasonably well correlated with GFR in children [4].

As with creatinine, cystatin C appears to have its limitations. Recent studies have shown that factors other than renal function, such as C-reactive protein (CRP) and smoking status, may influence serum cystatin C concentrations and the findings of cystatin C in the urine during glomerular and tubular injury also casts some doubt on the ability of serum cystatin C to accurately estimate GFR in certain circumstances. The major drawback however to cystatin C is its availability, as this is not a test that is routinely done in hospital laboratories [1–4].

In more stable patients, measures of glomerular filtration may be undertaken using radiologic means. Estimation of GFR by use of radioisotopes is becoming more commonplace. Though this is often not required in the intensive care setting, there is a place for this type of testing in critically ill hematology-oncology patient who require precise dosing of chemotherapeutics.

Measures (not estimates) of GFR can be made with diethylene triamine penta-acetic acid (^{99m}Tc-DTPA), ethylene diamine tetra-acetic acid ^{51}Cr-EDTA, and iothalamate. These techniques are known as single injection clearance techniques and rely on the theory that the renal clearance of a substance that is not metabolically produced or degraded, and that is excreted from the body completely or almost completely in the urine, can be used to calculate GFR [1]. Using the plasma disappearance of the substance, GFR can be calculated and normalized to 1.73 m^2. Because the entire dosed marker is excreted in the urine, the equation for this method essentially resembles the familiar $GFR = UV/P$. Timed blood draws are required for these methods; however, no urine collection is required. These methods have become quite useful given the limited availability and expertise with inulin and difficulties in collecting accurate timed urine in children. (The use of the clearance formula ($C_x = U_x V/P_x$) requires a timed urine collection and by standard this is a 24 h collection, which can be impractical in unstable ICU patients.)

Iothalamate can be utilized in its nonradioactive form. As before, a single injection is utilized and the plasma disappearance is measured. One caveat to the use of iothalamate is that it can be actively secreted by renal proximal tubular cells and may also undergo some tubular reabsorption, making GFR assessments potentially overestimated.

Finally, iohexol is a reliable alternative to inulin clearance, avoiding both the use of radioactivity and the problems related to timed urination and continuous infusion of marker. Iohexol is a nonionic, low osmolar, X-ray contrast medium that is safe and nontoxic and currently used in angiographic and urographic procedures. It is eliminated from plasma exclusively by glomerular filtration. Iohexol is distributed into the extracellular space and has less than 2% plasma protein binding. It is excreted completely unmetabolized in the urine, with 100% recovery within 24 h after injection. Extrarenal elimination of iohexol in a setting of reduced GFR is negligible. Iohexol is quantified in blood samples using HPLC or X-ray fluorescence. This may be limiting, as not all facilities will have the capability to do this. There is close agreement between GFR measured by inulin clearance and clearance of iohexol using a plasma disappearance method [1]. In a pilot study for the National Institutes of Health (NIH)-supported Chronic Kidney Disease in Children (CKiD) study, it was found that, even with low GFR, serum iohexol measures could be used to define GFR [5].

In the intensive care setting, patients are often unstable and cannot undergo accurate, radiologic assessment of renal function. Therefore, estimates such as the Schwartz formula and improved estimating formulas along with new renal biomarkers as they become available will be necessary to guide care based on renal status.

References

1. Work DF, Schwartz GJ (2008) Estimating and measuring glomerular filtration rate in children. Curr Opin Nephrol Hypertens 17:320–325
2. Stevens LA, Zhang Y, Schmid CH (2008) Evaluating the performance of equations for estimating glomerular filtration rate. J Nephrol 21:797–807
3. Schwartz GJ, Brion LP, Spitzer A (1987) The use of plasma creatinine concentration for estimating glomerular filtration rate in infants, children, and adolescents. Pediatr Clin North Am 34:571–590

4. Finney H, Newman DJ, Thakkar H, Fell JME, Price CP (2000) Reference ranges for plasma cystatin C and creatinine measurements in premature infants, neonates, and older children. Arch Dis Child 82:71–75

5. Schwartz GJ, Furth S, Cole SR, Warady B, Munoz A (2006) Glomerular filtration rate via plasma iohexol disappearance: pilot study for chronic kidney disease in children. Kidney Int 69:2070–2077

Creatinine Clearance, Measurement, Metabolism

ANDERS KALLNER

Department of Clinical Chemistry, Karolinska University hospital, Stockholm, Sweden

Origin, Structure, and Metabolism

Creatinine is a small, water-soluble compound with a molecular mass of 88.4. Creatinine is nonenzymatically formed from creatine, in vivo, and in vitro. Creatine plays a critical role in the energy production, storage, and transport in the cell through its high energy derivative the creatinphosphate. After a burst of activity the creatinphosphate can donate a high energy phosphate residue to ADP and thus anaerobically restore the ATP concentration in the cell. This reaction is reversible. Creatine is *de novo* synthesized in the liver from the amino acid glycine and arginine and also absorbed from the intestine.

Creatinine is mainly eliminated by filtration in the glomeruli of the kidneys but also by tubular excretion and to the gut, even in the healthy. The tubular excretion can be blocked by drugs, for example, cimetidine, but has been found to be stimulated when the glomerular filtration is impaired and the P-Creatinine increases. (In this text, the IFCC/IUPAC nomenclature for quantities is used, thus "P-Creatinine" refers to the plasma concentration of creatinine. For all practical purposes the S-Creatinine and P-Creatinine are exchangeable. Likewise, U-Creatinine is the creatinine concentration in urine. The unit, e.g., μmol/L or mg/dL will be given when appropriate and critical for the understanding.)

Creatinine is not a metabolic stable end-product but is further degraded to methyl guanidine and methyl urea through a long sequence of intermediary products. These are oxidative pathways and stimulated by reactive oxygen species (ROS). Accordingly this degradation increases in hyperbaric treatment of patients. It is unknown if they are nonenzymatic reactions or at least in some steps enzyme dependent. The oxidative pathways are favored in uremia. Methyl guanidine and methyl urea can potentially be nitrated to carcinogenic nitroso derivatives by endogenous nitric oxide (NO).

About 25% of creatinine ingested by healthy individuals will reach the colon. Creatinine that is present or excreted into the gut has been shown to be microbiologically converted to creatine by creatinase. The creatine can then be reabsorbed in an "enteric cycling" process and again metabolized to creatinine. In uremic patients the amount of creatinine in the stool increases.

Creatine and creatinine have been shown to form so-called amino-imidazo-azaarenes (AIA). These substances have been isolated from processed food, in particular broiled meat and other products that are cooked at high temperatures, for example, fried fish, eggs, and potatoes. They are regarded as highly mutagenic and there is experimental evidence that when occurring in the urine they are of dietary origin.

At least one of the mutagenic compounds has been shown to form at low temperatures, for example, 37°C. The endogenous production of AIA has been demonstrated in uremic patients with very high P-Creatinine and it is interesting to note the increased incidence of malignancies in uremic patients.

A comprehensive review of creatinine has recently been published [1].

Measurement of Creatinine Concentration in Serum, Plasma, and Urine

The concentration of creatinine in serum/plasma and urine are probably the most requested measurements from clinical laboratories.

Jaffe [2] observed in the late nineteenth century (1886) that creatinine reacted with an alkaline picrate solution to yield a colored product, often described as red-orange. There is no published evidence that Jaffe made any measurements of the concentration of creatinine in serum or urine based on the reaction; the colorimetric method that is referred to as the Jaffe method was introduced for urine by Otto Folin in 1914 and later applied to deproteinized serum [3, 4]. Already in his first paper on the method, Folin remarked that the reaction was not specific for creatinine and "the only substances I have found to give the reaction under the conditions of the experiment are acetoacetic ether, acetone, and hydrogen sulphide which can easily be removed by a few minutes heating with diluted hydrochloric acid." These substances thus interfere little with the reaction in urine but it is agreed that serum and plasma may contain several interfering substances (so-called matrix effects or non-creatinine chromogens) among which are α-keto acid salts, for example, acetoacetate and puryvate. Other interfering compounds are proteins, glucose, and ascorbate (vitamin C). A number of drugs have been reported to interfere with the reaction, for example, ascorbic acid and ciclosporin. Several modifications of the Jaffe method have been introduced both regarding the reagents and the measurement procedure. These reduce the matrix effects, for example, a widely used kinetic assay that determines the rate of color development a certain time after addition of the picrate and choosing a specific wavelength at which the readings are made.

Dietary intake of creatine that is popular among some athletes and used to increase physical performance falsely increases the serum creatinine but is metabolized and excreted. Any creatine that reaches the urine is nonenzymatically oxidized to creatinine and thus increases the concentration of creatinine in urine. However, freshly voided urine contains some endogenous creatine.

There are many variables in the measurement of substances in biological systems. Laboratories usually describe the performance in terms of precision and trueness, analytical specificity, and the detectability, that is, the lowest concentration that can be measured with a given precision. Equipment in modern laboratories produce results that are reproducible over time, that is, the precision of the measurements is high. The concentration of creatinine in serum and urine is high in relation to the detection limit, which allows the use of very small volumes of serum or urine for the measurement.

Calibration of a measuring system is always critical and is often thought to be the key to true results. However, in biological systems it is not always possible to calibrate the reactions with pure substances since there may be many confounding or interfering substances in the matrix. In the original method by Folin the developed color was compared with that of a suitable solution of potassium dichromate, which has a color that is close enough to that developed by creatinine and alkaline picrate. This is not satisfactory and modern methods use much more sophisticated materials and methods that are traceable to the concentration of well-defined reference materials. Lately, several calibrators are traceable to materials whose concentration has been determined using isotope-dilution-mass-spectrometric methods (ID-MS).

To improve the measurement of creatinine concentration in serum and urine the use of enzyme reactions have been employed. The original method is based on a series of enzyme reactions beginning with creatininase that hydrolyses creatinine to creatine, which is further degraded to sarcosine and urea using another enzyme, creatinase. Finally the sarcosine is oxidized using sarcosine oxidase that produces hydrogen peroxide, which can be measured by different color reactions or an amperometric assay. This sequence of reactions is specific for creatinine and not influenced by the matrix but needs correction for endogenous creatine.

The laboratories can thus offer an alternative to the Jaffe-based measurement procedure with a high precision and trueness. However, the reagents used in the Jaffe-based procedures are still much cheaper than those for the enzyme-based reactions and therefore still used in many, perhaps most laboratories.

Numerous comparison studies show that Jaffe-based assays give slightly higher results in the same samples than the enzyme-based procedures. This is attributed to unspecific reactions of the matrix. To improve the comparability of results several corrective procedures are employed in laboratories, for example, reducing the results obtained by a factor or a constant value to mimic the results of an enzymatic reaction. Other harmonization methods include adjusting the results as if the procedure had used an ID-MS measured calibrator. None of these procedures will eliminate the matrix effects of individual samples since they may be different from one sample to the next but the average output from the laboratories will be close to those of results using enzymatic procedures.

Reference Intervals and Biological Variation

In the use of biochemical markers for diagnosis of a disease the serum concentration of a marker is compared with a reference interval or reference values. These are often established by measuring the concentration of the marker in many individuals that are carefully defined, usually without the disease that the marker is intended to use for the diagnosis. By this definition the concept of normal values is abandoned and the reference interval can be linked to any condition, for example, age, gender, or even disease.

Creatine is thought to be converted to creatinine at an almost steady daily rate of about 2% of the total body creatine amount [1]. The latter is related to the muscle mass, which may explain the general observation that the P-Creatinine varies with the body size. Thus, in general men have higher serum concentrations than women, which may be attributed to the larger muscle mass of males. The P-Creatinine shows a remarkably small intra-individual variation, that is, the concentration varies comparatively little over time in the healthy, whereas the between individual variation is large. Fraser estimated the intra-individual variation to 4.9% and the inter-individual variation to 18.2% [5]. Large intakes of meat and extraordinary physical activity increase the P-Creatinine. Likewise, malnutrition causes a reduction of P-Creatinine. P-Creatinine increases slightly with age particularly accelerated above about 60 years of age for both men and women (about 5% between 20 and 60 years and about 12% between 60 and 80 years) [6].

P-Creatinine is a function of creatinine production and its elimination. Considering the general decrease of muscle mass by age the increase in P-Creatinine by age may be attributed to a general decrease in the kidney function, notably the glomerular filtration.

The reference intervals for P-Creatinine in healthy individuals varies for biological or physiological reasons. The reference intervals also vary from laboratory to laboratory depending on which measurement method is used, that is, reagents, calibrators, and calculation methods. It is therefore not possible or meaningful in a text like this to state the reference interval and each user should consider the local reference intervals. However, the upper limit of the reference interval for P-Creatinine is usually cited at about 110 μmol/L (0.11 mmol/L or 1.24 mg/dL) for men and 95 μmol/L (0.10 mmol/L or 1.07 mg/dL) for women. A modern laboratory can usually measure the P-Creatinine with a relative uncertainty of 4%. The minimal significant difference (MD) between two results (on a 95% probability level) is estimated to about 11%, that is, about 11 μmol/L (0.011 mmol/L or 0.12 mg/dL) at a concentration of 100 μmol/L (0.10 mmol/L or 1.13 mg/dL). In this figure the intraindividual biological variation or preanalytical errors are not considered.

Creatinine Clearance

There are different methods to estimate the glomerular filtration rate. One method is based on measuring the amount of a substance excreted in the urine during a certain time during which the concentration of the substance is kept constant in the plasma. The substance can be exogenous, for example, inulin, or endogenous, for example, creatinine or cystatin C. Another method is to administer an exogenous substance and measure the rate at which it disappears from the plasma. Both procedures give good estimates of the glomerular filtration rate provided the used substance used fulfills certain criteria. The most important is that the substance shall only be excreted through the glomeruli. There are also criteria of a technical nature, for example, the substance should be easily measured with a high precision and trueness. In the first case the plasma concentration should be kept constant during the observation period and the substance should not be metabolized. For instance intake of meat during the collection period of a creatinine clearance determination will jeopardize the results.

Diagnostic medicine often requires identifying a "gold method," which is the method that, at a given time, is regarded as that which best describes a condition or measures a substance or function. The gold method of estimating glomerular filtration is inulin clearance. Inulin is a polysaccharide that is an ideal substance because it is not metabolized and is only eliminated by filtration. The inulin clearance has been determined both after a single dose and estimating the elimination, and during constant administration and collection of the excreted amount during a period of time. However, the procedures are too complicated and cumbersome for routine purposes. All other methods of estimating glomerular filtration can be regarded as surrogate methods and compared with the inulin clearance.

Creatinine has long been a surrogate for inulin in the estimation of glomerular filtration in spite of the fact that its serum concentration is not constant during the day and creatinine is not only eliminated by filtration, for example, it is in a dynamic equilibrium with creatine in the intestine. This method also suffers from inherent problems, for example, collection and determination of the collection time.

The general formula for calculating clearance from plasma concentration of any suitable substance and the amount of the substance excreted in urine is here shown for creatinine.

$$Cl = \frac{1}{P - Crea} \times \frac{U - Crea \times U - Vol}{time}$$

Clearance is thus inversely proportional to the plasma concentration and directly proportional to the amount of substance (concentration times volume) excreted.

Clearance is usually expressed as mL/min, which is interpreted as the volume of plasma that is completely cleared from the substance in 1 min. This interpretation is classic but hardly understandable from a physiological point of view. Clearance can also be interpreted as amount of substance flux (mol/time) in relation to the concentration of the substance on the primary side of a membrane (mol/L). The implications are that the clearance – glomerular filtration rate – is influenced by the P-Creatinine and the substance flux. In kidney disease the flux is most likely impaired and consequently a new equilibrium established as recognized by the clearance and P-Creatinine.

As mentioned above the P-Creatinine is influenced by various demographic parameters, for example, gender and muscle mass. In particular it has been accepted that the glomerular filtration is related to the body surface (BSA).

To achieve comparable results, irrespective of the body size, the glomerular filtration is often normalized to the BSA. Randomly, the GFR is normalized to 1.73 m^2 based on BSA estimates according to du Bois and du Bois [7]. The normalized GRF is largely comparable between individuals of the same gender and therefore a reference value can be established.

Early on physicians tried to establish shortcuts to estimate the creatinine clearance from the P-Creatinine. A very interesting early suggestion was presented in the Lancet [8] who even created a nomogram including the age and weight. Before and after there have been innumerable algorithms presented to achieve the same goal. The most famous are the Cockroft–Gault (C-G) [9], the MDRD-eGFR [10], and the Mayo algorithms [11]. New algorithms are created and published [12]. The Cockroft–Gault differs from the other by including some demographic information in the formula, very similar to the nomogram of Molholm–Hansen. The algorithms are created by comparison of the P-Creatinine and glomerular filtration estimated by a gold method or surrogate, that is, Iohexol or ^{51}Cr-EDTA clearance. They have in common to be limited to a specific population and their advocates claim that the results can be used globally to set medical decision values.

There are serious theoretical and practical flaws in these procedures. Theoretically it is not acceptable to use epidemiological or population data for diagnosing individuals. It is however common practice to establish "population based reference intervals."

It is not acceptable to present the algorithms without information about the uncertainty of the results. It is reasonable to assume that the uncertainty of the analytical process is propagated by the uncertainty of the regression function.

Simplified, the algorithms are based on the P-Creatinine, age and some factors, or exponents. They all disregard the substance flux (see formula above) and the constitution of the patient and substitute this with information about gender and age except C-G algorithm that also includes the body mass (lean weight).

It is a major mistake to express the eGFR-MDRD as if normalized to BSA only because the algorithm was established in relation to a normalized iohexol clearance. It is erroneous because when the algorithm is used "backwards," that is, to estimate the GFR from the P-Creatinine, the demographics are lost and recalculation using the individual's BSA may give grossly erroneous results.

It has been shown that the MDRD-eGFR does not compensate for the age or the gender [13]; their influence is equal to that on P-Creatinine. It has also been shown

that the MDRD-eGFR does not add any diagnostic power to that of S-Creatinine [14].

It is symptomatic that new algorithms are designed also from the groups that have designed and advocated the initial MDRD-eGFR [12].

The most important take-away messages of this short review are that

- P-Creatinine is influenced by muscle mass, diet, and age.
- The intra-individual variation of P-Creatinine is small whereas the inter-individual variation is large. Consequently P-Creatinine and thus any "estimated GFR" varies much between individuals and cannot be used for diagnosis in a screening setting.
- All estimated GFR are liable to serious theoretical and practical flaws.

References

1. Wyss M, Kaddurah-Daouk R (2000) Creatine and creatinine metabolism. Physiol Rev 80(3):1108–1213
2. Jaffe M (1886) Ueber den Niederschlag, welchen Pikrinsäure in normalem Harn erzeugt und über eine neue Reaction des Kreatinins. Hoppe-Seyler's Z Physiol Chem 10:391–400
3. Folin O (1914) On the determination of creatinine and creatine in blood, milk and tissues. J Biol Chem 17:475–481
4. Folin O, Denis W (1914) On the creatinine and creatine content of blood. J Biol Chem 17:487–491
5. Fraser CG (2001) Biological variation: from principles to practice. AACC press, Washington, DC, ISBN 1-890883-49-2
6. Kallner A, Gustavsson E, Hendig E (2000) Can age and sex related reference intervals be derived for non-healthy and non-diseased individuals from results of measurements in primary health care? Clin Chem Lab Med 38(7):633–654
7. Du Bois D, du Bois E (1916) A formula to estimate the approximate surface area if height and weight be known. Arch Intern Med 17: 863–871
8. Siersbaek-Nielsen K, Mölholm-Hansen J, Kampmann J, Kristensen M (1971) Rapid evaluation of creatinine. Lancet 1133–1134
9. Cockcroft DW, Gault HM (1976) Prediction of creatinine clearance from serum creatinine. Nephron 16:31–41
10. Levey AS, Coresh J, Balk E, Kausz AT, Levin A, Steffes MW, Hogg RJ, Perrone RD, Lau J, Eknoyan G (2003) National Kidney Foundation Practice Guidelines for chronic kidney disease: evaluation, classification and stratification. Ann Intern Med 139:137–147
11. Rule AD, Larson TS, Bergstralh EJ, Slezak JM, Jacobsen SJ, Cosio FG (2004) Using serum creatinine to estimate glomerular filtration rate: accuracy in good health and in chronic kidney disease. Ann Intern Med 141:929–937
12. Levey A, Stevens LA, Schmid CH, Zhang YL, Castro AF III, Feldman A, Kusek JW, Eggers P, Van Lente F, Greene T, Coresh J (2009) A new equation to estimate glomerular filtration rate. Ann Intern Med 150:604–612
13. Kallner A, Ayling PA, Khatami Z (2008) Does eGFR improve the diagnostic capability of S-Creatinine concentration results? A retrospective population based study. Int J Med Sci 5:9–17
14. Pottel H, Martens F (2009) Are eGFR equations better than IDMS-traceable serum creatinine in classifying chronic kidney disease? Scand J Clin Lab Invest 69(5):550–561

Cretinism

This term refers to the congenital hypothyroidism.

Critical Illness Myopathy

▶ Critical Illness Polyneuropathy/Myopathy
▶ Mobility/Exercise, Early in ICU

Critical Illness Myopathy and/or Neuropathy (CRIMYNE)

▶ Weakness, Post ICU

Critical Illness Neuromuscular Abnormalities (CINMA)

▶ Mobility/Exercise, Early in ICU
▶ Weakness, Post ICU

Critical Illness Polyneuropathy (CIPN)

▶ Critical Illness Polyneuropathy/Myopathy
▶ Mobility/Exercise, Early in ICU
▶ Weakness, Post ICU

Critical Illness Polyneuropathy/ Myopathy

Brent P. Goodman
Mayo Clinic College of Medicine, Mayo Clinic Arizona, Scottsdale, AZ, USA

Synonyms

Critical illness myopathy; Critical Illness Polyneuropathy (CIPN); ICU-acquired weakness

Definition

Neuromuscular weakness is a frequent complication of critical illness, often resulting in prolongation of mechanical ventilation time and length of stay in the intensive care unit. Advancements in the care of patients with critical illness and improvements in survival have led to an increased recognition of this important problem and a greater understanding of the spectrum of neuromuscular disease associated with critical illness.

While severe muscle loss and atrophy in a patient with sepsis was reported by Osler in the later part of the nineteenth century, it was not until the pioneering work of Bolton and colleagues in 1984, that the clinical, morphologic, and electrodiagnostic features of neuromuscular weakness in patients with sepsis began to emerge [1]. These investigators introduced the term critical illness polyneuropathy (CIP), and described a peripheral neuropathy involving both motor and sensory fibers, characterized pathologically, and electrodiagnostically by axonal degeneration of peripheral nerve fibers. Patients with CIP characteristically have distal extremity weakness, and frequently have difficulty weaning from mechanical ventilation.

Over the past few decades, identification of a second, and likely more important cause of neuromuscular weakness in the critically ill patient has evolved – critical illness myopathy (CIM). CIM shares many of the same risk factors for development as CIP, particularly sepsis and the systemic inflammatory response syndrome (SIRS). Patients with CIM typically have generalized weakness involving limb, diaphragm, neck, and even facial muscles. Over the past several years, it has been increasingly recognized that patients with critical illness typically have clinical, electrodiagnostic, and even pathological features of both CIP and CIM. This has led some authors to suggest the term critical illness neuromyopathy might be most appropriate, recognizing that polyneuropathy and myopathy typically co-exist in patients with critical illness.

Epidemiology

The reported incidence of critical illness neuromyopathy is quite variable, and influenced by a number of factors including the study population, risk factors, timing of the diagnostic evaluation, and the diagnostic methods used. It is thought that 70–80% of critically ill patients develop CIP and/or CIM, and the reported incidence of neuromyopathy in patients with sepsis and multiorgan failure (MOF) is 100% [2]. It has been estimated that up to 77% of patients in the ICU for 7 or more days will develop a critical illness neuromyopathy. CIM has been reported in at least one-third of patients treated in an ICU for status asthmaticus, and has been a reported complication in 7% of patients who have undergone liver transplantation.

Risk Factors

Sepsis, SIRS, and MOF have long been recognized to be risk factors for the development of critical illness neuromyopathy. MOF in particular, seems to be a major risk factor for the development of neuromyopathy, and can occur in patients with not only sepsis, but also in patients with pancreatitis, burns, trauma, or following cardiac arrest. In fact, the neuromyopathy that develops in MOF could be viewed as another indicator of organ system failure, in addition to cardiac, respiratory, liver, circulatory, and renal systems.

It has been estimated that in healthy adults, muscle strength declines by 1% per day of bed rest. While immobilization in and of itself does not cause critical illness neuromyopathy, it could potentially contribute to more severe weakness. The duration of mechanical ventilation time, which can be viewed as a surrogate marker of immobilization time has consistently been associated with critical illness neuromyopathy, independent of MOF or other risk factors.

Considerable evidence implicates hyperglycemia as a risk factor for the development of critical illness neuromyopathy. These studies led to two randomized clinical trials of intensive insulin therapy in critically ill patients, which showed lower incidence of critical illness myopathy in the insulin treatment group. There are conflicting studies regarding the role of corticosteroids as a risk factor in the development of critical illness neuromyopathy. Some studies have suggested an increased risk of critical illness neuromyopathy in patients given corticosteroids, others have suggested no increase in risk, and one study even suggested that corticosteroids had a protective effect. Retrospective studies have suggested that neuromuscular junction blocking medications may be a risk factor for the development of critical illness myopathy. Liver or renal impairment in patients with MOF may affect neuromuscular blocking agent metabolism, increasing the risk of neurotoxicity in patients with critical illness. Other risk factors for the development of critical illness neuromyopathy include female gender, renal failure, hyperosmolality, low serum albumin, use of vasopressors, illness severity, duration of organ dysfunction, and parenteral nutrition.

Evaluation

Critical illness neuromyopathy characteristically manifests as failure to wean from mechanical ventilation and a generalized, flaccid weakness, typically with reduced or absent reflexes. Facial muscles may become weak, but the presence of opthalmoparesis should prompt consideration of an alternative diagnosis. Sensation may be reduced in the distal extremities. The majority of patients with critical illness neuromyopathy in the ICU will have a concomitant encephalopathy, manifesting as somnolence, agitation, confusion, or even coma. The presence of encephalopathy may considerably limit a patient's cooperation with the neurological examination and with electrodiagnostic testing.

Serum creatine kinase (CK) levels are normal in most patients with critical illness neuromyopathy. Electromyography (EMG) studies are helpful in the evaluation of suspected critical illness neuromyopathy. These studies include nerve conduction studies (NCS), which characteristically show low amplitude motor responses, and may show low amplitude sensory nerve amplitudes. The presence of low amplitude motor responses with prolonged action potential durations is highly specific for critical illness neuromyopathy [3]. This finding is helpful in confirming a diagnosis of critical illness neuromyopathy, and is not a characteristic finding in any other neuromuscular disorders. Needle EMG studies show fibrillation potentials and small, sometimes polyphasic motor unit potentials in affected muscles.

Nerve and muscle biopsies are not necessary in the routine evaluation of suspected critical illness neuromyopathy. These procedures should only be considered for research purposes, or for atypical presentations, where it is necessary to rule out other neuromuscular conditions. Nerve biopsy specimens performed in patients with CIP have shown axonal degeneration, without features of inflammation or primary demyelination. Muscle biopsy findings in CIM have been quite variable. Loss of thick filament myosin has been the most frequently reported pathological finding. Loss of type I, type II, or both fiber types has been reported in CIM. Rarely, patients with CIM have been reported to have widespread necrosis on muscle biopsy. Patients with a necrotizing CIM have historically been referred to as acute necrotizing myopathy of intensive care, and typically have severe quadriparesis, hyperCKemia, myoglobinura, and a poor prognosis for return of normal muscle strength.

Treatment

There is at this time no specific treatment for critical illness neuromyopathy. Aggressive treatment of sepsis and MOF is an obvious priority to not only improve patient survival but reduce the risk and severity of critical illness neuromyopathy. Use of corticosteroid and neuromuscular blocking medications should be avoided or minimized if at all possible. Nutritional interventions and supplements, growth hormone, testosterone derivatives, and immunoglobulins have been proposed, but have not been definitively shown to reduce the risk of developing critical illness neuromyopathy or hasten recovery.

As previously mentioned in this chapter, hyperglycemia has been shown consistently to be a risk factor for the development of critical illness neuromyopathy. Prospective, randomized, and controlled trials of intensive versus conventional insulin therapy in critically ill patients has shown a significant reduction in mechanical ventilation time and incidence of critical illness neuromyopathy from 49% to 25% in a surgical ICU cohort and 51% to 39% in a medical ICU cohort [4]. However, because these findings have not as of this time been replicated in a larger series, and given a number of concerns regarding safety and methodologic issues, intensive insulin therapy is not a recommended therapy for critical illness neuromyopathy. Further studies are necessary.

Physical, occupational, and respiratory therapy should be initiated early in a patient's course. Stretching and range of motion exercises should be initialized to prevent the development of contractures, skin protection measures are necessary to prevent the development of pressure ulcers, and early mobilization with progressive, submaximal resistance training should be pursued. There is evidence that early mobilization through physical and occupational therapy may improve outcome in patients with critical illness neuromyopathy.

Prognosis

Critical illness neuromyopathy is associated with prolonged ICU and hospitalization stays, and higher mortality rates. Spontaneous recovery of muscle strength may occur within several weeks or months, though patients with severe neuromuscular weakness may experience very little functional recovery and remain quadriparetic or paraparetic. In a long-term, prospective study of patients with critical illness neuromyopathy, 31% of patients had persistent muscular weakness [5]. Another study of 19 patients with CIP reported complete recovery in eight patients, persistent, severe weakness in four patients including two with complete quadriplegia, and death of four patients between months 2–9 following the diagnosis of CIP.

A number of poor prognostic factors have been suggested, including absent compound muscle action potentials on EMG studies, hyperCKemia, and necrosis on muscle biopsy. One small study suggested that patients with CIP may have a worse prognosis when compared with patients that have features of a purely or predominantly myopathic process.

After-care

Most patients with critical illness neuromyopathy will benefit from a transition into an inpatient rehabilitation unit once clinically stable. A multidisciplinary approach utilizing some combination of physical, occupational, speech, and neuropsychological therapies may offer patients the best opportunity to return to premorbid levels of function. Upon discharge to home patients may require assistive devices and adaptive equipment.

References

1. Bolton CF, Gilbert JJ, Hahn AF, Sibbald WJ (1984) Polyneuropathy in critically ill patients. J Neurol Neurosurg Psych 47:1223–1231
2. Zink W, Kollmar R, Schwab S (2009) Critical illness polyneuropathy and myopathy in the intensive care unit. Nat Rev Neurol 5:372–379
3. Goodman BP, Harper CM, Boon AJ (2009) Prolonged compound muscle action potential duration in critical illness myopathy. Muscle Nerve 40(6):1040–1042
4. Hermans G, De Jonghe B, Bruyinckx F, Van den Berghe G (2009) Interventions for preventing critical illness polyneuropathy and critical illness myopathy. Cochrane Database of Syst Rev 1: CD006832
5. Fletcher SN, Kennedy DD, Ghosh IR et al (2003) Persistent neuromuscular and neuropsychological abnormalities in long-term survivors of prolonged critical illness. Crit Care 31:1012–1016

Critical Illness Related Corticosteroid Insufficiency

▶ Adrenal Conditions, Insufficiency/Failure

Critical Illness–Related Corticosteroid Insufficiency (CIRCI)

The inadequate corticosteroid activity for the severity of the illness of a critically ill patient.

Crowning

Engagement of fetal head at cervical outlet.

Crush Injury

▶ Patterns of Injury

Crushed Limb

▶ Mangled Extremity

Cryptococcosis

Julie P. Chou[1], Tom Lim[1], Andrew G. Lee[2], Christopher H. Mody[3]
[1]Department of Internal Medicine, University of Calgary, Calgary, AB, Canada
[2]Department of Radiology, University of Calgary, AB, Canada
[3]Departments of Internal Medicine and Microbiology, Immunology and Infectious Disease, University of Calgary, Calgary, AB, Canada

Synonyms

Cryptococcus gattii; Torulosis

Definition

Cryptococcus gattii (formerly *C. neoformans* var. *gattii* or *C. neoformans* serotype B and C) is one of the two most common pathogenic species in the genus *Cryptococcus*. Cryptococcosis caused by both *C. neoformans* and *C. gattii* affects the lungs and central nervous system preferentially. The differences between the two species will be highlighted here. Please refer to the entry on *Cryptococcus neoformans*.

Cryptococcus gattii has emerged as a primary pathogen after outbreaks of infection associated with high mortality rates in otherwise healthy immunocompetent individuals on Vancouver Island and the neighboring Washington state, where cases were first described in 1999 and have continued to occur. *C. gattii* is classically found on eucalyptus trees in tropical and subtropical areas, including Australia, Papua New Guinea, South Africa, Mexico, Southern California, Brazil, and Zaire. However, on Vancouver Island, *C. gattii* is found on tree species native to the island, including red alder, Garry oak, and Douglas Fir. It has been speculated that this association with noneucalyptoid trees confers high virulence to the strains of *C. gattii* on Vancouver Island.

A retrospective study in Vancouver from 1997 to 2002 showed that *C. gattii* was 4.8 times more common in immunocompetent compared to immunosuppressed hosts, whereas *C. neoformans* is more common in the immunocompromised.

Cryptococcosis caused by both *C. neoformans* and *C. gattii* affects the lungs and central nervous system predominantly. During pulmonary infection, patients often present with cough, dyspnea, chest pain, and weight loss and can become critically ill (Fig. 1). Indeed, as of January 2009, 19 deaths have been associated with *C. gattii* infections on Vancouver Island. Remarkably, presentation can be delayed by up to 1 year from exposure, and meningitis with or without the involvement of the brain parenchyma is the most frequent CNS complication. In contrast to *C. neoformans*, cryptococcomas in the lungs and brain are more frequently observed with *C. gattii*. A higher frequency of neurological sequelae (and need for neurosurgical intervention) is noted with *C. gattii*.

Treatment

The current recommendation for therapy is similar for both *C. neoformans* and *C. gattii*. No specific guideline has been developed for *C. gattii*. However, the treatment duration is often extended for *C. gattii*, as mycological cure is often delayed. In addition, the use of corticosteroids has been advocated in *C. gattii* infections if there is risk of vision loss.

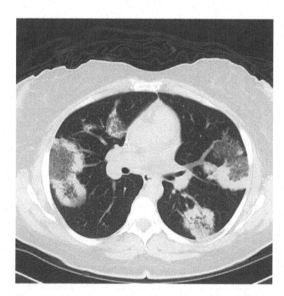

Cryptococcosis. Figure 1 *Cryptococcus gattii* pneumonia showing areas of dense consolidation and ground glass opacification

Echinocandins such as caspofungin are not active against *Cryptococcus* and should not be used.

Evaluation/Assessment
Serum antigen detection, or microscopy of bronchoalveolar lavage or cerebrospinal fluid, and histopathology of tissue specimens can provide a provisional diagnosis of *Cryptococcus* infection. To distinguish *C. gattii* from *C. neoformans*, growth on special media (canavanine-glycine-bromothymol blue (CGB) media) is employed. In addition, species identification can be achieved by molecular methods.

After-care
Mycological clearance is often slow, which extends the course of pharmacotherapy, and there is increased neurological morbidity and overall mortality. Consequently, a prolonged follow-up of patients infected with *C. gattii* is prudent.

Prognosis
Currently, on Vancouver Island where there is the highest endemic incidence reported worldwide, the case fatality rate was estimated to be 4.5% from 1999 to 2006.

References
1. Hoang LM, Magure JA, Doyle P et al (2004) Cryptococcus neoformans infections at Vancouver Hospital and Health Sciences Centre (1997–2002): epidemiology, microbiology and histopathology. J Med Microbiol 53:935–940

Cryptococcus gattii
▶ Cryptococcosis

Cryptogenic Subarachnoid Hemorrhage (SAH)
▶ Nonaneurysmal Subarachnoid Hemorrhage

Crystalloid Challenge
▶ Fluid Challenge

Crystalloids
▶ Intravenous Fluids

CST3
▶ Cystatin C

CT Coronary Angiography
▶ Coronary Computerized Tomographic Angiography

Cubozoa
▶ Jellyfish Envenomation

Cyanide Toxicity
RICHARD D. SHIH, OLIVER L. HUNG
Department of Emergency Medicine, Morristown Memorial Hospital, Morristown, NJ, USA

Synonyms
Nitril; Nitrile

Definition
Cyanide toxicity is the physiologic effect of cyanide salts or glycosides in inhibiting multiple enzymes processes in the body. The most commonly explained effect is its ability to inhibit cellular respiration by interrupting the electron transport chain. Cyanide induces cellular hypoxia by inhibiting cytochrome oxidase at the cytochrome a3 protein (also known as the cytochrome c oxidase). Cyanide also inhibits many other metalloenzymes such as succinate dehydrogenase, superoxide dismutase, aldolase, phosphatase, peroxidase, xanthine oxidase, and carbonic anhydrase; the physiologic effect of this inhibition is still unclear. Cyanide also activates the NMDA receptor, which leads to free radical

formation and lipid peroxidation. This is thought to be a potential causative factor for cyanide-induced neuronal injury.

Sources of cyanide toxicity include the following:

Cyanide salts: Cyanide salts are commonly used in industry and laboratories as a chemical reagant. In silver and gold mining, high-grade ore is mixed with cyanide forming a soluble complex. Cyanide is also found in the plating bath used for electroplating metals as well as metal cleaning solutions. Consequently, cyanide exposure is a very serious occupational hazard for jewelers. In photography, potassium cyanide is used in the photo lab to create the tintype photo process. It is also used to recover silver from x-ray film. In manufacturing, cyanide is used to make paper, plastics, and textiles. Cyanide gas (HCN) is used as a fumigant for ships/warehouses.

Fires: Cyanide is a by-product of the incomplete pyrrolysis of wool, silk, and plastics. Smoke inhalation victims are at risk for cyanide poisoning.

War agent and terrorism: Cyanide has previously been used as a mass casualty weapon by the Germans during World War II (HCN) and the Iraqis against the Kurds during the Iran–Iraq War; cults (Jamestown, KCN); and terrorist groups (Tylenol R US mass poisonings, Aum Shinrikyo, NaHCN).

Cyanogens: Natural or synthetic compounds that after absorption into the body are metabolized to release hydrocyanic acid (HCN). These include plants, nitroprusside, and nitriles (acetonitrile). Cyanogenic glycosides are found in a variety of plants including *Manihot* spp (cassava) (linamarin), *Prunus* species (prunes, apricots, cherries, peaches) (amygdalin), *Linum* spp, *Lotus* spp, *Sorghum* spp (dhurrin), *Phaseolus* spp. Toxicity occurs after the cyanogenic glycoside is ingested and hydrogen cyanide is slowly released during intestinal ingestion. The vasodilator sodium nitroprusside contains cyanide, which is slowly released following intravenous administration. High-dose (>2 mcg/kg/min) and/or prolonged nitroprusside infusion may result in cyanide poisoning. Patients with depleted sulfur stores including patients who are malnourished, critically ill, or post-surgery are at increased risk for developing cyanide poisoning. The active ingredient of artificial nail remover, acetonitrile, is metabolized by cytochrome P-450 enzymes in the liver to hydrogen cyanide. Ingestion of artificial nail remover may result in cyanide poisoning.

Chronic exposure to cyanide has been demonstrated to result in several unique toxicological sequelae. Tropical ataxic neuropathy is a demyelinating disorder that results from the consumption of improperly processed cassava, a cyanide-containing root. Tobacco amblyopia is a cyanide-induced cause of progressive vision loss in smokers.

Treatment

Treatment of cyanide toxicity includes prompt removal from the area of exposure, decontamination, supportive care, and the administration of a cyanide antidote (cyanide antidote package or hydroxocobalamin). Decontamination of cyanide victims depends on the type of exposure. Healthcare providers should receive the appropriate protection to prevent toxic exposure during the treatment of these patients. Dermal exposure decontamination includes the removal of clothing and irrigation of the skin with water. Gastrointestinal exposure includes the administration of activated charcoal (1/gkg) in patients with an intake airway. All patients should receive high-flow supplemental oxygen and appropriate airway control. IV crystalloids and vasopressors should be administered in hypotensive patients. IV sodium bicarbonate should be used to treat severe metabolic acidosis. Finally, seizures should be treated with an appropriate anticonvulsant (e.g., IV benzodiazepine or barbiturate). There are currently two available cyanide antidotes available in the USA, the cyanide antidote package (formerly the Lilly cyanide antidote kit) [containing amyl nitrite, sodium nitrite, and sodium thiosulfate] and hydroxocobalamin. Since hydroxocobalamin has only recently been approved by the FDA for the treatment of cyanide poisoning, there is much greater clinical experience with use of the cyanide antidote package. Although definitive studies are lacking, animal studies and human case reports suggest that hydroxocobalamin has a similar level of efficacy in treating cyanide poisoning compared to the cyanide antidote package. However, hydroxocobalamin has fewer side effects than the cyanide antidote package, whose nitrite component may produce excessive methemoglobinemia or cause significant hypotension.

Cyanide Antidotes

Cyanide antidote package: (amyl nitrite, sodium nitrite, sodium thiosulfate).

The cyanide antidote package consists of three constituents: amyl nitrite (12 ampules, 0.3 mL each), sodium nitrite (two 10 mL ampules of 3% solution), and sodium thiosulfate (two 50 mL 25% solution). The traditional method of action by which nitrites were thought to prevent cyanide toxicity is its ability to induce methemoglobinemia. Cyanide preferentially binds to methemoglobin over cytochrome a3 to form cyanomethemoglobin.

Cyanomethemoglobin is readily detoxified by the enzyme rhodanese to thiocyanate, which is then renally eliminated from the body. This method of action has been disputed for the following reasons. Nitrites are effective soon after administration before it is even able to induce a significant methemoglobinemia. Morever, even when blocked from inducing a methemoglobinemia by simultaneous methylene blue administration, nitrites have been demonstrated to be an effective cyanide therapy. The postulated true mechanism of action may instead be related to its reduction to nitric oxide and nitric oxide's ability to prevent free radial formation or its effect as a potent vasodilator and ability to modify cyanide's effect on local circulation. Nitrites (in particular sodium nitrite) possess two potentially serious adverse effects. It may produce an excessive amount of methemoglobinemia. As a potent vasodilator, nitrites may also cause significant hypotension. Nitrites are contraindicated in the setting of carbon monoxide poisoning because the combination of both nitrite-induced methemoglobinemia and carboxyhemoglobinemia may cause a critical impairment of oxygen delivery to the tissues. Consequently, the nitrite portions of the cyanide antidote package should be omitted in smoke inhalation patients without a measured carboxyhemoglobin level to exclude carbon monoxide poisoning. Finally, the final portion of the antidote package, sodium thiosulfate, should be administered immediately after IV sodium nitrite. Sodium thiosulfate acts as a sulfur donator, facilitating the ability of the enzyme rhodanese to detoxify cyanide to thiocyanate. Sodium thiosulfate has no significant adverse effects.

Amyl nitrite is intended to be used in patients who do not have IV access and cannot receive sodium nitrite (e.g., pre-hospital or initial ED resuscitation). Amyl nitrite ampules are broken in a handkerchief and held in front of the patient's mouth or introduced into the ventilator system for 15 s followed by a rest for 15 s with the process repeated until IV access is obtained and the sodium nitrite can be administered instead. Sodium nitrite is administered as an IV infusion over 2–4 min. The adult dose is 300 mg (10 mL) and the pediatric dose is 0.2 mL/kg not to exceed 10 mL. The normal adult dose rarely results in a methemoglobin level >10%. Another dose can be administered as a 1/2 initial dose if cyanide toxicity recurs or as a prophylactic measure. IV sodium thiosulfate 12.5 g or 50 mL in adults (or 400 mg/kg pediatrics) is administered immediately after sodium nitrite.

Hydroxocobalamin

Each hydroxocobalamin (pre-vitamin B12) molecule binds to one cyanide molecule to form cyanocobalamin (vitamin B12). Cyanocobalamin is either renally eliminated or releases the cyanide molecule slowly enough for detoxification by rhodanese. The recommended initial dose of 70 mg/kg (not to exceed 5 g initially) is administered over 15 min. In case of cardiac arrest, the same dose can be administered as a rapid IV push. A second 70 mg/kg dose, up to a total dose of 10 g (depending on the patient's clinical status over 15 min to 2 h period), may be administered as clinically necessary. Hydroxocobalamin is well tolerated without significant adverse reaction. The most common side effect is a transient red discoloration of the mucous membranes, plasma, and urine, which may last up to 12 h. This discoloration may interfere with the colorimetric measurement of a variety of laboratory tests including: carboxyhemoglobin and plasma/whole blood cyanide levels. Since sodium thiosulfate inactivates hydroxocobalamin, this should not administered through the same infusion site as sodium thiosulfate. Combination therapy with both hydroxocobalamin and sodium thiosulfate has been demonstrated to be efficacious in treating cyanide toxicity.

Other potential antidotes for cyanide toxicity exist including 4-dimethylaminophenol (4-DMAP), hydroxylamine, dicobalt ethylenediaminetetraacetic acid, cobinamide, stroma-free methemoglobin, alpha-ketoglurate, and hyperbaric oxygen therapy. However, these antidotes are either not available in the USA or demonstrate insufficient clinical efficacy and remain investigational.

Evaluation/Assessment

The signs and symptoms of cyanide toxicity are nonspecific; the diagnosis of cyanide poisoning is extremely difficult to make unless quickly entertained by the provider. In many cases, diagnosis is purely empiric based solely on strong clinical suspicion and usually in the setting of a critically ill patient who has sustained severe smoke inhalation. Onset of toxicity is dependent on both the type and route of exposure. Inhalation of gaseous HCN results in onset within several seconds. Ingestion of cyanide salt results in an onset within 30 min. Exposure to cyanogens usually results in a delayed onset of symptoms occurring several hours to 1 day post-ingestion and is dependent on the rate of biotransformation in the body. The estimated lethal oral dose for hydrocyanic acid [HCN] is 50 mg. The estimated lethal oral dose for the cyanide salts is 100–200 mg.

Symptoms of cyanide toxicity include:

General: weakness, malaise
Neurologic: headache, dizziness, vertigo, confusion, coma
Gastrointestinal: abdominal pain, nausea/vomiting

Cardiovascular: dyspnea, chest pain

Signs of cyanide toxicity include:

Vital signs: initial bradycardia and HTN followed by tachycardia and hypotension and finally bradycardia and hypotension. The measured pulse oximeter may be high due to impaired oxygen utilization.

Neurologic: confusion, ataxia, mydriasis, seizures, coma.

Skin: "cherry red" skin.

HEENT: bright red retinal arteries/veins and smell of bitter almonds. Redness or flushing of the skin as well as red retinal veins/arteries have been reported following cyanide poisoning and is attributed to the elevated venous oxygen content from decreased tissue oxygen extraction.

The smell of bitter almonds has been reported following cyanide poisoning with HCN concentrations >2–5 ppm. However, the classic bitter almond smell is not always present following cyanide exposure and 40–45% of the population have a specific anosmia for the bitter almond smell of cyanide.

Cardiovascular: pulmonary edema.

Laboratory testing for suspected cyanide-poisoned patients is limited because the definitive test to confirm cyanide toxicity, whole blood or plasma cyanide concentration, is not readily available and is not sufficiently fast enough to aid patient care. Surrogate testing have been used to detect the metabolic derangements caused by cyanide poisoning. These include arterial and venous gas measurement and serum lactate measurement. A reduced arterial-venous oxygen saturation difference (<10 mmHg) or a high central venous oxygen saturation (>90%) is suggestive of cyanide poisoning. A serum lactate level >10 mmol/L in smoke inhalation victims and >8 mmol/L after suspected cyanide poisonings also suggests significant cyanide exposure. Finally, a carboxyhemoglobin level should be obtained in all smoke inhalation victims to exclude the possibility of concurrent carbon monoxide poisoning.

After-care

All cyanide-poisoned patients should be admitted to the intensive care unit, for cardiac monitoring and supportive care. Patients poisoned with cyanogens may require a longer observation period because of prolonged cyanide toxicity from continued cyanogen biotransformation. In addition to the risk of developing anoxic encephalopathy, survivors of acute cyanide poisoning are at risk for developing a Parkinson's disease-like disorder (e.g., dystonia, rigidity, bradykinesia) several days to several months after

their exposure. Consequently, these patients should receive follow-up screening for long-term neurologic sequelae.

Prognosis

The prognosis of cyanide-poisoned patients is largely dependent on the quantity of cyanide absorbed by the patient as well as the timing of resuscitation and antidotal therapy. Measured whole blood cyanide concentrations of >2.5 mcg/mL and >3 mcg/mL have been associated with both coma and death, respectively.

References

1. Baud FJ, Barriot P, Toffis V et al (1991) Elevated blood cyanide concentrations in victims of smoke inhalation. New Engl J Med 325:1761–1766
2. Baud FJ, Borron SW, Mégarbane B et al (2002) Value of lactic acidosis in the assessment of the severity of acute cyanide poisoning. Crit Care Med 30:2044–2051
3. Bebarta VS, Tanen DA, Lairet J et al (2010) Hydroxocobalamin and sodium thiosulfate versus sodium nitrite and sodium thiosulfate in the treatment of acute cyanide toxicity in a swine (Sus scrofa) model. Ann Emerg Med 55:345–351
4. Hall AH, Saiers J, Baud F (2009) Which cyanide antidote? Crit Rev Toxicol 39:541–542

Cycling-off

The controller signal that terminates assist delivery.

Cystatin 3

▶ Cystatin C

Cystatin C

STEFAN HERGET-ROSENTHAL
Department of Nephrology, University of Duisburg-Essen, Duisburg, Germany

Synonyms

CST3; Cystatin 3; Gamma trace; Post-gamma protein

Definition

Cystatin C is a non-glycated, basic protein that is present in all human body fluids and belongs to the superfamily of cystatins. Cystatin C has a molecular weight of 13.3 kDa.

Characteristics

Physiology

Cystatin C functions as the most important endogenous inhibitor of cysteine proteinases and is produced by all types of nucleated cells at a constant rate low intraindividual variability [1, 2]. As cystatin C is not bound to plasma proteins, it is freely filtered in the glomerulus due to its characteristics as a low molecular weight protein. Like other low molecular weight proteins, it is reabsorbed and metabolized in the proximal tubule. The transmembrane receptor protein megalin mediates endocytic uptake of cystatin C in proximal tubular cells [1]. There is no tubular secretion and only minimal extrarenal elimination of cystatin C. Therefore, the blood concentration of cystatin C depends almost entirely on the glomerular filtration rate (GFR) [1, 2]. The correlation of serum cystatin C and GFR is hyperbolic and not linear alike to serum creatinine. However, the correlation curve is more favorable compared to creatinine, as cystatin C concentration increases already with mildly reduced GFR of 60–90 mL/min, that is, in the "creatinine-blind range" [2]. This can especially be attributed to the shorter half-life and the lower distribution volume of cystatin C compared to creatinine [2]. Consequently, changes in GFR are earlier and more accurately transferred into changes in serum cystatin C. As recently discovered, blood concentration of cystatin C is also minimally elevated by diabetes, high doses of glucocorticoids, hyperthyroidism, and inflammation, and mildly reduced by higher age and female gender [1, 2]. Cystatin C concentration is not substantially affected by diet, nutritional status, liver or malignant diseases, or other nonrenal factors.

Analytical Aspects

Cystatin C in serum and urine is stable for hours at room temperature, days at 4–8°C and months at −20°C or −80°C. These characteristics are helpful as no cumbersome preanalytical procedures are required to obtain correct cystatin C measurements. Presently, particle-enhanced nephelometric (PENIA) and turbidometric immunoassays (PETIA) are the most accurate, precise and established, automated and commercially available methods to measure cystatin C in serum, urine, and other body fluids [1, 2]. Analytical time is about 5 min and very large intra- and inter-assay precision have been described for both PENIA and PETIA [1]. As interfering factors with the measurement only excessively elevated bilirubin, rheumatoid factor and triglycerides in vitro have been described for cystatin C [1, 2]. Both methods provide consistent results in most comparative studies. However, measurements by PENIA are 10–15% lower compared to PETIA. Reference ranges are 0.50–0.95 mg/L for PENIA and 0.63–1.33 mg/L for PETIA. Reference values do not differ men or women and from the second year to the age of 70 years. In healthy children, the cystatin C concentration stabilizes from the second year of life and the reference range in pediatric populations is identical to adults. Higher cystatin C concentrations in infants and the elderly reflect the decreased kidney function in these age groups [2]. In healthy volunteer, urinary cystatin C concentrations are below the detection levels of PENIA and PETIA. Unfortunately, there is still no uniform cystatin C reference standard for the calibration of these two commercially available assays. In 2008, a reference preparation was produced using pure, recombinant cystatin C and further steps are currently taken to characterize this preparation and establish a reference standard. Besides PENIA and PETIA, several ELISA methods to measure serum cystatin C have been published. Compared to PENIA and PETIA, these ELISA kits perform poorly and may not be used on an automated biochemistry analyzer. This prevents accurate, precise, easy, rapid, and large-scale measurement by ELISA. At present, cystatin C in serum, urine, or other body fluids should only be measured by PENIA or PETIA methods.

Clinical Utility and Performance

Serum cystatin C has been demonstrated to be an accurate and precise marker of GFR especially in chronic kidney disease (CKD) but also in acute kidney injury (AKI) [1, 2]. Various cross-sectional studies have shown that cystatin C has greater sensitivity to detect reduced GFR in CKD than creatinine and other GFR markers. In particular, serum cystatin C permits to detect early stages of chronic kidney damage with mildly reduced GFR. These findings were confirmed by two meta-analyses [3]. The performance of cystatin C as a marker of GFR has been studied in numerous patient populations. Especially cohorts at risk of CKD and/or with limitations in regard to the use of serum creatinine such as children and elderly, type I and type II diabetics, mild to moderate CKD of nondiabetic origin, renal transplant recipients, patients with severe liver or neuromuscular disease, tumor patients, and pregnant women with preeclampsia profited most from serum cystatin C as a GFR marker [1, 2]. Virtually, all studies concluded that cystatin C performed even better than equations estimating GFR (eGFR) based on creatinine [2].

Several large epidemiological studies have observed an association between mild elevations of serum cystatin C and increased cardiovascular and overall morbidity and mortality [1, 2]. It still remains to be elucidated whether there is in fact a direct pathophysiological link between cystatin C and cardiovascular disease as studies suggest a protective role of cystatin C in the arterial vessel wall in atherosclerosis. Alternatively, this association could be due to the confounding effect of cardiovascular risk factors such as reduced GFR, microinflammation, older age, and male gender, all of which are demonstrated to be associated with minimally increased cystatin C concentrations. As none of these studies included a gold-standard measurement of GFR, it is presently unknown if the association between cystatin C and cardiovascular disease merely reflects early stages of CKD [1, 2].

Furthermore, recent longitudinal studies have shown that cystatin C concentrations rise earlier in AKI on intensive care unit, after liver transplantation, cardiac surgery, cisplatin chemotherapy and coronary angiography, and in acute renal transplant rejection [2, 4]. Especially its characteristics as the shorter half-life and the lower distribution volume may contribute to the superiority of serum cystatin C as a marker to detect rapid changes of GFR as in AKI [2]. In intensive care patients, serum cystatin C was a useful detection marker and detected AKI 1–2 days earlier than serum creatinine by the R-criteria of the RIFLE classification. This was confirmed insofar that serum cystatin C permitted to diagnose AKI post-cardiac surgery and 24 h earlier than serum creatinine again by the R-criteria of the RIFLE classification. This was equivalently compared to neutrophil gelatinase-associated lipocalin (NGAL). However, the excellent performance of serum cystatin C as an early marker of AKI is not as undisputed as its value in CKD, as only a limited number of studies are available and some showed that serum cystatin C was equal but not superior to serum creatinine [2]. Limitations in the use of serum cystatin C may arise in the renal impairment of systemic autoimmune disease or vasculitis, or solid organ transplantation when patients are treated by corticosteroids. Nonrenal factors are of no importance in patients with consecutive cystatin C measurements and continuous presence of these factors as in AKI.

Although cystatin C facilitates the recognition of incipient CKD without the need for correction for age and anthropometric data, several groups have recently developed eGFR equations from serum cystatin C using similar approaches as have been described, for example,

for serum creatinine in the MDRD equation. There have been numerous eGFR equations published from serum cystatin C [1, 2]. In difference to the MDRD equation, which was calculated from a large multicenter dataset, cystatin C-based equations were predominately generated and validated in smaller samples from single center settings. This partially explains the variation between individual equations. Cystatin C-based equations for eGFR seem to be a promising alternative to creatinine-based ones and the majority of studies found cystatin C-based equations to be superior to creatinine-based ones. Especially the bias was lower, and to a lesser extent precision and accuracy greater of cystatin C-based equations toward measured GFR compared to creatinine-based equations. Even after recalibration, the simple MDRD equation still requires three parameters in addition to serum creatinine whereas most cystatin C-based equations seem to perform at least equally well without additional covariates. At present, the available data is too preliminary to favor one equation over another and to permit a definite conclusion whether cystatin C-based equations are superior, and these equations need to be vigorously evaluated in large diverse populations in multicenter studies. Clinicians should not overestimate eGFR calculated from cystatin C-based equations, as many limitations of the creatinine-based equations, for example, moderate precision, may also apply. Recently, novel eGFR equations were generated which incorporate both serum creatinine and cystatin C, to improve bias, precision and accuracy [1, 2, 5]. Initial results demonstrate a better performance of these equations compared to the exclusively creatinine- or cystatin C-based ones. This may indicate that both serum cystatin C and creatinine could be complementary and not redundant in future equations estimating GFR.

Urinary cystatin C concentrations were elevated in conditions with functional or structural impairment of the proximal renal tubule. In these circumstances, level of urinary cystatin C may surpass those of serum cystatin C two or threefold. It has been demonstrated that in heavy proteinuria, albumin competes with low molecular weight protein absorption in the tubules leading to increased urinary cystatin C. Structural impairment of the renal tubule may be associated with acute or chronic renal disorders. In chronic tubulointerstitial disease, either primary or secondary to most renal disorders with fibrosis, tubular proteinuria with increased urinary cystatin C develops, independent of the degree of GFR reductions. In those forms of AKI in critically ill associated with tubular injury as acute tubular necrosis, elevated urinary cystatin C permitted prediction of AKI earlier than serum creatinine. In this study, urinary cystatin

C detected subsequent AKI within the first six after cardiac surgery, approximately 40 h prior to detection by serum creatinine, and performed as well as urinary NGAL and superior to plasma NGAL. Furthermore, increased urinary excretion of cystatin C accurately identified severe forms of AKI. Subsequent requirement of renal replacement therapy was predicted 4 days ahead of time and demonstrated a higher diagnostic value than alpha-1 and beta-2-microglobulin, other low molecular weight proteins and tubular enzymes. However, data about urinary cystatin C is still too limited to reach a definite conclusion.

References

1. Seronie-Vivien S, Delanaye P, Pieroni L, Mariat C, Froissart M, Cristol JP, Cystatin C (2008) Current position and future prospects. Clin Chem Lab Med 46:1664–1686
2. Herget-Rosenthal S, Bokenkamp A, Hofmann W (2007) How to estimate GFR – serum creatinine, serum cystatin C or equations? Clin Biochem 40:153–161
3. Roos JF, Doust J, Tett SE, Kirkpatrick CM (2007) Diagnostic accuracy of cystatin C compared to serum creatinine for the estimation of renal dysfunction in adults and children – a meta-analysis. Clin Biochem 40:383–391
4. Herget-Rosenthal S, Marggraf G, Husing J et al (2004) Early detection of acute renal failure by serum cystatin C. Kidney Int 66:1115–1122
5. Stevens LA, Coresh J, Schmid CH et al (2008) Estimating GFR using serum cystatin C alone and in combination with serum creatinine: a pooled analysis of 3418 individuals with CKD. Am J Kidney Dis 51:395–406

Cystic Echinococcosis (CE)

▶ Echinococcosis

Cystic Hydatidosis

▶ Echinococcosis

Cystitis

▶ Urinary Tract Infections

Printed by Printforce, the Netherlands